WITHDRAWN

SM01002859
3/22
£233.00
for 2 Vols.

✓

HNK VWP Q
(Lee)

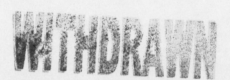

WITHDRAWN

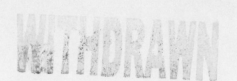

WITHDRAWN

CARLISLE LIBRARY
ST MARTINS SERVICES LTD.

M000568uSM

Computed Body Tomography

with MRI Correlation

Third Edition

Volume 2

Editors

Joseph K.T. Lee, M.D.
Ernest H. Wood, M.D.
Distinguished Professor
and Chairman
Department of Radiology
University of North Carolina
School of Medicine
Chapel Hill, North Carolina

Stuart S. Sagel, M.D.
Professor of Radiology
Co-Director, Body Computed
Tomography
Director, Chest Radiology
Mallinckrodt Institute of Radiology
Washington University School
of Medicine
St. Louis, Missouri

Robert J. Stanley, M.D.
Professor and Chairman
Department of Radiology
University of Alabama at Birmingham
Birmingham, Alabama

Jay P. Heiken, M.D.
Professor of Radiology
Director, Abdominal Imaging
Co-Director, Body Computed
Tomography
Mallinckrodt Institute of Radiology
Washington University School of
Medicine
St. Louis, Missouri

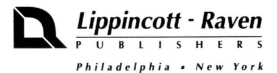

Lippincott - Raven
P U B L I S H E R S

Philadelphia • New York

Acquisitions Editor: James D. Ryan
Developmental Editor: Delois Patterson
Manufacturing Manager: Dennis Teston
Production Managers: Jodi Borgenicht and Maxine Langweil
Production Editors: Raeann Touhey and Jonathan Geffner
Cover Designer: Kevin Kall
Indexer: Kathy Garcia
Compositor: Tapsco, Inc.
Printer: Kingsport Press

© 1998, by Lippincott–Raven Publishers. All rights reserved. This book is protected by
copyright. No part of it may be reproduced, stored in a retrieval system, or transmitted, in any
form or by any means—electronic, mechanical, photocopy, recording, or otherwise—without the
prior written consent of the publisher, except for brief quotations embodied in critical articles and
reviews. For information write **Lippincott–Raven Publishers, 227 East Washington Square,
Philadelphia, PA 19106-3780.**

Materials appearing in this book prepared by individuals as part of their official duties as U.S.
Government employees are not covered by the above-mentioned copyright.

Printed in the United States of America

9 8 7 6 5 4 3 2 1

Library of Congress Cataloging-in-Publication Data

Computed body tomography with MRI correlation/[edited by] Joseph
  K. T. Lee . . . [et al].—3rd ed.
      p. cm.
  Includes bibliographical references and index.
  ISBN 0-7817-0291-7
  1. Tomography. 2. Magnetic resonance imaging. I. Lee, Joseph K. T.
  [DNLM: 1. Tomography, X-Ray Computed. 2. Magnetic Resonance Imaging.
WN 206 C7378 1996]
RC78.7. T6C6416 1998
616.07′57—DC20
DNLM/DLC
for Library of Congress

Care has been taken to confirm the accuracy of the information presented and to describe
generally accepted practices. However, the authors, editors, and publisher are not responsible for
errors or omissions or for any consequences from application of the information in this book and
make no warranty, express or implied, with respect to the contents of the publication.

The authors, editors, and publisher have exerted every effort to ensure that drug selection and
dosage set forth in this text are in accordance with current recommendations and practice at the
time of publication. However, in view of ongoing research, changes in government regulations,
and the constant flow of information relating to drug therapy and drug reactions, the reader is
urged to check the package insert for each drug for any change in indications and dosage and for
added warnings and precautions. This is particularly important when the recommended agent is a
new or infrequently employed drug.

Some drugs and medical devices presented in this publication have Food and Drug
Administration (FDA) clearance for limited use in restricted research settings. It is the
responsibility of the health care provider to ascertain the FDA status of each drug or device
planned for use in their clinical practice.

To our wives,
Christina, Beverlee, Sally, and Fran

and to our children,
Alexander, Betsy, and Catherine; Scott, Darryl, and Brett;
Ann, Robert, Catherine, and Sara; and Lauren

Contents

Contributing Authors

D. Claire Anderson, M.D.
Professor of Radiology
Washington University School of
    Medicine
St. Louis, Missouri

Ann Bagley Willms, M.D.
Clinical Instructor of Radiology
University of North Carolina School of
    Medicine
Chapel Hill, North Carolina
Currently, Costal Radiology
New Bern, North Carolina

Dennis M. Balfe, M.D.
Professor of Radiology
Director, Gastrointestinal Radiology
Washington University School of
    Medicine
St. Louis, Missouri

Gary T. Barnes, Ph.D.
Professor of Radiology
University of Alabama at Birmingham
Birmingham, Alabama

Harold F. Bennett, M.D.
Assistant Professor of Radiology
Washington University School of
    Medicine
St. Louis, Missouri

Joseph A. Borrello, M.D.
Assistant Professor of Radiology
Washington University School of
    Medicine
St. Louis, Missouri

Mark A. Brown, Ph.D.
Senior Technical Instructor
Siemens Medical Systems, Inc.
Training and Development Center
Cary, North Carolina

Mauricio Castillo, M.D.
Associate Professor of Radiology
Director, Neuroradiology
University of North Carolina School of
    Medicine
Chapel Hill, North Carolina

Matthew J. Fleishman, M.D.
Instructor of Radiology
Washington University School of
    Medicine
St. Louis, Missouri

David S. Gierada, M.D.
Assistant Professor of Radiology
Washington University School of
    Medicine
St. Louis, Missouri

Harvey S. Glazer, M.D.
Professor of Radiology
Washington University School of
    Medicine
St. Louis, Missouri

Fernando R. Gutierrez, M.D.
Associate Professor of Radiology
Washington University School of
    Medicine
St. Louis, Missouri

Stephen F. Hatem, M.D.
Assistant Professor of Radiology
Washington University School of
  Medicine
St. Louis, Missouri

Jay P. Heiken, M.D.
Professor of Radiology
Director, Abdominal Imaging
Co-Director, Body Computed
  Tomography
Washington University School of
  Medicine
St. Louis, Missouri

James N. Hiken, M.D.
Clinical Instructor of Radiology
University of North Carolina School of
  Medicine
Chapel Hill, North Carolina
Currently, Assistant Professor of
  Radiology
University of Louisville
Louisville, Kentucky

Paul S. Hsieh, M.D.
Assistant Professor of Radiology
Washington University School of
  Medicine
St. Louis, Missouri

Philip J. Kenney, M.D.
Professor of Radiology
University of Alabama at Birmingham
Birmingham, Alabama

Robert E. Koehler, M.D.
Professor of Radiology
Vice-Chairman
University of Alabama at Birmingham
Birmingham, Alabama

A. V. Lakshminarayanan, Ph.D.
Consultant
Atlanta, Georgia

Joseph K. T. Lee, M.D.
Ernest H. Wood, M.D.
Distinguished Professor of Radiology
Chairman
University of North Carolina School of
  Medicine
Chapel Hill, North Carolina

Matthew A. Mauro, M.D.
Professor of Radiology
Vice-Chairman
University of North Carolina School of
  Medicine
Chapel Hill, North Carolina

Bruce L. McClennan, M.D.
Professor of Radiology
Washington University School of
  Medicine
St. Louis, Missouri
Currently, Professor of Diagnostic
  Radiology
Chairman
Yale University School of Medicine
New Haven, Connecticut

Kevin W. McEnery, M.D.
Assistant Professor of Radiology
Director, Musculoskeletal Radiology
University of Texas
M.D. Anderson Cancer Center
Houston, Texas

David S. Memel, M.D.
Department of Medical Informatics
University of Utah School of Medicine
Salt Lake City, Utah

Paul L. Molina, M.D.
Associate Professor of Radiology
Director, Body Computed Tomography
University of North Carolina School of
  Medicine
Chapel Hill, North Carolina

Ernesto P. Molmenti, M.D.
Fellow, Transplant Surgery
University of Pittsburgh
Pittsburgh, Pennsylvania

Suresh K. Mukherji, M.D.
Assistant Professor of Radiology
University of North Carolina School of
  Medicine
Chapel Hill, North Carolina

Hrudaya Nath, M.D., D.M.R.,
  M.B.B.S.
Professor of Radiology
University of Alabama at Birmingham
Birmingham, Alabama

Jordan B. Renner, M.D.
Associate Professor of Radiology
Director, Musculoskeletal Radiology
University of North Carolina School of
*   Medicine*
Chapel Hill, North Carolina

Douglas D. Robertson, M.D., Ph.D.
Assistant Professor of Radiology and
*   Orthopedic Surgery*
Washington University School of
*   Medicine*
St. Louis, Missouri

Stuart S. Sagel, M.D.
Professor of Radiology
Director, Chest Radiology
Co-Director, Body Computed
*   Tomography*
Washington University School of
*   Medicine*
St. Louis, Missouri

Richard C. Semelka, M.D.
Associate Professor of Radiology
Director, Magnetic Resonance Imaging
University of North Carolina School of
*   Medicine*
Chapel Hill, North Carolina

Janice W. Semenkovich, M.D.,
Assistant Professor of Radiology
Washington University School of
*   Medicine*
St. Louis, Missouri

Marilyn J. Siegel, M.D.
Professor of Radiology
Washington University School of
*   Medicine*
St. Louis, Missouri

Richard M. Slone, M.D.
Assistant Professor of Radiology
Washington University School of
*   Medicine*
St. Louis, Missouri

J. Keith Smith, M.D., Ph.D.
Clinical Instructor of Radiology
University of North Carolina School of
*   Medicine*
Chapel Hill, North Carolina
Currently, Mid Carolina Radiology
*   Associates*
Sanford, North Carolina

Benigno Soto, M.D.
Professor of Radiology
University of Alabama at Birmingham
Birmingham, Alabama

Robert J. Stanley, M.D.
Professor of Radiology
Chairman
University of Alabama at Birmingham
Birmingham, Alabama

William G. Totty, M.D.
Professor of Radiology and
*   Orthopedic Surgery*
Washington University School of
*   Medicine*
St. Louis, Missouri

David M. Warshauer, M.D.
Associate Professor of Radiology
University of North Carolina School of
*   Medicine*
Chapel Hill, North Carolina

Steven S. Winn, M.D.
Instructor of Radiology
Washington University School of
*   Medicine*
St. Louis, Missouri

Franz J. Wippold II, M.D.
Associate Professor of Radiology
Washington University School of
*   Medicine*
St. Louis, Missouri

Pamela K. Woodard, M.D.
Assistant Professor of Radiology
Washington University School of
*   Medicine*
St. Louis, Missouri

Preface

Since the publication of the Second Edition of our textbook, *Computed Body Tomography with MRI Correlation* in 1989, significant technical advances have been made in both computed tomography (CT) and magnetic resonance imaging (MRI). The introduction of the helical (spiral) technique provides the unique opportunity to perform volumetric imaging and allows for further expansion of clinical applications of CT. Procedures such as CT angiography, virtual colonoscopy, and bronchoscopy have been developed because of helical scanning. The development of ultrafast CT scanning with electron beams has made imaging of the heart and pulmonary vasculature possible. These new advances have enabled CT to remain as the tomographic procedure of choice in evaluating most, if not all, thoracic and abdominal diseases.

During this same period of time, innovations and refinement in MR hardware and software technology have continued. The superiority of MRI over CT for evaluating many diseases of the central nervous system and the musculoskeletal and cardiovascular systems has been well established. The use of fast imaging sequences, fat saturation techniques, and intravenous contrast agents (e.g., gadolinium compounds) has made it possible to produce exquisite images of the abdomen and pelvis in a matter of seconds. Although MRI is not a screening procedure used for evaluating the abdomen and pelvis, it, nevertheless, has been used with increasing frequency as a problem-solving method in these areas. The role of MRI in thoracic imaging is still limited.

This edition has been prepared to present a comprehensive text on the application of CT and MRI to the extracranial organs of the body. Because of the large amount of information available for inclusion, we have elected to publish the Third Edition in two volumes. The book is intended primarily for the radiologist to use in either clinical practice or training. However, the internist, pediatrician, and surgeon can derive helpful information about the relative value and indications for CT and MRI of the body as well. As in the first two editions, anatomy in each area is emphasized initially, since such knowledge is basic to proper interpretation. The CT and MRI findings in a variety of pathologic conditions are described and illustrated. Instruction is provided to optimize the conduct, analysis, and interpretation of CT and MR images. Both technical and interpretative errors can occur in CT and MRI examinations and we hope the readers will benefit from our collective past experience.

Logical and cogent discussions of how CT and MRI are properly integrated with other clinical and radiological procedures, as well as with each other, for a variety of problems are included. Both radiologists and referring clinicians often face the dilemma of determining the best imaging approach for establishing a specific diagnosis given a set of clinical findings. With the increasing availability of a wide variety of imaging techniques, there is often a tendency to perform a large number of examinations before drawing a conclusion. This ''shot-gun'' or nondiscriminatory approach not only subjects the individual patient to unnecessary discomfort and risk, but also will be cost-prohibitive as managed care and capitation become more common methods of reimbursement in health care.

The task of deciding which diagnostic text is most appropriate for a given clinical problem has become an important part of our practice. An adequate understanding of clinical issues, as well as the advantages and limitations of each imaging technique, is essential for the radiologist to best help the referring clinician. Our recommended uses of CT and MRI have been developed through the cooperative

xiii

efforts of the diagnostic radiology staffs at our three medical centers. Each staff member has established an interest and expertise in a specific anatomic area. The proper sequencing of imaging tests for a variety of clinical entities has been discussed in numerous joint consultations and conferences during the past two decades, and from them, our current ideas have evolved. We are well aware that equally valid alternative imaging approaches to certain clinical problems are possible. Differences in available equipment and personal experience also could influence the selection of a particular imaging method. It is safe to predict that our recommendations on the optimal use of CT and MRI will have to be modified with further technologic improvements and increasing knowledge in both CT and MRI in the future.

J. K. T. L.
S. S. S.
R. J. S.
J. P. H.

Preface to the Second Edition

During the six years that have elapsed since the First Edition of our textbook, *Computed Body Tomography,* which was published in 1982, computed tomography (CT) has become the screening procedure of choice in evaluating many abdominal and spinal diseases. Improvements in scanning technology have resulted in better spatial resolution and faster data acquisition. This allowed a broader use of CT to areas such as the evaluation of bronchiectasis and articular abnormalities. Furthermore, CT is no longer used exclusively for detection and diagnosis, but to guide biopsy and treatment. To date, the strengths and weaknesses of CT are better defined, and its role in the evaluation of extracranial organs in relationship to other diagnostic techniques is more clearly established.

Concomitant with the maturation of CT technology, magnetic resonance imaging (MRI), described by Paul Lauterbur in 1973, has been introduced into clinical practice. The initial applications of MRI, like CT, focused on the brain because of its size and lack of respiratory or other physiologic motion. Developments of surface coil technology, cardiac triggering, various motion suppression techniques, and fast imaging sequences have made it possible to use MRI for other parts of the body. MRI has replaced CT as the imaging procedure of choice in evaluating many brain and spinal diseases because of its superior soft tissue contrast sensitivity and because of its direct multiplanar imaging capability. In addition, MRI is being used with increasing frequency in evaluating the musculoskeletal and cardio-vascular systems. Although MRI also can provide excellent anatomic information about the abdominal and pelvic organs, its role in these areas is less well established and more controversial.

This volume has been prepared to present a comprehensive text on the application of CT and MRI to the extracranial organs of the body. It is intended primarily for use by the radiologist in either clinical practice or training. The internist, pediatrician, and surgeon will also derive helpful information about the relative value and indications for CT and MRI of the body, their patients receiving the ultimate benefits. As in the First Edition, anatomy in each area is stressed initially, since such knowledge is basic to proper interpretation. The CT and MRI findings in a variety of pathologic conditions are described and illustrated. Instruction is provided to optimize the conduct, analysis, and interpretation of CT and MR images. Both technical and interpretative errors can occur in CT and MRI examinations, and, hopefully, the reader will benefit from our previous mistakes.

Logical and cogent discussions of how CT and MRI are properly integrated with other clinical and radiological procedures, as well as with each other, for a variety of problems are included. Both radiologists and referring clinicians often face the dilemma of determining the best radiologic approach toward documenting a specific diagnosis given a set of clinical findings. With the increasing availability of a wide variety of radiologic techniques, there is often a tendency to perform a large number of examinations before drawing a conclusion. This approach is extremely expensive and puts undue constraints on the total resources available for health care, aside from treating the individual patient unfairly by subjecting him or her to unnecessary discomfort and risk.

The task of deciding which diagnostic test is the most appropriate for a given clinical problem has become a substantial part of medical practice. An adequate understanding of clinical issues, as well as the advantages and limitations of each radiologic technique, is essential for the radiologist to best help the referring clinician. Our recommended uses of CT and MRI have been developed through the cooperative efforts of the diagnostic radiology staffs at the Mallinckrodt Institute and the University of Alabama at Birmingham. Each staff member has established an interest and expertise in a specific anatomic area. The proper sequencing of radiologic tests for a variety of clinical indications has been discussed in countless joint consultations and conferences during the past several years, and from this, our current ideas have evolved. We are well aware that equally valid alternative radiologic approaches to certain clinical problems are possible. Differences in available equipment and personal experience could modify the evaluation of any particular problem. Because of rapid technologic improvements in MRI, our recommendations on the optimal use of CT and MRI are by no means final, and enlightened physicians continually will need to update their ideas about how CT and MRI fit in with other imaging methods.

J. K. T. L.
S. S. S.
R. J. S.

Preface to the First Edition

Computed tomography (CT) was first developed for intracranial imaging in the late 1960s by Godfrey Hounsfield at the Central Research Laboratories of EMI Limited. Since that time, major technical advances have resulted in substantial improvements in image quality concomitant with a marked reduction in scanning time. In the past seven years, CT has become gradually accepted as an accurate and practical diagnostic technique, with its clinical applications broadened to include virtually every part of the body. This has occurred despite the initial skepticism of many regarding the value of extracranial CT in comparison to its cost. We have been fortunate to personally witness the germination and development of computed body tomography from its inception, to a technique that now has an enormous impact upon our practice of radiology. This radiological method has fulfilled the expectations of its early users and has proven to be an important and efficacious procedure for the evaluation of a myriad of pathologic problems.

In many cases, the information obtained by CT is unique. On occasion, data derived from CT have enabled reevaluation of traditional concepts of various disease processes. Body CT has supplanted or encroached upon other radiological procedures. Laryngography has been replaced. Lymphangiography for staging lymphoma and other neoplasms has declined drastically. Rapid, sequential, contrast-enhanced CT scans have been successfully substituted for angiography in many patients to diagnose or exclude suspected vascular lesions (e.g., aneurysm, dissection) or to assess the extent of a neoplastic process.

This volume has been prepared to present a comprehensive text on the application of CT to the extracranial regions of the body. It is intended primarily for use by the radiologist either in clinical practice or in training. The internist, pediatrician, and surgeon also will derive beneficial information about the relative value and indications for CT of the body, with their patients as the ultimate beneficiaries. Anatomy in each area is stressed initially, since such knowledge is basic to proper interpretation. Regions often are presented serially to portray the caudad progression of structures. The CT findings in a variety of pathologic conditions are described and illustrated. Instruction is provided to optimize the conduct, analysis, and interpretation of CT scans. Both technical and interpretative errors can occur in CT examinations, and hopefully the reader will benefit from our previous innumerable mistakes.

Comprehensive discussions of how CT is compatible with other clinical and radiological procedures for a variety of problems have been attempted. Both radiologist and referring clinician often are faced with the dilemma of determining the best radiologic approach toward documenting a specific diagnosis given a set of clinical findings. With the burgeoning availability of a wide variety of new radiologic techniques, there is often a tendency to perform a large number of examinations before drawing a conclusion. Such an approach, however, is extremely expensive and puts undue constraints on the total resources available for health care, besides being unfair to the individual patient who is subjected to unnecessary discomfort and risk.

The uses of CT we suggest have been developed through the cooperative efforts of the diagnostic radiology staff at the Mallinckrodt Institute. Each member has established an interest and expertise in a specific area. The proper sequencing of radiologic tests for a variety of clinical indications has been discussed in countless, joint consultations and conferences during the past several years. From this ongoing dialogue, our current ideas have evolved. We are well aware that equally valid alternative radiologic approaches to certain clinical problems are possible. It is obvious that available equipment and personal experience could modify the evaluation of any particular problem. Clearly our recommendations on the optimal use of CT are not final, and the enlightened physician continually will need to update his ideas about how CT fits in with other modalities as clinical research and technology continue to develop.

J. K. T. L.
S. S. S.
R. J. S.
1982

Acknowledgments

Providing recognition to everyone involved in the production of this edition is extremely difficult because of the large number of individuals from our three institutions who aided immeasurably in forming the final product. We graciously thank the various contributors who kindly provided chapters in their areas of expertise, in order to bring depth and completeness to the book.

A special note of gratitude goes to our secretaries, Sonia Bishop, Sue Day, Tracy Hall, Carol Keller, Sheila Wright, and Wilma Potts, who spent endless hours typing manuscripts and checking references. Bo Strain and Bert Fowler at the University of North Carolina Department of Radiology Photography Laboratory, as well as Thomas Murry and Michelle Wynn at the Mallinckrodt Institute Photography Laboratory, were extremely helpful in preparing the illustrative material. Tony Zagar in the University of Alabama Photography Laboratory was most helpful in preparing the illustrations for the University of Alabama contributors.

Our thanks go to our residents, fellows, and the many radiologic technologists who performed and monitored the CT and MRI studies. Their dedication is reflected in the high quality of images used throughout this book.

We also would like to express our appreciation to Lippincott–Raven Publishers, for their professionalism in handling this project. Most particularly, we would like to thank Jim Ryan and Delois Patterson for their timeless dedication and advice during each stage in the production of this book.

Computed Body Tomography

with MRI Correlation

Third Edition

Volume 2

CHAPTER 13

The Biliary Tract

David S. Memel, Dennis M. Balfe, and Richard C. Semelka

The most common indication for computed tomography (CT) and magnetic resonance imaging (MRI) of the biliary tract is the evaluation of patients with clinically suspected obstructive bile duct disease. The role of imaging in patients with suspected bile duct obstruction is not only to confirm the presence of biliary obstruction, but also to determine the level and cause of obstruction, and the extent or stage of the disease process (20,198). In determining the extent of the disease process, the goal of the radiologist is to provide information that will help determine whether treatment should be directed towards curative or palliative therapy, and whether the most appropriate treatment is operative, endoscopic, or percutaneous (87,96).

In patients with jaundice, it is important to differentiate obstructive from nonobstructive etiologies. The combination of clinical, laboratory, and imaging evaluation provides the optimal results in identifying the presence and precise etiology of obstruction of the biliary tree (193). History, physical examination, and laboratory evaluation can correctly differentiate obstructive from nonobstructive jaundice in 80% to 85% of icteric patients (156,221). The clinical presentation in patients with biliary obstruction is variable and will differ depending on whether the obstruction is partial or complete, and intermittent or constant, and depending on the length of time the obstruction has been present. Patients may present with painless jaundice and elevation of alkaline phosphatase or total bilirubin, with pain but normal laboratory tests, or with painful jaundice. If jaundice is determined to be obstructive in nature, a combination of noninvasive and invasive imaging techniques is necessary to determine the etiology of the bile duct obstruction.

Bile duct obstruction occurs in three phases: the functional phase, the anatomic phase, and the icteric phase (42). The initial phase is the functional phase. In this phase, serum alkaline phosphatase, total bilirubin, and aspartate aminotransferase (AST) begin to rise, but they remain within the normal range. Patients do not generally have clinical symptoms at this time and thus rarely come to the attention of a physician. Therefore, it is unusual to image patients in the functional phase of obstruction.

The anatomic phase follows the functional phase and has been reported to occur as early as 4 hours and as long as 4 days after obstruction (198,285). Early in the anatomic phase, dilatation of the extrahepatic ducts can be present without dilatation of the intrahepatic ducts (13). This phenomenon may be a reflection of Laplace's law which states that "the pressure or bursting force of a sphere or cylinder is proportional to its diameter" (57). In the case of the biliary tree, because the intrahepatic ducts have a smaller diameter than the extrahepatic ducts, they tend to have less bursting force and thus dilate later in the course of obstruction. Extrahepatic ductal dilatation without intrahepatic dilatation can be seen not only in early obstruction, but also in intermittent obstruction and in patients with obstruction and underlying liver disease (20,232,284). In patients with underlying liver disease, the abnormal hepatic parenchyma may prevent the distention of the obstructed intrahepatic bile ducts.

The last phase in the progression of bile duct obstruction is the icteric phase. In this phase, the total bilirubin levels are markedly elevated, and patients are clearly jaundiced. Imaging examinations performed during the icteric phase will show clearly identifiable biliary ductal dilatation.

False negative imaging exams can occur in patients with early obstruction who have no bile duct dilatation. The same may be true of patients with partial obstruction, such as that caused by the ball-valve effect sometimes

779

seen with distal common bile duct (CBD) stones. Unfortunately, imaging examinations can also yield false positive results in the presence of dilatation without obstruction. Nonobstructive dilatation can occur in patients with congenital anomalies of the biliary tree, or in patients who have had previous obstruction and ductal dilatation, but in whom the dilatation did not resolve after the obstruction was relieved. One example of the latter situation is the postcholecystectomy patient with a dilated CBD and no bile duct obstruction. The cause of nonobstructive dilatation of the bile duct after cholecystectomy has been debated in the literature for many years. There remains no consensus as to whether this is a real entity, and as to what the etiology of this finding is (55,187,236).

Indications for CT and MRI of the biliary tract, in addition to the evaluation of bile duct obstruction of uncertain etiology, include evaluation of postoperative complications from biliary tract surgery (particularly laparoscopic cholecystectomy), evaluation of patients with complicated biliary tract infections, evaluation of congenital anomalies of the gallbladder and bile ducts, and evaluation of known or suspected gallbladder and bile duct neoplasms. Furthermore, with the increasing use of laparoscopic techniques for biliary tract surgery, as noninvasive CT and MR cholangiography techniques improve, they may eventually be included in the preoperative evaluation of patients with gallstones and suspected associated CBD stones.

The development of helical CT, fast-scanning breathhold techniques for MRI, and organ-specific MRI contrast agents have contributed to the continuing evolution of the role of these modalities in imaging of the biliary tract. This chapter will discuss the current and possible future roles of CT and MRI in the evaluation of patients with suspected or known biliary tract disease.

GENERAL PRINCIPLES OF IMAGING BILIARY TRACT DISEASE

In addition to CT and MRI, the imaging techniques used for the evaluation of patients with suspected biliary tract disease include ultrasonography (US), radionuclide scintigraphy, endoscopic retrograde cholangiopancreatography (ERCP), and percutaneous transhepatic cholangiography (PTC). Each of these techniques has a role in the evaluation of the biliary tract; however, there are multiple factors that must be considered in selecting the appropriate imaging examination. The factors that should be taken into account include the patient's clinical presentation, the length of time the patient has been symptomatic, body habitus (obese patients may be difficult to evaluate with sonography, and patients with a paucity of intra-abdominal fat may be difficult to evaluate with CT), the presence or absence of a history of prior surgical procedures involving, or affecting access to, the biliary tract

(e.g., open or laparoscopic cholecystectomy, Billroth I or II gastrectomies, various biliary–enteric anastomoses, Whipple procedure, etc.), and the expertise of the radiologists and endoscopists at the institution evaluating the patient (12,193,235,246).

Sonography is the primary imaging modality in the evaluation of gallbladder disease, and it is the most commonly used screening modality in patients with suspected bile duct disease. It has a sensitivity of 87% to 90% (12,87,130) for detecting biliary obstruction. The use of a fatty meal or cholecystokinin (CCK) to stress the extrahepatic bile duct can be useful in cases in which sonography is normal or equivocal in the presence of laboratory evidence of obstruction (237,276). Sonography has been reported to be 60% to 95% and 39% to 88% accurate in determining the level and cause of obstruction, respectively (12,87,109,130). The accuracy of sonography for determining the extent of disease and the unresectability of primary and secondary tumors involving the bile ducts is in the range of 70% (87). With newer techniques, including intravascular, endoluminal, and laparoscopic sonography, accuracy in staging of malignancies involving the bile ducts will most likely improve.

Radionuclide scintigraphy is most often used in the evaluation of acute cholecystitis and has a sensitivity and specificity comparable to that of sonography (42). It is also useful in evaluating for bile leaks after biliary tract surgery (211,267,270)

Direct cholangiography (ERCP or PTC) provides the most precise delineation of the anatomy and pathology of the bile ducts. The morphology of duct abnormalities can be clearly demonstrated and can thus contribute significant information towards making a definitive diagnosis in some disease processes (e.g., primary sclerosing cholangitis). Both PTC and ERCP suffer from technical limitations, including the inability to access the bile ducts in 15% to 30% of PTCs in patients with normal caliber ducts, and in 5% to 10% of all ERCPs. In addition, there can be incomplete filling of the ducts due to tight strictures or intraductal debris. Complications of direct cholangiography include sepsis in patients with obstructed ducts, for both PTC and ERCP, and pancreatitis in 1% to 7% of diagnostic and therapeutic ERCPs. ERCP with sphincterotomy also can be complicated by duodenal perforation, retroperitoneal abscess, and pneumoperitoneum (127,197,234).

Computed tomography and MRI have complementary roles relative to the imaging modalities discussed, and to each other, in the evaluation of biliary tract disease. Computed tomography and MRI can aid in determining whether bile duct strictures found on ERCP or PTC result from intrinsic or extrinsic disease. In patients in whom direct cholangiography is contraindicated or could not be successfully performed, CT and MRI may be used in place of direct cholangiography to confirm or further delineate bile duct abnormalities detected with sonography.

Computed tomography and MRI also can provide information about extrabiliary spread of gallbladder and bile duct disease that cannot be obtained by sonography or direct cholangiography (182,213).

Semelka et al. (228) prospectively compared ERCP, CT, and MRI in the evaluation of bile duct disease and found ERCP to be the best technique for differentiating benign from malignant disease, CT the best technique for evaluation of the wall of the extrahepatic bile ducts, and MRI the best technique for showing the intrahepatic periportal tissue and determining the extent of tumor infiltration in malignant disease. In a study comparing MRI, CT, and cholangiography in the evaluation of malignant biliary obstruction, cholangiography was shown to be the most accurate technique for determining the precise level of obstruction (149). However, as noted, it was not as sensitive as CT or MRI for the detection of the extrabiliary extent of primary or metastatic bile duct malignancies, and thus it was limited in determining tumor resectability.

Computed tomography has been shown to have a 96% sensitivity and a 91% specificity for detecting the presence of biliary obstruction (12). The accuracy of CT in the determination of the level and cause of obstruction has been reported to be 88% to 92% and 63% to 70%, respectively (12,87,96). For evaluation of resectability of tumors involving the bile ducts, CT has been shown to have a positive predictive value of 89% for unresectability and 80% for resectability (96). Several studies have shown that MRI is equivalent to CT in the detection of biliary obstruction and the determination of the level and cause of obstruction (71,97,149).

Relative to MRI, CT has greater spatial resolution, it has the ability to acquire data from larger imaging volumes in a shorter period of time, it has more consistent image quality, and there are good oral contrast agents currently available for it. The advantages of MRI relative to CT include the greater safety of the current intravascular contrast agents, the availability (in the near future) of organ-specific contrast agents, the lack of ionizing radiation, its superior contrast resolution, and its ability for direct acquisition of multiplanar images. Furthermore, because of its ability to more quickly obtain rapid sequential images through a limited region of interest than CT, MRI also allows for greater resolution of organ, and tumor, contrast enhancement patterns over time (229).

Based on the pathophysiologic progression of biliary obstruction and the relative values of the various imaging techniques described, the following guidelines can be used to evaluate patients with suspected obstructive bile duct disease. In the evaluation of any patient with suspected bile duct obstruction, the first steps are a thorough history and physical exam, and the appropriate laboratory evaluation. If these examinations support the suspicion of biliary obstruction, the first imaging procedure should be sonography. If sonography shows normal bile ducts and the clinical suspicion of obstruction is high, the next

examination should be ERCP or PTC. The use of direct cholangiography as the second examination in the evaluation of patients with suspected obstructive jaundice and nondilated bile ducts on sonography was proposed 16 years ago (188) and is still considered to be appropriate today. If direct cholangiography is also normal, the workup should be redirected towards nonobstructive causes of the signs and symptoms of biliary tract disease (193).

If sonography shows evidence of bile duct dilatation and the suspected etiology of obstruction is stone disease, the next examination should be ERCP, which can be used both as a diagnostic and as a therapeutic procedure at the same time. If ERCP cannot be performed or is unsuccessful, CT is an acceptable alternative for the detection of bile duct stones. However, CT does not offer the same possibility of simultaneous diagnosis and therapy that ERCP affords. If the suspected etiology of obstruction is neoplastic, CT should be the examination performed after sonography. In these patients, CT is used to assess not only the level and cause of obstruction, but also the extent of extrabiliary disease. In some cases, ERCP is used in addition to CT to more precisely delineate the extent of tumors that are arising in or invading the bile duct. ERCP also can be used to place a bile duct stent in patients in whom a tumor causing the bile duct obstruction is deemed unresectable on the basis of the CT or ERCP findings. MRI should be reserved for patients in whom CT is contraindicated, or when proximal biliary obstruction is present and CT either does not show a mass or does not clearly delineate the extent of a potentially resectable tumor (149).

The role of CT and MRI in the evaluation of gallbladder disease is currently limited to patients with suspected complicated inflammatory or infectious processes, postoperative complications, or gallbladder neoplasms. As mentioned, both CT and MR cholangiography hold promise as noninvasive preoperative examinations in patients with cholelithiasis and suspected common duct stones.

TECHNIQUE

Computed Tomography

Optimal visualization of the normal and abnormal biliary tract requires modification of the examination technique according to the clinical history of the patient and the specific information being sought. The factors that can affect visualization of the different types of pathology include the use of oral and intravenous contrast agents, the use of axial versus helical scanning, retrospective reconstruction of raw data, slice collimation and spacing, milliampere second (mAs), and kilovolt peak [kV(p)].

Barium or iodinated oral contrast agents are routinely used in CT of the abdomen. Although also generally used in CT of the biliary tract, these positive contrast agents

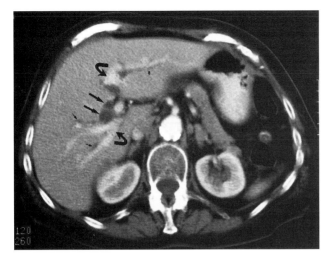

FIG. 1. Intrahepatic bile duct dilatation. Contrast-enhanced CT image of the liver shows obvious dilatation of the right and left hepatic ducts *(long arrows)*. The presence of intravenous contrast in the portal veins *(curved arrows)* aids in delineating the mildly dilated, more peripheral ducts *(short arrows)*.

can cause artifacts that may obscure important pathologic lesions in the bile ducts. Positive oral contrast in the duodenum can cause streak artifact across the CBD that obscures CBD stones (15,259). Therefore, when evaluating for stones in the CBD, scanning should initially be performed with no oral contrast or with water to distend the stomach and duodenum (7). Because gastric and duodenal peristalsis can also contribute to the production of

streak artifact across the CBD, using glucagon to decrease peristalsis can help improve image quality (259).

Intravenous contrast should be used routinely in CT examinations of the biliary tract unless it is medically contraindicated. The contrast volume used will vary depending on the concentration of the contrast agent and whether the contrast is a high osmolar or low osmolar solution. Regardless of the agent used, the total iodine dose should be 40 to 50 g. The entire volume should be administered as a rapid uniphasic (at least 2 to 3 ml/sec) or biphasic (e.g., 2 to 3 ml/sec for 50 ml, 1 ml/sec for 100 ml) injection, depending on the speed of the scanner. In the case of minimal dilatation of the intrahepatic bile ducts, intravenous contrast enhancement of the hepatic parenchyma and vasculature helps differentiate the low-attenuation bile ducts from the portal veins (Fig. 1). Enhancement of the bile duct walls, adjacent vascular structures, and pancreatic parenchyma aids in identification of the extrahepatic bile ducts (15,20) (Fig. 2). When evaluating for the presence of intrahepatic or CBD stones, scans should first be obtained without intravenous contrast. If precontrast scans are going to be obtained when looking for CBD stones, some authors advocate obtaining these images with 3 to 5 mm collimation at 3 to 5 mm intervals (259). In the case of intrahepatic bile duct stones, the enhancement of the liver parenchyma after intravenous contrast administration may obscure the high-attenuation stones (Fig. 3). Similarly, CBD stones, which often are only detected because of a rim of high attenuation, can be obscured if the high-attenuation rim cannot be differentiated from the enhancing bile duct wall. In addition, when

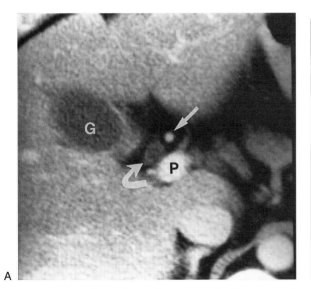

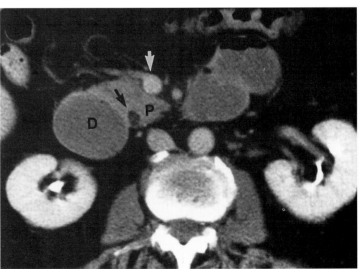

A   B

FIG. 2. Normal anatomy. **A:** Contrast-enhanced CT image at the level of the porta hepatis shows the normal relationships of the portal vein (P), hepatic artery *(arrow)*, and common duct *(curved arrow)*. The enhancement of the portal vein and hepatic artery aid in identifying the common duct in its normal location anterolateral to the portal vein. G, gallbladder. **B:** Contrast-enhanced CT image at the level of the head of the pancreas shows a normal caliber CBD *(black arrow)* surrounded by enhancing pancreatic parenchyma (P). D, duodenum; *white arrow*, superior mesenteric vein.

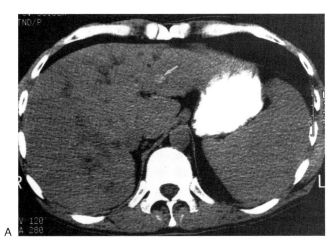
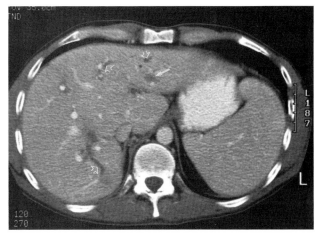

A

B

FIG. 3. Primary sclerosing cholangitis with intrahepatic stones. **A:** Noncontrast CT image through the liver shows a focal region of high attenuation *(arrow)* in the left lobe. This appearance is a result of intrahepatic biliary calculi that are higher attenuation than the unenhanced liver. Note the scattered areas of low attenuation in other areas of the liver. It is difficult to determine which of these are dilated intrahepatic bile ducts and which are unopacified blood vessels. **B:** Contrast-enhanced CT image at the same level shows the stones *(arrow)* are not readily recognizable as stones on this image because they appear lower in attenuation than the enhanced liver. Conversely, the scattered dilated intrahepatic bile ducts *(open arrows)* are easier to identify, because of the contrast enhancement of the liver parenchyma and portal veins.

scanning to evaluate for CBD stones, a maximal kV(p) [generally a 140 kV(p)] should be used because cholesterol, one of the major components of biliary stones, increases its attenuation with increasing kV(p) (17,20).

Although the use of oral and intravenous cholangiographic contrast agents in CT of the biliary tract has been described (59,92,189,204), before the advent of helical CT it never gained widespread acceptance. Because helical CT allows the collection of volumetric data sets without respiratory misregistration, it is now possible to produce high-quality multiplanar and three-dimensional (3-D) reconstructions of CT images. As a result, there has been renewed interest in noninvasive CT cholangiography with intravenous cholangiographic contrast agents (121,245,262) (Fig. 4). In a study by Maglinte and Dorenbusch (153), an intravenous cholangiographic contrast agent, iodipamide meglumine, was shown to be well tolerated and safer than previous agents. In this study of 113 patients, only one patient had an adverse reaction to the contrast agent, and this was only a mild skin rash. The studies performed to evaluate helical CT cholangiography (HCTC) have shown a close correlation between this technique and ERCP for common duct size, and a 94% accuracy rate for detection of CBD stones (245) (Fig. 5). There are some disadvantages to HCTC. For example, despite the study by Maglinte and Dorenbusch (153) showing the safety of iodipamide, the issue of the safety of intravenous cholangiographic contrast agents in general still requires further evaluation (89). In addition, although the contrast resolution of HCTC exceeds that of ERCP, the spatial resolution of ERCP is better. Furthermore, HCTC is not effective in patients with a serum bilirubin greater than

2 mg/dl, and image noise increases in obese patients and patients with ascites (38,245). The clinical applications that have been proposed for helical CT cholangiography include preoperative evaluation of patients who are to undergo laparoscopic cholecystectomy, evaluation for retained CBD stones after cholecystectomy, evaluation of patients with suspected biliary tract disease and normal liver function tests, and evaluation of those patients who are in need of cholangiography but who have altered anatomy from previous surgery such as a Billroth II gastrectomy (121,245). It is unlikely that HCTC will replace ERCP because of the limitations noted, and the fact that HCTC does not offer the possibility of therapeutic intervention that ERCP affords (89).

In general, on conventional dynamic incremental scans, slice collimation should be 5 mm at 8- to 10-mm intervals from the dome of the diaphragm through the pancreas. If these scans show a site of obstruction but the cause is not apparent, the zone of transition from dilated to normal duct caliber should be immediately rescanned with 3- to 5-mm collimation at 3- to 5-mm intervals with a small field of view (FOV). These "targeted" scans should be obtained with a higher mAs than the initial scans in order to decrease quantum mottle. The end result of obtaining the thin collimation images will be improved spatial resolution and thus potentially improved detection of small masses or obstructing stones not seen on the initial scans (Fig. 6), and improved visualization of abnormalities of the bile duct wall that may be helpful in arriving at a diagnosis (20).

In problematic cases in which obstruction is strongly suspected but there is no bile duct dilatation present on

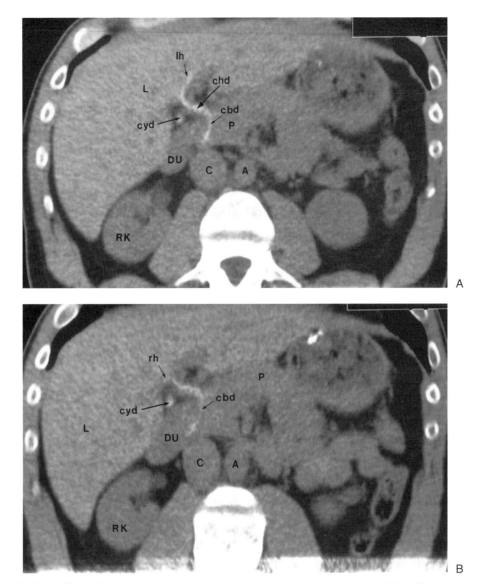

FIG. 4. Helical CT cholangiography performed with contrast enhancement of the biliary tree, in a normal subject. **A:** Oblique coronal volumetric data obtained during spiral CT shows the majority of the extrahepatic course of the biliary tree. The left hepatic duct (lh) joins the common hepatic duct (chd) immediately proximal to the hepatoduodenal ligament. A portion of the cystic duct (cyd) is also noted within the ligamentous fat. The common bile duct (cbd) exits the ligament to course posterior to the pancreatic head (P). **B:** Section obtained slightly posterior to (A) shows the distal portion of the common bile duct (cbd) as it enters the duodenum (DU). On this section, the central portion of the right hepatic duct (rh) is also observed. L, liver; DU, duodenum; C, inferior vena cava; A, aorta; RK, right kidney.

the CT scan, or in which bile duct dilatation is present but there is no clinical evidence of obstruction, one author has recommended rescanning the patient after stressing the bile duct with CCK or a fatty meal, using the same technique described for sonography (20). This technique involves scanning the patient approximately 45 minutes to 1 hour after a fatty meal, or 10 to 15 minutes after an intravenous injection of CCK. By stimulating the release of endogenous CCK with a fatty meal, or by administering CCK intravenously, the gallbladder is stimulated to contract, bile production by the liver is increased, and the

sphincter of Oddi relaxes. The net result is an increase in the flow of bile. In patients who have bile duct obstruction, ducts that appeared normal on the initial CT scan will be dilated on the poststress scan, and ducts that were dilated will remain dilated on the poststress scan. In patients without bile duct obstruction, ducts that were normal on the initial scan will not change or will decrease in size on the poststress scan, and ducts that were dilated on the initial CT scan will decrease in size on the poststress scan.

Helical CT scanning, if available, offers several advan-

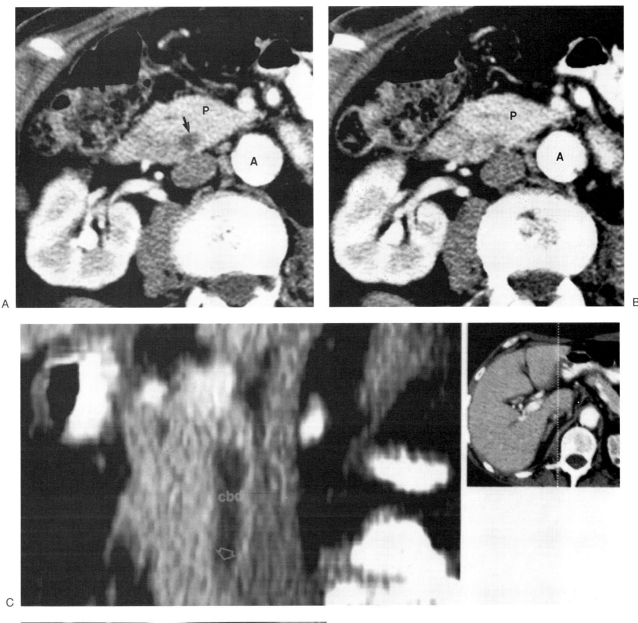

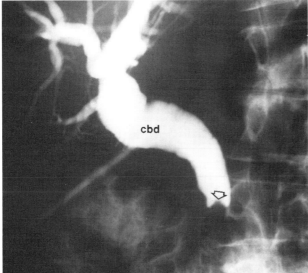

FIG. 5. Helical CT cholangiography performed without a cholangiographic contrast agent. Distally obstructing calculus in a 70-year-old woman with right upper quadrant pain and jaundice after an open cholecystectomy. **A:** Axial CT section through the head of the pancreas (P) shows dilatation of the distal CBD *(arrow)*. **B:** Axial CT section 5 mm inferior to (A) shows that the dilated duct is no longer identified; no mass or other pathologic process is observed to account for the biliary obstruction. **C:** Sagittal reformation of volumetric data obtained by helical CT shows the course of the dilated common bile duct (cbd). A high-attenuation structure *(open arrow)* with a convex superior border is observed at the lower margin of the dilated duct. **D:** Direct cholangiogram performed after the CT shows a calculus *(open arrow)* producing complete obstruction of the common bile duct (cbd). A, aorta; C, inferior vena cava.

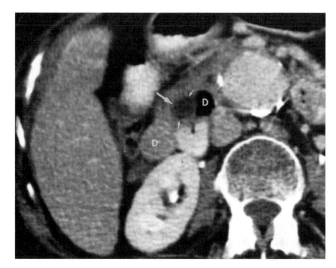

FIG. 6. Cholesterol stone. CT image at the level of the distal CBD shows a low-attenuation stone *(long arrow)* with a small amount of surrounding water density bile *(short arrows)*. Without the use of thin sections and visualization of the surrounding bile, this stone could easily be overlooked. D, fluid-filled second portion of the duodenum (to the right of the stone) and gas-filled diverticulum of the third portion of the duodenum (to the left of the stone).

tages over conventional axial scanning of the biliary tract. The continuous acquisition of data in helical scanning allows the examination of a longer segment (in the z axis) of the biliary tree during a single breath hold than can be obtained with conventional axial scanning. This results in scanning during optimal enhancement of vascular structures, decreased respiratory motion artifact and slice misregistration, and decreased examination time (74,114). The acquisition of a volumetric data set allows reconstruction of overlapping slices and the selection of slice locations other than those originally selected. This can provide more images through an area of interest without additional dose to the patient. In addition, this results in improved spatial and contrast resolution in the z axis and improved detection of small lesions (113,261). As mentioned, the lack of respiratory misregistration inherent in the volumetric data set also allows the production of high-quality multiplanar and 3-D reconstructions. This is useful not only for evaluation of the biliary tree itself, as described for HCTC, but also for evaluation of the vascular structures surrounding the biliary tree (CT angiography) (103,286). Helical CT scanning of the biliary tract is most commonly performed with 7-mm collimation at a pitch of 1 (table movement of 7 mm/sec). If targeted images are required, they can be obtained either by retrospective reconstruction of overlapping slices, or by rescanning the transition zone with a collimation of 3 to 5 mm at a pitch of 1 (table movement of 3 to 5 mm/sec).

Other techniques that can help improve the diagnostic yield of CT of the biliary tract include viewing the CT images directly on the monitor of independent CT con-

soles or workstations using different window and level settings, and the cine-paging technique (167). The cine-paging technique involves loading the images obtained through the bile ducts into the image buffer of the CT console or workstation and viewing the images sequentially in a cine-loop with the use of a trackball. As with tracing the course of the bowel in the case of suspected GI tract obstruction, this technique is helpful in following the course of the bile ducts and identifying sites of ductal obstruction.

Magnetic Resonance Imaging

Magnetic resonance techniques for imaging the biliary tree can be tailored to focus on either the bile duct walls or the fluid within the ducts. Imaging of the biliary lumen can be performed with either black-signal biliary fluid or bright-signal biliary fluid techniques. Optimal black fluid techniques generally include intravenous gadolinium chelate administration and image acquisition >2 minutes after contrast administration to ensure that all hepatic blood vessels contain gadolinium, so that only the bile ducts will appear as tubular structures with signal void (149,230). Spoiled gradient echo images can be obtained before contrast, immediately after contrast, and 5 to 10 minutes after contrast. The precontrast and immediate postcontrast images are used primarily for imaging the liver. The delayed postcontrast images aid in differentiating the low signal bile duct from the enhanced portal and hepatic veins (230) (Fig. 7). T1-weighted spoiled gradient

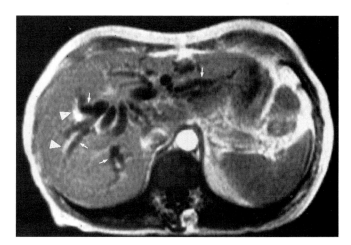

FIG. 7. Intrahepatic bile duct dilatation. Ten minutes after gadolinium, a spoiled gradient echo MR image demonstrates high-grade dilatation of the intrahepatic bile ducts *(arrows)*, which are seen as tubular areas of signal void adjacent to the enhancing portal veins *(arrowheads)*. Intrahepatic vessels are high in signal intensity at 10 minutes after contrast, so distinction between ducts and vessels is readily apparent. (Reproduced with permission from Semelka RC, Shoenut JP, Micflikier AB. The gallbladder and biliary tree. In: Semelka RC, Shoenut JP, eds. *MRI of the abdomen with CT correlation.* New York: Raven Press, 1993;43–52.)

echo (SGE) techniques are usually ideal sequences to employ because spin echo sequences frequently show mixed signal in blood vessels.

Recent descriptions of bright duct techniques have emphasized the inherent 3-D nature of MRI by reconstructing acquired data into 3-D data display, providing an MR cholangiogram effect (94,99,174,184,269). Both long echo time fast spin echo, with or without fat suppression, and steady-state gradient echo techniques have been employed in this fashion. The long T2 of biliary fluid is the underlying basis for the high signal of bile using these techniques. The high spatial resolution and relatively high S/N ratio obtained with the fast spin echo technique using a long echo time (TE 144 msec) has resulted in good image quality (94,174,249) (Fig. 8). Both fast spin echo and the gradient echo technique have the attractive feature of permitting 3-D data acquisition (184). One of the disadvantages of MR cholangiography is the inability of the current techniques to assess the length or asymmetry of bile duct strictures. These are characteristics that can be helpful in differentiating benign from malignant disease (99).

An alternative approach to obtaining bright biliary fluid is the use of T1-relaxation-enhancing, hepatocyte-specific intravenous contrast that is substantially excreted in the bile. Manganese-DPDP (dipyridoxal diphosphate), iron-HBED [bis(2-hydroxybenzyl)ethyl-

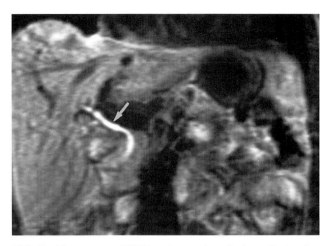

FIG. 9. Manganese-DPDP-enhanced spoiled gradient echo MR image (FLASH 140/4/80°). The CBD *(arrow)* is high in signal intensity because of excretion of manganese-DPDP in the bile.

enediaminediacetic acid], iron-EHPG [ethylenebis-(2-hydroxyphenylglycine)], and gadolinium-EOB (ethoxybenzyl)-DTPA (diethylene-triamine pentaacetic acid) are examples of these agents (28,75,100, 105,136–138, 145,223). The high signal of contrast-enhanced bile permits good visualization of the biliary tree (Fig. 9).

Sequences useful for the demonstration of the bile duct and gallbladder walls include T1-weighted, fat-suppressed spin echo with and without gadolinium chelates (230). Gadolinium-enhanced, T1-weighted, fat-suppressed spin echo images are also particularly well suited for the demonstration of abnormal ductal/periductal tissue as seen in ascending cholangitis and cholangiocarcinoma.

The liver, and therefore the bile ducts, are subject to a great deal of respiratory and cardiac motion artifact. These artifacts can be particularly problematic in spin echo pulse sequences after the administration of gadolinium chelates. Therefore, phase artifact suppression is very important when using spin echo techniques. Breath-hold techniques such as SGE or fat-suppressed SGE have an advantage over spin echo techniques because of the inherent absence of respiratory motion artifacts in SGE techniques, even without the use of phase artifact suppression (149).

NORMAL ANATOMY

Computed Tomography

Bile flows through the biliary tree from the periphery of the liver into the duodenum. The biliary tree is composed of the intrahepatic ducts, the common hepatic duct (CHD), and the CBD. The intrahepatic ducts course centrally from the periphery of the liver to the hepatic hilum, where they join to form the centrally located main left

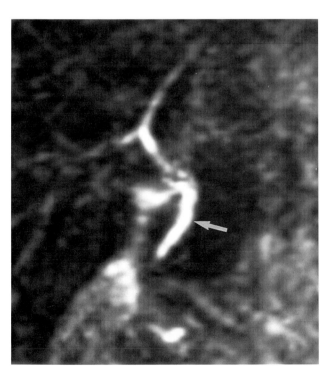

FIG. 8. Fast spin echo MR (8000/144) image of the normal CBD *(arrow)* in 3-D display. Fluid is high in signal on long TE, fast (turbo) spin echo techniques, resulting in good conspicuity of the bile in the biliary system. (Courtesy of Caroline Reinhold, M.D., Department of Radiology, Montreal General Hospital, Montreal, Quebec.)

and right hepatic ducts. The peripheral intrahepatic ducts are located adjacent to the portal veins and hepatic arteries as part of the portal triad. Originally these ducts were thought to occupy a constant anatomic position anterior to the portal veins. However, it is now known that the anatomic relationship of the intrahepatic bile ducts to the portal veins is variable (37). The ducts can be anterior or posterior to the portal veins, or they can even spiral around the portal veins. The high resolution of the currently available CT scanners enables the normal intrahepatic ducts to be visualized in 40% of patients. The mean diameter of the peripheral ducts is 1.8 mm, and that of the central ducts is 2 mm (range 1 to 3 mm) (141). The normal ducts are visualized more often in the right lobe of the liver than in the left lobe. When visualized, the normal intrahepatic ducts are seen as a few randomly scattered, nonconfluent, low-attenuation, circular or linear structures adjacent to the portal vein branches. This appearance, however, does not entirely exclude biliary abnormalities, as some disease processes, such as sclerosing cholangitis, can mimic this pattern (1,210,252).

The main right and left hepatic ducts join to form the proximal portion of the extrahepatic bile duct. This portion of the extrahepatic duct is called the common hepatic duct. The confluence of the main right and left ducts generally occurs either just outside the liver margin or inside the liver within 1.5 cm of the outer edge (236). The CHD is defined as that portion of the extrahepatic bile duct distal to the confluence of the main right and left hepatic ducts and proximal to the insertion of the cystic duct. The cystic duct and its entrance into the common duct are not commonly seen on CT. The location of the insertion of the cystic duct is variable, and therefore the length of the CHD is also variable. The cystic duct and CHD may travel caudally in a common sheath before joining to form the CBD (236). The CHD is located anterior to the portal vein and lateral to the hepatic artery as it courses from the hepatic hilum caudally through the hepatoduodenal ligament (Figs. 2 and 10). Before the advent of helical CT techniques, the normal CHD could be seen in 66% of patients; however, this number may be higher with helical techniques. The mean diameter of the CHD is generally around 2.8 mm, with a range of 1.3 to 8.0 mm (226).

The CBD is defined as that portion of the extrahepatic bile duct that extends from the junction of the cystic duct and CHD to the level of the ampulla of Vater, where it joins the main pancreatic duct. As with the CHD, the length of the CBD varies according to the level of insertion of the cystic duct. The CBD can be divided into suprapancreatic and intrapancreatic segments. The suprapancreatic segment initially courses caudally in the hepatoduodenal ligament with the hepatic artery and portal vein. The duct then begins to course away from the portal vein, posterior and medial to the duodenum, to become the intrapancreatic portion of the CBD. This segment of the duct courses through the pancreatic parenchyma or

along a groove on the posterior surface of the pancreas (Figs. 2,10) until it joins with the main pancreatic duct at the ampulla of Vater. The normal CBD can be seen in 82% of patients. As with the CHD, this number may be higher with helical techniques. The mean diameter of the CBD is 3.6 mm, with a range of 1.5 to 10.9 mm (231).

In addition to evaluating the caliber of the extrahepatic bile duct, it is also important to note the appearance of the bile duct wall. The normal CHD and CBD walls can be visualized in 59% and 52% of patients, respectively. The mean thickness of the CHD and CBD walls is 1 mm. The maximal normal wall thickness for all segments of the extrahepatic bile duct is 1.5 mm (226). The normal bile duct wall enhances to varying degrees after the administration of intravenous contrast; therefore, duct wall enhancement is an insensitive indicator of pathology. In the study by Schulte et al. (226) the duct wall enhancement in patients without biliary tract or pancreatic disease was similar to pancreatic enhancement in 51% of cases, slightly greater than pancreatic enhancement in 44% of cases, and markedly greater than pancreatic enhancement in 5% of cases.

The gallbladder is a near-water-density, round or oval structure most commonly located at the inferior margin of the liver in the region of the interlobar fissure (Fig. 10). The normal gallbladder wall is 1 to 3 mm thick and often enhances after administration of intravenous contrast. Bile in the gallbladder normally has an attenuation of 0 to 20 Hounsfield units (HU). Both obstruction of the cystic duct and chronic cholecystitis can lead to sludge formation and milk of calcium within the gallbladder, resulting in an increase in the attenuation of the gallbladder bile. Blood, pus, and excretion of contrast into the gallbladder also can cause an increase in the attenuation of bile (238,260).

To understand the pathology of the gallbladder and biliary tree, it is necessary to have a grasp of the anatomy of not only the gallbladder and bile ducts themselves, but also the perihepatic ligaments and nodal pathways by which hepatobiliary diseases spread (8,182,194). The perihepatic ligaments are peritoneal reflections that surround the liver. The ligaments most commonly involved in the spread of biliary tract disease are the gastrohepatic, hepatoduodenal, and falciform ligaments.

The gastrohepatic ligament attaches the lesser curvature of the stomach to the inferomedial aspect of the liver. The caudal continuation of the gastrohepatic ligament is the hepatoduodenal ligament. This structure passes from the inferomedial aspect of the liver to the duodenum. These two ligaments are continuous with each other and together constitute the lesser omentum (Fig. 11). The free edge of the hepatoduodenal ligament forms the anterior margin of the foramen of Winslow. The main portal vein, proper hepatic artery, and common bile and hepatic ducts course in the free edge of the hepatoduodenal ligament (275).

The ligamentum teres, a fibrous cord representing the

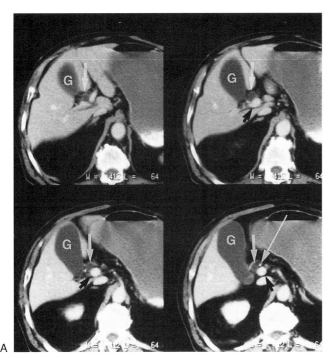

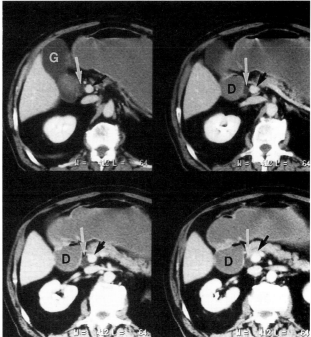

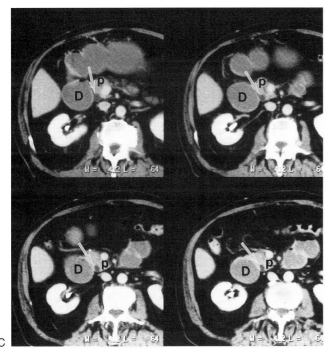

FIG. 10. Normal course of the extrahepatic bile duct. Sequential contrast-enhanced CT images **(A–C)** show the normal anatomy of the common duct as it courses through the hepatoduodenal ligament from the porta hepatis to the duodenum. Note the anterolateral relationship of the suprapancreatic portion of the duct *(thick white arrow)* to the portal vein *(black arrow)* in (A) and (B). As the duct courses more caudally, it can be seen medial to the duodenum (D). In (C), the intrapancreatic portion of the duct *(thick white arrow)* is seen coursing along the posterolateral aspect of the pancreatic head (p). G, gallbladder; *thin white arrow*, hepatic artery.

obliterated umbilical vein, passes cephalad from the umbilicus to the inferior surface of the liver into the fissure that separates the medial and lateral segments of the left lobe. This fibrous cord raises a peritoneal reflection from the anterior abdominal wall that extends from the umbilicus to the inferior surface of the diaphragm. This peritoneal reflection is the falciform ligament. The ligamentum teres travels in the posterior free edge of the falciform ligament. The falciform ligament passes, along with the ligamentum teres, into the fissure separating the medial and lateral segments of the left lobe of the liver (Fig. 12). The ligamentum teres and the gastrohepatic ligament are contiguous in the porta hepatis near the left portal vein (182). The falciform ligament is contiguous with the triangular ligaments over the dome of the liver (275). Through these ligaments, infectious, inflammatory, and neoplastic processes of the gallbladder and bile ducts can spread directly to the subdiaphragmatic space, anterior abdominal wall, retroperitoneum, transverse mesocolon, and duodenocolic ligament (182).

The lymphatic drainage pathways from the gallbladder and bile ducts include the following nodal sites: cystic duct nodes located anterior to the cystic duct, just lateral to the CHD; pericholedochal nodes located posteriorly and to the right of the CHD and CBD; posterosuperior pancreaticoduodenal nodes located between the duodenal sweep and the head of the pancreas; retroportal nodes located posterior to the portal vein and anterior to the inferior vena cava; right celiac nodes located on the posterior aspect of the common hepatic artery; hepatic nodes located adjacent to the proper hepatic artery or anterior to the common hepatic artery in the lesser omentum; superior mesenteric nodes located around the superior mesenteric artery; and aortocaval nodes located between the aorta and inferior vena cava (194).

Magnetic Resonance Imaging

The normal intrahepatic bile ducts are not generally visible on conventional T1- and T2-weighted images, but they are routinely visible on gadolinium-enhanced SGE images. The normal extrahepatic bile ducts, however, are frequently seen on routine T1-weighted and T2-weighted images, but they are best visualized on T2-weighted and gadolinium-enhanced SGE images (Figs. 13,14). In one study, the CBD could be identified in 50% of normal patients (244). The absence of motion-artifact-suppression techniques in the exams performed in that study presumably contributed to the relatively low frequency of visualization of the CBD. More recently, other authors have reported that in their experience, using flow-compensated spin echo or fast spin echo techniques, the distal CBD could be seen in almost all cases (171).

The mean diameter of the CBD on T1-weighted images is reported to be 6.4 mm, with a range of 4.5 to 10 mm. On T2-weighted images, the mean CBD diameter is reported to be 7.8 mm, with a range of 4.4 to 11.8 mm (244). The discrepancy between MRI and CT readings of the mean diameter of the CBD, and between the different MRI pulse sequences, may be accounted for by variation in patient populations, blurring of images, apparent enlargement of the duct because of respiratory motion artifact on spin echo images, and variation in the apparent size of anatomic structures on different MRI pulse sequences (203,244). Findings on breath-hold, gadolinium-enhanced, SGE images would be expected to be comparable to findings on CT images.

The MRI appearance of the gallbladder varies depending on the length of time between imaging and the patient's most recent meal. In a nonfasting patient with a normal gallbladder, bile is hypointense on T1-weighted images and hyperintense on T2-weighted images, relative to the signal intensity of the liver. This is because recently excreted bile is dilute and has a large amount of free water, resulting in long T1 and T2 values. In a patient with a normal gallbladder, up to 90% of the water in bile is absorbed by the mucosa in the first 4 hours of fasting. The resulting concentrated bile has a decreased amount of free water relative to the dilute fresh bile, and thus it has shorter T1 and T2 values. For this reason, bile

FIG. 11. Normal anatomic relationships of the gastrohepatic (gh) and hepatoduodenal (hd) ligaments. **A:** Coronal reformation of volumetric data obtained during spiral CT of the upper abdomen. Plane of section through the origin of the superior mesenteric artery (sma) and vein (smv). The superior mesenteric vein courses medial to the head and neck of the pancreas (P) at this level. The left gastric vessels (lg) run parallel to the medial border of the stomach (ST) within the gastrohepatic ligament. The posterior-most portion of the hepatoduodenal ligament is shown on this section. It is bounded by the liver (L), the duodenum (DU), the hepatic flexure (HF), and the gallbladder (gb), and it contains a portion of the left portal vein (lp). Gd, gastroduodenal artery. **B:** Coronal reformation 3 mm anterior to (A) shows the main portal vein (pv) coursing to the right. At this level, it remains within the retroperitoneum, medial to the duodenum and pancreas. The gastrohepatic ligament attaches to the liver within the fissure for the ligamentum venosum *(arrowhead)*, which separates the caudate lobe (seen on posterior sections) from the medial segment of the left lobe (seen on more anterior sections). **C:** Coronal reformation 3 mm anterior to (B) shows the portal vein exiting the retroperitoneum to lie in the inferior portion of the hepatoduodenal ligament. It is accompanied by the common hepatic duct (chd) on this section. Note the brightly enhancing left gastric, or coronary, vein (cor) within the gastrohepatic ligament.

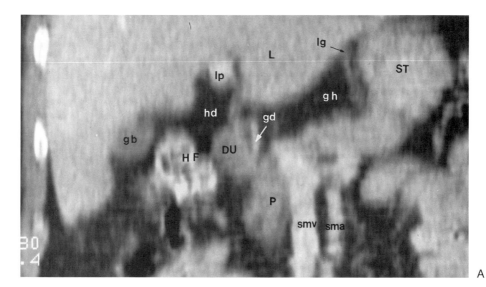

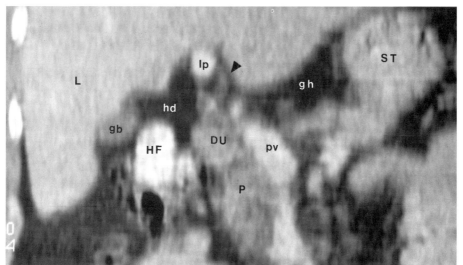

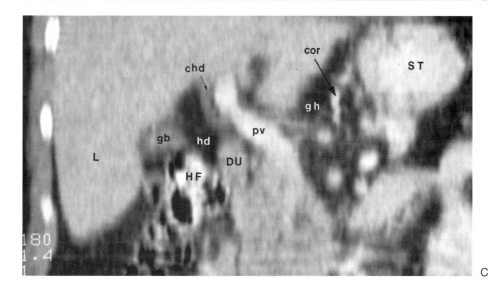

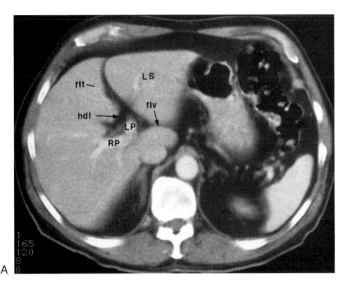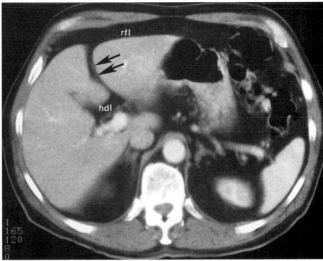

A

B

FIG. 12. Fissure for the ligamentum teres. **A:** Contrast-enhanced CT image obtained at the level of the porta hepatis shows the relationship between the fissure for the ligamentum venosum (flv), the hepatoduodenal ligament (hdl), and the fissure for the ligamentum teres (flt). The lateral segment (LS) of the left hepatic lobe lies to the left of the fissure for the ligamentum teres. RP, right portal vein; LP, left portal vein. **B:** CT image obtained 10 mm caudal to (A) more clearly shows the ligamentum teres *(arrows)*, a remnant of the umbilical vein, extending between the hepatoduodenal ligament and the extraperitoneal fat in the root of the falciform ligament (rfl).

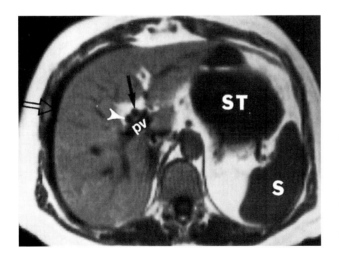

FIG. 13. Normal porta hepatis: MR image (SE 300/30). The fat in the ligamentum venosum and ligamentum teres has a high signal intensity, and the liver parenchyma has a homogeneous medium signal intensity. The portal vein (pv) and hepatic artery *(arrow)* yield low signal intensities because of the "flow-void" phenomenon. The CHD *(arrowhead)* also has a low signal intensity on this T1-weighted image because of the long T1 of bile. A small amount of ascites is present *(open arrow)*. ST, stomach; S, spleen. (From Lee JKT, Sagel SS, Stanley RJ, eds. *Computed body tomography with MRI correlation,* 2nd ed. New York: Raven Press, 1989.)

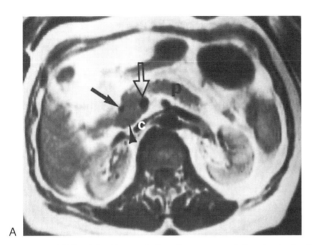
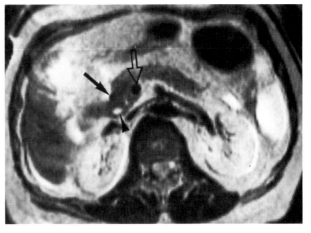

A   B

FIG. 14. Normal distal common bile duct. **A:** Balanced MR image (SE 2100/35). The distal CBD *(arrowhead)* is almost isointense with the pancreas (p). *Arrow,* gastroduodenal artery; *open arrow,* superior mesenteric vein; c, IVC. **B:** T2-weighted MR image (SE 2100/90). The distal CBD *(arrowhead)* has a much higher signal intensity and can be easily differentiated from the pancreas. Note that both the superior mesenteric vein *(open arrow)* and the gastroduodenal artery *(arrow)* still appear as areas of "flow void."

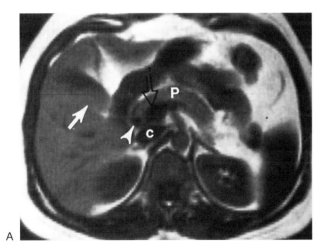
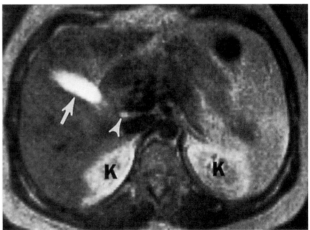

A   B

FIG. 15. Normal gallbladder. **A:** T1-weighted MR image (SE 300/15). The dependent portion of the gallbladder *(arrow)* has a medium signal intensity similar to that of the liver, whereas the top layer has a lower signal intensity. Note that the distal CBD *(arrowhead)* has a similar low signal intensity. P, pancreas; c, IVC; *open arrow,* superior mesenteric vein. **B:** T2-weighted MR image (SE 2100/90). Both the gallbladder *(arrow)* and the distal CBD *(arrowhead)* have high signal intensities. K, kidney.

in fasting patients, relative to the liver, is high in signal intensity on both T1- and T2-weighted images (66,106,118,119). It is noteworthy that the increased signal on the T1-weighted images results from the decreased amount of free water and not from an increased amount of lipids (66). Occasionally, on T1-weighted images, a layered appearance of the bile in the gallbladder can be seen (Figs. 15,16). This is because of fresh, dilute, low-signal-intensity bile floating on top of a layer of older, more concentrated, high-signal-intensity bile.

BILE DUCT OBSTRUCTION AND WALL ABNORMALITIES

Computed Tomography

In contrast to the randomly scattered, nonconfluent, circular or linear appearance of normal intrahepatic bile ducts, dilated intrahepatic bile ducts generally appear as a large number of confluent, circular or linear, branching structures that enlarge and join together as they approach the porta hepatis and form the main right and left hepatic ducts (Fig. 17) (20). Less frequently encountered patterns of intrahepatic bile duct dilatation include: pruning, defined as the presence on a single CT section of a 4-cm or longer segment of dilated duct (excluding the main right and left ducts) that lacks the expected side branch dilatation; beading, defined as at least three closely alternating regions of dilatation and stenosis in an intrahepatic duct on a single CT section; and skip dilatation, defined as isolated, dilated peripheral bile ducts with no visible connection to other dilated ducts on contiguous images (253) (Fig. 18). Pruning and beading are nonspecific patterns of intrahepatic bile duct dilatation that can be seen as a result of bile duct obstruction from a variety of etiologies. True pruning on direct cholangiography and CT is caused by narrowing and sclerosis of the bile duct side branches. However, the appearance of pruning can be simulated on CT by an obstructed bile duct with normal caliber side branches that have not yet dilated at the time of the CT scan. As with pruning, the appearance of beading can be simulated on CT. In the case of beading, the simulated appearance is caused by dilated tortuous ducts that meander in and out of the axial imaging plane.

Skip dilatations seen on CT are strongly suggestive of primary sclerosing cholangitis (PSC). Less frequently,

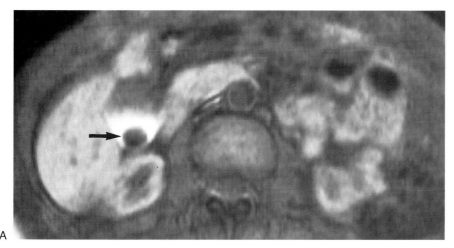

A

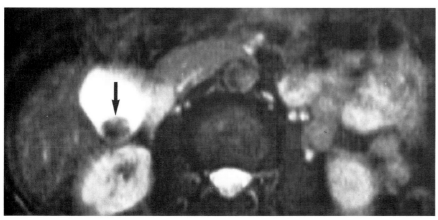

B

FIG. 16. MRI of gallbladder bile. T1-weighted, fat-suppressed spin echo (600/15) **(A)** and T2-weighted, fat-suppressed spin echo (2100/90) **(B)** images demonstrate a signal-void calculus *(arrow)* in the dependent portion of the gallbladder. Layering of low signal intensity bile on top of high signal intensity bile is apparent on the T1-weighted image. In this case the dependent layer of bile is higher in signal intensity than the liver on the T1-weighted image. Bile in the gallbladder may be either high or low signal intensity on T1-weighted images because of variations in bile composition. (Reproduced with permission from Semelka RC, Shoenut JP, Micflikier AB. The gallbladder and biliary tree. In: Semelka RC, Shoenut JP, eds. *MRI of the abdomen with CT correlation.* New York: Raven Press, 1993;43–52.)

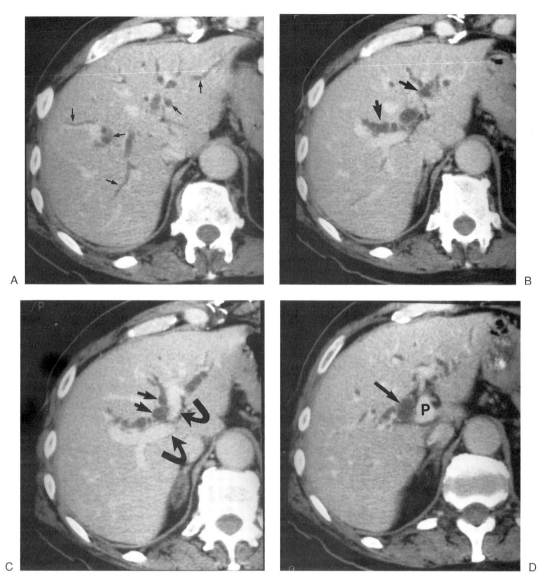

FIG. 17. Intrahepatic bile duct dilatation. Four contiguous contrast-enhanced CT images show a typical appearance of dilated intrahepatic bile ducts. **A:** The dilated ducts are seen as linear, low-attenuation, tubular and circular structures *(thin arrows)* paralleling the enhanced portal veins. Note that the ducts increase in diameter and appear to converge towards a common location as they course centrally. **B,C:** As the ducts course caudally and centrally, the peripheral ducts have joined to form the main left and right hepatic ducts *(thick arrows)* adjacent to the main trunk of the right and left portal veins *(curved arrows)*. **D:** The main right and left hepatic ducts have joined to form the CHD *(arrow)* anterolateral to the main portal vein (P).

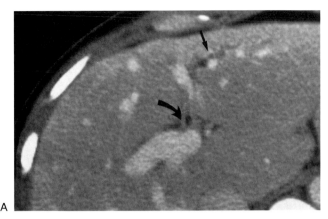
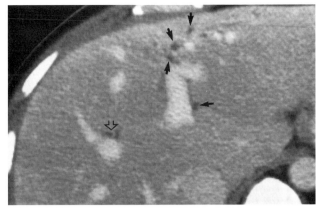

A   B

FIG. 18. Primary sclerosing cholangitis. **A:** Contrast-enhanced CT image shows a dilated duct with a "beaded" appearance *(arrow)* in the periphery of the left lobe of the liver. This appearance may be seen in PSC, but it is not specific for it. Also note the focal area of duct dilatation anterior to the right portal vein *(curved arrow)*. **B:** At the level 1 cm cephalad, irregular intrahepatic bile duct dilatation in the left lobe of the liver is seen as multiple small cystic-appearing structures *(arrows)*. This is the appearance of skip dilatations resulting from regions of mildly dilated ducts interspersed with short segmental strictures. Also note the focal area of duct dilatation in the right lobe *(open arrow)*.

skip dilatations can be caused by intrahepatic mass lesions or recurrent pyogenic cholangitis (RPC). The appearance of skip dilatation on CT can be simulated in a patient with intrahepatic bile duct dilatation from other causes if the axial CT images are not truly contiguous because of slice misregistration from patient respiration.

Lobar or segmental intrahepatic bile duct obstruction can be caused by tumor, inflammation, strictures, trauma, or intrahepatic bile duct stones (287). The distribution and extent of intrahepatic bile duct dilatation does not correlate with any one disease process (253). Some authors have reported a predilection for severe intrahepatic bile duct dilatation to involve the left lobe of the liver more often than the right lobe, regardless of the point of obstruction (3,43,198).

One of the pitfalls in the diagnosis of intrahepatic bile duct dilatation is perivascular lymphedema (Fig. 19). Perivascular lymphedema can occasionally mimic intrahepatic bile duct dilatation; however, with experience, these two entities can be differentiated from one another. While dilated intrahepatic bile ducts generally are seen on only one side of the portal vein branches at any one location, perivascular lymphedema tends to cause circumferential low attenuation around the veins (124). Infiltrating periductal neoplasms also have been reported as an abnormality that can mimic intrahepatic bile duct dilatation. The difference between the appearance of tumor and dilated bile ducts is that tumor is usually more lobular and irregular in appearance than dilated ducts (181).

Fatty infiltration of the liver is another pitfall in the diagnosis of intrahepatic bile duct dilatation. The low attenuation of the hepatic parenchyma in fatty infiltration decreases the attenuation difference between the dilated bile ducts and surrounding liver. This decrease in conspicuity of the dilated ducts can make their detection with CT much more difficult (Fig. 20) or obscure them completely (206).

The diagnosis of extrahepatic bile duct dilatation is based on the caliber of the CHD and CBD. On sequential axial CT images, the CHD and CBD appear as a series of water-attenuation, circular or oval structures. When determining the diameter of the extrahepatic bile ducts, the shortest axis of these circular or oval structures should be measured. Using this method the measurements are less likely to be subject to overestimation errors that result from oblique orientation of the duct in the axial imaging

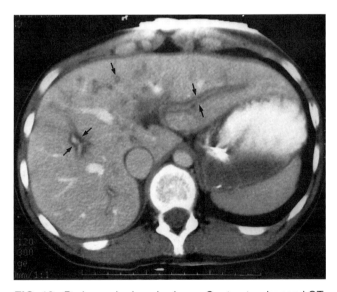

FIG. 19. Perivascular lymphedema. Contrast-enhanced CT of the liver shows a collar of low attenuation *(arrows)* completely surrounding the portal vein branches. This represents periportal lymphedema resulting from vigorous intravenous hydration with crystalloids in a trauma patient.

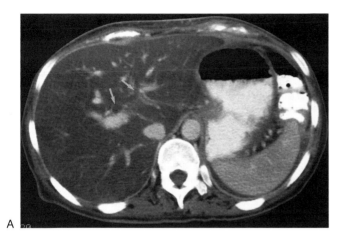

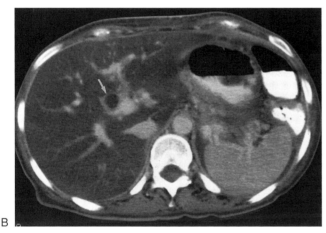

FIG. 20. Contiguous contrast-enhanced CT images in a patient with intrahepatic biliary ductal dilatation and diffuse hepatic fatty infiltration. **A:** At the level of the main right and left hepatic ducts *(arrows)*, it is difficult to distinguish the dilated ducts from the low attenuation of the surrounding liver. **B:** It is difficult to recognize the dilated CHD *(arrow)* 1 cm caudal to the confluence of the right and left hepatic ducts, because the low attenuation of the liver is nearly identical to the water attenuation of the bile.

plane. The anteroposterior (AP) diameter is generally more reliable than the transverse diameter (83). As discussed in the section on normal anatomy, the normal caliber of the CHD has been found to range from 1.3 to 8.0 mm, and that of the CBD from 1.5 to 10.9 mm (12,20,192). The diameter considered normal for the extrahepatic bile ducts varies, depending on the age of the patient and the imaging modality used for measurement (192,277). On CT, a common duct with a diameter of less than or equal to 7 mm should be considered normal, between 7 mm and 10 mm equivocal, and greater than 10 mm dilated.

When evaluating a dilated extrahepatic bile duct on CT, following the course of the duct on sequential axial images allows the principles of interpretation of the cholangiographic characteristics of normal and abnormal ducts to be applied to the interpretation of the axial CT images (20,198). Obstruction can be confirmed as the

cause of dilatation only if a transition zone between dilated and nondilated segments of the ducts can be identified. If a site of obstruction is identified, determination of the etiology of the obstruction requires detailed evaluation of the appearance of the transition zone (20,198). This often requires the use of high-resolution, thin-section (3 mm to 5 mm) CT techniques.

The appearance of the transition zone from dilated to nondilated duct can give important clues as to the cause of the obstruction (Fig. 21). The normal extrahepatic duct, or a duct with a benign distal stricture, gradually tapers as it approaches the ampulla of Vater (Fig. 22). In contrast, abrupt termination of the duct, with proximal dilatation, is most often a result of malignant obstruction (Fig. 23).

In their evaluation of the extrahepatic bile ducts, Schulte et al. (226) determined that wall thickness greater than 1.5 mm should be considered abnormal (Fig. 24). There are four general patterns of bile duct wall thickening: focal concentric, involving only the distal CBD; focal eccentric, involving any portion of the extrahepatic duct; diffuse concentric; and diffuse eccentric. Each pattern is associated with a specific group of diseases. The focal concentric pattern in the distal CBD is seen in pancreatitis, pancreatic carcinoma, and CBD stones. The focal eccentric pattern is most commonly seen with neoplasms. This pattern tends to have the greatest amount of wall thickening; in fact, any wall thickness greater than

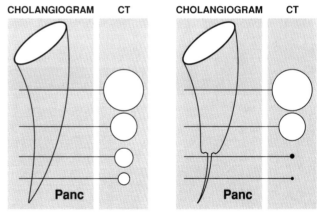

FIG. 21. Schematic drawing of cholangiographic and correlative CT appearance of normal and abnormal CBD. In a normal duct or a duct with a benign stricture *(left)*, the cholangiogram shows a smooth gradual tapering. The CT images of this duct show sequential water-attenuation circles with a progressively decreasing diameter, surrounded by the soft-tissue-attenuation pancreas. The cholangiogram of a duct with a malignant stricture *(right)* shows an abrupt change in caliber of the duct with complete occlusion of the lumen at the site of obstruction. The corresponding CT images would show water-attenuation circles that decrease in diameter to the level of the obstruction and then abruptly disappear. A mass may or may not be apparent at the site of obstruction. (Modified from Baron RL. Computed tomography of the biliary tree. *Radiol Clin North Am* 1991;29:1235–1250.)

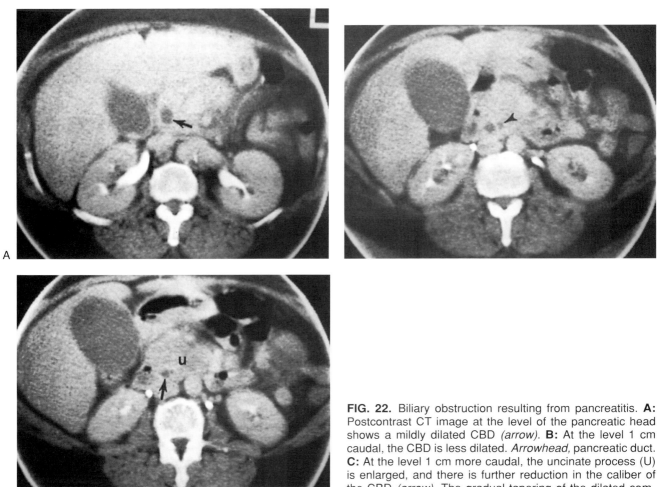

FIG. 22. Biliary obstruction resulting from pancreatitis. **A:** Postcontrast CT image at the level of the pancreatic head shows a mildly dilated CBD *(arrow)*. **B:** At the level 1 cm caudal, the CBD is less dilated. *Arrowhead,* pancreatic duct. **C:** At the level 1 cm more caudal, the uncinate process (U) is enlarged, and there is further reduction in the caliber of the CBD *(arrow)*. The gradual tapering of the dilated common duct is characteristic of a benign process.

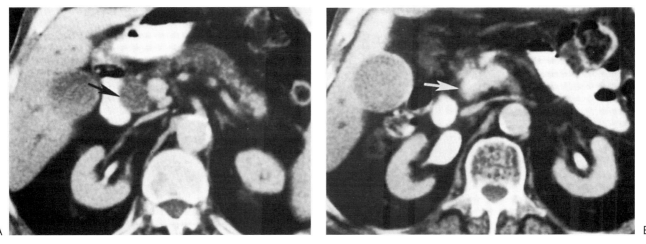

FIG. 23. CT of biliary obstruction caused by pancreatic carcinoma. **A:** Contrast-enhanced CT image shows a dilated CBD *(arrow)* in the pancreatic head. **B:** At the level 1 cm caudal, the CBD is not visible. Abrupt termination of a dilated common duct is highly suggestive of a malignant process. A small tumor was found in the uncinate process *(arrow)* at surgery.

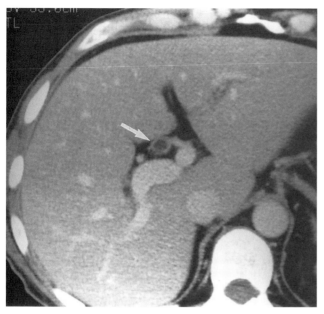

FIG. 24. Bile duct wall thickening. Contrast-enhanced CT image at the level of the right portal vein shows thickening of the wall of the CHD *(arrow)* in a patient with AIDS-related cholangiopathy.

5 mm should be considered neoplastic until proven otherwise. Diffuse concentric wall thickening is characteristic of acute cholangitis, and the diffuse eccentric pattern is most often seen in recurrent pyogenic cholangitis and PSC.

Gallbladder wall thickening is a nonspecific finding that can be caused by a variety of causes including hypoproteinemia, pancreatitis, hepatitis, acute or chronic cholecystitis, portal hypertension, autoimmune deficiency syndrome (AIDS) cholangiopathy, adeno-myomatosis, and gallbladder carcinoma (90,164,238, 241,273). The normal gallbladder wall should be no more than 3 mm thick. Benign gallbladder wall thickening appears as a thin rim of enhancing mucosa, surrounded by a thicker zone of near-water attenuation, representing submucosal edema (Fig. 25). Occasionally, there also may be small enhancing vessels within, and an outer rim of enhancement around, the low-attenuation edema. Benign gallbladder wall edema can simulate, and must be differentiated from, pericholecystic fluid. In general, pericholecystic fluid will not completely surround the gallbladder, and there will be no outer rim of enhancement. The presence of pericholecystic fluid is suggestive of acute cholecystitis with perforation and possible abscess formation (90).

Magnetic Resonance Imaging

The imaging appearance of bile duct obstruction on MRI differs from CT only in terms of the characteristics of the bile in the dilated ducts. Most commonly, dilated bile ducts appear hypointense relative to the liver on T1-weighted images, and hyperintense on T2-weighted images (71,97,149). However, because of the variable

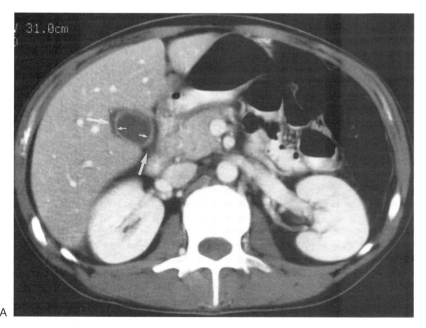

A

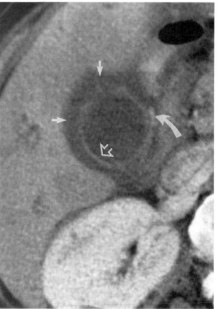

B

FIG. 25. Gallbladder wall edema. **A:** Contrast-enhanced CT scan in a patient with hepatitis shows the enhancing gallbladder mucosa *(short arrows)* surrounded by low-attenuation edema *(long arrows)* in the outer layers of the gallbladder wall. The wall edema in this patient was caused by hepatitis. **B:** In a different patient, low-attenuation gallbladder wall edema *(arrows)* is seen surrounding the enhancing gallbladder mucosa *(open arrows)*. An enhancing blood vessel is seen in the medial portion of the gallbladder wall *(curved arrow)*. The wall edema in this patient was secondary to biliary obstruction from pancreatic carcinoma.

composition of bile, the relative signal intensities of dilated intrahepatic ducts and the liver are not constant. This variability in bile duct–liver contrast on T1-weighted images necessitates the use of at least two pulse sequences when evaluating the bile ducts with MRI (119). In a comparison of CT and three different MR pulse sequences, Low et al. (149) found that the gadolinium-enhanced, T1-weighted SGE images were superior to fast spin echo and unenhanced T1-weighted spin echo images for the depiction of dilated bile ducts (Fig. 26). They found no significant difference between CT and the enhanced gradient echo pulse sequence.

In patients without biliary tract disease, the normal periportal fat is high in signal intensity on T1-weighted images. Abnormal periportal signal can be seen in pa-tients with biliary tract or diffuse hepatic disease (158). This abnormality, which results from edema, bile duct proliferation, dilated lymphatics, and inflammatory cell infiltrates, is low in signal intensity on T1-weighted images and high in signal intensity on T2-weighted images. Periportal signal abnormalities are seen in pa-tients with bile duct dilatation and obstructive jaundice or cholangitis, but not in patients with bile duct dilata-tion without obstruction or cholangitis.

Depiction of abnormalities of the bile duct and gall-bladder walls on MRI parallel those seen on CT. As stated in the technique section, gadolinium-enhanced, T1-weighted, fat-suppressed spin echo images are par-ticularly well suited for the demonstration of bile duct and gallbladder wall thickening.

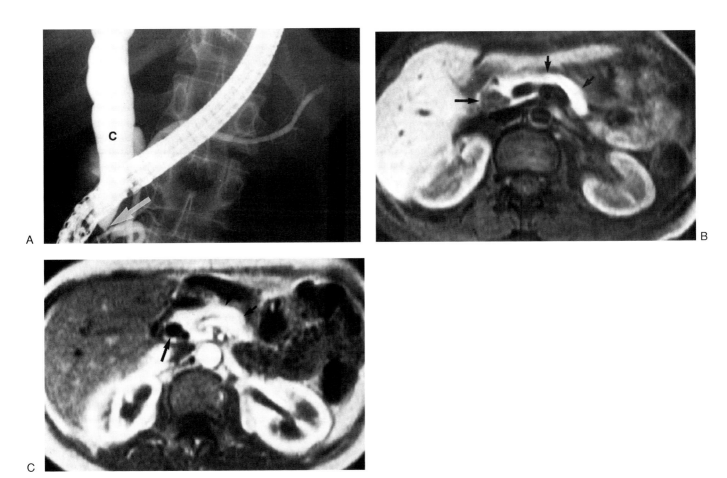

FIG. 26. Ampullary stenosis. **A:** ERCP image showing the typical smooth, tapered narrowing *(white arrow)* of the CBD (C) at the level of the ampulla of Vater. This appearance is characteristic of ampullary stenosis. **B:** Fat-suppressed, T1-weighted spin echo MR image (600/15) showing the normal high signal intensity pancreatic tissue *(short black arrows)* surrounding the dilated CBD *(long black arrow)*. On more caudal images (not shown) the duct narrowed in a smooth tapered fashion into the duodenum. **C:** Immediate-post-gadolinium-enhancement, spoiled gradient echo MR image (FLASH 130/4/80°) shows increased contrast between the high signal pancreatic tissue *(short black arrow)* and the signal-void CBD *(long black arrow)*. The strong contrast enhancement of normal pancreatic tissue on the spoiled gradient echo image is a consistent finding on immediate-post-gadolinium-enhancement images. (Reproduced with permission from Semelka RC, Shoenut JP, Kroeker MA, et al. Bile duct disease: prospective comparison of ERCP, CT and fat suppression MRI. *Gastrointest Radiol* 1992;17:347–352.)

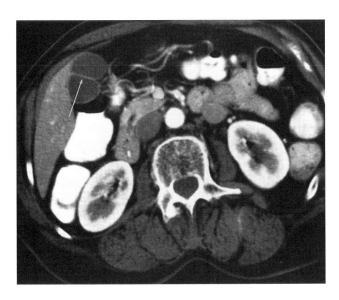

FIG. 27. Contrast-enhanced CT image shows a complete septation in the body of the gallbladder (arrow).

DISEASES OF THE GALLBLADDER

Congenital Anomalies

Congenital anomalies of the gallbladder include variations in location, number, and morphology. Although most of these anomalies are uncommon, they must be recognized and not mistaken for significant pathology. Intrahepatic, retrohepatic, retroperitoneal, and left subhepatic positions of the gallbladder are the most common variations in location. Agenesis and duplication of the gallbladder are less common than positional anomalies. Morphologic anomalies of the gallbladder include folds and septations (Fig. 27). In contrast to the majority of congenital anomalies, the phrygian cap is a relatively common normal variant, characterized by folding of the gallbladder fundus (165).

Adenomyomatosis

Adenomyomatosis is an abnormality of the gallbladder wall characterized by hyperplastic changes including overgrowth of the mucosa, thickening of the muscular layers, and formation of intramural crypts, sinus tracts, and diverticula (Rokitansky-Aschoff sinuses). It is found in approximately one fourth of all surgically removed gallbladders; however, the precise cause of this abnormality is unknown. Adenomyomatosis is neither neoplastic nor premalignant. The age range of patients found to have adenomyomatosis is 26 to 86 years, and men and women are affected equally. Adenomyomatosis is not known to cause clinical symptoms (25).

The gallbladder wall abnormalities in adenomyomatosis can be diffuse, segmental (annular), or focal. The focal form, called an adenomyoma, most often occurs in the fundus. Grossly it appears as a sessile, soft tissue mass

with a central umbilication. The diagnosis of adenomyomatosis is most often made with oral cholecystography or ultrasonography. Findings that may be seen on CT in adenomyomatosis include enlargement of the gallbladder with irregular wall thickening, a focal mass in the fundus, and proliferation of the subserosal fat of the gallbladder (86,175). The appearance of proliferation of the subserosal fat can be mimicked by the greater omentum wrapping around the gallbladder in the presence of chronic cholecystitis. Visualization of Rokitansky-Aschoff sinuses on CT has been reported only when the scan was performed in conjunction with oral cholecystography (33). Adenomyomatosis mimics gallbladder carcinoma when the only CT findings are gallbladder wall thickening or a focal mass in the fundus of the gallbladder.

Porcelain Gallbladder

Porcelain gallbladder is the term used to describe calcification of the gallbladder wall (Fig. 28). This condition is more common in women than in men and is believed to be the result of chronic inflammation (116,238). Two histologic types of calcification can be found in porcelain gallbladders: (a) a broad continuous band of calcification in the muscularis, and (b) multiple calcified microliths scattered throughout the mucosa and submucosa. Patients who have a porcelain gallbladder have an increased risk of developing gallbladder carcinoma. The incidence of gallbladder cancer in these patients is reported to be as high as 33%. The appearance of a porcelain gallbladder can be mimicked on CT by a contracted gallbladder containing a large stone with a calcified rim and a bile-attenuation center. Other causes of regions of high attenuation in the gallbladder wall, such as lipiodol deposition secondary to transarterial chemoembolization of hepatic

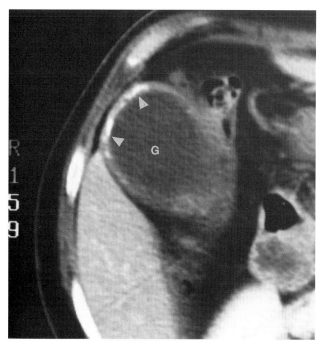

FIG. 28. Porcelain gallbladder. CT image through the fundus of the gallbladder (G) shows thickening and calcification of the wall *(arrowheads).*

tumors (Fig. 29), may occasionally be seen but are uncommon.

Hemobilia

Blood in the biliary tract can be caused by blunt trauma, traumatic venous– or arterial–biliary fistulas (usually iatrogenic), inflammatory disease, or tumor. The attenuation of normal bile varies between 0 and 20 HU. Blood raises the attenuation of the bile to a level generally greater than 50 HU. Initially, the bile may be diffusely increased in attenuation. As the blood clots, it settles in the dependent

portion of the gallbladder or bile ducts (Fig. 30). The high attenuation appearance of the bile can persist for several days (26,77,110,125).

Cholelithiasis

Gallstones are present in 10% to 20% of the U.S. population. The incidence of stones is greater in women than in men, and it increases with pregnancy and increasing age (111). The two primary types of calculi are cholesterol stones and pigment stones. Between 70% and 80% of gallstones in the United States are cholesterol stones. Pigment stones are more common in Asians, cirrhotics, and patients with chronic hemolytic anemia. Cholesterol stones contain between 25% and 90% cholesterol, whereas pigment stones generally contain 40% to 50% calcium bilirubinate and less than 25% cholesterol (21,36,39,230).

Approximately 20% of people with gallstones become symptomatic each year and require treatment (34). The most common therapy is open or laparoscopic cholecystectomy. Nonsurgical therapeutic options include gallstone dissolution therapy, percutaneous stone extraction, and biliary lithotripsy (35). The success of these nonsurgical treatments greatly depends on appropriate patient selection. The need for an accurate method for selecting patients has led to a multitude of studies correlating CT and MRI characteristics of gallstones (including attenuation, signal intensity, size, shape, and pattern of calcification) with successful dissolution therapy or lithotripsy (16,18,22,34,36,39,40,104,157,185). Although there appears to be some correlation between the appearance of gallstones on CT and the success of dissolution therapy, the precise role of CT and MRI in aiding appropriate patient selection is still being investigated. Moreover, as the role of laparoscopic cholecystectomy expands, there is diminishing need to perform selection studies for dissolution therapy.

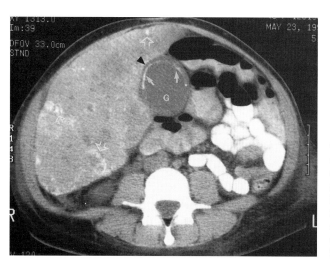

FIG. 29. CT scan at the level of the body of the gallbladder (G) shows a rim of high attenuation *(arrows)* in the gallbladder wall. This high-attenuation rim, which mimics the appearance of a porcelain gallbladder, is caused by lipiodol in the gallbladder wall. The outer low-attenuation rim of the gallbladder represents gallbladder wall edema *(arrowhead).* This patient had hepatic arterial chemoembolization for treatment of carcinoid metastases to the liver. The deposition of lipiodol in the gallbladder wall is uncommon. It is more common to see the lipiodol deposited as foci of high attenuation *(open arrows)* throughout the liver.

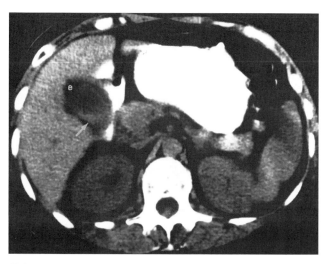

FIG. 30. Hemobilia. Noncontrast CT image shows high-attenuation material *(arrow)* in the dependent portion of the gallbladder. This represents blood in the gallbladder lumen resulting from an injury to the gallbladder wall during a percutaneous liver biopsy. Low-attenuation gallbladder wall edema, secondary to the injury, also is present (e).

Computed Tomography in Cholelithiasis

The most sensitive imaging modality for detecting gallstones is sonography, which has a sensitivity of 93% to 95% (58,157). Oral cholecystography and ultrasonography are equivalent in their ability to detect the number and size of gallstones. Computed tomography, however, which has a sensitivity of only 75% to 79% for the detection of gallstones, is the most sensitive imaging modality for detecting calcification within the stones (11,16,21,157). Stones less than 5 mm in size are less likely to be detected than larger stones, as a result of volume averaging. Furthermore, pure cholesterol stones are less likely to be detected than heavily calcified stones. Barakos et al. (11) found that visualization of gallstones is more dependent on the composition of the stones than the size.

Gallstones can have a variety of appearances on CT depending on their chemical composition and pattern of calcification (11,16,34,36,39,104). The calculi can be homogeneous or heterogeneous (Fig. 31). Homogeneous stones can be denser than soft tissue (generally >90 HU), equal in attenuation to soft tissue (30 to 89 HU), or lower in attenuation than soft tissue and isodense to bile (5 to 20 HU). Uncommonly, stones will appear to be homogeneously lower in attenuation than bile (Fig. 31). The CT attenuation of gallstones correlates more closely with the cholesterol content of the stones than with the calcium content (16,104). The negative correlation between the attenuation of gallstones on CT and the content of cholesterol in the stones is greater than the positive correlation between the attenuation of gallstones and the content of calcium.

Approximately 50% of gallstones have a central fissure. This fissure most often contains fluid; however, it can at times contain gas and create the so-called Mercedes Benz sign (23) (Fig. 31). Gallstones can be mimicked on CT by the enhancing mucosa of a contracted gallbladder with an edematous wall (Fig. 32), or by the gallbladder wall or neck, which often fold upon themselves, and, if cut in cross section, can be mistaken for a gallstone with a high-density rim and bile-attenuation center.

Magnetic Resonance Imaging in Cholelithiasis

Most gallstones produce little or no signal on MR images (Fig. 33). The absence of signal results from the restricted motion of the water and cholesterol molecules in the stones (119,179). Calculi are best demonstrated on MR images in which bile is high in signal intensity. Magnetic resonance imaging is superior to CT in the detection of small calculi because of the inherent high contrast, on bright biliary fluid techniques, between the low signal intensity calculi and the high signal intensity bile. Uncommonly, stones may be homogeneously high in signal intensity on T1-weighted images, or they may contain a central focus of increased signal intensity on T1- or T2-weighted images (Fig. 33). The correlation between signal intensity and chemical composition of gallstones is complex and has not yet been clearly defined. The variations in signal intensity have been attributed by different authors to increased amounts of fatty acids in the stones, decreased amounts of free water in the stones, and diffusion of dilute bile into fissures in the center of the stones (19,21,176,179,185). At the present time, no correlation between the signal intensity of gallstones and the success of dissolution therapy has been demonstrated (119).

Cholecystitis

Computed Tomography in Cholecystitis

Cholelithiasis is the cause of acute cholecystitis in approximately 95% of cases. Obstruction of the cystic duct by a stone leads to bile stasis and progressive distention of the gallbladder (hydrops). This eventually leads to vascular compromise of the gallbladder wall, with subsequent mucosal inflammation and necrosis, and bacterial contamination of the bile (255). CT plays little role in the initial evaluation of patients with acute cholecystitis. When the diagnosis of cholecystitis is made by CT, it is often in patients with confusing clinical pictures in whom the diagnosis of cholecystitis was not the primary consideration (255).

The most common CT findings in acute calculous cholecystitis are distention of the gallbladder (>5 cm in transverse or AP dimension), gallbladder wall thickening (>3 mm) and nodularity, stones in the gallbladder or cystic

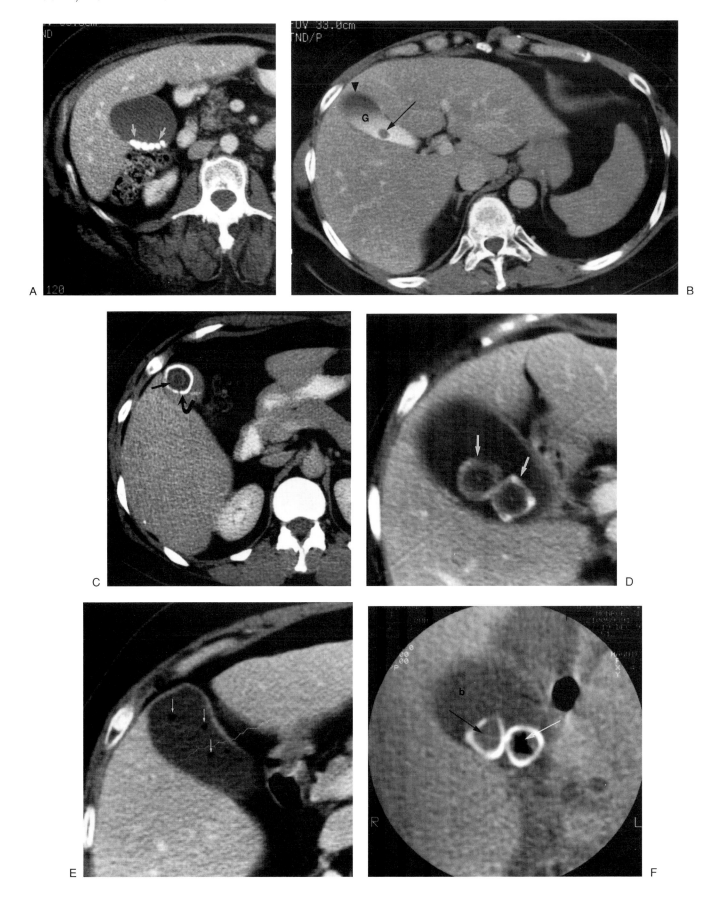

FIG. 31. CT appearance of gallstones. **A:** Multiple small, densely calcified, typical calcium bilirubinate stones *(arrows)* are layering in the dependent portion of the gallbladder. **B:** Contrast-enhanced CT image obtained 1 day after ERCP. The gallbladder (G) is filled with contrast material from the ERCP. A gallstone *(arrow)* appears as a round, low-attenuation filling defect in the contrast-filled gallbladder. This stone, which is isodense to the unenhanced portion of the bile *(arrowhead)*, would not have been seen without the presence of the ERCP contrast. **C:** Laminated gallstone. A densely calcified peripheral rim *(curved arrow)* surrounds a rim of low attenuation. The rim of low attenuation surrounds a faintly calcified ring *(straight arrow)*, which in turn surrounds a central region of low attenuation. **D:** Faceted gallstones *(arrows)* with densely calcified rims and a punctate central calcification. **E:** Multiple "pure" cholesterol gallstones *(arrows)* appear as foci of lower attenuation than the surrounding bile in the nondependent portion of the gallbladder. **F:** Note the rim calcification of the two stones in the gallbladder. The central portion of one of the stones *(black arrow)* is the same attenuation as the surrounding bile (b). The central portion of the adjacent stone *(white arrow)* contains gas, creating the "Mercedes Benz" sign.

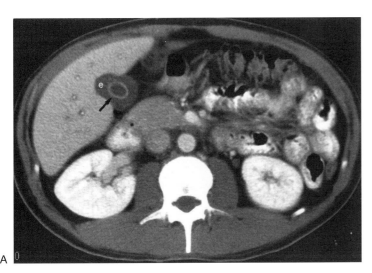

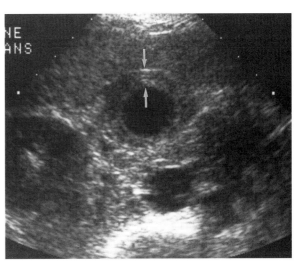

A

B

FIG. 32. Gallbladder wall edema mimicking a gallstone. **A:** Contrast-enhanced CT image shows low-attenuation edema (e) surrounding the enhancing gallbladder mucosa *(arrow)*, mimicking the appearance of a gallstone with a bile-attenuation center. **B:** Transverse sonographic image of the gallbladder, in the same patient, confirms the presence of marked wall thickening *(arrows)*. No stones were seen on sonography.

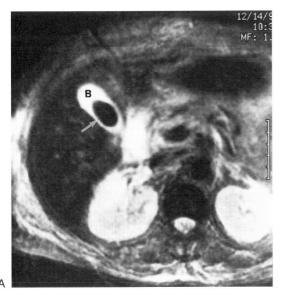

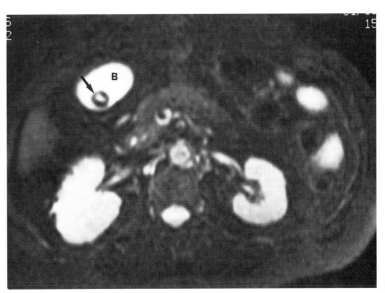

A

B

FIG. 33. MRI of gallstones. **A:** T2-weighted, fat-saturated fast spin echo MR image (4500/90) shows a gallstone *(arrow)* in the central portion of the gallbladder. Note the homogeneous low signal intensity of the stone surrounded by the high signal intensity bile (B). **B:** Conventional fat-saturated, T2-weighted spin echo MR image (2500/90) in a different patient shows a gallstone *(arrow)* in the dependent portion of the gallbladder. Note that this stone has a central focus of high signal intensity surrounded by a rim of low signal intensity. The high signal intensity in the central region of this stone is the same as the signal of the surrounding bile (B).

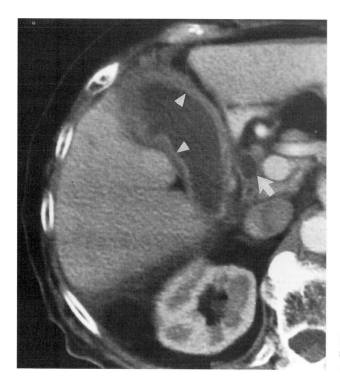

FIG. 34. Acute cholecystitis. Contrast-enhanced CT image shows diffuse thickening and edema of the gallbladder wall *(arrowheads)*. Note the dilated CHD *(arrow)*.

duct, poor definition of the gallbladder wall at the interface with the liver, a thin rim of pericholecystic fluid, inflammatory change in the pericholecystic fat, and increased density of the bile (>20 HU) (Figs. 34,35). The increased density of the bile does not appear to correlate

with the presence of empyema (115,240,255). Marked gallbladder wall enhancement on CT is not a specific finding for the diagnosis of acute cholecystitis. Yamashita et al. (280) described transient, focal, curvilinear areas of increased attenuation in the liver, adjacent to the gallblad-

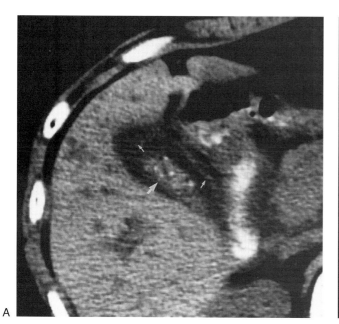

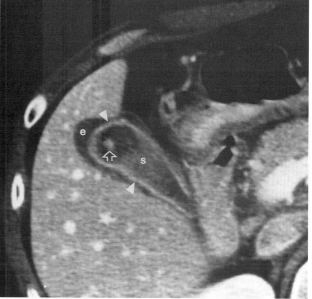

A

B

FIG. 35. Acute cholecystitis. **A:** Noncontrast CT image shows multiple small stones and high-attenuation sludge *(thick arrow)* within the gallbladder lumen. The gallbladder mucosa *(thin arrows)* is seen as a subtle linear area of high attenuation surrounded by lower-attenuation gallbladder wall edema. **B:** Gallbladder wall thickening is better demonstrated on contrast-enhanced CT images. This contrast-enhanced image, in the same patient as shown in (A), better delineates the gallbladder mucosa *(arrowheads)* and the low-attenuation edema (e). Again, note the presence of high-attenuation sludge (s) and a stone *(open arrow)* in the gallbladder lumen.

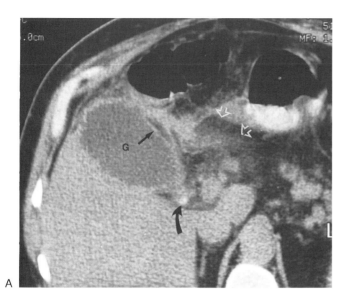 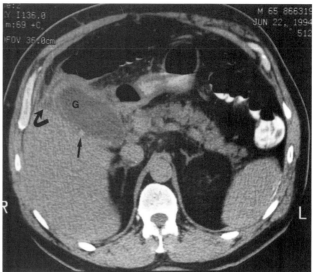

FIG. 36. Gangrenous cholecystitis. **A:** Noncontrast CT image shows a diffusely thickened and indistinct gallbladder wall containing a focal fluid collection *(straight black arrow)*. A high-attenuation gallstone is present in the cystic duct *(curved black arrow)*. There are inflammatory changes in the lesser omentum *(open white arrows)*. **B:** Several centimeters caudal to (A), the gallbladder wall adjacent to the liver cannot be identified. There is a high-attenuation stone in the dependent portion of the gallbladder *(arrow)*. A septated pericholecystic fluid collection is present around the fundus of the gallbladder *(curved arrow)*. At surgery, intramural and pericholecystic abscesses were found. G, gallbladder.

der fossa, in the late arterial or early portal venous phase of contrast enhancement in patients with acute cholecystitis. They attributed this finding to hepatic hyperemia secondary to the adjacent gallbladder inflammation.

Although acute cholecystitis subsides in the majority of patients with appropriate antibiotic therapy, in approximately 25% to 30% of patients complications will develop. Among the complications of acute cholecystitis are empyema, gangrene, and perforation of the gallbladder. The least well vascularized portion of the gallbladder and the most common site of perforation is the fundus (111). With perforation of the gallbladder, patients can develop pericholecystic or intrahepatic abscesses, cholecystoenteric fistulas, or bile peritonitis (238,255). The CT find-

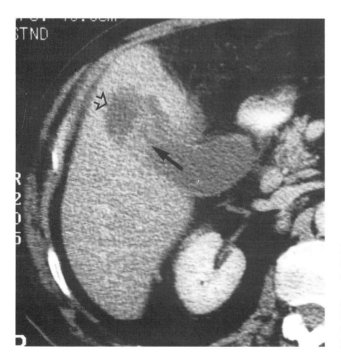

FIG. 37. Complicated cholecystitis. Contrast-enhanced CT image shows the wall of the fundus of the gallbladder to be thickened and indistinct *(arrow)*. A focal region of low attenuation *(open arrow)* is present in the adjacent liver. Sonography (not shown) demonstrated an intrahepatic fluid collection and membranes, consistent with necrotic gallbladder mucosa, within the thick-walled gallbladder. Surgery confirmed this to be a gangrenous gallbladder with perforation into the liver.

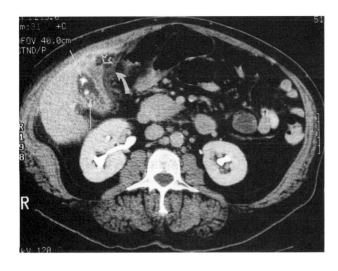

FIG. 38. Gangrenous cholecystitis. Contrast-enhanced CT image shows the gallbladder wall is thickened *(arrowhead)*, and high-attenuation stones and debris are present in the lumen *(straight arrows)*. A triangular high-attenuation fluid collection *(open arrow)* and inflammatory changes *(curved arrow)* are present in the pericholecystic fat. At surgery a perforated gangrenous gallbladder with a pericholecystic abscess was found.

ings corresponding to these complications include focal fluid collections in the gallbladder wall (Fig. 36), liver (Fig. 37), or pericholecystic soft tissues (Fig. 38), gas in the gallbladder and/or bile ducts, and free fluid in the abdomen with associated enhancing peritoneum.

Emphysematous cholecystitis is another complication of acute cholecystitis. This complication can be diagnosed when gas is present in the gallbladder lumen or wall (Fig. 39). Gas also can be seen in the bile ducts (pneumobilia) in these patients. This type of complicated acute cholecystitis is more common in diabetics and elderly men. Ischemia and bacterial overgrowth with *Clostridium perfringens* have been implicated as contributing factors in the development of emphysematous cholecystitis. Gallstones are not present in up to 50% of cases. Patients with this disease may have deceptively mild clinical symptoms; however, the gallbladder is five times more likely to perforate than in other types of acute cholecysti-

tis (42,111,163,238). Unfortunately, gas in the gallbladder lumen and bile ducts is not specific for emphysematous cholecystitis. These findings can also be seen in patients with postinflammatory or neoplastic cholecystoenteric fistulas, after endoscopic retrograde cholangiopancreatography, or as a result of a surgical biliary–enteric anastomosis (163,208) (Figs. 40,41). Therefore, a clear clinical history and careful examination of the imaging findings is important before making the diagnosis of emphysematous cholecystitis. It is also important to be aware that the appearance of the gallbladder on CT in patients with acute cholecystitis, with or without complications, can be normal.

Complicated cholecystitis must be differentiated from gallbladder carcinoma. Findings such as diffuse wall thickening, and infiltrative changes in the pericholecystic fat and lesser omentum are nonspecific and do not help in the differentiation. The presence of a low-attenuation

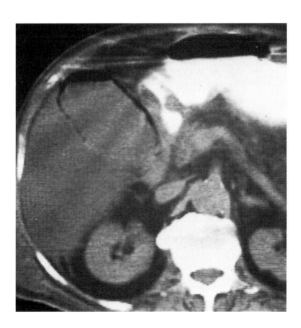

FIG. 39. Emphysematous cholecystitis in a diabetic man. CT image shows air is present in the wall, as well as in the lumen of the gallbladder.

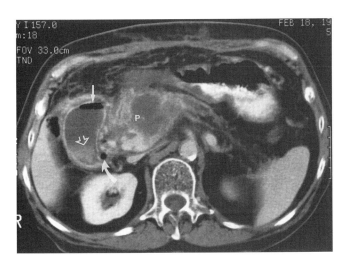

FIG. 40. Contrast-enhanced CT image in a patient with a biliary enteric bypass for palliation of pancreatic carcinoma. Gas *(straight arrow)* and high-attenuation debris *(open arrow)* are present in the gallbladder lumen. This appearance mimics the findings that may be seen in emphysematous cholecystitis. Also note the gas in the gallbladder neck *(curved arrow)* and the large pancreatic mass (P).

halo around the gallbladder is helpful in differentiating these two entities, as this is often present in complicated cholecystitis and is not seen in gallbladder carcinoma (239).

Acalculous cholecystitis accounts for 2% to 12% of all cases of acute cholecystitis (220). It occurs most commonly as a complication of sepsis, AIDS, hyperalimentation, major trauma, burns, and other prolonged critical illnesses. As with emphysematous cholecystitis, acute acalculous cholecystitis has an increased risk of perforation and mortality. The CT findings of gallbladder wall thickening and edema, pericholecystic soft tissue infiltrative changes, and gallbladder distention are no different

from those of calculous cholecystitis. However, unlike acute calculous cholecystitis, sonographic findings in patients with acalculous cholecystitis may be falsely negative (30,169,220).

Xanthogranulomatous cholecystitis is a rare inflammatory disease associated with gallstones and chronic infections. These two factors lead to stasis of bile and subsequent degeneration and necrosis of the gallbladder wall. The normal wall is eventually replaced with chronic inflammatory cells and xanthogranulomas causing marked gallbladder wall thickening. Patients with this condition have clinical signs and symptoms of chronic cholecystitis. The CT appearance is one of marked irregular wall thickening, often simulating a soft tissue mass. The abnormal soft tissue may rupture through the wall of the gallbladder and spread into the pericholecystic soft tissues, adhering to adjacent structures such as the liver, duodenum, or transverse colon. It is difficult to differentiate this entity from gallbladder carcinoma on the basis of the CT appearance alone (73,101).

Magnetic Resonance Imaging in Cholecystitis

The MRI findings in acute cholecystitis are similar to those seen on CT. The high sensitivity of gadolinium-enhanced, fat-suppressed spin echo images to inflammatory changes make this an optimal technique for assessing abnormalities of the gallbladder wall, pericholecystic fat, and intrahepatic periportal tissues (158,230). Patients with acute cholecystitis can have intense enhancement of the gallbladder wall as a result of severe inflammation (Fig. 42). The intramural inflammatory changes in the thickened gallbladder wall also cause increased signal intensity on T2-weighted images (173,272).

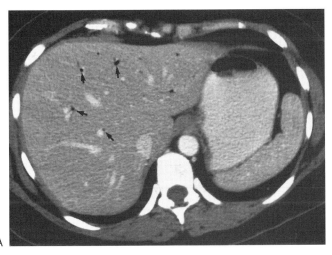
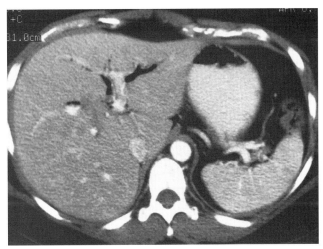

A
B

FIG. 41. Pneumobilia. **A:** Contrast-enhanced CT image shows air within multiple intrahepatic bile ducts *(arrows)*. **B:** At the level 2 cm caudal, the pneumobilia is more prominent in the left, nondependent portion of the biliary system than the right. This patient had a choledochoduodenostomy.

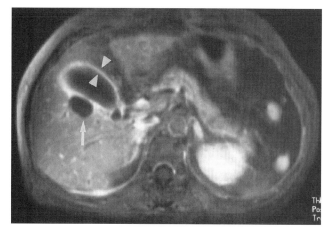

FIG. 42. Acute cholecystitis. Gadolinium-enhanced, T1-weighted, fat-suppressed spin echo MR image (600/15). The gallbladder wall *(arrowheads)* measures 5 mm in thickness and demonstrates substantial enhancement consistent with the inflammatory changes that can be seen in acute cholecystitis. A simple hepatic cyst is noted adjacent to the gallbladder fossa *(arrow)*. (Reproduced with permission from Semelka RC, Shoenut JP, Micflikier AB. The gallbladder and biliary tree. In: Semelka RC, Shoenut JP, eds. *MRI of the abdomen with CT correlation*. New York: Raven Press, 1993;43–52.)

Chronic cholecystitis appears as a small, irregular-shaped gallbladder with a thickened, mildly enhancing wall on gadolinium-enhanced, fat-suppressed images (Fig. 43). The degree of mural enhancement is a distinguishing feature between acute and chronic cholecystitis

on MR images. The milder enhancement in chronic cholecystitis likely reflects the milder nature of the inflammatory process.

If the gallbladder is inflamed, the mucosa may lose its ability to concentrate bile and actually allow the bile in a fasting patient to become progressively more dilute. Based on this premise, MRI was investigated as a diagnostic tool for detecting the presence of cholecystitis and differentiating between acute and chronic disease (147,161). However, Loflin et al. (147) demonstrated that the T1 and T2 relaxation times, and therefore the signal intensities, of bile could not reliably be used to diagnose cholecystitis or to differentiate acute from chronic disease.

Gallbladder Carcinoma

Gallbladder carcinoma is the most common malignant neoplasm of the biliary tract and the fifth most common cancer of the GI tract (4,50,111,128). It is found incidentally in 1% to 3% of cholecystectomy specimens, and 0.5% to 2.4% of autopsies (50,79). The peak incidence is in the sixth and seventh decades. Gallbladder cancer is 3 to 5 times more common in women than men, and it has a high incidence in Mexican-Americans and southwestern native Americans. The incidence of gallbladder cancer in Caucasians is 50% greater than in blacks (50,79,111). Gallstones are present in 65% to 95% of patients, and 40%

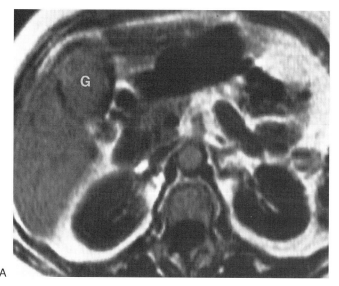

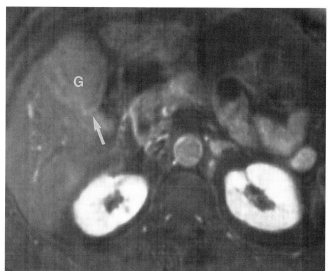

A   B

FIG. 43. Chronic cholecystitis. Precontrast spoiled gradient echo (FLASH 130/4/80°) **(A)** and gadolinium-enhanced, T1-weighted, fat-suppressed spin echo (600/15) **(B)** MR images. Gallbladder wall thickening is apparent on the spoiled gradient echo and contrast-enhanced, fat-suppressed images. There is minimal contrast enhancement of the gallbladder wall *(arrow)* on the gadolinium-enhanced, T1-weighted, fat-suppressed image confirming that active inflammation is not present. G, gallbladder. (Reproduced with permission from Semelka RC, Shoenut JP, Micflikier AB. The gallbladder and biliary tree. In: Semelka RC, Shoenut JP, eds. *MRI of the abdomen with CT correlation*. New York: Raven Press, 1993;43–52.)

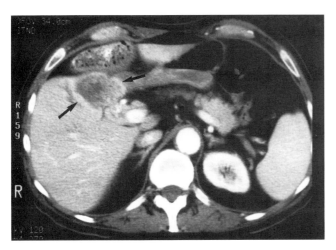

FIG. 44. Gallbladder carcinoma. Contrast-enhanced CT image at the level of the gallbladder fossa shows a heterogeneously enhancing mass *(arrows)* replacing the gallbladder. In the center of the mass there is a region of low attenuation, representing necrosis.

to 50% have a history of chronic cholecystitis. Porcelain gallbladder is also a risk factor for the development of gallbladder cancer (50,134,215,239,271). The histology of the tumor is adenocarcinoma in 80% to 90% of cases. Anaplastic carcinoma and squamous cell carcinoma are the tissue types found in the majority of other cases (50,215).

The vague nature and insidious onset of the symptoms in patients with gallbladder cancer make early diagnosis difficult. The symptoms include abdominal pain, jaundice, weight loss, anorexia, and vomiting. The clinical presentation is often confused with symptomatic cholelithiasis or chronic cholecystitis. The majority of patients are considered unresectable at the time of surgical exploration because of direct extension into adjacent organs, local lymph node metastases, or distant metastatic disease. The overall 5-year survival rate is less than 5% (4,50,79,111, 134,215,271).

Computed Tomography in Gallbladder Carcinoma

Gallbladder carcinoma has one of three morphologic patterns: a mass replacing the gallbladder, focal or diffuse gallbladder wall thickening, or a discrete intraluminal mass (79,84,134,215). The most common presentation is a large soft tissue mass, partially or completely replacing the gallbladder. This pattern occurs in 40% to 65% of cases. The tumors are generally low attenuation on unenhanced scans and heterogeneously enhance after the administration of intravenous contrast. The heterogeneous pattern of peripheral enhancement with central low attenuation is a result of the frequent presence of central tumor necrosis (Fig. 44). Calcifications within the tumor, thought to represent gallstones trapped within the mass, are often seen on CT (79,128,134,271).

Tumors presenting as focal or diffuse gallbladder wall

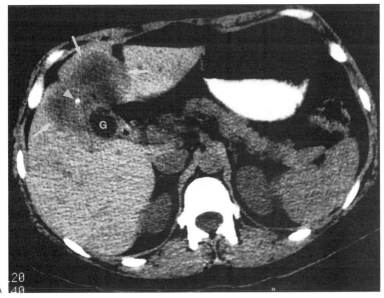
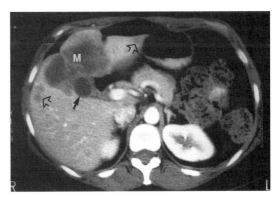

FIG. 45. Gallbladder carcinoma with direct invasion of the liver. **A:** Noncontrast CT image shows a low-attenuation mass *(arrows)* in the medial segment of the left lobe and anterior segment of the right lobe of the liver. A small calcification *(arrowhead)* is present in the mass. The mass is contiguous with the residual gallbladder lumen (G). **B:** Contrast-enhanced image at the same level shows the mass enhancing heterogeneously. In this case, the direct extension of the tumor mass (M) from the gallbladder fossa *(arrow)* into the liver is better delineated after the administration of intravenous contrast. Note the additional smaller lesions in the liver *(open arrows)*. These are metastatic foci.

thickening represent 20% to 30% of cases (134). These cases can be difficult to differentiate from complicated cholecystitis (108,271). Signs that are useful in making the diagnosis of tumor are the presence of a focal mass associated with the gallbladder wall thickening, invasion of the liver, and lymphadenopathy with associated bile duct obstruction in the porta hepatis (239). Tumors that present as an intraluminal mass represent 15% to 25% of cases (134). The intraluminal carcinomas are generally papillary in nature and well differentiated. These tumors tend to be less invasive than the other types described above (4).

The most common mode of spread of gallbladder carcinoma is direct extension into adjacent organs. Liver involvement is the most common; however, the stomach, duodenum, and hepatic flexure of the colon can also be involved. The frequency of liver involvement is reported to range from 34% to 89% in different surgical series (239). Direct extension to the liver can be observed pathologically as a solitary mass in the region of the primary tumor, a solitary mass with a few satellite nodules, or multiple masses throughout the liver (Fig. 45) (79,108, 128,134,271).

Lymphatic spread is also a common mode of tumor dissemination. The primary lymphatic drainage of the gallbladder is to the cystic and pericholedochal nodes. In addition to these nodes, common sites of nodal metastases in gallbladder carcinoma include the retroportal, right celiac, superior pancreaticoduodenal, and posterior pancreaticoduodenal chains (194). Metastatic lymphadenopathy often causes biliary obstruction in the region of the porta hepatis or around the distal CBD near the head of the pancreas (Fig. 46). A nodal mass in the region of the head of the pancreas will often be mistaken for a pancreatic carcinoma (271) (Fig. 47). Extension into the hepatoduodenal ligament, hematogenous dissemination, and spread through the bile ducts are additional pathways by which gallbladder carcinoma metastasizes.

Magnetic Resonance Imaging in Gallbladder Carcinoma

The morphology of gallbladder carcinoma on MRI is the same as that seen on CT (Fig. 48). Both the primary tumor and metastatic lesions are low signal intensity on

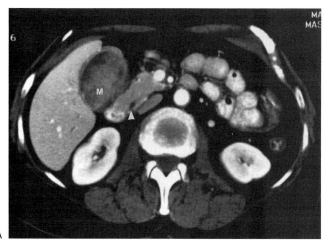

A

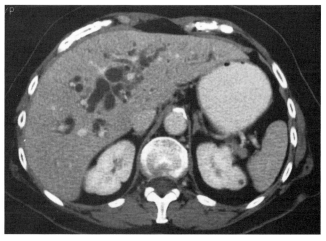

B

C

FIG. 46. Gallbladder carcinoma. **A:** Contrast-enhanced CT image shows a markedly abnormal gallbladder. There is a soft-tissue mass (M) nearly replacing the gallbladder lumen. The gallbladder wall is ill defined and thickened. Note the normal-sized CBD *(arrowhead)* and the absence of enlarged regional lymph nodes. **B:** Contrast-enhanced scan obtained 3 months after cholecystectomy shows marked intrahepatic bile duct dilatation. **C:** At a level several centimeters caudal to (B), a large nodal mass (m) is present in the peripancreatic region, causing obstruction of the common duct *(arrow)*. Note the dilated cystic duct remnant (C). P, pancreas.

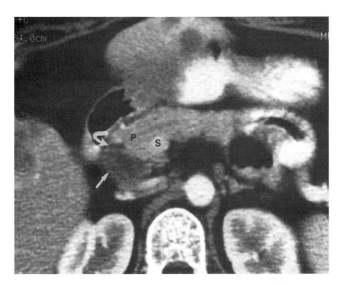

FIG. 47. Metastatic gallbladder carcinoma. Contrast-enhanced CT image shows low-attenuation metastatic lymph nodes *(arrow)* in the peripancreatic region. The nodal mass is adjacent to the CBD *(curved arrow)*, head and uncinate process of the pancreas (P), and superior mesenteric vein (S). This is a common location for lymph node metastases from gallbladder carcinoma, and the mass is often mistaken for a pancreatic head carcinoma. Note the metastatic lesions in the liver.

T1-weighted images and high signal intensity on T2-weighted images. Extension of tumor into the liver is well seen on T2-weighted images and dynamic gadolinium-enhanced, T1-weighted gradient echo images, while extension into the pancreas, hepatoduodenal ligament, and other adjacent tissues is best shown on T1-weighted, fat-suppressed spin echo images before and after gadolinium administration (215–217).

Metastatic Disease

Metastatic disease to the gallbladder is an uncommon occurrence. The most common tumor to metastasize to the gallbladder is melanoma, a hematogenous metastasis that most often appears as focal nodules protruding into the gallbladder lumen (Fig. 49). Metastatic disease to the gallbladder less commonly results from direct invasion by hepatic, pancreatic, or gastric neoplasms (250).

DISEASES OF THE BILE DUCTS

Congenital Anomalies: Choledochal Cysts

Cystic dilatation of the extrahepatic bile duct, with or without dilatation of the intrahepatic bile ducts, is an

uncommon congenital anomaly of the biliary tree. It is 3 to 4 times more common in female than in male patients, and two thirds of patients are clinically symptomatic before the age of 10 years. The classic clinical presentation is the triad of abdominal pain, jaundice, and a palpable right upper quadrant mass (178,219,231,282). This triad is present in 30% to 60% of patients presenting in the first decade of life, and only approximately 20% of patients diagnosed in adulthood (178,231).

The precise origin of this abnormality is unknown; however, Babbitt (5) proposed that the most likely etiology is bile duct injury resulting from the sequelae of an anomalous junction of the pancreatic and distal CBDs. The anomalous junction results in chronic reflux of pancreatic enzymes into the biliary tree, causing inflammation and weakening of the CBD wall with resultant scarring, stricture formation, and dilatation (231). Anomalous junction of the pancreatic and CBDs is found in 10% to 58% of patients with choledochal cysts (219).

The original classification of Alonzo-Lej has been modified and expanded by Todani et al. (258), who described five types of choledochal cysts (Fig. 50). Type I choledochal cysts, accounting for 80% to 90% of bile duct cysts, are subdivided into IA, IB, and IC. Type IA is cystic dilatation of the CBD, type IB is focal, segmental dilatation of the distal CBD, and type IC is fusiform dilatation of both the CHD and the CBD. Type II choledochal cysts, accounting for 2% of bile duct cysts, are true diverticula arising from the CBD. Type III cysts, defined as cystic dilatation involving only the intraduodenal portion of the CBD, are called choledochoceles and account for 1% to 5% of bile duct cysts. The clinical features and etiologic associations of this type of choledochal cyst differ from

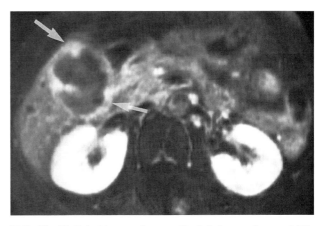

FIG. 48. Gallbladder carcinoma. Gadolinium-enhanced, T1-weighted, fat-suppressed MR image demonstrates irregular thickening and associated abnormal enhancement of the gallbladder wall *(arrow)*. These are features consistent with gallbladder carcinoma. (Reproduced with permission from Semelka RC, Shoenut JP, Micflikier AB. The gallbladder and biliary tree. In: Semelka RC, Shoenut JP, eds. *MRI of the abdomen with CT correlation.* New York: Raven Press, 1993;43–52.)

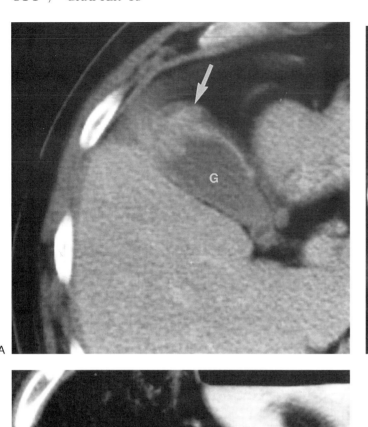

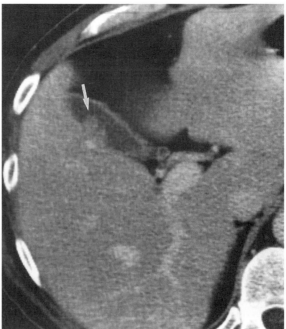

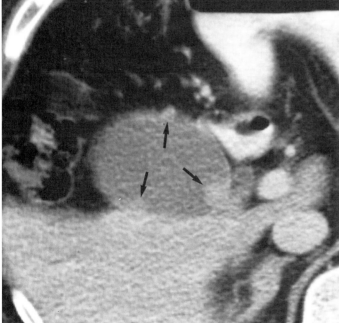

FIG. 49. Metastatic melanoma. Contrast-enhanced CT images through the gallbladder in three different patients shows a solitary soft tissue mass *(arrow)* involving the fundus of the gallbladder (G) in **(A)**, a focal mural mass *(arrow)* projecting into the mid portion of the gallbladder lumen in **(B)**, and several small enhancing mural nodules *(arrows)* distributed around the gallbladder wall in **(C)**.

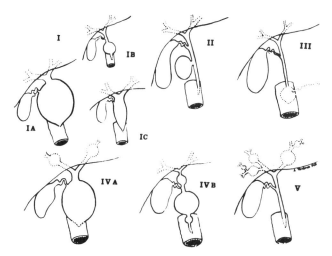

FIG. 50. Todani's classification scheme of choledochal cysts. (Reproduced with permission from Savader SJ, Beneati JF, Venbrux AC, et al. Choledochal cysts: classification and cholangiographic appearance. *AJR* 1991;156:327–331.)

the other types. Type IV choledochal cysts account for approximately 10% of bile duct cysts and are subdivided into types IVA and IVB. Type IVA has multiple intra- and extrahepatic cysts, and type IVB has multiple extrahepatic cysts only. Type V choledochal cysts comprise the remainder of bile duct cysts. This type generally involves only the intrahepatic ducts and may be single or multiple. When there are multiple intrahepatic bile duct cysts, the abnormality is called *Caroli disease* (59,219,227,231).

Complications associated with choledochal cysts include cholelithiasis, choledocholithiasis, cystolithiasis, ascending cholangitis, bile duct strictures, intrahepatic abscesses, biliary cirrhosis, portal hypertension, and hepatobiliary malignancy. Tumors occur in the intra- and extrahepatic ducts, both intra- and extracystic. Patients are also at increased risk for gallbladder carcinoma. Ninety percent of the malignant tumors that arise in the presence of a choledochal cyst are adenocarcinomas. The reported incidence of malignancy ranges from 3% to 40% (178,219,231). The risk increases with age, and the prognosis is poor because of the tendency for the tumors to be multicentric and to have extensive local and regional spread (178,282). The treatment for types I, II, and IV choledochal cysts is complete excision and subsequent biliary–enteric anastomosis for drainage. If treatment is attempted with internal drainage of the cyst, rather than complete excision, the risk of malignancy in the cyst is not reduced (31,231,282). The treatment for choledochoceles and type V cysts will be discussed later.

The role of imaging in the evaluation of choledochal cysts is to delineate the anatomy of the cysts, determine the relationship of the cysts to the rest of the intra- and extrahepatic biliary tree, evaluate associated biliary tract abnormalities (e.g., anomalous pancreaticobiliary junc-

tion), and identify complications, including stones, strictures, and neoplasms (219,231). The diagnosis of choledochal cyst can be made with radionuclide scintigraphy, sonography, CT, MRI, or direct cholangiography. Sonography is useful for assessing the full extent of biliary ductal dilatation and for identifying the connection of the cyst with the biliary tree. The presence of stones, strictures, or tumors also can be detected with sonography. Computed tomography and MRI are useful not only for delineating the anatomy of the cyst, the extent of biliary ductal dilatation, and the presence of stones, strictures, and tumors, but they have the added advantage of being able to define the extent of local and regional tumor spread (282).

On CT and MRI, a choledochal cyst appears as a right upper quadrant, fluid-filled structure in contiguity with the extrahepatic bile duct. Coronal imaging is helpful for delineating the communication of the cyst with the biliary tree. This can be accomplished with CT using multiplanar reformations, with or without the use of cholangiographic contrast agents. MRI, with or without the use of MR cholangiography techniques, allows direct imaging of the cyst in multiple planes (126,231). Coronal imaging with either CT or MRI demonstrates a dilated tubular structure that follows the expected course of the CBD (Fig. 51). The cysts must be differentiated from other cystic structures that may occur in this region, such as pancreatic pseudocysts and enteric duplication cysts (231,282). The presence of wall thickening, mural nodularity, and wall enhancement in a choledochal cyst, particularly in the absence of previous surgery, stones, or cholangitis, raises the possibility of the presence of tumor (178). Because direct cholangiography (PTC or ERCP) is the best method for complete evaluation of the biliary tree, whenever a choledochal cyst is detected with sonography, CT, or MRI, direct cholangiography should be performed before operative treatment. In addition to confirming the anatomy of the cyst and the presence of tumor masses, direct cholangiography is the most reliable method to diagnose the presence of an anomalous pancreaticobiliary junction.

The appearance of a choledochocele on CT differs from that of the other choledochal cysts. This abnormality appears as a fluid-filled mass that protrudes into the wall of the duodenum. The mass does not fill with GI tract oral contrast, but it can be opacified with the use of an oral biliary contrast agent (59,202). Unlike the other types of choledochal cysts, this abnormality has no predilection for either sex and there is no increased risk of hepatobiliary malignancy. For this reason, choledochoceles can be treated without complete surgical excision, by unroofing the cyst (266).

Congenital Anomalies: Caroli Disease

Caroli disease, also known as communicating cavernous ectasia of the biliary tract, was originally described

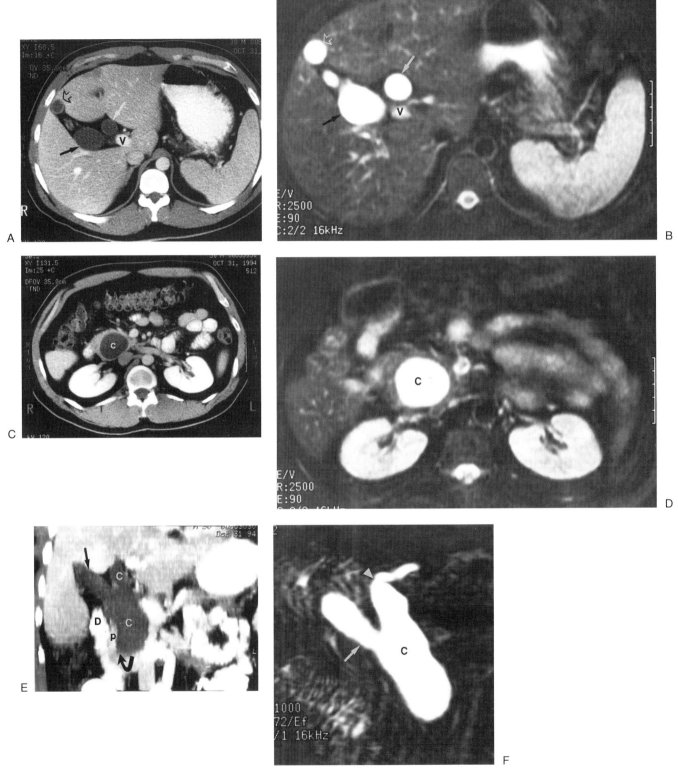

FIG. 51. Type IC choledochal cyst. Contrast-enhanced CT **(A)** and T2-weighted, fat-saturated MR image (SE 2500/90) **(B)** at the level of the porta hepatis show a markedly dilated CHD *(white arrow)* and cystic duct *(black arrow)*. The peripheral intrahepatic ducts are not dilated and the gallbladder *(open arrow)* is contracted. Contrast-enhanced CT **(C)** and T2-weighted, fat-saturated MR image **(D)** at the level of the pancreatic head show the dilated CBD (C), which tapers gradually to the ampulla. Coronal CT reformation **(E)** and noncontrast MR cholangiogram **(F)** show the entire length of the dilated common duct (C). The dilated cystic duct *(straight arrow)* is arising directly from the choledochal cyst. Note the tapering of the distal CBD *(curved arrow)* as it courses towards the duodenum (D). The transition *(arrowhead)* from the marked dilatation of the CHD to the minimal dilatation of the main left hepatic duct is demonstrated on the MR cholangiogram. V, portal vein; p, pancreas.

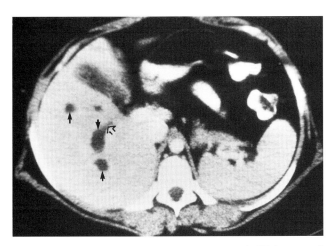

FIG. 52. Caroli disease. Contrast-enhanced CT image of the liver at the level of the gallbladder fossa shows multiple water-attenuation cystic structures *(arrows)* within the inferior segments of the right lobe. The largest of these cystic structures clearly connects to an adjacent tubular structure *(open arrow)* representing a mildly dilated bile duct.

as the combination of (a) segmental, saccular dilatation of the intrahepatic bile ducts; (b) a high incidence of bile duct stones, ascending cholangitis, and liver abscesses; (c) the absence of hepatic cirrhosis and portal hypertension; and (d) almost invariable association with renal cystic disease (31,44,54,112,189,227,242,243). The renal cystic abnormalities associated with Caroli disease include renal tubular ectasia (medullary sponge kidney), cortical cysts, and autosomal recessive polycystic kidney disease (54,227). The most common association is with medullary sponge kidney. Communicating cystic dilata-

tion of the intrahepatic bile ducts is now known to be a spectrum of congenital anomalies. The "pure" form of Caroli disease, as described, is one end of the spectrum and is very rare. Most cases of Caroli disease are actually at the other end of the spectrum, characterized by congenital hepatic fibrosis with associated cystic dilatation of the intrahepatic bile ducts, and renal cystic disease (54,155,189,242).

Patients with Caroli disease may be asymptomatic. When they do develop clinical symptoms, the symptoms are often nonspecific and depend on whether the predominant lesion is intrahepatic bile duct dilatation or hepatic fibrosis. The former group of patients generally present with episodic abdominal pain, fever, and jaundice secondary to biliary stone disease, ascending cholangitis, and liver abscesses. The latter group often present with signs and symptoms of portal hypertension, including hematemesis and lower GI tract bleeding (155,189,242). The cystic renal abnormalities associated with Caroli disease are generally asymptomatic. Caroli disease is most often diagnosed in children or young adults; however, patients may not present until their fifth decade. The male and female incidences are equal.

Before the emergence of cross-sectional imaging techniques, the diagnosis of Caroli disease was made at the time of surgical exploration and intraoperative cholangiography, or at autopsy. The diagnosis now can be made with noninvasive imaging techniques including sonography, CT, and MRI. Cross-sectional imaging examinations show nonobstructive, saccular or beaded dilatation of the intrahepatic bile ducts. This is displayed as multiple, intrahepatic, rounded cystic spaces of varying sizes communi-

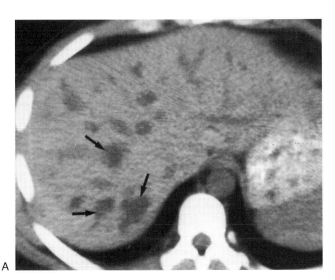
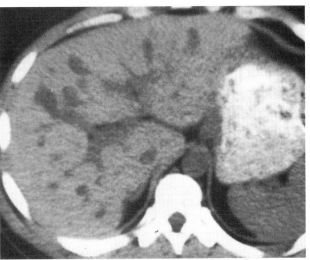

A   B

FIG. 53. Caroli disease. **A:** A cluster of near-water-density, cystic-appearing areas *(arrows)* is noted in the right lobe of the liver. **B:** At a level 3 cm caudal, several of the cystic areas appear to be arranged in a branching pattern similar to that of bile ducts, suggesting the diagnosis of Caroli disease.

cating with the branching, dilated, intrahepatic bile ducts (Figs. 52–54). These changes can be observed in a single segment, an entire lobe, or diffusely throughout the liver. The intrahepatic cystic spaces will often contain calculi and/or amorphous debris. There can also be bridging of the bile duct walls, causing the cystic dilatations to resemble septated hepatic cysts. One finding considered pathognomonic for Caroli disease is the central dot sign. This is characterized on unenhanced CT images by a small dot of slightly high attenuation in the dependent portion of the dilated bile duct. After the administration of intravenous contrast, these dots enhance intensely. The central dot sign is representative of portal venous radicles that are enveloped by, but not actually inside of, the markedly dilated bile ducts (54,112). The extrahepatic bile ducts in patients with Caroli disease can be normal, stenotic, slightly dilated, or associated with a choledochal cyst (31,54,112,155,189,242). Patients with hepatic fibrosis often have hepatosplenomegaly and dilated portal and splenic veins because of portal hypertension.

The appearance of Caroli disease on CT or MRI must be differentiated from polycystic liver disease and obstructive bile duct dilatation. Whereas the cystic spaces in Caroli disease are irregular in shape and communicate with the biliary tree, the cysts in polycystic liver disease are rounder and smoother, and they deform, but do not communicate with, the bile ducts. Moreover, in Caroli disease, the dilated bile ducts have a random, bizarre pattern, and there are focal areas of cystic ectasia. This differs from the appearance in obstructive bile duct dilatation where the dilatation is most marked centrally, tapers towards the periphery in an organized pattern, and lacks focal areas of cystic dilatation (112).

Because of the primarily intrahepatic nature of Caroli disease, patients with this congenital anomaly, unlike patients with choledochal cysts, do not have a specific abnormality that is treatable by surgical resection. Therefore, the treatment in these patients is primarily directed towards the associated complications of biliary calculi, cholangitis, and hepatic abscesses. Patients with Caroli disease, like those with choledochal cysts, are at an increased risk for developing cholangiocarcinoma (227).

Choledocholithiasis

Choledocholithiasis is present in 10% to 15% of all patients with acute or chronic cholecystitis (56). In the majority of cases, stones are formed within the gallbladder, and subsequently pass into the CBD. Nearly half of all patients over 65 years of age with cholecystolithiasis also have choledocholithiasis; however, common duct stones are present in only 12% to 15% of patients under 65 years of age with gallstones (82,91,111,133).

Primary bile duct calculi, including intrahepatic stones, are uncommon in Western countries. Most of these stones are pigment stones that develop as a result of bile duct strictures and bile stasis. Sclerosing cholangitis, recurrent pyogenic cholangitis, parasitic infections, choledochal cysts, Caroli disease, and posttraumatic bile duct strictures resulting from endoscopic or percutaneous biliary procedures, predispose patients to developing primary bile duct stones (168,224,225). In addition, 2% to 4% of patients who have had a cholecystectomy will subsequently develop choledocholithiasis (62,88).

Patients with CBD stones may be asymptomatic; however, the majority of patients have signs and symptoms of partial or complete bile duct obstruction, including cholangitis or pancreatitis. Between 20% and 42% of cases of biliary obstruction are caused by common duct stones (218). In 24% to 33% of patients with obstruction from common duct stones, there will be no bile duct

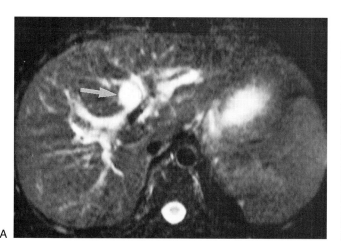
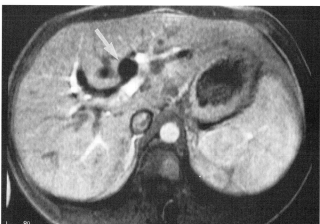

FIG. 54. Caroli disease. T2-weighted, fat-suppressed spin echo (2100/90) **(A)** and immediate-post-gadolinium-enhancement spoiled gradient echo (FLASH 130/4/80°) **(B)** MR images. Multiple areas of cystic dilatation of the intrahepatic biliary tree were present throughout the liver. One such area *(arrow)*, which is high in signal on the T2-weighted image and a signal void on the post-gadolinium-enhancement, T1-weighted spoiled gradient echo image, is present in the region of the left hepatic duct.

dilatation at the time of diagnostic imaging examination (63,93,131).

As discussed in the section on techniques, sonography should be the initial examination in patients suspected of having bile duct obstruction. The reported sensitivity of ultrasound for detecting CBD stones ranges from 12% to 80% (62,63,70,131–133). The stones that are not detected by sonography are usually in the distal CBD or the ampulla, and are obscured by overlying bowel gas. In the detection of common duct stones, CT is reserved for cases in which sonography is inconclusive and direct cholangiography is contraindicated or was technically unsuccessful. The sensitivity of CT for detecting choledocholithiasis ranges from 50% to 90% (12–14,109,170,199).

Computed Tomography in Choledocholithiasis

The detection of stones in the CBD depends on the attenuation of the stones, the position of the stones within the bile duct, and the plane of the stone and the duct relative to the plane of the CT image (Fig. 55). Because the majority of CBD stones have migrated from the gallbladder, their composition and CT attenuation parallel those of gallstones. Approximately 20% of CBD stones are homogeneously high in attenuation (>60 HU), 50% are soft tissue attenuation (20 to 60 HU), and the remainder are low attenuation (<20 HU) (20,91). The high-attenuation stones are easily visualized regardless of their location in the bile duct. These stones can be recognized as foci of homogeneous high attenuation in the expected location of the duct, with or without a surrounding rim of water-attenuation bile (Fig. 56).

In contrast, visualization of the soft-tissue-density and low-attenuation stones depends on the presence of a rim of surrounding water-attenuation bile (Figs. 6 and 57). If no rim of bile were present, the stones could not be separated from the surrounding bile duct wall and pancreatic soft tissue. In the presence of a common duct stone, the

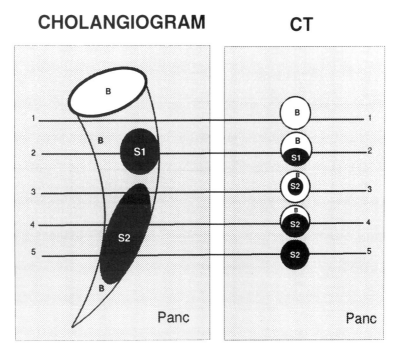

FIG. 55. Schematic representation of CT appearances of CBD stones. A line drawing of a cholangiogram *(left)* shows two stones in the common duct. The more proximal stone (S_1) is in the dependent portion of the duct, and the more distal stone (S_2) is impacted in the duct. On the *right* are line drawings of axial CT images at the levels indicated on the cholangiogram. Proximal to the stones, at level 1 on the CT image, the duct would appear as a bile-containing (B), water-density circle surrounded by the soft tissue of the pancreas. At level 2, the CT image through the stone in the dependent portion of the duct would show the stone (S_1) with the water-density bile (B) forming a crescent over its nondependent surface. Note that the same appearance can be seen at level 4, which is an image obtained obliquely through the impacted stone (S_2). At level 3, the axial CT image through the cephalad aspect of the impacted stone shows a central density (S_2) representing the stone surrounded by a complete rim of water-attenuation bile (B), creating a target appearance. At level 5, the impacted stone (S_2) is occupying the entire lumen of the duct, so an axial CT image at this level would show abrupt termination of the duct. There would be no bile surrounding the stone; therefore, if the stone is of soft-tissue attenuation, it may blend imperceptibly with the surrounding soft tissue of the pancreas. Occasionally, the enhancing bile duct wall may be seen as a rim of high attenuation surrounding the soft-tissue-density stone. (Modified from Baron RL. Computed tomography of the biliary tree. *Radiol Clin North Am* 1991;29:1235–1250.)

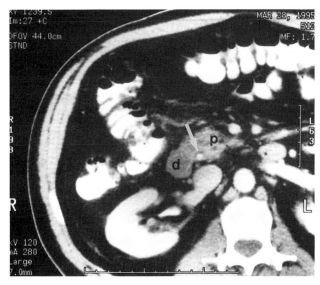

FIG. 56. Common bile duct stone. Contrast-enhanced CT image shows a homogeneously high-attenuation stone *(arrow)* in the distal CBD. The stone is higher in attenuation than the soft tissue of the surrounding pancreatic head (p), and, therefore, it is easily recognized. d, duodenum.

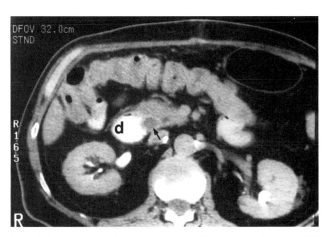

FIG. 58. Common bile duct stone. Contrast-enhanced CT image at the level of the pancreatic head shows an impacted soft-tissue density stone *(arrow)* in the intrapancreatic portion of the distal CBD. The subtle rim of high attenuation around the stone represents the normally enhancing bile duct wall. This should not be mistaken for a rim of calcification in the periphery of a stone. Note that no bile is seen around the impacted stone. d, duodenum.

bile duct wall can be thickened as the result of a surrounding inflammatory response. A high-attenuation rim in the course of the CBD also can be a clue to the presence of a stone; however, this is not specific, because it may simply represent the enhancing bile duct wall (Fig. 58). In fact, the presence of a high-attenuation rim in the distal CBD has a sensitivity of only 16% and a specificity of only 55% for the detection of stones (14).

The most specific and sensitive sign for the presence of a CBD stone is the target sign (14). This is character-

ized by the presence of a faintly visualized stone in the center of the duct lumen, surrounded by a complete rim of lower-attenuation bile (Fig. 59). The crescent sign, a variation of the target sign, is characterized by a soft-tissue-attenuation stone lying in the dependent portion of

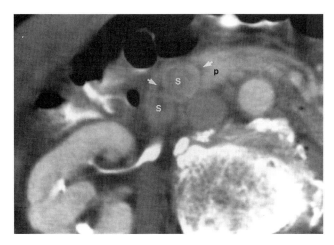

FIG. 57. Common bile duct stones. Contrast-enhanced CT image through the distal CBD shows two impacted soft-tissue-density stones (S) with a minimal amount of surrounding water-density bile *(arrows)* visible. Without the presence of the bile, the stones could not be clearly differentiated from the surrounding pancreatic tissue (p). Note the laminated appearance of the stones.

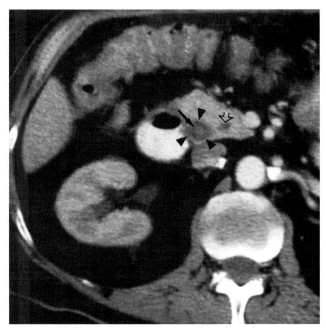

FIG. 59. Target sign. Contrast-enhanced CT image at the level of the pancreatic head shows a soft-tissue-density stone *(arrow)* in the central portion of the CBD. A complete rim of water-density bile *(arrowheads)* is surrounding the stone, creating a target appearance. Note the dilated pancreatic duct *(open arrow)* in the uncinate process.

the bile duct, with a crescent of lower-attenuation bile seen anterior to the stone (Fig. 60).

Occasionally, when a soft-tissue-density or low-attenuation stone occupies the entire lumen of the CBD, a dilated duct can appear to come to an abrupt termination without evidence of a surrounding mass. Some authors have suggested that this indicates the presence of a cholesterol stone (109). However, this appearance is present in 10% of patients with stones, as well as in 30% of patients with pancreatic head or ampullary tumors (14). Therefore, when there is abrupt termination of the duct without a surrounding mass, the most likely diagnosis is neoplasm (6,13,198,199). In these patients, direct cholangiography is indicated for confirmation.

Irregular, punctate densities within the lumen of the distal common duct can be a pitfall in the CT diagnosis of CBD stones. Although these may represent small foci of calcification within cholesterol stones, this same appearance can be seen in 25% of patients with pancreatic carcinoma and in 33% of normal patients (14). In the latter two groups of patients, the origin of these densities is not clear. Common duct stones also can be mimicked by pancreatic duct calculi, oral contrast in a duodenal diverticulum, and reflux of oral contrast from the duodenum into the CBD.

Magnetic Resonance Imaging in Choledocholithiasis

CBD stones have been found to have one of three appearances on MRI: signal void on both T1- and T2-weighted images, central high signal with a rim of signal void on T2-weighted images, and high signal on both T1- and T2-weighted images (97). The high contrast between a signal-void calculus and high-signal-intensity bile on T2-weighted images may allow MRI to be superior to CT in the detection of common duct stones. Fast spin echo images projected in a 3-D display can be an effective, noninvasive method of demonstrating the low-signal-intensity common duct stones within a background of high-signal-intensity bile (94) (Fig. 61). Review of the individual 2-D tomographic sections is essential, as stones may be masked by the reconstruction techniques.

Mirizzi Syndrome

The Mirizzi syndrome is an uncommon cause of obstructive jaundice that occurs in the setting of cholelithiasis and cholecystitis. The obstruction is caused by extrinsic compression of the CHD from an impacted stone in the gallbladder neck or cystic duct. The compression of the CHD can be caused by the impacted stone, or by the associated periductal inflammation (9,27,107,123). Low insertion of the cystic duct into the CHD has been proposed as the predisposing factor in the development of the Mirizzi syndrome. This anatomic arrangement is found in 18% to 49% of all patients having cholecystectomies. In these patients, the cystic duct and CHD are found to travel caudally in a long common sheath before joining together to form the CBD (123,186,200).

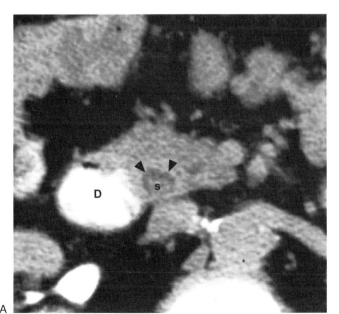
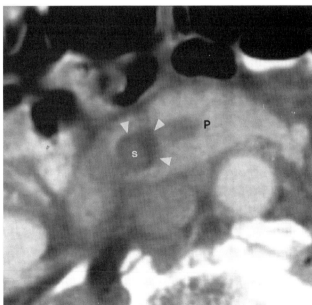

FIG. 60. Crescent sign. Contrast-enhanced CT images **(A,B)** through the pancreatic head in two different patients show a soft-tissue-attenuation stone (s) in the dependent portion of the common duct. A crescent-shaped rim of water-density bile *(arrowheads)* is present over the nondependent portion of the stone in each image. D, duodenum; P, pancreas.

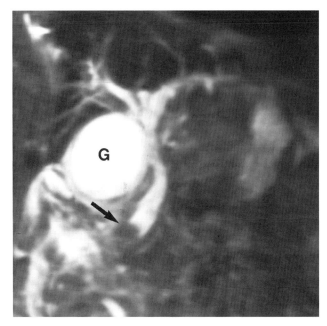

FIG. 61. Choledocholithiasis. Turbo (fast) spin echo (8000/91) MR image demonstrates a low-signal-intensity calculus *(arrow)* in the distal CBD. The dilated biliary tree is well demonstrated because of the high signal of bile using this technique. G, gallbladder.

The impacted calculus in the Mirizzi syndrome often erodes from the gallbladder neck or cystic duct into the periductal tissues, or directly into the CHD. In either case, this leads to the formation of a large cavity, and further regional inflammation and edema. The cavity, inflammation, and edema resulting from the erosion of the stone from the gallbladder neck or cystic duct can obscure the regional anatomy in the gallbladder fossa and hepatoduodenal ligament at the time of surgery. This can result in accidental ligation of the CHD or the CBD (27,107).

On cholangiography, the Mirizzi syndrome is demonstrated as a narrowing of the CHD, associated with adjacent cystic duct calculi. Unfortunately, the calculi are not always visible. Because of the anatomic relationship of the cystic duct and the CHD, the extrinsic compression of the CHD is most often on its posterior or lateral aspect. Entities that can cause extrinsic compression of the CHD and mimic the Mirizzi syndrome on cholangiography include hydrops of the gallbladder, carcinoma of the gallbladder or cystic duct, enlarged lymph nodes in the porta hepatis, pancreatic pseudocysts, and an enlarged cystic duct remnant in patients who have had a cholecystectomy (123,209). CT can be helpful in differentiating these abnormalities from a true Mirizzi syndrome. The findings that can be seen on CT in the Mirizzi syndrome include obstruction of the CHD, apparent widening of the gallbladder neck, an irregular cavity near the gallbladder

neck, and stones in the periductal or pericholecystic soft tissues (200) (Fig. 62).

Ascending Cholangitis

Bacterial infection of the biliary tree in the presence of complete or partial bile duct obstruction is called ascending cholangitis, acute cholangitis, bacterial cholangitis, or obstructive suppurative cholangitis. Gram-negative enteric bacteria are the most common causative organisms (10). Ascending cholangitis most often occurs in the presence of bile duct calculi, bile duct strictures, or papillary stenosis. Colonization of the bile ducts by bacteria in the absence of bile duct obstruction does not lead to the development of ascending cholangitis, nor does obstruction of the bile ducts in the absence of bacterial contamination (214).

Patients with ascending cholangitis can be variably symptomatic. Mild disease can be treated with antibiotics, but severe disease requires emergent biliary drainage. The classic signs and symptoms of acute ascending cholangitis are right upper quadrant pain, jaundice, and sepsis. These signs and symptoms, known as Charcot's triad, are present in only 60% to 70% of patients with ascending cholangitis. In fact, 20% of patients will not be jaundiced and will have a normal white blood cell count (10,212).

The role of CT in patients with suspected ascending cholangitis is to confirm the clinical diagnosis, identify the site and cause of biliary obstruction, and detect the presence of associated hepatic abnormalities (10). Although most patients with ascending cholangitis have abnormalities seen on CT, the absence of CT findings does not exclude the presence of infection. The CT findings that can be seen in patients with ascending cholangitis include dilatation of the intra- and extrahepatic bile ducts, increased attenuation of the bile because of the presence of intraductal debris, diffuse and concentric bile duct wall thickening, gas in the bile ducts or portal veins, and intrahepatic abscesses (seen as low-attenuation areas in contiguity with the intrahepatic bile ducts). MRI can show a similar spectrum of findings (Fig. 63). Because bile duct dilatation can be absent in patients with acute or partial obstruction, there is no correlation between the presence and degree of bile duct dilatation and the severity of acute cholangitis. However, the presence of hepatic abscesses, pneumobilia, and portal venous gas are indicative of a poor prognosis (10,20,67,226).

Oriental Cholangiohepatitis

Oriental cholangiohepatitis (OCH) is known by a variety of names including recurrent pyogenic cholangitis, intrahepatic pigmented stone disease, and biliary obstruction syndrome of the Chinese (49,78,81,144). This disease is endemic in Southeast Asia, and its prevalence in West-

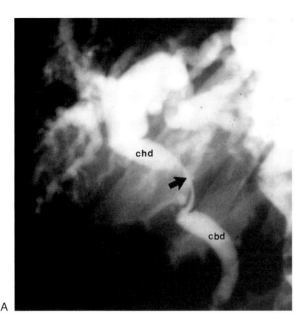
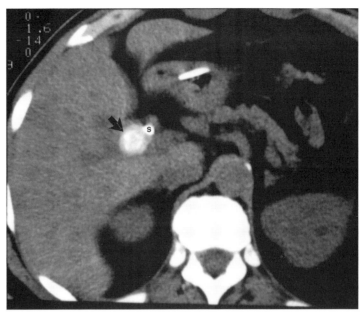

A   B

FIG. 62. Mirizzi syndrome. Elderly woman with right upper quadrant pain and jaundice. **A:** Cholangiogram performed during ERCP shows dilatation of the intrahepatic bile ducts. There is narrowing of the distal common hepatic duct (chd) and proximal common bile duct (cbd). The superior and medial displacement of the narrowed segment *(arrow)* suggests that its cause is an extrinsic mass. Note that the cystic duct and gallbladder are not opacified. **B:** Noncontrast CT image through the neck of the gallbladder shows a densely calcified "mass" *(arrow)* medially displacing the distal CHD and its contained stent (s). At cholecystectomy, the mass proved to be a gallstone lodged in the neck of the gallbladder. The impacted gallstone was the cause of the extrahepatic bile duct displacement and obstruction.

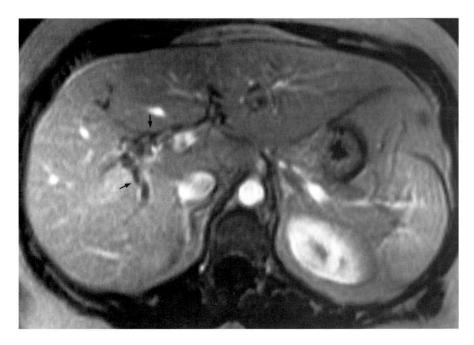

FIG. 63. Infectious cholangitis. The 90-sec-post-gadolinium-enhancement spoiled gradient echo MR image (FLASH 130/4/80°) demonstrates that the intrahepatic bile ducts *(arrows)* are dilated and there is thickening and abnormal enhancement of the bile duct walls.

ern countries, such as the United States, is increasing because of the growing number of Asian immigrants (144). OCH affects men and women equally. Patients are generally 20 to 40 years of age and often are of lower socioeconomic status. The clinical presentation of OCH includes recurrent attacks and remissions of abdominal pain, nausea, vomiting, fever, and shaking chills. Jaundice is present in up to 77% of patients, and gallstones are present in 15% to 70% of patients (81,144,264). The mortality rate in patients with acute exacerbations is as high as 28% (264). Patients with OCH are at increased risk for the development of hepatic cirrhosis and cholangiocarcinoma. Cholangiocarcinoma develops in 2% to 6% of these patients (81,129,144).

There are two theories regarding the etiology of OCH. One theory proposes that chronic infestation with parasites such as *Clonorchis sinensis* or *Ascaris lumbricoides* induces bile duct strictures, leading to bile stasis, intraductal stone formation, and suppurative cholangitis. The second theory suggests that poor eating habits and subsequent poor nutritional status predispose patients to repeated portal bacteremia with enteric organisms, the sequelae of which is manifested as OCH (49,144).

The pathology of OCH is centered around the bile ducts and portal tracts. There is proliferation of the ducts and thickening of the duct walls. The fibrous tissue in the portal tracts proliferates, and inflammatory cell infiltrates extend from the portal tracts into the hepatic parenchyma, causing hepatic necrosis. The intrahepatic bile ducts in patients with OCH are strictured and dilated in 35% to 79% of cases. The dilatation of the intrahepatic bile ducts is usually a result of strictures and intraductal stones. However, in up to 37% of patients, intrahepatic bile duct dilatation is present without strictures (129). Dilatation of the extrahepatic bile ducts is present in over 85% of cases. Strictures in the extrahepatic duct are generally absent, except at the level of the ampulla. The extrahepatic bile duct is frequently dilated both proximal and distal to intraductal stones, presumably as a result of the presence of these ampullary strictures, which are commonly present because of the passage of stones and subsequent fibrosis. Both the intra- and extrahepatic bile ducts contain primary pigmented stones in 75% to 80% of cases. The stones can be large and solid, have a sand-like consistency, or be very soft, resembling mud. The bile ducts also frequently contain necrotic debris and pus. The combination of the biliary mud, necrotic debris, and pus can form casts that fill the ducts (81,129,144,264).

The CT findings in OCH reflect these pathologic changes. There is irregular, segmental dilatation of the intrahepatic bile ducts, with a predilection for the lateral segment of the left lobe and posterior segment of the right lobe (81,144). The dilatation primarily involves the larger central ducts, which taper and end abruptly. The peripheral ducts frequently are not visualized. The dilatation can be fusiform, varicose, or cavitary. The extrahepatic

bile duct can be markedly dilated, even in the absence of dilatation of the intrahepatic ducts.

Intraductal stones can be detected by CT in 63% to 81% of patients. The stones can be in the intrahepatic ducts, in both the intra- and extrahepatic ducts, or only in the extrahepatic ducts (142). The stones are generally high in attenuation because of variable amounts of calcium and other inorganic components. Detection of the stones is easier on scans without intravenous contrast enhancement than with enhanced scans. On the enhanced scans, the high attenuation of the stones blends imperceptibly with the enhanced hepatic parenchyma. Additional abnormalities that suggest the presence of acute suppurative cholangitis include marked enhancement of the periductal tissues and pneumobilia. The pneumobilia is often a result of prior surgery (49) (Fig. 64).

In addition to the bile duct abnormalities, CT often demonstrates hepatic parenchymal disease. Early in the progression of the disease, the liver in patients with OCH can be enlarged and have multiple areas of scarring. The scarring is observed as segmental or lobar atrophy, and it is particularly likely to involve the lateral segment of the left lobe. Kusano et al. (129) found the hepatic atrophy to correlate with the presence of portal vein occlusion. After repeated attacks of cholangitis, the liver can become cirrhotic and diffusely decreased in size. In the presence of acute exacerbations, segmental or lobar areas of abnormally prolonged contrast enhancement can be seen. This finding suggests the presence of diffuse hepatic inflammation or pyogenic hepatitis. Occasionally, frank hepatic abscesses are present.

The goal of therapy in patients with OCH is to decrease the frequency of acute exacerbations and thus preserve hepatic parenchymal function. This is accomplished by removing as much of the intraductal debris as possible. In patients with OCH, multiple operations or interventional radiologic procedures are often required and are associated with high morbidity and mortality rates.

Bile Duct Parasites

A variety of parasites has been implicated as causative agents in biliary tract disease. The two most commonly noted are *Clonorchis sinensis* and *Ascaris lumbricoides.*

Clonorchis is found primarily in Southeast Asia. Humans are among the definitive hosts. The infection is acquired by eating raw fish, which are the second intermediate hosts. The larvae migrate from the duodenum into the CBD and enter the intrahepatic biliary tree. There the larvae develop into mature worms. The adult worms then live in the medium and small-sized intrahepatic bile ducts, and occasionally in the extrahepatic duct, gallbladder, and pancreatic duct. The worms cause mechanical obstruction of the bile ducts, and an inflammatory reaction involving the duct walls and periductal tissues. The inflammation

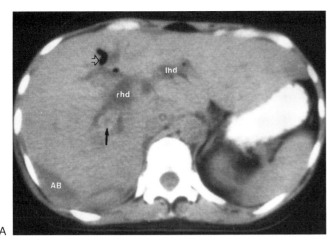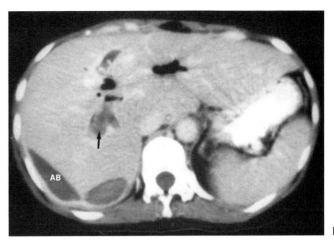

A   B

FIG. 64. Oriental cholangiohepatitis (recurrent pyogenic cholangitis) in a 31-year-old Asian man. The patient has a long history of multiple episodes of cholangitis and has undergone an operative biliary–enteric bypass (choledochojejunostomy). **A:** Noncontrast CT image obtained immediately above the liver hilus. There is moderate dilatation of the central right (rhd) and left (lhd) hepatic ducts. No obvious dilatation of the peripheral bile ducts is seen. Air in the left medial segmental duct *(open arrow)* is present due to the patent choledochojejunostomy. Note the high-density material *(arrow)* within the right posterior segmental duct. A perihepatic abscess (AB) resulted from a recent episode of cholangitis. **B:** CT section obtained at the same anatomic level as (A), after the intravenous administration of iodinated contrast material. The pigmented material in right posterior segmental duct *(arrow)* is less conspicuous than on the noncontrast image.

eventually leads to adenomatous hyperplasia of the bile duct walls. For this reason, *Clonorchis* infestation is not only associated with the development of OCH, but also cholangiocarcinoma.

Most patients have a chronic infection that is mild and asymptomatic. When symptoms of infestation develop, they include general malaise, abdominal discomfort, and diarrhea. The late stages of the disease can cause hepatomegaly, jaundice, and portal hypertension with associated splenomegaly and ascites. The CT findings are diffuse, minimal, uniform intrahepatic bile duct dilatation, especially in the periphery of the liver. The extrahepatic ducts are often not dilated. There may be intrahepatic bile duct calculi, or findings suggestive of suppurative cholangitis (52,143,152).

The pathology of ascariasis is similar to that caused by *Clonorchis*. The presence of worms in the bile ducts can lead to biliary colic, suppurative cholangitis, and acute acalculous cholecystitis. As the worms die and decompose, they may cause an inflammatory reaction that can result in bile duct strictures, liver abscesses, or the formation of intraductal calculi (207).

AIDS-Related Cholangiopathy

Biliary tract abnormalities in AIDS patients are often found in association with intestinal and biliary tract infection with *Cryptosporidium,* cytomegalovirus, *Mycobacterium avium-intracellulare,* and *Microsporida.* However, in 45% to 50% of patients, no pathogen can be identified.

In the patients in whom no infectious agent can be found, direct infiltration of the bile duct with human immunodeficiency virus (HIV) has been postulated as the mechanism of disease (42,48,238,254).

The spectrum of biliary tree abnormalities seen in AIDS patients includes papillary stenosis and sclerosing cholangitis, papillary stenosis alone, intrahepatic sclerosing cholangitis alone, and long, distal, extrahepatic bile duct strictures with or without intrahepatic sclerosing cholangitis (42,48,222,238). These patients present with right upper quadrant pain, nausea, vomiting, and fever. Jaundice is uncommon in the setting of AIDS-related cholangiopathy. Laboratory examination shows marked elevation of alkaline phosphatase, and only mild elevation of bilirubin and hepatic transaminases (69,254,257).

CT and sonography in patients with AIDS-related cholangiopathy can show CBD dilatation to the level of the papilla, asymmetric and irregular intrahepatic bile duct dilatation, dilatation of the pancreatic duct, thickening of the bile duct and gallbladder walls, and pericholecystic fluid (69,162,254) (Fig. 65). Unfortunately, a normal CT or sonogram does not exclude AIDS-related cholangiopathy. Cello (48) found that almost one third of patients with normal sonograms had abnormal cholangiograms. The cholangiographic findings in AIDS-related cholangiopathy include focal stricturing, irregular dilatation, and pruning of the intrahepatic bile ducts; uniform dilatation of the extrahepatic bile duct; long (up to 2.5 cm), smoothly tapering distal CBD strictures; irregularity and shagginess of the bile duct walls; and papillary stenosis.

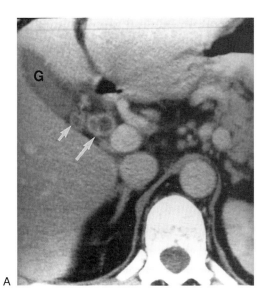 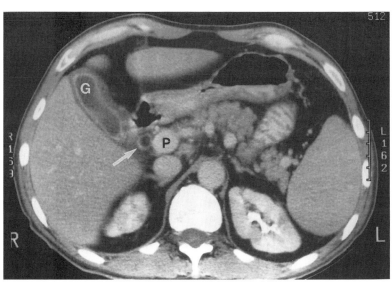

FIG. 65. AIDS cholangiopathy. **A:** Contrast-enhanced CT through the porta hepatis shows the wall of the CHD *(long arrow)* to be thickened. The cystic duct wall *(short arrow)* is also abnormal. **B:** Several centimeters caudal to (A) the CBD *(arrow)* and gallbladder (G) walls are also thickened. P, portal vein.

The bile duct abnormalities seen in AIDS patients can be difficult to distinguish from PSC; however, unlike in PSC, diverticular outpouchings and high-grade, segmental CBD strictures are uncommon in AIDS-related cholangiopathy. Furthermore, the long, tapering, distal CBD strictures seen in AIDS patients are uncommon in PSC (214).

The gallbladder abnormalities that can be seen in AIDS patients include nonspecific gallbladder wall thickening, acalculous cholecystitis, and Kaposi sarcoma of the gallbladder wall (222,254).

Primary Sclerosing Cholangitis

PSC is a chronic inflammatory disease of the biliary tract. It is characterized by progressive inflammation and fibrosis of the intra- and extrahepatic bile ducts, and of the periportal tissues. The inflammation and fibrosis lead to bile duct obliteration, cholestasis, and, eventually, biliary cirrhosis. The etiology of PSC is unknown. There appears to be a genetic predisposition to the development of this disease, as evidenced by the large percentage of patients with the human leukocyte antigens HLA-DRw52a, HLA-B8, and HLA-DR3. Although PSC can occur in the absence of coexisting diseases, there is a strong association between PSC and ulcerative colitis (UC). Although 25% to 72% of patients with PSC have UC, only 1% to 5% of patients with UC have PSC (51,60,98,135,139,152,195,205,274). There is no correlation between the time of onset of PSC and the length of time a patient has had UC. PSC can appear before the clinical onset of UC, or it may not manifest itself until after a total colectomy has been performed. Treatment of UC does not influence the activity of PSC.

There is, however, an association between the extent of colitis and the risk for developing PSC. Mild to moderate total colonic involvement by UC is present in 50% of patients with UC and PSC (42,60,195). The strong association between these two diseases has led some authors to suggest a pathogenetic relationship or a shared etiology (150). Disorders less commonly associated with PSC include Crohn's disease, Sjögren syndrome, retroperitoneal fibrosis, Riedel's thyroiditis, orbital pseudotumor, and sclerosing mediastinitis (47,274).

The diagnosis of PSC is made by a combination of clinical, biochemical, histologic, and radiologic evidence. PSC occurs twice as often in men as in women. Patients typically present in the third to fifth decade of life with progressive fatigue, right upper quadrant pain, pruritis, jaundice, and recurrent episodes of cholangitis. Laboratory examination characteristically shows marked elevation of serum alkaline phosphatase. Serum bilirubin levels also can be elevated. The absence of serum antimitochondrial antibody activity in patients with PSC is helpful in differentiating cirrhosis secondary to PSC, from primary biliary cirrhosis (135,139,152). The histologic changes seen in PSC are often highly suggestive of the diagnosis but are not pathognomonic. The findings include ductal and periductal fibrosis, formation of bile duct diverticula, fibrous cholangitis, and ductal obliteration. The extensive fibrosis in PSC can result in bile duct obstruction without evidence of significant bile duct dilatation. The intrahepatic ducts are involved in essentially all patients with PSC. In approximately 20% to 25% of cases, the abnormalities are limited to the intrahepatic ducts. The cystic duct is involved in 18% of cases and the pancreatic duct is involved in 8% of cases. In up to 15% of patients, there also may be fibrosis, chronic inflammation, and edema of the gallbladder wall (42,60,139).

The radiologic gold standard for the diagnosis of PSC is direct cholangiography (60). The most common findings seen on cholangiography are diffusely distributed, multifocal, short (1 to 2 mm), annular strictures involving both the intra- and extrahepatic bile ducts, in the absence of either choledocholithiasis or a history of bile duct surgery. The region of the junction of the right and left hepatic ducts is a common area for strictures in PSC. Strictures in this area often result in atrophy of one of the lobes of the liver. The segments of duct between the strictures generally have a normal caliber or are only mildly dilated. This pattern of alternating bandlike strictures and normal caliber segments of the bile ducts creates a ''beaded'' appearance. Diffuse bile duct dilatation is uncommon in PSC. The intrahepatic ducts also may show a decreased branching pattern creating the ''pruned tree'' appearance. The extrahepatic ducts often show multiple small outpouchings called diverticula. In addition to the caliber changes of the bile ducts, mucosal irregularities ranging from a fine brush border to a frankly nodular pattern can be present (95,98,135,150,152).

Computed Tomography in Sclerosing Cholangitis

In the evaluation of patients with PSC, CT has a role complementary to that of cholangiography. Computed tomography is not as sensitive as cholangiography for detecting the subtle mucosal abnormalities of the bile ducts, and therefore it should not be used as a screening examination in patients suspected of having PSC. However, the multiple, tight bile duct strictures in PSC can preclude adequate evaluation of the intrahepatic bile ducts with cholangiography; it is in this group of patients that CT can be helpful in evaluating the extent of disease (20,154).

The CT findings in PSC reflect the abnormalities seen on cholangiography. Intrahepatic bile duct abnormalities seen on CT include pruning, defined as the presence on a single CT section of a 4-cm or longer segment of dilated duct (excluding the main right and left ducts) that lacks the expected side branch dilatation; beading, defined as at least three closely alternating regions of dilatation and stenosis in an intrahepatic duct on a single CT section; and skip dilatation, defined as isolated, dilated peripheral bile ducts with no visible connection to other dilated ducts on contiguous images (210,252,253) (see the section on bile duct dilatation for further discussion of these findings). As mentioned previously, although pruning and beading can be present in PSC, they are not specific for this disease. Skip dilatations, on the other hand, when seen on CT, are strongly suggestive of PSC (253). The abnormalities of the intrahepatic bile ducts can have an irregular or asymmetric distribution; however, this also is not a specific finding for PSC (253). The CT findings of extrahepatic bile duct involvement by PSC include wall thickening (>2 mm and <5 mm), which can be focal or diffuse, and eccentric or concentric; bile duct dilatation; relative lack of dilatation proximal to an apparent bile duct stricture; and enhancing intraluminal mural nodules (>1 cm in diameter) seen on high-resolution, thin-section images (20,42,252) (Fig. 66). Enhancement of the bile duct wall is a nonspecific finding that can be seen in normal as well as abnormal bile ducts (253). Outwater et al. (196) showed that, in addition to the bile duct abnormalities, up to 65% of patients with PSC have benign enlargement of the celiac, gastrohepatic ligament, porta hepatis, periaortic, pancreaticoduodenal, and mesenteric lymph nodes. The nodes are generally homogeneous and isodense to the pancreas. Histologic examination of the enlarged lymph nodes shows reactive hyperplasia.

Computed tomography is helpful in the evaluation of the complications of PSC. Patients with PSC can develop intra- or extrahepatic bile duct calculi, cirrhosis, and portal hypertension. The cirrhosis and portal hypertension can be manifested on CT as a small, nodular liver, splenomegaly, varices, and ascites (20,252). In addition to these benign complications, PSC predisposes patients to the development of cholangiocarcinoma. This malignancy complicates PSC in about 6% to 12% of cases (80). When compared to patients with PSC alone, patients who develop cholangiocarcinoma in the setting of PSC tend to be older at the time of diagnosis of PSC, tend to have had UC longer, and tend to have more advanced PSC, often having already progressed to hepatic cirrhosis (151).

Patients with PSC who have a sudden worsening of jaundice should be suspected of having developed cholangiocarcinoma. Because there are no definitive cholangiographic features that allow the differentiation of uncomplicated PSC from PSC complicated by cholangiocarcinoma, CT may be more useful than cholangiography in detecting and staging this complication. The advantages of CT over cholangiography in this setting are its ability to evaluate not only the bile duct wall, but also the extraductal spread of disease, including local lymph node involvement and distant metastases. The CT findings suggestive of the development of cholangiocarcinoma include a polypoid mass larger than 1 cm, progressive stricture formation, or the development of large, nonsegmental areas of marked bile duct dilatation (20,60,152,154).

There is no effective medical treatment for PSC. Percutaneous biliary drainage and surgical biliary bypass procedures are palliative measures. Patients who develop cirrhosis can be treated with orthotopic liver transplantation.

Magnetic Resonance Imaging in Sclerosing Cholangitis

The use of T1-weighted, fat-suppressed spin echo pulse sequences, with or without intravenous gadolinium contrast agents, facilitates delineation of the bile duct wall

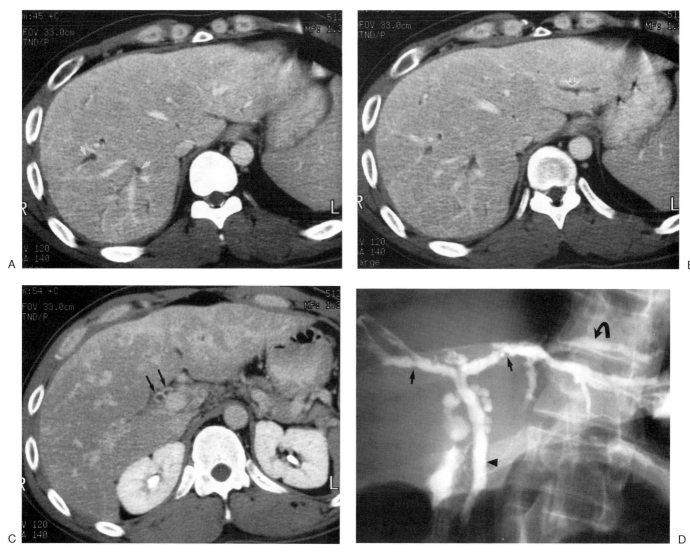

FIG. 66. Primary sclerosing cholangitis. **A:** Contrast-enhanced CT image of the liver shows nonuniform areas of intrahepatic bile duct dilation in both lobes *(arrows)* without any apparent connection to the central ducts. These represent skip dilatations that can be seen in sclerosing cholangitis. **B:** Several centimeters caudal to (A), in addition to the skip dilatations, there is a long segment of dilated duct *(open arrow)* without a normal branching pattern in the left lobe. This appearance is the CT equivalent of the cholangiographic "pruned tree" pattern. **C:** Contrast-enhanced image through the level of the porta hepatis shows thickening of the right and left hepatic duct walls *(arrows)*. Note the irregular areas of enhancement in both lobes of the liver. This appearance can be caused by fibrosis or periductal inflammation, both of which may be seen in PSC. **D:** ERCP in the same patient shows the irregular border of the CBD *(arrowhead)* and the band like strictures *(straight arrows)* of the intrahepatic ducts. Also note the long segment of the left hepatic duct *(curved arrow)* with the paucity of side branches corresponding to the appearance seen in (B).

(230). These techniques can be used to demonstrate abnormalities of the bile duct wall in sclerosing cholangitis (Fig. 67). On 2-D images, mild duct wall thickening, beading, and skip dilatations can be seen. In addition to the thickening of the bile duct walls, MR can show the scattered areas of bile duct dilatation and the changes caused by periportal inflammation. Periportal inflammation is seen as regions of low signal intensity on T1-weighted images, and signal intermediate between the liver and bile on T2-weighted images (172). On gadolinium-enhanced T1-weighted images, enhancement of inflammatory periportal tissue permits distinction from nonenhancing periportal edema. As they are refined, 3-D MR cholangiographic techniques may play a role in the noninvasive evaluation of patients with sclerosing cholangitis. It is possible that the mural and luminal abnormalities of the bile ducts will be better appreciated on 3-D data display than on 2-D tomographic images.

Hepatic-Artery-Infusion-Chemotherapy-Related Cholangitis

Secondary sclerosing cholangitis can develop in response to a variety of insults to the bile ducts. Prior biliary surgery, intraductal biliary calculi, suppurative cholangitis, AIDS, graft-versus-host disease, allograft rejection, and hepatic artery infusion chemotherapy (HAIC) all can result in diffuse bile duct injury (69,135,139). The bile duct abnormalities in secondary sclerosing cholangitis from many of these etiologies resemble those of PSC;

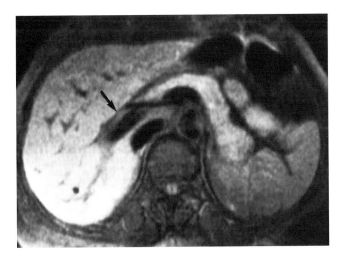

FIG. 67. Primary sclerosing cholangitis with minimal ductal dilatation and duct wall thickening. T1-weighted MR image demonstrates 4- to 5-mm thickening of the bile duct wall *(arrow)*. No substantial enhancement was present on post-gadolinium-enhancement images (not shown). This would be unusual for cholangiocarcinoma or infectious cholangitis. (Reproduced with permission from Semelka RC, Shoenut JP, Kroeker MA, et al. Bile duct disease: prospective comparison of ERCP, CT and fat suppression MRI. *Gastrointest Radiol* 1992;17:347–352.)

however, the bile duct abnormalities resulting from HAIC have a relatively characteristic distribution that helps in arriving at the correct diagnosis.

The chemotherapeutic agent responsible for causing secondary sclerosing cholangitis in patients receiving HAIC is almost always (5-flourodeoxyuridine (FUDR). The FUDR is extracted from the hepatic arterial blood by the liver and excreted through the biliary system (32,102,201). Injury to the bile ducts can result from either direct toxicity to the ductal epithelium, or chronic ischemia from compromise of the hepatic arterial blood flow. The histologic abnormalities seen in patients with HAIC-related cholangitis are obliterative endarteritis, necrosis and inflammation of the bile duct periluminal glands, absence of duct luminal epithelium, and fibrosis of the bile duct walls. The bile duct abnormalities are segmental, and usually they are most severe at the bifurcation of the CHD. There also may be involvement of the cystic duct and gallbladder (46). The intrahepatic ducts and the distal CBD are generally relatively spared (2,152,233). Often, there is also fibrosis around the chronically inflamed hepatic artery, which is usually patent (32,102,201).

Patients present with signs and symptoms of hepatic dysfunction, including jaundice. The average time to the onset of jaundice is 3 to 5 months, and the average time to the development of bile duct strictures is 12 months (2,32,233). It is important to recognize HAIC-related cholangitis as the cause of jaundice in these patients, because stopping the chemotherapy can arrest the progression of the bile duct abnormalities (2,32).

The cholangiographic changes in HAIC-related cholangitis range from minimal luminal and ductal contour irregularities to near obliteration of the duct lumen with proximal bile duct dilatation. The contour abnormalities can be eccentric and smoothly taper proximally and distally over a 2- to 3-cm segment. This appearance can mimic extrinsic compression of the bile duct by enlarged portal lymph nodes (2,233). CT is useful for excluding lymphadenopathy as the cause of bile duct narrowing. CT in patients with HAIC-related cholangitis shows wispy soft-tissue strands at the site of obstruction (Fig. 68). Intrahepatic bile duct dilatation is usually mild.

Cholangiocarcinoma

Cholangiocarcinoma accounts for 0.5% to 1% of all cancers in the United States annually, and it is found in approximately 1% of all patients undergoing biliary tract surgery. It is the most common primary malignancy of the bile ducts and accounts for 15% to 50% of obstructing bile duct tumors (152,191,281). Factors that predispose to the development of cholangiocarcinoma include UC, PSC, choledochal cysts, Caroli disease, polyposis syndromes of the colon, and *Clonorchis sinensis* infestation (42,281). The average age at the time of diagnosis is 60 to 65 years. When cholangiocarcinoma is associated with

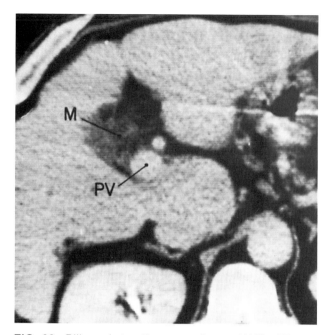

FIG. 68. Biliary obstruction secondary to HAIC. CT scan of the liver shows amorphous soft-tissue strands (M) in the porta hepatis surrounding the CHD in this patient who had received 5-fluorouracil treatment via an indwelling intra-arterial catheter, for colon metastases. Mild intrahepatic ductal dilatation was present on a higher image (not shown). Surgical biopsy of amorphous strands yielded only fibrosis.

UC, the age of onset is generally younger than in patients without UC. The frequency of occurrence in men is 1.5 times greater than in women (111,152,256,281). The most common clinical presentation is jaundice and weight loss. Patients with cholangiocarcinoma rarely present with bacterial cholangitis if they have not had prior endoscopic or percutaneous biliary tract procedures (256,281).

The histology in greater than 95% of cases of cholangiocarcinoma shows adenocarcinoma (281). The tumor arises from the extrahepatic bile ducts in up to 65% of cases, and from the intrahepatic bile ducts in up to 35% of cases. In 45% to 60% of cases, the tumor is limited to the confluence of the right and left hepatic ducts (Klatskin tumor), in 15% of cases it is limited to the middle third of the duct, in another 15% of cases it is limited to the distal third of the duct, and in 10% of cases it diffusely involves the extrahepatic bile duct. A small percentage of cholangiocarcinomas arise in the cystic duct (45,111,152,209,265). There are three morphologic patterns of extrahepatic cholangiocarcinoma: (a) infiltrative stenotic lesions, (b) bulky exophytic tumors, and (c) intraluminal papillary or polypoid masses. The infiltrating stenotic type is the most common pattern, occurring in up to 75% of cases (152,191,279).

The overall 5-year survival rate in patients with cholangiocarcinoma is 1% to 5%. The only chance for cure is complete resection of the tumor. Patients who have attempts at curative resection have a better prognosis, with 5-year survival rates of 10% to 50%. If the primary tumor is in the distal bile duct, the postoperative 5-year survival rate is 28% to 50%, and if the tumor is in the hilar region or middle third of the duct, the postoperative 5-year survival rate is less than 10% (42,111,191). The goal of the radiologic assessment of patients with cholangiocarcinoma is to identify patients who have clearly unresectable tumor, and to evaluate the extent of resection necessary for complete tumor removal in those patients considered resectable (6).

Computed Tomography in Cholangiocarcinoma

Direct cholangiography is the method of choice for detecting cholangiocarcinoma and assessing the extent of ductal involvement. Computed tomography is mainly used for assessing the extent of extrabiliary disease and for determining resectability of the primary tumor. The CT appearance of the primary tumor depends on its location and morphology. The primary tumor in extrahepatic cholangiocarcinoma can be seen by CT in 40% to 70% of cases (20,53,281). On unenhanced CT, the tumors most often appear isodense to the liver. Because cholangiocarcinomas are hypovascular and consist of abundant fibrous tissue in the central portion of the tumor, with the majority of the viable cells in the periphery, these tumors generally show no enhancement, or mild ring enhancement, in the portal venous phase of dynamic contrast-enhanced CT. Because of the nature of the vascularity of the fibrous tissue, the tumors show persistent diffuse enhancement on images obtained 10 to 15 minutes after injection. This finding is not specific for cholangiocarcinoma, but in the appropriate clinical setting it can help in confirming the diagnosis (248).

The infiltrative pattern of tumor occurs most commonly in the hilar region and appears as an ill-defined soft-tissue mass in the porta hepatis (Fig. 69). These tumors often directly invade the liver; however, the hepatic invasion can be difficult to detect with dynamic contrast-enhanced CT. If the findings are unclear, CT arterial portography can often give additional information regarding the presence and extent of hepatic invasion (20). Encasement of the vascular structures and spread to the regional lymph nodes is more common in the infiltrative pattern than the other morphologic types. The exophytic tumors more commonly arise from the intrahepatic ducts than the extrahepatic ducts. In either location, they appear as well-defined, nodular masses. The polypoid tumors are the least common pattern and appear as intraductal, soft-tissue masses greater than 1 cm in size (Fig. 70) (279).

If no tumor mass is seen, the diagnosis of a hilar cholangiocarcinoma can be made by noting the presence of high-grade intrahepatic bile duct dilatation and the apparent

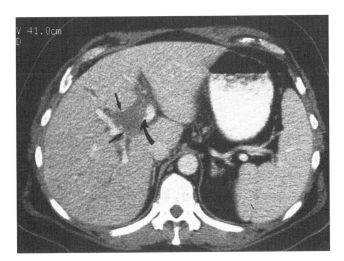

FIG. 69. Cholangiocarcinoma. Contrast-enhanced CT image shows mild intrahepatic bile duct dilatation. A diffusely infiltrating soft-tissue mass is present in the porta hepatis *(straight arrows)* and extends peripherally along the course of both the left and right hepatic ducts. Note the compression of the portal vein *(curved arrow)* by this mass. This was proven to be a cholangiocarcinoma with diffuse infiltration of the periportal tissues.

absence of the union of the right and left hepatic ducts. In the case of a hilar tumor, dilatation of the CHDs and CBDs usually will not be present. If the tumor is located in the mid or distal common duct, there will be dilatation of the duct down to the point of obstruction. At the point of obstruction, the duct will terminate abruptly, and there may be associated eccentric thickening of the bile duct wall, usually greater than 5 mm. Occasionally, the appearance of abrupt termination of the bile duct can be mimicked by cholesterol stones or benign bile duct strictures. However, bile duct wall thickening greater than 5 mm is seen only in the presence of biliary tumors (20,226).

Computed tomography is the most sensitive imaging technique for detecting unresectability of cholangiocarcinoma. In one report, CT accurately predicted unresectability in 78% of cases. In the study cases in which CT incorrectly predicted that a tumor was resectable, it failed to show portal vein infiltration without occlusion, metastases to duodenal lymph nodes, and small hepatic metastases (96,191,279). Cholangiocarcinoma most commonly spreads by direct extension into adjacent organs, or through lymphatic pathways to the periductal, peripancreatic, and periaortic lymph nodes (76,265). Hilar tumors result in nodal metastases more frequently than do distal CBD tumors. The decision as to whether or not the tumor is resectable depends mainly on the local extent of disease. The criteria for unresectability include: (a) invasion or occlusion of the main hepatic artery or portal vein, or both the right and left branches of the hepatic artery or portal vein; (b) involvement of second order or segmental bile ducts in both the left and right lobes of the liver; (c) regional metastases, including peritoneal deposits, lymph

node involvement outside of the hepatic hilum, or hepatic parenchymal disease involving both lobes; and (d) unilateral hepatic vascular occlusion with extensive contralateral intrahepatic bile duct involvement. All of these features are demonstrable on CT images. Lymphadenopathy, infiltration of fat planes adjacent to nonvascular structures, vascular compression, unilateral portal vein or hepatic artery occlusion, and unilateral hepatic metastases are not reliable indicators of unresectability, and they are not considered contraindications to exploration with the intent of curative resection (24,29,96,191).

Additional findings that can be seen on CT in patients with cholangiocarcinoma include hepatic lobar atrophy with associated crowding of the bile ducts, asymmetric intrahepatic bile duct dilatation, and segmental or lobar attenuation abnormalities (Figs. 70,71). Hepatic lobar atrophy can result from either portal venous obstruction or chronic bile duct obstruction and is more commonly associated with infiltrative tumors (45,148,190,247,279). The hepatic parenchymal attenuation abnormalities are believed to be related, most likely, to obstruction of the portal venous blood flow to the liver. The decreased portal blood flow results in decreased hepatic glycogen deposition, increased hepatic fat deposition, and a compensatory increase in arterial flow to the affected portion of the liver. The increased arterial flow results in increased hepatic parenchymal contrast enhancement on dynamic contrast-enhanced CT. This is particularly evident in the arterial phase of the examination in the portions of the liver supplied by the obstructed portal vein. Yamashita et al. (278) showed that these areas of increased contrast enhancement on dynamic CT correspond to segmental areas of abnormally high signal intensity on T2-weighted MRI images. The abnormal signal seen on MRI is believed to be a result of sinusoidal congestion. Mori et al. (183) described the presence of a dilated posterior superior pancreaticoduodenal artery as an indirect sign of portal venous invasion by pancreaticobiliary malignancies.

None of the preceding findings are specific for cholangiocarcinoma. They all can be seen in association with any disease process that causes portal venous obstruction or chronic biliary obstruction. In addition to vascular and bile duct obstruction, cholangiocarcinoma also can lead to obstruction of the stomach or duodenum. This is most often a late complication and can be the result of compression by a large peritoneal metastasis or local lymph nodes, direct tumor invasion of the duodenum, or scarring secondary to radiation therapy (76,177).

Magnetic Resonance Imaging in Cholangiocarcinoma

As described, the presence of high-grade obstruction of the biliary tree, and bile duct wall thickness >5 mm are CT findings consistent with cholangiocarcinoma (226). These features have also been observed on MR images

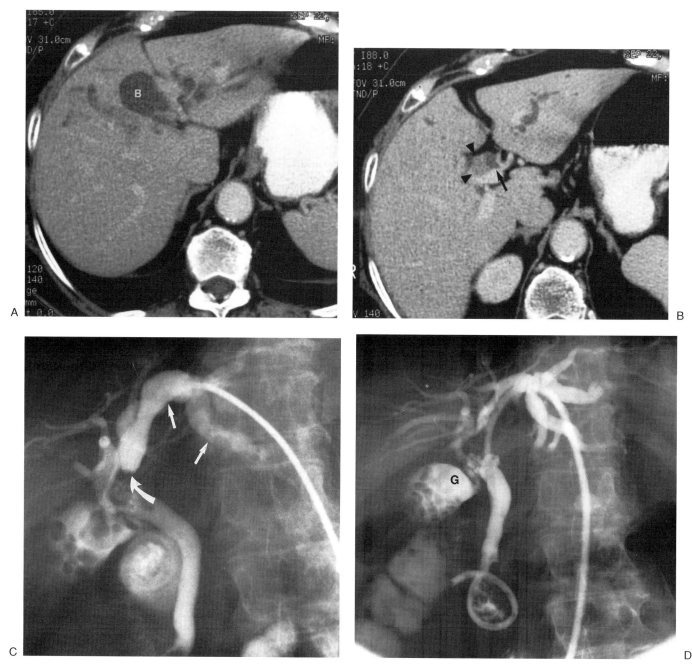

FIG. 70. Cholangiocarcinoma. **A:** Contrast-enhanced CT image shows dilated intrahepatic bile ducts primarily in the lateral segment of the left lobe. Small foci of ductal dilatation are present in the anterior segment of the right lobe and the medial segment of the left lobe. A biloma (B) is also present in the medial segment of the left lobe. **B:** At a level several centimeters caudal, again note the predominantly left lobe bile duct dilatation. Immediately anterior to the portal vein there is a soft-tissue mass *(arrowheads)* within the CHD. A small residual lumen *(arrow)* is present medial to the mass. **C:** Percutaneous transhepatic cholangiogram and drainage shows dilated left intrahepatic bile ducts *(straight arrows)*. Immediately proximal to the junction of the right and left ducts there is abrupt cut-off *(curved arrow)* of the left hepatic duct. Earlier images obtained in the cholangiogram showed that this was a mass extending from the CHD into the left hepatic duct. The right ductal system was only minimally dilated. **D:** At the completion of the procedure, a percutaneous biliary drainage catheter was passed through the small residual lumen of the CHD [seen in **(B)**] into the duodenum. Multiple filling defects representing gallstones are present in the gallbladder (G).

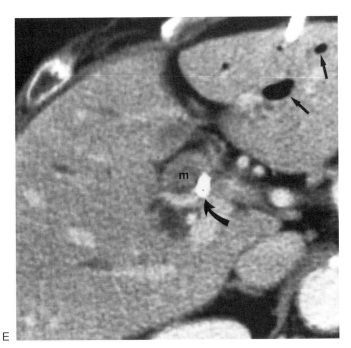

E

FIG. 70. (*Continued.*) **E:** Contrast-enhanced CT image obtained several days after the PTC shows pneumobilia *(arrows)* and the biliary catheter *(curved arrow)* passing through the residual lumen adjacent to the tumor mass (m).

(228). On T1-weighted spin echo images, cholangiocarcinoma is either isointense or low in signal intensity relative to the liver (Fig. 72). The tumor signal intensity on T2-weighted images ranges from markedly increased to mildly increased relative to the liver. The greater the fibrous content of the tumor, the lower the signal intensity on T2-weighted images (72).

On gadolinium-enhanced T1-weighted MR images, cholangiocarcinoma enhances to a moderate degree. When compared to CT, gadolinium-enhanced T1-weighted MRI permits better delineation of small primary hilar tumors, intrahepatic tumor extension, and periductal tumor infiltration. The primary tumor and the extent of hepatic invasion can be particularly well shown on contrast-enhanced T1-weighted breath-hold gradient echo images, with or without fat suppression, or fat-suppressed, T1-weighted contrast-enhanced spin echo images (149). When tumor extension is present in the periductal soft tissues, moderate enhancement of these tissues on gadolinium-enhanced T1-weighted fat-suppressed spin echo images facilitates accurate delineation of tumor from uninvolved surrounding tissues and structures (Fig. 73). Ductal tumors that arise in the intrapancreatic portion of the CBD are also well delineated on T1-weighted fat-suppressed images, with or without intravenous gadolinium-contrast enhancement. Tumors in this location are seen as low signal intensity masses against the background of the high signal intensity of the head of the pancreas (72,149).

Ampullary Carcinoma

Ampullary carcinomas are adenocarcinomas that arise from the intestinal-type mucosa lining the ampulla. They account for approximately 4% of periampullary tumors. They generally occur in the sixth and seventh decades of life and are two times more common in men than in women. Patients with UC and Gardner syndrome are at increased risk of developing this neoplasm. *Ascaris* infection also predisposes to the development of ampullary carcinoma.

The average size of these tumors is 3 cm or less. Patients present with signs and symptoms of obstruction of both the CBD and the pancreatic duct. Obstruction occurs earlier with these tumors than with pancreatic carcinomas because of their proximity to the lumen of the CBD. The prognosis for patients with ampullary carcinoma is much better than that for patients with pancreatic cancer. The 5-year survival rate varies from 10% to 70%, depending on the grade and stage of the tumor.

Ampullary tumors are often difficult to detect, even at endoscopy. CT, transabdominal ultrasound, and MRI may show the effects of the tumor on the bile duct and pancreatic duct, but they will frequently fail to demonstrate the actual tumor mass. In one series, CT showed the primary tumor in only 64% of cases (146). When seen on CT, the tumor is usually demonstrated as a soft-tissue mass protruding from the ampulla into the duodenum (Fig. 74). On MRI, T1-weighted fat-suppressed spin echo images show ampullary tumors as a low-signal-intensity mass in the region of the ampulla. Immediately after gadolinium enhancement, spoiled gradient echo sequences show mild heterogeneous enhancement of the tumor in the background of the higher signal intensity enhancing pancreatic parenchyma (Fig. 75). Delayed postcontrast, T1-weighted, fat-suppressed images show a greater degree of tumor enhancement than seen on the immediate postcontrast images.

Ampullary carcinomas can spread into the duodenal wall, pancreas, or regional lymph nodes. Distant metastases are uncommon. Endoscopic ultrasound is currently the most reliable technique for detecting and staging these tumors (41).

Miscellaneous Bile Duct Tumors

Malignant involvement of the bile ducts can be primary or secondary. Primary tumors of the bile duct other than cholangiocarcinoma are rare. Lymphoma, carcinoid, mucus-secreting papillary adenocarcinoma, and squamous cell carcinoma are some of the uncommon primary neoplasms of the bile duct that have been reported (85,120,251). Metastatic disease to the bile ducts can result from direct invasion by hepatocellular, gallbladder, or pancreatic carcinomas, or less com-

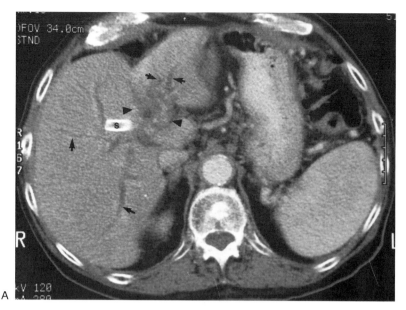

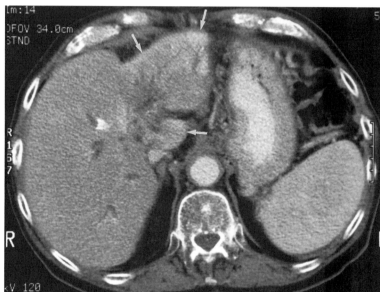

FIG. 71. Cholangiocarcinoma with left lobe atrophy. A: Contrast-enhanced CT image shows dilated intrahepatic bile ducts *(short arrows)* in both lobes of the liver with crowding of the ducts in the left lobe. The left lobe is atrophic. In the porta hepatis there is an ill-defined soft-tissue mass *(arrowheads)*, which represents the cholangiocarcinoma that is causing bile duct obstruction and occlusion of the left portal vein. s, metallic biliary stent. B: At a level 1 cm cephalad to (A), the atrophic left lobe of the liver and the caudate lobe *(arrows)* are enhanced to a slightly greater degree than the remainder of the liver. This is thought to be secondary to portal venous obstruction and subsequent increased arterial flow.

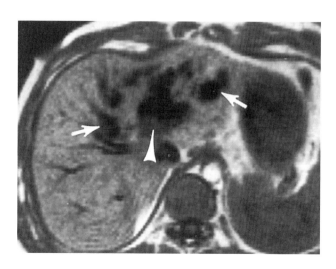

FIG. 72. Biliary obstruction secondary to cholangiocarcinoma. T1-weighted MR image (SE 300/15) shows marked dilatation of left intrahepatic ducts *(arrows)*. A mass *(arrowhead)* with signal intensity intermediate between that of liver and bile is seen near the origin of the left hepatic duct.

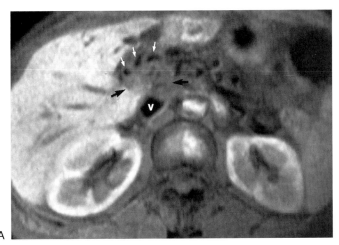
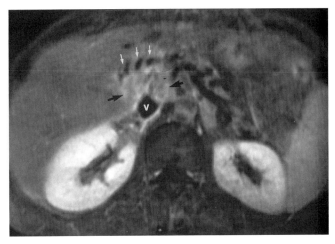

A   B

FIG. 73. Recurrent cholangiocarcinoma. Noncontrast, T1-weighted, fat-suppressed spin echo (SE 600/15) **(A)** and gadolinium-enhanced, T1-weighted, fat-suppressed spin echo **(B)** MR images. A soft-tissue mass that infiltrates along the hepatoduodenal ligament is present in the porta hepatis *(black arrows)*. This mass demonstrates moderate heterogeneous enhancement and also extends along the soft tissues anterior to the IVC (v). Multiple collateral vessels *(white arrows)* are present in the porta hepatis. This is a recurrent cholangiocarcinoma.

monly from hematogenous spread by tumors such as malignant melanoma. All of these tumors can cause bile duct obstruction and do not have a specific appearance on CT. They frequently mimic the CT appearance of primary cholangiocarcinomas.

Portal, hepatoduodenal, or gastrohepatic ligament lymph node metastases from extrabiliary primary tumors also can cause bile duct obstruction by extrinsic compression of the duct. It is uncommon for this to occur secondary to benign lymphadenopathy (213). Computed tomography is useful for differentiating intrinsic bile duct obstruction from extrinsic obstruction such as that caused by malignant portal lymphadenopathy.

Postoperative Complications of Hepatobiliary Surgery

Injury to the bile ducts can result from a variety of percutaneous (122) and operative hepatobiliary procedures. The increasing frequency of orthotopic liver transplantation and laparoscopic cholecystectomy has required that radiologists be familiar with the imaging appearance of the normal postoperative changes as well as the biliary complications associated with these procedures.

Biliary complications occur in 13% to 22% of liver transplant recipients (68,140,283). Complications have been reported to occur as soon as 1 day and as long as 4

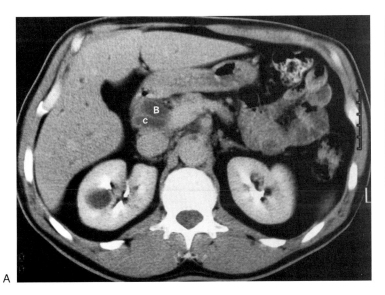

A

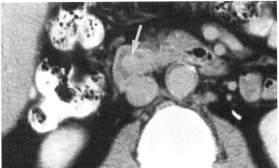

B

FIG. 74. Ampullary carcinoma. **A:** Contrast-enhanced CT image shows a dilated common bile duct (B) and cystic duct (c). Note the mildly dilated intrahepatic bile ducts. **B:** At a level 6 cm caudal to (A), a soft-tissue-attenuation mass *(arrow)* is seen bulging into the duodenum in the region of the ampulla. Endoscopic visualization and biopsy proved this to be an ampullary carcinoma.

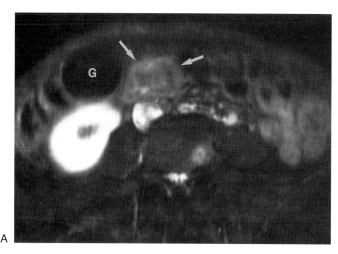
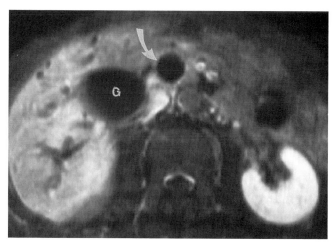

A
B

FIG. 75. Ampullary carcinoma. **A:** A 4-cm tumor mass *(arrows)* with mild heterogeneous enhancement is present in the periampullary region as seen on the immediate-post-gadolinium-enhanced, T1-weighted, fat-suppressed spin echo MR image (SE 600/15). **B:** T1-weighted, fat-suppressed post-gadolinium-enhancement spin echo image, at the level of the head of the pancreas, cephalad to (A), shows the CBD to be severely dilated *(curved arrow).* G, gallbladder.

years after transplantation; however, they most commonly manifest themselves within several weeks. The spectrum of biliary complications in liver transplant recipients includes bile duct strictures with resultant biliary obstruction, bile duct leaks, bile duct stones, bilomas, and cystic duct remnant mucoceles. Bile duct obstruction occurs more frequently than bile duct leaks. Obstruction resulting from biliary strictures usually occurs at the site of the bile duct anastomosis. The most common cause of bile duct strictures in transplant patients is ischemia. This re-

sults from hepatic artery stenosis or thrombosis (68,140). The injury caused by ischemia can range from mild mucosal injuries producing irregularity of the bile duct contour, to complete bile duct necrosis with resultant bile leak, bile peritonitis, and intrahepatic biloma formation. In transplant patients with bile duct injuries from ischemia, CT can show bile duct dilatation, free fluid in the abdomen and pelvis, and intrahepatic fluid collections representing bilomas.

Mucoceles in liver transplant recipients result from mu-

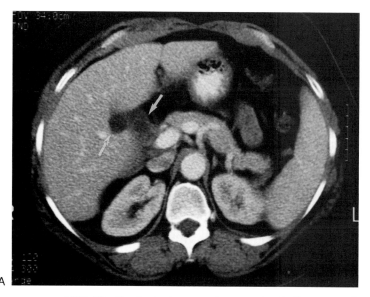
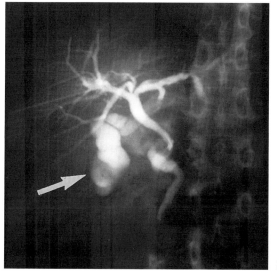

A
L
B

FIG. 76. Cystic duct remnant mucocele. **A:** Contrast-enhanced CT image of a patient after orthotopic liver transplant shows a dilated tubular structure *(arrows)* in the expected location of the common duct. **B:** Percutaneous transhepatic cholangiogram shows normal intrahepatic biliary radicals and a normal common duct. The dilated tubular structure seen on CT was directly punctured and opacified and proven to be a mucocele of the donor cystic duct remnant *(arrow).*

cus accumulation in a donor or recipient cystic duct remnant that has been obstructed as a result of incorporation of the orifice of the cystic duct into the suture line of the CBD anastomosis. In patients with cystic duct remnant mucoceles, CT shows a well-defined fluid-attenuation mass in the region of the porta hepatis, adjacent to the CHD (Fig. 76) (283). The differential diagnosis of this appearance includes loculated ascites, lymphocele, biloma, abscess, and a fluid-filled Roux-en-Y jejunal loop. Mucoceles of the cystic duct remnant can become clinically significant if they cause bile duct obstruction.

There are two major categories of complications associated with laparoscopic cholecystectomy. The first category is laparoscopy related injuries to the bowel, bladder, ureter, abdominal wall vessels, and solid viscera. These injuries can be manifested on CT as abdominal wall or rectus sheath hematomas, peritoneal hemorrhage, persistent pneumoperitoneum and ascites, or liver lacerations (211).

The second category is cholecystectomy-related complications including retained CBD stones, bile duct injury, incomplete resection of the gallbladder, and infection (180). Injury to the bile ducts is the most significant postoperative complication. Bile duct injuries occur 3 to 5 times more often in laparoscopic cholecystectomy than in open cholecystectomy (263). The most common symptoms are abdominal pain and distention, and a low-grade fever as a result of bile leaks associated with bile peritonitis or infected bilomas. Patients can also present with mildly abnormal liver function tests from biliary obstruction due to bile duct ligation, or bile duct strictures resulting from laser or cautery injuries (64,65,268). The diagnosis is usually made 1 to 2 weeks after the cholecystectomy in the case of bile leaks, and 2 weeks to 4 months postoperatively in the case of bile duct strictures (65).

The rate of biliary complications for laparoscopic cholecystectomy is in the range of 0.5% to 1.5%. This is significantly higher than the reported biliary complication rate of 0.2% to 0.4% for open cholecystectomy. As experience with laparoscopic cholecystectomy has increased, the complication rate has decreased (35,61,180). The expected postoperative findings after laparoscopic cholecystectomy include pneumoperitoneum, subcutaneous emphysema, a small amount of fluid in the gallbladder fossa, adynamic ileus, pleural effusions, and lower lobe atelectasis, all of which generally resolve within the first postoperative week. Patients also may have ascites, which most often resolves by the 12th postoperative day (117,159, 160,166,268).

Bile duct injuries classically result from mistaking the CHD for the cystic duct. A portion of the CHD then gets resected or ligated. These injuries are often associated with injuries to the right hepatic artery. Another source of complications in laparoscopic cholecystectomy is an aberrant right hepatic duct. The anomalous duct can be mistaken for the cystic duct at the time of surgery, and

thus be ligated, with resultant impaired drainage of a portion of the right lobe of the liver. Anatomic variations of the extrahepatic bile ducts are present in up to 25% of people (227).

Bile leaks, which usually originate from the cystic duct stump or gallbladder remnant, result in gallbladder fossa or perihepatic fluid collections, and often ascites (Fig. 77). The CT findings in patients with bile duct injuries are nonspecific, because the gallbladder fossa or perihepatic fluid collections also could represent seromas, lymphoceles, hematomas, or abscesses (267). The presence of a bile leak can be confirmed with ERCP or radionuclide scintigraphy (Fig. 78).

In addition to fluid collections, CT also may demonstrate retained stones in the CBD or stones that have dropped into the peritoneal space. Routine operative cholangiography is recommended by some authors to delineate the bile duct anatomy and thus decrease the likelihood of bile duct injury. Operative cholangiography also enables the surgeon to detect CBD stones that can be treated either by converting the laparoscopic procedure to an open cholecystectomy, or by endoscopic retrieval at a later time. The success of operative cholangiography during laparoscopic cholecystectomy is 71% to 90% (267,270). Because of the invasive nature of direct cholangiography, it is not currently routinely used as part of the preoperative work-up for patients who are to undergo laparoscopic cholecystectomy. However, the role of noninvasive techniques such as helical CT cholangiography and MR cholangiography in the preoperative evaluation

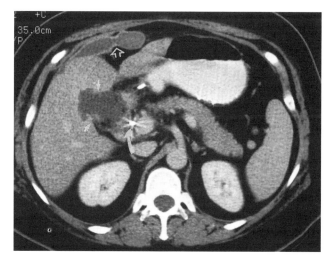

FIG. 77. Biloma. Contrast-enhanced CT image in a patient after laparoscopic cholecystectomy shows an ill-defined fluid collection *(arrows)* in the region of the porta hepatis. A stent *(curved arrow)* is present in the CBD. Anterior to the liver, adjacent to the abdominal wall, there is a second fluid collection *(open arrow)* which has an enhancing rim. This patient was known to have a bile duct injury and subsequent bile leak from the cholecystectomy. These fluid collections were proved by percutaneous aspiration to be infected bilomas.

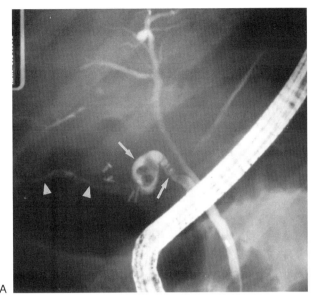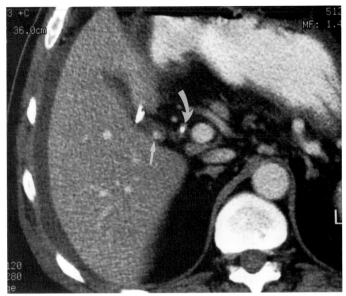

A   B

FIG. 78. A: ERCP in a patient after laparoscopic cholecystectomy shows filling of the cystic duct and a gallbladder remnant *(arrows)*. There are filling defects in the gallbladder remnant which proved to be retained gallstones. Note the contrast leaking from the gallbladder remnant *(arrowheads)*. **B:** Contrast-enhanced CT image in the same patient obtained after the ERCP shows the high-attenuation stones in the gallbladder remnant *(straight arrow)* medial to the cholecystectomy clips. Also note the stent in the CBD *(curved arrow)* and the fluid collection around the liver caused by the bile leak demonstrated on ERCP.

of these patients may grow as these techniques are further refined.

REFERENCES

1. Ament AE, Haaga JR, Wiedenmann SD, Barkmeier JD, Morrison SC. Primary sclerosing cholangitis: CT findings. *J Comput Assist Tomogr* 1983;7:795–800.
2. Anderson SD, Holley HC, Berland LL, Van Dyke JA, Stanley RJ. Causes of jaundice during hepatic artery infusion chemotherapy. *Radiology* 1986;161:439–442.
3. Araki T, Itai Y, Tasaka A. Computed tomography of localized dilatation of the intrahepatic bile ducts. *Radiology* 1981;141:733–736.
4. Araki T, Hihara T, Karikomi M, Kachi K, Uchiyama G. Intraluminal papillary carcinoma of the gallbladder: prognostic value of computed tomography and sonography. *Gastrointest Radiol* 1988;13:261–265.
5. Babbitt DP. Congenital choledochal cyst: new etiological concept based on anomalous relationships of common bile duct and pancreatic bulb. *Ann Radiol (Paris)* 1969;12:231–240.
6. Baer HU, Stain SC, Dennison AR, Eggers B, Blumgart LH. Improvements in survival by aggressive resections of hilar cholangiocarcinoma. *Ann Surg* 1993;217:20–27.
7. Baert AL, Roex L, Marchal G, Hermans P, Dewilde D, Wilms G. CT of the stomach with water as an oral contrast agent: technique and preliminary results. *J Comput Assist Tomogr* 1989;13:633–636.
8. Balfe DM, Mauro MA, Koehler RE, et al. Gastrohepatic ligament: normal and pathologic CT anatomy. *Radiology* 1984;150:485–490.
9. Balthazar EJ. The Mirizzi syndrome: inflammatory stricture of the common hepatic duct. *Am J Gastroenterol* 1975;64:144–148.
10. Balthazar EJ, Birnbaum BA, Naidich M. Acute cholangitis: CT evaluation. *J Comput Assist Tomogr* 1993;17:283–289.
11. Barakos JA, Ralls PW, Lapin SA, et al. Cholelithiasis: evaluation with CT. *Radiology* 1987;162:415–418.
12. Baron RL, Stanley RJ, Lee JKT, Koehler RE, Melson GL, Balfe DM, Weyman PJ. A prospective comparison of the evaluation of biliary obstruction using computed tomography and ultrasonography. *Radiology* 1982;145:91–98.
13. Baron RL, Stanley RJ, Lee JKT, Koehler RE, Levitt RG. Computed tomographic features of biliary obstruction. *AJR* 1983;140:1173–1178.
14. Baron RL. Common bile duct stones: reassessment of criteria for CT diagnosis. *Radiology* 1987;162:419–424.
15. Baron RL. CT diagnosis of choledocholithiasis. *Semin Ultrasound CT MR* 1987;8:85–102.
16. Baron RL, Rohrmann CA Jr, Lee SP, Shuman WP, Teefey SA. CT evaluation of gallstones in vitro: correlation with chemical analysis. *AJR* 1988;151:1123–1128.
17. Baron RL, Schulte SJ, Goodsitt MM, Lee SP. *Factors determining CT appearances of gallstones: answers from dual-energy CT.* Presented at the annual meeting of the Society of Gastrointestinal Radiologists, Palm Desert, CA; February 19–23, 1989.
18. Baron RL, Kuyper SJ, Lee SP, et al. In vitro dissolution of gallstones with MTBE: correlation with characteristics at CT and MR imaging. *Radiology* 1989;173:117–121.
19. Baron RL, Shuman WP, Lee SP. MR appearance of gallstones in vitro at 1.5T: correlation with chemical composition. *AJR* 1989;153:497–502.
20. Baron RL. Computed tomography of the biliary tree. *Radiol Clin North Am* 1991;29:1235–1250.
21. Baron RL. Gallstone characterization: the role of imaging. *Semin Roentgenol* 1991;26:216–225.
22. Baron RL. Role of CT in characterizing gallstones: an unsettled issue (comment). *Radiology* 1991;178:635–636.
23. Becker CD, Vock P. Apperance of gas-containing gallstones on sonography and computed tomography. *Gastrointest Radiol* 1984;9:323–328.
24. Bengmark S, Ekberg H, Evander A, Klofver-Stahl B, Tranberg KG. Major liver resection for hilar cholangiocarcinoma. *Ann Surg* 1988;207:120–125.

25. Berk R, van der Vegt JH, Lichtenstein JE. The hyperplastic cholecystoses: cholesterolosis and adenomyomatosis. *Radiology* 1983; 146:593–601.

26. Berland LL, Doust BD, Foley WD. Acute hemorrhage into the gallbladder diagnosed by computerized tomography and ultrasonography. *J Comput Assist Tomogr* 1980; 4:260–262.

27. Berland LL, Lawson TL, Stanley RJ. CT appearance of Mirizzi syndrome. *J Comput Assist Tomogr* 1984; 8:165–166.

28. Bernardino ME, Young SW, Lee JKT, Weinreb JC. Hepatic MR imaging with Mn-DPDP: safety, image quality, and sensitivity. *Radiology* 1992; 183:53–58.

29. Bismuth H, Castaing D, Traynor O. Resection or palliation: priority of surgery in the treatment of hilar cancer. *World J Surg* 1988; 12:39–47.

30. Blankenberg F, Wirth R, Jeffrey RB Jr, Mindelzun R, Francis I. Computed tomography as an adjunct to ultrasound in the diagnosis of acute acalculous cholecystitis. *Gastrointest Radiol* 1991; 16: 149–153.

31. Bloustein PA. Association of carcinoma with congenital cystic conditions of the liver and bile ducts. *Am J Gastroenterol* 1977; 67:40–46.

32. Botet JF, Watson RC, Kemeny N, Daly JM, Yeh S. Cholangitis complicating intraarterial chemotherapy in liver metastases. *Radiology* 1985; 156:335–337.

33. Boukadoum M, Siddiky MA, Zerhouni EA, Stitik RP. CT demonstration of adenomyomatosis of the gallbladder. *J Comput Assist Tomogr* 1984; 8:177–180.

34. Bova JG, Schwesinger WH, Kurtin WE. In vivo analysis of gallstone composition by computed tomography. *Gastrointest Radiol* 1992; 17:253–256.

35. Bowen JC. Gallstone disease: current therapy. *Semin Ultrasound CT MR* 1993; 14:321–324.

36. Brakel K, Lameris JS, Nijs HGT, Terpstra OT, Steen G, Blijenberg BC. Predicting gallstone composition with CT: in vivo and in vitro analysis. *Radiology* 1990; 174:337–341.

37. Bret PM, deStempel JV, Atri M, Lough JO, Illecas FF. Intrahepatic bile duct and portal vein anatomy revisited. *Radiology* 1988; 169: 405–407.

38. Brink JA, Heiken JP, Balfe DM, et al. Noninvasive cholangiography with spiral CT. *Radiology* 1992; 185(P):141.

39. Brink JA, Kammer B, Mueller PR, Balfe DM, Prien EL, Ferrucci JT. Prediction of gallstone composition: synthesis of CT and radiographic features in vitro. *Radiology* 1994; 190:69–75.

40. Brink JA, Kammer B, Mueller PR, Prien EL, Ferrucci JT. Dissolution of calcified gallstones. Part I. Correlation of in vitro dissolution kinetics in methyl tert-butyl ether with patterns of calcification by computed tomography. *Invest Radiol* 1994; 29:448–453.

41. Buck JL, Elsayed AM. Ampullary tumors: radiologic-pathologic correlation. *Radiographics* 1993; 13:193–212.

42. Burrell MI, Zeman RK, Simeone JF, et al. The biliary tract: imaging for the 1990's. *AJR* 1991; 157:223–233.

43. Buxton-Thomas M, Chisholm R, Dixon AK. Intrahepatic bile duct dilatation shown by computed tomography—predilection for the left lobe? *Br J Radiol* 1985; 58:499–502.

44. Caroli J, Couinaud C. Une affection nouvelle sans doute congenitale des voies biliaires: la dilatation kystique unioibaire des canaux hepatiques. *Semin Hosp Paris* 1958; 496:136–142.

45. Carr DH, Hadjis NS, Banks LM, Hemingway AP, Blumgart LH. Computed tomography of hilar cholangiocarcinoma: a new sign. *AJR* 1985; 145:53–56.

46. Carrasco CH, Freeny PC, Chuang VP, Wallace S. Chemical cholecystitis associated with hepatic artery infusion chemotherapy. *AJR* 1983; 141:703–706.

47. Carroll BA, Oppenheimer DA. Sclerosing cholangitis: sonographic demonstration of bile duct wall thickening. *AJR* 1982; 139:1016–1018.

48. Cello JP. Acquired immunodeficiency syndrome cholangiopathy: spectrum of disease. *Am J Med* 1989; 86:539–546.

49. Chan FL, Man SW, Leong LL, Fan ST. Evaluation of recurrent pyogenic cholangitis with CT: analysis of 50 patients. *Radiology* 1989; 170:165–169.

50. Chao TC, Greager JA. Primary carcinoma of the gallbladder. *J Surg Oncol* 1991; 46:215–221.

51. Chapman RWG, Marborgh BAM, Rhodes JM, et al. Primary sclerosing cholangitis: a review of its clinical features, cholangiography, and hepatic histology. *Gut* 1980; 21:870–877.

52. Choi BI, Kim HJ, Han MC, Do YS, Han MH, Lee SH. CT findings of clonorchiasis. *AJR* 1989; 152:281–284.

53. Choi BI, Lee JH, Han MC, Kim SH, Yi JG, Kim CW. Hilar cholangiocarcinoma: comparative study with sonography and CT. *Radiology* 1989; 172:689–692.

54. Choi BI, Yeon KM, Kim SH, Han MC. Caroli disease: central dot sign in CT. *Radiology* 1990; 174:161–163.

55. Co CS, Shea WJ, Goldberg HI. Evaluation of common bile duct diameter using high resolution computed tomography. *J Comput Assist Tomogr* 1986; 10:424–427.

56. Coelho JC, Buffara M, Pozzobon CE, Altenburg FL, Artigas GV. Incidence of common bile duct stones in patients with acute and chronic cholecystits. *Surg Gynecol Obstet* 1984; 158:76–80.

57. Compton RA. Bursting forces within the human body. *Radiology* 1973; 107:77–80.

58. Cooperberg PL, Gibney RG. Imaging of the gallbladder, 1987. *Radiology* 1987; 163:605–613.

59. Cory DA, Don S, West KW. CT cholangiography of a choledochocele. *Pediatr Radiol* 1990; 21:73–74.

60. Craig DA, MacCarty RL, Wiesner RH, Grambsch PM, LaRusso NF. Primary sclerosing cholangitis: value of cholangiography in determining the prognosis. *AJR* 1991; 157:959–964.

61. Crist DW, Gadacz TR. Complications of laparoscopic surgery. *Surg Clin North Am* 1993; 73:265–289.

62. Cronan JJ, Mueller PR, Simeone JF, et al. Prospective diagnosis of choledocholithiasis. *Radiology* 1983; 146:467.

63. Cronan JJ. US diagnosis of choledocholithiasis: a reappraisal. *Radiology* 1986; 161:133–134.

64. Davidoff AM, Pappas TN, Murray EA, et al. Mechanisms of major biliary injury during laparoscopic cholecystectomy. *Ann Surg* 1992; 215:196–202.

65. Davidoff AM, Branum GD, Meyers WC. Clinical features and mechanisms of major laparoscopic biliary injury. *Semin Ultrasound CT MR* 1993; 14:328–345.

66. Demas BE, Hricak H, Moseley M, et al. Gallbladder bile: an experimental study in dogs using MR imaging and proton MR spectroscopy. *Radiology* 1985; 157:453–455.

67. Dennis MA, Pretorius D, Manco-Johnson ML, Bangert-Burroughs KB. CT detection of portal venous gas associated with suppurative cholangitis and cholecystitis. *AJR* 1985; 145:1017–1018.

68. Dodd GD III, Orons PD, Campbell WL, Zajko AB. Imaging of hepatic transplantation. In: Taveras JM, Ferrucci JT, eds. *Radiology: diagnosis, imaging, intervention,* vol 4. Philadelphia: JB Lippincott, 1994; 1–11.

69. Dolmatch BL, Laing FC, Federle MP, Jeffrey RB, Cello J. AIDS-related cholangitis: radiographic findings in nine patients. *Radiology* 1987; 163:313–316.

70. Dong B, Chen M. Improved sonographic visualization of choledocholithiasis. *J Clin Ultrasound* 1987; 15:185–190.

71. Dooms GC, Fisher MR, Higgins CB, Hricak H, Goldberg HI, Margulis AR. MR imaging of the dilated biliary tract. *Radiology* 1986; 158:337–341.

72. Dooms GC, Kerlan RK Jr, Hricak H, Wall SD, Margulis AR. Cholangiocarcinoma: imaging by MR. *Radiology* 1986; 159:89–94.

73. Duber C, Storkel S, Wagner P-K, Muller J. Xanthogranulomatous cholecystitis mimicking carcinoma of the gallbladder: CT findings. *J Comput Assist Tomogr* 1984; 8:1195–1198.

74. Dupuy DE, Costello P, Ecker CP. Spiral CT of the pancreas. *Radiology* 1992; 183:815–818.

75. Elizondo G, Fretz C, Stark DD, et al. Preclinical evaluation of MnDPDP: new paramagnetic hepatobiliary contrast agent for MR imaging. *Radiology* 1991; 178:73–78.

76. Engels JT, Balfe DM, Lee JK. Biliary carcinoma: CT evaluation of extrahepatic spread. *Radiology* 1989; 172:35–40.

77. Erb RE, Mirvis SE, Shanmuganathan K. Gallbladder injury secondary to blunt trauma: CT findings. *J Comput Assist Tomogr* 1994; 18:778–784.

78. Fan ST, Choi TK, Chan FL, Lai EC, Wong J. Role of computed tomography in the management of recurrent pyogenic cholangitis. *Aust N Z J Surg* 1990; 60:599–605.

79. Fanquet T, Montes M, de Azua YR, et al. Primary gallbladder

carcinoma: imaging findings in 50 patients with pathologic correlation. *Gastrointest Radiol* 1991;16:143–148.

80. Farrant JM, Hayllar KM, Wilkinson ML, et al. Natural history and prognostic variables in primary sclerosing cholangitis. *Gastroenterology* 1991;100:1710–1717.

81. Federle MP, Cello JP, Laing FC, Jeffrey RBJ. Recurrent pyogenic cholangitis in Asian immigrants: use of ultrasonography, computed tomography, and cholangiography. *Radiology* 1982;143:151–156.

82. Flickinger FW, Sathyanarayana, Stincer EJ. Common bile duct calculus: MRI findings. *South Med J* 1993;86:242–244.

83. Foley WD, Wilson CR, Quiroz FA, Lawson TL. Demonstration of the normal extrahepatic biliary tract with computed tomography. *J Comput Assist Tomogr* 1980;4:48–52.

84. Franquet T, Montes M, Ruiz de Azua Y, Jimenez FJ, Cozcolluela R. Primary gallbladder carcinoma: imaging findings in 50 patients with pathologic correlation. *Gastrointest Radiol* 1991;16:143–148.

85. Gembala RB, Arsuaga JE, Friedman AC, et al. Carcinoid of the intrahepatic ducts. *Abdom Imaging* 1993;18:242–244.

86. Gerard PS, Berman D, Zafaranloo S. CT and ultrasound of gallbladder adenomyomatosis mimicking carcinoma. *J Comput Assist Tomogr* 1990;14:490–491.

87. Gibson RN, Yeung E, Thompson JN, et al. Bile duct obstruction: radiologic evaluation of level, cause, and tumor resectability. *Radiology* 1986;160:43–47.

88. Glenn F. Postcholecystectomy choledocholithiasis. *Surg Gynecol Obstet* 1972;134:249–252.

89. Goldberg HI. Helical cholangiography: complementary or substitute study for endoscopic retrograde cholangiography? *Radiology* 1994;192:615–616.

90. Goldstein RB, Wing VW, Laing FC, Jeffrey RB. Computed tomography of thick-walled gallbladder mimicking pericholecystic fluid. *J Comput Assist Tomogr* 1986;10:55–56.

91. Gore RM, Nemcek AA, Vogelzang RL. Choledocholithiasis. In: Gore RM, Levine MS, Laufer I, eds. *Textbook of gastrointestinal radiology,* vol 2. Philadelphia: WB Saunders, 1994;1670–1674.

92. Greenberg M, Rubin JM, Greenberg BM. Appearance of the gallbladder and biliary tree by CT cholangiography. *J Comput Assist Tomogr* 1983;7:788–794.

93. Gross BH, Harter LP, Gore RM, et al. Ultrasonic evaluation of common bile duct stones: prospective comparison with endoscopic retrograde cholangiopancreatography. *Radiology* 1983;146:471–474.

94. Guibaud L, Bret PM, Reinhold C, Atri M, Barkun ANG. Diagnosis of choledocholithiasis: value of MR cholangiography. *AJR* 1994;163:847–850.

95. Gulliver DJ, Baker ME, Putnam W, Baillie J, Rice R, Cotton PB. Bile duct diverticula and webs: nonspecific cholangiographic features of primary sclerosing cholangitis. *AJR* 1991;157:281–285.

96. Gulliver DJ, Baker ME, Cheng CA, Meyers WC, Pappas TN. Malignant biliary obstruction: efficacy of thin-section dynamic CT in determining resectability. *AJR* 1992;159:503–507.

97. Gupta RK, Kakar AK, Jena A, Mishra PK, Khushu S. Magnetic resonance in obstructive jaundice. *Australasian Radiol* 1989;33:245–251.

98. Hadjis NS, Adam A, Blenkharn I, Hatzis G, Benjamin IS, Blumgart LH. Primary sclerosing cholangitis associated with liver atrophy. *Am J Surg* 1989;158:43–47.

99. Hall-Craggs MA, Allen CM, Owens CM, et al. MR cholangiography: clinical evaluation in 40 cases. *Radiology* 1993;189:423–427.

100. Hamm B, Vogl TJ, Branding G, et al. Focal liver lesions: MR imaging with Mn-DPDP—initial clinical results in 40 patients. *Radiology* 1992;182:167–174.

101. Hanada K, Nakata H, Nakayama T, Tsukamoto Y, Terashima H, Kuroda Y, Okuma R. Radiologic findings in xanthogranulomatous cholecystitis. *AJR* 1987;148:727–730.

102. Haq MM, Valdes LG, Peterson DF, Gourley WK. Fibrosis of extrahepatic biliary system after continuous hepatic artery infusion of floxuridine through an implantable pump (Infusaid pump). *Cancer* 1986;57:1281–1283.

103. Heiken JP, Brink JA, Vannier MW: Spiral (helical) CT. *Radiology* 1993;189:647–656.

104. Hickman MS, Schwesinger WH, Bova JD, Kurtin WE. Computed tomographic analysis of gallstones. *Arch Surg* 1986;121:289–291.

105. Hoener B, Engelstad BL, Ramos EC, et al. Comparison of Fe-HBED and Fe-EHPG as hepatobiliary MR contrast agents. *J Magn Reson Imaging* 1991;1:357–362.

106. Hricak H, Filly RA, Margulis AR, et al. Work in progress: nuclear magnetic resonance imaging of the gallbladder. *Radiology* 1983;147:481–484.

107. Htoo MM. Surgical implications of stone impaction in the gallbladder neck with compression of the common hepatic duct (Mirizzi's syndrome). *Clin Radiol* 1983;3:651–655.

108. Itai Y, Araki T, Yoshikawa K, Furui S, Yashiro N, et al. Computed tomography of gallbladder carcinoma. *Radiology* 1980;137:713–718.

109. Jeffrey RB, Federle MP, Laing FC, et al. Computed tomography of choledocholithiasis. *AJR* 1983;140:1179.

110. Jenkins PF, Golding RH, Cooperberg PL. Sonography and computed tomography of hemorrhagic cholecystitis. *AJR* 1983;140:1197–1198.

111. Kahng KU, Roslyn JJ. Surgical issues for the elderly patient with hepatobiliary disease. *Surg Clin North Am* 1994;74:345–373.

112. Kaiser JA, Mall JC, Salmen BJ, Parker JJ. Diagnosis of Caroli disease by computed tomography: report of two cases. *Radiology* 1979;132:661–664.

113. Kalendar WA, Polacin A, Süss C. A comparison of conventional and spiral CT: an experimental study on the detection of spherical lesions. *J Comput Assist Tomogr* 1994;18:167–176.

114. Kalendar WA. Technical foundations of spiral CT. *Semin Ultrasound CT MR* 1994;15:81–89.

115. Kane RA, Costello P, Duszlack E. Computed tomography in acute cholecystitis: new observations. *AJR* 1983;141:697–701.

116. Kane RA, Jacobs R, Katz J, P. Porcelain gallbladder: ultrasound and CT appearance. *Radiology* 1984;152:137–141.

117. Kang EH, Middleton WD, Balfe DM, et al. Laparoscopic cholecystectomy: evaluation with sonography. *Radiology* 1991;181:439–442.

118. Kang YS, Pope CF, Gore JC. Alterations in MR relaxation of normal canine gallbladder bile during fasting. *Magn Reson Imaging* 1986;4:399–406.

119. Kanzer GK, Weinreb JC. Magnetic resonance imaging of diseases of the liver and biliary system. *Radiol Clin North Am* 1991;29:1259–1284.

120. Khan TF, Sherazi ZA, Alias NA, Mahmood Z. Multifocal mucus secreting papillary adenocarcinoma of the bile duct causing obstructive jaundice. *Ann Acad Med Singapore* 1993;22:251–253.

121. Klein HM, Wein B, Truong S, Pfingsten FP, Guenther RW. CT cholangiography with spiral scanning and 3D image processing. *Br J Radiol* 1993;66:762–767.

122. Koda M, Okamoto K, Miyoshi Y, Kawasaki H. Hepatic vascular and bile duct injury after ethanol injection therapy for hepatocellular carcinoma. *Gastrointest Radiol* 1992;17:167–169.

123. Koehler RE, Melson GL, Lee JKT, Long J. Common hepatic duct obstruction by cystic duct stone: Mirizzi syndrome. *AJR* 1979;132:1007–1009.

124. Koslin DB, Stanley RJ, Berland LL, Shin MS, Dalton SC. Hepatic perivascular lymphedema: CT appearance. *AJR* 1988;150:111–113.

125. Krudy AG, Doppman JL, Bissonette MB, Girton M. Hemobilia: computed tomographic diagnosis. *Radiology* 1983;148:785–789.

126. Kubo S, Kinoshita H, Higaki I, Nishio H. Choledochal cyst detected by MR cholangiopancreatography. *AJR* 1995;164:513–514.

127. Kuhlman JE, Fishman EK, Milligan FD, Siegelman SS. Complications of endoscopic retrograde sphincterotomy: computed tomographic evaluation. *Gastrointest Radiol* 1989;14:127–132.

128. Kumar A, Aggarwal S. Carcinoma of the gallbladder: CT findings in 50 cases. *Abdom Imaging* 1994;19:304–308.

129. Kusano S, Okada Y, Endo T, Yokoyama H, Ohmiya H, Atari H. Oriental cholangiohepatitis: correlation between portal vein occlusion and hepatic atrophy. *AJR* 1992;158:1011–1014.

130. Laing FC, Jeffrey RB Jr, Wing VW, Nyberg DA. Biliary dilatation: defining the level and cause by real-time US. *Radiology* 1986;160:39–42.

131. Laing FC, Jeffrey RB Jr. Choledocholithiasis and cystic duct ob-

struction: difficult ultrasonographic diagnosis. *Radiology* 1983; 146:475–479.

132. Laing FC, Jeffrey RB, Wing VW. Improved visualization of choledocholithiasis by sonography. *AJR* 1984;143:949–952.

133. Laing FC. Ultrasound diagnosis of choledocholithiasis. *Semin Ultrasound CT MR* 1987;8:103–113.

134. Lane J. Primary carcinoma of the gallbladder: a pictorial essay. *Radiographics* 1989;9:209–228.

135. LaRusso NF, Wiesner RH, Ludwig J, MacCarty RL. Primary sclerosing cholangitis. *N Engl J Med* 1984;310:899–903.

136. Lauffer RB, Greif WL, Stark DD, et al. Iron-EHPG as an hepatobiliary MR contrast agent: initial imaging and biodistribution studies. *J Comput Assist Tomogr* 1985;9:431–438.

137. Lauffer RB, Vincent AC, Padmanabhan S, et al. Hepatobiliary MR contrast agents: 5-substituted iron-EHPG derivatives. *Magn Reson Med* 1987;4:582–590.

138. Leander P, Golman K, Klaveness J, et al. MRI contrast media for the liver efficacy in conditions of acute biliary obstruction. *Invest Radiol* 1990;25:1130–1134.

139. Lefkowitch JH. Primary sclerosing cholangitis. *Arch Intern Med* 1982;142:1157–1160.

140. Letourneau JG, Hunter DW, Payne WD, Day DL. Imaging of and intervention for biliary complications after hepatic transplantation. *AJR* 1990;154:729–733.

141. Liddell RM, Baron RL, Ekstrom JE, Varnell RM, Shuman WP. Normal intrahepatic bile ducts: CT depiction. *Radiology* 1990; 176:633–635.

142. Lim JH, Ko YT, Lee DH, Hong KS. Oriental cholangiohepatitis: sonographic findings in 48 cases. *AJR* 1990;155:511–514.

143. Lim JH. Radiologic findings of clonorchiasis. *AJR* 1990;155: 1001–1008.

144. Lim JH. Oriental cholangiohepatitis: pathologic, clinical, and radiologic features. *AJR* 1991;157:1–8.

145. Lim KO, Stark DD, Leese PT, Pfefferbaum A, Rocklage SM, Quay SC. Hepatobiliary MR imaging: first human experience with Mn-DPDP. *Radiology* 1991;178:79–82.

146. Lim JH, Lee DH, Ko YT, Yoon Y. Carcinoma of the ampulla of Vater: sonographic and CT diagnosis. *Abdom Imaging* 1993;18: 237–241.

147. Loflin TG, Simeone JF, Mueller PR, et al. Gallbladder bile in cholecystitis: in vitro MR evaluation. *Radiology* 1985;157:457–459.

148. Lorigan JG, Charnsangavej C, Carrasco CH, Richli WR, Wallace S. Atrophy with compensatory hypertrophy of the liver in hepatic neoplasms: radiographic findings. *AJR* 1988;150:1291–1295.

149. Low RN, Sigeti JS, Francis IR, et al. Evaluation of malignant biliary obstruction: efficacy of fast multiplanar spoiled gradient-recalled MR imaging vs spin-echo MR imaging, CT, and cholangiography. *AJR* 1994;162:315–323.

150. MacCarty RL, LaRusso NF, Wiesner RH, Ludwig J. Primary sclerosing cholangitis: findings on cholangiography and pancreatography. *Radiology* 1983;149:39–44.

151. MacCarty RL, LaRusso NF, May GR, et al. Cholangiocarcinoma complicating primary sclerosing cholangitis: cholangiographic appearances. *Radiology* 1985;156:43–46.

152. MacCarty RL. Diseases of the bile ducts. In: Taveras JM, Ferrucci JT, eds. *Radiology: diagnosis, imaging, intervention,* vol 4. Philadelphia: JB Lippincott, 1994;1–16.

153. Maglinte D, Dorenbusch M. Intravenous infusion cholangiography: an assessment of its role relevant to laparoscopic cholecystectomy. *Radiol Diagn* 1993;34:91–96.

154. Majoie CBLM, Reeders JWAJ, Sanders JB, Huibregtse K, Jansen PLM. Primary sclerosing cholangitis: a modified classification of cholangiographic findings. *AJR* 1991;157:495–497.

155. Mall JC, Ghahremani GG, Boyer JL. Caroli's disease associated with congenital hepatic fibrosis and renal tubular ectasia. *Gastroenterology* 1974;66:1029–1035.

156. Martin WB, Apostolakos PC, Roazen H. Clinical versus actuarial prediction in the differential diagnosis of jaundice. *Am J Gastroenterol* 1979;71:168–176.

157. Marzio L, Innocenti P, Genovesi N, Di Felice F, Napolitano AM, Contantini R, Di Giandomenico E. Role of oral cholecystography, real-time ultrasound, and CT in evaluation of gallstones and gallbladder function. *Gastrointest Radiol* 1992;17:257–261.

158. Matsui O, Kadoya M, Takashima T, Kamayam T, Yoshikawa J, Tamura S. Intrahepatic periportal abnormal intensity on MR images: an indication of various hepatobiliary diseases. *Radiology* 1989;171:335–338.

159. McAllister JD, D'Altorio RA, Snyder A. CT findings after uncomplicated percutaneous laparoscopic cholecystectomy. *J Comput Assist Tomogr* 1991;15:770–772.

160. McAllister JD, D'Altorio RA, Rao V. CT findings after uncomplicated and complicated laparoscopic cholecystectomy. *Semin Ultrasound CT MR* 1993;14:356–367.

161. McCarthy S, Hricak H, Cohen M, et al. Cholecystitis: detection with MR imaging. *Radiology* 1986;158:333–336.

162. McCarty M, Choudhri AH, Helbert M, Crofton ME. Radiologic features of AIDS related cholangitis. *Clin Radiol* 1989;40:582–585.

163. McMillin K. Computed tomography of emphysematous cholecystitis. *J Comput Assist Tomogr* 1985;9:330–332.

164. Meanock CI, Saverymuttu SH, Maxwell JD, Joseph AEA. Gallbladder wall thickening in chronic liver disease: a sign of portal hypertension (abstract). *Br J Radiol* 1988;61:770.

165. Meilstrup JW, Hopper KD, Thieme GA. Imaging of gallbladder variants. *AJR* 1991;157:1205–1208.

166. Millitz K, Moote DJ, Sparrow RK, Girotti MJ, Holliday RL, McLarty TD. Pneumoperitoneum after laparoscopic cholecystectomy: frequency and duration as seen on upright chest radiographs. *AJR* 1994;163:837–839.

167. Memel DS, Berland LL. CT of bowel obstruction: interpretation using cine-paging. *AJR* 1995;164:766–767.

168. Menu Y, Lorphelin J-M, Scherrer A, Grenier P, Nahum H. Sonographic and computed tomographic evaluation of intrahepatic calculi. *AJR* 1985;145:579–583.

169. Mirvis SE, Whitley NO, Miller JW. CT diagnosis of acalculous cholecystitis. *J Comput Assist Tomogr* 1987;11:83–87.

170. Mitchell SE, Clark RA. A comparison of computed tomography and sonography in choledocholithiasis. *AJR* 1984;142:729–733.

171. Mitchell DG, Stark DD. Normal anatomy and MRI appearance. In: Mitchell DG, Stark DD, eds. *Hepatobiliary MRI: a text-atlas at mid and high field.* St. Louis: Mosby Year Book, 1992;47–59.

172. Mitchell DG, Stark DD. Inflammatory disease. In: Mitchell DG, Stark DD, eds. *Hepatobiliary MRI: a text-atlas at mid and high field.* St. Louis: Mosby Year Book, 1992;153–158.

173. Mitchell DG, Stark DD. Biliary system. In: Mitchell DG, Stark DD, eds. *Hepatobiliary MRI: a text-atlas at mid and high field.* St. Louis: Mosby Year Book, 1992;213–226.

174. Mitchell DG, Outwater EK, Vinitski S. Hybrid RARE: implementations for abdominal MRI. *J Magn Reson Imaging* 1994;4:109–117.

175. Miyake H, Aikawa H, Hori Y, Mori H, Sakamoto I, Matsuoka Y, Himeno K, Yamashita H. Adenomyomatosis of the gallbladder with subserosal fatty proliferation: CT findings in two cases. *Gastrointest Radiol* 1992;17:21–23.

176. Moeser PM, Julian S, Karstaedt N, et al. Unusual presentation of cholelithiasis on T1-weighted MR imaging. *J Comput Assist Tomogr* 1988;12:150–152.

177. Mogavero GT, Jones B, Cameron JL, Coleman J. Gastric and duodenal obstruction in patients with cholangiocarcinoma in the porta hepatis: increased prevalence after radiation therapy. *AJR* 1992;159:1001–1003.

178. Montana MA, Rohrmann CA. Cholangiocarcinoma in choledochal cyst: preoperative diagnosis. *AJR* 1986;147:516–517.

179. Moon KL Jr, Hricak H, Margulis AR, et al. Nuclear magnetic resonance imaging characteristics of gallstones in vitro. *Radiology* 1983;148:753–756.

180. Moran J, Del Grosso E, Wills JS, Hagy JA, Baker R. Laparoscopic cholecystectomy: imaging of complications and normal postoperative CT appearance. *Abdom Imaging* 1994;19:143–146.

181. Morehouse H, Leibman AJ, Biempica L, Hoffman J. Infiltrating periductal neoplasm mimicking biliary ductal dilatation on computed tomography. *J Comput Assist Tomogr* 1983;7:721–723.

182. Mori H, Hisayuki A, Koichi H, et al. Exophytic spread of hepatobiliary disease via perihepatic ligaments: demonstration with CT and US. *Radiology* 1989;172:41–46.

183. Mori H. Dilated posterior superior pancreaticoduodenal vein: rec-

ognition with CT and clinical significance in patients with pancreaticobiliary carcinomas. *Radiology* 1991;181:793.

184. Morimoto K, Shimoi M, Shirakawa T, et al. Biliary obstruction: evaluation with three-dimensional MR cholangiography. *Radiology* 1992;183:578–580.

185. Moriyasu F, Ban N, Nishida O, et al. Central signals of gallstones in magnetic resonance imaging. *Am J Gastroenterol* 1987;82:139–142.

186. Moult RG, Wilczynski M, Mullangi U, Mehta H. Mirizzi syndrome (hepatic duct obstruction). *J Am Osteopath Assoc* 1992;92:930–932.

187. Mueller PR, Ferrucci JT, Simeone JF, et al. Post cholecystectomy bile duct dilatation: myth or reality? *AJR* 1981;136:355–358.

188. Muhletaler CA, Gerlock AJ Jr, Fleischer AC, James AE Jr. Diagnosis of obstructive jaundice with nondilated bile ducts. *AJR* 1980;134:1149–1152.

189. Musante F, Derchi LE, Bonati P. CT cholangiography in suspected Caroli's disease. *J Comput Assist Tomogr* 1982;6:482–485.

190. Myracle MR, Stadalnik RC, Blaisdell FW, Farkas JP, Matin P. Segmental biliary obstruction: diagnostic significance of bile duct crowding. *AJR* 1981;137:169–171.

191. Nesbit GM. Cholangiocarcinoma: diagnosis and evaluation of resectability by CT and sonography as procedures complementary to cholangiography. *AJR* 1988;151:933–938.

192. Niederau C, Sonnenberg A, Mueller J. Comparison of the extrahepatic bile duct size measured by ultrasound and by different radiographic methods. *Gastroenterology* 1984;87:615–621.

193. O'Connor KW, Snodgrass PJ, Swonder JE, et al. A blinded prospective study comparing four current noninvasive approaches in the differential diagnosis of medical versus surgical jaundice. *Gastroenterology* 1983;84:1498–1504.

194. Ohtani T, Shirai Y, Tsukada K, Hatakeyama K, Muto T. Carcinoma of the gallbladder: CT evaluation of lymphatic spread. *Radiology* 1993;189:875–880.

195. Olsson R, Danielsson Å, Järnerot G, et al. Prevalence of primary sclerosing cholangitis in patients with ulcerative colitis. *Gastroenterology* 1991;100:1319–1323.

196. Outwater E, Kaplan MM, Bankoff MS. Lymphadenopathy in sclerosing cholangitis: pitfall in the diagnosis of malignant biliary obstruction. *Gastrointest Radiol* 1992;17:157–160.

197. Outwater EK, Gordon SJ. Imaging the pancreatic and biliary ducts with MR. *Radiology* 1994;192:19–21.

198. Pedrosa CS, Casanova R, Rodiquez R. Computed tomography in obstructive jaundice. Part I: The level of obstruction. *Radiology* 1981;139:627–634.

199. Pedrosa CS, Casanova R, Lezana AH, Fernandez MC. Computed tomography in obstructive jaundice. Part II: The cause of obstruction. *Radiology* 1981;139:635–645.

200. Pedrosa CS, Casanova R, Torre SDE, Villacorta J. CT findings in Mirizzi syndrome. *J Comput Assist Tomogr* 1983;7:419–425.

201. Pien EH, Zeman RK, Benjamin SB, et al. Iatrogenic sclerosing cholangitis following hepatic arterial chemotherapy infusion. *Radiology* 1985;156:329–330.

202. Pollack M, Shirkhoda A, Charnsangavej C. Computed tomography of choledochocele. *J Comput Assist Tomogr* 1985;9:360–362.

203. Posin JP, Ortendahl DA, Hylton NM, et al. Variable magnetic resonance imaging parameters: effect on detection and characterization of lesions. *Radiology* 1985;155:719–725.

204. Pretorius DH, Gosink BB, Olson LK. CT of the opacified biliary tract: use of calcium ipodate. *AJR* 1982;138:1073–1075.

205. Prochazka EJ, Terasaki PI, Park MS, Goldstein LI, Busuttil RW. Association of primary sclerosing cholangitis with HLA-DRw52a. *N Engl J Med* 1990;322:1842–1844.

206. Quint LE, Glazer GM. CT evaluation of the bile ducts in patients with fatty liver. *Radiology* 1984;153:755–756.

207. Radin DR, Vachon LA. CT findings in biliary and pancreatic ascariasis. *J Comput Assist Tomogr* 1986;10:508–509.

208. Radin DR, Santiago EM. Cholecystoduodenal fistula due to pancreatic carcinoma: CT diagnosis. *J Comput Assist Tomogr* 1986;10:149–150.

209. Radin DR, Chandrasoma P, Ralls PW. Carcinoma of the cystic duct. *Gastrointest Radiol* 1990;15:49–52.

210. Rahn NH III, Koehler RE, Weyman PJ, Truss CD, Sagel SS,
Stanley RJ. CT appearance of sclerosing cholangitis. *AJR* 1983;141:549–552.

211. Ray CE. Complications after laparoscopic cholecystectomy: imaging findings. *AJR* 1993;160:1029–1032.

212. Rege RV. Adverse effects of biliary obstruction: implications for treatment of patients with obstructive jaundice. *AJR* 1995;164:287–293.

213. Reiman TH, Balfe DM, Weyman PJ. Suprapancreatic biliary obstruction: CT evaluation. *Radiology* 1987;163:49–56.

214. Rohrmann CA, Kimmey MB. Benign conditions of the bile ducts. In: Silvis SE, Rohrmann CA, Ansel HJ, eds. *Text and atlas of endoscopic retrograde cholangiopancreatography*. New York: Igaku-Shoin, 1995;193–244.

215. Rooholamini SA, Tehrani NS, Razavi MK, et al. Imaging of gallbladder carcinoma. *Radiographics* 1994;14:291–306.

216. Rossman MD, Friedman AC, Radecki PD, et al. MR imaging of gallbladder carcinoma. *AJR* 1987;148:143–144.

217. Sagoh T, Itoh K, Togashi K, et al. Gallbladder carcinoma: evaluation with MR imaging. *Radiology* 1990;174:131–136.

218. Sauerbrei EE. Ultrasound of the common bile duct. *Ultrasound Annu* 1983;1–45.

219. Savader SJ, Beneati JF, Venbrux AC, et al. Choledochal cysts: classification and cholangiographic appearance. *AJR* 1991;156:327–331.

220. Savoca PE, Longo WE, Zucker KA, et al. The increasing prevalence of acalculous cholecystitis in outpatients: results of a 7-year study. *Ann Surg* 1990;211:433–437.

221. Schenker S, Balint J, Schiff L. Differential diagnosis of jaundice: report of a prospective study of 61 proved cases. *Am J Dig Dis* 1962;7:449–463.

222. Schneiderman DJ. Hepatobiliary abnormalities of AIDS. *Gastroenterol Clin North Am* 1988;17:615–630.

223. Schuhmann-Giampieri G, Schmitt-Willich H, Press W-R, Negishi C, Weinmann H-J, Speck U. Preclinical evaluation of Gd-EOB-DTPA as a contrast agent in MR imaging of the hepatobiliary system. *Radiology* 1992;183:59–64.

224. Schulman A. Non-western pattern of biliary stones and the role of ascariasis. *Radiology* 1987;162:425–430.

225. Schulman A. Intrahepatic biliary stones: imaging features and a possible relationship with ascaris lumbricoides. *Clin Radiol* 1993;47:325–332.

226. Schulte SJ, Baron RL, Teefey SA, et al. CT of the extrahepatic bile ducts: wall thickness and contrast enhancement in normal and abnormal ducts. *AJR* 1990;154:79–85.

227. Schulte SJ. Embryology and congenital anomalies of the bile and pancreatic ducts. In: Silvis SE, Rohrmann CA, Ansel HJ, eds. *Text and atlas of endoscopic retrograde cholangiopancreatography*. New York: Igaku-Shoin, 1995;114–145.

228. Semelka RC, Shoenut JP, Kroeker MA, et al. Bile duct disease: prospective comparison of ERCP, CT and fat suppression MRI. *Gastrointest Radiol* 1992;17:347–352.

229. Semelka RC, Shoenut JP. General considerations for conducting abdominal magnetic resonance imaging examinations. In: Semelka RC, Shoenut JP, eds. *MRI of the abdomen with CT correlation*. New York: Raven Press, 1993;7–11.

230. Semelka RC, Shoenut JP, Micflikier AB. The gallbladder and biliary tree. In: Semelka RC, Shoenut JP, eds. *MRI of the abdomen with CT correlation*. New York: Raven Press, 1993;43–52.

231. Shanley DJ, Gagliardi JA, Daum-Kowalski R. Choledochal cyst complicating pregnancy: antepartum diagnosis with MRI. *Abdom Imaging* 1994;19:61–63.

232. Shanser JD, Korobkin M, Goldberg HI, Rohlfing BM. Computed tomographic diagnosis of obstructive jaundice in the absence of intrahepatic ductal dilatation. *AJR* 1978;131:389–392.

233. Shea WJ Jr, Demas BE, Goldberg HI, Horn DC, Ferrell LD, Kerlan RK. Sclerosing cholangitis associated with hepatic arterial FUDR chemotherapy: radiographic-histologic correlation. *AJR* 1986;146:717–721.

234. Sherman S, Lehman G. ERCP- and endoscopic sphincterotomy-induced pancreatitis. *Pancreas* 1991;3:350–367.

235. Silvis ST, Meier PB. Techniques for endoscopic retrograde cholangiopancreatogaphy. In: Silvis SE, Rohrmann CA, Ansel HJ, eds. *Text and atlas of endoscopic retrograde cholangiopancreatography*. New York: Igaku-Shoin, 1995;22–50.

236. Silvis ST. The normal bile duct. In: Silvis SE, Rohrmann CA, Ansel HJ, eds. *Text and atlas of endoscopic retrograde cholangiopancreatography.* New York: Igaku-Shoin, 1995;168–192.

237. Simeone JF, Butch RJ, Mueller PR. The bile ducts after a fatty meal: further sonographic observations. *Radiology* 1985;154:763–768.

238. Simeone JF, Brink JA. The gallbladder: pathology. In: Taveras JM, Ferrucci JT eds. *Radiology: diagnosis, imaging, intervention,* vol 4. Philadelphia: JB Lippincott, 1994;1–17.

239. Smathers R, Lee JKT, Heiken JP. Differentiation of complicated cholecystitis from gallbladder carcinoma by computed tomography. *AJR* 1984;143:255–259.

240. Solomon A, Kreel L, Pinto D. Contrast-computed tomography in diagnosis of acute cholecystitis. *J Comput Assist Tomogr* 1979;3:585–588.

241. Somer K, Kivisaari L, Standertskjold-Nordenstam C-G, Kalima TV. Contrast-enhanced computed tomography of the gallbladder in acute pancreatitis. *Gastrointest Radiol* 1984;9:31–34.

242. Sood GK, Mahapatra JR, Khurana A, Chaudhry V, Sarin SK, Boor SL. Caroli disease: computed tomographic diagnosis. *Gastrointest Radiol* 1991;16:243–244.

243. Sorensen KW, Glazer GM, Francis IR. Diagnosis of cystic ectasia of intrahepatic bile ducts by computed tomography. *J Comput Assist Tomogr* 1982;6:486–489.

244. Spritzer C, Kressel HY, Mitchell D, Axel L. MR imaging of normal extrahepatic bile ducts. *J Comput Assist Tomogr* 1987;11:248–252.

245. Stockberger SM Jr, Wass JL, Sherman S, Lehman GA, Kopecky KK. Intravenous cholangiography with helical CT: comparison with endoscopic retrograde cholangiography. *Radiology* 1994;192:675–680.

246. Sugawa C, Luca CE. The role of endoscopic retrograde cholangiopancreatography in surgery of the pancreas and biliary ducts. In: Silvis SE, Rohrmann CA, Ansel HJ, eds. *Text and atlas of endoscopic retrograde cholangiopancreatography.* New York: Igaku-Shoin, 1995;3–21.

247. Takayasu K, Muramatsu Y, Shima Y, et al. Hepatic lobar atrophy following obstruction of the ipsilateral portal vein from hilar cholangiocarcinoma. *Radiology* 1986;160:389–393.

248. Takayasu K, Ikeya S, Mukai K, Muramatsu Y, Makuuchi M, Hasegawa H. CT of hilar cholangiocarcinoma: late contrast enhancement in six patients. *AJR* 1990;154:1203–1206.

249. Takehara Y, Ichijo K, Tooyama N, et al. Breath-hold MR cholangiopancreatography with a long-echo-train fast spin-echo sequence and a surface coil in chronic pancreatitis. *Radiology* 1994;192:73–78.

250. Tamura S, Kihara Y, Kakitsubata Y, Kakitsubata S, Iwata K, Higashi H, Setoguchi T, Watanabe K. Hepatocellular carcinoma invading the gallbladder: CT, arteriography and MRI findings. *Clin Imaging* 1993;17:109–111.

251. Tartar VM, Balfe DM. Lymphoma in the wall of the bile ducts: radiologic imaging. *Gastrointest Radiol* 1990;15:53–57.

252. Teefey SA, Baron RL, Rohrmann CA, Shuman WP, Freeny PC. Sclerosing cholangitis: CT findings. *Radiology* 1988;169:635–639.

253. Teefey SA, Baron RL, Schulte SJ, Patten RM, Molloy MH. Patterns of intrahepatic bile duct dilatation at CT: correlation with obstructive disease processes. *Radiology* 1992;182:139–142.

254. Teixidor HS, Godwin TA, Ramirez EA. Cryptosporidiosis of the biliary tract in AIDS. *Radiology* 1991;180:51–56.

255. Terrier F, Becker CD, Stoller C, Triller JK. Computed tomography in complicated cholecystitis. *J Comput Assist Tomogr* 1984;8:58–62.

256. Thorsen MK, Quiroz F, Lawson TL, Smith DF, Foley DW, Stewart ET. Primary biliary carcinoma: CT evaluation. *Radiology* 1984;152:479–483.

257. Thuluvath PJ, Connolly GM, Forbes A, Gazzard BD. Abdominal pain in HIV infection. *Q J Med* 1991;78:275–285.

258. Todani T, Watanabe Y, Narusue M, et al. Congenital bile duct cysts: classification, operative procedure, and review of thirty-seven cases including cancer arising from choledochal cyst. *Am J Surg* 1977;134:263–269.

259. Turner MA. Examination techniques and normal anatomy. In: Gore RM, Levine MS, Laufer I, eds. *Textbook of gastrointestinal radiology,* vol 2. Philadelphia: WB Saunders, 1994;1570–1593.

260. Ueda J, Kobayashi Y, Nishida T. Computed tomography evaluation of high-density bile in the gallbladder. *Gastrointest Radiol* 1990;15:22–26.

261. Urban BA, Fishman EK, Kuhlman JE, Kawashima A, Hennessey JG, Siegelman SS. Detection of focal hepatic lesions with spiral CT: comparison of 4- and 8-mm interscan spacing. *AJR* 1993;160:783–785.

262. Van Beers BE, Lacrosse M, Trigaux JP, de Cannière L, De Ronde T, Pringot J. Noninvasive imaging of the biliary tree before or after laparoscopic cholecystectomy: use of three-dimensional spiral CT cholangiography. *AJR* 1994;162:1331–1335.

263. Van Campenhout I, Prosmanne O, Gagner M, Pomp A, Deslandres E, Lévesque HP. Routine operative cholangiography during laparoscopic cholecsytectomy: feasibility and value in 107 patients. *AJR* 1993;160:1209–1211.

264. VanSonnenberg E, Casola G, Cubberley DA, et al. Oriental cholangiohepatitis: diagnostic imaging and interventional management. *AJR* 1986;146:327–331.

265. Vazquez JL, Thorsen MK, Dodds WJ, Foley WD, Lawson TL. Atrophy of the left hepatic lobe caused by cholangiocarcinoma. *AJR* 1985;144:547–548.

266. Venu RP, Geenen JE. Periampullary region: physiology and pathophysiology. In: Silvis SE, Rohrmann CA, Ansel HJ, eds. *Text and atlas of endoscopic retrograde cholangiopancreatography.* New York: Igaku-Shoin, 1995;146–167.

267. Walker AT, Shapiro AW, Brooks DC, Braver JM, Tumeh SS. Bile duct disruption and biloma after laparoscopic choelcystectomy: imaging evaluation. *AJR* 1992;158:785–789.

268. Walker AT, Brooks DC, Tumeh SS, Braver JM. Bile duct disruption after laparoscopic cholecystectomy. *Semin Ultrasound CT MR* 1993;14:346–355.

269. Wallner BK, Schumacher KA, Weidenmaier W, Friedrich JM. Dilated biliary tract: evaluation with MR cholangiography with a T2-weighted contrast-enhanced fast sequence. *Radiology* 1991;181:805–808.

270. Ward EM, Leroy AJ, Bender CE, Donohue JH, Hughes RW. Imaging of complications of laparoscopic cholecystectomy. *Abdom Imaging* 1993;18:150–155.

271. Weiner SN, Koenigsberg Morehouse H, Hoffman J. Sonography and computed tomography in the diagnosis of carcinoma of the gallbladder. *AJR* 1984;142:735–739.

272. Weissleder R, Stark DD, Compton C, et al. Cholecystitis: diagnosis by MR imaging. *Magn Reson Imaging* 1988;6:345–348.

273. West MS, Garra BS, Horii SC, Hayes WS, Cooper C, Silverman PM, Zeman RK. Gallbladder varices: imaging findings in patients with portal hypertension. *Radiology* 1991;179:179–182.

274. Williams LF Jr, Schoetz DJ Jr. Primary sclerosing cholangitis. *Surg Clin North Am* 1981;61:951–962.

275. Williams PL, Warwick R. Splanchnology: the peritoneum. In: Williams PL, Warwick R, eds. *Gray's anatomy,* 36th ed. Philadelphia: WB Saunders, 1980:1321–1333.

276. Wilson SA, Gosink BB, van Sonnenberg E. Unchanged size of a dilated common bile duct after a fatty meal: results and significance. *Radiology* 1986;160:29–31.

277. Wu CC, Ho YH, Chen CY. Effect of aging on common bile duct diameter: a real-time ultrasonographic study. *J Clin Ultrasound* 1984;12:473–478.

278. Yamashita Y, Takahashi M, Kanazawa S, Charnsangavej C, Wallace S. Parenchymal changes of the liver in cholangiocarcinoma: CT evaluation. *Gastrointest Radiol* 1992;17:161–166.

279. Yamashita Y, Takahashi M, Kanazawa S, Charnsangavej C, Wallace S. Hilar cholangiocarcinoma. An evaluation of subtypes with CT and angiography. *Acta Radiol* 1992;33:351–355.

280. Yamashita K, Jin MJ, Hirose Y, et al. CT finding of transient focal increased attenuation of the liver adjacent to the gallbladder in acute cholecystitis. *AJR* 1995;164:343–346.

281. Yeo CJ, Pitt HA, Cameron JL. Cholangiocarcinoma. *Surg Clin North Am* 1990;70:1429–1447.

282. Yoshida H, Itai Y, Minami M, Kokubo T, Ohtomo K, Kuroda A. Biliary malignancies occurring in choledochal cysts. *Radiology* 1989;173:389–392.

283. Zajko AB, Bennett MJ, Campbell WL, Koneru B. Mucocele of the cystic duct remnant in eight liver transplant recipients: findings at cholangiography, CT, and US. *Radiology* 1990;177:691–693.

284. Zeman RK, Dorfman GS, Burrell MI, Stein S, Berg GR, Gold JA. Disparate dilatation of intrahepatic and extrahepatic bile ducts in surgical jaundice. *Radiology* 1981;138:129–136.

285. Zeman RK, Taylor KJW, Rosenfield AT, Schwartz A, Gold JA. Acute experimental biliary obstruction in the dog: sonographic findings and clinical implications. *AJR* 1981;136:965–967.

286. Zeman RK, Fox SH, Silverman PM, et al. Helical (spiral) CT of the abdomen. *AJR* 1993;160:719–725.

287. Zeman RK, Simeone JF. The biliary ducts: anatomy, examination technique, and pathophysiologic considerations. In: Taveras JM, Ferrucci JT, eds. *Radiology: diagnosis, imaging, intervention,* vol 4. Philadelphia: JB Lippincott, 1994;1–17.

CHAPTER 14

Spleen

David M. Warshauer and Robert E. Koehler

The spleen is well seen on computed tomography (CT) and magnetic resonance (MR) images of the abdomen in virtually every patient. Normally, it appears as an oblong or ovoid organ in the left upper abdomen. The contour of the superior lateral border of the spleen is convex, conforming to the shape of the adjacent abdominal wall and left hemidiaphram. The margins of the spleen are smooth, and the parenchyma is sharply demarcated from the adjacent fat. The hilum usually is directed anteromedially, and the splenic artery and vein and their branches can be seen entering the spleen in this region (Fig. 1). The posteromedial surface of the spleen behind the hilum often is concave where it conforms to the shape of the adjacent left kidney. The medial surface anterior to the hilum is in contact with the stomach, and it assumes a shallow concave shape in some patients (Fig. 2). On images performed without intravenous injection of contrast material, the normal spleen appears homogeneous in density, with CT attenuation values in the range of 55 to 65 Hounsfield units (HU), equal to or slightly less than those for the normal liver (139).

Like the liver, the spleen ordinarily has a small area that is not covered by peritoneum, a so-called bare area (224). Smaller than the bare area of the liver, this corresponds to an approximately 2- by 3-cm portion of the spleen's surface contained between the anterior and posterior leaves of the splenorenal ligament. This area overlies the renal fascia covering the anterior aspect of the upper pole of the left kidney. Ascites and other intraperitoneal, left upper abdominal fluid collections tend to surround all surfaces of the spleen except this small area. Recognition of this feature is occasionally helpful in determining whether fluid lies in the peritoneal space or the left pleural space.

The splenic vessels are seen even on noncontrast-enhanced CT images in most individuals. The splenic vein follows a fairly straight course toward the splenic hilum, running transversely along the posterior aspect of the body and tail of the pancreas. Unlike the splenic vein, the splenic artery often is tortuous, especially in older patients. On any given section, it may appear as a single curvilinear structure, or it may wander in and out of the plane of the section and appear as a series of round densities, each of which represents a cross-sectional image of a portion of the artery. In older individuals, it is common to see calcified atheromas within the wall of the splenic artery.

USE OF CONTRAST MATERIAL

It is useful to administer iodinated contrast material intravenously when examining the spleen by CT. Dy-

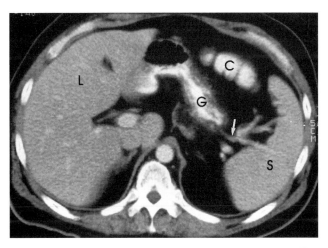

FIG. 1. Computed tomographic image of normal spleen (S). The outer border is convex and conforms to the shape of the adjacent body wall. The medial surface is concave. The splenic artery *(arrow)* enters the hilum. C, colon; G, stomach; L, liver.

845

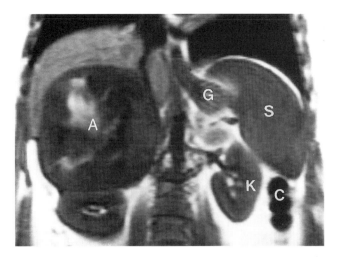

FIG. 2. Coronal T1-weighted FLASH MR image (140/4/80°) of normal spleen (S). Note the intimate relationship of the spleen to the left hemidiaphragm. G, gastric fundus; K, left kidney; C, colon. Note is also made of a large right adrenal carcinoma (A).

namic scans performed during a bolus injection are optimal for clarifying the nature of soft-tissue structures in the splenic hilar and retropancreatic regions that can mimic abnormalities of the pancreas or left adrenal gland, but that may, in fact, result from normal splenic vasculature. The splenic artery and vein and their branches undergo dense contrast enhancement during bolus injection and are easily identified. Splenic parenchymal opacification also occurs and may be used to improve the detectability of focal mass lesions within the spleen. When contrast material is given by rapid intravenous injection and scans are obtained early in the injection, the splenic parenchyma appears initially heterogeneous (Fig. 3). Arciform and

wavelike patterns can be seen during this phase. This heterogeneous enhancement is thought to reflect the variable blood flow within different compartments of the spleen (73). Only after a minute or more passes does the splenic parenchyma achieve uniform, homogeneous enhancement. Care must be taken not to misinterpret this early postinjection heterogeneity of splenic density as an indication of focal abnormality.

No significant difference in splenic parenchymal enhancement has been shown between ionic and nonionic contrast material (83,139). After administration of 180 ml of iothalamate-60%, iopamidol-300, or iohexol-300 at 2 ml/sec, mean enhancement of splenic parenchyma ranges from 75 HU to 97 HU (139).

Contrast agents taken up specifically by the reticuloendothelial system have been investigated for several years. Ethiodized oil emulsion 13 (EOE-13), an aqueous emulsion of iodinated esters of poppyseed oil developed at the National Institutes of Health, has been noted to increase the attenuation of normal splenic tissue by 50 HU, whereas it enhances tumor tissue by an average of only 3 HU (127). Significant complications have precluded release of this agent for general use. Particulate iodipamide ethyl ester (110,179) and proliposomes incorporating water-soluble contrast material (153) have also been investigated in animal models as splenic contrast agents. It remains to be determined whether a clinically acceptable agent of this type can be developed for human use.

MAGNETIC RESONANCE IMAGING

The spleen has relatively long T1 and T2 relaxation times. Its signal intensity on T1-weighted images is less (i.e., darker) than that of liver and is similar to that of

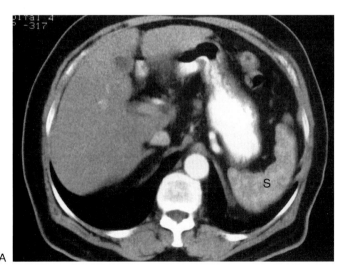

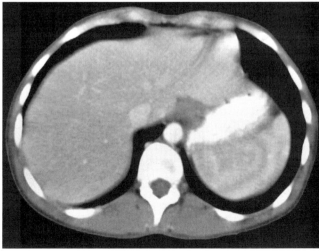

FIG. 3. Computed tomographic appearance of the normal spleen (S) in two patients during bolus intravenous injection of contrast material. **A:** Patchy pattern of early splenic parenchymal enhancement. The aorta and splenic vessels are densely opacified. **B:** Arciform pattern of splenic parenchymal opacification.

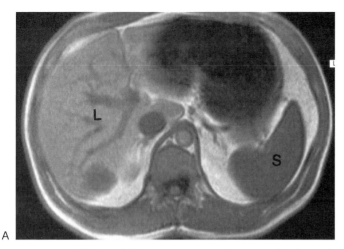 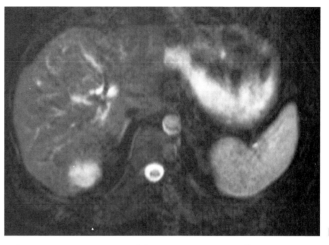

FIG. 4. MRI appearance of the normal spleen (S). **A:** On this T1-weighted FLASH image (140/4/80°), the signal intensity of the spleen is less than that of the liver (L) and much less than that of the surrounding fat. **B:** On this fat-saturated, T2-weighted MR image (2400/90) there is reversal of the relative signal intensities of the spleen and liver.

renal cortex. On T2-weighted images, the spleen appears brighter than liver, reflecting its greater free water content (Fig. 4). Breathhold spoiled gradient echo techniques [e.g., fast low-angle shot (FLASH)] have proven useful in splenic evaluation by decreasing time of acquisition and hence respiratory-motion artifact. The flow void produced by moving blood allows the major splenic vessels to be seen well, without the use of intravenous contrast material. Because the tissue relaxation times of splenic parenchyma and many tumors of the spleen are similar (80), the use of intravenous contrast material for evaluating the spleen has become important (128,185). Gadolinium-DTPA (diethylene-triamine penta-acetic acid) is the most

common agent used. Multisection T1-weighted spoiled gradient echo sequences can be employed at various times after contrast material injection to image the spleen in perfusion, nonequilibrium, equilibrium, and washout phases (Fig. 5). Using this technique, approximately 80% of patients demonstrate normal heterogeneous or arciform enhancement on the perfusion images; 15% show a uniform high signal. Although the significance of the early uniform high signal is unclear, it has been suggested that this may represent alteration of splenic blood flow in response to a coexisting inflammatory or neoplastic process (185).

Superparamagnetic iron oxide and gadolinium-labeled

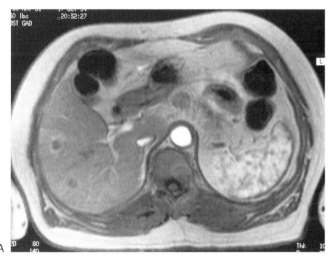 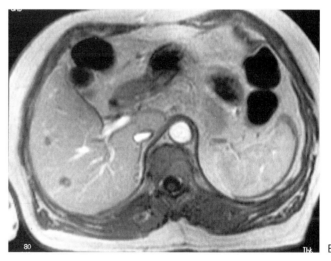

FIG. 5. MRI appearance of the normal spleen (S). **A:** On this T1-weighted FLASH image (140/4/80°) performed during the perfusion phase of intravenous gadolinium-DTPA administration, the splenic parenchyma shows heterogeneous enhancement. **B:** The spleen has assumed a more homogeneous appearance 45 sec later.

liposomes have also been investigated as contrast agents for evaluation of the splenic parenchyma (97,236). Whether these reticuloendothelium-specific agents will find general release is uncertain.

At present, intravenous contrast-enhanced MR appears to be as sensitive or slightly more sensitive than CT for evaluation of the splenic parenchyma. The ability of MR to directly image in the coronal and sagittal planes is advantageous in showing the relationship of the spleen to the adjacent left kidney, adrenal, and hemidiaphram. Although respiratory-motion artifact and the increased cost and time involved in an MR study remain difficulties, the future of MR in splenic imaging appears promising.

SPLENIC SIZE

The spleen measures from 12 to 15 cm in length, 4 to 8 cm in width and 3 to 4 cm in thickness (7). Because of its irregular shape and oblique orientation within the left upper quadrant, these measurements are of very limited use as a guide to normal splenic size on CT. Most observers judge splenic volume by subjective evaluation of the CT based on experience. Rounding of the normally crescentic spleen, and extension of the spleen anterior to the aorta or below the right hepatic lobe or rib cage are further clues to splenomegaly.

A more accurate approach to the assessment of splenic volume is the splenic index (108,207), which is the product of the length, width, and thickness of the spleen as seen on CT (Fig. 6). Splenic length is determined by summing the number of contiguous CT slices on which the spleen is visible. The width is the longest splenic diameter that can be drawn on any transverse image. The thickness is measured at the level of the splenic hilum and is the distance between the inner and outer (peripheral) borders of the spleen. When the thicknesses of the anterior and posterior portions of the spleen differ significantly, two or three measurements of thickness are averaged. When determined in this way, normal splenic size corresponds to an index of 120 to 480 cm^3 (108).

The correlation between the splenic index, essentially a rough estimate of splenic volume, and the weight of the surgically excised spleen is an imperfect one. It has been demonstrated that the weight of the excised spleen in grams averages from one third to one half of the splenic index (71,207). This is not surprising, because the size and weight of the excised spleen are affected by the amount of blood that drains from the specimen before it is weighed. The splenic index as determined by CT is probably a better indicator of splenomegaly than is the weight of the spleen as determined in the operating room or pathology laboratory.

Most accurate of all are computer programs for calculating actual splenic volume from a series of CT or MR images. However, even this method is limited in clinical

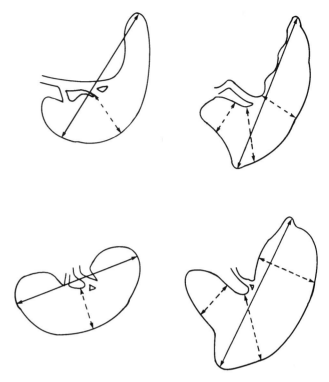

FIG. 6. Diagrammatic representation of the measurements used in calculating the splenic index from transverse CT or MR images of spleens of various shapes. The width *(solid lines)* and thickness *(dashed lines)* are shown. (See text for details.)

usefulness, because the splenic volume varies so greatly from one normal person to another.

NORMAL VARIANTS AND CONGENITAL ANOMALIES

The spleen forms from multiple mesenchymal cell aggregates in the dorsal mesogastrium. As the dorsal mesentery bows to the left with the developing stomach, these aggregates coalesce. The left side of the dorsal mesentery fuses with the parietal peritoneum covering the left adrenal and kidney to form Gerota's fascia. This fusion brings the developing dorsal pancreas and splenic vasculature into the retroperitoneum. The spleen, however, remains intraperitoneal, with its vasculature running in the splenorenal ligament. The gastrosplenic ligament represents the remaining anterior portion of the dorsal mesogastrium and connects the spleen to the greater curvature of the stomach. The combination of both splenorenal and gastrosplenic ligaments forms the deep margins of the lesser sac (52).

In light of this fairly complex development, it should not be surprising that the shape and position of the normal spleen vary considerably from one individual to another. Commonly, there is a bulge or lobule of splenic tissue

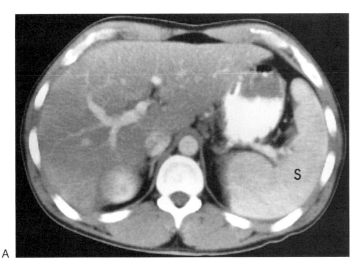 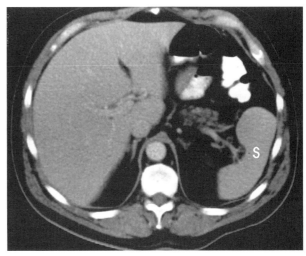

FIG. 7. Normal variation in splenic shape. **A:** Prominent lobule of splenic tissue extends medially from the posterior margin of the spleen (S). **B:** Prominent splenic lobule is noted extending off the anterior margin of the spleen (S).

that extends medially from the posterior portion of the spleen to lie anterior to the upper pole of the left kidney (76,104,159) (Fig. 7). This can simulate the appearance of a left renal or adrenal mass on excretory urography, but it is usually identifiable without difficulty by CT. Less commonly, a bulge from the anterior margin of the spleen also occurs and can simulate an intrasplenic mass. Occasionally, a lobule of splenic tissue can lie partially behind the left kidney and displace it anteriorly. Residual clefts between adjacent lobulations can be sharp and occasionally are as deep as 2 to 3 cm (Fig. 8). They tend to occur on the superior diaphragmatic portion of the spleen and may mimic lacerations (52).

The spleen is sufficiently soft and pliable in texture

that left upper quadrant abdominal masses or organ enlargement can cause considerable displacement and deformity in its shape. When this happens, the spleen conforms to the shape of the adjacent mass, and the resulting deformity can be quite striking (Fig. 9). Likewise, changes in the position of the spleen occur when adjacent organs are surgically removed (Fig. 10). This is particularly true in patients who have undergone left nephrectomy, in which case the spleen can occupy the left renal fossa. Occasionally, there is sufficient laxity in the ligamentous attachments of the spleen that it lies in an unusual position in the absence of an abdominal mass or previous operation. The upside-down spleen (48,237) is a variant in which the splenic hilum is directed superiorly toward the

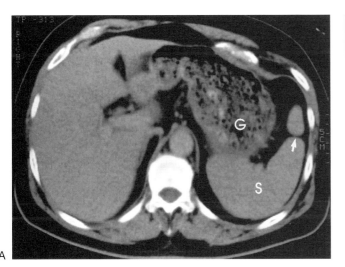 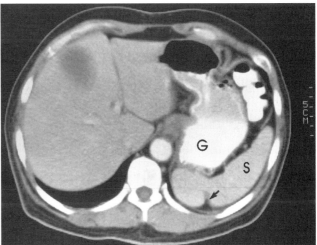

FIG. 8. Prominent splenic clefts between adjacent splenic lobulations. This anatomic variation can simulate a splenic laceration. **A:** Prominent cleft *(arrow)* along anterior margin of spleen. **B:** Splenic cleft *(arrow)* along posterior splenic margin. S, spleen; G, stomach.

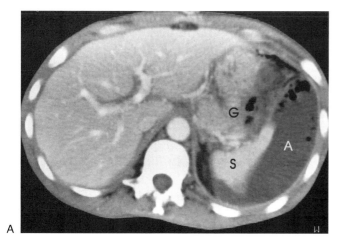

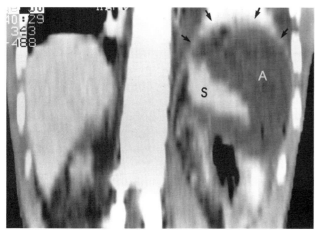

FIG. 9. Marked alteration in splenic shape and position resulting from compression by left subphrenic abscess (A). **A:** Axial slice. S, spleen; A, subphrenic abscess; G, stomach. **B:** Coronal reconstruction. S, spleen; A, subphrenic abscess; *arrows*, hemidiaphragm.

medial, or occasionally the lateral, portion of the left hemidiaphram.

"Wandering" Spleen

The "wandering" spleen is another congenital variant that sometimes causes diagnostic difficulties. In this rare condition, most common in women, there is striking laxity of the suspensory splenic ligaments, which permits the spleen to move about in the abdomen (5,29,77) The CT findings consist of an abdominal soft-tissue-density "mass" with a size appropriate for the spleen, plus the absence of a spleen in the normal location (Fig. 11). It may be possible to recognize the characteristic shape of the spleen and to trace the splenic vasculature back to its origin. The density and pattern of enhancement after bolus injection of contrast material may also lend support to the diagnosis. When there is uncertainty whether the mass truly represents an ectopically located spleen, radionuclide imaging with technetium-99m (^{99m}Tc) sulfur colloid can resolve the dilemma. The most common clinical presentation is that of a mass, with intermittent abdominal pain. Less commonly, an asymptomatic mass is discovered in the abdomen or pelvis. An acute abdominal presentation is least common but most worrisome and indicates torsion and compromise of the vascular supply (29,93,187,194). With infarction, the radionuclide study can be falsely negative (187). Although splenic enhancement is absent with complete infarction, the remaining CT findings should still allow for correct diagnosis (87,140). Ascites can also be present (87,187). In addition, if the pancreatic tail is involved in the torsion, CT can demonstrate a whorled appearance of the pancreatic tail and

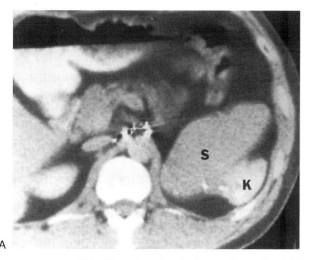

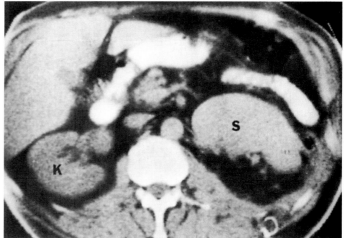

FIG. 10. Altered splenic position after left upper abdominal operation. **A:** Postoperative excretory urogram showed lateral displacement of the left kidney (K), but CT shows that this is due to a shift in the relative positions of spleen and kidney. **B:** In another patient, an image after left nephrectomy shows that spleen has shifted into the position formerly occupied by the left kidney. Splenic hilum is now directed posterosuperiorly.

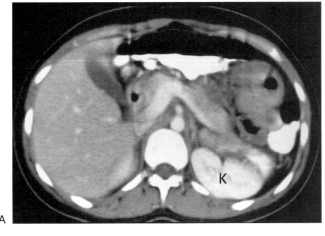

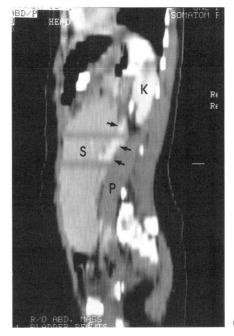

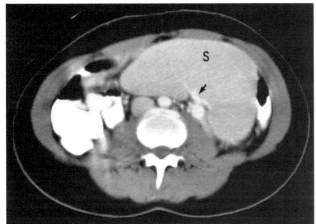

FIG. 11. Wandering spleen. **A:** No splenic shadow is seen in the left upper abdomen. K, kidney. **B:** The spleen (S) is seen in the lower mid abdomen and mimics the appearance of an abdominal tumor. *Arrow,* splenic hila. **C:** Sagittal reconstruction shows splenic vein *(arrows)* running cephalad. Marked splenomegaly in this case is secondary to mononucleosis. K, kidney; P, psoas muscle.

adjacent fat (151). A thick, enhancing pseudocapsule representing omental and peritoneal adhesions has been described in one case in which torsion and infarction were missed for several weeks (188). Chronic torsion also has been reported to lead to the development of splenomegaly (178), hypersplenism (234), and gastric varices (197).

Accessory Spleens

In autopsy series, accessory spleens are noted in 10% to 20% of individuals (82,229). They are also common findings on CT and probably arise as a result of failure of fusion of some of the multiple buds of splenic tissue in the dorsal mesogastrium during embryonic life. Although accessory spleens are usually single, approximately 10% of patients with one have a second focus. More than two deposits are seen infrequently (5%) (82,229). Studies on patients who have undergone splenectomy show an increased prevalence of both single and multiple accessory spleens, probably because the underlying pathology has made microscopic deposits clinically apparent (47,58).

Accessory spleens usually occur near the hilum of the spleen, but they are sometimes found in its suspensory ligaments or in the tail of the pancreas (Fig. 12). Rarely, they occur elsewhere in the abdomen or retroperitoneum. They vary in size from microscopic deposits that are not visible on CT or MRI, to nodules that are 2 to 3 cm in diameter (16,82,229). In patients with pathologic splenic findings or in those who have previously undergone splenectomy, accessory spleens can hypertrophy and reach a size of 5 cm or more (16,96). The typical accessory spleen has a smooth, round or ovoid shape. Its blood supply is usually derived from the splenic artery, with drainage occurring into the splenic vein.

In most patients, accessory spleens represent an incidental finding of no clinical significance. Occasionally, it is important to identify accessory splenic tissue, particularly when it is confused with a mass of another type. For instance, an accessory spleen can mimic the findings of a gastric (96), pancreatic (86), left adrenal (205), or other intra-abdominal or retroperitoneal mass (11,45,205). Identification is particularly crucial in patients in whom a splenectomy was initially performed for a hematologic disorder resulting in hypersplenism. In these patients, the growth of accessory splenic tissue can lead to a return of splenic hyperactivity, with resultant relapse (6).

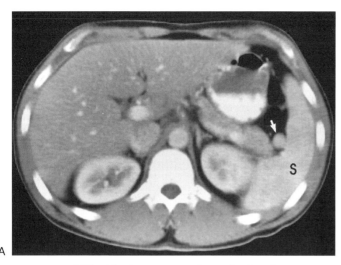 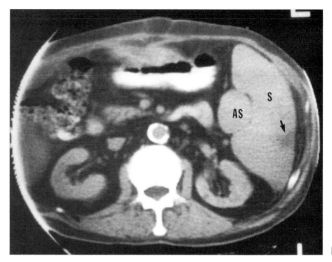

A B

FIG. 12. Accessory spleen. **A:** Small accessory spleen *(arrow)* adjacent to the splenic hilum. S, spleen. **B:** Enlarged accessory spleen (AS) in a patient with myeloid metaplasia. S, spleen; *arrow*, small infarct.

When there is uncertainty whether a nodule seen on CT represents an accessory spleen, one can compare the CT attenuation number of the structure in question with that of the spleen before and after intravenous injection of contrast material. Accessory splenic tissue tends to exhibit the same pattern of contrast enhancement as does the spleen itself (73). In problematic cases, a radionuclide study (^{99m}Tc sulfur colloid scan or heat-damaged tagged red blood cell study) may prove useful (16,84). Ultrasound (US) also has been used to document that the vessels supplying a presumed accessory spleen arise from the splenic artery and vein (208).

RARE CONGENITAL CONDITIONS

Splenic Gonadal Fusion

Splenic gonadal fusion is a rare congenital anomaly in which functioning splenic tissue is located in close proximity to gonadal tissue This entity is found predominantly in men, with a male:female ratio of 17:1 (33). The functioning splenic tissue, which usually appears as an encapsulated mass, may lie in the epididymis, along the spermatic cord, or within the tunica albuginea. It is hypothesized that this anomaly arises from adhesion between the developing gonadal primordia and the splenic anlage prior to gonadal descent. A fibrous band that can contain additional splenic tissue is found extending to the main spleen in slightly over half of patients. This *continuous* type of splenic gonadal fusion is associated with other congenital anomalies including limb defects, micrognathia, and cardiac defects. Hernia and undescended testis are associated in 15% to 20% of patients (33). The *discontinuous* type, in which there is no connection to the main spleen, is usually not associated with

other congenital anomalies. Although the mass is usually asymptomatic, confusion with testicular malignancy can occur and may lead to unnecessary orchiectomy (17,33).

Polysplenia

Polysplenia is a rare combination of congenital anomalies characterized by multiple aberrant splenic nodules and malformations in other organ systems. Although frequently referred to as left isomerism (bilateral left-sidedness), the associated abnormalities are complex and characterized by no single pathognomonic anomaly (Table 1) (156,241). In most cases, the spleen is divided into 2 to 16 masses of equal size (Fig. 13). These are located in either the right or left upper quadrant along the greater curve of the stomach. Less commonly, there are one or two large spleens along with several small splenules. There may be only a single bilobed spleen (156). Anomalous positions of other abdominal viscera also can occur. In one study of 146 cases of polysplenia (156), a symmetric midline position of the liver was noted in 57%, with 21% having full situs inversus. In 65% of patients, interruption of the inferior vena cava with azygous continuation was noted. A short pancreas in which the body and tail are truncated also has been observed (79,88). Abnormal rotation of the bowel was common and usually characterized as either reverse rotation or nonrotation of the midgut loop. Genitourinary tract anomalies, including renal agenesis or hypoplasia, and multiple ureters are also observed.

Associated thoracic anomalies include bilateral morphologic left lungs (i.e., with two lobes and hyparterial bronchus) in 58%. Bilateral superior vena cava, right-sided aortic arch, and partial anomalous pulmonary venous return occur in 40% to 50% of patients. Cardiac anomalies are common

TABLE 1. *Summary of anomalies in asplenia and polysplenia*

Anomaly	Asplenia (right isomerism)	Polysplenia (left isomerism)
Lungs	Bilateral trilobed lungs (69%)	Bilateral bilobed lungs (58%)
Superior Vena Cava (SVC)	Bilateral SVC (53%)	Bilateral SVC (47%)
Inferior Vena Cava (IVC)	Normal IVC—atrial communication	Azygous continuation of IVC (65%)
Cardiac	Single atrioventricular valve (87%)	Atrial septal defect (78%)
	Absent coronary sinus (85%)	Ventricular septal defect (63%)
	Pulmonary stenosis or atresia (78%)	Right sided aortic arch (44%)
	Total anomalous pulmonary venous return (72%)	Partial anomalous pulmonary venous return (39%)
	Transposition of great vessels (72%)	Mal- or transposition of great vessels (31%)
	Atrial septal defect (66%)	Pulmonary valvular stenosis (23%)
	Single ventricle (44%)	Subaortic stenosis (8%)
Spleen	Absent	Multiple spleens
Gastrointestinal tract	Abdominal heterotaxia (38%)	Abdominal heterotaxia (57%)
	Situs inversus (15%)	Situs inversus (21%)
	Partial situs inversus (15%)	
	Situs solitus (31%)	Situs solitus (21%)
Genitourinary tract	Miscellaneous anomalies (15%)	Miscellaneous anomalies (17%)

From ref. 156 (polysplenia) and ref. 175 (asplenia).

and are the usual cause of death, with half of patients succumbing before 6 months of age. The most common cardiac anomalies are atrial septal defect, ventricular septal defect, malposition or transposition of the great vessels, and pulmonary stenosis or atresia (156). Although only 10% of patients survived to mid adolescence in one reported series (156), it is important to note that the polysplenia syndrome occasionally can exist without significant cardiac anomalies and may be discovered as an incidental finding on CT (198,241). CT or MRI may be used to characterize the visceral anomalies (94,227).

Asplenia

The congenital asplenia syndrome (right isomerism or Ivemark syndrome) is characterized by an absent spleen

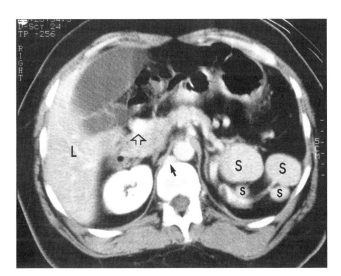

FIG. 13. Polysplenia. Multiple splenules (S) are seen in the left upper quadrant. The azygos vein *(solid arrow)* is prominent and the inferior vena cava is absent. *Open arrow,* portal vein; L, liver.

and multiple anomalies in both the abdomen and thorax (Table 1). The inferior vena cava–right atrial communication is usually normal; however, abnormal visceral position is frequently observed. In one study of 39 cases of asplenia (175), total or partial situs inversus was noted in 31%, with abdominal heterotaxy seen in 38%. Associated intestinal malrotation is common (129), genitourinary tract anomalies are seen in 15% (175), and bilateral morphologic right lungs are noted in 69% (175). The most serious associated anomalies are cardiovascular. These typically are more complex malformations than those seen with polysplenia. In the series of 39 patients cited (175), 87% had a single atrioventricular valve; a single ventricle was seen in 44%. Transposition of the great vessels and total anomalous pulmonary venous drainage were also common. These serious anomalies account for much of the high mortality, with 80% of patients dead by the end of the first year (175). Sepsis related to asplenia also contributes to this mortality figure.

Although the majority of patients with asplenia present with cyanosis or cardiorespiratory problems, a few present with bowel obstruction (129). In both groups, CT or MR can be helpful in suggesting the diagnosis and fully characterizing the disorder (217).

PATHOLOGIC CONDITIONS

Splenomegaly

Confusion sometimes arises as to whether a mass felt in the left upper abdomen truly represents an enlarged spleen. In such cases, CT, US, or MRI can provide a definite answer as to whether the spleen is enlarged or whether there is a separate abdominal mass. When the spleen is enlarged, its visceral surface often becomes convex as the spleen assumes a more globular shape.

When splenomegaly is present, there often are CT findings that indicate its cause. Neoplasm, abscess, or cyst may be seen within the spleen. Abdominal lymph node enlargement may suggest lymphoma or sarcoidosis. Cirrhotic patients with splenomegaly on the basis of portal hypertension often show characteristic alterations in the size and shape of the liver and prominence of the venous structures in the splenic hilum and gastrohepatic ligament (see Chapter 12, The Liver). The CT attenuation value of the spleen (as well as of the liver) is increased in some patients with hemochromatosis of either the primary or secondary type.

Cysts

Three types of nonneoplastic cysts are known to occur in the spleen (49,70): hydatid cysts due to *Echinococcus granulosa* infection, congenital epithelial cysts, and posttraumatic pseudocysts (Fig. 14).

On a worldwide basis, echinococcal infection is thought to be responsible for two thirds of all splenic cysts (66). This is despite the fact that splenic involvement occurs in less than 5% of cases of echinococcosis (24). In approximately 75% of patients with echinococcal involvement of the spleen, other structures also are involved, the liver being most common (24,66). In North America, echinococcal disease is unusual, with fewer than 200 cases diagnosed yearly. More than 90% of these are acquired on other continents (240). Symptoms generally are related to the large size of the cyst. Fever is not usually present unless secondary infection of a cyst has developed (240). When present, echinococcal cysts are well-circumscribed, low-density lesions that enlarge the spleen. In one study (68), cyst wall calcification was noted in 4 of 7 cases.

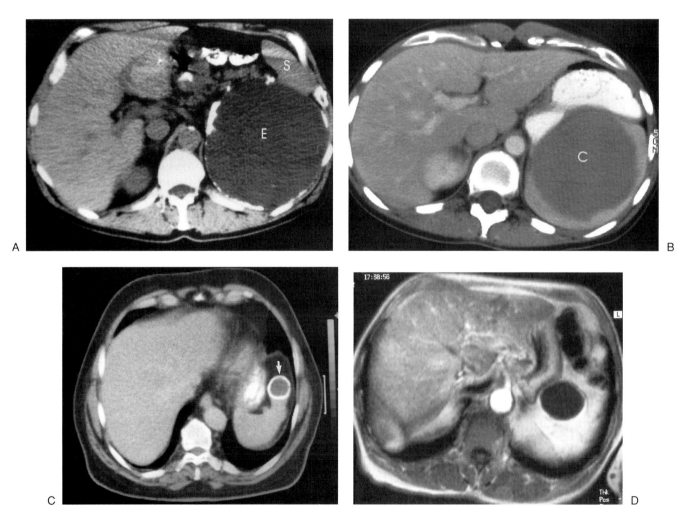

FIG. 14. Splenic cysts. **A:** Echinococcal cyst. A large, low-density lesion with peripheral calcification (E) is noted in the spleen (S). **B:** In another patient, a large unilocular low-density lesion is noted. After removal, this was shown to be an epithelial cyst (C). **C:** This round and sharply circumscribed cyst *(arrow)* with a calcified rim was presumed to be secondary to trauma. **D:** T1-weighted FLASH image (130/4/80°) performed during the perfusion phase of intravenous gadolinium-DTPA administration shows a hypointense, well-circumscribed lesion consistent with a posttraumatic cyst.

Two of 7 patients had multilocular cysts formed by the budding of daughter cysts from their outer walls (68). No enhancement of the lesions was observed on CT (68), although prior studies with angiography have shown enhancement of the outer cyst wall (173). On MR, hydatid cysts are hypointense compared to liver parenchyma on T1-weighted images, and hyperintense on T2-weighted images. In 75% of cases, the signal intensity is heterogeneous. Daughter cysts typically give a slightly lower signal than the main cyst on T1-weighted sequences. A continuous 4- to 5-mm-thick, low-intensity rim surrounding the cyst usually is evident. This rim corresponds to a dense fibrous capsule encasing the parasitic membranes (120,226). Treatment is by surgical removal. Percutaneous aspiration should be avoided because of the risk of allergic reaction to cyst contents and spread of infection (95).

Epithelial (also called epidermoid, mesothelial, or primary) cysts are congenital in origin (78). Pathologically, they are true cysts with an epithelial lining, thought by some investigators to originate from peritoneal mesothelial cells that have become trapped within the splenic parenchyma during development (31,49,148). In most series, epithelial cysts make up approximately 20% of nonparasitic cysts. They are usually discovered in childhood or in the early adult years (49,57,70), and they are more common in female than in male patients (49). Although the vast majority of cases are sporadic, familial occurrence has been reported (2,72,170). In 80% of cases, congenital splenic cysts are unilocular and solitary. On CT, they appear as spherical, sharply circumscribed, water-density lesions that show no central or rim enhancement after administration of intravenous contrast material (49). Computed tomography may show cyst wall trabeculation or peripheral septation. The wall of an epidermoid cyst occasionally calcifies (49).

Most splenic cysts encountered in the United States [approximately 80% in a series from the Armed Forces Institute of Pathology (70)] are posttraumatic in origin and are thought to represent the final stage in the evolution of splenic hematomas (49,53). Histologically, they are not lined by epithelium and thus are referred to as pseudocysts. Like epithelial cysts, they appear on CT as sharply demarcated lesions, are almost always unilocular, show no enhancement, and contain fluid of a density similar to or slightly above that of water (49). In one series, the average greatest dimension was 13 cm with no significant size difference noted between pseudocysts and true cysts (49). Computed tomography-visible calcification was more common in pseudocysts than epithelial cysts (50% versus 14%). Cyst wall trabeculation or peripheral septation was more common in epithelial cysts (86% versus 17%). Splenic pseudocysts can also occur as a result of the trauma and fluid related to a ventriculoperitoneal shunt catheter (123).

Although usually asymptomatic, a nonparasitic splenic cyst of either type may present as a left upper quadrant mass, causing a sense of epigastric fullness or intermittent dull pain (49,70). An acute abdominal presentation may occur with rupture or infection (49,170,171) Compression of the left kidney may lead to renal colic or, rarely, to hypertension (166).

The differential diagnosis of a splenic cyst includes abscess, acute hematoma, intrasplenic pancreatic pseudocyst (147), cystic neoplasm (lymphangioma or hemangioma), and cystic metastasis (49,59).

SPLENIC TUMORS

Lymphoma

Lymphoma is the most common primary malignancy of the spleen. Primary splenic lymphoma is rare and makes up approximately 1% to 2% of all lymphomas (3,116,200). When it occurs, it is usually non-Hodgkin lymphoma (NHL) of the small cell type, with evidence of B cell origin (136,200). Secondary splenic involvement in both Hodgkin and non-Hodgkin lymphoma is frequent, with lymphomas as a group being the most common splenic malignancy. It is estimated that at the time of diagnosis, splenic involvement is present in one fourth to one third of patients with Hodgkin or non-Hodgkin lymphoma (36,63,69,223,242). In patients with NHL, splenic involvement is associated with infiltrated para-aortic nodes in approximately 70% of patients (223).

Splenic involvement in lymphoma can take several forms: (a) homogeneous enlargement, (b) miliary nodules, (c) multifocal, 1- to 10-cm lesions, and (d) a single solitary mass (3,63) (Figs. 15–17). As a general rule, large cell lymphomas produce either solitary or multiple masses. Small cleaved and mixed cell types and lymphocytic lymphomas commonly produce a miliary pattern.

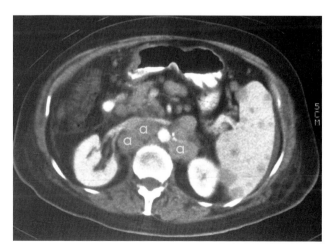

FIG. 15. Non-Hodgkin lymphoma. Splenomegaly with multiple hypodense nodules and extensive retroperitoneal adenopathy (a) in a patient with small cleaved cell lymphoma.

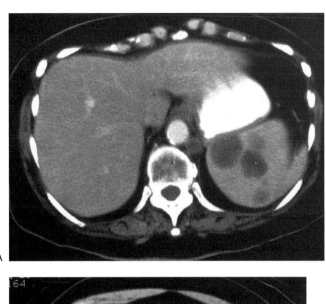

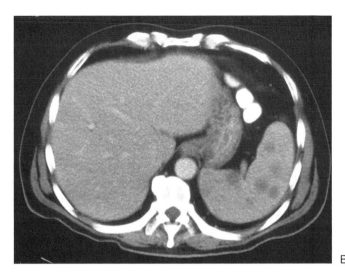

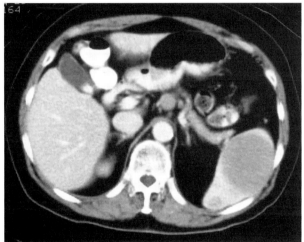

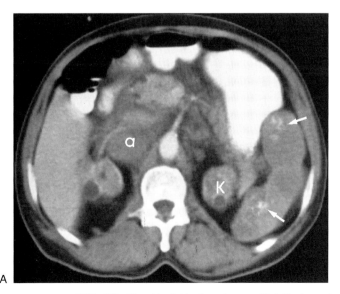

FIG. 16. Non-Hodgkin lymphoma. Hypodense nodules of varying sizes in three patients. **A:** Mixed large and small cell lymphoma. Also noted is an enlarged left retrocrural lymph node. **B:** Large cell type of T cell lymphoma **C:** Follicular large cell lymphoma.

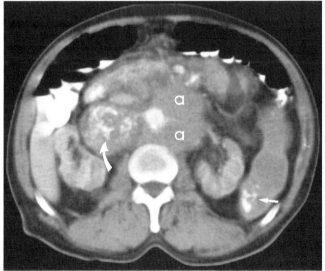

FIG. 17. Non-Hodgkin lymphoma. Faintly hypodense nodules with scattered punctate calcification *(arrows)* are noted in the spleen in a patient with untreated diffuse large cell lymphoma. Note extensive retroperitoneal adenopathy (a), which also demonstrates calcification *(curved arrow)*. **A:** At the level of the superior mesenteric artery takeoff. K, Kidney. **B:** At the level of the renal arteries.

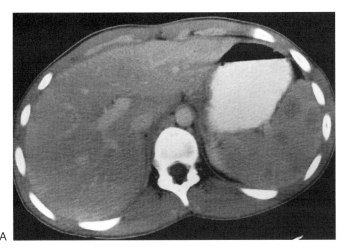 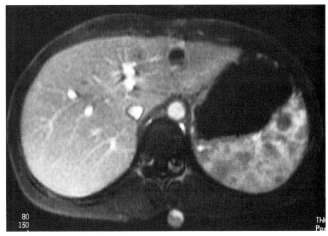

FIG. 18. Hodgkin disease. **A:** Multiple, faint, hypodense splenic nodules are noted on contrast-enhanced CT. **B:** T1-weighted FLASH image (140/4/80°) performed during the intravenous administration of gadolinium-DTPA also demonstrates multiple hypointense nodules of varying size.

Low grade lymphomas with associated blood involvement typically cause homogeneous enlargement. Hodgkin disease can cause solitary or multiple masses or a miliary pattern (242) (Figs. 18,19). Necrosis of large lesions has been reported and can give an irregular cystic appearance (23,85). In a patient with lymphoma-associated fever, this appearance may mimic a splenic abscess. Radiologically visible calcification has also been reported in aggressive lesions and after therapy (121) (Fig. 17). Although splenic lymphoma most often is confined by the splenic capsule, local extension with invasion into adjoining structures has been reported (85,99).

On CT, focal lymphomatous lesions show lower attenuation than normal splenic parenchyma. On unenhanced MR, no significant change has been noted in T1 or T2 values for spleens involved with lymphoma (145,214,235). Focal lesions are frequently isointense with splenic parenchyma on T1- and T2-weighted images. If seen, portions of lesions can be either low or high in signal intensity, depending on variations in the amount of necrosis, hemorrhage, fibrosis, and edema (80,144,145). In a study comparing MR, CT, and US for detecting splenic infiltration in patients with Hodgkin and non-Hodgkin lymphoma, MR and US were better than CT in demonstrating infiltration in patients with Hodgkin lymphoma, although no major difference was noted with NHL. All three imaging techniques failed to detect the majority of cases of NHL infiltration (144).

The use of intravenous contrast material on MR may improve its ability to detect focal splenic lesions (128). Agents specific for reticuloendothelial tissue may be useful for either MR or CT. Superparamagnetic iron oxide has been shown to improve significantly the ability of MR to distinguish normal spleen from diffuse

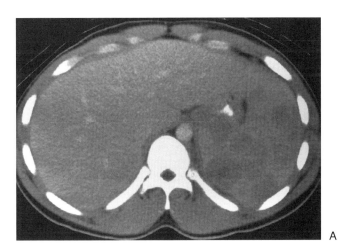

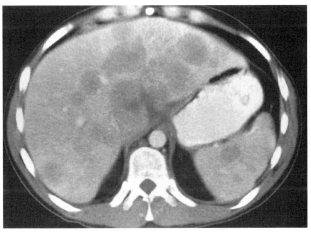

FIG. 19. Hodgkin disease. **A:** Splenomegaly with multiple hypodense splenic nodules in a patient with nodular sclerosing Hodgkin disease. **B:** Multiple hypodense nodules in the liver and spleen in a patient with advanced Hodgkin disease.

splenic lymphoma (235). Similarly improved detection of splenic lymphoma has been demonstrated on CT after administration of EOE-13 (213).

The reported accuracy of CT as a predictor of splenic involvement by lymphoma ranges from a low sensitivity and specificity of 30% and 71%, respectively (37,71,126), to a high sensitivity and specificity of approximately 90% (206,207). The lower figures are more in line with extensive clinical literature that demonstrates both that normal-sized spleens frequently show microscopic involvement and that mildly to moderately enlarged spleens are often uninvolved (60,98,101,242). However, markedly enlarged spleens (weighing more than 400 to 500 g) almost always show lymphomatous involvement (36,223).

Other Primary Splenic Tumors

Malignancies arising from the mesenchymal components of the spleen occur but are quite rare (25,51, 103,134,238). Most are tumors of vascular origin, such as angiosarcomas of varying degrees of differentiation. Some authors have used the term *hemangioendothelioma* to refer to vascular tumors of borderline malignant potential (242). Symptoms include abdominal pain, left upper quadrant mass, fever, weight loss, anemia, and consumptive coagulopathy. Splenic rupture is reported to occur in approximately one third of patients (8,193,238). On CT, such neoplasms generally appear as focal, rounded or irregular areas of heterogeneous low attenuation (112,193,216) (Fig. 20). Cystic and necrotic areas may be evident within the mass. Areas of enhancement may also be shown. At angiography, multiple vascular lakes have been observed, which may mimic the appearance of cavernous hemangiomata (103).

Angiosarcoma has been caused by exposure to Thorotrast, a colloidal suspension of thorium dioxide used

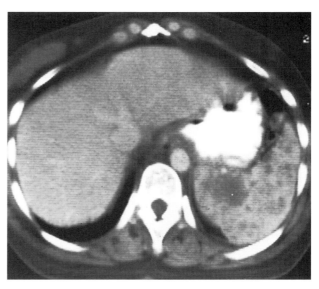

FIG. 21. Diffuse cavernous hemangiomatosis of the spleen.

until the 1950s as an angiographic contrast agent (112). In these patients, CT shows a striking increase in the attenuation of the splenic parenchyma due to chronic retention of the radiopaque material in reticuloendothelial cells of the spleen. Although Thoratrast-associated angiosarcoma has occurred much more commonly in the liver, a primary case in the spleen has been reported (112). Vinyl chloride and arsenic exposure, although associated with hepatic angiosarcoma, have not been shown to predispose to splenic angiosarcoma (22,172,242).

Other primary mesenchymal malignancies that have been reported in the spleen include fibrosarcoma, leiomyosarcoma, malignant teratoma, and malignant fibrous histiocytoma (MFH) (132,238). The CT appearance of these lesions is not specific. MFH has been described as a large mass with extensive areas of necrosis (28). Mucinous cystadenocarcinoma also has been reported in the spleen and is thought to arise either from invaginated capsular mesothelium or from embryonic rests of pancreatic or enteric tissue. On CT, mucinous cystadenocarcinoma has the appearance of a large multicystic mass. Mural calcification can be observed (133).

Benign splenic tumors are uncommon. Hemangiomas and lymphangiomas are the two most frequent, with hemangiomas seen in 0.01% to 0.14% of patients at autopsy (25,106,160,180). They are usually asymptomatic. Less frequently, they present as an abdominal mass or pain. Rupture and hemorrhage are reported in up to 25% in some series (92). Anemia, thrombocytopenia, and a consumptive coagulopathy (Kasabach-Merritt syndrome) have been noted (186,231). Portal hypertension with esophageal varices also has been infrequently reported (163,211). Splenic hemangiomas can be multiple or associated with hemangiomas in other organs (149,161) (Figs. 21,22). They range in size from a few millimeters to over

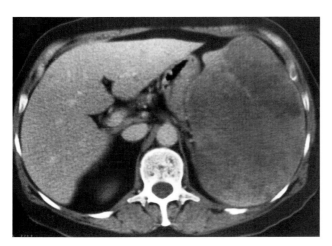

FIG. 20. Large, partially enhanced angiosarcoma of the spleen.

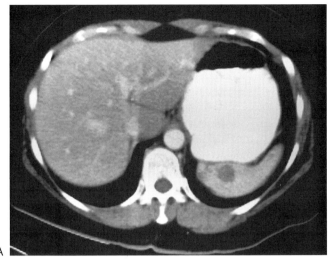

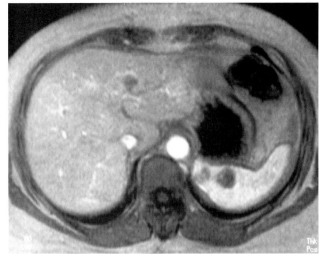

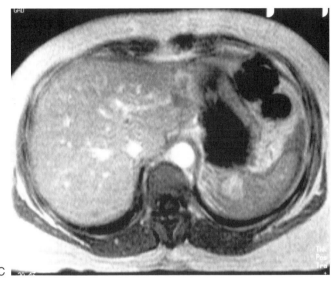

FIG. 22. Presumed splenic hemangioma. **A:** Contrast-enhanced CT shows a hypodense mass in the spleen. **B,C:** T1-weighted FLASH image (140/4/80°) performed during the perfusion (B) and equilibrium (C) phases of intravenous gadolinium-DTPA administration. The lesion is hypointense on the initial perfusion image but demonstrates full enhancement on the equilibrium image, 7 min later.

15 cm (174). In the spleen, cavernous hemangiomas are more common than capillary-type hemangiomas (132).

The imaging characteristics of splenic hemangioma are similar to those in the liver. On unenhanced CT, they appear as a well-defined, hypodense mass that may contain cystic components. With contrast injection, the lesion may remain hypodense, or it may enhance from its periphery (55,135,149,155,167,174). Calcification can occur as scattered, punctate, curvilinear densities, or as dense rays radiating from a central point (81,149,174). On MR, these lesions appear hypo- or isointense with respect to the rest of the spleen on T1-weighted images, and hyperintense on T2-weighted sequences. Heterogeneous signal is sometimes noted on T2-weighted images, reflecting the presence of cystic and solid components with varying amounts of fibrosis, necrosis, and hemorrhage (55,155,167). Injection of intravenous gadolinium-DTPA causes enhancement similar to that observed with iodinated contrast material on CT.

Lymphangiomas can occur as single or multiple lesions (132). Although most common in the neck and axilla, they do occur rarely in the abdominal viscera. Disseminated lymphangiomatosis affecting multiple areas also has been reported (10). Lymphangiomas are categorized as capillary, cavernous, or cystic, depending on the size of the abnormal lymphatic channels. In the spleen, the cystic type is most common. Splenic lymphangiomas are usually asymptomatic or discovered as a left upper quadrant mass. CT demonstrates multiple, thin-walled, well-marginated cysts, often in a subcapsular location. No enhancement is noted after intravenous contrast material administration. CT attenuation measurements from the cysts vary from 15 to 35 HU (162,164,221). Curvilinear calcifications have been reported (162).

Splenic hamartomas (also called splenomas, or nodular hyperplasia of the spleen) are rare, benign splenic lesions (70). They are composed of an anomalous mixture of normal splenic elements, with red pulp predominating. A

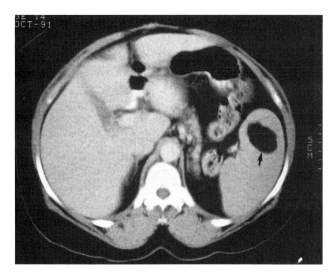

FIG. 23. Splenic lipoma. Contrast-enhanced CT shows a well-defined fat density mass *(arrow)*.

mixture of red and white pulp, or white pulp alone, occurs less commonly. The hamartomas occur singly or, less commonly, as multiple nodules (204). Their diameter ranges from less than 1 cm to greater than 15 cm (131,204). Like most other benign splenic lesions, they are usually discovered incidentally or because of a mass-related symptomatology. Splenic hamartomas are reported as a rare manifestation of tuberous sclerosis (50). On CT, splenic hamartomas appear iso- or hypodense on precontrast images, with occasional lesions showing cystic components (26,243). They usually show slow enhancement and fill in after intravenous contrast material administration. Lesions that are isodense to normal spleen on both pre- and postcontrast images also have been reported (143). Prolonged enhancement similar to that seen with hemangiomas has been noted with both enhanced CT and MR. On unenhanced MR, the lesions are often isointense on T1-weighted images and hyperintense on T2-weighted images relative to the background spleen (26,146).

Inflammatory pseudotumors are rare, benign lesions consisting of a polymorphous inflammatory cell infiltrate with varying amounts of granulomatous reaction, fibrosis, and necrosis (177). They have been described in virtually every organ system, including lung, esophagus, liver, lymph nodes, and spleen (13,130,158,177,201,242). They can be asymptomatic or present as a mass accompanied by vague constitutional symptoms (e.g., fever, malaise). Their etiology is uncertain, although there has been speculation that they have an infectious or autoimmune origin. In the spleen, inflammatory pseudotumors appear as well-circumscribed encapsulated masses. They usually are solitary, but multiple lesions have been reported in the liver and spleen (74). They range from 1.5 cm to more than 14 cm in diameter (130,177). On CT, they appear as a nonspecific heterogeneous hypodense mass. Peripheral

calcification may be present (67,239). After intravenous contrast material administration, there is progressive enhancement, although persistent areas of hypodensity corresponding to areas of fibrosis may be noted. The presence of a central stellate area of hypodensity (a central scar) is thought to suggest splenic inflammatory pseudotumor (67). On MR, these lesions show slight hyperintensity on T1-weighted images, with more marked hyperintensity relative to normal spleen on T2-weighted images. Mild-to-moderate enhancement is noted after intravenous gadolinium administration (74).

Other benign lesions that have been noted in the spleen include lipomas and fibromas (Fig. 23). These are extremely rare (25,56,106,242).

Metastatic Disease

Metastatic deposits in the spleen are unusual. They occur most commonly from hematogenous spread and are almost always seen in patients with widespread carcinoma (i.e., metastasis to three or more organs) (232). In autopsy series, they are noted in approximately 1% to 9% of patients with carcinoma (1,19,232). Of these, one third to one half are found only on microscopic examination (19,122,232). The lack of afferent splenic lymphatics, the periodic changes in spleen size, and the filtering of blood by liver and lung have all been suggested to explain the relative infrequency of gross splenic metastasis (34,232). The most common primary sites of splenic metastases are breast and lung (19,122). Melanoma has the highest frequency of splenic involvement on a per primary basis, with 34% of melanoma patients showing splenic metastasis at autopsy (19). Splenic metastases most frequently appear as multiple nodules, although diffuse infiltration occurs in 8% to 10% of affected patients. The splenic deposits are usually asymptomatic.

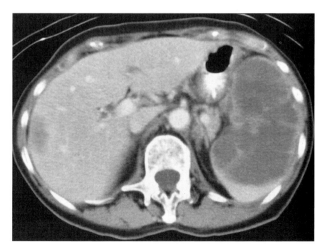

FIG. 24. Endometrial carcinoma metastatic to the spleen. Contrast-enhanced CT demonstrates large, complex, low density metastasis.

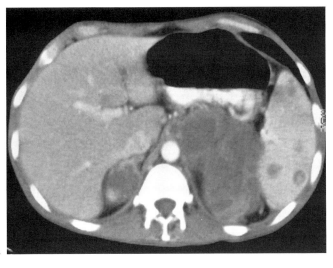

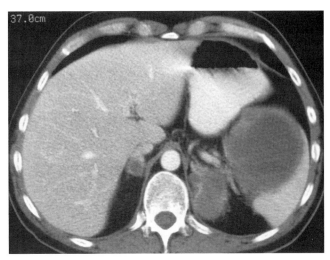

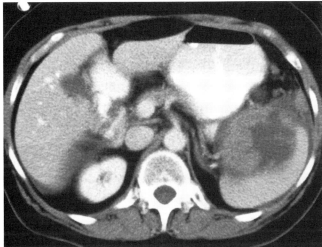

FIG. 25. Carcinoma metastatic to the spleen. **A:** Small, low density lesions in the spleen with bilateral adrenal metastases in a patient with squamous cell carcinoma of the lung. **B:** Hypodense mass within the spleen with bilateral adrenal masses in a patient with malignant melanoma. **C:** Complex mass in the splenic hilum in a patient with ovarian carcinoma.

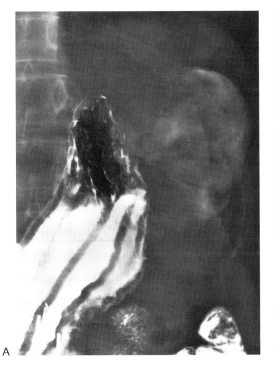

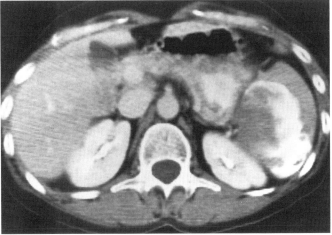

FIG. 26. Ovarian carcinoma metastatic to the spleen. **A:** On upper GI, a large, partially calcified mass is seen in the left upper quadrant, deforming the adjacent stomach. **B:** CT demonstrates hypodense mass with extensive calcification in the spleen.

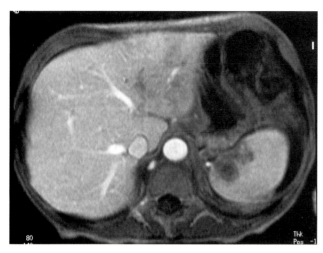

FIG. 27. Ovarian carcinoma metastatic to the spleen. An irregular hypointense mass is seen in the spleen on this T1-weighted FLASH image (140/4/80°) performed during intravenous administration of gadolinium-DTPA.

On CT, nodular metastases appear as rounded, hypodense lesions (Figs. 24–27). Cystic lesions may occur with metastasis from ovary, breast, and endometrium, and from melanoma (34,62,105,106,132,141,159). Calcification is uncommon but does occur in patients with a mucinous adenocarcinoma primary (167) (Fig. 26). Peritoneal implants in patients with an ovarian, gastrointestinal, or pancreatic cancer can cause scalloping of the capsular surface of the spleen (62). Direct splenic invasion is unusual but can occur from adjacent primaries in the stomach, colon, pancreas, or kidney (105,132).

SPLENIC INFECTION

Splenic infection can occur either as a single focus or as part of a diffuse or miliary process. Although splenic infection is uncommon, the increasing prevalence of immunosuppression in cancer, transplant, and acquired immunodeficiency syndrome (AIDS) patients has placed a greater population at risk (35,138).

Splenic infection is usually the result of hematogenous dissemination, with predisposing primary infections occurring in 68% of patients in one series (44). [In series reported after 1977, this rate is significantly lower, probably because of antibiotic use (138).] In the series by Chun et al. (44), endocarditis was the most common associated infection, occurring in 12%. Other associated infections included urinary tract infection, surgical wound infections, appendicitis, and pneumonia. Abscess in other organs occurs in 15% to 20% of patients (44,215). Direct spread of infection from adjacent organs has been reported in cases of gastric ulcer and carcinoma, carcinoma of the descending colon, and perihepatic abscess. Noninfectious predisposing factors include diabetes, immunosuppression, and sickle cell disease. Disruption of the

normal splenic parenchyma by trauma or infarction also predisposes to subsequent infection (35,44).

Patients with splenic abscess present clinically with fever and pain. The latter can localize in either the left upper quadrant or the left side of the chest, or it can be referred to the shoulder. Although this presentation is typical for a solitary splenic abscess in a normal host, the immunosuppressed patient with multiple splenic abscesses often shows no localizing signs (35). Splenomegaly is noted on physical examination in about half of patients with splenic abscess (44). The most common organisms are *Staphylococcus* and *Streptococcus,* each occurring in approximately 10% to 20% of patients. *Salmonella* and *Escherichia coli* are also frequent. Anaerobic organisms are noted in 5% to 17% of patients (44,138). Mycobacteria, *Candida* species, and *Pneumocystis carinii* infection also occur (42,154). With the increasing prevalence of immunosuppression, fungal infection has become more frequent and in some series now causes approximately 25% of splenic abscesses (35,138).

On CT, splenic abscess appears as a nonenhancing area of decreased attenuation (Figs. 28,29). The rim of the abscess often is isodense with the surrounding spleen, but it may be enhanced when iodinated contrast material is injected intravenously (189). Although intravenous contrast medium administration usually aids in demonstrating splenic abscesses, lesions that are more easily seen on unenhanced studies have been reported. Some authors recommend performance of both pre- and postcontrast

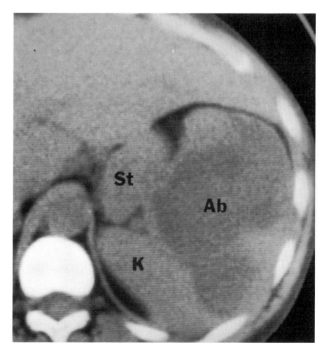

FIG. 28. Splenic abscess (Ab) in an alcoholic patient with fever. The spleen is enlarged, and the abscess appears as a lobulated, low density region within it. K, kidney; St, stomach.

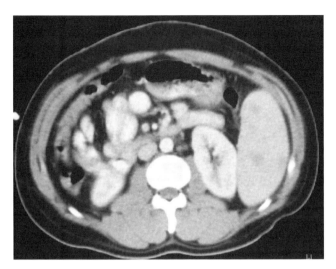

FIG. 29. Splenomegaly with multiple, small, faintly visualized, hypodense nodules in a patient with brucellosis.

scans, particularly when the miliary abscesses typical of fungal infection are suspected (152). Size may vary from less than 1 cm in the patient with multifocal or miliary abscess, to 14 cm in diameter (4,15,35,215). Fungal infection in the spleen is most likely to appear as a miliary, multifocal, or multilocular process (40,65,189). Whereas 64% of multilocular abscesses have a fungal etiology, unilocular abscesses have a bacterial etiology in 94% of cases (138). Gas occasionally is noted within splenic abscesses but usually is absent. Calcification has been seen in treated *Candida* microabscess and in lesions caused by other fungi (most notably *Histoplasma*), mycobacteria, and *Pneumocystis carinii* (61,64,117,189,190,218) (Figs. 30,31). The overall sensitivity of CT for splenic abscess is significantly higher than that of US or radionuclide scintigraphy (138). It should be noted, however, that a CT scan without focal abnormality does not exclude the possibility of early infection, particularly in hematogenously disseminated fungal disease (189).

On MR, hepatosplenic candidiasis appears as low signal on T1-weighted and high signal on T2-weighted images relative to the normal splenic parenchyma (41). After intravenous administration of gadolinium, the lesions show no enhancement (Fig. 32). Early postcontrast T1-weighted spoiled gradient echo imaging appears to be the most sensitive MR imaging sequence for detecting lesions, even more sensitive than contrast-enhanced CT (184).

SPLENIC TRAUMA

Please refer to Chapter 21 (Thoracoabdominal Trauma) for a full discussion of splenic trauma.

MISCELLANEOUS SPLENIC DISORDERS

Sarcoidosis

Studies using percutaneous splenic aspiration have demonstrated splenic involvement in 24% to 59% of patients with sarcoidosis (182,210). Splenic sarcoidosis usually is asymptomatic. However, with marked involvement, abdominal discomfort, fever, malaise, hypersplenism, and even rupture may occur (102). The presentation and appearance of the spleen may mimic lymphoma, resulting in unnecessary splenectomy. In one review of the CT findings in 59 patients with sarcoidosis (233), marked splenic enlargement was noted in 6% of patients, with mild-to-moderate splenomegaly seen in 27% (Fig. 33). Hypodense nodules, corresponding to aggregated granulomata, were seen in the spleen in 15% of patients (Fig. 34). Coexistent abdominal lymphadenopathy was noted frequently in patients with splenomegaly. The chest radiograph, however, was normal in 25% of patients with splenomegaly or discrete nodules (233).

Splenic Artery Aneurysm

Splenic artery aneurysm is the most common abdominal visceral artery aneurysm. Its incidence in autopsy series generally has been 0.01% to 0.2%, although, when specifically looked for, they have been found in up to 10% of autopsies (18,32,181,199). The latter figure includes lesions less than 0.5 to 1 cm in diameter (18). Predisposing conditions include pregnancy and multiparity, portal hypertension, and arteriosclerotic disease (32,202,219). Because of the association with pregnancy, splenic artery aneurysms are significantly more common in women, with fewer than 15% being seen in men (219). Most

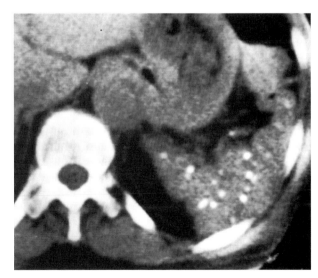

FIG. 30. Multiple calcified splenic granulomata, presumed to be due to histoplasmosis.

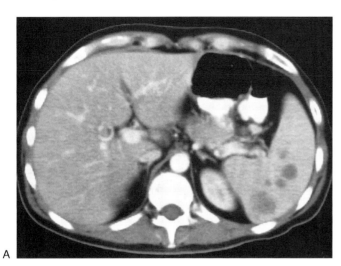
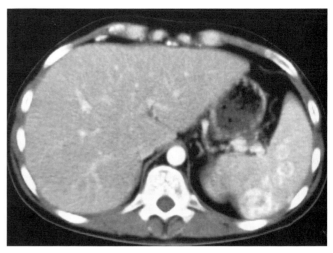

A   B

FIG. 31. *Pneumocystis carinii* infection. **A:** Lesions initially appear as multiple hypodense nodules. **B:** After 10 weeks of therapy, lesions show peripheral and some central calcification.

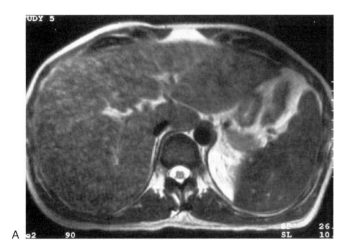

A

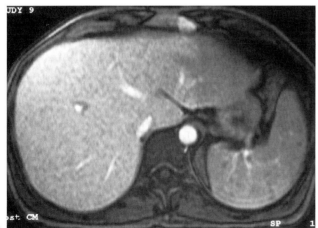

B

FIG. 32. Hepatosplenic candidiasis. **A:** T2-weighted MR (3800/90) shows multiple, small, high-signal-intensity lesions in liver and spleen. **B:** Gadolinium-DTPA-enhanced T1-weighted MR (130/4/80°). Abscesses appear as multiple, small, hypointense lesions. (Case courtesy of Dr. Susan M. Ascher, Georgetown University.)

aneurysms are saccular, and over 75% occur in the distal third of the splenic artery. Thirty percent to 40% are multiple. Size ranges from less than 1 cm to 30 cm (32,219). Although most patients are asymptomatic, a pulsatile mass, left upper quadrant pain, and rupture have been reported (32,202,219). Embolization or resection is recommended if the aneurysm is found in pregnant women or in women of childbearing age, is symptomatic, is greater than 1.5 to 2.0 cm in diameter, or is increasing in size (12,32).

Occasionally, a specific cause can be cited for the development of splenic artery pseudoaneurysms. Acute and chronic pancreatitis, penetrating gastric ulcer, trauma, and septic emboli have all been implicated (30,32, 124,150,202). Mycotic aneurysms involving the intrasplenic branches of the splenic artery also have been reported (9).

On unenhanced CT, a low-density lesion with peripheral calcification is observed along the course of the splenic artery. Bright enhancement is observed after intravenous contrast material administration unless the lesion is thrombosed (30,222) (Figs. 35,36).

Splenic Infarcts

Splenic infarction can occur with embolic disease of cardiac or atherosclerotic origin and in patients with arteritis, myeloproliferative disease, pancreatitis, pancreatic mass, and sickle cell anemia (14,142). If they are small, splenic infarcts are frequently asymptomatic. Large infarcts can cause left upper quadrant pain, fever, and diaphragmatic irritation. On CT, infarcts classically appear as sharply marginated, low-density regions that are wedge-shaped, with the base at the splenic capsule and

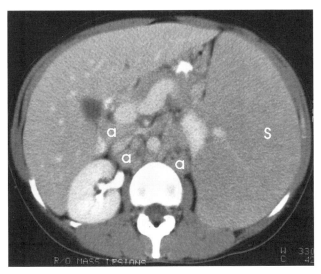

FIG. 33. Sarcoidosis with marked splenomegaly (S), and para-aortic and portacaval adenopathy (a).

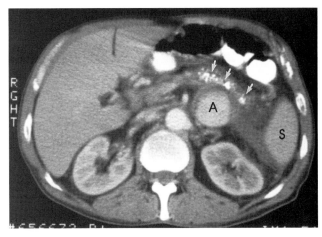

FIG. 35. Splenic artery aneurysm (A) in a patient with a history of pancreatitis. Note pancreatic calcifications *(arrowheads)*. S, spleen.

apex toward the hilum (14,69,137,191) (Fig. 37). Not uncommonly, however, infarcts appear as multiple, poorly marginated, hypodense lesions, indistinguishable from other forms of focal splenic pathology (14). When the entire spleen is infarcted, such as after occlusion or avulsion of the splenic artery, there is failure of contrast enhancement of all but the parenchyma immediately subjacent to the capsule (Fig 38). This peripheral enhancement, the so-called rim sign, is due to arterial supply from capsular vessels.

Lack of splenic parenchymal enhancement without infarction also occurs in the setting of profound hypotension (21). This can mimic splenic arterial disruption after blunt abdominal trauma. In the setting of massive splenic in-

farction, gas bubbles can appear even in uninfected splenic parenchyma, and they may be confused with splenic abscess formation (54,113). Splenic infarction also can be seen with MR imaging. Hemorrhagic infarcts have a high signal intensity on both T1- and T2-weighted images (89).

Patients with sickle cell anemia usually have repeated episodes of splenic infarction that eventually result in a shrunken spleen containing diffuse, microscopic deposits of calcium and iron (119) (Fig. 39). CT has been helpful in establishing that a focal area of uptake of ^{99m}Tc diphosphonate seen in the left upper abdomen on radionuclide scintigraphy a result of uptake in a calcified spleen rather than in a focus of osteomyelitis in the overlying rib (157). Acute splenic sequestration crisis is characterized by sud-

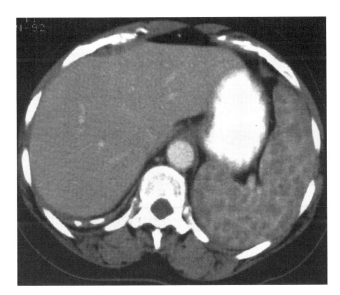

FIG. 34. Sarcoidosis with splenomegaly and multiple hypodense nodules.

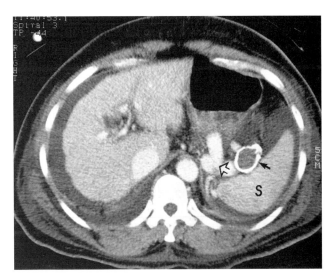

FIG. 36. Thrombosed splenic artery aneurysm *(arrow)*. Note peripheral calcification. Ascites and right pleural effusion are also present. S, spleen; *open arrow,* spontaneous splenorenal shunt.

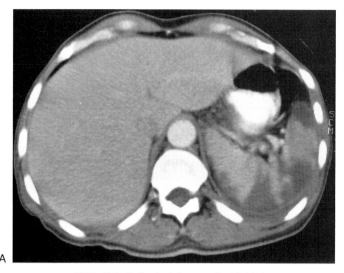
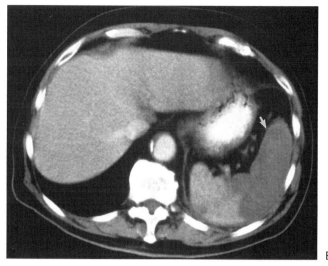

A   B

FIG. 37. Splenic infarcts. **A:** Multiple wedge-shaped hypodensities are noted, with the apex of the wedge pointing toward the splenic hila. **B:** Infarction involving more than half the spleen. Note preservation of some capsular enhancement *(arrow)*.

den massive splenic enlargement, accompanied by an abrupt decline in hematocrit. CT demonstrates splenomegaly with multiple peripheral areas of low attenuation. These low-attenuation regions are thought to represent areas of subacute hemorrhage and show high signal on both T1- and T2-weighted sequences (176). Splenic rupture also can complicate sickle cell disease and can be readily diagnosed with CT (118).

Hemochromatosis

Hemochromatosis is categorized into primary and secondary forms. The latter form, usually seen in patients receiving multiple blood transfusions, causes reticuloendothelial deposition of iron, which sometimes can be identified on CT as an increase in splenic density (90,115). Primary hemochromatosis, caused by an inappropriately high iron absorption from the gastrointestinal tract, results in parenchymal iron deposition in liver, pancreas, heart, and other organs. In this setting, splenic density is usually unchanged. When severe, secondary hemochromatosis can cause parenchymal iron deposition. Similarly, primary hemochromatosis can occasionally result in reticuloendothelial involvement. Magnetic resonance imaging is more sensitive than computed tomography for demonstrating iron deposition. The paramagnetic

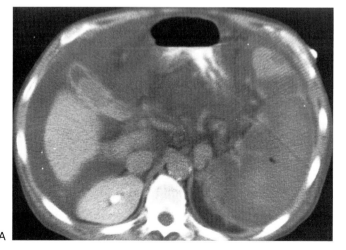
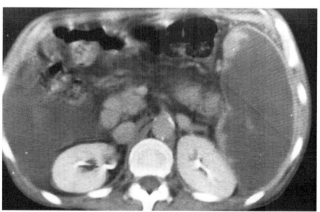

A   B

FIG. 38. A: Splenic infarction 1 week after therapeutic embolization of the splenic artery in a patient with portal hypertension and bleeding esophageal varices. There is extensive liquefactive necrosis and hemorrhage, and a tiny gas bubble, introduced during the procedure, lies near the center of the spleen. Note the rim of enhanced splenic capsule. **B:** Three weeks after the therapeutic infarction, the gas is gone and the density of the hemorrhagic fluid in the spleen has decreased. Rim enhancement persists.

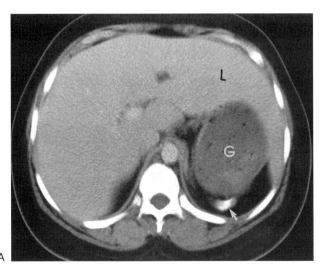 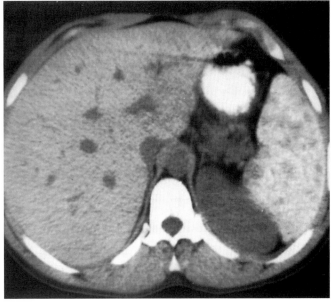

FIG. 39. A: Tiny calcified infarcted spleen *(arrow)* in an adult with sickle cell anemia. **B:** In another patient with sickle cell disease, unenhanced CT image demonstrates the spleen to be almost completely calcified, with few residual areas of normal parenchyma. This is undoubtedly the result of multiple episodes of infarction. G, stomach; L, liver.

properties of deposited iron result in a marked decrease in signal intensity on T2-weighted spin echo and gradient echo sequences (75,192,203) (Fig. 40).

Amyloidosis

Amyloidosis results from the deposition of extracellular fibrillar material in a wide variety of tissues and organs. It occurs commonly with multisystem involve-

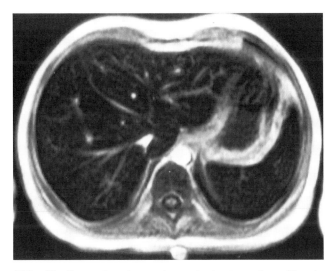

FIG. 40. Secondary hemochromatosis. Iron deposition in the reticuloendothelial system has caused loss of signal in both liver and spleen on this T1-weighted MR image (140/4/80°).

ment, although an unusual localized form is reported. Systemic amyloidosis can be divided into two main types based on the biochemistry of the amyloid fibril. In type AL (primary) amyloidosis, the amyloid protein is produced by a monoclonal population of plasma cells, either with or without clinical signs of multiple myeloma. In type AA, or secondary amyloidosis, amyloid deposition is secondary to chronic inflammatory disease such as rheumatoid arthritis (27,107). Splenic involvement occurs in both types and usually is homogeneous and diffuse. Focal tumorlike lesions also have been reported and can occur as part of either a systemic or a localized disease (39,114). Decreased splenic attenuation and enhancement have been observed on CT, either diffusely or focally (114,209). Extensive splenic calcification has been reported in a case of primary amyloidosis (100). Spontaneous splenic rupture has been noted in cases of splenic amyloidosis and is felt to be secondary to vascular and/or splenic capsular fragility from amyloid deposition (91). On MR, decreased signal intensity on T2-weighted images has been reported in cases of splenic amyloidosis (169).

Peliosis

Peliosis is a rare condition in which multiple, blood-filled spaces form in the liver, spleen, and, rarely, other parts of the reticuloendothelial system. It has been associated with the use of anabolic steroids and oral contraceptives, and it also is seen in patients with human immuno-

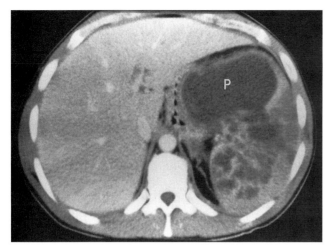

FIG. 41. Large pancreatic pseudocyst (P) in the splenic hilum extends into the splenic parenchyma.

deficiency virus (HIV) infection or chronic wasting states (168,212,220). Splenic rupture has been reported in patients with peliosis (220). On unenhanced CT, peliosis usually appears as small, hypodense lesions (125), which occasionally can coalesce to form large, muliloculated masses with well-defined septa (46). Enhancement varies, with some lesions becoming isodense and others demonstrating no enhancement (46,125,168). On MR, the lesions in peliosis have a variety of signal characteristics depending on the state of the contained blood (125).

Splenic Involvement in Pancreatitis

In patients with pancreatitis, fluid can collect around the spleen, particularly laterally (225). Pseudocysts arising in the tail of the pancreas adjacent to the splenic hilum (147) occasionally extend beneath the splenic capsule or even into the splenic parenchyma (230) (Fig. 41). Pancreatic pseudocysts consist of low-density material surrounded by a well-defined wall, which may enhance after intravenous administration of contrast material. Splenic subcapsular hematoma, rupture, infarction, splenic artery pseudoaneurysm, and splenic vein thrombosis all have been reported in patients with complicated pancreatitis (109,124,228).

SPLENIC BIOPSY AND ASPIRATION

Diagnostic splenic aspiration has been used in the evaluation of sarcoidosis and to evaluate focal lesions in the spleen (165,182,183,195,196,210). The complication rate with fine-needle (20- to 22-gauge) aspiration is low (183,196,210). Core biopsy using a fine needle (22- or 21-gauge Surecut) has also been undertaken for staging of lymphoma, with no significant complications encountered in 46 patients (38).

Multiple reports have shown that splenic abscess can be treated with aspiration or percutaneous drainage with a success rate up to 68% in one study (20,43,111, 138,165). This procedure may aid in splenic salvage.

REFERENCES

1. Abrams HL, Spiro R, Goldstein N. Metastases in carcinoma: analysis of 1000 autopsied cases. *Cancer* 1950;3:74–85.
2. Ahlgren LS, Beardmore HE. Solitary epidermoid splenic cysts: occurrence in sibs. *J Pediatr Surg* 1984;19:56–58.
3. Ahmann DL, Kiely JM, Harrison EG, Payne WS. Malignant lymphoma of the spleen: a review of 49 cases in which the diagnosis was made at splenectomy. *Cancer* 1966;19:461–469.
4. Allal R, Kastler B, Gangi A, et al. Splenic abscesses in typhoid fever: US and CT studies. *J Comput Assist Tomogr* 1993;17:90–93.
5. Allen KB, Gay BB, Skandalakis JE. Wandering spleen: anatomic and radiologic considerations. *South Med J* 1992;85:976–984.
6. Ambriz P, Munoz R, Quintanar E, Sigler L, Aviles A, Pizzuto J. Accessory spleen compromising response to splenectomy for idiopathic thrombocytopenia purpura. *Radiology* 1985;155:793–796.
7. Amenta PS, Amenta II PS. The anatomy of the spleen. In: Bowdler AJ, ed. *The spleen: structure, function and clinical significance*. London: Chapman and Hall Medical, 1990;3–7.
8. Autry JR, Weitzner S. Hemangiosarcoma of spleen with spontaneous rupture. *Cancer* 1975;35:534–539.
9. Avery GR, Wildson JB, Mitchell L. Case report: CT and angiographic appearances of intrasplenic mycotic aneurysm. *Clin Radiol* 1991;44:271–272.
10. Avigad S, Jaffe R, Frand M, Yakov I, Rotem Y. Lymphangiomatosis with splenic involvement. *JAMA* 1976;236:2315–2317.
11. Azar GB, Awwad JT, Muffarij IK. Accessory spleen presenting as adnexal mass. *Acta Obstet Gynecol Scand* 1993;72:587–588.
12. Babb RR. Aneurysm of the splenic artery. *Arch Surg* 1976;111:924–925.
13. Bahadori M, Liebow AA. Plasma cell granulomas of the lung. *Cancer* 1973;31:191–208.
14. Balcar I, Seltzer SE, Davis S, Geller S. CT patterns of splenic infarction: a clinical and experimental study. *Radiology* 1984;151:723–729.
15. Balthazar EJ, Hilton S, Naidich D, Megabow A, Levine R. CT of splenic and perisplenic abnormalities in septic patients. *AJR* 1985;144:53–56.
16. Beahrs JR, Stephens DH. Enlarged accessory spleens: CT appearance in postsplenectomy patients. *AJR* 1980;135:483–486.
17. Bearss RW. Splenic-gonadal fusion. *Urology* 1980;16:277–279.
18. Bedford PD, Lodge B. Aneurysm of the splenic artery. *Gut* 1960;1:312–320.
19. Berge T. Splenic metastasis: frequencies and patterns. *Acta Pathol Microbiol Scand* 1974;82:499–506.
20. Berkman WA, Harris SA, Bernardino M. Nonsurgical drainage of splenic abscesses. *AJR* 1983;141:395–396.
21. Berland L, Van Dyke JA. Decreased splenic enhancement of CT in traumatized hypotensive patients. *Radiology* 1985;156:469–471.
22. Block JB. Angiosarcoma of the liver following vinyl chloride exposure. *JAMA* 1974;229:53–54.
23. Bloom RA, Freund U, Perkes EH, Weiss Y. Acute Hodgkin disease masquerading as splenic abscess. *J Surg Oncol* 1981;17:279–282.
24. Bonakdarpour A. *Echinococcus* disease: report of 112 cases from Iran and a review of 611 cases from the United States. *AJR* 1967;99:660–667.
25. Bostick WL. Primary splenic neoplasm. *Am J Pathol* 1945;21:1143–1165.
26. Brinkley A, Lee J. Cystic hamartoma of the spleen: CT and sonographic findings. *J Clin Ultrasound* 1981;9:136–138.
27. Browning M, Banks R, Tribe C, et al. Ten years' experience of an amyloid clinic—a clinicopathological survey. *Q J Med* 1985;54:213–227.
28. Bruneton JN, Drouillard J, Rogopoulos A, et al. Extraretroperito-

neal abdominal malignant fibrous histiocytoma. *Gastrointest Radiol* 1988;13:299–305.

29. Buehner M. Wandering spleen. *Surg Gynecol Obstet* 1992;175:373–387.

30. Burke JW, Erickson SJ, Kellum CD, Tegtmeyer CJ, Williamson BRJ, Hansen MF. Pseudoaneurysms complicating pancreatitis: detection by CT. *Radiology* 1986;161:447–450.

31. Burrig K-F. Epithelial (true) cysts: pathogenesis of the mesothelial and so-called epidermoid cyst of the spleen. *Am J Surg Path* 1988;12:275–281.

32. Busuttil RW, Brin BJ. The diagnosis and managment of visceral artery aneurysms. *Surgery* 1980;88:619–624.

33. Carragher AA. One hundred years of splenogonadal fusion. *Urology* 1990;35:471–475.

34. Carrington BM, Thomas NB, Johnson RJ. Intrasplenic metastases from carcinoma of the ovary. *Clin Radiol* 1990;41:418–20.

35. Caslowitz PL, Labs JD, Fishman EK, Siegelman SS. Changing spectrum of splenic abscess. *Clin Imaging* 1989;13:201–207.

36. Castellino RA. Hodgkin disease: practical concepts for the diagnostic radiologist. *Radiology* 1986;159:305–310.

37. Castellino RA, Hoppe RT, Blank N, et al. Computed tomography, lymphography, and staging laparotomy: correlations in initial staging of Hodgkin disease. *AJR* 1984;143:37–41.

38. Cavanna L, Civardi G, Fornari F, et al. Ultrasonically guided percutaneous splenic tissue core biopsy in patients with malignant lymphomas. *Cancer* 1992;69:2932–2936.

39. Chen K, Flam M, Workman R. Amyloid tumor of the spleen. *Am J Surg Pathol* 1987;11:723–725.

40. Chew FS, L SP, Barboriak D. Candidal splenic abscesses. *AJR* 1991;156:474.

41. Cho J-S, Kim EE, Varma DGK, Wallace S. MR imaging of hepatosplenic candidiasis superimposed on hemochromatosis. *J Comput Assist Tomogr* 1990;14:774–776.

42. Choi BI, Im J-G, Han MC, Lee HS. Hepatosplenic tuberculosis with hypersplenism: CT evaluation. *Gastrointest Radiol* 1989;14:265–267.

43. Chou Y-H, Hsu C-C, Tiu C-M, Chang T. Splenic abscess: sonographic diagnosis and percutaneous drainage or aspiration. *Gastrointest Radiol* 1992;17:262–266.

44. Chun CH, Raff MJ, Contreras L, et al. Splenic abscess. *Medicine* 1980;59:50–65.

45. Clark RE, Korobkin M, Palubinskas AJ. Angiography of accessory spleens. *Radiology* 1972;102:41–44.

46. Cochrane LB, Freson M. Peliosis of the spleen. *Gastrointest Radiol* 1991;16:83–84.

47. Curtis GM, Movitz D. The surgical significance of the accessory spleen. *Ann Surg* 1946;123:276–298.

48. D'Altorio RA, Canno JY. Upside-down spleen as cause of suprarenal mass. *Urology* 1978;11:422–424.

49. Dachman AH, Ros PF, Marari PJ, Olmsted WW, Lichtenstein JE. Nonparasitic splenic cysts: a report of 52 cases with radiologic-pathologic correlation. *AJR* 1986;147:537–542.

50. Dardin JW, Teeslink R, Parrish RA. Hamartoma of the spleen: a manifestation of tuberous sclerosis. *Am Surg* 1975;41:564–566.

51. Das Gupta T, Coombes B, Brasfield RD. Primary malignant neoplasm of the spleen. *Surg Gynecol Obstet* 1965;120:947–960.

52. Dodds WJ, Taylor AJ, Erickson SJ, Stewart ET, Lawson TL. Radiologic imaging of splenic anomalies. *AJR* 1990;155:805–810.

53. Dourthe O, Maquin P, Pradere B, Railhac J-J. Splenic cyst: demonstration of the relationship between subcapsular hematoma and false cyst by imaging. *Br J Radiol* 1992;65:541–542.

54. Downer WR, Peterson MS. Massive splenic infarction and liquefactive necrosis complicating polycythemia vera. *AJR* 1993;161:79–80.

55. Duddy MJ, Calder CJ. Cystic haemangioma of the spleen: findings on ultrasound and computed tomography. *Br J Radiol* 1989;62:180–182.

56. Easler RE, Dowlin WM. Primary lipoma of the spleen. *Arch Pathol* 1969;88:557–559.

57. Ehrlich P, Jamieson CG. Nonparasitic splenic cysts: a case report and review. *Can J Surg* 1990;33:306–308.

58. Eraklis AJ, Filler RM. Splenectomy in childhood: review of 1413 cases. *J Pediatr Surg* 1972;7:382–388.

59. Faer MJ, Lynch RD, Lichtenstein JE, Feigin DS. Traumatic splenic cysts, RPC from the AFIP. *Radiology* 1980;134:371–376.

60. Farrer-Brown G, Bennett MH, Harrison CV, Millett Y, Jelliffe AM. The diagnosis of Hodgkin's disease in surgically excised spleens. *J Clin Pathol* 1972;25:294–300.

61. Feverstein IM, Francis P, Raffeld M, Pluda J. Widespread calcification in disseminated *Pneumocystis carinii* infection: CT characteristics. *J Comput Assist Tomogr* 1990;14:149–151.

62. Fishman EK, Kawashima A. Infections and diffuse diseases. In: Dachman AH, Friedman AC, eds. *Radiology of the spleen.* Baltimore: Mosby, 1993;138–170.

63. Fishman EK, Kuhlman JE, Jones RJ. CT of lymphoma: spectrum of disease. *Radiographics* 1991;11:647–669.

64. Fishman EK, Magid D, Kuhlman JE. *Pneumocystis carinii* involvement of the liver and spleen: CT demonstration. *J Comput Assist Tomogr* 1990;14:146–148.

65. Fitzgerald EJ, Coblentz C. Fungal microabscesses in immunosuppressed patients—CT appearances. *J Can Radiol Assoc* 1988;39:10–12.

66. Fowler RH. Collective review: hydatid cysts of the spleen. *Int Abstr Surg* 1953;96:105–116.

67. Franquet T, Montes M, Aizcorbe M, Barberena J, Ruiz De Azua Y, Cobo F. Inflammatory pseudotumor of the spleen: ultrasound and computed tomographic findings. *Gastrointest Radiol* 1989;14:181–183.

68. Franquet T, Montes M, Lecumberri FJ, Esparza J, Bescos JM. Hydatid disease of the spleen: imaging findings in nine patients. *AJR* 1990;154:525–528.

69. Frick MP, Feinberg SB, Loken MK. Noninvasive spleen scanning in Hodgkin's disease and non-Hodgkin's lymphoma. *Comput Tomogr* 1980;5:73–80.

70. Garvin DF, King FM. Cysts and nonlymphomatous tumors of the spleen. *Pathol Annu* 1981;16:61–80.

71. Gilbert T, Castellino RA. Critical review of the spleen in Hodgkin disease: diagnostic value of CT. *Invest Radiol* 1986;21:437–439.

72. Gilmartin D. Familial multiple epidermoid cyst of the spleen. *Conn Med* 1978;42(5):297–300.

73. Glazer GM, Axel L, Goldberg HI, Moss AA. Dynamic CT of the normal spleen. *AJR* 1981;137:343–346.

74. Glazer M, Lally J, Kanzer M. Inflammatory pseudotumor of the spleen: MR findings. *J Comput Assist Tomogr* 1992;16:980–983.

75. Gomori JM, Grossman RI, Drott HR. MR relaxation times and iron content of thalassemic spleens: an in vitro study. *AJR* 1988;150:567–569.

76. Gooding GAW. The ultrasonic and computed tomographic appearance of splenic lobulations: a consideration in the ultrasonic differential of masses adjacent to the left kideny. *Radiology* 1981;126:719–720.

77. Gordon DH, Burrell MI, Levin DC, Mueller CF, Becker JA. Wandering spleen—the radiological and clinical spectrum. *Radiology* 1977;125:39–46.

78. Griscom NT, Hargreaves HK, Schwartz MZ, Reddish JM, Colodny AH. Huge splenic cyst in a newborn: comparisons with 10 cases in later childhood and adolescence. *AJR* 1977;129:889–891.

79. Hadar H, Gadoth N, Herskovitz P, et al. Short pancreas in polysplenia syndrome. *Acta Radiol* 1991;32:299–301.

80. Hahn PF, Weissleder R, Stark DD, Saini S, Elizondo G, Ferrucci JT. MR imaging of focal splenic tumors. *AJR* 1988;150:823–827.

81. Halgrimson CG, Rustad DG, Zeligman BE. Calcified hemangioma of the spleen. *JAMA* 1984;252:2959–2960.

82. Halpert B, Gyorkey F. Lesions observed in accessory spleens of 311 patients. *Am J Clin Pathol* 1959;31:165–168.

83. Halvorsen RA, Dunnick NR, Thompson WM. Contrast agent enhancement in abdominal computed tomography: ionic vs. nonionic agents. *Invest Radiol* 1984;19:S234–S243.

84. Hansen S, Jarhult J. Accessory spleen imaging: radionuclide, ultrasound and CT investigations in a patient with thrombocytopenia 25 years after splenectomy for ITP. *Scand J Haematol* 1986;37:74–77.

85. Harris NL, Aisenberg AC, Meyer JE, Ellman L, Ellman A. Diffuse large cell (histiocytic) lymphoma of the spleen: clinical and pathologic characteristics of ten cases. *Cancer* 1984;54:2460–2467.

86. Hayward I, Mindelzeun RE, Jeffrey RB. Intrapancreatic accessory

spleen mimicking pancreatic mass on CT. *J Comput Assist Tomogr* 1992;16:984–985.

87. Herman TE, Siegel MJ. CT of acute spleen torsion in children with wandering spleen. *AJR* 1991;156:151–153.

88. Herman TE, Siegel MJ. Polysplenia syndrome with congenital short pancreas. *AJR* 1991;156:799–800.

89. Hess CF, Griebel J, Schmiedl U, Kurtz B, Koelbel G, Jaehde E. Focal lesions of the spleen: preliminary results with fast MR imaging at 1.5 T. *J Comput Assist Tomogr* 1988;12:569–574.

90. Housman JF, Chezmar JL, Nelson RC. Magnetic resonance imaging in hemochromatosis: extrahepatic iron deposition. *Gastrointest Radiol* 1989;14:59–60.

91. Hurd W, Katholi R. Acquired functional asplenia: association with spontaneous rupture of the spleen and fatal spontaneous rupture of the liver in amyloidosis. *Arch Intern Med* 1980;140:844–845.

92. Husni EA. The clinical course of splenic hemangioma. *Arch Surg* 1961;83:681–688.

93. Isikoff MB, White DW, Diaconis JN. Torsion of the wandering spleen, seen as a migratory abdominal mass. *Radiology* 1977;123:36.

94. Jelinek JS, Stuart PL, Done SL, Ghaed N, Rudd SA. MRI of polysplenia syndrome. *Magn Reson Imaging* 1989;7:681–686.

95. Jones TC. Cestodes (Tapeworms). In: Mandell GL, Douglas RG, Bennett JE, eds. *Principles and practice of infectious disease*, 3rd ed. New York: Churchill Livingston, 1990;2155–2156.

96. Joshi SN, Wolverson MK, Cusworth RB, Nair SG, Perrillo RP. Complementary use of computerized tomography and technetium scanning in the diagnosis of accessory spleen. *Dig Dis Sci* 1980;25:888–892.

97. Kabalka G, Buonocore E, Hubner K, Moss T, Norley N, Huang L. Gadolinium-labeled liposomes: targeted MR contrast agents for the liver and spleen. *Radiology* 1987;163:255–258.

98. Kadin ME, Glatstein E, Dorfman RF. Clinicopathologic studies of 117 untreated patients subjected to laparotomy for the staging of Hodgkin's disease. *Cancer* 1971;27:1277–1294.

99. Karpeh MS, Hicks DG, Torosian MH. Colon invasion by primary splenic lymphoma: a case report and review of the literature. *Surgery* 1992;111:224–227.

100. Kennan N, Evans C. Case report: hepatic and splenic calcifications due to amyloid. *Clin Radiology* 1991;44:60–61.

101. Kim H, Dorfman RF. Morphological studies of 84 untreated patients subjected to laparotomy for the staging of non-Hodgkin's lymphomas. *Cancer* 1974;33:657–674.

102. Kimbrell Jr OC. Sarcoidosis of the spleen. *New Engl J Med* 1957;257:128–131.

103. Kishikawa T, Numaguchi Y, Tokunaga M, Matsuura K. Hemangiosarcoma of the spleen with liver metastases: angiographic manifestations. *Radiology* 1977;123:31–35.

104. Koehler RE, Evens RG. The spleen. In: Teplick JG, Haskin MD, eds. *Surgical radiology*. Philadelphia: WB Saunders, 1981;1064–1088.

105. Krause R, Larsen CR, Scholz FJ. Gastrosplenic fistula: complication of adenocarcinoma of stomach. *Comput Med Imaging Graph* 1990;14:273–276.

106. Krumbhaar EB. The incidence and nature of splenic neoplasm. *Ann Clin Med* 1927;5:833–860.

107. Kyle R, Gertz M. Systemic amyloidosis. *Crit Rev Oncol Hematol* 1990;10:49–87.

108. Lackner K, Brecht G, Janson R, Scherholz K, Lutzeler A, Thurn P. Wertigkeit der Computertomographie bei der Stadieneinteilung primarer Lymphknotenneoplasien. *Fortschr Roentgenstr* 1980;132:21–30.

109. Lankisch PG. The spleen in inflammatory pancreatic disease. *Gastroenterology* 1990;98:509–516.

110. Lauteala L, Kormano M, Violante MR. Uptake and dissolution of particulate iodipamide ethyl ester in the spleen: a morphologic study. *Invest Radiol* 1987;22:829–835.

111. Lerner RM, Spataro RF. Splenic abscess: percutaneous drainage. *Radiology* 1984;153:643–645.

112. Levy DW, Rindsbert S, Friedman AC, et al. Thorotrast-induced hepatosplenic neoplasia: CT identification. *AJR* 1986;146:997–1004.

113. Levy DW, Wasserman PI, Weiland DE. Nonsuppurative gas for-mation in the spleen after transcatheter splenic infarction. *Radiology* 1981;139:375–376.

114. Liu T-Y, Chen S-C, Wang L-Y, Chuang W-L, Chang W-Y, Liu L-Y. Systemic amyloidosis presenting as splenic tumor. *Gastrointest Radiol* 1991;16:137–138.

115. Long JA, Doppman JL, Nienhus AW, Mills SR. Computed tomographic analysis of beta-thalassemic syndromes with hemochromatosis: pathologic findings with clinical and laboratory correlations. *J Comput Assist Tomogr* 1980;4:159–165.

116. Long JC, Aisenberg AC. Malignant lymphoma diagnosed at splenectomy and idiopathic splenomegaly: a clinicopathologic comparison. *Cancer* 1974;33:1054–1061.

117. Lubat E, Megibow AJ, Balthazar EJ, Goldenberg AS, Birnbaum BA, Bosniak MA. Extrapulmonary *Pneumocystis carinii* infection in AIDS: CT findings. *Radiology* 1990;174:157–160.

118. Magid D, Fishman EK, Charache S, Siegelman SS. Abdominal pain in sickle cell disease: the role of CT. *Radiology* 1987;163:325–328.

119. Magid D, Fishman EK, Siegelman SS. Computed tomography of the spleen and liver in sickle cell disease. *AJR* 1984;143:245–249.

120. Marani SA, Canossi GC, Nicoli FA, Alberti GP, Monni SG, Casolo PM. Hydatid disease: MR imaging study. *Radiology* 1990;175:701–706.

121. Marti-Bonmati L, Ballesta A, Chirivella M. Unusual presentation of non-Hodgkin lymphoma of the spleen. *J Can Assoc Radiol* 1989;40:49–50.

122. Marymont JGJ, Gross S. Patterns of metastatic cancer in the spleen. *Am J Clin Pathol* 1963;40:58–66.

123. Mata J, Alegret X, Llauger J. Splenic pseudocyst as a complication of ventriculoperitoneal shunt: CT features. *J Comput Assist Tomogr* 1986;10:341–342.

124. Mauro MA, Schiebler ML, Parker LA, Jaques PF. The spleen and its vasculature in pancreatitis: CT findings. *Am Surg* 1993;59:155–159.

125. Maves CK, Caron KH, Bisset III GS. Splenic and hepatic peliosis: MR findings. *AJR* 1992;158:75–76.

126. Mendenhall NP, Cantor AB, Williams JL, et al. With modern imaging techniques, is staging laparotomy necessary in pediatric Hodgkin's disease? A pediatric oncology group study. *J Clin Oncol* 1993;11:2218–2225.

127. Miller DL, Vermess M, Doppman JL, et al. CT of the liver and spleen with EOE-13: review of 225 examinations. *AJR* 1984;143:235–243.

128. Mirowitz S, Brown J, Lee J, Heiken J. Dynamic gadolinium-enhanced MR imaging of the spleen: normal enhancement patterns and evaluation of splenic lesions. *Radiology* 1991;179:681–686.

129. Mishalany H, Mahnovski V, Woolley M. Congenital asplenia and anomalies of the gastrointestinal tract. *Surgery* 1982;91:38–41.

130. Monforte-Mujnoz H, Ro JY, Manning JT, et al. Inflammatory pseudotumor of the spleen: report of two cases with a review of the literature. *Am J Clin Pathol* 1991;96:491–495.

131. Morgenstern L, McCaffertry L Jr, Michel SL. Hamartomas of the spleen. *Arch Surg* 1984;119:1291–1294.

132. Morgenstern L, Rosenberg J, Geller SA. Tumors of the spleen. *World J Surg* 1985;9:468–476.

133. Morinaga S, Ohyama R, Koizumi J. Low grade mucinous cystadenocarcinoma in the spleen. *Am J Surg Pathol* 1992;16:903–908.

134. Morissette JJ, Viamonte M, Viamonte M, Rolfs H. Primary spindle cell sarcoma of the spleen with angiographic demonstration. *Radiology* 1973;106:549–550.

135. Moss CN, Van Dyke JA, Koehler RE, Smedberg CT. Multiple cavernous hemangiomas of the spleen: CT findings. *J Comput Assist Tomogr* 1986;10:338–340.

136. Narang S, Wolf BC, Neiman RS. Malignant lymphoma presenting wth prominent splenomegaly: a clinicopathologic study with special reference to intermediate cell lymphoma. *Cancer* 1985;55:1948–1957.

137. Nebesar RA, Rabinov KR, Potsaid MA. Radionuclide imaging of the spleen in suspected splenic injury. *Radiology* 1974;110:609–614.

138. Nelken N, Ignathius J, Skinner M, Christensen N. Changing spectrum of splenic abscess: multicenter study and review of the literature. *Am J Surg* 1987;154:27–34.

139. Nelson RC, Chezmar JL, Peterson JE. Contrast-enhanced CT of the liver and spleen: comparison of ionic and nonionic contrast agents. *AJR* 1989;153:973–976.

140. Nemcek Jr AA, Miller FH, Fitzgerald SW. Acute torsion of a wandering spleen: diagnosis by CT and duplex Doppler and color flow sonography. *AJR* 1991;157:307–309.

141. Newmark H. Breast cancer metastasizing to the spleen seen on computerized tomography. *Comput Radiol* 1982;6:53–55.

142. Nguyen VD. Rare cause of splenic infarct and fleeting pulmonary infiltrates: polyarteritis nodosa. *Comput Med Imaging Graph* 1991;15:61–65.

143. Norowitz DG, Morehouse HT. Isodense splenic mass: hamartoma, a case report. *Comput Med Imaging Graph* 1989;13:347–350.

144. Nyman R, Rehn S, Glimelius B, et al. Magnetic resonance imaging, chest radiography, computed tomography, and ultrasonography in malignant lymphoma. *Acta Radiol* 1987;28:253–262.

145. Nyman R, Rhen S, Ericsson A, et al. An attempt to characterize malignant lymphoma in spleen, liver and lumph nodes with magnetic resonance imaging. *Acta Radiol* 1987;28:527–533.

146. Ohtomo K, Fukuda H, Mori K, Minami M, Itai Y, Inoue Y. CT and MR appearances of splenic hamartoma. *J Comput Assist Tomogr* 1992;16:425–428.

147. Okuda K, Taguchi T, Ishihara K, Konno A. Intrasplenic pseudocyst of the pancreas. *J Clin Gastroenterol* 1981;3:37–41.

148. Ough YD, Nash R, Wood DA. Mesothelial cysts of the spleen with squamous metaplasia. *Am J Clin Pathol* 1981;76:666–669.

149. Pakter RL, Fishman EK, Nussbaum A, Giargiana F, Zerhouni E. CT findings in splenic hemangiomas inthe Klippel-Trenaunay-Weber syndrome. *J Comput Assist Tomogr* 1987;11:88–91.

150. Pantongrag-Brown L, Suwanwela N, Arjhansiri K, Chetpukdeechit V, Kitisin P. Demonstration on computed tomography of two pseudoaneurysms complicating chronic pancreatitis. *Br J Radiol* 1991;64:754–757.

151. Parker LA, Mittelstaedt CA, Mauro MA, Mandell VS, Jaques PF. Torsion of a wandering spleen: CT appearance. *J Comput Assist Tomogr* 1984;8:1201–1204.

152. Pastakia B, Shawker TH, Thaler M, O'Leary T, Pizzo PA. Hepatosplenic candidiasis: wheels within wheels. *Radiology* 1988;166:417–421.

153. Payne NI, Whitehouse GH. Delineation of the spleen by a combination of proliposomes with water soluble contrast media: an experimental study using computed tomography. *Br J Radiol* 1987;60:535–541.

154. Pedro-Botet J, Maristany MT, Miralles R, Lopez-Colomes JL. Splenic tuberculosis in patients with AIDS. *Rev Infect Dis* 1991;13:1069–1071.

155. Peene P, Wilms G, Stockx L, Rigauts H, Vanhoenacker P, Baert AL. Splenic hemangiomatosis: CT and MR features. *J Comput Assist Tomogr* 1991;15:1070–1073.

156. Peoples WM, Moller JH, Edwards JE. Polysplenia: a review of 146 cases. *Pediatr Cardiol* 1983;4:129–137.

157. Perlmutter S, Jacobstein JG, Kazam E. Splenic uptake of 99m Tc-diphosphonate in sickle cell disease associated with increased splenic density on computerized transaxial tomography. *Gastrointest Radiol* 1977;2:77–79.

158. Perrone T, DeWolf-Peeters C, Frizzera G. Inflammatory pseudotumor of lymph nodes. *Am J Surg Pathol* 1988;12:351–361.

159. Piekarski J, Federle MP, Moss AA, London SS. CT of the spleen. *Radiology* 1980;135:683–689.

160. Pines B, Rabinovitch J. Hemangioma of the spleen. *Arch Pathol* 1942;33:487–503.

161. Pinkhas J, De Vries A, Safra D, Dollberg L. Diffuse angiomatosis with hypersplenism: splenectomy followed by polycythemia. *Am J Med* 1968;45:795–801.

162. Pistoia F, Markowitz SK. Splenic lymphangiomatosis: CT diagnosis. *AJR* 1988;150:121–122.

163. Pitlik S, Cohen L, Hadar H, Srulijes C, Rosenfield JB. Portal hypertension and esophageal varices in hemangiomatosis of the spleen. *Gastroenterology* 1977;72:937–940.

164. Pyatt RS, Williams ED, Clark M, Gasking R. CT diagnosis of splenic cystic lymphangiomatosis. *J Comput Assist Tomogr* 1981;5:446–448.

165. Quinn SF, vanSonnenberg E, Casola G, Wittich GR, Neff CC. Interventional radiology in the spleen. *Radiology* 1986;161:289–291.

166. Qureshi MA, Hafner CD. Clinical manifestations of splenic cysts: study of 75 cases. *Am Surg* 1965;31:605–608.

167. Rabushka LS, Kawashima A, Fishman EK. Imaging of the spleen: CT with supplemental MR examination. *Radiographics* 1994;14:307–322.

168. Radin DR, Kanel GC. Peliosis hepatis in a patient with human immunodeficiency virus infection. *AJR* 1991;156:91–92.

169. Rafal RB, Jennis R, Kosovsky PA, Markisz JA. MRI of primary amyloidosis. *Gastrointest Radiol* 1990;15:199–201.

170. Ragozzino MW, Singletary H, Patrick R. Familial splenic epidermoid cyst. *AJR* 1990;155:1233–1234.

171. Rathaus V, Zissin R, Goldberg E. Spontaneous rupture of an epidermoid cyst of spleen: preoperative ultrasonographic diagnosis. *J Clin Ultrasound* 1991;19:235–237.

172. Regelson W, Kim U, Ospina J, Holland JF. Hemangioendothelial sarcoma of liver from chronic arsenic intoxication by Fowler's solution. *Cancer* 1968;21:514–522.

173. Rizk GK, Tayyarah KA, Ghandur-Mnaymneh L. The angiographic changes in hydatid cysts of the liver and spleen. *Radiology* 1971;99:303–309.

174. Ros PR, Moser Jr RP, Dachman AH, Murari PJ, Olmsted WW. Hemangioma of the spleen: radiologic-pathologic correlation in ten cases. *Radiology* 1987;162:73–77.

175. Rose V, Izukawa T, Moes CAF. Syndromes of asplenia and polysplenia: a review of 60 cases with special reference to diagnosis and prognosis. *Br Heart J* 1975;37:840–852.

176. Roshkow JE, Sanders LM. Acute splenic sequestration crisis in two adults with sickle cell disease: US, CT, and MR imaging findings. *Radiology* 1990;177:723–725.

177. Safran D, Welch J, Rezuke W. Inflammatory pseudotumor of the spleen. *Arch Surg* 1991;126:904–908.

178. Salomonowitz E, Frick MP, Lund G. Radiologic diagnosis of wandering spleen complicated by spenic volvulus and infarction. *Gastrointest Radiol* 1984;9:57–59.

179. Sands MS, Violante MR. Computed tomographic enhancement of liver and spleen in the dog with iodipamide ethyl ester particulate suspensions. *Invest Radiol* 1987;22:408–416.

180. Schottenfeld LE, Wolfson WL. Cavernous hemangioma of the spleen. *Arch Surg* 1937;35:867–877.

181. Seids JV, Hauser H. Aneurysm of the splenic artery. *Radiology* 1941;36:171–180.

182. Selroos O. Fine needle aspiration biopsy of the spleen in diagnosis of sarcoidosis. *Ann N Y Acad Sci* 1976;278:517–521.

183. Selroos O, Koivunen E. Usefulness of fine-needle aspiration biopsy of spleen in diagnosis of sarcoidosis. *Chest* 1983;83:193–195.

184. Semelka RC, Shoenut JP, Greenberg HM, Bow EJ. Detection of acute and treated lesions of hepatosplenic candidiasis: comparison of dynamic contrast enhanced CT and MR imaging. *J Magn Reson Imaging* 1992;2:341–345.

185. Semelka RC, Shoenut JP, Lawrence PH, Greenberg HM, Madden TP, Kroeker MA. Spleen: dynamic enhancement patterns on gradient-echo MR images enhanced with gadopentetate dimeglumine. *Radiology* 1992;185:479–482.

186. Shanberge JN, Tanaka K, Gruhl MC. Chronic consumptive coagulopathy due to hemangiomatous transfromation of the spleen. *Am J Clin Pathol* 1971;56:723–729.

187. Sheflin JR, Lee CM, Kretchman KA. Torsion of wandering spleen and distal pancreas. *AJR* 1984;142:100–101.

188. Shiels WE, Johnson JF, Stephenson SR, Huang YC. Chronic torsion of the wandering spleen. *Pediatr Radiol* 1989;19:465–467.

189. Shirkhoda A. CT findings in hepatosplenic and renal candidiasis. *J Comput Assist Tomogr* 1987;11:795–798.

190. Shirkhoda A, Lopez-Berestein G, Holbert JM, Luna MA. Hepatosplenic fungal infection: CT and pathologic evaluation after treatment with liposomal amphotericin B. *Radiology* 1986;159:349–353.

191. Shirkhoda A, Wallace S, Sokhandan M. Computed tomography and ultrasonography in splenic infarction. *J Can Assoc Radiol* 1985;36:29–33.

192. Siegelman ES, Mitchell DG, Rubin R, et al. Parenchymal versus

reticuloendothelial iron overload in the liver: distinction with MR imaging. *Radiology* 1991;179:361–366.

193. Smith VC, Eisenberg BL, Mc Donald EC. Primary splenic angiosarcoma: case report and literature review. *Cancer* 1985;55:1625–1627.

194. Smulewicz JJ, Clement AR. Torsion of the wandering spleen. *Dig Dis* 1975;20:274–279.

195. Soderstrom N. How to use cytodiagnostic spleen puncture. *Acta Med Scand* 1976;199:1–5.

196. Solbiati L, Bossi MC, Bellotti E, Ravetto C, Montali G. Focal lesions in the spleen: sonographic patterns and guided biopsy. *AJR* 1983;140:59–65.

197. Sorgen RA, Robbins DI. Bleeding gastric varices secondary to wandering spleen. *Gastrointest Radiol* 1980;5:25–27.

198. Spencer JA, Golding SJ. Case of the month: not another case of aortic dissection! *Br J Radiol* 1993;66:565–566.

199. Sperling L. Aneurysm of the splenic artery. *Surgery* 1940;8:633–638.

200. Spier CM, Kjeldsberg CR, Eyre HJ, Behm FG. Malignant lymphoma with primary presentation in the spleen: a study of 20 patients. *Arch Pathol Lab Med* 1985;109:1076–1080.

201. Standiford SB, Sobel H, Dasmahaptra KS. Inflammatory pseudotumor of the liver. *J Surg Oncol* 1989;40:283–287.

202. Stanley JC, Fry WJ. Pathogenesis and clinical significance of splenic artery aneurysm. *Surgery* 1974;76:898–909.

203. Stark D. Hepatic iron overload: paramagnetic pathology. *Radiology* 1991;179:333–335.

204. Steinberg JJ, Suhrland MJ, Valensi QJ. The association of splenoma with disease. *Lab Invest* 1985;52:65A.

205. Stiris MG. Accessory spleen versus left adrenal tumor: computed tomographic and abdominal angiographic evaluation. *J Comput Assist Tomogr* 1980;4:543–544.

206. Strijk SP, Boetes C, Bogman MJJT, De Pauw BE, Wobbes T. The spleen in non-Hodgkin lymphoma: diagnostic value of computed tomography. *Acta Radiol* 1987;28:139–144.

207. Strijk SP, Wagener DJT, Bogman MJJT, de Pauw BE, Wobbes T. The spleen in Hodgkin disease: diagnostic value of CT. *Radiology* 1985;154:753–757.

208. Subramanyam BR, Balthazar EJ, Horii SC. Sonography of the accessory spleen. *AJR* 1984;143:47–49.

209. Suzuki S, Takizawa K, Nakajima Y, Katayama M, Sagawa F. CT findings in hepatic and splenic amyloidosis. *J Comput Assist Tomogr* 1986;10:332–334.

210. Taavitsainen M, Koivuniemi A, Helminen J, et al. Aspiration biopsy of the spleen in patients with sarcoidosis. *Acta Radiol* 1987;28:723–725.

211. Tada S, Shin M, Takashina T, et al. Diffuse capillary hemangiomatosis of the spleen as a cause of portal hypertension. *Radiology* 1972;104:63–64.

212. Taxy JB. Peliosis: a morphologic curiosity becomes an iatrogenic problem. *Hum Pathol* 1978;9:331–340.

213. Thomas JL, Bernardino ME, Vermess M, et al. EOE-13 in the detection of hepatosplenic lymphoma. *Radiology* 1982;145:629–634.

214. Thomsen C, Josephsen P, Karle H, Juhl E, Sorensen PG, Henriksen O. Determination of T1 and T2 relaxation times in the spleen of patients with splenomegaly. *Magn Reson Imaging* 1990;8:39–42.

215. Tikkakoski T, Siniluoto T, Paivansalo M, et al. Splenic abscess: imaging and intervention. *Acta Radiol* 1992;33:561–565.

216. Tiu CM, Chou YH, Wang HT, Chang T. Epitheloid hemangioendothelioma of spleen with intrasplenic metastasis: ultrasound and computed tomography appearance. *Comput Med Imaging Graph* 1992;16:287–290.

217. Tonkin ILD, Tonkin AK. Visceroatrial situs abnormalities: sonographic and computed tomographic appearance. *AJR* 1982;136:509–515.

218. Towers MJ, Withers CE, Hamilton PA, Kolin A, Walmsley S. Visceral calcification in patients with AIDS may not always be due to *Pneumocystis carinii*. *AJR* 1991;156:745–747.

219. Trastek VF, Pairolero PC, Joyce JW, Hollier LH, Bernatz PE. Splenic artery aneurysms. *Surgery* 1982;91:694–699.

220. Tsuda K, Nakamura H, Murakami T, et al. Peliosis of the spleen with intraperitoneal hemorrhage. *Abdom Imaging* 1993;18:283–285.

221. Tsurui N, Ishida H, Morikawa P, Ishii N, Hoshino T, Masamune O. Splenic lymphangioma: report of two cases. *J Clin Ultrasound* 1991;19:244–249.

222. Ueda J, Kobayashi Y, Hara K, Kawamura T, Ohmori Y, Uchida H. Giant aneurysm of the splenic artery and huge varix. *Gastrointest Radiol* 1985;10:55–57.

223. Veronesi U, Musumeci R, Pizzeti F, Gennari L, Bonadonna G. The value of staging laparotomy in non-Hodgkins lymphomas (with emphasis on histiocytic type). *Cancer* 1974;33:446–459.

224. Vibhakar SD, Bellon EM. The bare area of the spleen: a constant CT feature of the ascitic abdomen. *AJR* 1984;1412:953–955.

225. Vick CW, Simeone JF, Ferrucci JT, Wittenberg J, Mueller PR. Pancreatitis-associated fluid collections involving the spleen: sonographic and computed tomographic appearance. *Gastrointest Radiol* 1981;6:247–250.

226. von Sinner W, te Strake L, Clark D, Sharif H. MR imaging in hydatid disease. *AJR* 1991;157:741–745.

227. Vossen PG, Van Hedent EF, Degryse HR, De Schepper AM. Computed tomography of the polysplenia syndrome in the adult. *Gastrointest Radiol* 1987;12:209–211.

228. Vyborny CJ, Merrill TN, Reda J, Geurkiwk RE, Smith SJ. Subacute subcapsular hematoma of the spleen complicating pancreatitis: successful percutaneous drainage. *Radiology* 1988;169:161–162.

229. Wadham BM. Incidence and location of accessory spleens. *N Engl J Med* 1981;304:111.

230. Wang SJ, Chen J-J, Changchien C-S, et al. Sequential invasions of pancreatic pseudocysts in pancreatic tail, hepatic left lobe, caudate lobe and spleen. *Pancreas* 1993;8:133–136.

231. Warrell RP, Kempin SJ, Benua RS, Reiman RE, Young CW. Intratumoral consumption of indium-111 labeled platelets in a patient with hemangiomatosis and intravascular coagulation (Kasabach-Merritt syndrome). *Cancer* 1983;52:2256–2260.

232. Warren S, Davis AH. Studies on tumor metastasis: the metastases of carcinoma to the spleen. *Am J Cancer* 1981;21:517–533.

233. Warshauer DM, Dumbleton SA, Molina PL, Yankaskas BC, Parker LA, Woosley JT. Abdominal CT findings in sarcoidosis: radiologic and clinical correlation. *Radiology* 1994;192:93–98.

234. Weinreb N, Bauer J, Dikman S, Forte FA. Torsion of the spleen as a rare cause of hypersplenism. *JAMA* 1974;230:1015–1016.

235. Weissleder R, Elizondo G, Stark DD. Diagnosis of splenic lymphoma by MR imaging: value of superparamagnetic iron. *AJR* 1989;152:175–180.

236. Weissleder R, Hahn PF, Stark DD, et al. Superparamagnetic iron oxide: enhanced detection of focal splenic tumors with MR imaging. *Radiology* 1988;169:399–403.

237. Westcott JL, Krufky EL. The upside-down spleen. *Radiology* 1972;105:517–521.

238. Wick MR, Smith SL, Scheithauer BW, Beart RW. Primary nonlymphoreticular malignant neoplasm of the spleen. *Am J Surg Pathol* 1982;6:229–242.

239. Wiernik PH, Rader M, Becker NH, Morris SF. Inflammatory pseudotumor of spleen. *Cancer* 1990;66:597–600.

240. Wilson ME. *A world guide to infections: disease, distribution, diagnosis.* New York: Oxford University Press, 1991.

241. Winer-Muram HT, Tonkin ILD, Gold RE. Polysplenia syndrome in the asymptomatic adult: computed tomography evaluation. *J Thorac Imaging* 1991;6:69–71.

242. Wolf BC, Neiman RS. Disorders of the spleen. In: Bennington JL, ed. *Major problems in pathology,* vol 20. Philadelphia: WB Saunders, 1989.

243. Zissin R, Lishner M, Rathaus V. Case report: unusual presentation of splenic hamartoma; computed tomography and ultrasonic findings. *Clin Radiol* 1992;45:410–411.

CHAPTER 15

Pancreas

Robert J. Stanley and Richard C. Semelka

Computed tomography (CT) and ultrasonography are the most commonly used diagnostic imaging methods for the evaluation of the pancreas. Magnetic resonance imaging (MRI) has been shown to be comparable to CT, and in some instances superior, in the evaluation of certain aspects of pancreatic disease. However, it is not in widespread clinical use at the present time. Furthermore, calcifications that appear as nonspecific low to medium signal intensities on MRI cannot be confidently diagnosed as such. Other imaging methods, including endoscopic retrograde pancreatography, plain film radiography, contrast examinations of the gastrointestinal tract, angiography, endoscopic ultrasonography, and portal venous sampling (for the detection of hormone gradients in endocrine tumors of the pancreas), all have definite but lesser roles in the overall evaluation of pancreatic disease.

Implementation of new MR techniques that limit artifacts in the abdomen have increased the role of MRI to detect and characterize pancreatic disease. Breath holding and fat suppression techniques, and dynamic administration of gadolinium chelate have resulted in images of the pancreas of sufficient quality to detect and characterize pancreatic mass lesions as small as 1 cm in diameter (164,221,225,227). The combination of sequences also provides information on lesion characterization that was not formerly obtainable in a noninvasive fashion. MR cholangiography further increases the comprehensive nature of imaging investigation of pancreatic disease by MRI (165,240,243).

CT AND MRI TECHNIQUES

Standard routines for performing CT examinations of the abdomen are covered elsewhere in this text. If the pancreas is the primary organ of interest, whether for inflammatory or neoplastic disease, more specific, tailored protocols should be developed. A variety of techniques exist depending on whether dynamic sequential or helical scanning is used. The goals of the different techniques are similar, namely, to optimize the contrast enhancement of the pancreas, minimize motion and misregistration artifacts, and improve the detection of abnormalities, whether large or small (27,97).

With respect to the evaluation of a known or suspected pancreatic mass, the general goals of CT are to confirm the diagnosis, localize the mass, and evaluate for extent of disease, vascular involvement, and local or distant metastases. Suggested technical factors for both helical and incremental scanning equipment are listed in Table 1. If intravenous contrast medium is not contraindicated, a bolus intravenous (IV) contrast injection (3 ml/sec 180 ml high osmolar or 150 ml low osmolar) may be used. Oral contrast (approx. 750 to 1000 ml 3% iodine water solution) is highly desirable.

For the initial CT study of a mass, noncontrast images through the pancreas may be helpful. If one is using a nonhelical (incremental) scanner, it may be helpful to start at the bottom of the pancreas or at the iliac crest and scan upward to reach the pancreas earlier in the enhancement phase in order to provide more contrast between enhancing parenchyma and hypo-enhancing carcinoma or hyper-enhancing neuroendocrine tumors. With a helical scanner, a set of images can be obtained during the arterial phase of contrast enhancement (after a 30 to 35 sec delay) followed by images during the venous phase (70-sec total delay) (27). Contiguous 5-mm axial images or 5-mm helical images are obtained through the pancreas to decrease volume averaging effects. During the arterial phase of a helical scan, 3-mm images may be obtained

TABLE 1. *CT techniques for pancreatic mass*

Initial CT of mass:	Helical	Incremental
Mode:	Helical	Dynamic (2 sec with ~4 sec interscan delay)
Delay:	30–35 sec for arterial images 70 sec for venous images	20–30 sec
kVp:	120	120
mAs:	220–330	280–340 (140–170 mA for 2 sec)
Slice thickness:	3–5 mm for arterial images 5 mm for venous images Pitch 1:1–2:1	5 mm at 5-mm interval
Comments:	Precontrast 7–10 mm axial scans	Precontrast 7- to 10-mm axial scans. Start below the pancreas and scan upward to reach the pancreas earlier in its enhancement

on most patients (unless the patient is exceptionally large) to further decrease volume averaging. In order to provide adequate volume of coverage for these 3- and 5-mm thickness scans during a single breath-hold, and to minimize tube heating, the pitch may have to be increased up to 2:1.

For the follow-up of most pancreatic masses a routine abdominal scan is usually adequate. This would involve no noncontrast images and, with an incremental scanner, would start at the top of the liver with a 45-sec delay. However, for precise, presurgical evaluation, the same protocol as used for the initial evaluation of the mass should be used.

When pancreatitis is the clinical concern, the general goals of the CT examination are occasionally to confirm an uncertain diagnosis, but more often to evaluate for complications such as hemorrhage, infection, fluid collections, pancreatic necrosis, vascular thrombosis, or pseudoaneurysms. Technical factors for helical and incremental units in the initial evaluation of pancreatitis are listed in Table 2. Regarding intravenous and oral contrast media, the same protocol as is used for a pancreatic mass applies. For the initial CT evaluation of known or suspected pancreatitis, when there is a question of hemorrhagic pancreatitis, noncontrast images through the pancreas may be advisable for baseline assessment of attenuation values. For the initial evaluation of suspected

pancreatic necrosis, one should start at the bottom of the pancreas or at the iliac crest and scan upward to reach the pancreas earlier in the enhancement phase to provide more contrast between enhancing and nonenhancing parenchyma. Because this is not as significant a concern with a helical scanner, which can scan through the region of the pancreas very quickly, scanning may start at the top of the liver and proceed caudally. If the question is simply to confirm the diagnosis of pancreatitis, it may be helpful to perform 5-mm helical images through the pancreas or 5-mm contiguous axial images to maximize sensitivity to the more subtle findings of pancreatitis. However, this is usually not required.

For the follow-up of pancreatitis a routine abdominal scan is usually adequate (no noncontrast images and, with an incremental scanner, starting at the top of the liver with a 45-sec delay). Suggested technical factors for both helical and incremental units are shown in Table 3.

A standard MR protocol includes T1-weighted fat-suppressed imaging (T1FS) and spoiled gradient refocused echo (GRE) sequences (225). T2-weighted imaging of the pancreas is not routinely performed, but is used for the investigation of associated liver metastases or for patients with pancreatic endocrine tumors (221). Limitations of routine use of T2-weighted imaging of the pancreas include motion artifact from breathing and peristalsis, poor contrast resolution between pancreatic parenchyma and

TABLE 2. *CT techniques for pancreatitis*

Initial CT of episode:	Helical	Incremental
Mode:	Helical	Dynamic (2 sec with ~4 sec interscan delay)
Delay:	70 sec	20–30 sec
kVp:	120	120
mAs:	240–330	280–340 (140–170 mA for 2 sec)
Slice thickness:	7 mm, 1:1 pitch	5 mm at 10-mm interval
Comments:	Precontrast 7- to 10-mm axial scans	Precontrast 7- to 10-mm axial scans. Start below the pancreas and scan upward to reach the pancreas earlier in its enhancement

TABLE 3. *CT techniques for follow-up of pancreatitis*

Follow-up pancreatitis (routine abdomen):	Helical	Incremental
Mode:	Helical	Dynamic (2 sec with ~4 sec interscan delay)
Delay:	70 sec	45 sec
kVp:	120	120
mAs:	240–330	280–340 (140–170 mA for 2 sec)
Slice thickness:	7 mm, 1:1 pitch	5 mm at 10-mm interval
Comments:	Can increase pitch up to 2:1 as needed to increase coverage or decrease tube heating	

surrounding tissues, poor contrast resolution between pancreatic parenchyma and carcinoma, and the prolonged length of the study. T2-weighted fat-suppressed spin echo (T2FS) is a good T2-weighted technique in that removal of fat signal improves the conspicuity of high signal intensity diseased tissue such as pancreatic endocrine tumors. The implementation of breathing-independent T2-weighted sequences such as Half-Fourier single shot turbo spin-echo (HASTE) may increase the role of T2-weighted images for the investigation of pancreatic diseases. Reproducible high image quality is achieved with this for the investigation of abdominal disease (224).

Various bright bile MR cholangiographic techniques have been recently introduced that generate three-dimensional (3-D) datasets allowing reconstructions of the biliary and pancreatic ducts. In the future, MR cholangiography may provide diagnostic information when endoscopic retrograde cholangiopancreatography (ERCP) fails because high-grade ductal obstruction in the head of the pancreas does not interfere with the MR technique.

Spoiled gradient echo images are acquired precontrast and immediately following rapid bolus injection of intravenous gadolinium while the patient is positioned in the bore of the magnet. The sequence is initiated immediately

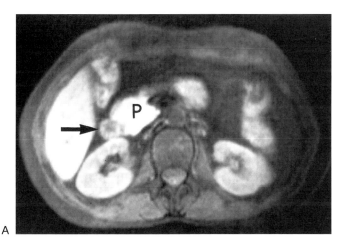

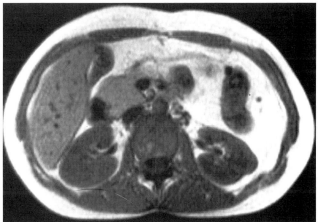

FIG. 1. Normal pancreatic head. T1FS (SE 500/15) (**A**), FLASH (140/4/80°) (**B**) and immediate postgadolinium FLASH (**C**). Normal pancreatic tissue (p) is high in signal on noncontrast T1FS images and is clearly separated from bowel, which has a lower signal with a feathery appearance (*arrow,* A). Pancreas is of approximately similar signal to liver on FLASH images (B) and enhances substantially immediately following gadolinium administration (C).

following a rapid normal saline flush. A T1-weighted fat-suppressed sequence is repeated at 40-sec postcontrast, and a spoiled GRE sequence (FLASH) is repeated at 5 to 10 min. The normal pancreas is isointense relative to liver on spoiled GRE (FLASH) and hyperintense relative to liver on T1FS images due to the presence of aqueous protein in the glandular elements of the pancreas. On immediate postcontrast images, the pancreas demonstrates a uniform capillary blush that renders it higher in signal intensity than liver and adjacent fat (225) (Fig. 1). On 10-min post-contrast spoiled GRE (FLASH) images, the pancreas has diminished signal intensity relative to fat.

MR imaging of the pancreas performed at high field (>1.0 Tesla) allows good signal-to-noise (S/N) ratio for breath-hold imaging and adequate fat–water frequency shift for chemically selective, excitation spoiling fat suppression. A study comparing six T2-weighted sequences for the evaluation of the pancreas, using quantitative and qualitative measures, found that chemically selective fat suppression was useful and that a spoiled gradient refocused echo (GRE) technique, fast low-angle shot (FLASH), was a good breath-hold technique (228).

NORMAL ANATOMY

As experience with various cross-sectional imaging methods has grown, so too has our knowledge and understanding of normal and pathologic pancreatic anatomy. Considerable variation exists in the size, shape, and location of the normal pancreas, depending on differences in body habitus as well as the normal or abnormal size and positioning of contiguous organs. In the most common normal configuration, the long axis of the body and tail of the pancreas lies in an oblique orientation, extending from the hilum of the spleen, at its lateral and most cephalad extent, toward the midline of the body, where it passes anterior to that portion of the portal vein where it is being formed by the confluence of the superior mesenteric vein and splenic vein (Fig. 2). At this point the pancreas turns caudally in a more vertical orientation ending in the uncinate process, its most caudal extent. The main pancreatic duct in most people represents the fusion of the dorsal duct (Santorini) and the ventral duct (Wirsung), and empties into the duodenal lumen through the major papilla. In a third or slightly more of normal individuals, a separate drainage site for the continuation of the ventral duct is located in the medial wall of the duodenum proximal to the major papilla, referred to as the minor papilla. Details of the development of the pancreatic duct system, including normal variations and congenital anomalies, can be found in a 1994 comprehensive report (218). High-quality CT and MRI can define the anatomy of the pancreas, including its duct system, with great precision, affording information on the integrity of the pancreatic parenchyma, the caliber of the duct system, and the intimate relationships of the pancreas to surrounding anatomic structures (Fig. 3).

FORM

Modern real-time ultrasound, CT, and MRI consistently show that the thickness of the normal pancreatic parenchyma, measured perpendicular to its long axis on the cross-sectional view, varies depending on whether the head, neck, body, or tail is measured. The thickness of the head averages approximately 2 cm; the neck of the pancreas, just anterior to the portal vein, is the thinnest portion, ranging in thickness from 0.5 to 1.0 cm; the body and tail range from 1.0 to 2.0 cm, with many normal glands tapering slightly toward the tail (Fig. 2). The cephalocaudal dimension of the body and tail ranges from 3.0 to 4.0 cm in most individuals, whereas the cephalocaudal dimension of the head is more variable, and portions of the head can be seen over distances ranging from 3 cm to as much as 8 cm. With respect to size and shape, the most reliable indicator of a pancreatic mass has been the presence of an abrupt focal change rather than generalized variations from the range of normal dimensions. However, with the use of high-quality, contrast-enhanced helical CT imaging, subtle focal changes in the pancreatic parenchyma, indicative of the presence of a tumor, which do not change the size or shape of the pancreas can be defined (142). Recent detailed analyses of normal variations in the lateral contour of the head and neck of the pancreas, obtained with helical CT scanners, have shown three general categories of variation from the normal flat interface of the lateral border of the head of the pancreas to the medial wall of the duodenum which could be misinterpreted as a focal mass (208). In each instance, the character of the enhancement of the focal variation was identical to the adjacent normal pancreatic parenchyma, studied during its arterial and capillary phase, allowing a correct interpretation. Newer techniques with MRI also allow for detection of subtle lesions that do not alter the size or shape of the pancreas.

The surface contour of the pancreatic parenchyma can be either smooth or lobular, the latter being more frequently seen when there is abundant peripancreatic, retroperitoneal fat. Although the pancreas is totally invested in fine connective tissue, it does not have a true fibrous capsule. Therefore, the lobular architecture of the pancreas is well defined by the interdigitating peripancreatic fat. Fatty replacement of much of the pancreatic substance is a common degenerative process seen in the elderly. However, marked interdigitation of peripancreatic fat can simulate this late degenerative process in obese individuals (Fig. 4). As will be discussed in more detail later, fatty replacement may be associated with alterations in pancreatic function and may be a late sequel to various forms of chronic pancreatitis.

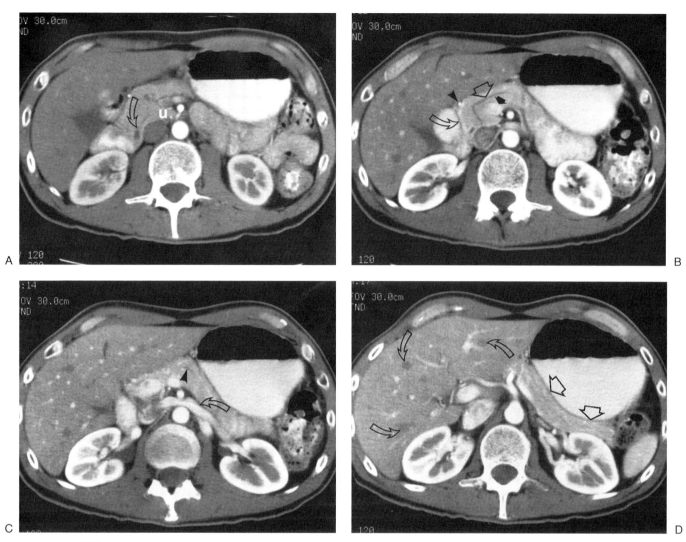

FIG. 2. Normal pancreas studied with contrast-enhanced helical CT. Because of the paucity of perivisceral fat, the surface of the pancreas has a smooth rather than lobular appearance. All portions of the pancreas are clearly defined in the early arterial and capillary phase of this dynamic study. **A:** At the level of the pancreatic head and uncinate process (u), the junction of the main pancreatic duct and common bile duct (*curved arrow*) is clearly defined. The brightly enhancing superior mesenteric artery lies directly anterior to the aorta and posterior to the junction of the neck and body of the pancreas. **B:** At the level of the neck of the pancreas, a normal caliber main pancreatic duct (*open arrow*) is visible over several centimeters of its length. The portal vein, only partially enhanced in this early phase (*black arrow*), lies immediately posterior to the neck of the pancreas and lateral to the superior mesenteric artery. The tissue plane separating the lateral surface of the pancreatic head and medial wall of the duodenum (*curved arrow*) is well seen at this level. *Arrowhead,* Anterior superior pancreaticoduodenal artery, which is also visible in Fig. 2A. **C:** More cephalad at the level of the body of the pancreas, a short segment of the main pancreatic duct (*arrowhead*) is visible. As the contrast reaches the early venous phase, the left renal vein (*curved arrow*) is well opacified. **D:** At this most cephalad level the body and tail of the pancreas are now seen to be uniformly enhanced and sharply defined by the posterior wall of the stomach (*arrows*). The hepatic veins (*curved arrows*) are not yet enhanced at this phase.

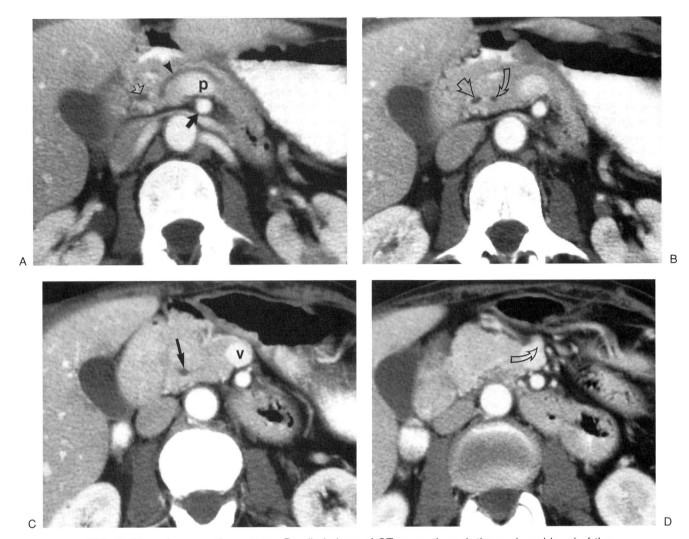

FIG. 3. Normal pancreatic anatomy. Detailed views of CT scans through the neck and head of the pancreas. **A:** The main pancreatic duct lies in the plane of the CT scan as it passes through the neck of the pancreas (*arrowhead*). The enhancing portal vein (p) lies immediately posterior to the neck. The superior mesenteric artery lies posterior to the portal vein at this level and anterior to the left renal vein (*black arrow*). The caliber of the main pancreatic duct at this level is approximately 2.5 mm. A normal caliber common bile duct (*open arrow*) lies lateral to the main pancreatic duct. **B:** At this level both the normal caliber common bile duct (*arrow*) and main pancreatic duct (*curved arrow*) are seen in cross-section as they approach the ampulla. **C:** 5 mm caudal, the main pancreatic duct and common bile duct have joined to form the ampulla (*arrow*). Note that in this patient, the head of the pancreas lies directly anterior to the aorta rather than to the right of it. The superior mesenteric artery lies posterior to the superior mesenteric vein (v). **D:** CT section just caudal to the entry of the ampulla into the major papilla. No ducts are visible at this level, which is through the most caudal portion of the head of the pancreas and uncinate process. Note the gastrocolic trunk (*curved arrow*) as it enters the anterior aspect of the superior mesenteric vein.

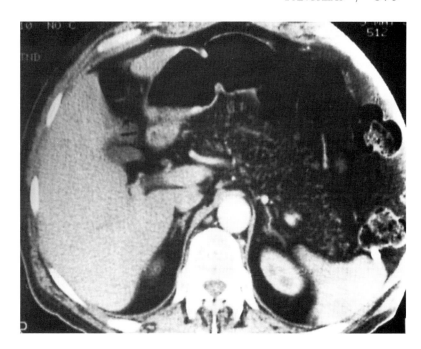

FIG. 4. Fatty replacement. In this elderly patient with no clinical evidence of pancreatic insufficiency, the individual lobules of the pancreas are so widely separated one from another by extensive fatty infiltration that it is difficult to differentiate the body and tail of the pancreas from the surrounding retroperitoneal fat. There was no prior history of pancreatic disease.

Part or all of the normal main pancreatic duct can be seen in nearly all patients studied, if high-detail CT technique is employed. With such high-resolution, contrast-enhanced, thin section technique, the portion of the duct within the head of the pancreas, perpendicular to the plane of the slice, is most conspicuous (see Fig. 3). Such technique also greatly increases the chances of demonstrating that portion of the duct in the body and tail of the pancreas, which lies generally parallel to the plane of the CT image (see Fig. 2).

ANATOMIC RELATIONSHIPS

The splenic vein lies on the dorsal surface of the body and tail of the pancreas, caudal to the splenic artery. In comparison with the more tortuous course of the splenic artery, the vein runs closely parallel to the longitudinal orientation of the pancreas. Depending upon how much retroperitoneal fat is present, a thin fat plane may separate the anterior surface of the splenic vein from the posterior surface of the pancreatic parenchyma. The left adrenal gland lies posteromedial to the splenic vein and the pancreas at the junction of the body and tail.

The tail of the pancreas extends to the splenic hilum, entering the splenorenal ligament and becoming intraperitoneal for a short distance. Although generally located anterior to the splenic vein, the tail of the pancreas occasionally may be imaged in the same plane as, or even posterior to, the splenic vein or a tributary. The body and tail of the pancreas normally are located anterior or anterolateral to the left kidney. However, in a patient lacking a left kidney (surgically removed or congenitally absent), or in a patient with an ectopic left kidney, the body and tail will be displaced posteromedially, lying adjacent to the spine and occupying the empty renal fossa. Usually, there is an accompanying posteromedial rotation in the position of the spleen.

The body of the pancreas arches anteriorly over the superior mesenteric artery, close to its origin from the aorta, separated by a distinct fat plane, which encircles the superior mesenteric artery in all but the leanest individuals. The superior mesenteric vein runs parallel and to the right of the superior mesenteric artery and usually is larger in diameter. At the point where the superior mesenteric vein joins the splenic vein to form the portal vein, the neck of the pancreas, the thinnest segment of the pancreas in the anteroposterior (AP) dimension, is seen to pass immediately ventral to the portal vein. Generally, there is no intervening fat plane between the neck of the pancreas and the portal vein. The presence of a fat plane between the lateral surface of the superior mesenteric vein and the medial aspect of the uncinate process of the pancreatic head is variable.

The head of the pancreas lies medial to the second portion of the duodenum, to the right of the superior mesenteric vein, and anterior to the inferior vena cava (IVC). Generally, a thin, distinct fat plane separates the posterior surface of the head of the pancreas from the anterior surface of the IVC. The uncinate process of the pancreatic head is a curving, beak-like inferior and medial extension of the head that originates lateral to the superior mesenteric vein and curves posteriorly behind it, approximately at the level of the left renal vein.

With the improvement in techniques afforded by helical CT scanners, finer details of arterial and venous anatomy can be defined. The arterial and venous structures that lie anterior and posterior to the pancreatic head can now be identified in a significant percentage of patients. A recent study evaluated the appearance of the normal gastrocolic trunk, which courses over the anterior surface of the head of the pancreas. The gastrocolic trunk is formed by veins that lie in the transverse mesocolon, one of which is the right gastroepiploic vein, as well as an anterior pancreaticoduodenal vein (167). The authors reported being able to identify a normal gastrocolic trunk (2.6 to 4.7 mm diameter) in approximately half of a control group, when the CT scans were obtained with 10-mm-thick sections, and in 90% of CT scans obtained with 5-mm-thick sections (see Fig. 3). They also noted abnormal dilatation of the gastrocolic trunk in cases where the superior mesenteric vein or portal vein, downstream from the junction of the gastrocolic trunk and superior mesenteric vein, were involved by disease resulting in stenosis, occlusion, or thrombosis (167).

In a small percentage of patients, the head of the pancreas may lie in a position that is completely to the left of the aorta. Although this situation may develop because of an enlarging mass in the liver or peripancreatic area, displacing the pancreas to the left, it has also been seen in patients with no relevant abdominal disease. In these instances, despite the fact that the head of the pancreas is completely to the left of the aorta, the pancreas still bears the normal relationship to the superior mesenteric vein and artery. It has been suggested that the left-sided pancreas may be an acquired positional variation due to increasing laxity of retroperitoneal tissues occurring with age, as well as tortuosity of the abdominal aorta, causing it to swing farther to the right than usual. In one study, all of the patients who had a left-sided pancreas and no associated abdominal disease were over the age of 50 years (63).

The normal-sized common bile duct, varying in diameter from 3 to 6 mm, can be seen in cross-section within the head of the pancreas, close to its lateral and posterior surface, appearing as a circular or oval near water density structure. Its detectability is improved if the surrounding substance of the pancreatic parenchyma is enhanced by intravenous contrast material. Under optimal imaging conditions, the vertically oriented segment of the main pancreatic duct lying in the head can be seen running parallel and medial to the common bile duct, ranging in diameter from 1 to 3 mm (see Figs. 2 and 3).

The pancreas lies in the anterior pararenal space and is related to the second segment of the duodenum along the lateral surface of the head and to the third and fourth segments of the duodenum along the inferior surface of the head, body, and tail. The stomach lies anterior to the pancreas and is separated from it by the parietal peritoneum and the lesser sac, a potential space. The transverse mesocolon, which forms the inferior boundary of the lesser sac, is formed by the fusion of the parietal peritoneal leaves as they fuse and extend anteriorly from the

ventral surface of the pancreas along its entire length. The significance of this anatomic relationship between the transverse colon and the pancreas via the transverse mesocolon becomes important in acute pancreatitis because this peritoneal communication serves as a pathway for the flow of inflammatory exudates associated with pancreatitis.

When retroperitoneal perivisceral fat is abundant, the pancreas will be well defined. However, even in lean patients, the pancreas can be accurately delineated by the use of ample quantities of oral contrast material to opacify the lumen of contiguous loops of bowel and intravenous contrast material to delineate the intra- and peripancreatic vascular structures.

DEVELOPMENTAL VARIANTS AND ANOMALIES

Pancreas divisum, the most common anatomic variant of the human pancreas, is defined as a completely separate pancreatic ductal system in a grossly undivided gland. It results from failure of fusion of the dorsal and ventral pancreatic ducts, which normally occurs in the second month in utero. The main portion of the pancreas, including the superior-anterior part of the head, the body, and the tail, is drained by the dorsal pancreatic duct through the accessory papilla. The posterior-inferior part of the head and uncinate process is drained by the short, narrow ventral pancreatic duct that joins the common bile duct in the ampulla. In autopsy series, pancreas divisum has an incidence of 5% to 10%; as an ERCP finding, its incidence is approximately 4% (169). In a series of patients with pancreatitis, however, there was a 16% incidence of pancreas divisum, and the incidence of the abnormality increased to 25% in idiopathic pancreatitis (49). Therefore, it appears as though pancreas divisum is associated with pancreatitis.

The diagnosis of pancreas divisum can be suggested with high- detail CT and MRI when an isolated ventral duct is identified or if separate dorsal and ventral pancreatic moieties can be defined (Fig. 5). Although the overall size of the pancreas may be normal in this developmental variant, the cranial caudal extent or the AP thickness of the pancreatic head may be increased. Additionally, the ventral and dorsal pancreatic moieties may be distinctly visible, separated by a fat plane (285).

Annular pancreas, a rare developmental anomaly with only three cases reported among 20,000 autopsies reported (107,198), may be suggested on CT by apparent thickening of the anterior, lateral, and posterior aspect of the descending duodenum caused by tissue having a density and enhancement characteristics identical to that of the pancreatic parenchyma in the head (Fig. 6) (2,102,107). The diagnosis of annular pancreas on CT will be reinforced by the typical changes on an upper

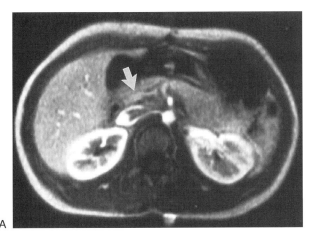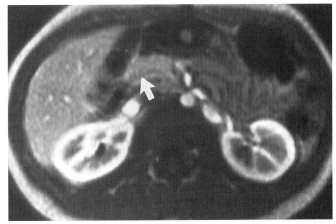

A B

FIG. 5. Pancreas divisum. Gadolinium enhanced FLASH images show normal pancreatic enhancement (**A, B**). Separate entry into the duodenum of the ducts of Santorini (*arrow,* A) and Wirsung (*arrow,* B) can be identified with no continuity between the ducts. (Reproduced with permission from ref. 226.)

gastrointestinal examination and confirmed by successful demonstration of that portion of the pancreatic duct system within the annular component by ERCP (Fig. 6E).

Agenesis of the dorsal pancreatic moiety has been reported (229). In this developmental anomaly, only the head of the pancreas is visible on CT. No pancreatic parenchyma can be identified in the expected locations of the neck, body, and tail. In contrast to pancreas divisum, dorsal pancreas agenesis is an extremely rare anomaly. Because most of the islet cells are located in the tail of the pancreas, the absence of the body and tail may contribute to the development of diabetes. Most of the reported cases of complete agenesis of the dorsal pancreas were in patients with diabetes mellitus (273). A case of dorsal pancreas passing through a posterior defect in the diaphragm immediately lateral to the right crus, presenting as a mass in the right cardiophrenic angle, has been reported (47).

PATHOLOGIC CONDITIONS

Neoplasia

Adenocarcinoma

Cancer of the pancreas is currently the ninth most common malignancy, but it represents the fourth most common cause of cancer-related death. Between 24,000 and 27,000 new cases will be diagnosed in the United States annually (170,276). In this country, pancreatic cancer has a peak incidence in the seventh and eighth decades. Adenocarcinoma accounts for between 90% and 95% of all primary pancreatic malignant neoplasms. With respect to risk factors, there is evidence to indicate an increased risk of pancreatic cancer associated with diabetes and with cigarette smoking, but the relationship to alcohol intake and to chronic pancreatitis is less clear (28,69,86,141).

The signs and symptoms of pancreatic cancer are varied and nonspecific. Other diseases may cause features identical to those experienced by patients with pancreatic cancer. Weight loss and pain are common features for patients with pancreatic cancer, whether in the head, body, or tail. One distinguishing sign is the presence of jaundice, which will be present in >80% of patients with a tumor in the head, whereas it is most unusual for this to be present in patients with body and tail neoplasms. The jaundice of pancreatic cancer is almost always associated with pain and the concept of painless jaundice being typical for cancer of the pancreas should be abandoned (60,81,101,115).

The majority (60% to 65%) of pancreatic carcinomas occur in the head, whereas approximately 20% and 10% occur in the body and tail, respectively. Between 5% and 10% involve the pancreas diffusely (42,73). Because of the pancreatic head's intimate involvement with the common bile duct and duodenum, tumors that arise there tend to present clinically at an earlier stage than those that occur in the body or tail (Figs. 7 and 8). Consequently, they tend to be smaller at the time of discovery than those in the body or tail. However, on rare occasion, very large tumors arising in the head may be present without causing jaundice (Fig. 9).

Recent studies continue to support the view that CT should be the initial diagnostic procedure in any patient who is suspected of having a pancreatic neoplasm. The report of the Radiology Diagnostic Oncology Group, in which the relative values of CT versus MRI in the imaging of pancreatic adenocarcinoma were compared, concluded that CT is recommended for initial imaging assessment (154). While ultrasonography is widely used as an initial screening procedure, it has not been found to be as sensi-

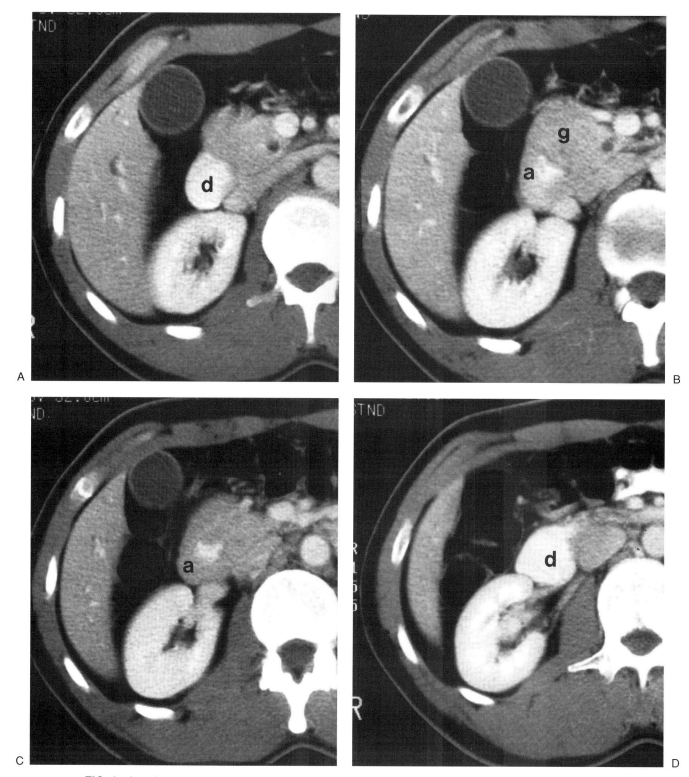

FIG. 6. Annular pancreas in a patient with a glucagonoma. **A–D:** Images of the head of the pancreas moving in a cephalocaudal direction show the normal caliber lumen of the second duodenum (d) above and below an annular pancreas (a) incidentally discovered in a patient being evaluated for a suspected glucagonoma (g), which produces a prominent anterior bulge in the surface of the head of the pancreas without an appreciable difference in enhancement compared to the normal parenchyma.

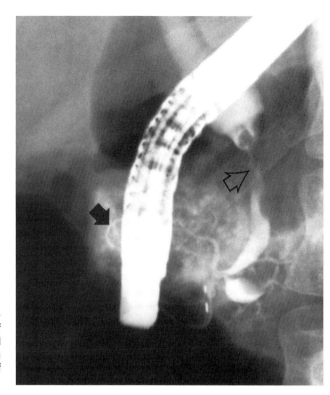

E

FIG. 6. (*Continued.*) **E:** Detailed view of an endoscopic retrograde cholangiopancreatography (ERCP) shows that portion of the pancreatic duct (*black arrow*) draining the annular ventral moiety. The glucagonoma is shown to be partially obstructing the distal common bile duct (*curved arrow*). (ERCP courtesy of Dr. Todd Baron, Birmingham, Alabama.)

tive in defining the entire constellation of important findings related to pancreatic malignancies including local nodal spread or involvement of the major arterial and venous structures. CT is of value in the staging of the neoplasm as well as the determination of resectability of the tumor (11,72,73,78,154,209,267).

Recent reports on the role of endoscopic ultrasonography indicate that this diagnostic method may have considerable value in cases where a mass is not readily apparent (137,207,239). However, this diagnostic method is limited in its availability to a few centers in Europe, Japan, and the United States.

The CT appearance of pancreatic adenocarcinomas is variable. If intravenous contrast medium is not administered, the attenuation value of the tumor generally is very similar to that of normal parenchyma, unless extensive necrosis or cystic change is present. Therefore, without intravenous contrast medium, these tumors usually will be recognized only when they become large enough to cause a focal distortion in the expected pancreatic contour. If intravenous contrast medium is administered, using bolus technique and rapid, thin section scanning, especially with helical CT, most adenocarcinomas will be hypoenhancing with respect to the surrounding uninvolved pancreatic parenchyma (Figs. 9 and 10). With such techniques, small tumors that do not produce a visible mass or alter the contour of the gland will nevertheless be detectable as a focal area of diminished enhancement (see Fig. 8) (5,11,73,98,99,153).

Conventional spin-echo MR images are generally of limited value in the detection of pancreatic cancer (245).

However, T1-weighted images, either spin-echo or GRE, are useful to evaluate extension of tumor into peripancreatic tissue (185,263). Tumor tissue is low in signal and contrasts well with high-signal peripancreatic fat. Fat-suppressed T1-weighted spin-echo images have inherently high contrast resolution for imaging of the pancreas and may be well suited for the detection of small, non-organ-deforming tumors (80). Detection of cancer with MRI is best performed by T1FS and immediate post-gadolinium spoiled GRE images (Fig. 11) (225). Normal pancreatic tissue is well delineated from tumors and the interface between the two can be well demonstrated on MR images (Fig. 12). MRI is particularly well suited for the detection or exclusion of small pancreatic cancers in patients who demonstrate enlargement of the pancreatic head without clear definition of tumor on helical CT examination (223). Staging of pancreatic cancer requires the addition of noncontrast T1-weighted spin echo or spoiled GRE for local tumor extension (263) and T2FS for detection of liver metastases. Thin image section thickness is also helpful; however, 8- mm sections may be sufficiently thin to detect small cancers due to the high contrast resolution.

In an evaluation of the conspicuity of pancreatic tumors using two-phase helical CT techniques, pancreatic tumors were better seen during the pancreatic phase (40 to 70 sec after infusion of IV contrast material) than during the hepatic phase (70 to 100 sec after infusion) (142). Factors considered included mean pancreatic enhancement, mean tumor enhancement, and tumor–pancreas contrast. In addition, peripancreatic arterial and venous enhancement

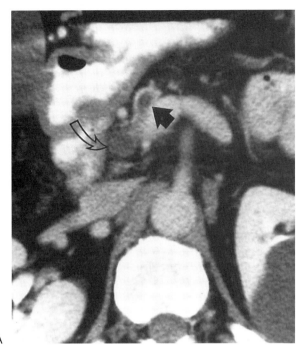

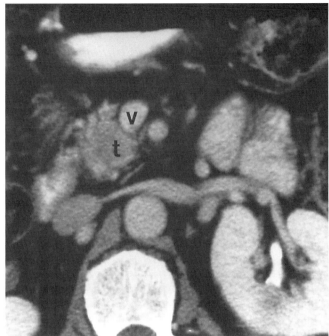

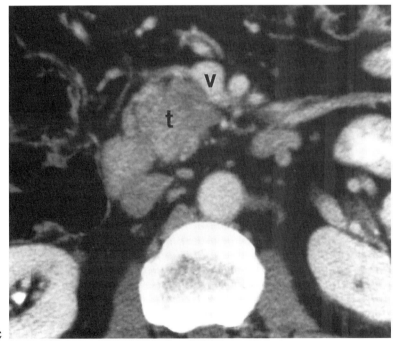

FIG. 7. Small, resectable carcinoma of the head of the pancreas (**A–C**). The most cephalad level (A) shows a dilated common bile duct (*curved arrow*) and a dilated main pancreatic duct (*black arrow*) within a markedly atrophic pancreatic neck. In B the lumen of the common bile duct is obliterated by a poorly marginated infiltrating tumor (t) in the head of the pancreas. Note that the tumor does not appreciably enlarge the head. At the time of a Whipple procedure the tumor was found to be adjacent to but not invading the wall of the superior mesenteric vein (v).

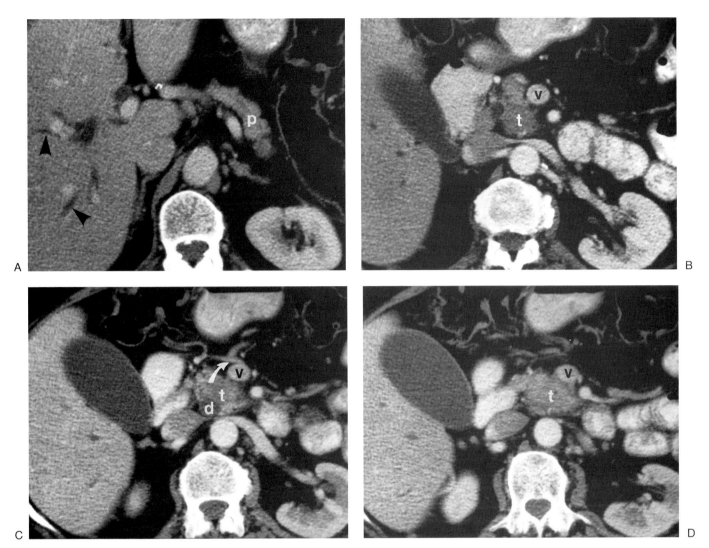

FIG. 8. Small carcinoma of the head of the pancreas obstructing the distal common bile duct (**A–D**). A–D: In the most cephalad image, atrophy of the body and tail of the pancreas is seen (p). Minimal intrahepatic biliary dilation (*black arrows*) reflects the distal obstruction. In B and C a discrete plane separates the superior mesenteric vein (v) from the centrally located tumor (t); however, in D focal adherence of the tumor to the superior mesenteric vein is noted. Note the abrupt change in caliber of the distal common bile duct (d). At the time of a Whipple procedure, the tumor replaced most of the head of the pancreas without significantly enlarging it. A short segment of SMV had to be resected (*curved white arrow,* gastrocolic trunk).

was substantially greater during the pancreatic phase than during the hepatic phase. The improved conspicuity of the primary tumor during the pancreatic parenchymal phase was also matched by better recognition of local tumor spread (142).

There are several other CT findings that can indicate the presence of a neoplasm when a contour-altering mass is not identified. First, because with aging the pancreas may become heterogeneous in its attenuation value, with diffuse fatty infiltration, a focal region of homogeneous soft-tissue density within such a gland should be viewed with suspicion (134,272). Second, the presence of both a dilated common bile duct and dilated main pancreatic duct in the absence of an obstructing calculus suggests an ampullary or pancreatic head neoplasm (Fig. 13). However, on rare occasions, this finding can be seen in benign disease (130). Third, the finding of a dilated main pancreatic duct (MPD) in the body and tail, but not in the head or neck, also suggests the presence of a neoplasm (Figs. 14 and 15). A fourth suggestion of the presence of a

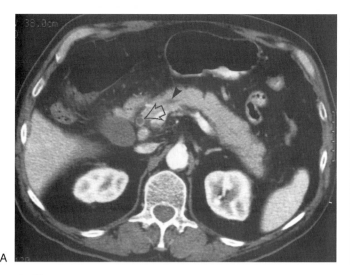

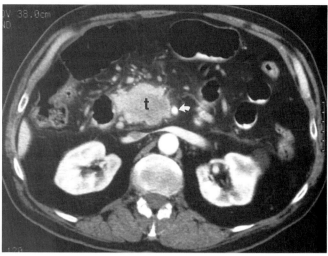

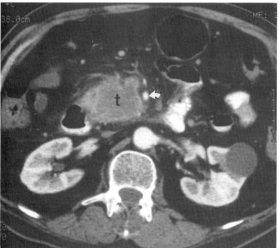

FIG. 9. Large carcinoma of the head of the pancreas (**A, B**). Images of the pancreas in a cephalocaudad direction show minimal dilatation of the main pancreatic duct (*arrowhead*) and a normal caliber common bile duct (*open arrow*) in A. A large, relatively hypovascular lesion (t) enlarges the head of the pancreas and completely obliterates the superior mesenteric vein but does not involve the superior mesenteric artery (*curved white arrow*).

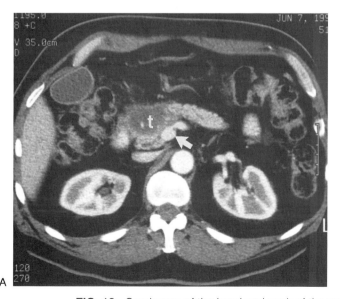

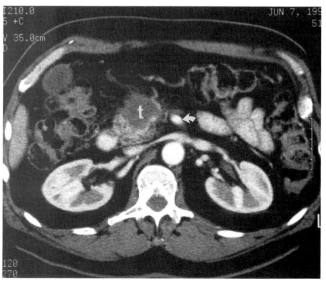

FIG. 10. Carcinoma of the head and neck of the pancreas. **A, B:** Images at the level of the neck and head of the pancreas show a 3-cm-diameter markedly hypovascular neoplasm (t). Although the superior mesenteric vein is patent at its junction with the splenic vein (*white arrow*), its lumen is obliterated by the tumor 15 mm more caudal. Unresectable tumor. *Curved white arrow,* superior mesenteric artery.

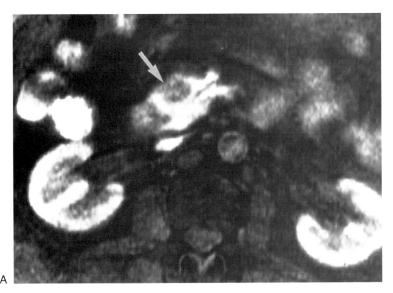

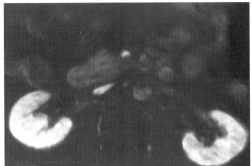

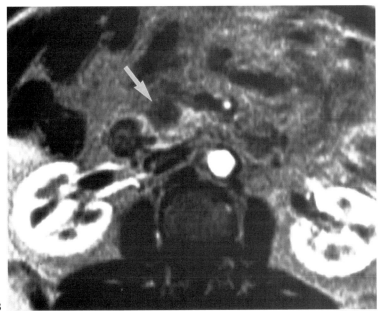

FIG. 11. Small, non-organ-deforming pancreatic cancer. T1FS (**A**), immediate postgadolinium FLASH (**B**), and delayed post- gadolinium T1FS (**C**) images. The small cancer appears as a well-defined low-signal mass in the head of the pancreas on T1FS (*arrow,* A) and immediate postgadolinium FLASH (*arrow,* B) images. On later post-contrast images, the tumor is higher in signal than background pancreas (C). T1-weighted fat-suppressed FLASH (D) and immediate post- gadolinium FLASH (E) images in a second patient with a small, non-organ-deforming pancreatic cancer. The tumor (*arrow,* D, E) is lower in signal than background pancreas on the precontrast fat-suppressed image and immediate postgadolinium image.

FIG. 12. Small pancreatic head cancer. The immediate postgadolinium FLASH image shows good contrast resolution between tumor (*arrow*) and pancreas. Contrast resolution was suboptimal on T1FS images (*not shown*) due to low signal of normal pancreas presumably secondary to distal changes of chronic pancreatitis.

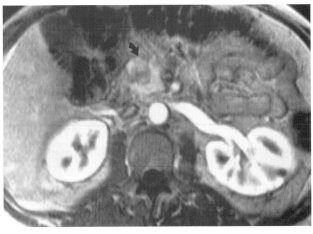

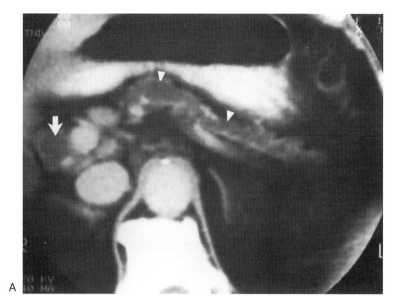

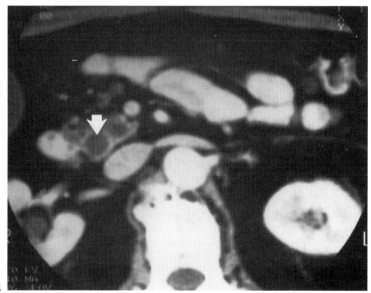

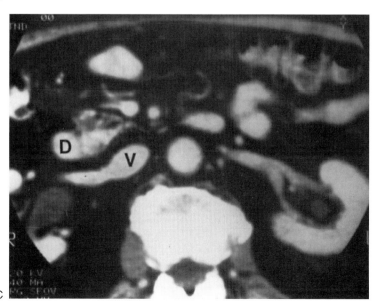

FIG. 13. Small carcinoma of the ampulla. **A:** CT image through the level of the body and tail of the pancreas shows a markedly dilated main pancreatic duct (*arrowheads*), with associated atrophy of the pancreatic parenchyma. A dilated common bile duct (*arrow*) is seen immediately lateral to the portal vein. **B:** At the level of the pancreatic head, the dilated common bile duct (*arrow*) lies parallel and lateral to the dilated main pancreatic duct, indicating a point of obstruction caudal to this. **C:** One centimeter more caudal, at the level of the uncinate process, the dilated ducts are no longer visible, indicating an abrupt obliteration of their respective lumens. No mass is discernible either in the head of the pancreas or in the adjacent duodenum (**D**). Note that the fat plane separating the head of the pancreas from the vena cava (**V**) remains intact. The absence of evidence of local invasion or hepatic metastases indicated resectability. A 1-cm-diameter carcinoma of the ampulla was found at the time of operation.

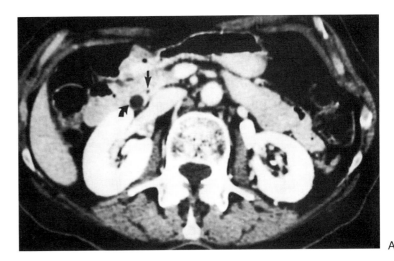

A

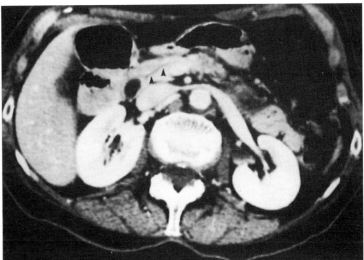

B

FIG. 14. Multifocal adenocarcinoma involving the body and tail. **A:** The head of the pancreas is unremarkable, and a normal caliber main pancreatic duct (*arrow*) is visible. An incidental finding is a nonobstructed, moderately dilated distal common bile duct (*curved arrow*) in this postcholecystectomy patient. **B:** Two centimeters cephalad, the normal caliber main pancreatic duct (*arrowheads*) extends to the region of the neck of the pancreas. **C:** At a level 1 cm cephalad to B, an abrupt transition in the caliber of the main pancreatic duct occurs (*white arrow*), although a discrete mass is not apparent at the point of transition. Necrotic tumor (*arrowheads*) replaces a portion of the pancreatic tail. At operation, a small focus of tumor in the neck of the pancreas obstructed the main pancreatic duct, and extensive tumor involved the remainder of the body and tail.

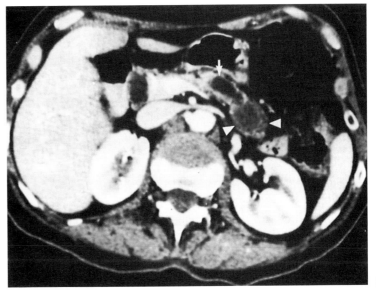

C

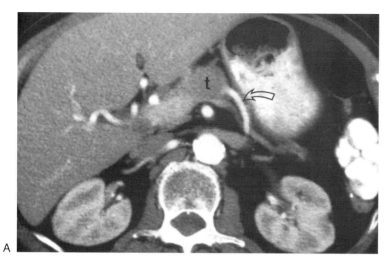

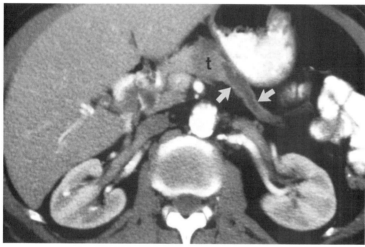

FIG. 15. Infiltrating carcinoma of the body of the pancreas. **A:** The tumor (t) was seen to displace but not encase the splenic artery (*curved arrow*) on more cephalad images. **B:** The tumor (t) replaced the normal parenchyma of the body with resultant obstruction of the main pancreatic duct and associated marked atrophy of the parenchyma of the tail (*white arrows*).

neoplasm is the finding of rounded convex borders of both the anterior and posterior surfaces of the uncinate process (Fig 16).

A carcinoma in the head or distal body of the pancreas may produce changes in the more proximal body and tail that are definable on CT. These changes include pancreatic duct dilatation (Fig. 17), cyst due to obstruction (Fig. 18), typical changes of acute pancreatitis, and atrophy (21,44,138,278). A dilated pancreatic duct is a sensitive indicator of pancreatic disease, but it is not specific for carcinoma and it can occur in pancreatitis or in duodenal inflammatory disease (22,117,130,138). In a patient without a history of pancreatitis, a dilated pancreatic duct implies the presence of a distal obstructing neoplasm. If the neoplasm is not identified on the CT examination, ERCP will frequently clarify the nature of the obstruction. The obstruction of the pancreatic duct may cause elevated intraductal pressure, resulting in small-duct rupture and subsequent enzyme release associated with focal pancreatitis. Central necrosis of large body and tail cancers may

occasionally show communication with the MPD on ERCP (Fig. 19).

That portion of a pancreas which is proximal to a duct-obstructing cancer will also show changes on MRI indicative of the increased fluid content, changes of subacute or chronic pancreatitis, duct dilatation, and parenchymal atrophy. In these cases immediate post-gadolinium spoiled GRE images are better able to define the size and extent of cancers that will appear as low-signal-intensity mass lesions in a background of slightly greater enhancing, chronically inflamed pancreas (see Fig. 12). Although pancreatic cancers are lower in signal intensity than normal pancreatic parenchyma on immediate postgadolinium images, the appearance of cancers on >1-min post-gadolinium images is variable. The enhancement of cancer relative to pancreas reflects the volume of extracellular space and venous drainage of cancers compared to adjacent pancreatic tissue.

Although a focal mass is the primary CT finding of a pancreatic adenocarcinoma, not all masses are carcino-

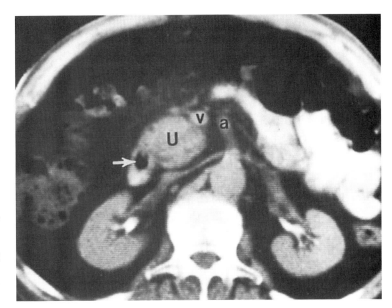

FIG. 16. Carcinoma in the uncinate process. Rounding of the normally slender hook-like configuration of the uncinate process (U) as it extends posteromedial to the superior mesenteric vein (v) indicates abnormality of this portion of the pancreatic head. Convex borders to both the anterior and posterior surfaces of the uncinate process should always be viewed with suspicion; (*arrow*) duodenum; (a) superior mesenteric artery.

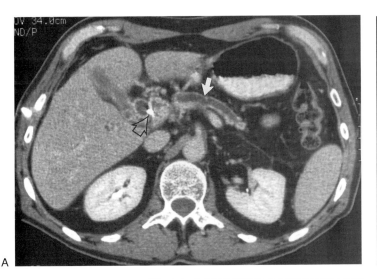

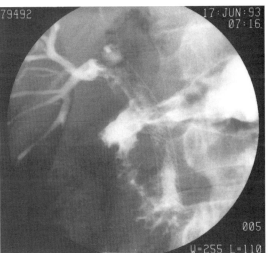

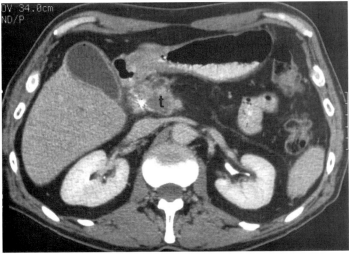

FIG. 17. Carcinoma of the head of the pancreas obstructing the common bile duct and main pancreatic duct. **A:** Marked dilatation of the main pancreatic duct (*white arrow*) with associated atrophy of the parenchyma of the body and tail reflects the longstanding obstruction. A biliary catheter (*open arrow*) decompresses the obstructed bile duct. **B:** An infiltrating, hypovascular tumor (t) replaces most of the pancreatic head. Because the tumor was unresectable, a biliary wall stent (**C**) was used for palliation.

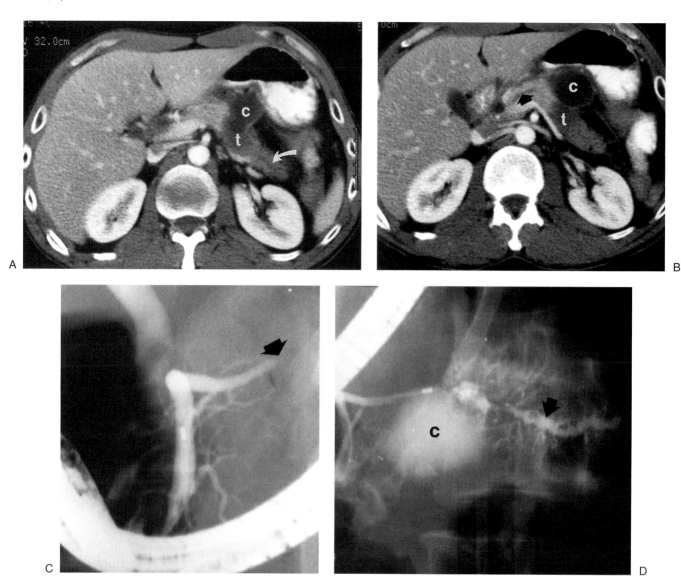

FIG. 18. Small carcinoma of the body of the pancreas with an associated obstructive cyst in a 38-year-old male patient. **A:** CT scan at the level of the body of the pancreas shows a focal area of diminished enhancement in the body of the pancreas (t). Because the tail of the pancreas is also not well enhanced, the dilated main pancreatic duct (*curved arrow*) is not easily appreciated. An obstructive retention cyst (c) arises from the anterior aspect of the body of the pancreas. **B:** One centimeter caudal to A, the retention cyst (c) is more well defined, a normal caliber main pancreatic duct is visible (*black arrow*) in the neck of the pancreas, and the focal area of hypoenhancement (t) is again noted just anterior to the normal appearing splenic vein. **C:** Detailed view from an ERCP shows a normal caliber main pancreatic duct in the head and neck with abrupt termination (*black arrow*) in the midportion of the body. **D:** Following the successful cannulation of the strictured segment, the dilated, irregular main pancreatic duct in the proximal body and tail is seen (*black arrow*). Filling of the previously noted retention cyst (c) is also shown. Following resection of the body and tail of the pancreas, a 1.5-cm-diameter locally infiltrating adenocarcinoma of the mid body of the pancreas was identified without evidence of nodal spread. (ERCP courtesy of Dr. Todd Baron, Birmingham, Alabama.)

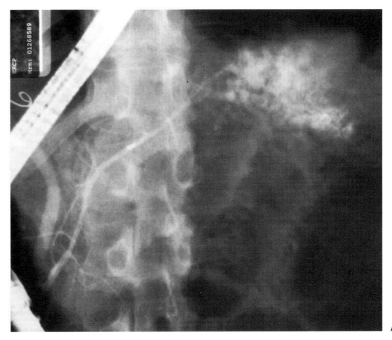

A

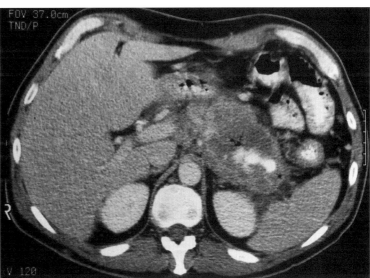

B

FIG. 19. Large necrotic carcinoma of the tail of the pancreas in a 44-year-old male patient who presented with pain and fever. **A:** Detailed view of the left upper quadrant from an ERCP shows communication of the main pancreatic duct with an irregular space in the left upper abdomen. **B:** CT scan shortly after the ERCP shows contrast within a centrally necrotic area of a huge tumor in the tail of the pancreas. (ERCP courtesy of Dr. Todd Baron, Birmingham, Alabama.)

mas, and not all carcinomas present as masses. Differentiating between carcinoma and inflammatory disease occasionally can be difficult because the pancreas may be diffusely enlarged by an extensive cystic and necrotic tumor or secondary to a carcinoma-induced pancreatitis (Fig. 20). Additionally, pancreatitis can present as a focal mass (42,130,171). Secondary signs of pancreatic carcinoma, when present, may permit this distinction to be made. These secondary signs include hepatic and lymph node metastases, contiguous organ invasion, and vascular encasement (18,117,199,279). The most common sites of metastases, in order of decreasing frequency, are liver,

regional lymph nodes, other retroperitoneal and intraperitoneal structures, and lungs (Figs. 21 and 22). Because of the pancreas's rich lymphatic supply and lack of a fibrous capsule, metastases to regional nodes (peripancreatic, periaortic, pericaval, and periportal) and direct spread to contiguous structures tend to occur early; however, lymph node enlargement occasionally can be seen in patients with pancreatitis or unrelated conditions such as chronic active hepatitis (279). Not uncommonly, enlarged, contiguous peripancreatic lymph nodes may be indistinguishable from the substance of the pancreas itself and appear as a large pancreatic mass. Differing contrast-

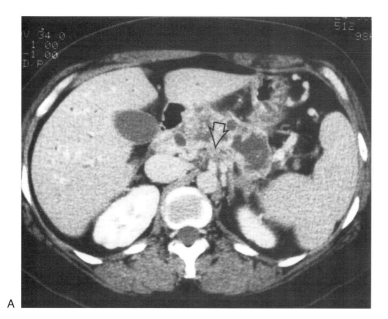

A

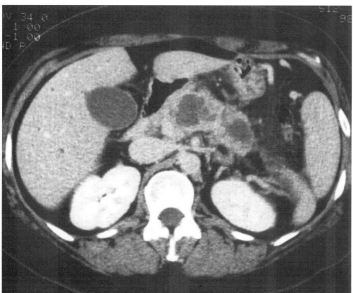

B

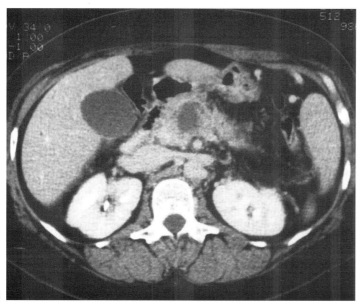

C

FIG. 20. Extensive carcinoma of the entire pancreas presenting clinically and radiologically like pancreatitis. **A–C:** Three levels through the body, neck, and head of the pancreas show an enlarged appearing gland with multiple low-density areas within it. Although this pattern suggests the appearance of necrotizing pancreatitis, the lack of inflammatory change in the surrounding peripancreatic fat as well as the loss of the normal fat plane anterior to the origin of the superior mesenteric artery (*open arrow,* A) should suggest the correct diagnosis of a diffuse carcinoma of the pancreas.

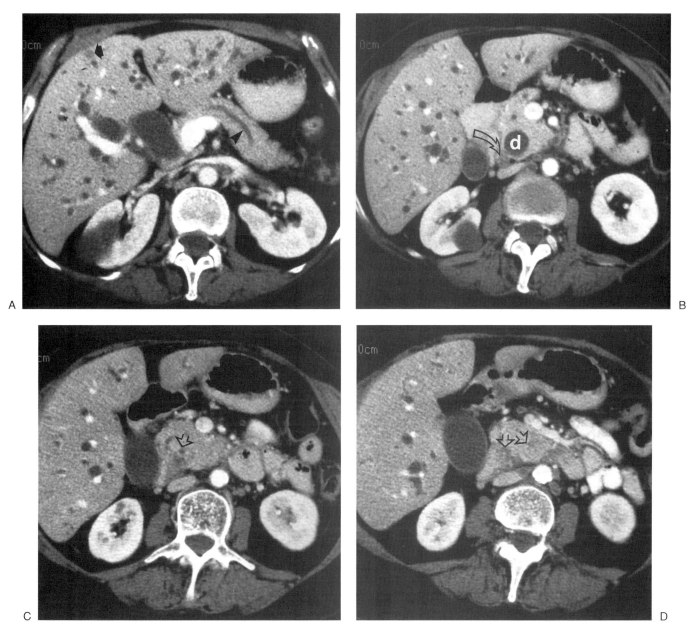

FIG. 21. Carcinoma of the head of the pancreas. **A–D:** Scans oriented cephalocaudad show marked intrahepatic biliary dilatation extending to the peripheral third in association with a 16- mm-diameter common bile duct (d). Moderate dilatation of the main pancreatic duct (*arrowheads*) is seen in the body and head of the pancreas. Abrupt obliteration of the lumen of the distal common bile duct is caused by a poorly defined hypovascular neoplasm (*open arrows*) in the head and uncinate process (C, D). An enlarged lymph node (*curved arrow*) due to metastasis is shown in B and one of several small hepatic metastases (*black arrow*) is seen in A.

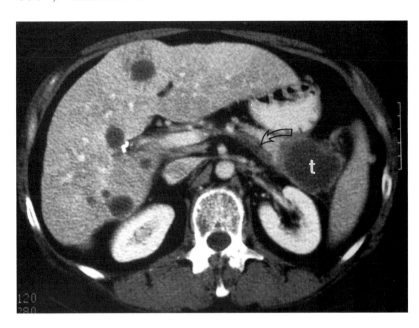

FIG. 22. Large, 3 × 5 cm, hypovascular, possibly necrotic carcinoma of the tail of the pancreas (t) is associated with numerous, similarly hypovascular metastases in the liver at the time of initial evaluation. The splenic vein (*curved arrow*) was found to be thrombosed. Distinction between bland thrombosis and tumor thrombus could not be made based on the CT appearance.

enhancement characteristics following intravenous contrast medium often will allow distinction between the nodes and the pancreatic parenchyma.

Local extension of cancer and lymphatic and vascular involvement can be demonstrated on nonsuppressed T1-weighted images (Fig. 23) (185,263). Vascular patency may be evaluated by either a flow-sensitive gradient echo technique (184) or by dynamic gadolinium- enhanced spoiled GRE technique. Liver metastases from pancreatic cancers are generally of a low signal intensity on conventional or fat-suppressed T1-weighted images, minimally hyperintense on T2-weighted images, and demonstrate a faint, irregular rim of enhancement on immediate post-contrast GRE images. The low-signal-intensity centers of metastatic lesions presumably reflect the hypovascular, fibrotic nature of the parent tumor or, possibly, central necrosis (Fig. 24) (227).

Recent experience with thin section contrast-enhanced CT indicates that the question of vascular involvement by tumor can be achieved with greater accuracy. Helical CT in particular allows for better delineation of the peripancreatic vasculature due to its capacity to provide thin sections through a significant volume of tissue in a short period of time when the arteries and veins are optimally enhanced (Figs. 9, 25, 26) (142). CT has been shown to accurately define the extent of vascular involvement and correctly predict resectability in over 85% of patients (73,78). If the tumor can be shown to be separated from the adjacent vessels by a plane of fat, vascular involvement is unlikely. If the tumor encircles the superior mesenteric vein or superior mesenteric artery, unresectability is virtually assured. However, when the tumor is shown

to abut the superior mesenteric artery or vein, it is difficult to predict whether the tumor is attached to the wall of the vessel or is simply contiguous (see Fig. 7). In situations where the remainder of the findings would suggest resectability, it is felt prudent to give the patient the benefit of the doubt and make the determination of vascular involvement operatively. When the tumor is invading the peripancreatic vasculature extensively, the contrast-enhanced CT images will often show the constricted or obliterated lumen of the encased vessel (Figs. 26 to 28). Although experience is limited, MRI can show similar changes of vascular involvement (Fig. 29).

The appearances of the dilated common bile duct and main pancreatic duct can assist in the differentiation between malignant and benign disease. Abrupt termination of either the common bile duct or the pancreatic duct favors the presence of malignant disease (18,199). In one large series, abrupt termination of the bile duct was seen in all patients with obstruction caused by a malignant neoplasm and in only 20% of patients with benign disease. Smooth, gradual tapering of the common bile duct was present in 80% of the patients with benign disease and in none of the patients with malignant disease (18). Early results with MR cholangiography techniques show that details of the presence, level, and probable cause of ductal obstruction can be well shown (Fig. 30) (250).

The obstructed main pancreatic duct can dilate in three different forms: smooth, beaded, and irregular. Smooth or beaded dilatation was seen in 85% of patients with carcinoma and 27% of patients with chronic pancreatitis (117). Irregular dilatation was seen in 73% of patients with chronic pancreatitis and only 15% of patients with

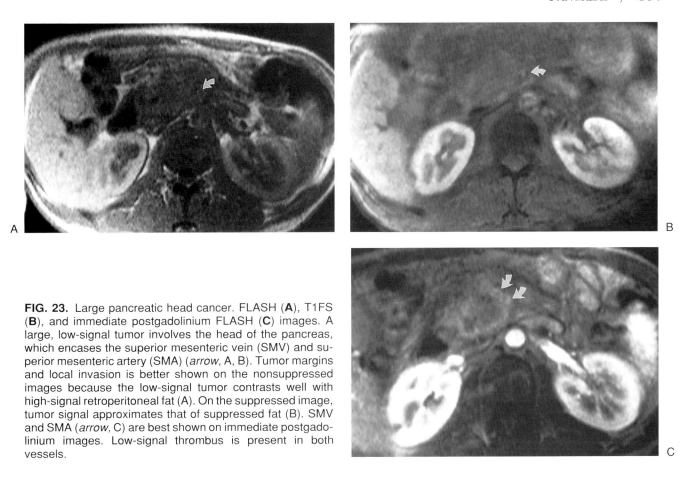

FIG. 23. Large pancreatic head cancer. FLASH (**A**), T1FS (**B**), and immediate postgadolinium FLASH (**C**) images. A large, low-signal tumor involves the head of the pancreas, which encases the superior mesenteric vein (SMV) and superior mesenteric artery (SMA) (*arrow, A, B*). Tumor margins and local invasion is better shown on the nonsuppressed images because the low-signal tumor contrasts well with high-signal retroperitoneal fat (A). On the suppressed image, tumor signal approximates that of suppressed fat (B). SMV and SMA (*arrow, C*) are best shown on immediate postgadolinium images. Low-signal thrombus is present in both vessels.

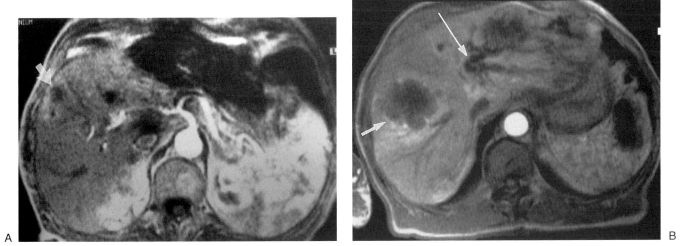

FIG. 24. Liver metastases from pancreatic cancer. **A:** Immediate postgadolinium FLASH image demonstrates irregular peripheral enhancement with low-signal-intensity center (*arrow*). The central low signal intensity reflects the hypovascular, fibrotic composition of the primary tumor. **B:** Immediate postgadolinium FLASH in a second patient shows liver metastases with a similar appearance (*arrow*). Dilated intrahepatic biliary ducts in the left lobe are also appreciated (*long arrow*).

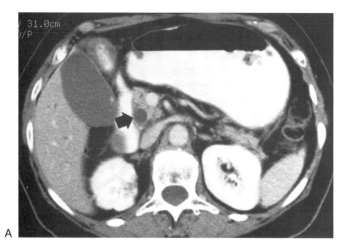

A

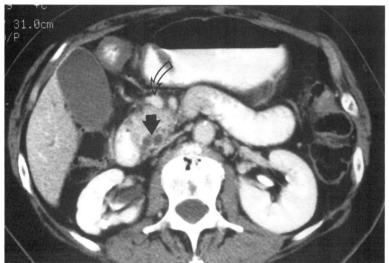

B

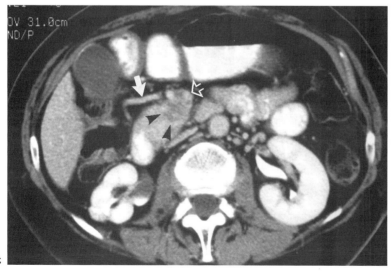

C

FIG. 25. Carcinoma of the head of the pancreas with obstruction of the distal common bile duct and invasion of the superior mesenteric vein. **A:** Most cephalad level in the pancreatic head shows a 10-mm-diameter common bile duct (*black arrow*). **B:** The most distal ends of the common bile duct and main pancreatic duct are seen (*black arrow*). The gastrocolic trunk (*curved arrow*) is slightly prominent. **C:** A poorly margin-ated hypovascular lesion (*arrowheads*) involves the uncinate process and partially obliterates the lumen of the superior mesenteric vein. The tumor abuts the superior mesenteric artery (*open arrow*). The prominent right gastroepiploic vein (*white arrow*) may reflect increased collateral flow due to the obstruction of the superior mesenteric vein caudal to the junction of the gastrocolic trunk. Note the cortical scarring of atrophic pyelo-nephritis in the right kidney.

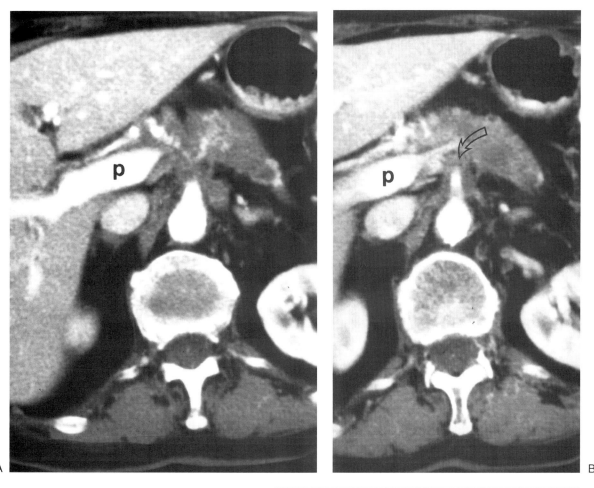

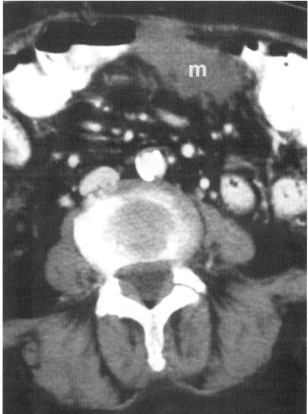

FIG. 26. Carcinoma of the body of the pancreas with spread to blood vessels and bowel (**A–C**). A, B: Detailed views at the level of the celiac axis show encasement of the hepatic and splenic arteries by extensive tumor. The portal vein (p) in (A and B) shows tapering due to surrounding tumor. Encasement without obliteration of the superior mesenteric artery (*curved arrow*) is present in B. C: Site of focal metastasis to the serosal surface of the midtransverse colon (m) is secondary to spread along the transverse mesocolon.

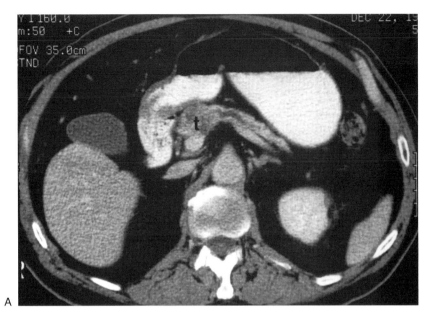

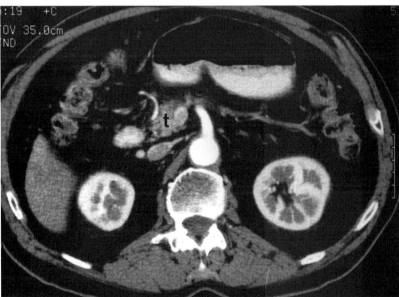

FIG. 27. Nine-month interval growth of unresectable cancer in the head of the pancreas. **A, B:** Initial study shows a hypovascular tumor (t) in the neck of the pancreas producing obstruction of the main pancreatic duct.

carcinoma. When the ratio of pancreatic duct diameter to pancreatic gland width is >0.5, the presence of carcinoma is favored (see Figs. 15 and 17). When the ratio is <0.5, benign disease is more likely. In fact, carcinoma was present approximately 90% of the time when the ratio exceeded 0.5 (117).

If secondary signs of malignant disease are not present it may not be possible to distinguish between a carcinoma and focal pancreatitis. If the mass is thought to represent focal inflammation, follow-up studies should be performed to confirm that resolution occurs. In equivocal, nonresolving, or indeterminate cases, ERCP or direct percutaneous fine-needle aspiration may aid in diagnosis. Although there has been some experience in the role of

MRI in the evaluation of pancreatitis, the value of MRI in differentiating subtle tumor from focal pancreatitis has not been established (226). In a small percentage of cases, nothing short of surgically obtained histologic material will resolve the issue.

Other potentially useful aids for distinguishing between neoplastic pancreatic disease and inflammatory disease are recently developed tumor markers including the monoclonal antibodies CA-19-9 and CA-125 (180). In the detection of pancreatic cancer, both CA-19-9 and CA-125 had approximately the same sensitivity, about 75%, which is somewhat better than that of carcinoembryonic antigen (CEA), which ranges from 25% to 62% (202). In a study of more than 5000 patients (201), CA-19-9 was

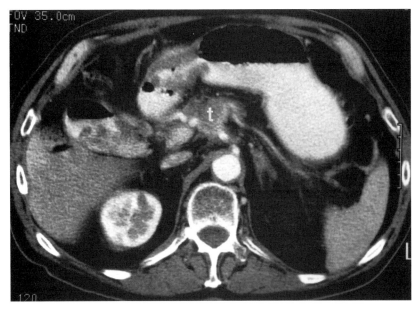

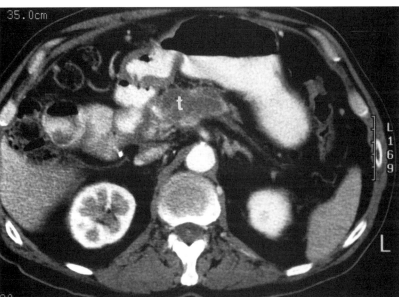

FIG. 27. (*Continued.*) **C, D:** Nine months following a diverting cholecystojejunostomy, the tumor now has extended into the body of the pancreas (t) and has encased portions of the celiac axis as shown in C.

positive in 100% of resectable lesions, whereas it was positive in only 53% of patients with advanced pancreatic cancer. It is also positive, however, in the presence of other neoplasms of the gastrointestinal tract, such as gastric cancer, and has a false positive rate of 11% in patients with pancreatitis and 2% in healthy subjects.

Other tumor markers include CA-50, DU-PAN-2, 47D10, SPAN-1, RA-96, PCAA, and PaA; the use of these tumor markers is summarized in a National Cancer Institute Tumor Marker Conference report (158). Serum markers "might be useful in confirming a diagnosis of pancreatic cancer and, in some instances, would be helpful in distinguishing benign from malignant pancreatic disease. However, their lack of tumor specificity and pan-

creas organ specificity made these serum markers unreliable for diagnosis when used by themselves" (158).

Besides being used for tumor detection, CT also plays an important role in the staging of pancreatic neoplasms and in the determination of their resectability. A report from the Radiology Diagnostic Oncology Group (154) showed that, using dynamic IV bolus contrast-enhanced CT scanning with 5-mm-thick slices, the positive predictive value for nonresectability was 89%, but the technique is poor in predicting that the tumor will be truly resectable with a negative predictive value of 28%. The results from MRI were similar, i.e., 88% and 23%, respectively. Some of the reasons for this relative inaccuracy include low sensitivity for detecting small hepatic metas-

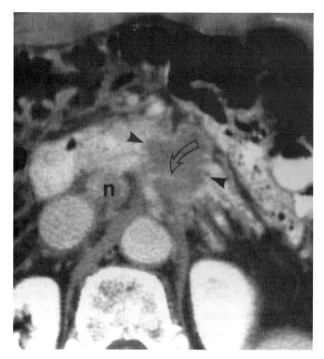

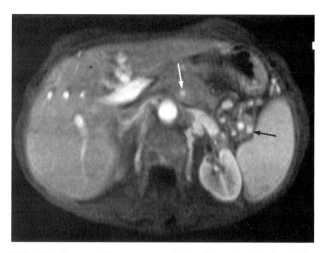

FIG. 28. Posteriorly infiltrating carcinoma of the body of the pancreas. CT scan at the level of the body of the pancreas reveals a hypoenhancing infiltrating tumor (*arrowheads*) of the body of the pancreas with posterior extension and encasement of the nearly obliterated splenic artery (*curved arrow*). Metastatic enlargement of a paracaval lymph node (n) is also apparent at this level.

FIG. 29. Pancreatic cancer arising from the body of the pancreas. A 45-sec postgadolinium FLASH image demonstrates a large tumor mass involving the body and tail of the pancreas with encasement of the SMA (*white arrow*). Multiple varices are present in the splenic hilum (*black arrow*) and along the greater curvature of the stomach due to thrombosis of the splenic vein.

tases or small metastatic lesions on the surface of the liver or growing on the peritoneal lining. More recent experience with two-phase helical CT techniques (142) suggests that further improvements can be made in the determination of resectability. Similarly, the outcomes of current MR techniques are substantially superior to those of the techniques described in that report (223).

Pancreatic cancer tends to be disseminated at the time of diagnosis. When initially evaluated, only approximately 15% of patients have tumor confined to the pancreas, whereas 65% of them have advanced local dissemination or distant metastases, and the remaining 20% have localized disease, with spread to the regional lymph nodes (see Fig. 21) (62). CT is able to show hepatic or distant metastases, regional lymphadenopathy, and high-attenuation-value (hemorrhagic or malignant) ascites in a significant percentage of these cases. It is also able to reveal vascular encasement or invasion of contiguous organs. The neoplasm is considered unresectable if there are distant metastases, major vessel encasement, or contiguous organ invasion other than directly into the wall of the duodenum (20). Recent refinements in surgical technique, management of anesthesia, preoperative and postoperative care, along with experience being concentrated in large referral centers have resulted in significant improvements in morbidity and operative mortality

(52,160,186,258). Although the 5-year survival after curative resection has been generally dismal, several centers have recently reported encouraging results with improved actuarial 5-year survivals after curative resection approaching 20% to 25% (39,186,258).

Pancreatic Endocrine Tumors

Pancreatic endocrine tumors are uncommon, having a prevalence of <10 per million population (111). Insulinomas and gastrinomas are the most common of these rare

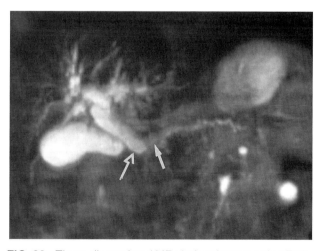

FIG. 30. Three-dimensional MR cholangiogram using Turbo (fast) spin echo (8000/94). Pancreatic cancer causes high-grade obstruction of the common bile duct (*hollow arrow*) and high-grade obstruction of the pancreatic duct (*solid arrow*).

tumors, whereas glucagonomas, VIPomas (tumors that secrete vasoactive intestinal polypeptide), and somatostatinomas are much more rare. GRFomas (tumors that secrete growth hormone–releasing factor) are extremely rare. PPomas, which secrete pancreatic polypeptide, have no known symptoms due to hypersecretion and are much like nonfunctioning (hormonally quiescent) pancreatic endocrine tumors. In surgical studies, nonfunctioning pancreatic endocrine tumors are reported to compose 15% to 20% of all pancreatic endocrine tumors removed (36), and in a large surgical pathology series, the nonfunctioning tumors accounted for 36% of all pancreatic endocrine tumors (124).

Although commonly referred to as islet cell tumors, the bulk of the evidence suggests a non–islet cell ductular origin (55). The tumors are thought to originate from cells that are part of the diffuse neuroendocrine cell system (88). These neuroendocrine cells share cytochemical properties and, together with pheochromocytomas, melanomas, carcinoid tumors, and medullary carcinoma of the thyroid, have been called APUDomas. APUD is an acronym for *a*mine *p*recursor *u*ptake and *d*ecarboxylation. This would account for several different hormones not present in normal islet cells being present in the various tumors under this category. The benign or malignant nature of these tumors is sometimes difficult to establish unless metastatic tumor has been documented. In order to establish that one of these tumors is benign, long-term follow-up is required. In general, 5% to 10% of insulinomas are reported as malignant, whereas in various series 50% to 90% of the other tumors are reported as malignant (25,50,95,110).

Nonfunctioning pancreatic endocrine tumors are clini-cally silent until they cause symptoms due to their size or to metastases. As a consequence, they are usually large at the time of discovery, ranging in size from 3 to 24 cm in diameter with 30% being >10 cm (64,173). With the exception of rare cystic forms, the endocrine tumors of the pancreas are vascular tumors which enhance prominently with intravenous contrast on CT (Fig. 31). Hepatic metastases share the same vascular properties.

It is important to differentiate between nonfunctioning endocrine tumors of the pancreas and ductal adenocarcinomas because patients with endocrine tumors often respond favorably to surgery and specific chemotherapy and consequently have a better prognosis than patients with adenocarcinomas (111). Of the various imaging methods available, contrast-enhanced CT (helical preferred) and ultrasonography are the most commonly used initial methods for detection or localization. When a nonfunctioning endocrine tumor is encountered on CT, three features that aid in the differentiation of this from an adenocarcinoma are the presence of calcification, the lack of vascular encasement, and the absence of central necrosis or cystic degeneration. Approximately 20% of pancreatic endocrine tumors contain calcification, whereas <2% of adenocarcinomas do. Encasement of the celiac artery or superior mesenteric artery, which is commonly seen in adenocarcinomas, is rarely seen in the endocrine tumors; however, encasement of the superior mesenteric vein or portal vein has been reported (26,64). Pancreatic endocrine tumors, even when large, rarely undergo central necrosis or cystic degeneration because of their rich vascularity, which continues to grow as the mass grows (254). Although 60% of pancreatic endocrine tumors occur in the body and tail, location is not a useful differenti-

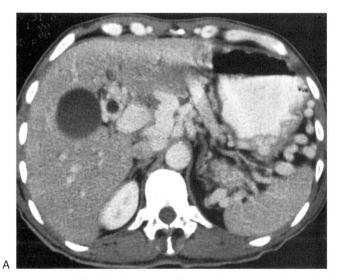
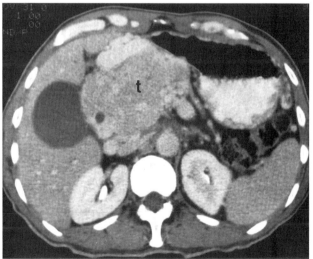

A

B

FIG. 31. Large, nonfunctioning pancreatic endocrine tumor. **A, B:** The numerous dilated arteries and veins in the region of the porta hepatis reflect the marked hypervascularity of this large, nonfunctioning endocrine tumor (t) of the head of the pancreas. The increased arterial flow through the tumor acts like an arteriovenous fistula into the portal venous system. Compression by the tumor also causes dilatation of the venous return from the spleen.

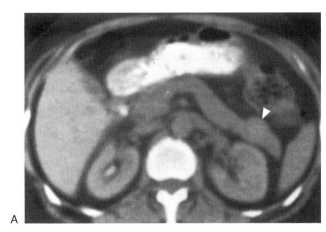 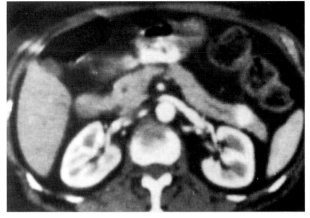

FIG. 32. Insulinoma. **A:** A subtle alteration in the contour of the anterior surface of the tail of the pancreas (*arrowhead*) is apparent in this patient suspected of having an insulinoma. **B:** Postcontrast bolus technique. A 1.5-cm densely enhancing lesion is visible in the areas of contour irregularity. This pattern of enhancement is typical for an islet cell tumor.

ating feature in individual cases. In summary, the diagnosis of a nonfunctioning (hormonally quiescent) endocrine tumor should be considered when a large, nonuniformly enhancing, calcified pancreatic mass without cystic areas and with hyperdense areas is identified on a contrast-enhanced CT examination (64).

The presenting symptoms of a functioning endocrine tumor depend on the hormone secreted. Insulinomas are the most common symptomatic endocrine tumor and are essentially always confined to the pancreas (Fig. 32). Gastrinomas occur most frequently in the general vicinity of

the head of the pancreas, including the pancreatic head itself as well as the wall of the duodenum and stomach, and lymph nodes in an area termed the "gastrinoma triangle" (Fig. 33). Ninety percent of the extrapancreatic gastrinomas occur in this area bounded by the junction of the cystic and common hepatic ducts superiorly, the second and third portions of the duodenum inferiorly, and the junction between the neck and body of the pancreas medially (168,242).

These two neoplasms usually are small (90% are <2 cm in diameter) and may be multiple (gastrinomas and

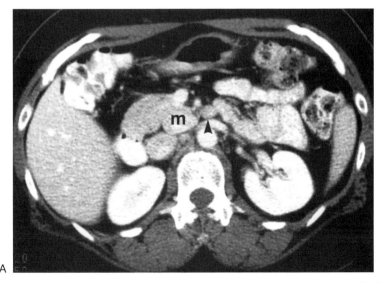 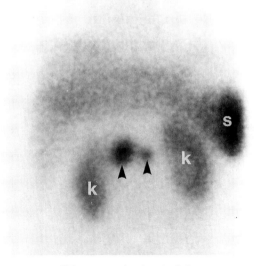

FIG. 33. Surgically proven extrapancreatic gastrinoma. **A:** Post contrast CT scan at the level of the head of the pancreas shows a 2 × 3 cm mass (m) posterior to the uncinate process. A second separate mass, presumed to be within a lymph node (*arrowhead*), lies directly anterior to the left renal vein. No intrapancreatic mass was identified in this patient with the Zollinger-Ellison syndrome who had been managed medically up to this point. **B:** Anterior view of an Indium 111 octreotide scintigram shows that both lesions seen on CT accumulate the radionuclide (*arrowheads*) consistent with multiple gastrinomas. The radionuclide agent normally accumulates in the spleen (s) and is excreted by the kidneys (k). Surgically proven.

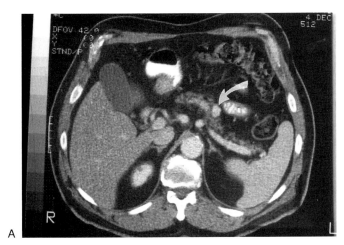

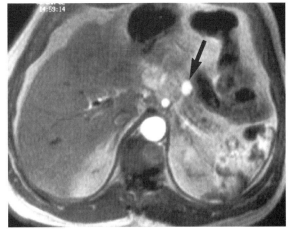

FIG. 34. Insulinoma. Dynamic contrast-enhanced CT (**A**) and immediate postgadolinium FLASH (**B**) images demonstrate good conspicuity of the 1.5-cm enhancing tumor arising from the body of the pancreas (*white arrow*). More intense enhancement is present on the MR image. (Reproduced with permission from ref. 222.)

insulinomas are multiple 60% and 10% of the time, respectively) (67,90,91,111,192,254). VIPomas, glucagonomas, and somatostatinomas are frequently larger, many being >5 cm in diameter, due to the nonspecificity of their symptoms and resultant delay in diagnosis (25,110,264). Because of the typically small size of insulinomas and gastrinomas, they seldom alter the contour of the pancreas; therefore, contrast-enhanced dynamic CT techniques, occasionally using intra-arterial contrast delivery, must be used to maximize the chances of detecting them (1). Endocrine tumors of the pancreas enhance to a greater degree than normal pancreatic parenchyma during the arterial and capillary phase of bolus contrast enhancement (Figs. 32 and 33). Additionally, the use of thin section techniques or helical CT will also improve the conspicuity of the tumors. Calcification, which may occur in these

endocrine tumors, is more common in malignant than in benign neoplasms (34,280).

Because ultrasound and CT are readily available, these imaging methods are most often used for the detection and localization of functioning endocrine tumors of the pancreas. However, there is evidence to show that MRI is at least as effective as CT. In the MRI evaluation of pancreatic endocrine tumors, T1FS, immediate postgadolinium spoiled GRE images (Fig. 34), and T2-weighted fat-suppressed (T2FS) images may be useful (163,221,222). The tumors are low in signal intensity on T1FS, demonstrate homogeneous or ring enhancement on immediate postgadolinium spoiled GRE, and are high in signal intensity on T2FS images (Fig. 35). The MRI features that distinguish endocrine tumors from ductal adenocarcinomas include high signal intensity on T2FS, in-

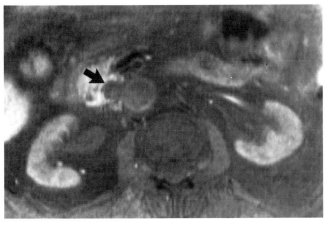

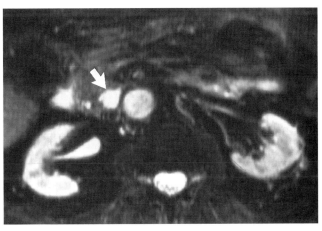

FIG. 35. Gastrinoma. T1FS (**A**) and T2FS (**B**) images demonstrate a 2-cm well-defined mass (*arrows*) arising from the uncinate process of the pancreas, which is low in signal on T1FS (**A**) and high in signal on T2FS (**B**). The high signal on T2FS distinguishes this mass from pancreatic ductal carcinoma, which is low in signal on T2-weighted images. (Reproduced with permission from ref. 221.)

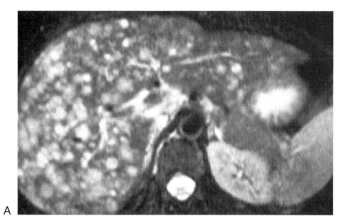
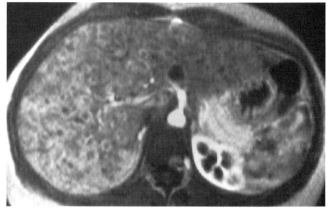

A   B

FIG. 36. Gastrinoma liver metastases. T2FS (**A**) and immediately postgadolinium SGE (**B**) images demonstrate well-defined small metastases that are high in signal on T2FS (A) and possess distinct ring enhancement immediately following contrast (B). (Reproduced with permission from ref. 222.)

creased homogeneous enhancement on immediate post-gadolinium images, and hypervascular liver metastases (Figs. 36 and 37). Morphologic features include lack of vascular encasement and absence of central necrosis in large tumors, as is similarly shown on CT examinations. Recent literature provides conflicting information on the relative merits of MRI, ultrasound, CT, or angiography. One study demonstrated that MRI was more sensitive than the other imaging methods for detecting metastatic disease to the liver (Fig. 38), but the role of MRI remains unclear for detecting primary pancreatic endocrine tumors with the same study cited above demonstrating that it has a low sensitivity (22%), equal to that of ultrasound and CT and less than that of angiography (189). Another study demonstrated that MRI with gadolinium enhancement and fat suppression techniques demonstrated 91% of all pri-

mary pancreatic endocrine tumors (222). The striking difference in sensitivity in these two studies largely reflects differences in MR technique; however, it may also reflect the size of the primary tumors. In the latter study, 90% of the tumors were at least 2 cm in diameter. It appears that the ability of the various imaging methods to detect pancreatic endocrine tumors depends on the size of the tumor. Using any of the imaging methods, whether US, CT, MRI, or angiography, <10% of tumors smaller than 1 cm, 30% to 40% of tumors 1 to 3 cm, and 70% to 80% of tumors >3 cm were detected (6,7,77,111,149,189,268). Selective portal venous sampling for localizing the hormone gradient and intraoperative ultrasound at the time of surgery are techniques having the greatest sensitivity with detection results superior to standard imaging methods (172,174).

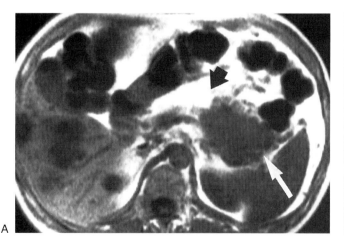
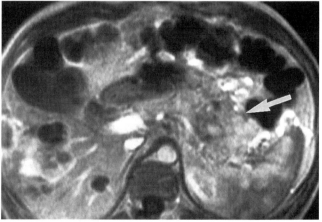

A   B

FIG. 37. Glucagonoma. FLASH (**A**) and immediate postgadolinium FLASH (**B**) images demonstrate a 5-cm tumor arising from the tail of the pancreas (*white arrow*, A). Extensive fatty replacement of the remainder of the pancreas (*black arrow*, A) is present as shown by high signal intensity identical to subcutaneous fat. Multiple liver metastases are also present. The primary tumor possesses heterogeneous enhancement immediately following contrast (*arrow*, B) and the liver metastases demonstrate irregular rim enhancement. The appearance of the liver metastases is typical for liver metastases from neuroendocrine tumors. (Reproduced with permission from ref. 221.)

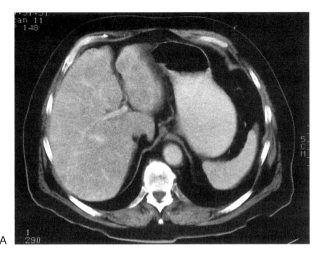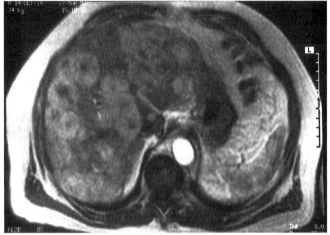

A

B

FIG. 38. Dynamic contrast-enhanced CT (**A**) and immediate postgadolinium FLASH MRI (**B**) images of hepatic metastases from a pancreatic endocrine tumor demonstrate that ring-like enhancement of multiple metastases are better shown on the enhanced MR image. (Reproduced with permission from ref 222.)

Cystic Neoplasms

Cystic neoplasms of the pancreas are uncommon, accounting for 5% to 15% of all cystic pancreatic masses (37,105,287). These neoplasms are divided into two groups—microcystic adenoma (sometimes referred to as serous cystadenoma) and mucinous cystic neoplasm (also called macrocystic adenoma and adenocarcinoma)—which have significantly different therapeutic and prognostic implications.

Microcystic adenoma has typical CT and pathologic appearances (Fig. 39) (45,106). This tumor is found in an elderly population. Approximately 80% of patients are 60 years of age or older at the time of diagnosis, with a weak sexual predilection (female-to- male ratio is 3:2) (37,75,106). The tumor can vary in size from 1 to 12 cm, with an average diameter of approximately 5 cm. It is a benign tumor with no malignant potential (37,75,106,114). These masses may occur in any part of the pancreas with a relatively equal distribution throughout the head, body, and tail. On CT, this neoplasm has a smooth or lobulated contour, with a spectrum of appearances of the tumor tissue itself ranging from a nearly solid appearance due to the presence of innumerable minute cysts, to many small but visible cysts, to a more multilocular-appearing mass having thin septa and thin walls (Fig. 39). When there are multiple small but visible cysts, the tumor has a honeycomb appearance (37,105,106). It is not always well demarcated from surrounding pancreatic parenchyma as its capsule is not well developed. The soft-tissue components of this tumor are enhanced following intravenous administration of contrast media, in keeping with its angiographic hypervascular appearance (105). Occasionally a central scar is present and its spoke-like strands of connective tissue may calcify in a stellate or sunburst appearance (Fig. 40) (37,75,105,287). Based solely on its CT appearance, it may be difficult at times to distinguish it from other cystic pancreatic processes or, in the case of the tumor that contains innumerable minute cysts, from a solid pancreatic mass. However, on histologic examination, its cytoplasm is rich in glycogen, with little or no mucin, a distinguishing feature (45,75,106). When examined with ultrasound, the appearance of the tumor may range from very echogenic to a relatively hypoechoic mass that appears septated and composed of only a few cysts. On MR images the tumors are well defined and do not demonstrate invasion of fat or adjacent organs (162). Breathing independent HASTE images are particularly effective at demonstrating the thin septations within microcystic adenomas (Fig. 41). Delayed enhancement of the central scar may occasionally be observed (227).

It has been reported that ''microcystic adenomas'' may have macrocystic variants. Five cases of macrocystic serous cystadenoma of the pancreas, two of which were of the unilocular type, exhibited distinctly different macroscopic features from typical microcystic adenomas, which created diagnostic problems both radiologically and pathologically (136). These authors suggested that microcystic and macrocystic serous tumors represent morphologic variants of the same benign pancreatic neoplasm and felt that ''serous cystadenoma'' should once again be used to encompass all variants of this benign neoplasm.

Mucinous cystic pancreatic neoplasms, sometimes referred to as macrocystic adenoma and macrocystic adenocarcinoma, should be considered malignant neoplasms because there appears to be a continuous evolution of these lesions from benign to malignant over time (46,59,75). These tumors occur more commonly in women with a 6:1 female-to-male ratio and present be-

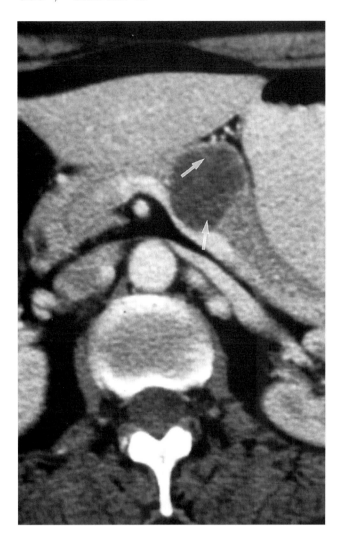

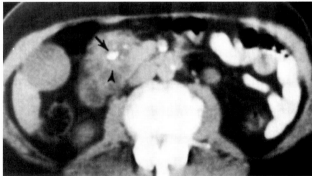

FIG. 39. Microcystic adenoma of the body of the pancreas in a 61-year-old female patient. Because the multiple cysts are so small within this lesion, it appears almost homogeneous in its architecture. Faint linear structures within the lesion suggest septations (*arrows*). The gross specimen consisted of multiple cysts in the 2- to 3-mm range with thin septations. Although the splenic vein appears compressed by the posterior aspect of the cystic tumor in this image, the narrowing did not appear to be hemodynamically significant.

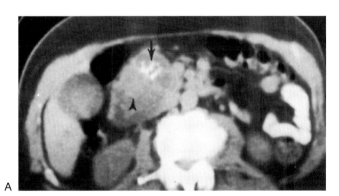

A   B

FIG. 40. Microcystic adenoma. Two serial images at a 1-cm interval show a multicystic tumor in the head of the pancreas, with central soft-tissue density (*arrowheads*) cysts varying in size from 2 mm to 10 mm in diameter, and calcifications (*arrows*) arranged in a radial pattern.

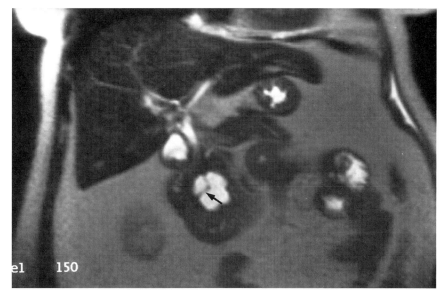

FIG. 41. Microcystic adenoma. Coronal HASTE image demonstrates a well-defined high-signal-intensity cystic mass arising in the head of the pancreas. Thin internal septations (*arrow*) are sharply defined on this image acquired in a breathing-independent fashion.

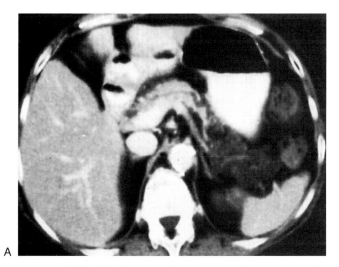

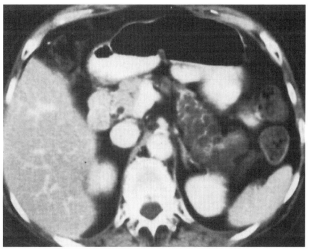

A   B

FIG. 42. Macrocystic adenoma. Two images, 2 cm apart, show a low-density mass in the body and tail of the pancreas composed of multiple cysts in the range of 1 to 2 cm in diameter, with visible septa. Because of the preponderance of cysts, minimal contrast enhancement is seen. (Courtesy of Dr. Arthur Bishop, Peoria, Illinois.)

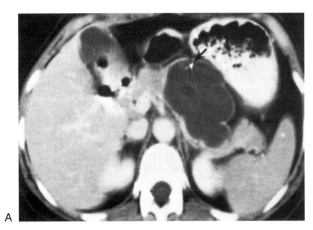 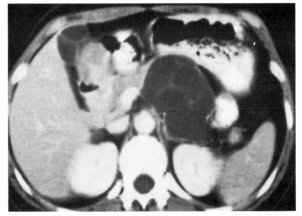

FIG. 43. Macrocystic adenoma. Two images, 2 cm apart, show a large, cystic-appearing mass with minimal septation and a very sharply defined wall. A small septal calcification is noted anteriorly (*arrow*). As the cysts become larger in a macrocystic adenoma, it is more difficult to define the internal septal architecture on CT. (Courtesy of Dr. Arthur Bishop, Peoria, Illinois.)

tween the ages of 40 and 60 years (46,59,75). They are most often located in the body or tail of the pancreas, are large (mean diameter of 10 cm), encapsulated, and multiloculated (Fig. 42). Stromal elements (septa) separate the cystic areas, which typically are >2 cm in size (Fig. 43). The septa themselves are thicker than those found in microcystic adenomas and may infrequently calcify. The walls of these cystic tumors are thick and often nodular (46,105,114). The amount of stroma varies and, when small, the septa may not be apparent on CT. In that case, the tumor appears unilocular and resembles a pseudocyst. Pathologically, these neoplasms contain mucin and all have malignant potential (Fig. 44). They should be resected because the outcome is very favorable. In comparison with usual ductal carcinomas, 5-year survival rates may be as high as 50% (46,59,75).

Concerning MR evaluation of these tumors, on T2-weighted HASTE images or gadolinium-enhanced T1FS images, large, irregular cystic spaces separated by thick septa are demonstrated (Fig. 45). The mucin produced by these tumors may result in high signal intensity on T1- and T2-weighted images of the primary tumor and metastases (Fig. 46).

In a review of images from ERCP performed in patients with cystic pancreatic neoplasms, obstruction of the main pancreatic duct occurred in 60% of malignant tumors and was seen in only 1 of 23 patients with benign lesions (4%). Although this finding did not prove to be an absolute indicator of benign or malignant disease, it was nevertheless felt to be a valuable differential point (82).

A tumor that may represent a subcategory of mucinous cystadenomas and cystadenocarcinomas is referred to as

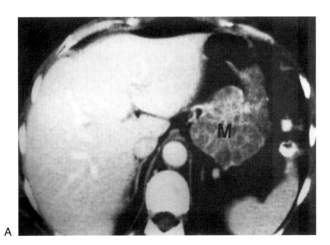 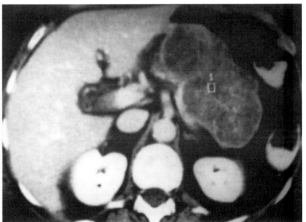

FIG. 44. Macrocystic adenocarcinoma (formerly termed mucinous cystadenocarcinoma). **A:** A large, heterogeneous mass (M) with internal cysts and septations is identified in a retrogastric location. **B:** At a level 3 cm caudal to A, the same mass replaces the body and tail of the pancreas. The margins of the tumor are well defined, and the fat plane posterior to the pancreas is not invaded. The tumor was found to be resectable at the time of surgery. (Courtesy of Dr. Arthur Bishop, Peoria, Illinois.)

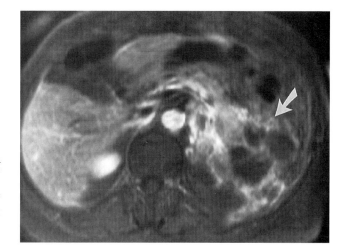

FIG. 45. Mucinous cystic neoplasm (macrocytic adenocarcinoma). Gadolinium-enhanced T1FS image demonstrates a large, low-signal-intensity tumor mass arising from the tail of the pancreas (*arrow*). Multiple large irregular signal void defects are noted in the mass consistent with cysts. Invasion of the spleen and multiple liver metastases were also present (*not shown*) confirming the malignant nature of this tumor. (Reproduced with permission from ref. 227.)

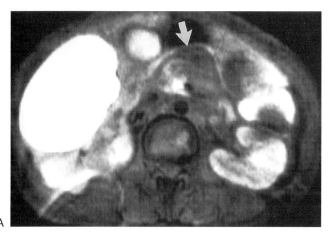

A

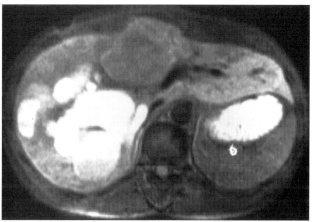

B

FIG. 46. Macrocystic adenocarcinoma with liver metastases. T1FS (**A, B**) and T2FS (**C**) images demonstrate a tumor arising from the midbody of the pancreas (*arrow,* A) and multiple liver metastases (A–C). T1-weighted image (B) and T2-weighted image (C) from the same tomographic section demonstrate that many metastases are high in signal on both sequences consistent with the presence of mucin. Layering of proteinaceous material is observed in some metastases on the T2FS (C) image. (Reproduced with permission from ref. 227.)

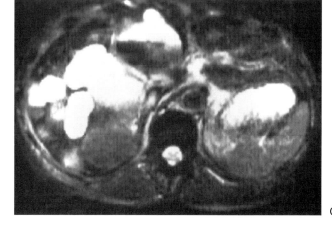

C

a mucin-producing tumor and in a few reports as "duct-ectatic mucinous tumor" (59,79,176,177,282). A primary characteristic of these mucin-producing tumors is that a papillary tumor is present in the dilated main or branch ducts of the pancreas (Fig. 47). In the benign lesion the tumor consists of hyperplastic epithelium, whereas in the malignant cases the tumor usually consists of papillary and atypical hyperplasia with only small areas of adenocarcinoma. These papillary lesions produce copious mu-

cin which on endoscopy is often seen being extruded through the wide-open orifice of the papilla (282). The age incidence is similar to the mucinous cystic tumors of the pancreas (median age of the benign cases 63 years and median age of the malignant cases 69 years). However, the sex predilection is reversed with men predominating and the tumors are most often located in the head of the pancreas (282). Compared to typical pancreatic cancer, the prognosis is better for patients with mucin-

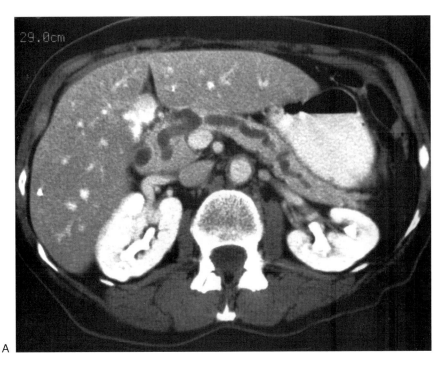

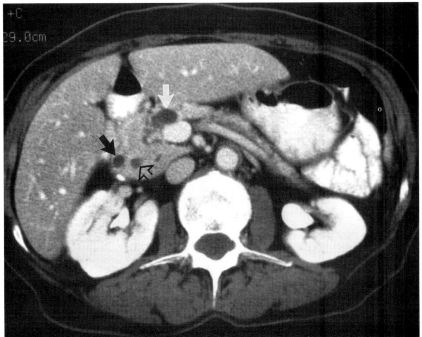

FIG. 47. Mucinous carcinoma of the duct-ectatic type. **A, B:** The entire duct system of the pancreas appears dilated due to the presence of copious mucin. A prominently ectatic side branch (**white arrow**) is present in the neck of the pancreas. Note the subtle difference in the attenuation value of the common bile duct (*black arrow*) and the mucin within the ectatic pancreatic duct (*open black arrow*). The mucin measured approximately 10 Hounsfield units higher. The diagnosis was established with endoscopy and ERCP.

producing tumors as well as mucinous cystic neoplasms. From a therapeutic standpoint, it is important to detect and diagnose this lesion, which can present simply as pancreatitis due to the obstruction produced by the excessive amount of mucin filling the main pancreatic duct. The diagnosis of a mucin-producing tumor of the pancreatic ducts is best established with ERCP. The observation of copious mucin exiting the papilla along with the demonstration of characteristic filling defects within the main pancreatic duct or within dilated side branches is key to the establishment of the diagnosis of this tumor. The CT findings will reflect the morphologic changes with cystic areas in the head of the pancreas and uncinate process as well as varying degrees of dilatation of the main pancreatic duct, in some instances extending to the body and tail (Fig. 47).

The major pathologic entities to be differentiated from the mucinous cystic neoplasms and mucin-producing variants are focal pancreatitis, with an associated pseudocyst, and a necrotic adenocarcinoma (287). A history of pancreatitis or trauma usually is present in patients with focal pancreatitis or an isolated pseudocyst; however, based on CT findings alone, it may be impossible to distinguish a cystadenoma from a pseudocyst. Necrotic

adenocarcinoma characteristically has a thick irregular wall without calcification on CT (see Fig. 19). The uncommon mucinous adenocarcinoma may be difficult to distinguish from a cystadenoma (Fig. 48) (92,104, 238,283,287). The rare pancreatic lymphangioma, a benign tumor originating from lymphatic vessels, also may be indistinguishable from a cystadenoma (58,179,214). Finally, pancreatic lesions may be the only abdominal manifestation of von Hippel-Lindau disease and they include cysts, microcystic adenomas, and neuroendocrine tumors (Fig. 49) (40,100).

Other Neoplastic Lesions

The solid and papillary epithelial neoplasm (SPEN) of the pancreas is an uncommon low-grade malignant tumor that occurs chiefly in young women (mean age 25 years) (38). These tumors are generally large with a mean transverse diameter of 9 cm and, while predominating in the tail, can be found in any portion of the pancreas. CT and MRI of SPEN will commonly show hemorrhagic degeneration with typical fluid–debris levels indicating blood products in areas of cystic degeneration and necro-

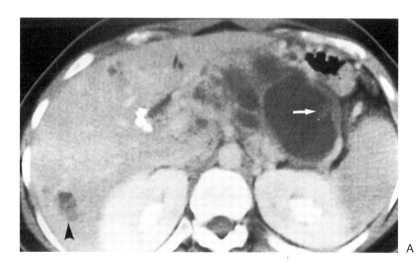

A

B

FIG. 48. Mucinous adenocarcinoma of the body and tail of the pancreas. **A, B:** Two images, 3 cm apart, show a large multicystic mass occupying the area of the body and tail of the pancreas. Papillary projections (*white arrows*) arise from the thick-walled cystic portions of the tumor. One of several hepatic metastases is indicated by the arrowhead. Incidental gallstones were noted in the body and neck of the gallbladder. The findings are characteristic of an extensive mucinous adenocarcinoma.

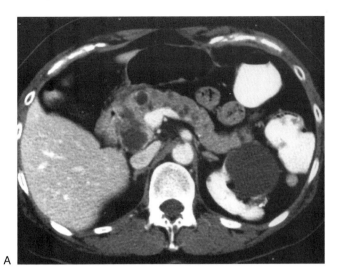
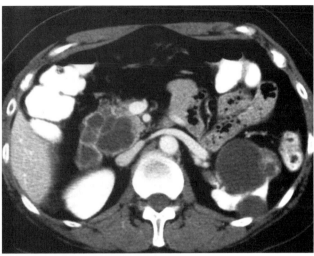

A   B

FIG. 49. A 44-year-old woman with von Hippel-Lindau disease and a history of renal cell carcinoma, multiple pancreatic cysts, and a cerebellar hemangioblastoma. **A, B:** Two levels through the body and head of the pancreas reveal numerous, variable-sized cysts within the body, neck, and head of the pancreas that were not adversely affecting either exocrine or endocrine function. Note the cysts within the midportion of the left kidney.

sis (Fig. 50). In a review of six patients with SPEN studied with MRI, the authors found that all tumors were well-demarcated lesions containing central high signal intensity on T1-weighted images consistent with hemorrhagic necrosis (178). The differential diagnosis includes cystic neoplasms and endocrine tumors of the pancreas (15,38,76,122,212).

Pleomorphic carcinoma is an uncommon malignant neoplasm that has a fulminant clinical course. It metastasizes early to the liver, lung, adrenal, kidney, thyroid, and bone. This tumor shows irregular enhancement after intravenous contrast material and it may be cystic, with thick irregular walls and a lobulated contour. The presence of extensive retroperitoneal lymphadenopathy helps to differentiate it from adenocarcinoma (281). A variety of other rare neoplasms of the pancreas have been reported including acinar cell carcinoma, malignant giant cell tumor, sarcoma, plasmacytoma, lipoma, oncocytoma, and small cell carcinoma (56,57,166,175,220,275).

Pancreatic tumors are rare in infants and children. The CT, MRI, and ultrasound imaging characteristics of pancreatoblastomas, a rare pancreatic tumor of acinar cell origin in children between the ages of 1 and 8, have recently been reported (108,145,246).

Although lymphoma can involve the pancreas and peripancreatic lymph nodes and can be confused with a primary pancreatic neoplasm, usually it is a systemic disease with retroperitoneal and mesenteric lymphadenopathy also present (191,230,270). The two most reliable signs to distinguish peripancreatic lymphadenopathy from a primary neoplasm are intact fat planes between the nodes and the pancreas and anterior displacement of the pancreas; however, these findings are seen less than half of the time (Fig. 51) (286). Lymphoma often is larger than adenocarcinoma. In one study it was reported that no adenocarcinoma was larger than 10 cm, and 60% were between 4 and 6 cm (251). On MRI, intermediate signal intensity peripancreatic lymph nodes are readily distinguished from high-signal-intensity pancreatic parenchyma on T1FS images. Invasion of the pancreas is shown by loss of the usual signal intensity of the pancreatic parenchyma on the T1FS images (Fig. 52).

Pancreatic metastases, which are rarely diagnosed clinically, most commonly arise from melanoma and carcinomas of the breast, lung, kidney, prostate, and gastrointestinal tract (Fig. 53). Isolated metastases to the pancreas from primary bone tumors have also been reported (210). When multiple masses are present in the pancreas in a patient with a known primary carcinoma, metastases can be presumed; however, when solitary, it may be indistinguishable from primary pancreatic carcinoma (211). MRI may be useful in the evaluation of pancreatic metastases by showing features such as increased vascularity in the context of a hypervascular primary malignancy (121). The majority of metastases are low signal in a background of high-signal pancreas on T1FS images (Fig. 54). Melanoma has a typical high signal intensity on T1-weighted images due to the paramagnetic properties of melanin.

Benign Inflammatory Diseases

Acute Pancreatitis

Acute pancreatitis is a complex disease with a broad spectrum of presentations ranging from mild biochemical and anatomic derangements that may not even be symptomatic to a catastrophic, fatal outcome. Our understand-

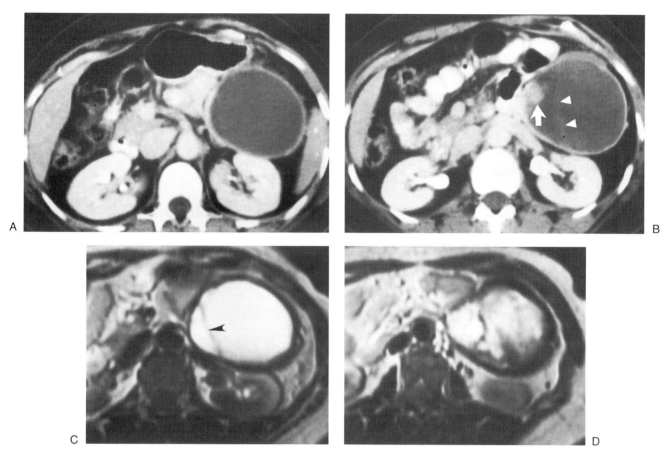

FIG. 50. Solid and papillary epithelial neoplasm of the pancreas. **A, B:** Two images, 2 cm apart, in this 41-year-old female patient with a left upper quadrant mass show a well-defined cystic-appearing mass with a uniformly thick wall and a papillary projection (*arrow*) arising from the medial wall. A suggestion of a septation is also seen (*arrowheads*). In this case, the most likely diagnosis would be macrocystic adenoma. However, this also falls into the spectrum of solid and papillary epithelial neoplasms. (Courtesy of Dr. Arthur Bishop, Peoria, Illinois.) **C:** T2-weighted MR image (SE, TR = 1500 msec, TE = 70 msec) at a similar level as A shows a cystic structure with a single septation (*arrowhead*) and a thick, low-intensity wall. **D:** Three centimeters more caudal, the mass has mixed medium- to-low-signal-intensity areas representing solid components of this tumor.

ing of the disease, from an imaging standpoint, continues to evolve as advancements are made in the application of ultrasound, CT, MRI, and endoscopic techniques to the evaluation of this disease. In efforts to describe the morphologic changes demonstrated with these various imaging techniques, a variety of terms have evolved that are sometimes confusing or not well defined. In an effort to bring some consistency to the terminology used in this disease, an international symposium on acute pancreatitis was held in September 1992 (30). By consensus of a diverse group of 40 international authorities, a classification system was proposed. The following are the definitions and characteristics agreed upon:

Acute pancreatitis—Acute pancreatitis is an acute inflammatory process of the pancreas, with variable involvement of other regional tissues or remote organ systems.

Clinical manifestations—Most often, acute pancreatitis has a rapid onset, is accompanied by upper abdominal pain, and is associated with variable abdominal findings ranging from mild tenderness to rebound. Acute pancreatitis is often accompanied by vomiting, fever, tachycardia, leukocytosis, and elevated pancreatic enzyme levels in the blood and/or urine.

Pathologic findings—Findings range from microscopic interstitial edema and fat necrosis of the pancreatic parenchyma to macroscopic areas of pancreatic and peripancreatic necrosis and hemorrhage. These pathologic changes in acute pancreatitis represent a continuum, with interstitial edema and minimal histologic evidence of necrosis at the minor end of the scale and confluent macroscopic necrosis at the other extreme (30).

For clarity mild and severe forms of acute pancreatitis were further defined:

Mild acute pancreatitis—Mild acute pancreatitis is associated with minimal organ dysfunction and an unevent-

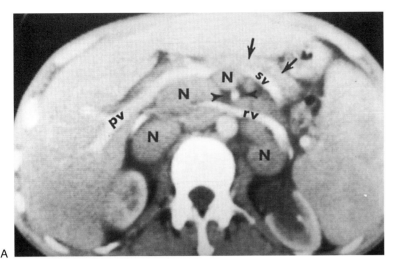

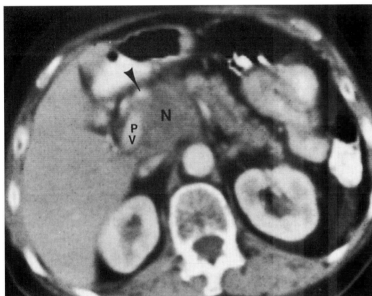

FIG. 51. Peripancreatic lymphoma. **A:** After intravenous bolus enhancement, the splenic, portal, and left renal veins are densely enhanced, and the pancreas (*arrows*) is seen to be anteriorly displaced by the lymph nodes (N) enlarged by lymphoma. Note that the fat plane surrounding the superior mesenteric artery (*arrowheads*) remains intact. This would not be the case in the presence of a similar-sized adenocarcinoma of the pancreas. **B:** In another patient, postcontrast CT image shows a large nodal mass (N) in the region of the pancreatic head. It would be unusual for a pancreatic carcinoma to achieve this size without causing biliary obstruction. The pancreatic body and tail are normal; (pv) portal vein; (*arrowhead*) gastroduodenal artery; (sv) splenic vein; (rv) renal vein.

ful recovery, and it lacks the described features of severe acute pancreatitis.

Severe acute pancreatitis—Severe acute pancreatitis is associated with organ failure and/or local complications such as necrosis, abscess, or pseudocyst.

In most cases mild acute pancreatitis rapidly responds to supportive, conservative medical therapy. It is a rare occurrence for mild acute pancreatitis to progress to the severe form. If a satisfactory clinical response has not been obtained within 48 to 72 hours, dynamic, contrast-enhanced CT should be performed for further assessment.

On the other hand, severe acute pancreatitis most often progresses very rapidly, manifesting the characteristic symptoms, signs, and laboratory findings within 24 to 72 hours of admission.

In an effort to objectively quantify the degree of severity, Ranson and colleagues developed a list of 11 risk factors (5 on admission and 6 within the first 48 hours

after admission) to help make this assessment (14, 194,195). These criteria are shown in Table 4. Modifications to the Ranson criteria, such as the modified Glasgow criteria (Table 5) as well as evaluation systems combining these criteria with findings on CT, have evolved since the mid-1970s (243).

A more recent prognostic index called the Acute Physiology and Chronic Health Evaluation score (APACHE II) has come into use. The APACHE II score is based on a weighted index of 12 routine physiologic measurements, age, and previous health status to provide a general measure of severity of disease. Under this system, the maximum possible score is 71 although in actual use a patient will rarely exceed a score of 55. In the presentation of acute pancreatitis, scores in the mid-20s to mid-30s would indicate severe disease (125).

This same symposium established definitions for pancreatic necrosis, acute fluid collections, pseudocysts, and pan-

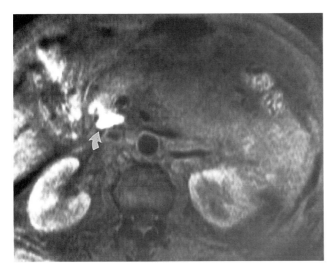

FIG. 52. Lymphoma. T1FS image demonstrates extensive lymphomatous involvement of the pancreas, which causes diffuse signal loss of the pancreas. Sparing of the head and uncinate process is present, demonstrated by retention of the normal high signal of pancreatic tissue (*white arrow*). Periaortic and paracaval adenopathy is also apparent. (Reproduced with permission from ref. 227.)

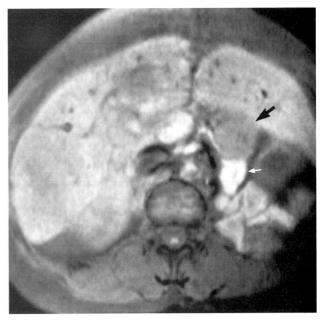

FIG. 54. Metastases to pancreas. T1FS image demonstrates a low signal mass (*black arrow*) arising from the midbody of the pancreas that has a normal high signal intensity (*white arrow*). Multiple large low-signal masses are present in the liver, which represent liver metastases.

creatic abscess. Pancreatic necrosis is defined as a diffuse or focal area of nonviable pancreatic parenchyma, which is typically associated with peripancreatic fat necrosis (30).

As a means of biochemically assessing pancreatic necrosis, a variety of laboratory tests have been devised. Serum methemalbumin rises significantly in the presence of extensive pancreatic necrosis (243). Several studies have shown that quantitative determination of the C-

reactive protein can discriminate between mild and severe acute pancreatitis. The data from these studies suggest that this laboratory test is as reliable a predictor as the multiple criteria of Ranson or Glasgow.

Trypsinogen-activated peptide (TAP) is liberated from trypsinogen upon activation to trypsin. TAP is rapidly excreted in the urine where it can be measured by a specific immunoassay. One study compared urinary TAP, blood CRP, and the modified Glasgow criteria in differentiating mild from severe pancreatitis. TAP was found to be superior to the other two criteria upon admission to the hospital as well as at 24 hours later (89).

From an imaging standpoint, dynamic contrast-enhanced CT has been shown to be quite accurate in diagnosing and quantitating pancreatic necrosis. Scoring systems that incorporate the degree of pancreatic necrosis have been shown to be of value in predicting outcome. A CT severity index that combines an earlier grading system relating to pancreatic and peripancreatic morphology and fluid collections with one of three categories for percentages of pancreatic necrosis provided statistically significant differences in the incidence of morbidity and mortality when the CT severity index was used to create three separate groups of patients (14). Those in the highest severity index range had a 17% mortality and a 92% complication rate. Based on a number of studies evaluating the role of CT in pancreatic necrosis, it would appear that dynamic, contrast-enhanced CT should play a major role in predicting the outcome of cases of severe acute pancreatitis.

Acute fluid collections were defined as occurring early in the course of acute pancreatitis, located in or near the

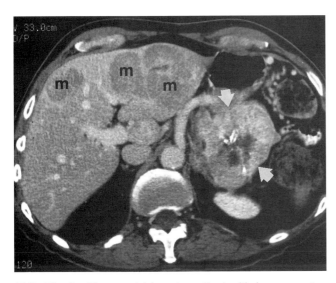

FIG. 53. An 80-year-old female patient with known metastatic colon carcinoid to the pancreas and liver. A large centrally necrotic and calcified lesion (*white arrows*) arises within the body and tail of the pancreas and displaces the proximal celiac axis anteriorly. At least three metastases (m) are present in the liver. The largest of the three, in the lateral segment of the left lobe, shows signs of central necrosis similar to its counterpart in the pancreas.

TABLE 4. *Ranson criteria*

At admission:	(1) Age over 55 years
	(2) White blood cell count >16,000 cells/mm^3
	(3) Blood glucose >11 mmol/L (no history of prior hyperglycemia)
	(4) Serum LDH >350 IU/L (normal, up to 225 IU/L)
	(5) AST (SGOT) >250 U/L (normal, up to 40 U/L)
During initial 48 hours:	(6) Hematocrit drop >10 percentage points
	(7) BUN rise >1.8 mmol/L as urea
	(8) Arterial Po$_2$ <60 mm Hg
	(9) Base deficit >4 mEq/L
	(10) Serum calcium <2.0 mmol/L
	(11) Estimated fluid sequestration >6 L

LDH, lactic dehydrogenase; IU, international units; AST, aspartate aminotransferase; BUN, blood urea nitrogen.
From ref. 193.

pancreas. These fluid collections always lacked a wall of granulation or fibrous tissue. Such acute fluid collections occur in approximately 30% to 50% of cases but more than half of these collections regress spontaneously (29,233).

Pseudocyst is defined as a collection of pancreatic juice enclosed by a wall of fibrous or granulation tissue that arises as a consequence of acute pancreatitis, pancreatic trauma, or chronic pancreatitis (30). It evolves from acute fluid collections in about 30% to 50% of patients with acute pancreatitis (233). The evolution of an acute fluid collection into a pseudocyst requires at least 4 weeks. Interestingly, a significant number of nonoperatively managed patients with pseudocysts will show spontaneous, complete resolution within a year. In one study in which 36 patients with documented pseudocysts were managed nonoperatively, 60% had complete resolution of the pseudocyst and 40% had pseudocysts that remained stable or decreased size, followed for an average of 1 year (196). In this study, operative management was used only for patients with persistent abdominal pain or enlargement or complications of the pseudocyst. The size of the pseudocyst was a significant predictor of the need for operative

drainage. Those pseudocysts <6 cm in diameter were most often managed nonoperatively (126,265,284).

Pancreatic abscess was defined as circumscribed intra-abdominal collections of pus, usually in proximity to the pancreas, containing little or no pancreatic necrosis, arising as a consequence of acute pancreatitis or pancreatic trauma. An "infected pseudocyst" in earlier terminology was included under the category of pancreatic abscess by members of the symposium. Infected necrosis was defined as infected pancreatic and/or peripancreatic necrotic tissue (30). If gas bubbles are not present within the collection on a CT scan, direct percutaneous needle aspiration is necessary to quickly establish this crucial diagnosis.

Role of CT and MRI in Acute Pancreatitis

The use of CT now enables us to show the morphologic changes in this disease, ranging from minimal edema of the pancreatic parenchyma in the interstitial inflammation of mild pancreatitis (Fig. 55) to the extensive fluid collections, necrosis, and hemorrhage that develop in fulminant severe pancreatitis.

The above-mentioned acute fluid collections arise from the exudation of fluid into the interstitium of the pancreas and subsequent leakage of this fluid, containing activated proteolytic enzymes, into the surrounding tissue spaces. The pancreatic enzyme trypsin is suspected to be the agent in the ensuing coagulative necrosis (51,61,133). Although much has been learned concerning the pathophysiology of pancreatitis, the pathogenetic mechanism of autodigestion remains unclear (83,152).

The diagnosis of mild acute pancreatitis generally is established by the clinical presentation and biochemical tests without the need for diagnostic imaging. However, biochemical abnormalities are not always evident at the time of initial presentation (253). The serum amylase level may initially be normal in up to one-third of patients clinically suspected of having acute pancreatitis associated with alcohol abuse who have CT or ultrasound findings consistent with pancreatitis (241).

TABLE 5. *Glasgow criteria*

Any time during first 48 hr after hospitalization:
(1) White blood cell count >15,000 cells/mm^3
(2) Blood glucose >10 mmol/L (no history of prior hyperglycemia)
(3) BUN >16 mmol/L as urea (after adequate hydration)
(4) Arterial Po$_2$ <60 mm Hg
(5) Serum calcium <2.0 mmol/L
(6) Serum albumin <32 g/L
(7) Serum LDH >600 U/L (normal, up to 250 U/L)
(8) AST (SGOT) at ALT (SGPT) >200 U/L (normal, up to 40 U/L)

LDH, lactic dehydrogenase; AST, aspartate aminotransferase; BUN, blood urea nitrogen; ALT, alanine aminotransferase.
From ref. 236.

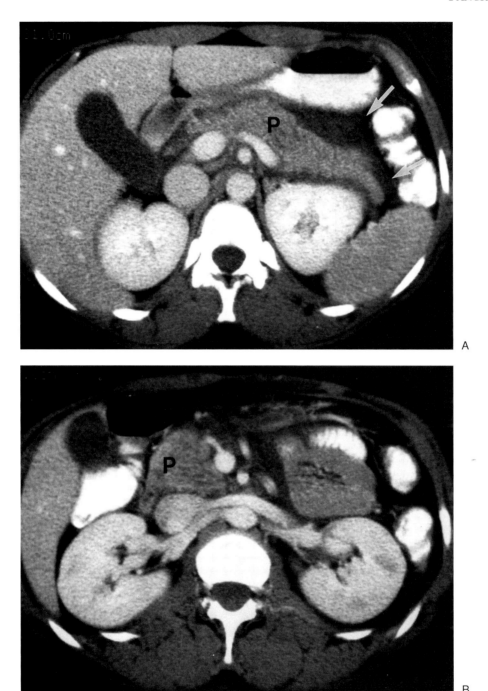

FIG. 55. Mild acute pancreatitis in a 23-year-old female patient with rheumatoid arthritis on prednisone; 4-day history of abdominal pain with elevated serum lipase and amylase. **A, B:** Two scans through the body and head of the pancreas (p) show diffuse mild swelling of the gland which enhances uniformly and blurring of the pancreatic-peripancreatic fat interface. A zone of inflammatory change is present in the peripancreatic fat (*arrows*), recognized by an increase in the attenuation value of this fat compared with the perinephric fat.

Thus, although CT is not necessary in all cases of mild acute pancreatitis, it is quite valuable when the diagnosis has not been firmly established clinically or when complications are suspected. CT imaging should be used to evaluate for pancreatitis in acutely ill patients with severe abdominal pain, hypotension, and leukocytosis (Fig. 56) (93,156). In former years, exploratory laparotomy was performed on many such patients to exclude a ruptured viscus, vascular occlusion, or other abdominal catastrophe. The mortality among such patients after unnecessary surgery varied from 20% to 80% (10).

In some patients, the inflammatory process in acute pancreatitis results in no more than transient edema of the gland, followed by full recovery. CT will show a normal appearing gland in one third or more of patients with acute pancreatitis (61,156,235). The changes of acute pancreatitis recognizable with CT include diffuse or focal glandular enlargement, contour irregularity, focal irregular areas of decreased attenuation presumably secondary to edema or focal necrosis, and changes in the peripancreatic areolar tissues, fat, and parietal peritoneal planes (Figs. 57 to 59) (61,156,233,235).

The MR signal intensity features of the pancreas in uncomplicated acute pancreatitis resemble those of nor-

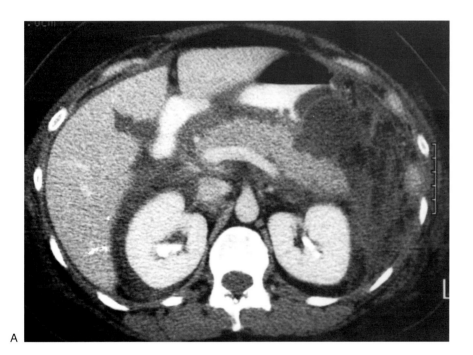

A

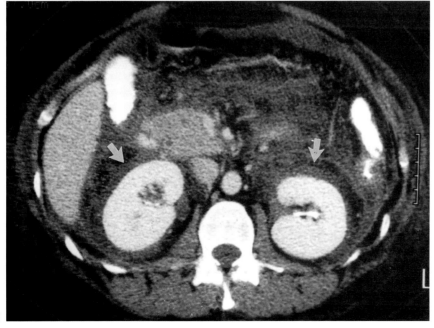

B

FIG. 56. Post-ERCP severe acute pancreatitis. **A, B:** Two scans through the level of the body and head of the pancreas show extensive inflammatory and exudative expansion of the entire anterior pararenal space. In this case, Gerota's fascia has failed to serve as a protective barrier. Note the diffuse inflammatory change within the perinephric fat bilaterally (*arrows*).

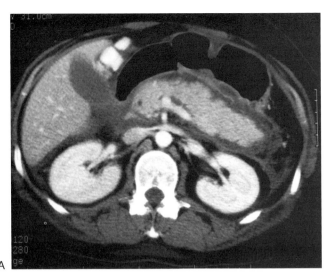

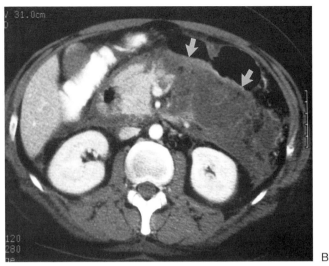

FIG. 57. Acute complicated pancreatitis. **A, B:** Two levels through the body and head of the pancreas in this middle-aged woman with acute complicated pancreatitis shows a uniformly enhancing, slightly swollen pancreas. The pancreatic fluid and inflammatory exudate expands the anterior pararenal space (*arrows*) predominantly on the left side.

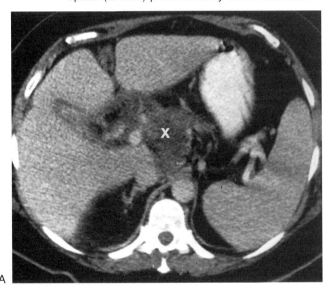

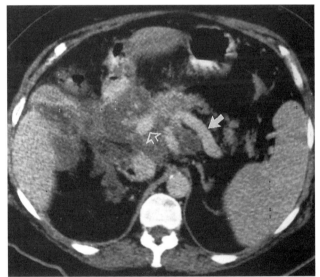

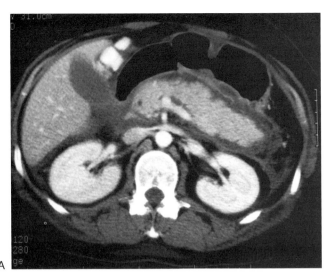

FIG. 58. Severe acute pancreatitis. **A–C:** Pancreatic fluid and inflammatory exudate (x) expands the hepatoduodenal ligament and extends to the porta hepatis superiorly, while remaining predominantly right-sided around the head of the pancreas (p), separating the head from the inferior vena cava (v) posteriorly. (white arrow) Splenic vein; (open white arrow) portal vein; (curved white arrow) right gastroepiploic vein.

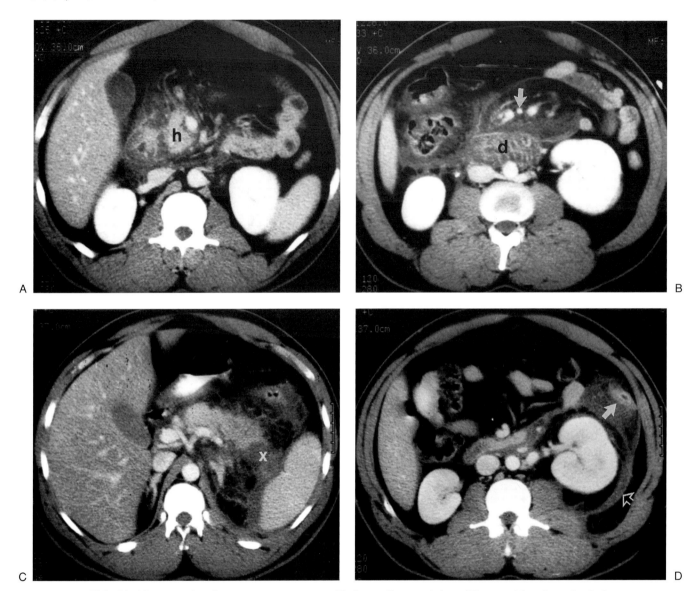

FIG. 59. Two attacks of severe acute pancreatitis,3 months apart, in a 36-year-old male patient. **A, B:** Images through the head (h) and uncinate process show involvement of the midline and right side of the anterior pararenal space by an extensive inflammatory process. Note the effect on the third/fourth duodenum (d) and the widening of the space between the aorta and the superior mesenteric artery (*arrow*). **C, D:** Three months later another attack of acute pancreatitis now affects predominately the left side of the anterior pararenal space. Note the more normal relationships of the aorta and superior mesenteric artery and vein at this time. The inflammatory, exudative process (x) now involves the descending colon (*arrow*). The fluid of the inflammatory process also dissects into the layers of the posterior portion of Gerota's fascia (*open arrow*).

mal pancreatic tissue. The pancreas is high in signal intensity on T1FS images and possesses a uniform capillary blush. In cases of more severe acute pancreatitis, variable diminished signal is present on T1FS and immediate postgadolinium spoiled GRE images (Fig. 60). The diagnosis of acute pancreatitis on MR images relies on the presence of morphologic changes, much the same as CT (221). Morphologically, the pancreas shows either focal or diffuse enlargement that may be subtle. Peripancreatic fluid is best shown on noncontrast spoiled GRE images which appears as low-signal-intensity strands of fluid collections on a background of high-signal-intensity fat.

The initial changes that are shown by CT include blurring of the outline of a swollen-appearing pancreas by edematous and inflammatory changes in the contiguous peripancreatic fat. Changes will also be recognizable in the anterior pararenal space because of dissection of fluid, initially limited in quantity into the left lateral extent of this space, resulting in the appearance of thickening of the anterior perinephric fascia (Gerota's fascia). As the inflammatory and exudative process continues, the space fills with fluid, spreading superiorly and inferiorly in this anterior compartment of the retroperitoneum. Small acute fluid collections can develop within the pancreas as well

as in the immediate peripancreatic space. Early in the evolution of severe acute pancreatitis, the barrier provided by the parietal peritoneum overlying the pancreas may be disrupted and inflammatory fluid will enter the lesser sac. From this location, the fluid may enter the main peritoneal cavity through the foramen of Winslow or may enter directly by disrupting the peritoneum in the anterior surface of the lesser sac. It has been noted that there appears to be an inverse relationship between the degree of autodigestion of the gland and the volume of peripancreatic fluid (233). Large collections of fluid often are accompanied by relative preservation of the pancreas, whereas cases involving severe parenchymal damage, including pancreatic necrosis, are more apt to be associated with lesser amounts of peripancreatic fluid.

Based on earlier generation CT images, it was believed that the posterior pararenal space was also commonly involved in the inflammatory process of severe acute pancreatitis. However, a subsequent study showed that the posterior collections actually represented extension of pancreatitis from the anterior pararenal space to a potential space between the laminae of the posterior renal fascia (see Fig. 59) (196). Among 40 patients with posterior extension of the fluid and inflammatory process, interfas-

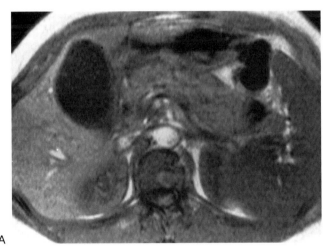

A

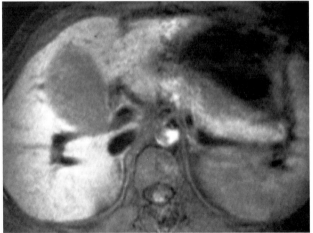

B

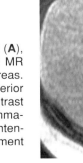

C

FIG. 60. Moderately severe acute pancreatitis. FLASH (**A**), T1FS (**B**), and immediate postgadolinium FLASH (**C**) MR images demonstrate diffuse enlargement of the pancreas. A thin layer of low-signal fluid is present along the anterior surface of the pancreas, best shown on the postcontrast image (*arrow,* C). The severity of the pancreatic inflammation has resulted in heterogeneous diminished signal intensity on the T1FS image (B) and diminished enhancement on immediate postgadolinium images (C).

cial involvement was observed in all 40 and was bilateral in 9 (23%). True involvement of the posterior pararenal space was uncommon, as was extension into the perirenal space. These investigators noted that the posterior renal fascia was thicker than the anterior and had at least two layers which could be separated. The lateroconal fascia was shown to be continuous with the posterior lamina of the posterior renal fascia, thereby serving to direct the inflammatory exudate between the fascial layers, producing an appearance that simulated extension into the posterior pararenal space.

Pathways of dissection commonly followed by the peri-pancreatic fluid and inflammatory process include the gastrohepatic, gastrosplenic, and gastrocolic ligaments (Fig. 61). Fluid will also dissect into the transverse mesocolon and along the root of the mesentery (Fig. 62). Large extrapancreatic fluid collections can extend superiorly into the mediastinum and even into the pericardial space (140,150). Following the pathways provided by the root of the mesentery and the anterior pararenal space, large collections can extend to and around segments of the cecum, ascending colon, and descending colon (Fig. 61), as well as extending inferiorly into the lumbar, pelvic, and inguinal regions (109). The Grey Turner sign of flank

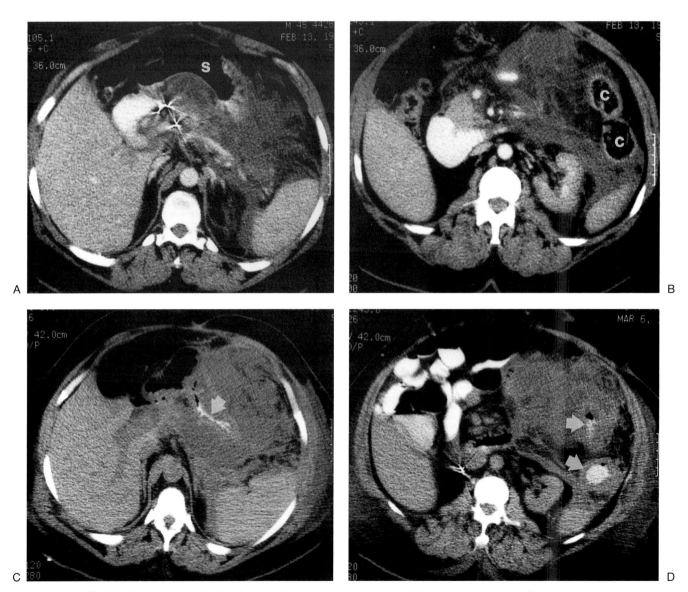

FIG. 61. Gastric and colic involvement by severe acute pancreatitis developing over a 3-week period. **A, B:** Initial CT study shows extensive inflammatory and exudative involvement of the anterior pararenal space extending into the lesser sac. The process is contiguous with the posterior surface of the stomach (s) and is approaching the splenic flexure (c). **C, D:** At approximately the same levels, 3 weeks later, the more extensive process now significantly compromises the lumen of the stomach outlined by oral contrast (*arrow,* C). The same process now surrounds and compromises the lumen of the transverse and descending colon (*arrows,* D).

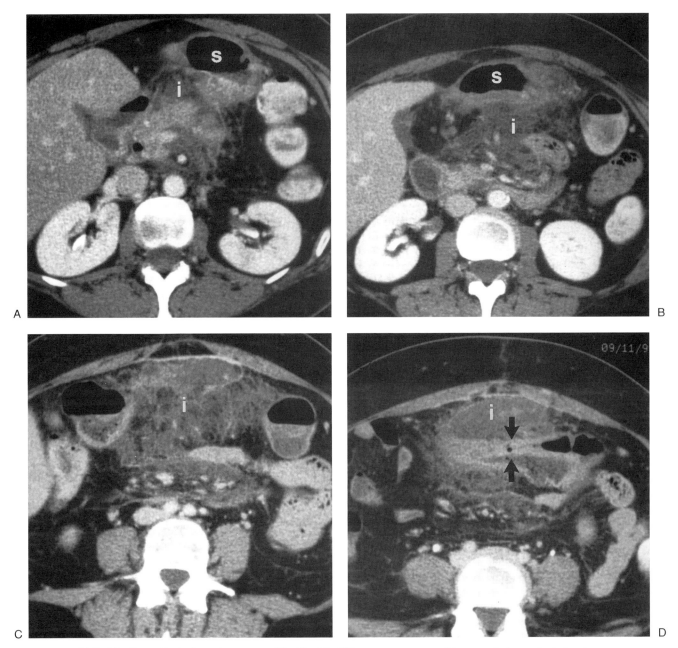

FIG. 62. Complicated acute pancreatitis (**A–D**). CT scans sequenced in a cephalocaudad direction in a middle-aged woman with acute complicated pancreatitis show spread of the inflammatory process (i) into the gastrocolic ligament and transverse mesocolon with secondary narrowing of the transverse colon (*arrows*), which is circumferentially surrounded by the inflammatory, exudative process; (s) stomach.

discoloration is produced by spread from the anterior pararenal space to between the two leaves of the posterior renal fascia and subsequently to the lateral edge of the quadratus lumborum muscle. The Cullen sign of periumbilical staining is secondary to the tracking of liberated pancreatic enzymes to the anterior abdominal wall from the inflamed gastrohepatic ligament and across the falciform ligament. Another more direct pathway would be extension of inflammatory changes in the small bowel mesentery or greater omentum to the round ligament and then to properitoneal fat beneath the umbilicus (159).

Involvement of the ascending or descending colon in the inflammatory process of severe acute pancreatitis can lead to hemorrhage, necrosis, perforation, and stricture formation (248). A pancreatic inflammatory mass involving the colon may be difficult to distinguish from a primary colonic neoplasm with local spread, based on the CT images alone (Fig. 63).

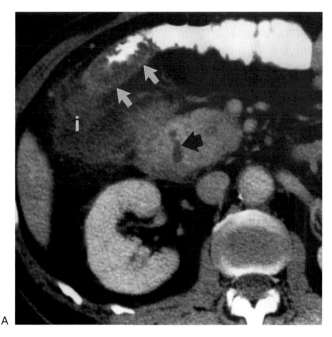

A

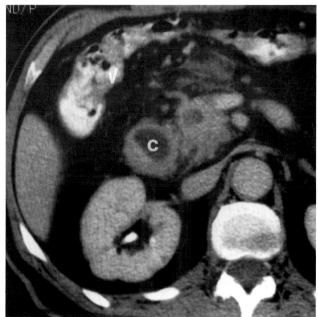

B

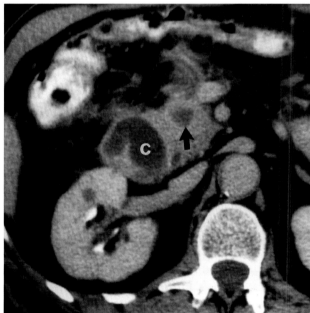

C

FIG. 63. Complication of pancreatitis—extension to right colic flexure and subsequent development of duodenal intramural pseudocyst. **A:** CT scan at the level of the head of the pancreas shows extension of the inflammatory process (i) through the transverse mesocolon to the right colic flexure. Note the marked thickening (*white arrows*) of the wall of the proximal transverse colon. Also, note the cleft of low-attenuation material (*black arrow*) within the head of the pancreas. Its relationship to the medial wall of the duodenum is not apparent at this time. **B, C:** Two contiguous CT images at approximately the same level as in A, obtained 3 months later, show relative clearing of the inflammatory process, which had extended to the right colic flexure. The colon now appears unremarkable. Previously noted cleft of fluid within the head of the pancreas now has evolved into an intramural pseudocyst (c) affecting the medial wall of the second duodenum. At this time the patient had symptoms of partial obstruction of the duodenum endoscopically confirmed. A smaller cystic area (*black arrow*) in the head of the pancreas has enlarged slightly over the interval.

In severe acute pancreatitis, an increase in the attenuation value of the peripancreatic fat is commonly observed. However, for reasons not fully understood, a cylindrical envelope of fat surrounding the superior mesenteric artery (SMA) and superior mesenteric vein (SMV) usually remains unaltered by inflammatory process (Fig. 64). In some complex cases this observation may be helpful in the distinction between inflammatory and neoplastic diseases. But exceptions to this general rule have been reported in which suspected posteriorly spreading pancreatic cancer was proven to be changes secondary to pancreatitis (143).

In contrast to the acute fluid collections, and as previously defined, pseudocysts have a thick, well-defined capsule composed of dense fibrous connective tissue and usually are round or oval in shape. Evolution of an acute fluid collection into a pseudocyst usually will occur over a period of 4 weeks or longer. Some smaller pseudocysts will ultimately spontaneously resolve whereas the majority of larger pseudocysts (>6 cm in diameter) require some form of intervention (Figs. 65 and 66) (284).

Usually the fluid in a pseudocyst is homogeneous in attenuation value near that of water. When the contents of a pseudocyst are either heterogeneous or uniformly increased in attenuation value, intracystic hemorrhage or infection may be present. If discrete areas of high-density material can be seen within a pseudocyst, clot formation

secondary to hemorrhage should be strongly suspected (Fig. 67). These same changes can occur in peripancreatic acute fluid collections secondary to hemorrhage within the substance of the pancreas or secondary to erosion of an extrapancreatic blood vessel (93).

Pseudocysts in the bowel wall have been reported in the duodenum, stomach, and colon (151,161). The rarity of intramural pseudocysts suggests that the bowel wall is a relatively strong barrier to proteolytic pancreatic enzymes. However, once the barrier is crossed, expansion of the pseudocysts within the wall is capable of producing obstruction of the bowel lumen, most typically involving the posterolateral wall of the second portion of the duodenum. Two CT features distinctive of the intramural location are (a) the extension of the pseudocyst along the wall of the duodenum, resulting in a tubular shape conforming to the course of the duodenum, and (b) abrupt flattening of the otherwise tubular or spherical pseudocyst at the border of the duodenal lumen (see Fig. 63). Circumferential involvement of the duodenum may occur.

A report of the association of duodenal duplication in the adult with pancreatitis shows that an intramural dissection of a pancreatic pseudocyst into the wall of the duodenum could be simulated by the appearance of a duodenal duplication, which can be both tubular and spherical (193). Based on imaging characteristics alone, it may be impossible to differentiate duodenal duplication

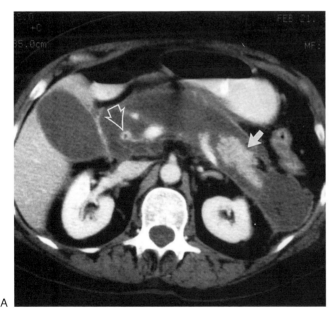 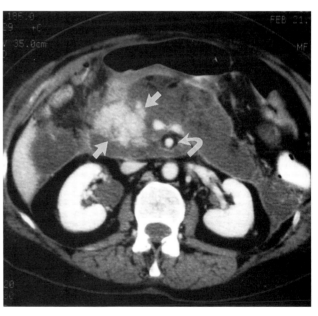

A   B

FIG. 64. Two weeks post onset of gallstone pancreatitis with severe necrosis. **A:** CT scan through the level of the body of the pancreas shows enhancement in only a small portion of the tail of the pancreas (*arrows*). The skeletonized common bile duct (*open arrow*) courses through this loculated collection. **B:** Enhancement of the pancreatic head (*arrows*) is preserved. No other portions of the pancreas, besides the small portion of the tail, remained vascularized. Note the heterogeneous composition of the material within the distended anterior pararenal space, reflecting the process of necrosis. Note also the preservation of the sleeve of fat (*curved arrow*) surrounding the enhancing superior mesenteric artery. This patient remained severely symptomatic for an additional month before being successfully decompressed by an endoscopic method.

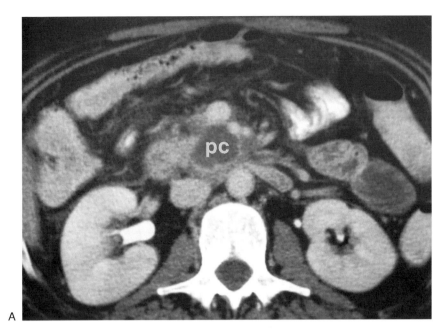

A

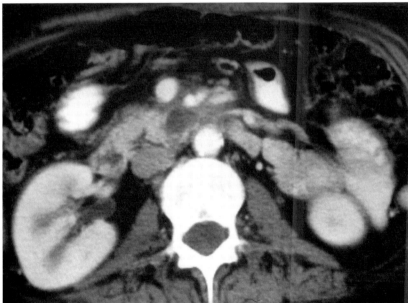

B

FIG. 65. Pseudocyst of the uncinate process resolving without intervention, followed over a 6-month period. **A, B:** A 3 × 2 cm pseudocyst (pc) is present in the uncinate process of the head of the pancreas with associated inflammatory change in the peripancreatic fat. On a 6-month follow-up, shown in B, this same pseudocyst now measures 1.5 × 1 cm and the associated peripancreatic inflammatory change has cleared.

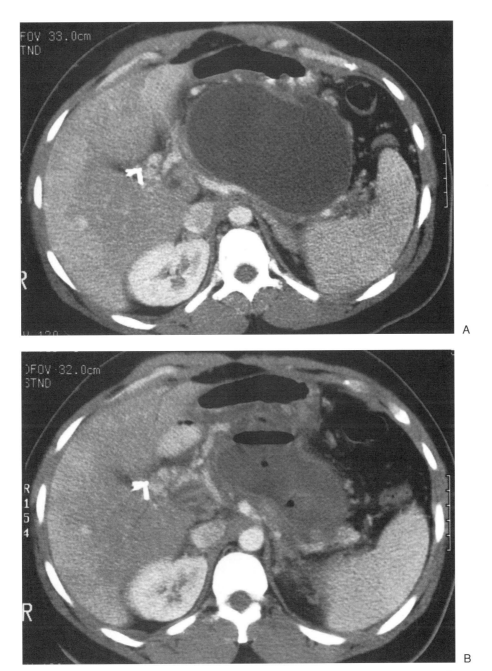

FIG. 66. Pre- and postsurgical cystogastrostomy of large pseudocyst. **A:** A large, $12 \times 7\frac{1}{2}$ cm pseudocyst compresses the body of the pancreas posteriorly. **B:** 24 hours post cystogastrostomy, significant decompression has occurred. A gas–fluid level is now present and the attenuation value of the fluid has risen reflecting a change in its composition.. Note the reduction in the compression of the body of the pancreas posterior to the collection.

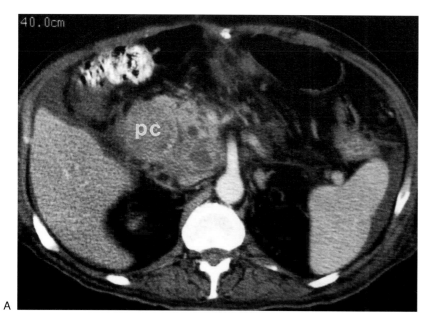

A

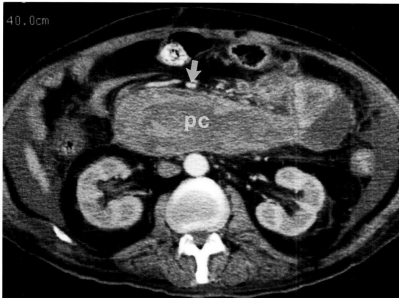

B

FIG. 67. Complication of chronic pancreatitis: hemorrhagic pseudocyst (pc) of the head of the pancreas dissecting intramurally in the second, third, and fourth portions of the duodenum. **A, B:** At the levels of the head of the pancreas and the third and fourth duodenum, a pseudocyst of the head has dissected into the wall of the duodenum expanding the space between the aorta and superior mesenteric artery (*arrow*) and obliterating the lumen of the duodenum. The scattered high-density material within the pseudocyst represents hemorrhage/hematoma.

in the setting of pancreatitis with the development of the pancreatic pseudocyst dissecting into the wall of the second duodenum. One differential feature in the cases reported was that the duplications were located most often on the mesenteric border or on its anterior border and in some cases internal septa were also detectable.

Pancreatic abscess continues to be a lethal complication of severe acute pancreatitis with mortality rates ranging from 5% to 18% in recent reports (31,148,187,268). However, not all of these studies clearly differentiated between pancreatic abscess and infected pancreatic necrosis as more recently defined. CT and ultrasound-guided fine needle aspiration of pancreatic fluid collections suspected of being infected as well as percutaneous catheter drainage have enjoyed increasing use and success in the past decade (Fig. 68) (71,244,247,262).

Although there has been some success in the percutaneous management of pseudocysts (Fig. 69) and infected pseudocysts or abscesses (12), there has been very little success in the percutaneous management of gross pancreatic necrosis (Fig. 70). Recent studies (32,118) suggest that surgical debridement is not always necessary in the absence of infected necrosis. Conversely, there is uniform agreement that infected necrosis requires surgical debridement (Fig. 71) (32,74,112,197). When patients remain systemically ill, even in the absence of infection, surgical debridement of the pancreatic necrosis is recommended by some investigators. A series of patients with symptomatic extensive organized pancreatic necrosis successfully treated with endoscopic drainage have been reported. Transgastric or transduodenal drainage was ac-complished with the addition of intrapancreatic naso-biliary lavage. The use of dynamic contrast-enhanced CT allowed the initial determination of pancreatic necrosis and also served as a guide for precise localization of these very large (mean diameter of 16 cm) collections with respect to the choice of the proper access site, either transgastric or transduodenal (Fig. 72) (19). MRI may be useful in the evaluation of encapsulated pancreatic collections. On T2-weighted images, necrotic material appears as irregular low-signal-intensity substance in the dependent portion of the encapsulated collection (Fig. 73) (213).

Determination of Prognosis

In addition to the clinical and physiologic evaluation methods described earlier, an important CT criterion is to determine whether or not pancreatic necrosis is present. The systemic hypotension that frequently follows the outpouring of fluids in pancreatitis may cause stasis within the microcirculation of the pancreas, leading to intensification of the pancreatic inflammation and ultimate ischemia and necrosis. In order to determine if necrosis is present, several investigators have used the relative degree of enhancement of the pancreatic parenchyma following a large intravenous bolus of contrast material as a determinant of the presence of necrosis (see Figs. 64, 70, 72). In a study from 1985 of 58 patients with alcohol-induced acute pancreatitis, all 36 patients with mild acute pancreatitis showed increased or normal contrast enhancement during the first 2 min following an intravenous

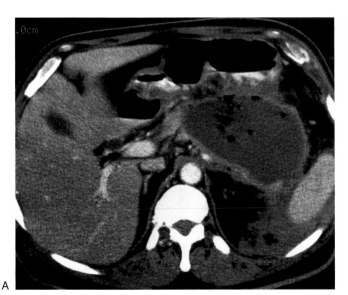
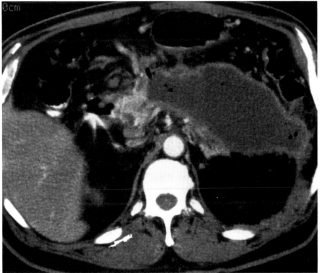

A   B

FIG. 68. Pancreatic abscess. **A, B:** Two scans at a level inferior to the body and tail of the pancreas show a well-defined fluid collection with typical changes of an abscess. Gas bubbles are noted throughout the high-viscosity pus, which was subsequently drained percutaneously successfully.

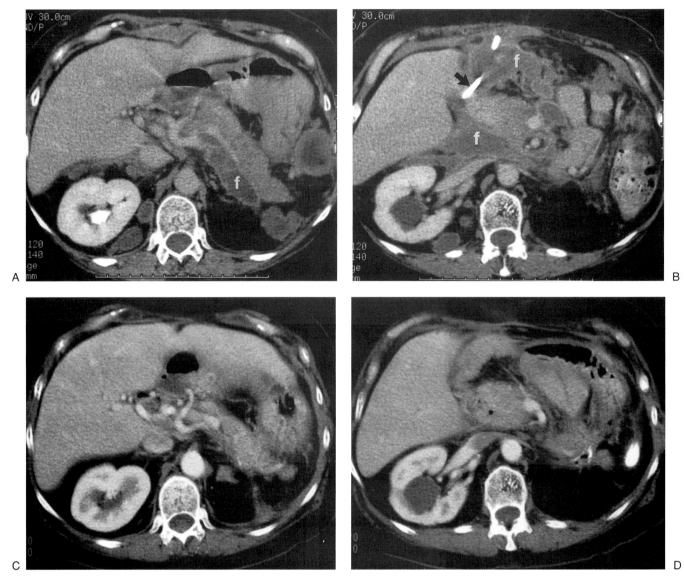

FIG. 69. One-year follow-up of severe, complicated acute pancreatitis in a 64-year-old woman. **A, B:** Scans through the body and head of the pancreas reveal extensive changes of severe acute pancreatitis. Peripancreatic fluid collections (f) are well defined. An anterior extension of the inflammatory and exudative process had required drainage through a percutaneous catheter (*arrow*). **C, D:** Images through the same levels as above, 1 year later, show the remarkable capacity for the severe inflammatory process to heal.

bolus of contrast material, whereas all those with severe acute pancreatitis (22 patients with hemorrhagic necrosis proved at laparotomy) showed decreased contrast enhancement of the pancreas (217). This same group reevaluated the methodology 8 years later, having an experience of 168 severely ill patients (123). Patients with what they termed ''hemorrhagic-necrotizing pancreatitis'' (HP) showed significantly lower contrast enhancement during the first minute after bolus injection of contrast material than patients with either a normal pancreas or those who

had ''oedematous pancreatitis'' (OP). Only 4 of 65 patients with HP showed normal (>40 Hounsfield units enhancement) and 8 of 103 patients with OP showed low (<30 Hounsfield units) contrast enhancement. These authors concluded that the method of pre- and postcontrast enhancement evaluation of the pancreas in pancreatitis seems to be the most reliable method available to differentiate the two categories of acute pancreatitis, which they called hemorrhagic-necrotizing pancreatitis from edematous (roughly the equivalent of severe and

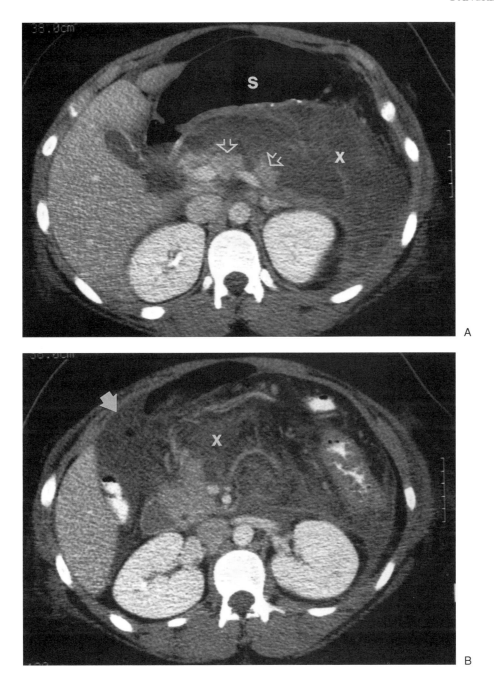

FIG. 70. Gallstone pancreatitis—severe, necrotizing. **A, B:** Two scans through the expected level of the pancreatic body and head show only fragments of enhancing pancreas (*open white arrows*) in the region of the body. No other portions of the body and tail of the pancreas were seen to enhance, indicating necrosis. The pancreatic fluid and inflammatory exudate (x) not only expands the anterior pararenal space but fills the lesser sac, displacing the stomach (s) anteriorly, and reaches the anterior abdominal wall within the peritoneal cavity (*short white arrow*).

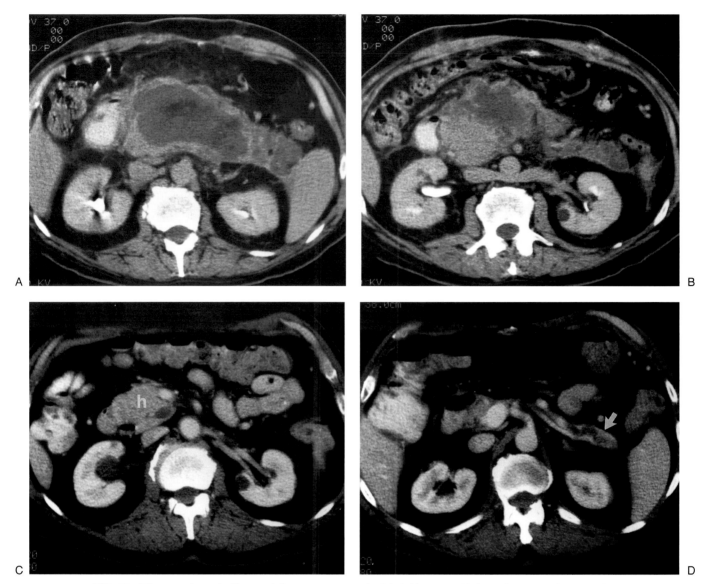

FIG. 71. Three and one-half years follow-up post surgical debridement of infected pancreatic necrosis. **A, B:** Two scans at the level of the body and head of the pancreas show marked destruction of the body and tail of the pancreas. The clinical course as well as the results of a percutaneous aspiration led to surgical debridement of this infected, post pancreatitis necrosis. **C, D:** Three and one-half year follow-up shows an intact pancreatic head (h) but only a trace of pancreatic parenchyma remaining in the tail (*arrow*) surrounding a dilated main pancreatic duct. The patient manifested no evidence of endocrine or exocrine deficiency.

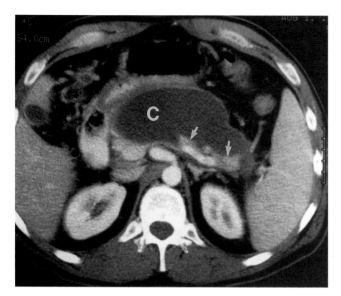

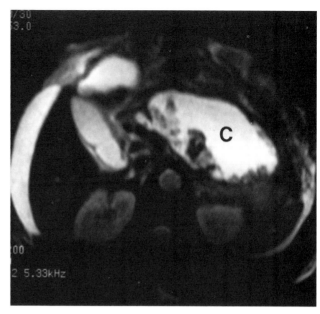

FIG. 72. Idiopathic pancreatitis complicated by necrosis. CT, obtained 7 weeks post onset of symptoms, through the level of the body of the pancreas shows absence of an enhancing pancreas in the region of the neck and distal body. A small amount of enhancing parenchyma is seen in the tail and proximal body (*white arrows*). A large, well-defined fluid collection (c) has developed and the patient has remained symptomatic with upper abdominal pain and loss of appetite. This collection was successfully drained transduodenally by an endoscopic method.

FIG. 73. MRI of pancreatic necrosis, loculated collection, 7 weeks post onset of acute, necrotizing pancreatitis associated with pancreas divisum. Cross-sectional T2FS through a fluid collection (C) associated with pancreatic necrosis shows increased signal intensity of the fluid containing lower signal intensity amorphous, semisolid necrotic debris.

mild acute pancreatitis, respectively (Figs. 74 and 75) (123). Several other studies varying in patient population size and protocol all tend to support the usefulness of dynamic, contrast-enhanced CT studies in the evaluation of acute pancreatitis (33,43,132,139,249). With regard to the role of MRI in the determination of necrosis, dynamic gadolinium-enhanced MRI may be useful for this determi-

nation as it is sensitive to the presence or absence of enhancement. Complications of acute pancreatitis such as hemorrhage or pseudocyst formation are well examined by MRI (Fig. 76). Pseudocysts are either areas of low signal intensity or signal void defects in a background of normal-signal-intensity pancreatic tissue on both spoiled GRE and T1FS images. Hemorrhagic fluid collections, in contrast, are high in signal intensity.

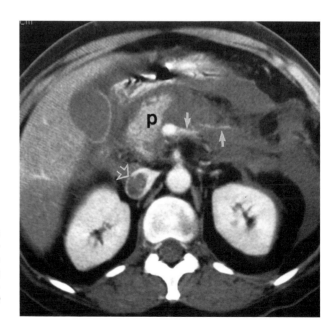

FIG. 74. Fatal necrotizing pancreatitis. Only a portion of the head of the pancreas (p) enhances, indicating extensive necrosis of the remainder of the gland. Skeletonized-appearing patent veins (*arrows*) pass through the poorly organized necrotic and inflammatory material, which dissects through the pararenal space. Note the chronic, nonocclusive thrombus (*open arrow*) within the inferior vena cava.

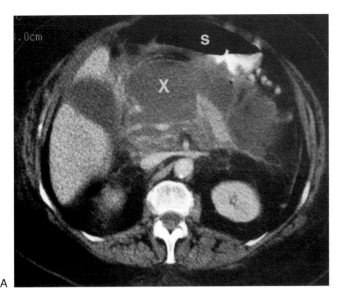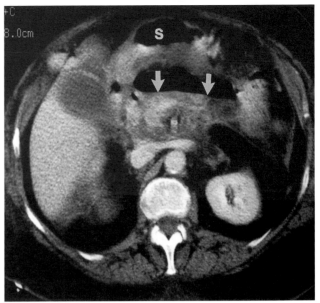

A   B

FIG. 75. Severe hemorrhagic necrotizing pancreatitis with spontaneous decompression into the stomach causing significant clinical improvement. **A:** Huge collection of fluid (x) and necrotic debris bulges into the lesser sac and compresses the stomach (s) anteriorly. **B:** Study performed 1 week later, 24 hours after the patient showed remarkable clinical improvement, shows that the collection is now substantially decompressed with a gas–fluid level being present (*arrows*). Further evaluation revealed that the patient had spontaneously communicated with the lumen of the stomach (s).

Association of Acute Pancreatitis with End-stage Renal Disease

Various reports in the literature have suggested an association between acute pancreatitis and end-stage renal disease (ESRD), including patients on maintenance dialysis (16,85,204). The association of acute pancreatitis with renal transplantation also has been emphasized (48,65,70,113,188,261). Because the patients are compromised hosts, they have an increased risk for morbidity and mortality from the disease. Furthermore, acute pancreatitis may be underdiagnosed in this category of patients, in whom elevated serum amylase levels are of limited diagnostic value. Abdominal pain in patients with ESRD should signal the possibility of acute pancreatitis and the need for appropriate imaging studies (261).

Association of Acute Pancreatitis with Pancreas Divisum

Although some investigators consider pancreas divisum as nothing more than an anatomic variant of no clinical significance (54), others believe that it has a higher than expected association with idiopathic recurrent pancreatitis (49,87,127). The latter postulate that the association of pancreas divisum with pancreatitis occurs because most of the functioning pancreatic tissue coming from the dorsal pancreas has to discharge its exocrine secretions into the duodenum through the relatively small ori-

fice at the minor papilla (Fig. 77). Of relevance is a case report in which the spared area of pancreatic tissue in the head, drained by the ventral duct, created a "pseudomass" in contrast with the diffusely fat-replaced neck, body, and tail drained by the dorsal duct (234). A separate case report described isolated ventral pancreatitis in an alcoholic patient with pancreas divisum. In this patient, the body and tail of the gland appeared normal on ultrasound, CT, and by endoscopic retrograde pancreatography. However, the changes in the ventral duct draining the head were characteristic of chronic pancreatitis producing a focal mass with some areas of calcification (35). Finally, a 5-year review of patients with pancreas divisum and documented acute or chronic pancreatitis revealed a subset of patients who appeared to benefit from endotherapeutic procedures (e.g., stenting of orifice of accessory duct) aimed at improving flow in the dorsal duct (127).

Chronic Pancreatitis

According to the revised classification of pancreatitis from the Marseille Symposium of 1984, acute and chronic pancreatitis are very different diseases and only rarely does acute pancreatitis lead to chronic pancreatitis. Chronic pancreatitis, a disease of prolonged pancreatic inflammation and fibrosis, is characterized by irreversible morphologic and/or functional abnormalities (216,236).

In one study, the average age of onset for acute pancreatitis (51 years) was 13 years greater than that for chronic

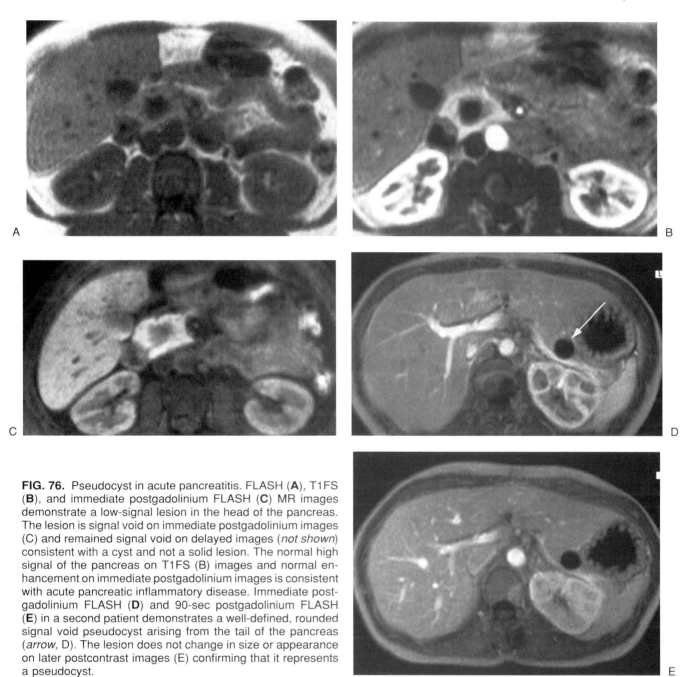

FIG. 76. Pseudocyst in acute pancreatitis. FLASH (**A**), T1FS (**B**), and immediate postgadolinium FLASH (**C**) MR images demonstrate a low-signal lesion in the head of the pancreas. The lesion is signal void on immediate postgadolinium images (C) and remained signal void on delayed images (*not shown*) consistent with a cyst and not a solid lesion. The normal high signal of the pancreas on T1FS (B) images and normal enhancement on immediate postgadolinium images is consistent with acute pancreatic inflammatory disease. Immediate postgadolinium FLASH (**D**) and 90-sec postgadolinium FLASH (**E**) in a second patient demonstrates a well-defined, rounded signal void pseudocyst arising from the tail of the pancreas (*arrow,* D). The lesion does not change in size or appearance on later postcontrast images (E) confirming that it represents a pseudocyst.

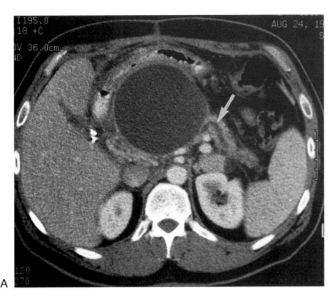

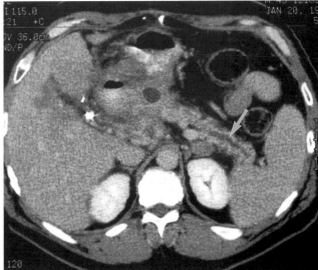

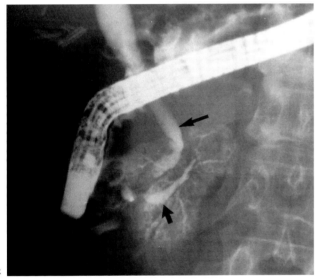

FIG. 77. Before and after cystogastrostomy in a patient with a pseudocyst and pancreas divisum. **A:** A 9-cm-diameter, well-formed pseudocyst compresses the neck and head of the pancreas posteriorly and the antrum of the stomach anteriorly. The dilated main pancreatic duct (*arrow*) is prominently visible. **B:** CT study performed 5 months following surgical cystogastrostomy reveals significant decompression of the pseudocyst with only a 10 × 12 mm collection persisting. The main pancreatic duct (*arrow*) remains dilated, but the body and tail of the pancreas are no longer compressed by the mass. **C:** ERCP shows the characteristic changes of pancreas divisum with only the common bile duct (*long arrow*) and the ventral duct (*short arrow*) of the pancreas being opacified through the major papilla. The minor papilla could not be cannulated. (ERCP courtesy of Dr. Todd Baron, Birmingham, Alabama.)

calcifying pancreatitis (38 years) (215). Most cases of true acute pancreatitis, such as recurring bouts of acute pancreatitis secondary to biliary disease, do not result in chronic pancreatitis. There is a strong association of alcohol abuse with chronic pancreatitis. It is postulated that when the first bout of clinical pancreatitis occurs in patients who are alcoholics of 6 years duration or greater, the pancreas is already diffusely scarred, and the initial bout of alcoholic pancreatitis actually heralds the onset of chronic pancreatitis (135,194,215).

In support of the concept that acute pancreatitis and chronic pancreatitis are separate diseases, a long-term follow-up of 27 patients who were treated with conservative surgery for severe acute pancreatitis, involving hemorrhagic necrosis, showed that almost complete recovery of exocrine function was achieved within 4 years after discharge, whereas about half of these patients still showed abnormal endocrine function (3). The morphologic sequelae remained relatively unchanged during the

follow-up period and the data appeared to exclude an evolution of severe pancreatitis, associated with necrosis and hemorrhage, toward chronic pancreatitis (see Fig. 71). Laboratory tests showed defective pancreatic secretion in 40% of the patients at the first follow-up evaluation, but only 7% at a later follow-up evaluation. Assessment of endocrine function, however, showed an increased incidence of diabetes at the time of the follow-up evaluation, from 11% initially to 47% of subjects after 4 years. The clinical correlation agreed with the laboratory data in that during the 4 years of the follow-up, none of the 27 patients complained of symptoms suspicious for chronic recurrent pancreatitis (3).

In addition to chronic alcoholic pancreatitis, chronic pancreatitis is found with familial occurrence in kindreds with hyperlipidemia, hyperparathyroidism, cystic fibrosis, and cholelithiasis (119). Additionally, there is a distinct group of patients with a familial form of pancreatitis in whom precipitating factors are not identified. This form

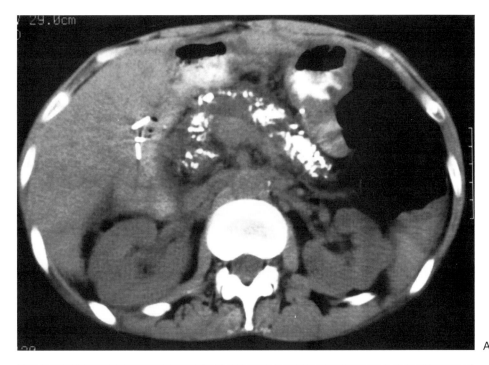

A

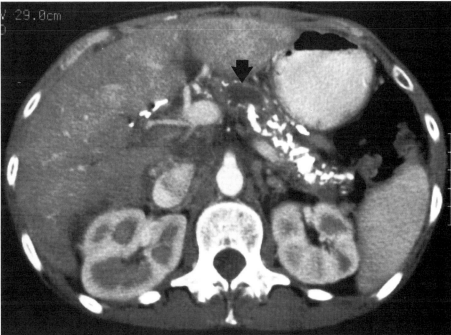

B

FIG. 78. Chronic calcifying pancreatitis. **A:** A pre-contrast CT scan through the neck and body of the pancreas shows extensive ductal calcification. **B:** Post intravenous contrast at the level of the body and tail shows minimal enhancement of pancreatic parenchyma and a prominently dilated main pancreatic duct (*arrow*). The changes are characteristic of chronic pancreatitis.

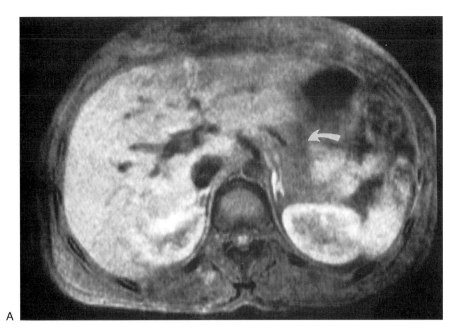

A

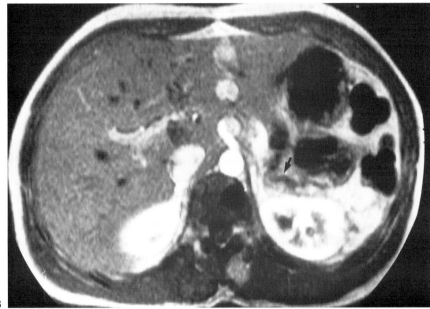

B

FIG. 79. Chronic pancreatitis. T1FS (**A**), immediate postgadolinium FLASH (**B**), and gadolinium-enhanced T1FS (**C**) images demonstrate a pancreas that is low in signal on T1FS (*arrow,* A), and enhances in a diminished, heterogeneous fashion on immediate postgadolinium images.

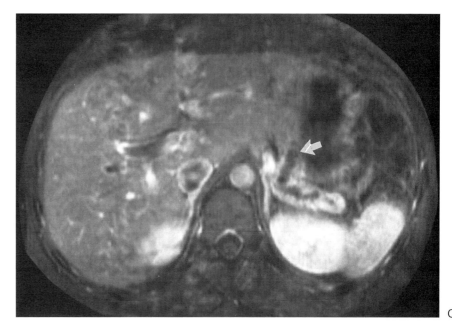

C

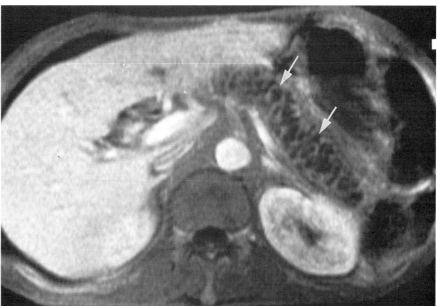

FIG. 79. (*Continued.*) Dilatation of the pancreatic duct (*arrow,* B, C) is apparent associated with atrophy of the gland, which are common features in chronic pancreatitis. Ninety-second postgadolinium FLASH (**D**) in a second patient demonstrates numerous signal void foci throughout the pancreas (*arrows*) that represent extensive calcifications in chronic pancreatitis.

D

of familial pancreatitis, termed *hereditary pancreatitis,* is thought to be inherited in an autosomal dominant fashion with variable penetrance. The typical clinical features include an early age of onset, with varying degrees of abdominal pain and disability. Complications of endocrine and exocrine pancreatic insufficiency, pseudocyst formation, and adenocarcinoma of the pancreas may develop. The hallmark finding in this form of pancreatitis is the presence of very large calculi within dilated pancreatic ducts, visible on plain radiographs of the abdomen in childhood (119,206).

Idiopathic fibrosing pancreatitis is a chronic process of unknown etiology, occurring in childhood, characterized by extensive infiltration of the pancreatic parenchyma by fibrous tissue (8). On rare occasion it has been found to be the cause of obstructive jaundice. Unlike acute pancreatitis, histologic examination of these patients demonstrates no evidence of pancreatic or fat necrosis. Of the few reported cases, follow-ups varying from 9 months to 15 years have shown no evidence of progressive pancreatic disease or development of pancreatic insufficiency (84,103,157,274).

In a retrospective analysis of 56 patients with documented chronic pancreatitis studied with contrast-enhanced CT examinations, dilatation of the main pancreatic duct was seen in 68% of cases, parenchymal atrophy in 54%, pancreatic calcifications in 50%, fluid collections in 30%, focal pancreatic enlargement in 30%, biliary ductal dilatation in 29%, and alterations in peripancreatic fat or fascia in 16% (Fig. 78) (144). In only 7% of the patients were no abnormalities detected. Also lacking, compared with earlier descriptions, was generalized pancreatic enlargement.

In theory, MRI may be better suited to detect the fibrosis of chronic pancreatitis than CT. In the presence of fibrosis MRI will show a diminished signal intensity of the gland on T1FS images and diminished heterogeneous enhancement on immediate postgadolinium spoiled GRE images (Figs. 79 and 80) (226). In a report on 22 patients, including 13 with chronic calcifying pancreatitis and 9 with presumed acute recurrent pancreatitis, differences between these groups were observed on T1FS and immediate postgadolinium MR images. All patients with pancreatic calcifications had a diminished signal intensity of the pancreatic parenchyma on T1FS and abnormally low percent contrast enhancement on postgadolinium images. In patients with acute recurrent pancreatitis the involved pancreas had signal intensity comparable to normal pancreatic parenchyma. Because fibrosis may precede the development of calcification, MRI may be capable of detecting the onset of fibrosis in chronic pancreatitis at a stage earlier than CT. However, CT is much more sensi-

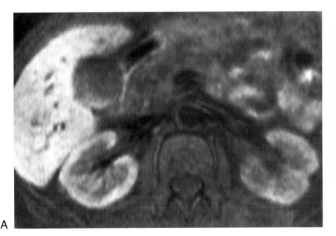

A

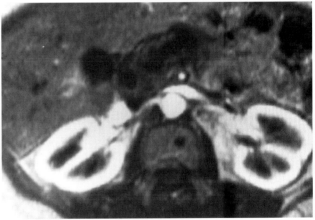

B

C

FIG. 80. Chronic pancreatitis with focal glandular enlargement. T1FS (**A**), immediate postgadolinium FLASH (**B**), and postgadolinium T1FS (**C**) images. Low signal intensity of pancreas on fat-suppressed images (A) and diminished gadolinium enhancement (B) are findings of chronic pancreatitis. Signal void rounded and tubular structures in the pancreas represent a combination of calcifications and common bile and pancreatic ducts (A–C). (Reproduced with permission from ref. 227.)

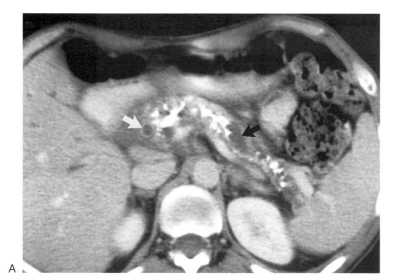

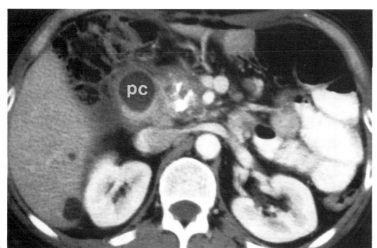

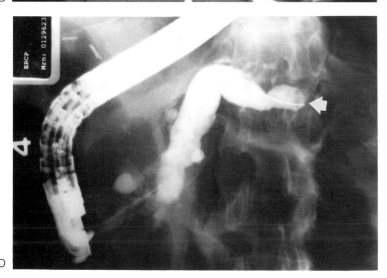

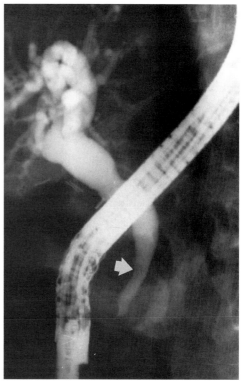

FIG. 81. Chronic pancreatitis with biochemical evidence of intermittent bile duct obstruction. **A, B:** CT scans at the level of the body and head of the pancreas in a 45-year-old male patient with known chronic pancreatitis show characteristic, extensive ductal calcification associated with a prominently dilated main pancreatic duct (*black arrow*). Although the biliary tract was significantly dilated within the liver, the bile duct (*white arrow*) within the substance of the pancreas tapered progressively toward the ampulla. A pseudocyst (pc)) adds to the degree of obstruction by its compressive effect. **C, D:** Images of the biliary tract and main pancreatic duct from an ERCP show a dilated intrahepatic and proximal extrahepatic biliary tract with tapered narrowing of that portion of the bile duct within the substance of the pancreas (*arrow,* C). The markedly dilated main pancreatic duct with associated side branch dilatation and irregularity are characteristic changes of chronic obstructive, calcifying pancreatitis. The guidewire is halted by a completely obstructing calculus (*arrow,* D). Other calculi are obscured by the contrast in the opacified portion of the duct. (ERCP courtesy of Dr. Todd Baron, Birmingham, Alabama.)

tive than MRI in detecting calcifications. In cases where the differential diagnosis is between pancreatic cancer and focal chronic pancreatitis, MRI may be capable of showing diffuse low signal intensity of the entire pancreas, including the area of focal enlargement on T1FS and immediate postgadolinium spoiled GRE images, lending support for a diagnosis of chronic pancreatitis. Small pseudocysts are well shown on gadolinium-enhanced T1FS images (Fig. 76).

As stated previously, smooth or beaded dilatation of the main pancreatic duct is most commonly associated with carcinoma, whereas irregular dilatation is more frequently seen in chronic pancreatitis. Furthermore, a ratio of duct width to total gland width <0.5 favors the diagnosis of chronic pancreatitis (117). Chronic pancreatitis occasionally can present as a focal, noncalcified mass that by all CT criteria would be indistinguishable from a carcinoma (130,171). Despite appropriate follow-up periods and the performance of transhepatic cholangiography and/or ERCP and percutaneous needle biopsy, many of these cases remain indeterminate and direct surgical assessment is required.

Chronic pancreatitis also can be associated with ob-struction of the biliary tree. In most instances, the lumen of the obstructed common bile duct tapers gradually, in contrast to an abrupt transition commonly associated with neoplasm (Fig. 81). In an analysis of 51 patients with chronic alcoholic pancreatitis and common duct obstruction, an elevated serum alkaline phosphatase level was the most common abnormal laboratory finding (4). The elevation in serum bilirubin level was never progressive; a rising and falling pattern was most often encountered. The combination of CT evaluation and cholangiography by either the percutaneous or endoscopic route, correlated with the clinical and laboratory findings, generally will permit differentiation of this type of bile duct obstruction secondary to fibrosis from that due to neoplasm.

Pseudocysts can occur in both acute pancreatitis and chronic pancreatitis. When pseudocysts are found in association with ductal dilatation and intraductal calcification, chronic pancreatitis is the underlying disease (Figs. 82 and 83). Along with hemorrhage and superinfection, as previously discussed, another major complication of pseudocyst formation is spontaneous rupture. Pseudocysts may rupture into the peritoneal cavity (with the development of ascites), into the extraperitoneal spaces, the pleu-

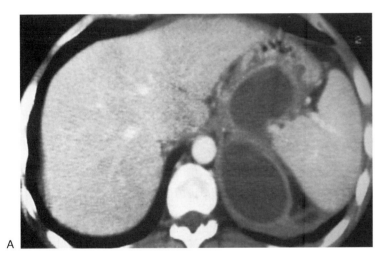

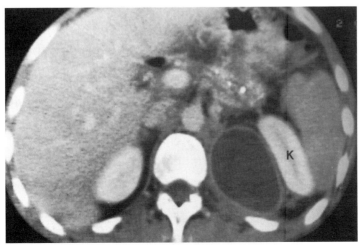

FIG. 82. Pancreatic pseudocyst. **A:** A biloculated pseudocyst displaces the spleen laterally and the stomach anteriorly. The uniform low density of the fluid and the well-defined wall are characteristic of a mature pseudocyst. **B:** The inferior extension of the posterior component of the pseudocyst displaces and compresses the left kidney (K) between itself and the spleen. Flecks of calcification are present in the body of the pancreas, consistent with the patient's known chronic pancreatitis.

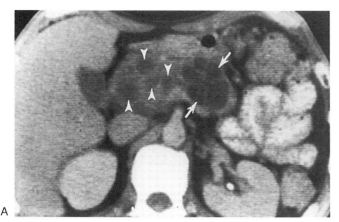

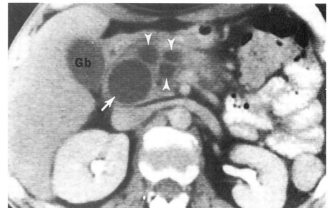

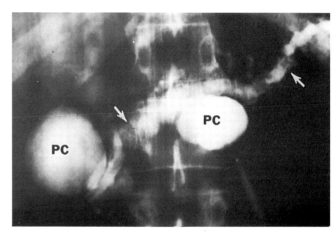

FIG. 83. Multiple pseudocysts in a patient with chronic pancreatitis. **A:** A large septated pseudocyst (*arrows*) and smaller cystic areas (*arrowheads*) are present in an enlarged pancreatic body. **B:** An image 2 cm caudad shows several other small pseudocysts (*arrowheads*) in addition to a large unilocular pseudocyst (*arrow*) in the head of the pancreas; (Gb) gallbladder. **C:** An intraoperative pancreatogram shows an enlarged pancreatic duct (*arrows*), with contrast material filling the two dominant pseudocysts (PC). The smaller pseudocysts either are not adequately filled with contrast material or are not in free communication with the main pancreatic duct.

ral cavity, or the gastrointestinal tract (see Fig. 75) (128,269,271). Pancreaticopleural fistulas are most often associated with chronic alcoholic pancreatitis and in these cases the patients present more often with chest symptoms than with abdominal symptoms. Endoscopic retrograde pancreatography combined with CT can generally delineate the cause for the recurring pleural effusion (205,260). When communication with the lumen of the bowel is established, gas may be seen within the pseudocyst and will not necessarily be an indication of a gas-forming infection (155,156,257).

Pseudocysts can be confused with cystic or necrotic tumors, a markedly dilated and tortuous pancreatic duct, or a true or false aneurysm of an intrapancreatic or peripancreatic artery (Fig. 84) (116). Cystic tumors usually occur in patients without a history of pancreatitis and may show some characteristic CT findings, as previously described. Necrotic tumors generally have thick and irregular walls that rarely, if ever, calcify, compared with the uniform and occasionally calcified walls of pseudocysts. Aneurysms or false aneurysms characteristically will be enhanced following an intravenous bolus of contrast material (Figs. 85 to 87). Even prior to administration of contrast material, the similarity between the density of the fluid in the false aneurysm and the density of the blood in the aorta or vena cava will be a clue to its nature.

Aneurysms or false aneurysms can also be diagnosed by MRI and pulsed Doppler ultrasound without the use of intravenous contrast agents.

Chronic pancreatitis has been shown to be associated with splenic and portal venous obstruction. In a review of 266 patients with chronic pancreatitis who were followed up for a mean time of 8.2 years, splenic and portal venous obstruction was found in 35 patients (13.2%) but was symptomatic in only two. Initial obstruction involved the splenic vein in 22 patients, the portal vein in 10, and the superior mesenteric vein in 3. The authors concluded that in chronic pancreatitis, splenic and portal venous obstruction should be systematically sought in patients with acute problems or pseudocysts, especially if therapeutic decisions would be modified by a diagnosis of venous obstruction. The data also showed that the risk of gastrointestinal variceal bleeding is lower than previously reported (23).

Chronic pancreatitis frequently results in pancreatic insufficiency of both the exocrine and endocrine functions. However, some patients may initially present in a state of pancreatic insufficiency without a clear cause being apparent in the patient's previous medical history. In one retrospective review of patients diagnosed as having pancreatic insufficiency, CT was found to be a key diagnostic tool in understanding the cause of the problem. Previously

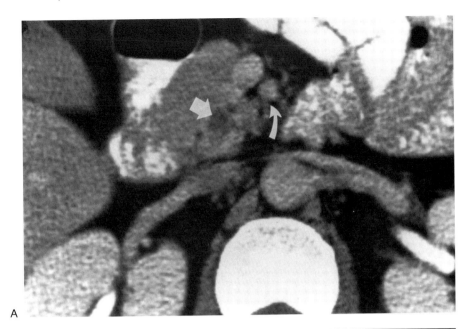

A

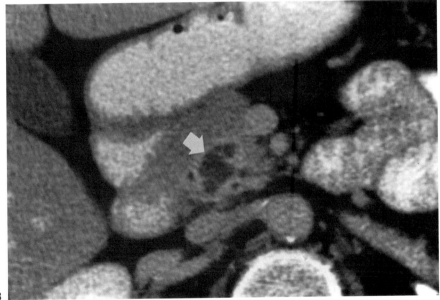

B

FIG. 84. Slowly enlarging area of chronic fibrosis with cystic change mimicking a cystic tumor. **A:** An ill-defined low-density area is present in the uncinate process of the head of the pancreas (*straight arrow*) with some focal inflammatory change extending toward the superior mesenteric artery (*curved arrow*). **B:** Thirteen-month follow-up shows a larger, more well-defined cystic mass, raising the question of a cystic tumor. The surgical specimen revealed a focal area of chronic pancreatitis with fibrotic and cystic change. Inflammatory adhesions to the wall of the superior mesenteric artery were noted by the surgeon.

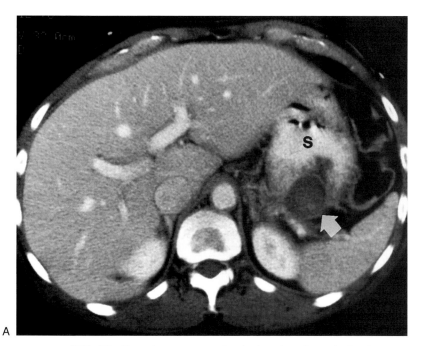
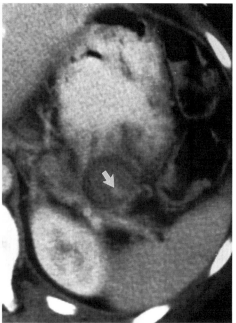

A   B

FIG. 85. Pseudoaneurysm of splenic artery branch due to pancreatitis. **A:** A cystic structure (*arrow*) is seen lying between the tail of the pancreas and the posterior aspect of the stomach (s). The center of the cystic structure appears to have material of higher attenuation value than the periphery. **B:** Detailed view of the pseudocyst shows a slightly eccentric focus of enhancement (*arrow*) surrounded by a nonenhancing hematoma within the larger cavity containing lower attenuation value serum. These findings indicated the true nature of this surgically proven pseudoaneurysm.

undiagnosed carcinoma, classic changes of chronic pancreatitis, confirmation of complete surgical removal, and evidence of complete idiopathic atrophy were some of the diagnostic findings described. Because pancreatic insufficiency often is a difficult clinical diagnostic problem, CT should be used if abdominal radiographs or sonograms are nondiagnostic (231).

Pancreatic Changes in Cystic Fibrosis and Associated Diseases

Cystic fibrosis (CF) is a dysfunction of exocrine glands characterized by chronic bronchopulmonary infections, malabsorption secondary to pancreatic insufficiency, and an increased sweat sodium concentration. Complete fatty replacement of the pancreatic parenchyma has been shown both by CT and by ultrasound to occur in cystic fibrosis (53,183). MRI has been able to demonstrate similar changes in the pancreas and the lack of ionizing radiation may be of value in this young patient population. Three patterns of pancreatic abnormality have been described: lobulated enlarged pancreas with complete fatty replacement, small atrophic pancreas with partial fatty replacement, and diffusely atrophic pancreas without fatty replacement (252). Fatty replacement is well shown on T1-weighted images as high- signal-intensity tissue. The fatty nature of the tissue may be confirmed with

T1FS by demonstrating suppression of the signal from the gland (Fig. 88). A less common manifestation of cystic fibrosis has been complete replacement of the pancreas by multiple macroscopic cysts. This form of pancreatic cystosis is considered an inflammatory process in which complete cystic transformation of the pancreas occurs, possibly related to ductal protein hyperconcentration, inspissation, and ductal ectasia (41,96).

The Schwachman-Diamond syndrome, which occurs 100 times less commonly than cystic fibrosis, is considered second only to cystic fibrosis as a cause of exocrine pancreatic insufficiency in children. The absence of abnormal sweat electrolytes and the tendency to improvement distinguishes this disease from cystic fibrosis. On CT examination in this disease, the pancreas commonly is totally replaced by fat. Lipomatosis of the pancreas is the typical pathologic feature of this syndrome (203).

The Johanson-Blizzard syndrome, which consists of congenital aplasia of the alae nasi, deafness, hypothyroidism, dwarfism, absent permanent teeth, and malabsorption, presents with pancreatic insufficiency as a nearly uniform finding, and the severe degree of malabsorption is often fatal in infancy. If enzyme supplements successfully correct the malabsorption, the affected individuals can reach adulthood. Total lack of a normal pancreas and fatty replacement in the pancreatic bed is the characteristic CT finding. In contrast to the Schwachman-Diamond syndrome, in which the pancreatic defect is restricted to exo-

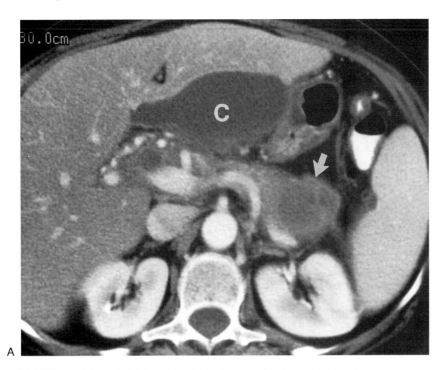

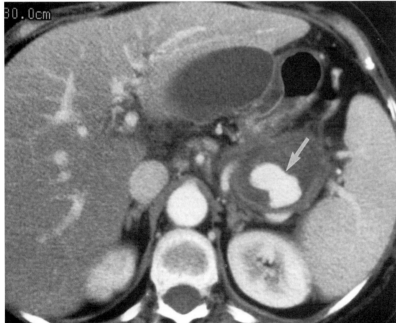

FIG. 86. Post pancreatitis pseudoaneurysm of splenic artery. **A:** CT scan at the level of the pancreatic body and tail shows the presence of a cystic appearing mass (*white arrow*) in the tail of the pancreas. A more low-attenuation value pseudocyst (c) lies wedged between the posterior surface of the left lobe of the liver and the stomach. **B:** CT scan 2 cm cephalad to the level in Figure A shows enhancement of the center of this mass (*arrow*) equal to the enhancement of the aortic lumen. The findings are diagnostic of a pseudoaneurysm arising from the splenic artery. Low-attenuation clot surrounds the enhancing lumen.

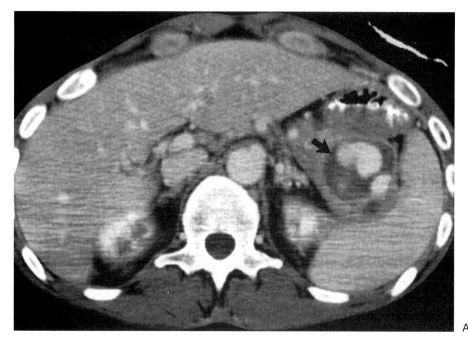

A

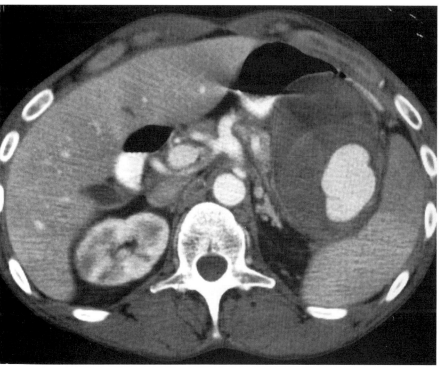

B

FIG. 87. Expanding pseudoaneurysm secondary to acute pancreatitis. **A:** Initial contrast-enhanced CT reveals a $4\frac{1}{2}$ cm in diameter pseudoaneurysm in the region of the tail of the pancreas (*arrow*) with enhancement of the central portions equivalent to the enhancement of the aorta. For overriding clinical reasons, this pseudoaneurysm was not initially treated. **B:** Follow-up examination, 70 days after the initial study, shows marked expansion of the pseudoaneurysm with several layers reflecting various ages of hematoma visible. The lumen of the pseudoaneurysm has tripled in size over this period of time. Surgically resected. (Courtesy of Dr. Rob Wise, South Georgia Medical Center, Valdosta, Georgia).

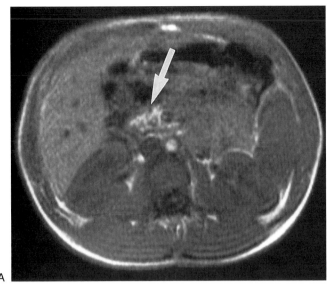 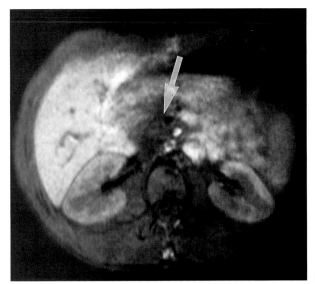

A   B

FIG. 88. Pancreas in cystic fibrosis. FLASH (**A**) and T1FS (**B**) images. The pancreas is fatty replaced as shown by high signal on FLASH images (*arrow,* A), which diminishes in signal on fat-suppressed images (*arrow,* B).

crine dysfunction, diabetes mellitus will develop in patients with the Johanson-Blizzard syndrome (259).

Primary Hemochromatosis

Primary hemochromatosis is a hereditary disease in which iron is deposited in the parenchyma of various organs. The liver, pancreas, and heart are primarily affected. On MR images, the iron deposition results in loss of signal on T2-weighted sequences (Fig. 89). Iron deposition is predominantly in the liver. Deposition of iron in

the pancreas tends to occur later, after liver damage is irreversible (232).

Pancreatic Trauma

Because of its relatively fixed extraperitoneal location just anterior to the spine, the pancreas occasionally is affected in blunt upper abdominal trauma. Either blunt or sharp abdominal trauma may cause pancreatic ductal disruption, with subsequent escape of pancreatic enzymes and the potential for development of the entire spectrum

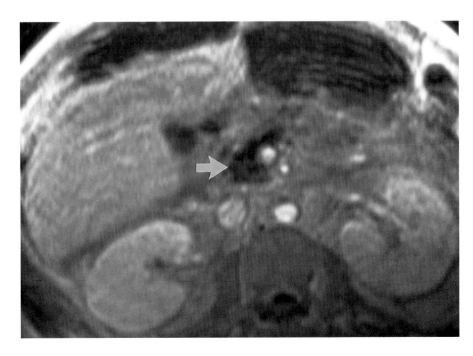

FIG. 89. Pancreas in primary hemochromatosis. The pancreas (*arrow*) is near signal void on 90-sec postgadolinium FLASH image consistent with iron deposition in the pancreas. The liver appears more normal in signal because it is a transplanted liver.

of acute pancreatitis (Fig. 90). The appearances of traumatic pancreatitis on CT are the same as with a nontraumatic cause (256). However, a recent study of 10 patients with surgical or autopsy-proved pancreatic injury after blunt abdominal trauma who were all evaluated with CT scan showed the presence of fluid interdigitating between the splenic vein and the pancreatic parenchyma in nine patients. The authors concluded that this was a very helpful CT finding for the diagnosis of traumatic pancreatic injury (131).

Complete transection of the pancreas can be diagnosed by CT (Fig. 91). The two ends of the transected gland generally are separated by a variable quantity of low-density fluid that will remain relatively confined to the anterior pararenal space in the immediate postinjury period (9,237). Intraoperative injury of the pancreas occasionally will be seen following splenectomy. The diagnosis can be established by CT in the early postoperative period (13,277). A more detailed description of CT findings in pancreatic trauma can be found in Chapter 21.

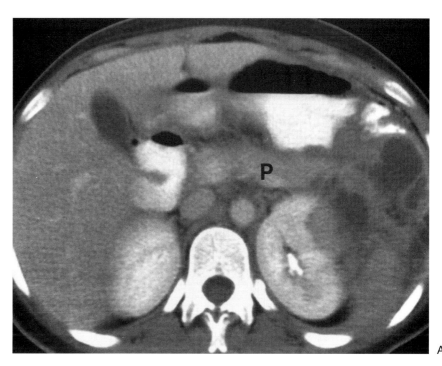

A

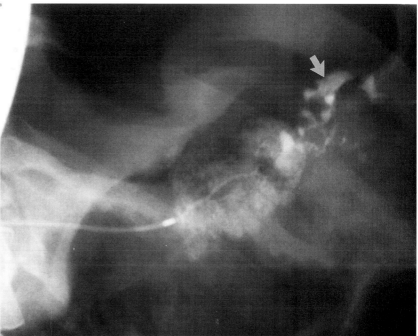

B

FIG. 90. Delayed recognition of traumatic injury to tail of the pancreas secondary to motor vehicle accident injury. **A:** CT scan through the level of the kidneys and tail of the pancreas (P) shows an area of diminished nephrogram involving the lateral aspect of the left kidney and loculations of fluid anterolateral to the left kidney. An assumption was made that the fluid was related to the renal injury. **B:** Continued left upper quadrant pain led to the patient's transfer. A review of her outside CT suggested posttraumatic pseudocyst. This detailed view of the tail of the pancreas from an ERCP shows extravasation of the contrast medium (*arrow*) from the injured pancreatic tail. The patient was successfully treated with a main pancreatic duct stent, resulting in complete resolution of the left upper quadrant inflammatory process. (Case courtesy of Dr. Todd Baron, Birmingham, Alabama.)

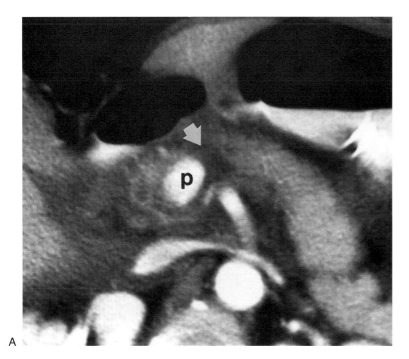

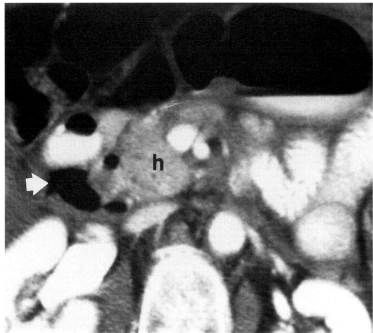

FIG. 91. Traumatic transection of the neck of the pancreas with associated perforation of the second duodenum. **A:** Detailed CT view at the junction of the body and neck of the pancreas shows complete transection (*arrow*) of the neck of the pancreas. The entire area is surrounded by a combination of clotted blood and pancreatic fluid. The portal vein (p) is partly skeletonized. **B:** At the level of the head (h), extraluminal, retroperitoneal gas (*arrow*) is detected behind the second duodenum. At the time of operation, the neck and head of the pancreas were badly crushed. A small perforation of the posterior wall of the duodenum was also found.

POSTOPERATIVE EVALUATION

In patients who have either partial or total pancreatectomy, most often for neoplastic disease, frequently it is difficult to opacify with oral contrast material those segments of bowel used for the anastomosis to the biliary tree or remaining segment of pancreas because of the direction of flow in these Roux-en-Y loops. Administration of glucagon prior to CT imaging facilitates opacification of the afferent jejunal loop with oral contrast material, thus helping to define the structures in the right upper quadrant and to distinguish the unopacified loop of bowel from possible recurrent tumor in the region of the head of the pancreas (Fig. 92) (94). In postoperative patients, the lymph node–bearing region between the aorta and the SMV and SMA, previously occupied by the uncinate process of the pancreas, is an important area to evaluate for tumor recurrence. Because radical pancreatectomy usually leaves this area free of tissue having the attenuation value of either pancreatic tissue or lymph nodes, tumor recurrence will be readily detectable by CT.

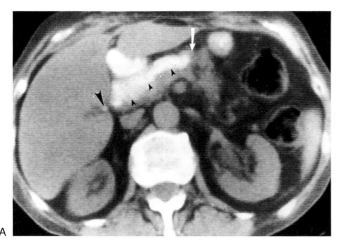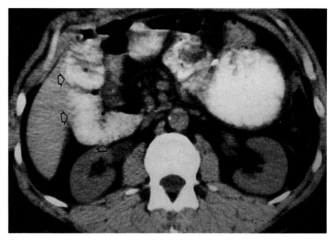

FIG. 92. Normal post-Whipple CT appearance. **A:** Pancreaticojejunal anastomosis (*white arrow*) is seen anterior to the superior mesenteric artery at the level of the splenic vein. Jejunal loop filled with oral contrast material (*small arrowheads*) courses rightward to porta hepatis, where contrast material has refluxed into the common hepatic duct (*large arrowhead*). **B:** CT images from a different patient who was given intravenous glucagon prior to imaging. The afferent jejunal loop (*arrows*) has filled with oral contrast material, probably as a result of paralysis of antegrade peristalsis. (From ref. 94.)

PANCREAS TRANSPLANTATION

Most pancreas transplants are performed in combination with renal transplants and as such account for at least 86% of all pancreas transplants performed in the United States (190,219). Pancreatic graft survival rates have been shown to be highest when kidney-pancreas transplants are performed rather than isolated pancreatic grafts (1-year graft survival, 74% versus 50%; 5-year graft survival, 65% versus 20%) (190). The improvement in survival presumably relates to the practice of biopsying the renal transplant for signs of rejection. When these signs were present, they were often concomitant with rejection of the pancreas transplant, thus providing a stimulus for more aggressive therapy to combat rejection.

The pancreas transplants usually are anastomosed to either the right or left common iliac vessels, resulting in a soft-tissue mass in the upper pelvis slightly to the right or left of midline. The major value of CT in the assessment of pancreas transplantation is in the identification and management of perigraft abdominal fluid collections in transplant patients with abdominal pain and fever. The fluid represents the exocrine secretion of the transplant. During the initial development of techniques for performing pancreas transplantation, either the pancreas was allowed to drain openly into the peritoneum or the pancreatic duct was ligated, injected with polymers, or internally drained via a Roux-en-Y pancreaticojejunostomy. A more recent surgical technique has been to anastomose a cuff of accompanying duodenum to the dome of the urinary bladder, allowing drainage of pancreatic secretions into the lumen of the bladder. In such cases, good CT technique, with complete opacification of the bowel lumen, as well as precise knowledge of the surgical technique

employed, is necessary for adequate evaluation of these complex cases. CT has not been particularly valuable in determining the presence or absence of transplant rejection (147), but it can be helpful in revealing subtle anastomotic leaks (24).

A growing body of experience indicates that pulsed Doppler ultrasonography will play a larger role in the evaluation of pancreas transplants, with assessment of the arterial inflow and venous outflow as well as other indications of vascularity within the pancreatic parenchyma (68,181,182,255). MRI of the pancreas transplant is still at an investigational level. One study showed that although MRI was capable of producing excellent images of the in situ pancreatic transplant, the imaging method was unable to reliably distinguish the normal from the abnormal transplant with unenhanced MRI scans (120). A separate brief report suggested that enhanced MRI studies could differentiate normal pancreatic transplants from dysfunctional ones based on the percent enhancement (66). In a more recent series with time-of-flight MR angiographic sequences (breath-hold gradient-recalled acquisition in the steady state and spoiled gradient-recalled echo imaging), signal void within a vascular pedicle had a sensitivity of 100% and a specificity of 93% for acute vascular thrombosis of pancreas transplants (129).

CLINICAL ROLES OF CT AND MRI

At the present time, CT and ultrasound should remain the first-line imaging methods in the evaluation of pancreatic disease primarily because of greater availability and more extensive experience with these imaging methods. Patients may be considered for MR studies in the following clinical settings: (a) patients with impaired renal function, allergy to iodinated contrast media, or other contraindications for iodine contrast administration; (b) symptomatic patients with focal enlargement of the pancreas in which no definable mass can be identified on CT; (c) patients in whom the clinical history is worrisome for malignancy and the findings on CT are equivocal or difficult to interpret; (d) where a distinction cannot be made between chronic pancreatitis with focal enlargement and pancreatic carcinoma; and (e) patients with biochemical evidence of pancreatic endocrine tumors but indeterminate findings on CT.

REFERENCES

1. Ahlström H, Magnusson A, Grama D, Eriksson B, Öberg K, Lörelius L-E. Preoperative localization of endocrine pancreatic tumours by intra-arterial dynamic computed tomography. *Acta Radiol* 1990;31:171–175.
2. Ahmed A, Chan KF, Song IS. Annular pancreas. *J Comput Assist Tomogr* 1982;6:409–411.
3. Angelini G, Pederzoli P, Caliari S, et al. Long-term outcome of acute necrohemorrhagic pancreatitis: a 4-year follow-up. *Digestion* 1984;30:131–137.
4. Aranha GV, Prinz RA, Freeark RJ, Greenlee HB. The spectrum of biliary tract obstruction from chronic pancreatitis. *Arch Surg* 1984;119:595–600.
5. Ariyama J, Suyama M, Ogawa K, et al. The detection and prognosis of small pancreatic carcinoma. *Int J Pancreatol* 1990;7:37–47.
6. Aspestrand F, Kolmannskog F. CT compared to angiography for staging of tumors of the pancreatic head. *Acta Radiol* 1992;33:556–560.
7. Aspestrand F, Kolmannskog F, Jacobsen M. CT, MR imaging and angiography in pancreatic apudomas. *Acta Radiol* 1993;34:468–473.
8. Atkinson GO Jr, Wyly JB, Gay BB Jr, Ball TI, Winn KJ. Idiopathic fibrosing pancreatitis: a cause of obstructive jaundice in childhood. *Pediatr Radiol* 1988;18:28–31.
9. Baker LP, Wagner EJ, Brotman S, Whitley NO. Transection of the pancreas. *J Comput Assist Tomogr* 1982;6:411–412.
10. Baker RJ. Acute surgical diseases of the pancreas. *Surg Clin North Am* 1972;52:239–256.
11. Balthazar EJ, Chako AC. Computed tomography of pancreatic masses. *Am J Gastroenterol* 1990;85:343–349.
12. Balthazar EJ, Freeny PC, vanSonnenberg E. Imaging and intervention in acute pancreatitis. *Radiology* 1994;193:297–306.
13. Balthazar EJ, Megibow A, Rothberg M, Lefleur RS. CT evaluation of pancreatic injury following splenectomy. *Gastrointest Radiol* 1985;10:139–144.
14. Balthazar EJ, Robinson DL, Megibow AJ, Ranson JH. Acute pancreatitis: value of CT in establishing prognosis. *Radiology* 1990;174:331–336.
15. Balthazar EJ, Subramanyam BR, Lefleur RS, Barone CM. Solid and papillary epithelial neoplasm of the pancreas: radiographic, CT, sonographic, and angiographic features. *Radiology* 1984;150:39–40.
16. Barcenas CG, Gonzalez-Molina M, Hull AR. Association between acute pancreatitis and malignant hypertension with renal failure. *Arch Intern Med* 1978;138:1254–1256.
17. Barish MA, Yucel EK, Soto JA, Chuttani R, Ferrucci JT. MR cholangiopancreatography: efficacy of three-dimensional turbo spin-echo technique. *AJR* 1995;165:295–300.
18. Baron RL, Stanley RJ, Lee JKT, Koehler RE, Levitt RG. Computed tomographic features of biliary obstruction. *AJR* 1983;140:1173–1178.
19. Baron TH, Thaggard WG, Morgan DE, Stanley RJ. Endoscopic

20. management of organized pancreatic necrosis. *Gastroenterology* 1996;111:755–764.
20. Beahrs OH, Henson DE, Hutter RVP, Kennedy BJ. *Manual for staging of cancer,* 4th ed. Philadelphia: JB Lippincott, 1992.
21. Berk T, Friedman LS, Goldstein SD, Marks GP, Rosato FE. Relapsing acute pancreatitis as the presenting manifestation of an ampullary neoplasm in a patient with familial polyposis coli. *Am J Gastroenterol* 1985;80:627–629.
22. Berland LL, Lawson TL, Foley WD, Geenen JE, Stewart ET. Computed tomography of the normal and abnormal pancreatic duct: correlation with pancreatic ductography. *Radiology* 1981;141:715–724.
23. Bernades P, Baetz A, Levy P, Belghiti J, Menu Y, Fekete F. Splenic and portal venous obstruction in chronic pancreatitis. A prospective longitudinal study of a medical-surgical series of 266 patients. *Dig Dis Sci* 1992;37:340–346.
24. Bischof TP, Thoeni RF, Melzer JS. Diagnosis of duodenal leaks from kidney-pancreas transplants in patients with duodenovesical anastomoses: value of CT cystography. *AJR* 1995;165:349–354.
25. Boden G. Glucagonomas and insulinomas. *Gastroenterol Clin North Am* 1989;18:831–845.
26. Bok EJ, Cho KJ, Williams DM, Brady TM, Weiss CA, Forrest ME. Venous involvement in islet cell tumors of the pancreas. *AJR* 1984;142:319–322.
27. Bonaldi VM, Bret PM, Atri M, Garcia P, Reinhold C. A comparison of two injection protocols using helical and dynamic acquisitions in CT examinations of the pancreas. *AJR* 1996;167:49–55.
28. Boyle P, Hsieh CC, Maisonneuve P, et al. Epidemiology of pancreas cancer (1988). *Int J Pancreatol* 1989;5:327–346.
29. Bradley EL, Gonzalez AC, Clements JL Jr. Acute pancreatic pseudocysts: incidence and implications. *Ann Surg* 1976;184:734–737.
30. Bradley EL III. A clinically based classification system for acute pancreatitis. *Arch Surg* 1993;128:586–590.
31. Bradley EL III. Management of infected pancreatic necrosis by open drainage. *Ann Surg* 1987;206:542–550.
32. Bradley EL III, Allen K. A prospective longitudinal study of observation versus surgical intervention in the management of necrotizing pancreatitis. *Am J Surg* 1991;161:19–24.
33. Bradley EL III, Murphy F, Ferguson C. Prediction of pancreatic necrosis by dynamic pancreatography. *Ann Surg* 1989;210:495–504.
34. Breatnach ES, Han SY, Rahatzad MT, Stanley RJ. CT evaluation of glucagonomas. *J Comput Assist Tomogr* 1985;9:25–29.
35. Brinberg DE, Carr MF Jr, Premkumar A, Stein J, Green PH. Isolated ventral pancreatitis in an alcoholic with pancreas divisum. *Gastrointest Radiol* 1988;13:323–326.
36. Broughan TA, Leslie JD, Soto JM, Hermann RE. Pancreatic islet cell tumors. *Surgery* 1986;99:671–678.
37. Buck JL, Hayes WS. From the Archives of the AFIP. Microcystic adenoma of the pancreas. *RadioGraphics* 1990;10:313–322.
38. Buetow PC, Buck JL, Pantongrag-Brown L, Beck KG, Ros PR, Adair CF. Solid and papillary epithelial neoplasm of the pancreas: imaging-pathologic correlation in 56 cases. *Radiology* 1996;199:707–711.
39. Cameron JL, Crist DW, Sitzmann JV, et al. Factors influencing survival after pancreaticoduodenectomy for pancreatic cancer. *Am J Surg* 1991;161:120–125.
40. Choyke PL, Glenn GM, Walther MM, Patronas NJ, Linehan WM, Zbar B. von Hippel-Lindau disease: genetic, clinical, and imaging features. *Radiology* 1995;194:629–642.
41. Churchill RJ, Cunningham DG, Henkin RE, Reynes CJ. Macroscopic cysts of the pancreas in cystic fibrosis demonstrated by multiple radiological modalities. *JAMA* 1981;245:72–74.
42. Clark LR, Jaffe MH, Choyke PL, Grant EG, Zeman RK. Pancreatic imaging. *Radiol Clin North Am* 1985;23:489–501.
43. Clavien PA, Hauser H, Meyer P, Rohner A. Value of contrast-enhanced computerized tomography in the early diagnosis and prognosis of acute pancreatitis. A prospective study of 202 patients. *Am J Surg* 1988;155:457–466.
44. Cohen DJ, Fagelman D. Pancreas islet cell carcinoma with complete fatty replacement: CT characteristics. *J Comput Assist Tomogr* 1986;10:1050–1051.
45. Compagno J, Oertel JE. Microcystic adenomas of the pancreas

(glycogen-rich cystadenomas). *Am J Clin Pathol* 1978;69:289–298.

46. Compagno J, Oertel JE. Mucinous cystic neoplasms of the pancreas with overt and latent malignancy (cystadenocarcinoma and cystadenoma): a clinicopathologic study of 41 cases. *Am J Clin Pathol* 1978;69:573–580.
47. Coral A, Jones SN, Lees WR. Dorsal pancreas presenting as a mass in the chest. *AJR* 1987;149:718–720.
48. Corrodi P, Knoblauch M, Binswanger U, Scholzel E, Largiander F. Pancreatitis after renal transplantation. *Gut* 1975;16:285–289.
49. Cotton PB. Congenital anomaly of pancreas divisum as cause of obstructive pain and pancreatitis. *Gut* 1980;21:105–114.
50. Creutzfeldt W. Endocrine tumors of the pancreas. In: Volk BW, Arquilla ER, eds. *The diabetic pancreas,* 2nd ed. New York: Plenum Press 1985;543–586.
51. Creutzfeldt W, Schmidt H. Aetiology and pathogenesis of pancreatitis. *Scand J Gastroenterol* 1970;5:47–62.
52. Dalton RR, Sarr MG, van Heerden JA, Colby TV. Carcinoma of the body and tail of the pancreas: is curative resection justified? *Surgery* 1992;111:489–494.
53. Daneman A, Gaskin K, Martin DJ, Cutz E. Pancreatic changes in cystic fibrosis: CT and sonographic appearances. *AJR* 1983;141:653–655.
54. Delhaye M, Engelholm L, Cremer M. Pancreas divisum: congenital anatomic variant or anomaly? Contribution of endoscopic retrograde dorsal pancreatography. *Gastroenterology* 1985;89:951–958.
55. Delvalle J, Yamada T. Secretory tumors of the pancreas. In: Sleisenger MH, Fordtran JS, eds. *Gastrointestinal disease: pathophysiology, diagnosis, management,* 4th ed. Philadelphia: WB Saunders, 1990;1884–1900.
56. Di Maggio EM, Solcia M, Dore R, et al. Intrapancreatic lipoma: first case diagnosed with CT. *AJR* 1996;167:56–57.
57. di Sant'Agnese PA. Acinar cell carcinoma of the pancreas. *Ultrstruct Pathol* 1991;15:573–577.
58. DiCorato MP, Schned AR. A rare lymphoepithelial cyst of the pancreas. *Am J Clin Pathol* 1992;98:188–191.
59. DiMagno EP. Pancreatic adenocarcinoma. In: Yamada T, ed. *Textbook of gastroenterology,* 2nd ed, vol 2. Philadelphia: JB Lippincott, 1995;2113–2131.
60. DiMagno EP, Malagelada JR, Taylor WF, Go VL. A prospective comparison of current diagnostic tests for pancreatic cancer. *N Engl J Med* 1977;297:737–742.
61. Donovan PJ, Sanders RC, Siegelman SS. Collections of fluid after pancreatitis: evaluation by computed tomography and ultrasonography. *Radiol Clin North Am* 1982;20:653–665.
62. Douglass HO Jr, Tepper J, Leichman L. Neoplasms of the exocrine pancreas. In: Holland JF, Frei E III, Bast RC Jr, Kufe DW, Morton DL, Weichselbaum RR, eds. *Cancer medicine.* Philadelphia: Lea and Febiger, 1993;1466–1484.
63. Dunn GD, Gibson RN. The left-sided pancreas. *Radiology* 1986;159:713–714.
64. Eelkema EA, Stephens DH, Ward EM, Sheedy PF II. CT features of nonfunctioning islet cell carcinoma. *AJR* 1984;143:943–948.
65. Fernandez JA, Rosenberg JC. Post-transplantation pancreatitis. *Surg Gynecol Obstet* 1976;143:795–798.
66. Fernandez MP, Bernardino ME, Neylan JF, Olson RA. Diagnosis of pancreatic transplant dysfunction: value of gadopentetate dimeglumine-enhanced MR imaging. *AJR* 1991;156:1171–1176.
67. Fink IJ, Krudy AG, Shawker TH, Norton JA, Gorden P, Doppman JL. Demonstration of an angiographically hypovascular insulinoma with intraarterial dynamic CT. *AJR* 1985;144:555–556.
68. Finlay DE, Letourneau JG, Longley DG. Assessment of vascular complications of renal, hepatic, and pancreatic transplantation. *RadioGraphics* 1992;12:981–996.
69. Fontham ET, Correa P. Epidemiology of pancreatic cancer. *Surg Clin North Am* 1989;69:551–567.
70. Freeny PC, Lawson TL. *Radiology of the pancreas.* New York: Springer-Verlag, 1982;170–171.
71. Freeny PC, Lewis GP, Traverso LW, Ryan JA. Infected pancreatic fluid collections: percutaneous catheter drainage. *Radiology* 1988;167:435–441.
72. Freeny PC, Marks WM, Ryan JA, Traverso LW. Pancreatic ductal adenocarcinoma: diagnosis and staging with dynamic CT. *Radiology* 1988;166:125–133.
73. Freeny PC, Traverso LW, Ryan JA. Diagnosis and staging of pancreatic adenocarcinoma with dynamic computed tomography. *Am J Surg* 1993;165:600–606.
74. Frey CF. Hemorrhagic pancreatitis. *Am J Surg* 1979;137:616–623.
75. Friedman AC, Lichtenstein JE, Dachman AH. Cystic neoplasms of the pancreas: radiological–pathological correlation. *Radiology* 1983;149:45–50.
76. Friedman AC, Lichtenstein JE, Fishman EK, Oertel JE, Dachman AH, Siegelman SS. Solid and papillary epithelial neoplasm of the pancreas. *Radiology* 1985;154:333–337.
77. Frucht H, Doppman JL, Norton JA, et al. Gastrinomas: comparison of MR imaging with CT, angiography, and US. *Radiology* 1989;171:713–717.
78. Fuhrman GM, Charnsangavej C, Abbruzzese JL, et al. Thin-section contrast-enhanced computed tomography accurately predicts the resectability of malignant pancreatic neoplasms. *Am J Surg* 1994;167:104–113.
79. Furuta K, Watanabe H, Ikeda S. Differences between solid and duct-ectatic types of pancreatic ductal carcinomas. *Cancer* 1992;69:1327–1333.
80. Gabata T, Matsui O, Kadoya M, et al. Small pancreatic adenocarcinomas: efficacy of MR imaging with fat suppression and gadolinium enhancement. *Radiology* 1994;193:683–688.
81. Gambill EE. Pancreatic and ampullary carcinoma: diagnosis and prognosis in relationship to symptoms, physical findings, and elapse of time as observed in 255 patients. *South Med J* 1970;63:1119–1122.
82. Gazelle GS, Mueller PR, Raafat N, Halpern EF, Cardenosa G, Warshaw AL. Cystic neoplasms of the pancreas: evaluation with endoscopic retrograde pancreatography. *Radiology* 1993;188:633–636.
83. Geokas MC, Baltaxe HA, Banks PA, Silva J Jr, Frey CF. Davis conference. Acute pancreatitis. *Ann Intern Med* 1985;103:86–100.
84. Ghishan FK, Greene HL, Avant G, O'Neill J, Neblett W. Chronic relapsing pancreatitis in childhood. *J Pediatrics* 1983;102:514–518.
85. Gilboa N, Largent JA, Urizar RE. Acute pancreatitis in an anephric child maintained on chronic hemodialysis. *Int J Pediatrics Nephrol* 1980;1:64–65.
86. Gold EB, Cameron JL. Chronic pancreatitis and pancreatic cancer. *N Engl J Med* 1993;328:1485–1486.
87. Gold RP, Berman H, Fakhry J, Heier S, Rosenthal W, DelGuercio L. Pancreas divisum with pancreatitis and pseudocyst. *AJR* 1984;143:1343–1344.
88. Grizzle WE. Silver staining methods to identify cells of the dispersed neuroendocrine system. *J Histotechnol* 1996;19:225–234.
89. Gudgeon AM, Heath DI, Hurley P, et al. Trypsinogen activation peptides assay in the early prediction of severity of acute pancreatitis. *Lancet* 1990;335:4–8.
90. Günther RW, Klose KJ, Rückert K, Beyer J, Kuhn F-P, Klotter H-J. Localization of small islet-cell tumors. Preoperative and intraoperative ultrasound, computed tomography, arteriography, digital subtraction angiography, and pancreatic venous sampling. *Gastrointest Radiol* 1985;10:145–152.
91. Günther RW, Klose KJ, Rückert K, et al. Islet-cell tumors: detection of small lesions with computed tomography and ultrasound. *Radiology* 1983;148:485–488.
92. Gustafson KD, Karnaze GC, Hattery RR, Scheithaur BW. Pseudomyxoma peritonei associated with mucinous adenocarcinoma of the pancreas: CT findings and CT-guided biopsy. *J Comput Assist Tomogr* 1984;8:335–338.
93. Hashimoto BE, Laing FC, Jeffrey RB Jr, Federle MP. Hemorrhagic pancreatic fluid collections examined by ultrasound. *Radiology* 1984;150:803–808.
94. Heiken JP, Balfe DM, Picus D, Scharp DW. Radical pancreatectomy: postoperative evaluation by CT. *Radiology* 1984;153:211–215.
95. Heitz PU, Kasper M, Polak JM, Kloppel G. Pancreatic endocrine tumors. *Hum Pathol* 1982;13:263–271.
96. Hernanz-Schulman M, Teele RL, Perez-Atayde A, et al. Pancreatic cystosis in cystic fibrosis. *Radiology* 1986;158:629–631.

97. Herts BR, Baker ME, Davros WJ, et al. Helical CT of the abdomen: comparison of image quality between scan times of 0.75 and 1 sec per revolution. *AJR* 1996;167:58–60.

98. Hollett MD, Jorgensen MJ, Jeffrey RB Jr. Quantitative evaluation of pancreatic enhancement during dual-phase helical CT. *Radiology* 1995;195:359–361.

99. Hosoki T. Dynamic CT of pancreatic tumors. *AJR* 1983;140:959–965.

100. Hough DM, Stephens DH, Johnson CD, Binkovitz LA. Pancreatic lesions in von Hippel-Lindau disease: prevalence, clinical significance, and CT findings. *AJR* 1994;162:1091–1094.

101. Howard JM, Jordan CL Jr. Cancer of the pancreas. *Curr Probl Cancer* 1977;2:5–52.

102. Inamoto K, Ishikawa Y, Itoh N. CT demonstration of annular pancreas: case report. *Gastrointest Radiol* 1983;8:143–144.

103. Ingomar CJ, Terslev E. A case of chronic pancreatitis in early childhood. *Dan Med Bull* 1965;12:91–92.

104. Itai Y, Kokubo T, Atomi Y, Kuroda A, Haraguchi Y, Terano A. Mucin-hypersecreting carcinoma of the pancreas. *Radiology* 1987;165:51–55.

105. Itai Y, Moss AA, Ohtomo K. Computed tomography of cystadenoma and cystadenocarcinoma of the pancreas. *Radiology* 1982;145:419–425.

106. Itai Y, Ohhashi K, Furui S, et al. Microcystic adenoma of the pancreas: spectrum of computed tomographic findings. *J Comput Assist Tomogr* 1988;12:797–803.

107. Itoh Y, Hada T, Terano A, Itai Y, Harada T. Pancreatitis in the annulus of annular pancreas demonstrated by the combined use of computed tomography and endoscopic retrograde cholangiopancreatography. *Am J Gastroenterol* 1989;84:961–964.

108. Jaksic T, Yaman M, Thorner P, Wesson DK, Filler RM, Shandling B. A 20-year review of pediatric pancreatic tumors. *J Pediatr Surg* 1992;27:1315–1317.

109. Jeffrey RB, Federle MP, Laing FC. Computed tomography of mesenteric involvement in fulminant pancreatitis. *Radiology* 1983;147:185–188.

110. Jensen RT, Gardner JD. Gastrinoma. In: Go VW, DiMagno EP, Gardner JD, et al., eds. *The pancreas: biology, pathobiology and disease,* 2nd ed. New York: Raven Press, 1993;931–978.

111. Jensen RT, Norton JA. Endocrine neoplasms of the pancreas. In: Yamada T, ed. *Textbook of gastroenterology,* 2nd ed, vol 2. Philadelphia: JB Lippincott, 1995;2131–2160.

112. Jimenez H, Aldrete JS. Clinical implications derived from the morphological classification of 89 patients with acute pancreatitis. *J Clin Gastroenterol* 1983;5:137–142.

113. Johnson WC, Nabseth DC. Pancreatitis in renal transplantation. *Ann Surg* 1970;171:309–314.

114. Kalmar JA, Merritt CRB, Matthews CC. CT demonstration of cystadenocarcinoma of the pancreas with calcified lymphadenopathy. *South Med J* 1983;76:1042–1044.

115. Kalser MH, Barkin J, MacIntyre JM. Pancreatic cancer. Assessment of prognosis by clinical presentation. *Cancer* 1985;56:397–402.

116. Kaplan JO, Isikoff MB, Barkin J, Livingstone AS. Necrotic carcinoma of the pancreas: ''the pseudo-pseudocyst''. *J Comput Assist Tomogr* 1980;4:166–167.

117. Karasawa E, Goldberg HI, Moss AA, Federle MP, London SS. CT pancreatogram in carcinoma of the pancreas and chronic pancreatitis. *Radiology* 1983;148:489–493.

118. Karimgani I, Porter KA, Langevin RE, Banks PA. Prognostic factors in sterile pancreatic necrosis. *Gastroenterology* 1992;103:1636–1640.

119. Kattwinkel J, Lapey A, di Sant'Agnese PA, Edwards WA, Jufty MP. Hereditary pancreatitis: three new kindreds and a critical review of the literature. *Pediatrics* 1973;51:55–69.

120. Kelcz F, Sollinger HW, Pirsch JD. MRI of the pancreas transplant: lack of correlation between imaging and clinical status. *Magn Reson Med* 1991;21:30–38.

121. Kelekis NL, Semelka RC, Siegelman ES. MRI of pancreatic metastases from renal cancer. *JCAT* 1996; 20(2):249–253.

122. Kingsnorth AN, Galloway SW, Lewis-Jones H, Nash JRG, Smith PA. Papillary cystic neoplasm of the pancreas: presentation and natural history in two cases. *Gut* 1992;33:421–423.

123. Kivisaari L, Schroder T, Sainio V, Somer K, Standertskjöld-Nordenstam CG. CT evaluation of acute pancreatitis: 8 years clinical experience and experimental evidence. *Acta Radiol (Suppl)* 1991;377:20–24.

124. Kloppel G, Heitz PU. Pancreatic endocrine tumors. *Pathol Res Pract* 1988;183:155–168.

125. Knaus WA, Draper EA, Wagner DP, Zimmerman JE. APACHE II: a severity of disease classification system. *Crit Care Med* 1985;13:818–829.

126. Kourtesis G, Wilson SE, Williams RA. The clinical significance of fluid collections in acute pancreatitis. *Am Surg* 1990;56:796–799.

127. Kozarek RA, Ball TJ, Patterson DJ, Brandabur JJ, Raltz SL. Endoscopic approach to pancreas divisum. *Dig Dis Sci* 1995;40:1974–1981.

128. Kravetz GW, Cho KC, Baker SR. Radiologic evaluation of pancreatic ascites. *Gastrointest Radiol* 1988;13:163–166.

129. Krebs TL, Daly B, Wong JJ, Chow CC, Bartlett ST. Vascular complications of pancreatic transplantation: MR evaluation. *Radiology* 1995;196:793–798.

130. Lammer J, Herlinger H, Zalaudek G, Hofler H. Pseudotumorous pancreatitis. *Gastrointest Radiol* 1985;10:59–67.

131. Lane MJ, Mindelzun RE, Sandhu JS, McCormick VD, Jeffrey RB. CT diagnosis of blunt pancreatic trauma: importance of detecting fluid between the pancreas and the splenic vein. *AJR* 1994;163:833–835.

132. Larvin M, Chalmers AG, McMahon MJ. Dynamic contrast enhanced computed tomography: a precise technique for identifying and localising pancreatic necrosis. *BMJ* 1990;300:1425–1428.

133. Lawson TL. Acute pancreatitis and its complications: computed tomography and sonography. *Radiol Clin North Am* 1983;21:495–513.

134. Levitt RG, Stanley RJ, Sagel SS, Lee JKT, Weyman PJ. Computed tomography of the pancreas: 3 second scanning vs 18 second scanning. *J Comput Assist Tomogr* 1982;6:259–267.

135. Levy P, Mathurin P, Roqueplo A, Rueff B, Bernades P. A multidimensional case-control study of dietary, alcohol, and tobacco habits in alcoholic men with chronic pancreatitis. *Pancreas* 1995;10:231–238.

136. Lewandrowski K, Warshaw A, Compton C. Macrocystic serous cystadenoma of the pancreas: a morphologic variant differing from microcystic adenoma. *Hum Pathol* 1992;23:871–875.

137. Lightdale CJ, Botet JF, Woodruff JM, Brennan MF. Localization of endocrine tumors of the pancreas with endoscopic ultrasonography. *Cancer* 1991;68:1815–1820.

138. Lin A, Feller ER. Pancreatic carcinoma as a cause of unexplained pancreatitis: report of ten cases. *Ann Intern Med* 1990;113:166–167.

139. London NJ, Leese T, Lavelle JM, et al. Rapid-bolus contrast-enhanced dynamic computed tomography in acute pancreatitis: a prospective study. *Br J Surg* 1991;78:1452–1456.

140. Louie S, McGahan JP, Frey C, Cross CE. Pancreatic pleuropericardial effusions: fistulous tracts demonstrated by computed tomography. *Arch Intern Med* 1985;145:1231–1234.

141. Lowenfels AB, Maisonneuve P, Cavallini G, et al. Pancreatitis and the risk of pancreatic cancer. International Pancreatitis Study Group. *N Engl J Med* 1993;328:1433–1437.

142. Lu DSK, Vedantham S, Krasny RM, Kadell B, Berger WL, Reber HA. Two-phase helical CT for pancreatic tumors: pancreatic versus hepatic phase enhancement of tumor, pancreas, and vascular structures. *Radiology* 1996;199:697–701.

143. Luetmer PH, Stephens DH, Fischer AP. Obliteration of periarterial retropancreatic fat on CT in pancreatitis: an exception to the rule. *AJR* 1989;153:63–64.

144. Luetmer PH, Stephens DH, Ward EM. Chronic pancreatitis: reassessment with current CT. *Radiology* 1989;171:353–357.

145. Lumkin B, Anderson MW, Ablin DS, McGahan JP. CT, MRI, and color Doppler ultrasound correlation of pancreatoblastoma: a case report. *Pediatr Radiol* 1993;23:61–62.

146. Macaulay SE, Schulte SJ, Sekijima JH, et al. Evaluation of a non-breath-hold MR cholangiography technique. *Radiology* 1995;196:227–232.

147. Maile CW, Crass JR, Frick MP, Feinberg SB, Goldberg ME, Sutherland DER. CT of pancreas transplantation. *Invest Radiol* 1985;20:609–612.

148. Malangoni MA, Richardson JD, Shallcross JC, Seiler JG, Polk HC Jr. Factors contributing to fatal outcome after treatment of pancreatic abscess. *Ann Surg* 1986;203:605–613.

149. Maton PN, Miller DL, Doppman JL, et al. Role of selective angiography in the management of patients with Zollinger-Ellison syndrome. *Gastroenterology* 1987;92:913–918.

150. McCarthy S, Pellegrini CA, Moss AA, Way LW. Pleuropancreatic fistula: endoscopic retrograde cholangiopancreatography and computed tomography. *AJR* 1984;142:1151–1154.

151. McCowin MJ, Federle MP. Computed tomography of pancreatic pseudocysts of the duodenum. *AJR* 1985;145:1003–1007.

152. Mechanism of pancreatic autodigestion. *N Engl J Med* 1970;283:487–488.

153. Megibow AJ. Pancreatic adenocarcinoma: designing the examination to evaluate the clinical questions. *Radiology* 1992;183:297–303.

154. Megibow AJ, Zhou XH, Rotterdam H, Francis IR, Zerhouni EA, Balfe DM, et al. Pancreatic 4denocarcinoma: CT versus MR imaging in the evaluation of resectability-report of the Radiology Diagnostic Oncology Group. *Radiology* 1995;195:327–332.

155. Mendez G Jr, Isikoff MB. Significance of intrapancreatic gas demonstrated by CT: a review of nine cases. *AJR* 1979;132:59–62.

156. Mendez G Jr, Isikoff MB, Hill MC. CT of acute pancreatitis: interim assessment. *AJR* 1980;135:463–469.

157. Meneely RL, O'Neill J, Ghishan FK. Fibrosing pancreatitis—an obscure cause of painless obstructive jaundice: a case report and review of the literature. *Pediatrics* 1981;67:136–139.

158. Metzgar RS, Asch HL. Antigens of human pancreatic adenocarcinomas: their role in diagnosis and therapy. *Pancreas* 1988;3:352.

159. Meyers MA, Feldberg MA, Oliphant M. Grey Turner's sign and Cullen's sign in acute pancreatitis. *Gastrointest Radiol* 1989;14:31–37.

160. Miedema BW, Sarr MG, van Heerden JA, Nagorney DM, McIlrath DC, Ilstrup D. Complications following pancreaticoduodenectomy. Current management. *Arch Surg* 1992;127:945–950.

161. Milici LP, Markowitz SK. Gastric intramural pseudocyst: computed tomographic diagnosis. *Gastrointest Radiol* 1989;14:113–114.

162. Minami M, Itai Y, Ohtomo K, Yoshida H, Yoshikawa K, Iio M. Cystic neoplasms of the pancreas: comparison of MR imaging with CT. *Radiology* 1989;171:53–56.

163. Mitchell DG, Cruvella M, Eschelman DJ, Miettinen MM, Vernick JJ. MRI of pancreatic gastrinomas. *J Comput Assist Tomogr* 1992;16:583–585.

164. Mitchell DG, Vinitski S, Saponaro S, Tasciyan T, Burk DL Jr, Rifkin MD. Liver and pancreas: improved spin-echo T1 contrast by shorter echo time and fat suppression at 1.5T. *Radiology* 1991;178:67–71.

165. Miyazaki T, Yamashita Y, Tsuchigame T, Yamamoto H, Urata J, Takahashi M. MR cholangiopancreatography using HASTE (Half-fourier acquisition single-shot turbo spin-echo) sequences. *AJR* 1996; 166:1297–1303.

166. Morant R, Bruckner HW. Complete remission of refractory small cell carcinoma of the pancreas with cisplatin and etoposide. *Cancer* 1989;64:2007–2009.

167. Mori H, McGrath FP, Malone DE, Stevenson GW. The gastrocolic trunk and its tributaries: CT evaluation. *Radiology* 1992;182:871–877.

168. Mozell E, Stenzel P, Woltering EA, Rösch J, O'Dorisio TM. Functional endocrine tumors of the pancreas: clinical presentation, diagnosis, and treatment. *Curr Probl Surg* 1990;27:301–386.

169. Mulholland MW, Moossa AR, Liddle RA. Pancreas: anatomy and structural anomalies. In: Yamada T, ed. *Textbook of gastroenterology,* 2nd ed, vol 2. Philadelphia: JB Lippincott, 1995;2051–2064.

170. Murr MM, Sarr MG, Oishi AJ, van Heerden JA. Pancreatic cancer. *Ca Cancer J Clin* 1994;44:304–318.

171. Neff CC, Simeone JF, Wittenberg J, Mueller PR, Ferrucci JT Jr. Inflammatory pancreatic masses: problems in differentiating focal pancreatitis from carcinoma. *Radiology* 1984;150:35–38.

172. Norton JA, Cromack DT, Shawker TH, et al. Intraoperative ultrasonographic localization of islet cell tumors: a prospective comparison to palpation. *Ann Surg* 1988;207:160–168.

173. Norton JA, Levin B, Jensen RT. Cancer of the endocrine system. In: DeVita VT Jr, Hellman S, Rosenberg SA, eds. *Cancer: principles and practice of oncology,* vol 2, 4th ed. Philadelphia: JB Lippincott, 1993;1333–1435.

174. Norton JA, Shawker TH, Doppman JL, et al. Localization and surgical treatment of occult insulinomas. *Ann Surg* 1990;212:615–620.

175. Nozawa Y, Abe M, Sakuma H, et al. A case of pancreatic oncocytic tumor. *Acta Pathol Jpn* 1990;40:367–370.

176. Obara T, Maguchi H, Saitoh Y, et al. Mucin-producing tumor of the pancreas: a unique clinical entity. *Am J Gastroenterol* 1991;86:1619–1625.

177. Ohta T, Nagakawa T, Akiyama T, et al. The "duct-ectatic" variant of mucinous cystic neoplasm of the pancreas: clinical and radiologic studies of seven cases. *Am J Gastroenterol* 1992; 87:300–304.

178. Ohtomo K, Furui S, Onoue M, et al. Solid and papillary epithelial neoplasm of the pancreas: MR imaging and pathologic correlation. *Radiology* 1992;184:567–570.

179. Pandolfo I, Scribano E, Gaeta M, Fiumara F, Longo M. Cystic lymphangioma of the pancreas: CT demonstration. *J Comput Assist Tomogr* 1985;9:209–213.

180. Pasanen PA, Eskelinen M, Partanen K, Pikkarainen P, Penttila I, Alhava E. A prospective study of the value of imaging, serum markers and their combination in the diagnosis of pancreatic carcinoma in symptomatic patients. *Anticancer Res* 1992;12:2309–2314.

181. Patel B, Markivee CR, Mahanta B, Vas W, George E, Garvin P. Pancreatic transplantation: scintigraphy, US, and CT. *Radiology* 1988:167:685–687.

182. Patel B, Wolverson MK, Mahanta B. Pancreatic transplant rejection: assessment with duplex US. *Radiology* 1989;173:131–135.

183. Patel S, Bellon EM, Haaga J. Fat replacement of the exocrine pancreas. *AJR* 1980;135:843–845.

184. Patt R, Zeman RK, Nauta R, et al. Vascular encasement by pancreatobiliary neoplasms: assessment with dynamic CT, spin-echo MR imaging, and gradient-echo MR imaging. *Radiology* 1991; 181(p):259.

185. Pavone P, Occhiato R, Michelini O, et al. Magnetic resonance imaging of pancreatic carcinoma. *Eur Radiol* 1991;1:124–130.

186. Pellegrini CA, Heck CF, Raper S, Way LW. An analysis of the reduced morbidity and mortality rates after pancreaticoduodenectomy. *Arch Surg* 1989;124:778–781.

187. Pemberton JH, Nagorney DM, Becker JM, Ilstrup D, Dozois RR, Remine WH. Controlled open lesser sac drainage for pancreatic abscess. *Ann Surg* 1986;203:600–604.

188. Penn I, Durst AL, Machado M, et al. Acute pancreatitis and hyperamylasemia in renal homograft recipients. *Arch Surg* 1972;105:167–172.

189. Pisegna JR, Doppman JL, Norton JA, Metz DC, Jensen RT. Prospective comparative study of ability of MR imaging and other imaging modalities to localize tumors in patients with Zollinger-Ellison syndrome. *Dig Dis Sci* 1993;38:1318–1328.

190. Pozniak MA, Propeck PA, Kelcz F, Sollinger H. Imaging of pancreas transplants. *Radiol Clin North Am* 1995;33:581–594.

191. Prayer L, Schurawitzki H, Mallek R, Mostbeck G. CT in pancreatic involvement of non-Hodgkin lymphoma. *Acta Radiol* 1992;33:123–127.

192. Price J, Cockram CS, McGuire LJ, Crofts TJ, Stewart IET, Metreweli C. Uptake of 99mTc-methylene diphosphonate by pancreatic insulinoma. *AJR* 1987;149:69–70.

193. Procacci C, Portuese A, Fugazzola C, et al. Duodenal duplication in the adult: its relationship with pancreatitis. *Gastrointest Radiol* 1988;13:315–322.

194. Ranson JH. Acute pancreatitis—where are we? *Surg Clin North Am* 1981;61:55–70.

195. Ranson JH, Rifkind KM, Roses DF, Fink SD, Eng K, Spencer FC. Prognostic signs and the role of operative management in acute pancreatitis. *Surg Gynecol Obstet* 1974;139:69–81.

196. Raptopoulos V, Kleinman PK, Marks S Jr, Snyder M, Silverman PM. Renal fascial pathway: posterior extension of pancreatic effusions within the anterior pararenal space. *Radiology* 1986;158:367–374.

197. Rattner DW, Legermate DA, Lee MJ, Mueller PR, Warshaw AL. Early surgical debridement of symptomatic pancreatic necrosis is beneficial irrespective of infection. *Am J Surg* 1992;163:105–110.

198. Ravitch MM, Woods AC. Annular pancreas. *Ann Surg* 1950;132: 1116–1127.

199. Reiman TH, Balfe DM, Weyman PJ. Suprapancreatic biliary obstruction: CT evaluation. *Radiology* 1987;163:49–56.

200. Reinhold C, Bret PM. Current status of MR cholangiopancreatography. *AJR* 1996;166:1285–1295.

201. Ritts R Jr, Jacobsen D, Ilstrup D, et al. A prospective evaluation of MoAb CA 19-9 to detect GI cancer in a high risk clinic population. *Cancer Detect Prev* 1984;7:525.

202. Ritts R Jr, Klug T, Jacobsen D, et al. Multiple tumor marker tests enhance sensitivity of pancreatic carcinoma detection. *Cancer Detect Prev* 1984;7:459.

203. Robberecht E, Nachtegaele P, Van Rattinghe R, Afschrift M, Kunnen M, Verhaaren R. Pancreatic lipomatosis in the Shwachman-Diamond syndrome: identification by sonography and CT scan. *Pediatr Radiol* 1985;15:348–349.

204. Robinson DO, Alp MH, Grant AK, Lawrence JR. Pancreatitis and renal disease. *Scand J Gastroenterol* 1977;12:17–20.

205. Rockey DC, Cello JP. Pancreaticopleural fistula. Report of 7 patients and review of the literature. *Medicine* 1990;69:332–344.

206. Rohrmann CA, Surawicz CM, Hutchinson D, Silverstein FE, White TT, Marchioro TL. The diagnosis of hereditary pancreatitis by pancreatography. *Gastrointest Endosc* 1981;27:168–173.

207. Rösch T, Braig C, Gain T, et al. Staging of pancreatic and ampullary carcinoma by endoscopic ultrasonography. Comparison with conventional sonography, computed tomography, and angiography. *Gastroenterology* 1992;102:188–199.

208. Ross BA, Jeffrey RB Jr, Mindelzun RE. Normal variations in the lateral contour of the head and neck of the pancreas mimicking neoplasm: evaluation with dual-phase helical CT. *AJR* 1996;166: 799–801.

209. Ross CB, Sharp KW, Kaufman AJ, Andrews T, Williams LF. Efficacy of computerized tomography in the preoperative staging of pancreatic carcinoma. *Am Surg* 1988;54:221–226.

210. Rubin E, Dunham WK, Stanley RJ. Pancreatic metastases in bone sarcomas: CT demonstration. *J Comput Assist Tomogr* 1985;9: 886–888.

211. Rumancik WM, Megibow AJ, Bosniak MA, Hilton S. Metastatic disease to the pancreas: evaluation by computed tomography. *J Comput Assist Tomogr* 1984;8:829–834.

212. Rustin RB, Broughan TA, Hermann RE, Grundfest-Broniatowski SF, Petras RE, Hart WR. Papillary cystic epithelial neoplasms of the pancreas: a clinical study of four cases. *Arch Surg* 1986;121: 1073–1076.

213. Saifuddin A, Ward J, Ridgeway J, Chalmers AG. Comparison of MR and CT scanning in severe acute pancreatitis: initial experiences. *Clin Radiol* 1993; 48:111–116.

214. Salimi Z, Fishbein M, Wolverson MK, Johnson FE. Pancreatic lymphangioma: CT, MRI, and angiographic features. *Gastrointest Radiol* 1991;16:248–250.

215. Sarles H. Chronic calcifying pancreatitis–chronic alcoholic pancreatitis. *Gastroenterology* 1974;66:604–616.

216. Sarner M. Pancreatitis: definitions and classification. In: Go VLW, ed. *The exocrine pancreas: biology, pathobiology, and diseases.* New York: Raven Press, 1986;459–464.

217. Schröder T, Kivisaari L, Somer K, Standertskjöld-Nordenstam C-G, Kivilaakso E, Lempinen M. Significance of extrapancreatic findings in computed tomography (CT) of acute pancreatitis. *Eur J Radiol* 1985;5:273–275.

218. Schulte SJ. Congenital anomalies of the biliary system and pancreas. In: Taveras JM, Ferrucci JT, eds. *Radiology: diagnosis, imaging, intervention,* vol. 4. Philadelphia: Lippincott-Raven, 1995:1–23.

219. Scott GC, Boudreaux JP, Letourneau JG. Imaging of pancreas transplants. In *Categorical Course Syllabus of the American Roentgen Ray Society,* 96th Annual Meeting, May 5–10, 1996, San Diego;205–210.

220. Scott R, Jersky J, Hariparsad G. Case report: malignant giant cell tumour of the pancreas presenting as a large pancreatic cyst. *Br J Radiol* 1993;66:1055–1057.

221. Semelka RC, Ascher SM. MR imaging of the pancreas. *Radiology* 1993;188:593–602.

222. Semelka RC, Cumming MJ, Shoenut JP, et al. Islet cell tumors: comparison of dynamic contrast-enhanced CT and MR imaging with dynamic gadolinium enhancement and fat suppression. *Radiology* 1993;186:799–802.

223. Semelka RC, Kelekis NL, Molina PL, Sharp TJ, Calvo B. Pancreatic masses with inconclusive findings on spiral CT: is there a role for MRI? *JMRI* 1996; 6:585–588.

224. Semelka RC, Kelekis NL, Thomasson D, Brown MA, Laub GA. HASTE MR imaging: description of technique and preliminary results in the abdomen. *JMRI* 1996; 6:698–699.

225. Semelka RC, Kroeker MA, Shoenut JP, Kroeker R, Yaffe CS, Micflikier AB. Pancreatic disease: prospective comparison of CT, ERCP, and 1.5-T MR imaging with dynamic gadolinium enhancement and fat suppression. *Radiology* 1991;181:785–791.

226. Semelka RC, Shoenut JP, Kroeker MA, Micflikier AB. Chronic pancreatitis: MR imaging features before and after administration of gadopentetate dimeglumine. *JMRI* 1993;3:79–82.

227. Semelka RC, Shoenut JP, Kroeker MA, Micflikier AB. The pancreas. In: Semelka RC, Shoenut JP, eds. *MRI of the abdomen with CT correlation.* New York: Raven Press, 1993;59–76.

228. Semelka RC, Simm FC, Recht M, Deimling M, Lenz G, Laub GA. MRI of the pancreas at high field strength/a comparison of six sequences. *J Comput Assist Tomogr* 1991;15(6):966–971.

229. Shah KK, DeRidder PH, Schwab RE, Alexander TJ. CT diagnosis of dorsal pancreas agenesis. *J Comput Assist Tomogr* 1987;11: 170–171.

230. Shtamler B, Bickel A, Manor E, Shahar MB, Kuten A, Suprun H. Primary lymphoma of the head of the pancreas. *J Surg Onc* 1988; 38:48–51.

231. Shuman WP, Carter SJ, Montana MA, Mack LA, Moss AA. Pancreatic insufficiency: role of CT evaluation. *Radiology* 1986;158: 625–627.

232. Siegelman ES, Mitchell DG, Outwater E, Munoz SJ, Rubin R. Idiopathic hemochromatosis: MR imaging findings in cirrhotic and precirrhotic patients. *Radiology* 1993;188:637–641.

233. Siegelman SS, Copeland BE, Saba GP, Cameron JL, Sanders RC, Zerhouni EA. CT of fluid collections associated with pancreatitis. *AJR* 1980;134:1121–1132.

234. Silverman PM, McVay L, Zeman RK, Garra BS, Grant EG, Jaffe MH. Pancreatic pseudotumor in pancreas divisum: CT characteristics. *J Comput Assist Tomogr* 1989;13:140–141.

235. Silverstein W, Isikoff MB, Hill MC, Barkin J. Diagnostic imaging of acute pancreatitis: prospective study using CT and sonography *AJR* 1981;137:497–502.

236. Singer MV, Gyr K, Sarles H. Revised classification of pancreatitis. Report of the Second International Symposium on the Classification of Pancreatitis in Marseille, France, March 28–30, 1984. *Gastroenterology* 1985;89:683–685.

237. Smith DR, Stanley RJ, Rue LW III. Delayed diagnosis of pancreatic transection after blunt abdominal trauma. *J Trauma* 1996;40: 1009–1013.

238. Smith E, Matzen P. Mucus-producing tumors with mucinous biliary obstruction causing jaundice: diagnosed and treated endoscopically. *Am J Gastroenterol* 1985;80:287–289.

239. Snady H, Cooperman A, Siegel J. Endoscopic ultrasonography compared with computed tomography with ERCP in patients with obstructive jaundice or small peripancreatic mass. *Gastrointest Endosc* 1992;38:27–34.

240. Soto JA, Barish MA, Yucel EK, et al. Pancreatic duct: MR cholangiopancreatography with a three-dimensional fast spin-echo technique. Radiology 1995; 196:459–464.

241. Spechler SJ, Dalton JW, Robbins AH, et al. Prevalence of normal serum amylase levels in patients with acute alcoholic pancreatitis. *Dig Dis Sci* 1983;28:865–869.

242. Stabile BE, Morrow DJ, Passaro E Jr. The gastrinoma triangle: operative implications. *Am J Surg* 1984;147:25–31.

243. Steinberg WM. Predictors of severity of acute pancreatitis. *Gastroenterol Clin North Am* 1990;19:849–861.

244. Steiner E, Mueller PR, Hahn PF, et al. Complicated pancreatic abscesses: problems in interventional management. *Radiology* 1988;167:443–446.

245. Steiner E, Stark DD, Hahn PF, et al. Imaging of pancreatic neoplasms: comparison of MR and CT. *AJR* 1989;152:487–491.

246. Stephenson CA, Kletzel M, Seibert JJ, Glasier CM. Pancreatoblastoma: MR appearance. *J Comput Assist Tomogr* 1990;14:492–493.

247. Stiles GM, Berne TV, Thommen VD, Molgaard CP, Boswell WD. Fine needle aspiration of pancreatic fluid collections. *Am Surg* 1990;56:764–768.

248. Strax R, Toombs BD, Rauschkolb EN. Correlation of barium enema and CT in acute pancreatitis. *AJR* 1981;136:1219–1220.

249. Takada T, Yasuda H, Uchiyama K, Hasegawa H, Shikata J, Nagai J. CT score and the severity of acute pancreatitis. *Int Surg* 1988;73:94–98.

250. Takehara Y, Ichijo K, Tooyama N, et al. Breath-hold MR cholangiopancreatography with a long-echo-train fast spin-echo sequence and a surface coil in chronic pancreatitis. *Radiology* 1994;192:73–78.

251. Teefey SA, Stephens DH, Sheedy PF II. CT appearance of primary pancreatitis lymphoma. *Gastrointest Radiol* 1986;11:41–43.

252. Tham RTO, Heyerman HGM, Falke THM, et al. Cystic fibrosis: MR imaging of the pancreas. *Radiology* 1991;179:183–186.

253. Thoeni RF, Fell SC, Goldberg HI. CT detection of asymptomatic pancreatitis following ERCP. *Gastrointest Radiol* 1990;15:291–295.

254. Thompson NW, Eckhauser FE, Vinik AI, Lloyd RV, Fiddian-Green RG, Strodel WE. Cystic neuroendocrine neoplasms of the pancreas and liver. *Ann Surg* 1984;199:158–164.

255. Tobben PJ, Zajko AB, Sumkin JH, et al. Pseudoaneurysms complicating organ transplantation: roles of CT, duplex sonography, and angiography. *Radiology* 1988;169:65–70.

256. Toombs BD, Lester RG, Ben-Menachem Y, Sandler CM. Computed tomography in blunt trauma. *Radiol Clin North Am* 1981;19:17–35.

257. Torres WE, Clements JL, Sones PJ, Knopf DR. Gas in the pancreatic bed without abscess. *AJR* 1981;137:1131–1133.

258. Trede M, Schwall G, Saeger HD. Survival after pancreatoduodenectomy. 118 consecutive resections without an operative mortality. *Ann Surg* 1990;211:447–458.

259. Trellis DR, Clouse RE. Johanson-Blizzard syndrome. Progression of pancreatic involvement in adulthood. *Dig Dis Sci* 1991;36:365–369.

260. Uchiyama T, Suzuki T, Adachi A, Hiraki S, Iizuka N. Pancreatic pleural effusion: case report and review of 113 cases in Japan. *Am J Gastroenterol* 1992;87:387–391.

261. Van Dyke JA, Rutsky EA, Stanley RJ. Acute pancreatitis associated with end-stage renal disease. *Radiology* 1986;160:403–405.

262. vanSonnenberg E, Wittich GR, Casola G, et al. Percutaneous drainage of infected and noninfected pancreatic pseudocysts: experience in 101 cases. *Radiology* 1989;170:757–761.

263. Vellet AD, Romano W, Bach DB, Passi RB, Taves DH, Munk PL. Adenocarcinoma of the pancreatic ducts: comparative evaluation with CT and MR imaging at 1.5T. *Radiology* 1992;183:87–95.

264. Vinik AI, Strodel WE, Eckhauser FE, Moattari AR, Lloyd R. Somatostatinomas, PPomas, neurotensinomas. *Semin Oncol* 1987;14:263–281.

265. Vitas GJ, Sarr MG. Selected management of pancreatic pseudocysts: operative versus expectant management. *Surgery* 1992;111:123–130.

266. Wank SA, Doppman JL, Miller DL, et al. Prospective study of the ability of computed axial tomography to localize gastrinomas in patients with Zollinger-Ellison syndrome. *Gastroenterology* 1987;92:905–912.

267. Warshaw AL, Gu Z, Wittenberg J, Waltman AC. Preoperative staging and assessment of resectability of pancreatic cancer. *Arch Surg* 1990;125:230–233.

268. Warshaw AL, Jin GL. Improved survival in 45 patients with pancreatic abscess. *Ann Surg* 1985;202:408–417.

269. Weaver DW, Walt AJ, Sugawa C, Bouwman DL. A continuing appraisal of pancreatic ascites. *Surg Gynecol Obstet* 1982;154:845–848.

270. Webb TH, Lillemoe KD, Pitt HA, Jones RJ, Cameron JL. Pancreatic lymphoma. Is surgery mandatory for diagnosis or treatment? *Ann Surg* 1989;209:25–30.

271. Weiner SN, Das K, Gold M, Stollman Y, Bernstein RG. Demonstration of an internal pancreatic fistula by computed tomography. *Gastrointest Radiol* 1984;9:123–125.

272. Weyman PJ, Stanley RJ, Levitt RG. Computed tomography in evaluation of the pancreas. *Semin Roentgenol* 1981;16:301–311.

273. Wildling R, Schnedl WJ, Reisinger EC, et al. Agenesis of the dorsal pancreas in a woman with diabetes mellitus and in both of her sons. *Gastroenterology* 1993;104:1182–1186.

274. Williams TE Jr, Sherman NJ, Clatworthy HW Jr. Chronic fibrosing pancreatitis in childhood: a cause of recurrent abdominal pain. *Pediatrics* 1967;40:1019–1023.

275. Wilson TE, Korobkin M, Francis IR. Pancreatic plasmacytoma: CT findings. *AJR* 1989;152:1227–1228.

276. Wingo PA, Tong T, Bolden S. Cancer statistics, 1995. *CA Cancer J Clin* 1995;45:8–30.

277. Winsett MZ, Kumar R, Balachandran S, Bedi DG, Gallagher P, Fagan CJ. Pseudocyst following splenectomy: impact of CT and ultrasound on its diagnosis and management. *Gastrointest Radiol* 1988;13:177–179.

278. Wise RH Jr, Stanley RJ. Carcinoma of the ampulla of Vater presenting as acute pancreatitis. *J Comput Assist Tomogr* 1984;8:158–161.

279. Wittenberg J, Simone JF, Ferrucci JT Jr, Mueller PR, van Sonnenberg E, Neff CC. Non-focal enlargement in pancreatic carcinoma. *Radiology* 1982;144:131–135.

280. Wolf EL, Sprayregen S, Frager D, Rifkin H, Gliedman ML. Calcification in an insulinoma of the pancreas. *Am J Gastroenterol* 1984;79:559–561.

281. Wolfman NT, Karstaedt N, Kawamoto EH. Pleomorphic carcinoma of the pancreas: computed-tomographic, sonographic, and pathologic findings. *Radiology* 1985;154:329–332.

282. Yamada M, Kozuka S, Yamao K, Nakazawa S, Naitoh Y, Tsukamoto Y. Mucin-producing tumor of the pancreas. *Cancer* 1991;68:159–168.

283. Yamaguchi K, Hirakata R, Kitamura K. Mucinous cystic neoplasm of the pancreas. *Acta Chir Scand* 1990;156:553–564.

284. Yeo CJ, Bastidas JA, Lynch-Nyhan A, Fishman EK, Zinner MJ, Cameron JL. The natural history of pancreatic pseudocysts documented by computed tomography. *Surg Gynecol Obstet* 1990;170:411–417.

285. Zeman RK, McVay L, Silverman PM, et al. Thin section CT of pancreas divisum (abstract). In: *Syllabus of the Society of Gastrointestinal Radiologists,* 17th Annual Meeting and Postgraduate Course, January 16–20, 1988, Nassau, Bahamas;31.

286. Zeman RK, Schiebler M, Clark LR, et al. The clinical and imaging spectrum of pancreaticoduodenal lymph node enlargement. *AJR* 1985;144:1223–1227.

287. Zirinsky K, Abiri M, Baer JW. Computed tomography demonstration of pancreatic microcystic adenoma. *Am J Gastroenterol* 1984;79:139–142.

CHAPTER 16

Abdominal Wall and Peritoneal Cavity

Jay P. Heiken and Steven S. Winn

ABDOMINAL WALL

Normal Anatomy

The normal anatomy of the abdominal wall is discussed in Chapter 10.

Pathologic Conditions

Hernias

Although the diagnosis of hernia almost always can be established clinically, CT may be useful in selected instances in differentiating between a hernia and a mass within the abdominal cavity or abdominal wall (158). In addition, CT may identify clinically unsuspected incisional hernias in patients undergoing postoperative CT examinations and ventral hernias in patients who have sustained blunt or penetrating abdominal trauma (56, 104,162). Herniation of intraperitoneal fat and bowel through fascial defects in the abdominal wall is easily demonstrated on CT. When bowel herniation is present, CT can often detect complications such as ischemia and obstruction. A ventral hernia is produced when the linea alba is disrupted and fat and/or bowel herniate anteriorly through the defect (Fig. 1). A Spigelian hernia results from weakness in the internal oblique and transversus aponeuroses, allowing peritoneal contents to herniate beneath an intact external oblique muscle. Computed tomography (CT) can establish the diagnosis by demonstrating a peritoneal and muscular defect at the lateral border of the rectus sheath (11) (Fig. 2). Lumbar hernias can occur at two weak points in the posterolateral abdominal wall (103,226). The lower of the two weak points, called

the inferior lumbar triangle, or Petit's triangle, lies just above the iliac crest between the external oblique and latissimus dorsi muscles (7,103). The larger superior lumbar triangle, or Grynfelt's triangle, is bounded by the twelfth rib, the serratus posticus muscle, the internal oblique muscle, and the erector spinae muscles. These rare posterior abdominal wall hernias may contain intraperitoneal or extraperitoneal contents.

The indirect inguinal hernia, the most common type of external abdominal hernia, results from herniation of peritoneal contents through the deep inguinal ring (Fig. 3). If sufficiently large, the hernia sac may extend into the scrotum in men or into the labium majorus in women. A femoral hernia results when peritoneal contents enter the femoral canal adjacent to the femoral artery and vein. In this type of hernia, the sac protrudes lateral to the inguinal canal between the external oblique muscle insertion on the superior pubic ramus and the superior pubic ramus itself (185). The most common type of obturator hernia results when intraperitoneal or extraperitoneal contents protrude between the pectineus and external obturator muscles (135). Less commonly, herniation occurs between the external and internal obturator muscles (Fig. 4) or between the fasciculi of the external obturator muscle.

Masses

Hematoma

Abdominal wall hematomas occur most commonly within the sheath of the rectus abdominis muscle and are most often secondary to anticoagulant therapy, although they may occur with various disease states, abdominal wall trauma, and severe exertion (17,169). Clinical find-

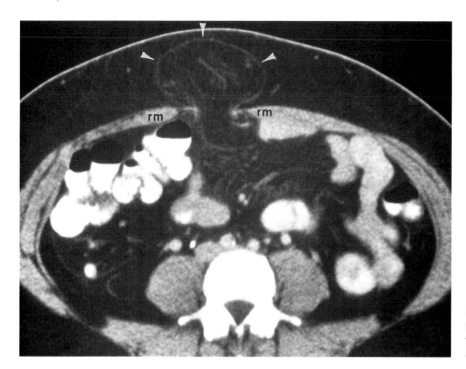

FIG. 1. Ventral hernia. Omental fat has herniated anteriorly through a defect in the linea alba (*arrowheads*); (rm) rectus abdominis muscle.

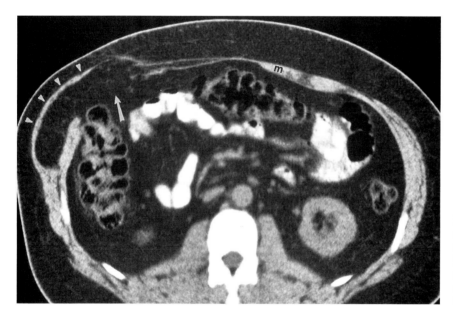

FIG. 2. Spigelian hernia. A defect (*arrow*) in the aponeurosis of the internal oblique and transversus muscles allows intraperitoneal fat to herniate into the abdominal wall beneath an intact external oblique muscle (*arrowheads*); (m) rectus abdominis muscle.

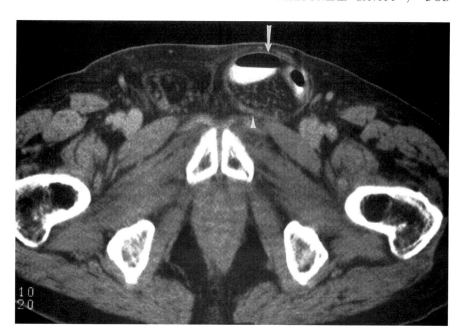

FIG. 3. Left inguinal hernia. Bowel opacified with oral contrast material has herniated into the left inguinal canal. The aponeurosis of the external oblique muscle (*arrow*) forms the anterior wall, and the aponeurosis of the transversus muscle (*arrowhead*) forms the posterior wall of the canal.

ings that suggest an abdominal wall hematoma include acute onset of abdominal pain in association with a palpable mass, discoloration of the skin overlying the mass, and a decreasing hematocrit. Often the clinical presentation is one of acute abdominal pain alone, and CT can make the diagnosis of hematoma, excluding other intraperitoneal etiologies. Computed tomography may accurately assess the extent of hematoma and determine if a concomitant intraabdominal or retroperitoneal hematoma is present.

The CT appearance of abdominal wall hematoma is that of an abnormal mass, often elliptical or spindle-shaped, in one or more layers of the abdominal wall, enlarging, obliterating, or displacing normal structures (Fig. 5). Rectus sheath hematomas are usually limited to one side of the abdomen by the linea alba. Large hematomas may, however, dissect inferiorly along fascial planes and extend into the pelvis, compressing viscera and crossing to the contralateral side (160). An acute abdominal wall hematoma has a density equal to or greater than the density of the abdominal muscles due to the high protein content of hemoglobin. Seventy-five percent of body wall hematomas scanned within the first 2 weeks after hemorrhage are hyperdense and often heterogeneous (197). On occasion, a fluid–fluid level can be seen due to the settling of cellular elements within the hematoma ("the hematocrit effect") (Fig. 5). As the hematoma matures, the progressive breakdown and removal of protein within red blood cells reduces the attenuation value of the hematoma (145). The process of clot lysis often occurs in a centripetal fashion, producing a low-attenuation halo at the periphery that widens as lysis progresses. By 2 to 4 weeks after the initial bleeding episode, the density of the hematoma may approach that of serum (20 to 30 HU) and then remains serum density for the duration of its existence. With time a fibroblastic and vascular membrane (pseudo-

capsule) grows around the hematoma, producing a dense rim on CT images. On occasion, the periphery of a chronic hematoma (seroma) may calcify.

The MRI appearance of abdominal wall hematoma undergoes an evolution similar to that seen on CT. In addition to age, the MRI appearance of a hematoma depends on the magnetic field strength at which it is imaged and the pulse sequence used. When examined at high magnetic field strength (1.5 T), an acute hematoma has a signal intensity similar to that of muscle on T1-weighted images with marked hypointensity on T2-weighted images (175). The prominent hypointensity on T2-weighted images implies preferential T2 proton relaxation enhancement (60). It has been proposed that the high concentration of Fe^{2+}-deoxyhemoglobin inside intact red blood cells in acute hematomas creates local heterogeneity of magnetic susceptibility, resulting in preferential T2 proton relaxation enhancement (60). This T2 shortening of fat is more pronounced with a gradient echo sequence than with a spin-echo technique. Large acute hematomas may demonstrate a fluid–fluid level on MR images, similar to that seen on CT scans. On CT, the dependent portion of the hematoma is high in attenuation. On T1-weighted MR images the dependent portion is hyperintense compared to the supernatant, whereas on T2-weighted images this signal intensity relationship is reversed (69).

Subacute hematomas (older than 1 week) have a more characteristic MRI appearance on T1-weighted images, consisting of a medium-signal-intensity (slightly greater than muscle) central area corresponding to the high-attenuation area on CT, surrounded by a high-intensity ring corresponding to the area of low attenuation on CT, which in turn is surrounded by a thin rim of very low signal intensity (69,175,204). On T2-weighted images, the signal intensity of the central core is similar to that

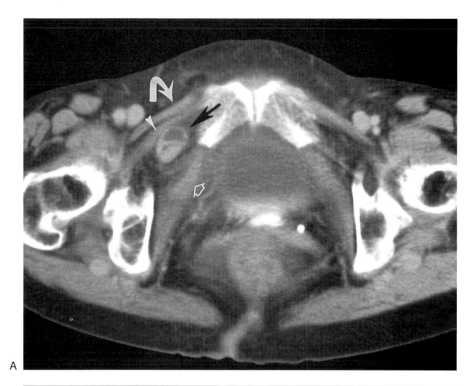

A

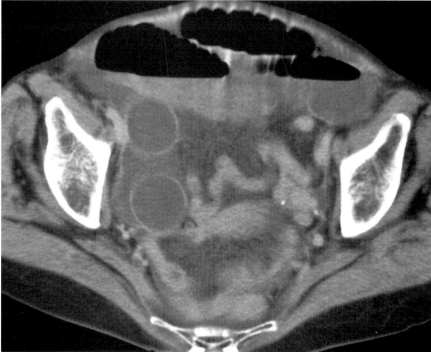

B

FIG. 4. A: Obturator hernia causing small bowel obstruction. A: In most obturator hernias, the hernia sac (*arrow*) passes between the pectineus muscle (*curved arrow*) and the external obturator muscle (*arrowhead*). In this patient it passes between the external and internal (*open arrow*) obturator muscles. **B:** A more cephalad image demonstrates dilated fluid-filled obstructed small bowel loops.

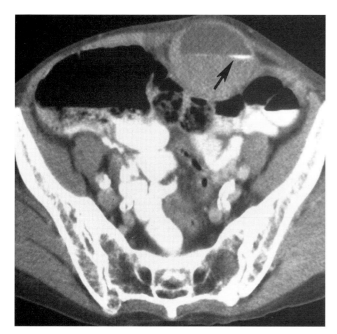

FIG. 5. Acute abdominal wall hematoma. A contrast-enhanced image demonstrates a round fluid collection with a hematocrit level in the left rectus abdominis muscle. The very high attenuation material (*arrow*) represents extravasated IV contrast medium indicating active hemorrhage.

of the peripheral zone. The thin outer rim remains very low in signal intensity. The high signal intensity of subacute hematomas is due to T1 shortening caused by the presence of extracellular methemoglobin resulting from oxidative denaturation of hemoglobin (19).

Inflammation/Infection

Inflammation in the abdominal wall is most often the result of infection, most commonly postoperative wound infection (224). Other less common causes include trauma, direct extension from intraabdominal inflammatory processes, and altered host defense (186). Clinical diagnosis of an abdominal wall infection is often difficult, especially in early postoperative or obese patients. The extent of tissue involvement is often underestimated by physical examination. Computed tomography can be useful in differentiating abscess from cellulitis, diagnosing or excluding infection in patients with postoperative wound tenderness, delineating the size and extent of an abscess when present, and determining whether or not the peritoneal cavity is involved.

The CT findings of abdominal wall inflammation are nonspecific and include streaky soft tissue densities, loss of normal intermuscular fat planes, enlargement of abdominal wall muscles, localized masses of varying density, and masses that dissect along fascial planes. An abdominal wall abscess appears as an abnormal mass that frequently has a low-attenuation central zone (Fig. 6). The peripheral zone or wall of the abscess may enhance after administration of intravenous iodinated contrast material. Occasionally, gas, resulting from gas-producing organisms, may be present in an abdominal wall abscess (Fig. 7). However, the presence of gas within the abdominal wall is not a specific sign of abscess, as gas in a partially open abdominal wound or gas in a fistula connecting bowel to the skin surface may appear similar. Because the CT appearance of abscess is not specific, needle aspiration may be necessary to confirm the

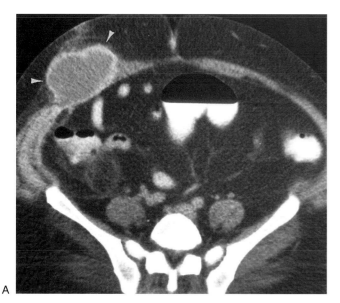

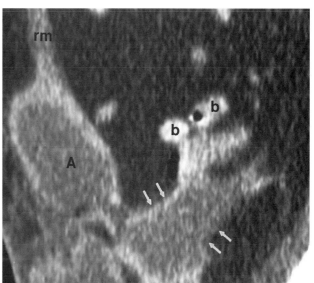

FIG. 6. A: Abdominal wall abscess. The right rectus abdominis muscle contains a low attenuation fluid collection with an enhancing wall (*arrowheads*). **B:** Sagittally reformatted spiral CT image demonstrates the abdominal wall abscess (A) with intraperitoneal extension (*arrows*). (b) bowel loops, (rm) rectus abdominis muscle.

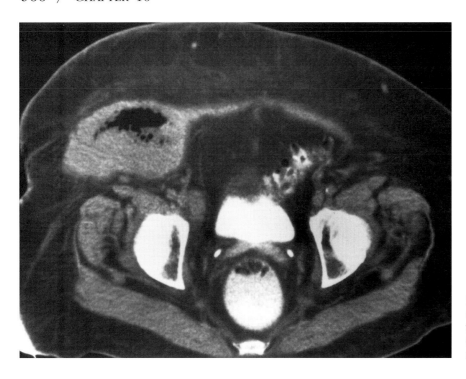

FIG. 7. Gas-containing abdominal wall abscess. High-attenuation fluid collection in the right rectus abdominis muscle contains multiple gas bubbles and a gas–fluid level.

diagnosis. Although both MRI and CT are effective in detection and characterization of abdominal wall infections, CT is preferable whenever percutaneous biopsy and/or drainage are considered (186). The multiplanar capability of CT and MRI can be of particular help in defining intraperitoneal extension and in surgical planning (78,186) (see Fig. 6).

Other Nonneoplastic Entities

Endometrial implants in the abdominal wall can occur in laparotomy incisions or in the tracts of instrument ports

from laparoscopy (Fig. 8). Although they usually result from procedures that expose the endometrial cavity, such as cesarean section (219), seeding also can occur from adnexal or peritoneal endometriosis. CT may demonstrate a soft tissue attenuation mass that is difficult to differentiate from the adjacent abdominal wall musculature. Magnetic resonance imaging may show high signal intensity on T1- and T2-weighted images due to hemorrhage (Fig. 9).

Heterotopic ossification, a form of myositis ossificans traumatica, can occur in midline abdominal surgical incisions. The osseous, cartilaginous, and, less commonly,

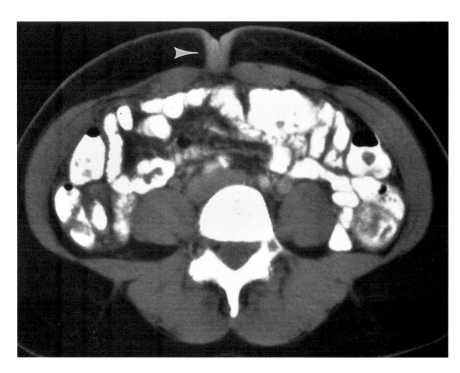

FIG. 8. Umbilical endometriosis. Soft tissue attenuation prominence of the umbilicus (*arrowhead*) represents seeding of a laparoscopy tract by endometriosis. This patient experienced cyclic umbilical bleeding, corresponding to her menstrual cycle.

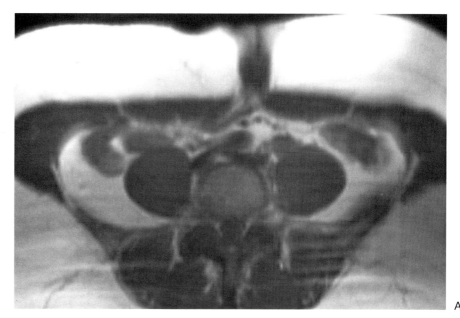

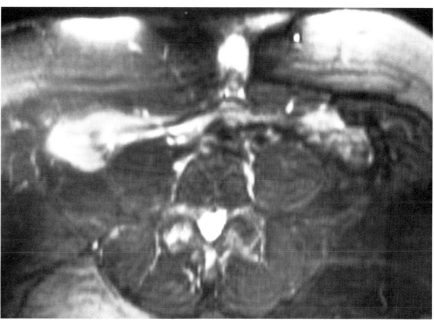

FIG. 9. Umbilical endometriosis. MRI demonstrates thickening of the umbilicus which is intermediate in signal intensity on T1-weighted (**A**) and high in signal intensity on T2-weighted (**B**) images.

A

B

marrow elements are responsible for the predictable CT appearance of soft tissue, bone, and sometimes fat attenuation components. Recognition of this lesion allows distinction from other entities such as postoperative hematoma or infection, retained foreign body, and primary or metastatic malignancy (84).

Diffuse lipomatosis of the abdominal wall is a benign condition that may be impossible to differentiate from a well-differentiated liposarcoma with CT or MRI, requiring histologic diagnosis (35).

Neoplasm

Both primary and secondary neoplasms can involve the abdominal wall. Although large masses generally are discovered by inspection and palpation, small tumors may be difficult to detect clinically, particularly in obese patients or in those with surgical scars or indurated tissue. Computed tomography is capable of demonstrating small abdominal wall tumors and may be valuable in defining the extent of palpable lesions for the purpose of placing radiotherapy ports and assessing the effectiveness of chemotherapy. Computed tomography is also helpful in detecting tumor recurrence after surgical excision (46).

Lipomas are common, benign tumors that can be found throughout the body, including the subcutaneous fat or muscle layers of the abdominal wall (Fig. 10). They are well-defined, homogeneous, fat attenuation (−40 to −100 HU) masses that may contain thin soft tissue septa and vessels.

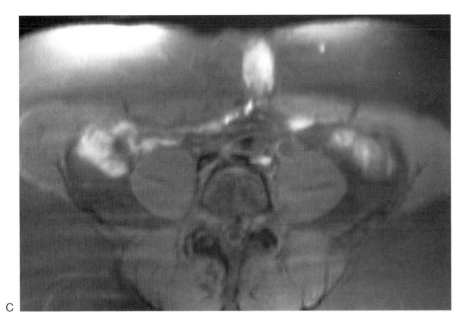

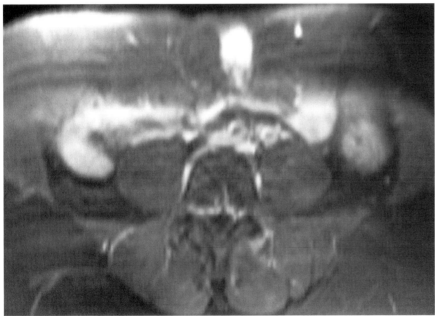

FIG. 9. (*Continued.*) Pre- (**C**) and post-gadolinium-enhanced (**D**) T1-weighted images with fat suppression demonstrate that the umbilical lesion is high in signal intensity and undergoes contrast enhancement.

Desmoid tumors are locally aggressive, benign fibrous tissue neoplasms that occur most commonly in the musculoaponeurotic fascia of the anterior abdominal wall, usually in the rectus abdominis and internal oblique muscles and their fascial coverings. Approximately three fourths of abdominal wall desmoids occur in women, predominantly during the childbearing years (20). On precontrast CT images, desmoids have an attenuation value similar to that of muscle, but they may enhance on postcontrast CT scans to become hyperdense relative to muscle (Fig. 11) (80). On MR images, desmoids commonly appear isointense to muscle on T1-weighted images, variable in signal intensity on T2-weighted images, and demonstrate diffuse enhancement after intravenous administration of gadolinium (172). Extensive fibrosis is suggested by areas

of low signal intensity on both T1- and T2-weighted images (83). These MR signal characteristics are nonspecific, but suggestive in the proper clinical setting. The multiplanar capability of MRI is helpful in defining the connection of the mass to the abdominal wall muscle or fascia (83).

The most common primary malignant neoplasms of the abdominal wall are sarcomas, followed in frequency by lymphomas. Hematogenously spread metastases may involve either the abdominal wall muscles (Figs. 12 and 13) or the subcutaneous fat. Metastatic involvement of muscle produces enlargement of the muscle, often with an associated alteration in normal attenuation value. Subcutaneous metastases usually are nodular (Fig. 14), and are readily detected by CT as soft

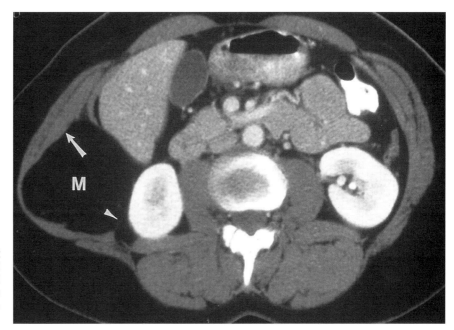

FIG. 10. Abdominal wall lipoma. Fat attenuation mass (M) in the right lateral abdominal wall displaces the internal and external oblique muscles (*arrow*) laterally, and the fascia of the transversus muscle (*arrowhead*) medially.

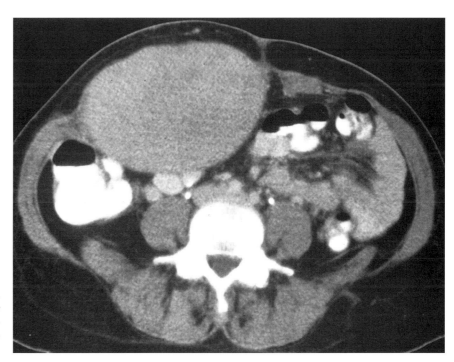

FIG. 11. Desmoid tumor in a postpartum woman. A large homogeneously enhancing mass involving the right rectus abdominis muscle displaces intraperitoneal structures.

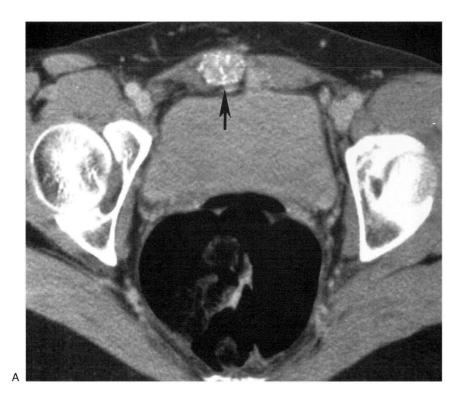

A

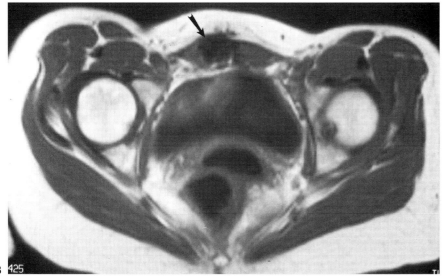

B

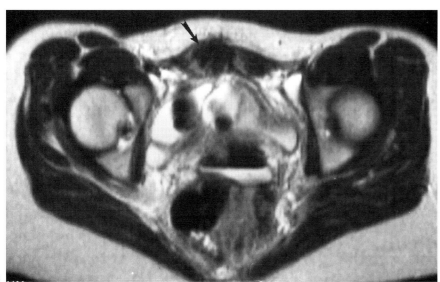

C

FIG. 12. Metastatic ovarian carcinoma. **A:** CT demonstrates a calcified ovarian carcinoma metastasis (*arrow*) to the right rectus abdominis muscle. T1-weighted (**B**) and T2-weighted (**C**) MR images of the same lesion (*arrow*) demonstrate low signal intensity due to the absence of free protons in the calcification.

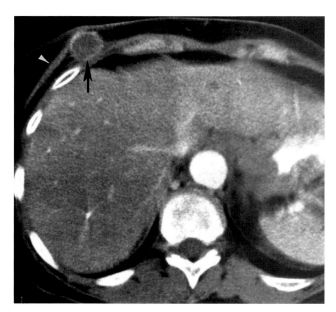

FIG. 13. Metastatic breast carcinoma. Metastatic nodule (*arrow*) with low attenuation center and enhancing rim elevates the external oblique muscle (*arrowhead*).

tissue attenuation masses in the lower attenuation subcutaneous fat (161). Direct spread to the abdominal wall by an intraabdominal neoplasm appears as a thickening of the muscles with loss of the intermuscular and perimuscular fat planes (158). Malignant neoplasms that spread intraperitoneally, such as ovarian and gastrointestinal (GI) carcinoma, have a tendency to involve the umbilical region, producing periumbilical masses

(Fig. 15). Abdominal wall metastases of colon, ovarian, gastric, and gallbladder carcinoma have been reported in incisions and port sites after laparoscopy (14,23,32, 57,85,87). Differentiation of abdominal wall neoplasm from abscess or hematoma may not be possible using CT criteria alone and clinical correlation is often necessary. Percutaneous needle biopsy under CT guidance may be required to differentiate among these entities.

PERITONEAL CAVITY

Anatomy

The peritoneal cavity contains a series of communicating but compartmentalized potential spaces that are not visualized on CT scans unless they are distended by fluid. Knowledge of the anatomy of these spaces and of the ligaments that define them is important in our understanding of pathologic processes involving the peritoneal cavity.

The walls of the peritoneal cavity, as well as the abdominal and pelvic organs contained within, are lined with peritoneum, an areolar membrane covered by a single row of mesothelial cells (64). Folds of peritoneum, called ligaments, connect and provide support for structures within this cavity. The name of a particular ligament usually reflects the two major structures that it joins, e.g., the gastrocolic ligament extends between the greater curvature of the stomach

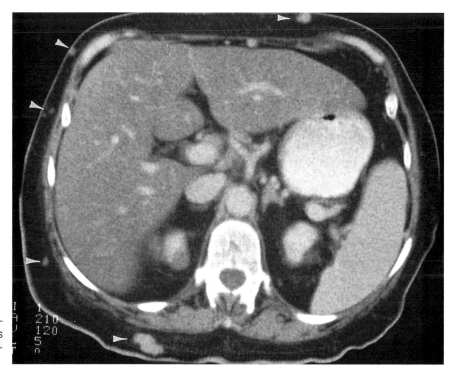

FIG. 14. Metastatic melanoma. Multiple small soft tissue attenuation nodules (*arrowheads*) are present in the subcutaneous fat.

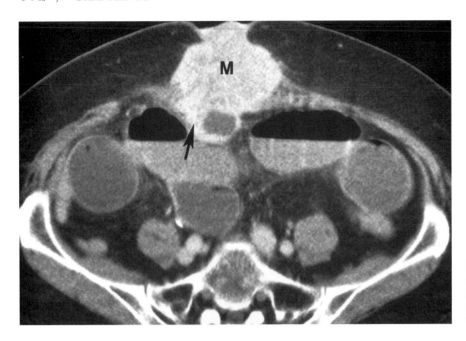

FIG. 15. Metastatic squamous cell carcinoma. A densely enhancing mass (M) involves the umbilicus and anterior abdominal wall, with intraperitoneal extension (*arrow*).

and the transverse colon. A ligament that connects the stomach to other structures is called an omentum. The greater omentum joins the greater curvature of the stomach to the colon and then continues downward anterior to the small bowel. The lesser omentum (also called the gastrohepatic ligament) joins the lesser curvature of the stomach to the liver. A mesentery is a fold of peritoneum connecting either the small bowel or portions of the colon to the posterior abdominal wall. Normally, these peritoneal folds are not directly imaged by CT, but fat, lymph nodes, and vessels contained within them can be identified (191). When the peritoneal folds become thickened by edema, inflammation, or neoplastic infiltration, they can be directly visualized on CT scans. Ligaments, omenta, and mesenteries can serve as routes of spread of benign and malignant pathologic processes within the peritoneal cavity, as well as between the peritoneum and the retroperitoneum. The mode of spread can be by direct extension or via the lymphatics, vessels, or nerves in the areolar tissue enclosed by peritoneum (4, 28,29,42,134,153–157). Knowledge of these structures is important in image interpretation.

The major barrier dividing the peritoneal cavity is the transverse mesocolon, which separates the cavity into supramesocolic and inframesocolic compartments (130). An understanding of the anatomy of the supramesocolic compartment is aided by familiarity with the embryologic development of this space (see Chapter 10).

Supramesocolic Compartment

In the following discussion, the left and right peritoneal spaces are arbitrarily divided into a number of subspaces.

Although these spaces freely communicate, they often become separated by fibrous adhesions when inflammatory or neoplastic processes cause fluid to collect in these spaces. (For a complete discussion of the anatomy of the peritoneal spaces, see Chapter 10.)

Left Peritoneal Space

The left peritoneal space can be divided into anterior and posterior perihepatic and anterior and posterior subphrenic spaces. The *left anterior perihepatic space* can be affected by pathology emanating from the left lobe of the liver or the anterior wall of the body and antrum of the stomach (Figs. 16 and 17). In addition, it may be involved by extension of pathologic processes from other portions of the left peritoneal space.

The *left posterior perihepatic space* is also referred to as the gastrohepatic recess. This space may be affected by pathologic processes arising in any of the structures to which it is closely related, including the left lobe of the liver, the lesser curvature of the stomach, the anterior wall of the duodenal bulb, and the anterior wall of the gallbladder (211) (Figs. 17 and 18).

The *left anterior subphrenic space* is in direct continuity with the left anterior perihepatic space inferomedially and with the left posterior subphrenic space dorsally (80,195) (Figs. 19 and 20). Fluid collections in this region may result from perforation of the splenic flexure of the colon or of the fundus or upper body of the stomach. In addition, left anterior subphrenic space collections may result from extension of disease processes involving the left perihepatic spaces or the left posterior subphrenic space.

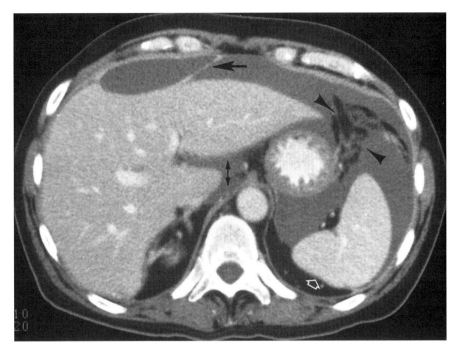

FIG. 16. Malignant ascites in a woman with metastatic ovarian carcinoma. Anteriorly the falciform ligament (*arrow*) separates the right and left peritoneal spaces. Fat in the gastrocolic ligament (*arrowheads*) defines the left margin of the left anterior perihepatic space. A small amount of fluid is present in the lesser sac (*double arrow*). Along the posterior border of the spleen, fluid is limited medially by the spleen's peritoneal reflection (the bare area of the spleen) (*open arrow*).

The *left posterior subphrenic (perisplenic) space* is the posterior continuation of the anterior subphrenic space (Fig. 21). Common sources of pathology involving the left posterior subphrenic space include splenic surgery (i.e., postoperative abscess or hematoma), splenic trauma, and extension of disease processes involving the anterior subphrenic space. In addition, pathology involving the tail of the pancreas can affect the left subphrenic space. Uncommonly, disease processes arising in retroperitoneal organs such as the left kidney or left adrenal gland can extend into this peritoneal space.

Right Peritoneal Space

The right peritoneal space includes both the lesser sac and the right portion of the greater peritoneal space surrounding the liver, i.e., the right perihepatic space. These two spaces communicate via the epiploic foramen (foramen of Winslow).

Right Perihepatic Space

The right perihepatic space consists of a subphrenic and a subhepatic space (Fig. 22), which are partially sepa-

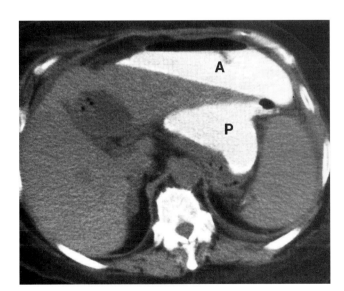

FIG. 17. Gastric perforation has allowed oral contrast material and air to fill the anterior (A) and posterior (P) perihepatic spaces.

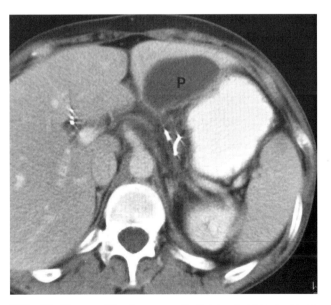

FIG. 18. Pancreatitis. A pancreatic fluid collection involves the left posterior perihepatic space (P). Note that the walled-off collection appears to be intrahepatic.

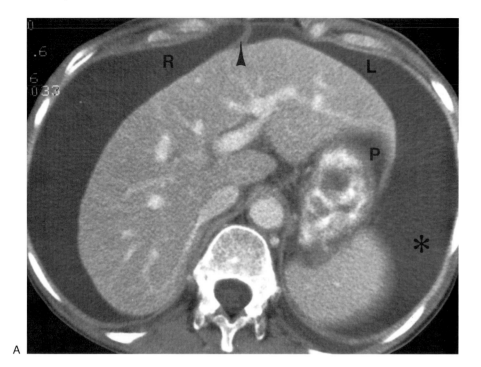

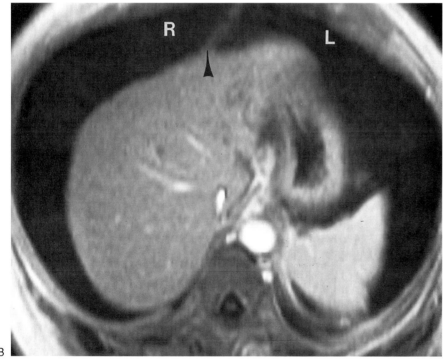

FIG. 19. Ascites in two different patients. CT (**A**) and MR (**B**) images demonstrate ascites in the right (R) and left (L) anterior perihepatic spaces, separated by the falciform ligament (*arrowhead*). The left anterior and posterior (P) perihepatic spaces are in continuity with the left subphrenic space (∗).

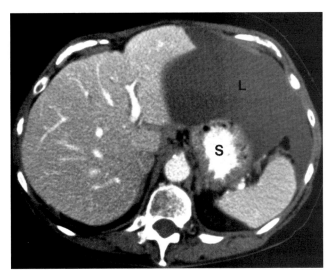

FIG. 20. Malignant ascites from metastatic ovarian carcinoma. Loculated ascites in the left subphrenic space (L) displaces the left lobe of the liver and the stomach (S).

rated by the right coronary ligaments. The posterior subhepatic space projects cephalad into the recess between the liver and the right kidney (Fig. 23). This recess, known as the hepatorenal fossa or Morison's pouch, is the most dependent part of the subhepatic space when the body is in the supine position and is therefore important in the spread and localization of intraperitoneal fluid collections. Common sources of pathology causing fluid collections in the right perihepatic space include the gallbladder, the descending portion of the duodenum (Figs. 24 to 26), the right lobe of the liver, and the right colon. Another

important cause of a right perihepatic fluid collection is cephalad extension of pelvic fluid via the right paracolic gutter. Occasionally, retroperitoneal disease processes arising in the right kidney, right adrenal gland, or head of pancreas can extend into the right perihepatic space.

Lesser Sac

The lesser sac communicates with the remainder of the right peritoneal space through a narrow inlet between the inferior vena cava and the free margin of the hepatoduodenal ligament called the epiploic foramen (of Winslow). In patients with intraperitoneal inflammation, this foramen may seal, separating the lesser sac from the greater peritoneal cavity (130). A prominent fold of peritoneum, elevated from the posterior abdominal wall by the left gastric artery, divides the lesser sac into two compartments—a large lateral compartment on the left and a smaller medial compartment on the right (130) (Fig. 27). The medial compartment contains a superior recess that wraps around the caudate lobe of the liver (Fig. 28).

Disease processes producing generalized ascites or those involving the pancreas, transverse colon, posterior wall of the stomach, posterior wall of the duodenum, and caudate lobe of the liver can produce pathologic changes in the lesser sac (Figs. 29 and 30). The most common lesser sac collection is ascites (45). Whereas patients with benign, transudative ascites tend to have large greater sac collections with little fluid in the lesser sac, patients with peritoneal carcinomatosis often have proportional fluid volumes in the two spaces (62). The largest fluid collec-

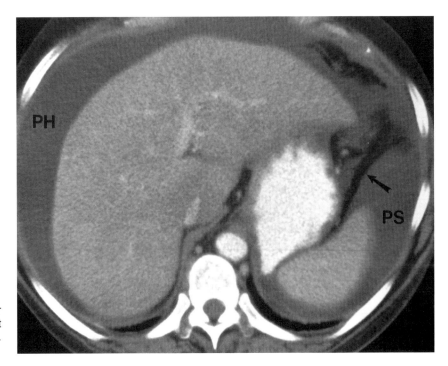

FIG. 21. Ascites fills the left posterior subphrenic (perisplenic) (PS) and right subphrenic (perihepatic) space (PH). Gastrosplenic ligament (*arrow*).

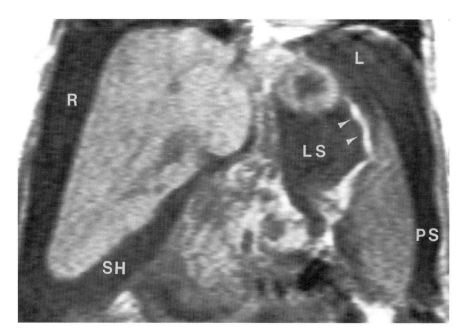

FIG. 22. Coronal T1-weighted MR image demonstrates ascitic fluid in the right perihepatic (R), subhepatic (SH), left subphrenic (L), and perisplenic (PS) spaces. Ascites in the lesser sac (LS) is separated from the left subphrenic fluid by the gastrosplenic ligament (*arrowheads*).

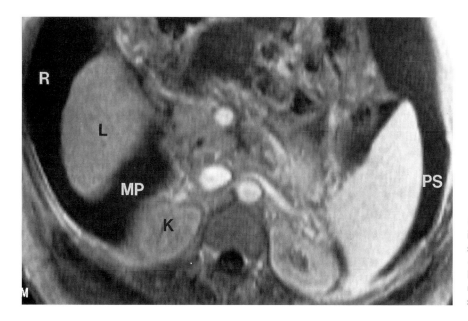

FIG. 23. T1-weighted transaxial MR image demonstrates low-signal-intensity ascites in the hepatorenal fossa (Morison's pouch) (MP), between the liver (L) and right kidney (K). It is contiguous with fluid in the right perihepatic space (R). Perisplenic space (PS).

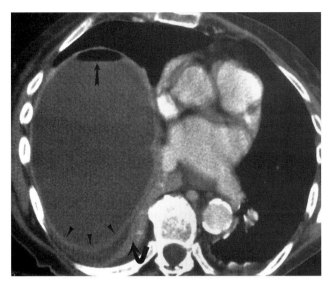

FIG. 24. Right subphrenic abscess after gastrojejunostomy. A large fluid collection with an air—fluid level (*arrow*) fills the right subphrenic space. The diaphragm (*arrowheads*) separates the abscess from a right pleural effusion posteriorly. Atelectatic lung (*curved arrow*).

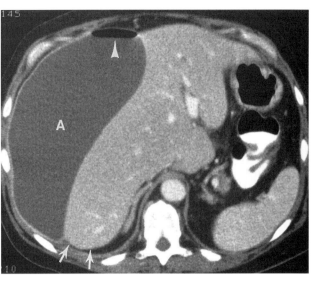

FIG. 25. Abscess in right perihepatic space secondary to perforated duodenal ulcer. A near-water-density collection (A) with an air—fluid level (*arrowhead*) in the right perihepatic (subphrenic) space is limited posteriorly by the bare area of the liver (*arrows*).

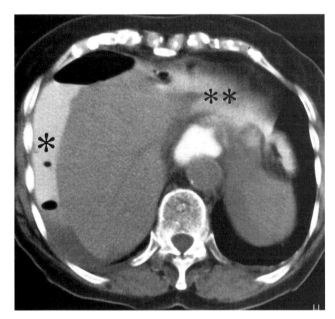

FIG. 26. Perforated duodenal ulcer. Fluid, air and high density oral contrast material (∗) fill the right perihepatic space. Air and oral contrast material are also identified in the left peritoneal space (∗∗).

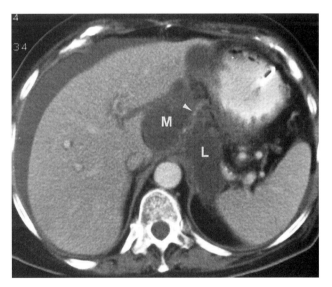

FIG. 27. Ascites in the lesser sac. The lateral (L) and medial (M) compartments of the lesser sac are divided by a fold of peritoneum through which passes the left gastric artery (*arrowhead*). Ascites is also present in the left and right greater peritoneal spaces.

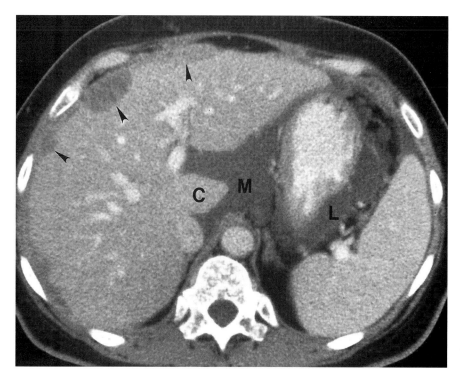

FIG. 28. Metastatic ovarian carcinoma. Malignant ascites fills the medial (M) and lateral (L) compartments of the lesser sac. The superior recess of the medial compartment wraps around the caudate lobe of the liver (C). Perihepatic serosal metastatic implants (*arrowheads*) are present.

tions to occupy the lesser sac occur in patients with disease processes involving organs directly bordering this space. Although pancreatitic fluid collections located anterior to the pancreas are generally considered to be within the lesser sac, a recent anatomic study suggests that such

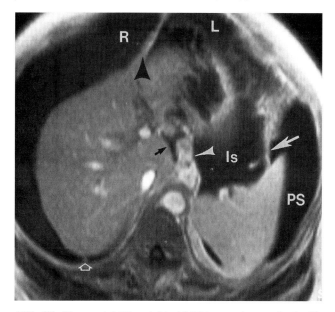

FIG. 29. Transaxial T1-weighted MR image in a patient with ascites delineates the peritoneal spaces. The falciform ligament (*black arrowhead*) separates fluid in the left (L) and right (R) peritoneal spaces anteriorly. Fluid in the lateral compartment of the lesser sac (Is) is separated from that in the perisplenic space (PS) by the gastrosplenic ligament (*white arrow*), and from the superior recess of the medial compartment of the lesser sac (*black arrow*) by the left gastric artery (*white arrowhead*). The triangular ligament (*open arrow*) can be seen in this patient because it is surrounded by peritoneal fluid.

collections are more likely located within retroperitoneal fascial planes (137). Fluid collections involving the lateral compartment of the lesser sac displace the stomach anteriorly (Fig. 30) and sometimes medially, whereas medial compartment collections may cause lateral displacement of the stomach. Collections extending below the level of the pancreatic body displace the transverse colon and mesocolon caudally. Less commonly, a lesser sac collection may extend ventral and caudal to the transverse colon due to a persistent inferior lesser sac recess in the leaves of the greater omentum (45). Occasionally, inflammation involving the medial compartment may extend via the aortic or diaphragmatic hiatus into the lower mediastinum (45).

Inframesocolic Compartment

The inframesocolic compartment is divided into two unequal spaces by the obliquely oriented small bowel mesentery (Fig. 31). The smaller right inframesocolic space is restricted inferiorly by the junction of the distal small bowel mesentery with the cecum, whereas the larger left inframesocolic space is open to the pelvis inferiorly except where it is bounded by the sigmoid mesocolon.

The paracolic gutters are located lateral to the attachments of the peritoneal reflections of the ascending and descending colon. The right paracolic gutter is continuous superiorly with the right perihepatic space. On the left, however, the phrenicocolic ligament forms a partial barrier between the left paracolic gutter and the left subphrenic space. The most dependent portion of the peritoneal cavity in both the erect and supine positions is in

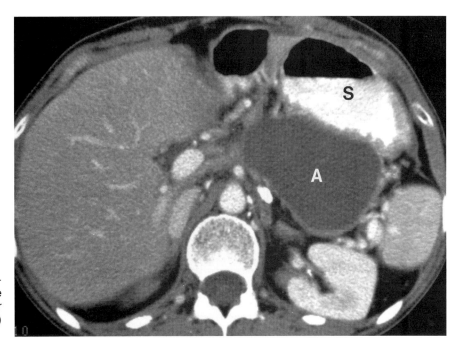

FIG. 30. Metastatic ovarian carcinoma. Malignant ascites distends the lateral compartment of the lesser sac (A) displacing the stomach (S) anteriorly.

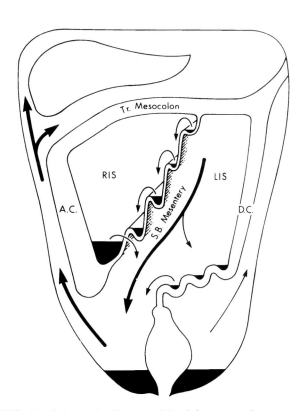

FIG. 31. Schematic diagram of the inframesocolic compartment of the peritoneal cavity. The small bowel mesentery divides the inframesocolic compartment into two unequal spaces. The arrows indicate the natural flow of ascites within the peritoneal cavity. RIS, right infracolic space; LIS, left infracolic space; AC, ascending colon; DC, descending colon.

the pelvis and consists of lateral paravesical spaces and the midline pouch of Douglas (rectovaginal space in women, rectovesical space in men).

The natural flow of intraperitoneal fluid is directed by gravity and variations in intraabdominal pressure due to respiration along pathways determined by the anatomic compartmentalization of the peritoneal cavity (130) (Fig. 31). Abscesses usually form and metastases usually grow in sites where natural flow permits pooling of infected fluid or malignant ascites. The most common sites of pooling of infected peritoneal fluid and thus for abscess formation are the pelvis, right subhepatic space, and right subphrenic space (130) (see Fig. 24). Similarly, the most common sites for pooling of malignant ascites and subsequent fixation and growth of peritoneal metastases are the pouch of Douglas, the lower small bowel mesentery near the ileocecal junction, the sigmoid mesocolon, and the right paracolic gutter (129). Fluid in the inframesocolic compartment rapidly seeks the pelvis, where it first fills the pouch of Douglas and then the lateral paravesical fossae. Fluid in the right infracolic space flows along the recesses of the small bowel mesentery until it pools at the confluence of the mesentery with the colon near the ileocecal junction, with subsequent overflow into the pouch of Douglas. Fluid in the left infracolic space is frequently arrested by the sigmoid mesocolon before descending into the pelvis. From the pelvis, fluid can ascend both paracolic gutters with changes in intraabdominal pressure during respiration. Flow along the left paracolic gutter is slow and weak, and cephalad extension is usually limited by the phrenicocolic ligament (127,128). The major flow is along the right paracolic gutter into the right subhepatic space, particularly the posterior extension of this space, Morison's pouch (127). From the right subhepatic space, fluid may ascend further into the right subphrenic space. Direct spread from the right subphrenic space across the midline to the left subphrenic space is prevented by the falciform ligament.

Pathologic Conditions

Ascites

Ascites is the accumulation of fluid in the peritoneal cavity resulting from either increased fluid production or impaired removal. The etiologies of ascites include congestive heart failure, hypoalbuminemia, cirrhosis, venous or lymphatic obstruction, inflammation, and neoplasm. Computed tomography can accurately demonstrate and localize even small amounts of free peritoneal fluid. Localized collections of ascites are frequently seen in the right perihepatic space, Morison's pouch, or the pouch of Douglas. Peritoneal fluid in the paracolic gutter is easily distinguished from retroperitoneal fluid by the preservation of the retroperitoneal fat posterior to the ascending or descending colon (89,92) (Fig. 32). When a large amount of ascites is present, the small bowel loops usually are located centrally within the abdomen and fluid often accumulates in triangular configurations within the leaves of the small bowel mesentery or adjacent to bowel loops

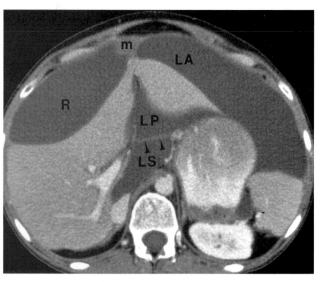

FIG. 33. Ovarian carcinoma. A metastatic implant (m) on the falciform ligament separates malignant ascites in the right perihepatic (R) and left anterior (LA) perihepatic spaces. The right perihepatic fluid is loculated and deforms the liver margin. The gastrohepatic ligament (*arrowheads*) separates ascites in the left posterior perihepatic space (LP) and the medial compartment of the lesser sac (LS).

(176) (Fig. 32). Loculated ascites, secondary to postoperative, inflammatory, or neoplastic adhesions, may appear as a well-defined fluid attenuation mass that displaces adjacent structures (Fig. 33). Occasionally, peritoneal fluid collections can become loculated within the four normal or accessory fissures of the liver and can mimic intrahepatic cysts, abscesses, or hematomas (6) (Fig. 34). Peritoneal metastases in these locations also can be mistaken for intrahepatic lesions (6).

The attenuation of ascitic fluid generally ranges from 0 to 30 HU but may be higher in cases of exudative ascites, with the density of the fluid increasing with increasing protein content (24). However, attenuation values of ascitic fluid are nonspecific, and infected or malignant ascites cannot reliably be distinguished from uncomplicated transudative ascites based on the attenuation value alone. Relatively acute intraperitoneal hemorrhage often can be distinguished from other fluid collections because it results in peritoneal fluid with an attenuation value of >30 HU (50). However, acute traumatic hemoperitoneum can commonly have attenuation values of <20 HU and should not be assumed to be ascites in the proper clinical setting (106). Conversely, ascitic fluid may show enhancement on delayed CT imaging after the intravenous administration of iodinated contrast material (37). This increase in the attenuation value of ascites on delayed postcontrast images is a nonspecific finding that should not be confused with high-attenuation fluid resulting from hemorrhage or perforation of the GI or urinary tract.

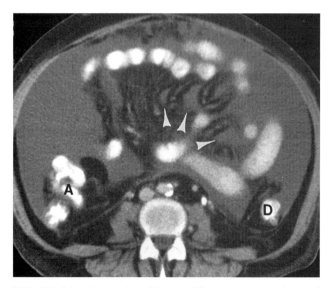

FIG. 32. Massive ascites. The small bowel loops are located centrally within the abdomen. The pleated nature of the small bowel mesentery can be appreciated as fluid outlines several of the mesenteric leaves. Fluid accumulating between leaves of the mesentery takes on a triangular configuration (*arrowheads*). Note that the retroperitoneal fat posterior to the ascending (A) and descending (D) colon is preserved.

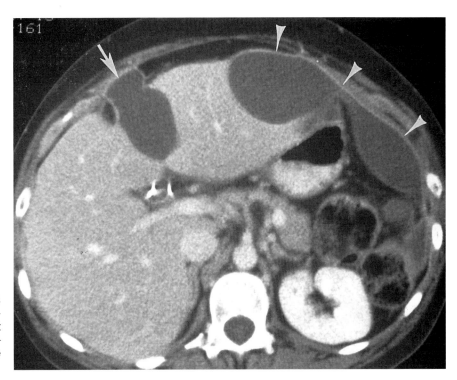

FIG. 34. Biloma. Intraperitoneal bile is loculated in the fissure for the ligamentum teres (*arrow*) and in the left anterior perihepatic space (*arrowheads*) in a patient who had undergone laparoscopic cholecystectomy.

The distribution of ascitic fluid in the peritoneal cavity may suggest the nature of the fluid. Patients with benign transudative ascites tend to have large greater sac collections with little fluid in the lesser sac, whereas patients with malignant ascites often have proportional volumes of fluid in these peritoneal spaces (33) (Fig. 35). Large lesser sac collections may be seen in patients with disease processes in organs that border this space (62). However, these CT features are not specific and needle aspiration may be necessary to differentiate transudative from exudative ascites.

Magnetic resonance imaging also can be used to evaluate intraabdominal fluid collections. Transudative ascites appear low in signal intensity on T1-weighted images,

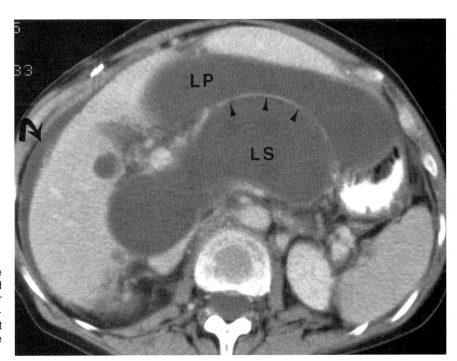

FIG. 35. Ovarian carcinoma. Large collections of malignant ascites distend the lesser sac (LS) and left posterior perihepatic space (LP), which are separated by the gastrohepatic ligament (*arrowheads*). Right perihepatic space fluid (*curved arrow*).

where it is seen best, and high in signal intensity on T2-weighted images because of its long T1 and T2 relaxation (33,212) (Fig. 36). The T1 relaxation of fluid collections decreases with increasing protein concentration (202). Thus exudative fluid collections demonstrate intermediate to short T1 and long T2 values. These collections are best seen on T2-weighted images where they appear high in signal intensity (33). The MRI appearance and relaxation times are not specific enough to obviate diagnostic needle aspiration. In addition, the lack of a reliable GI contrast agent for MRI makes it difficult to distinguish small extraluminal fluid collections from dilated fluid-filled bowel loops. Additionally, lesser sac collections are more difficult to demonstrate on MR images, possibly due to the effect of peristaltic and respiratory motion artifact (33).

Intraperitoneal Abscess

The epidemiology of intraabdominal abscess has changed in recent decades. In the first half of the twentieth century, perforated ulcer, appendicitis, and biliary tract disease were the most common causes (48,152). However, over the past several decades, intraabdominal abscess has occurred most commonly after surgery, particularly surgery involving the stomach, biliary tract, and colon (71,178,187,213). Despite advances in surgical technique and antimicrobial therapy, intraabdominal abscess remains a serious diagnostic and therapeutic problem. Even with treatment, mortality rates can reach 30% (164).

Although most patients present with fever, leukocytosis, and abdominal pain, patients with chronic, walled-off abscesses may present with few overt clinical signs or symptoms. Furthermore, some symptoms may be masked by the administration of antibiotics or corticosteroids (3).

Computed tomography is the most accurate single imaging modality for diagnosing intraabdominal abscess (44). When examining a patient for a suspected abscess, careful attention to technique is crucial for correct diagnosis. The entire abdomen from the diaphragm to the pubic symphysis should be scanned and adequate oral contrast material should be administered to avoid mistaking a fluid-filled bowel loop for an abscess.

The CT appearance of an abscess is variable depending on its age and location. In its earliest stage, an abscess consists of a focal accumulation of neutrophils in a tissue or organ seeded by bacteria and thus appears as a mass with an attenuation value near that of soft tissue. As the abscess matures, it undergoes liquefactive necrosis. At the same time, highly vascularized connective tissue proliferates at the periphery of the necrotic region. At this stage, the abscess has a central region of near-water attenuation surrounded by a higher attenuation rim that usually enhances after administration of intravenous contrast material (5) (Fig. 37). Approximately one third of abscesses contain variable amounts of air, appearing on CT scans as either multiple small bubbles or an air–fluid level (5,25, 70,86,99,221) (Figs. 37 and 38). The presence of a long air–fluid level suggests communication with the GI tract (86). Ancillary findings include displacement of surrounding structures, thickening or obliteration of adjacent fascial planes, and increased density of adjacent mesenteric fat (Fig. 39). Whereas most abscesses are round or oval in shape, those adjacent to solid organs, such as the liver, may have a crescentic or lenticular configuration (see Fig. 25).

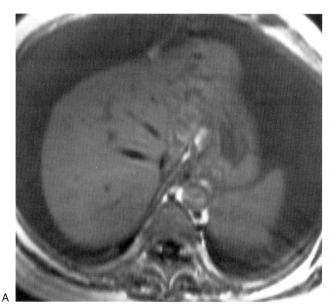
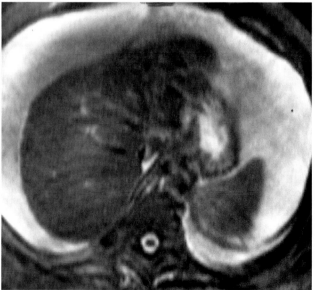

A   B

FIG. 36. Transudative ascites. Because of its long T1 and T2 relaxation, ascites appears low in signal intensity on T1-weighted (**A**) and high in signal intensity on T2-weighted (**B**) MR images.

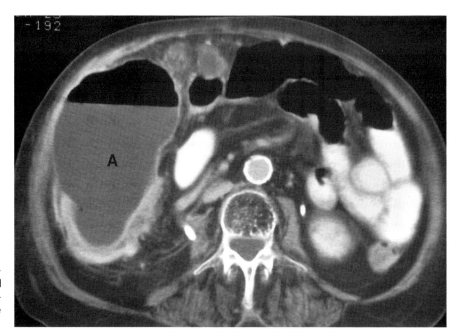

FIG. 37. Abscess. Large low-attenuation fluid collection (A) with air–fluid level and enhancing rim in the right midabdomen. The patient had undergone recent right hemicolectomy.

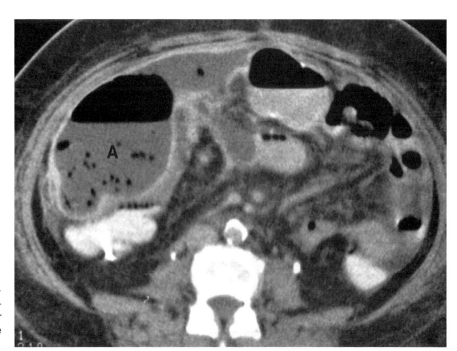

FIG. 38. Abscess after right hemicolectomy. Right mid-abdominal fluid collection (A) contains multiple small air bubbles and an air–fluid level. Note the enhancing rim.

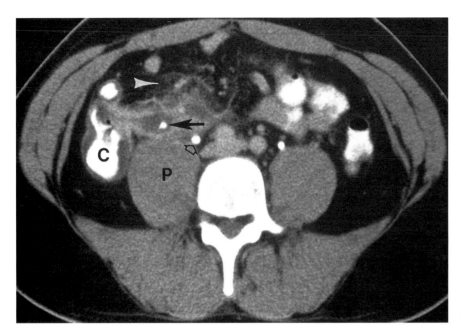

FIG. 39. Appendiceal abscess. Calcified appendicolith (*arrow*) is demonstrated just anterior to the psoas muscle (P), surrounded by low-attenuation fluid with a higher attenuation rim and surrounding streaky soft tissue densities extending into the adjacent mesenteric fat (*arrowhead*). Cecum (C); ureter (*open arrow*).

In some cases, the CT appearance of an abscess can suggest its etiology. A low-density right lower quadrant mass containing a round calcific density is highly suggestive of an appendiceal abscess with an appendicolith (Fig. 39). Elsewhere in the abdomen, a low-density mass containing a high-density object suggests a foreign body abscess.

Although the above CT findings are highly suggestive of abscess, they are not specific. Other masses that can have a central low attenuation value include a cyst, pseu-docyst, hematoma, urinoma, lymphocele, biloma, loculated ascites, thrombosed aneurysm, and necrotic neoplasm. In addition, normal structures such as unopacified bladder, stomach, and bowel can mimic the appearance of an abscess (Fig. 40). Thickening of adjacent fascial planes is also non-specific and can be seen with intraabdominal hematoma and neoplastic infiltration. Even the presence of gas within a mass is nonspecific for abscess because a necrotic noninfected neoplasm and a mass that communicates with bowel can also contain gas. Because

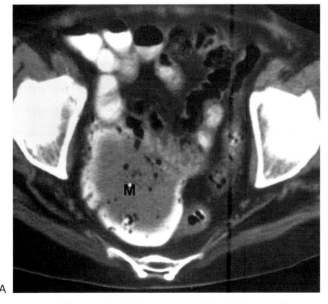

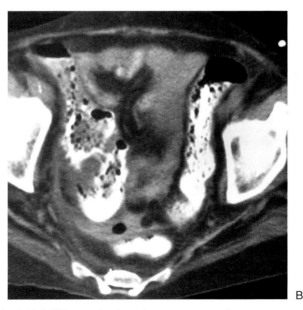

A

B

FIG. 40. Fluid-filled cecum simulating an abscess. **A:** Initial CT examination demonstrates a low-attenuation pelvic mass (M) with multiple air bubbles simulating an abscess. **B:** Follow-up examination 1 day later demonstrates marked change in appearance of the now less distended cecum containing stool and oral contrast material.

a specific diagnosis of abscess based on CT findings alone is not possible, correlation with clinical history is important. Percutaneous needle aspiration may be necessary to make a definitive diagnosis. In this regard, CT can be very helpful in identifying a plane of access for aspiration that is both safe and free of contamination from bowel. The presence or absence of an abscess can be established by obtaining a specimen for Gram stain and culture. In most instances, if an abscess is present, a catheter can be inserted percutaneously for definitive drainage (194,207). Percutaneous abscess drainage has proven to be a safe and effective approach to the diagnosis and treatment of intraabdominal abscess (179,206). Although it was originally thought that only well-defined, unilocular abscesses with safe drainage routes should be drained percutaneously, the criteria for percutaneous drainage have been expanded to include ill-defined and multiseptated abscesses, as well as those communicating with the GI tract or located deep to major abdominal organs (55,140). Even potentially complicated abscesses such as appendiceal, diverticular, and interloop abscesses secondary to Crohn disease can be drained without complications (12,91, 144,148,177,209). In the case of periappendiceal abscesses, percutaneous drainage may completely eliminate the need for surgery (12,91,148,209), whereas percutaneous drainage of diverticular abscesses often converts complex two- or three-stage surgical procedures to safer one-stage colonic resections (144). The only factor of value in predicting the eventual outcome of percutaneous drainage is location, with subphrenic and hepatic abscesses being more likely to have a successful outcome than those in other locations (86). Because no specific CT features of an abscess (other than location) provide predictive value, all intraabdominal abscesses should be considered candidates for percutaneous drainage (55,86). The technical details of CT-guided abscess drainage are described in Chapter 3.

The MRI appearance of intraabdominal abscess is also non-specific. Therefore, MRI does not eliminate the need for aspiration in establishing a diagnosis. Because of its short to intermediate T1 and long T2, an abscess demonstrates intermediate to high signal intensity on T1-weighted images and high signal intensity on T2-weighted images (33,212). It is usually best seen on T1-weighted images (33,212). In a study of percutaneously obtained normal and abnormal body fluids, the mean T1 value of abscess contents was found to be significantly shorter and the mean T2 value significantly longer than those of bile, ascitic fluid, urine collections, cysts and pseudocyst fluid, and pleural fluid (22).

Accuracy of CT in Intraperitoneal Abscess

The accuracy of CT in detecting intraabdominal abscess is approximately 95% (5,68,70,98–101,180,221).

Most false positive diagnoses are due to mistaking unopacified fluid-filled stomach, bowel, or bladder for an abscess. If a question exists as to the nature of a fluid-filled structure, additional oral, rectal, or intravenous contrast material can be administered (Fig. 41).

Comparison of CT with Other Imaging Techniques

Other imaging techniques also have been shown to be accurate in the detection of intraabdominal abscess, particularly ultrasound and radionuclide imaging. In a number of published studies, sensitivity and overall accuracy for ultrasound have ranged from 90% to 96% (100, 119,201), although one study reported an accuracy of only 44% (117). Ultrasound images can be obtained in multiple anatomic planes and a thorough examination can be performed in a relatively short time. In addition, if a patient is too unstable to be moved, an ultrasound study can be done at the patient's bedside. The areas of the abdomen best suited to ultrasound diagnosis of abscess are the right and left upper quadrants and the pelvis (208). In these areas, the liver, spleen, and distended urinary bladder can be used as acoustic windows for transmission of the ultrasonic beam into the abdomen. However, abscesses located in the midabdomen may be difficult to detect with ultrasound due to interruption of the ultrasonic beam by bowel gas and mesenteric fat (21). In addition, other patient factors such as obesity or the presence of open wounds, drainage tubes, and large dressings may hamper the ultrasound examination. In comparison to the potential limitations of ultrasound, CT is capable of providing high-quality images of all areas of the abdomen and pelvis, including the retroperitoneum, regardless of body habitus and despite the presence of open wounds, drainage tubes, overlying dressings, and large amounts of bowel gas. Computed tomography is thus better able to detect and define the extent of intraabdominal fluid collections and to aid in the planning of either percutaneous or surgical abscess drainage by clearly delineating the relationship of the abscess to surrounding structures.

Radionuclide imaging using [67]gallium citrate (^{67}Ga)– and [111]indium (^{111}In)–labeled leukocytes also has been effective in detecting and localizing intraabdominal abscesses. Various studies have reported sensitivities ranging from 80% to 92% (100,108,125). The major advantage of radionuclide scintigraphy is that it provides images of the entire body, thus occasionally displaying unsuspected extraabdominal sites of infection (181). The major disadvantage of ^{67}Ga imaging is that 48 to 72 hours frequently is required before the study can be properly interpreted (98). In addition, uptake of ^{67}Ga is nonspecific in that it accumulates in certain tumors, postsurgical beds, healing wounds, and other areas of simple inflammation (98,108). Because it is excreted by the colon, difficulty can be encountered in differentiating an abdominal ab-

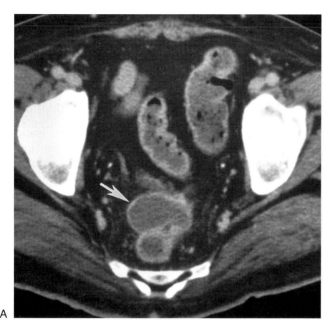 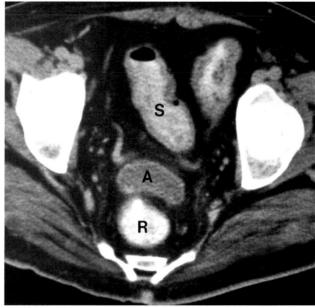

FIG. 41. Cul-de-sac abscess after cholecystectomy. **A:** A small fluid collection (*arrow*) with enhancing rim is difficult to distinguish from unopacified adjacent rectum and sigmoid colon. **B:** After administration of rectal contrast material, the abscess (A) is easily distinguishable from the now opacified rectum (R) and sigmoid colon (S).

scess from normal colonic activity (100). [111]In imaging avoids some of the problems of ^{67}Ga imaging because it does not take as long, is not excreted by the colon, and does not accumulate in tumors. However, ^{111}In is a cyclotron-produced isotope whose preparation requires care to maintain function of the leukocytes (98). In addition, the distribution of the labeled leukocytes and their accumulation at sites of inflammation may be altered by splenectomy, bone marrow radiation, hyperalimentation, hemodialysis, hyperglycemia, and antibiotic therapy (98). Furthermore, chronic abscesses may have a well-defined wall without significant inflammatory response and therefore may not be detected by ^{111}In leukocyte studies (98). Other limitations include obscuration of upper abdominal abscesses by activity in the liver and spleen and nonspecific uptake of ^{111}In leukocytes by other inflammatory and some noninflammatory processes (123). Another limitation of radionuclide imaging in the evaluation of a suspected abdominal abscess is that when an abnormal accumulation of radiotracer is identified, an additional imaging study usually is needed to provide more specific anatomic localization.

Approach to Imaging a Suspected Intraabdominal Abscess

In patients who are acutely ill or who have localized clinical findings, CT is the initial imaging procedure of choice for detecting and defining the extent of intraabdominal abscesses. If the CT examination is equivocal,

ultrasonography may provide valuable information. Ultrasound can be used as the initial examination if a right upper quadrant, left upper quadrant, or pelvic abscess is suspected. However, a negative ultrasound examination should be followed by CT because ultrasound does not optimally evaluate the midabdomen and retroperitoneum. If the CT examination of the entire abdomen and pelvis is unequivocally normal, abscess can be confidently excluded.

In patients with a suspected abdominal abscess who are not acutely ill and have no localizing signs, radionuclide imaging with ^{67}Ga citrate- or ^{111}In-labeled leukocytes can be considered as the initial screening technique. If the radionuclide examination is normal, no further radiologic evaluation is indicated. If the examination demonstrates one or more areas of increased activity, a CT or ultrasound examination is then performed to document and further evaluate the area of possible abscess. Magnetic resonance imaging, because of its more limited availability, stringent patient requirements, relatively high cost, and relatively long examination time, plays only a limited role in the detection of intraabdominal abscesses.

Other Intraperitoneal Fluid Collections

Intraperitoneal hemorrhage may result from overanticoagulation; bleeding diathesis; trauma to the liver, spleen, or mesentery; spontaneous rupture of a vascular neoplasm; hemorrhagic cyst or ectopic pregnancy; perforation of a duodenal ulcer; or acute mesenteric ischemia

(Fig. 42B). In addition, intraperitoneal blood is frequently seen after abdominal surgery. CT has been shown to be highly sensitive and specific for diagnosing hemoperitoneum (50), with the diagnosis being based on the high attenuation value of the peritoneal fluid (Fig. 42B). However, it is important to keep in mind that acute hemoperitoneum can have attenuation values of <20 HU (106). The CT appearance of intraperitoneal hemorrhage depends on the location, age, and extent of the bleeding. Immediately after hemorrhage, intraperitoneal blood has the same attenuation as circulating blood. However, within hours the attenuation increases as hemoglobin is concentrated during clot formation (145,146). In most

cases, the attenuation begins to decrease within several days as clot lysis takes place (16). The attenuation value decreases steadily with time and often approaches that of water (0 to 20 HU) after 2 to 4 weeks (101). During the hyperdense phase, the attenuation value of intraperitoneal blood ranges from 20 to 90 HU (50,110,197,220). In one large study, all patients with hemoperitoneum <48 hours old had fluid collections containing areas of attenuation >30 HU (50). The morphologic characteristics of recent intraperitoneal hemorrhage are variable. The fluid collection may be homogeneously hyperdense or may be heterogeneous with nodular or linear areas of high attenuation surrounded by lower attenuation fluid. The heterogeneity

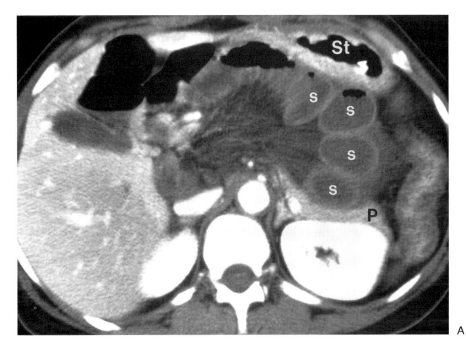

A

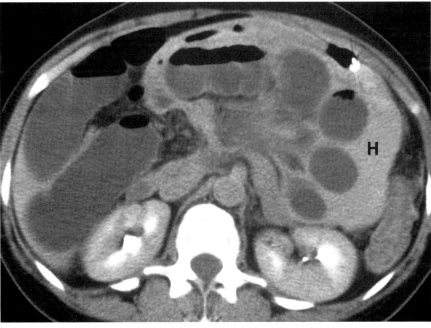

B

FIG. 42. Strangulated lesser sac hernia. **A:** Dynamic contrast-enhanced CT demonstrates dilated, fluid-filled small bowel loops (s) in the lesser sac. Mesenteric edema is manifested as a diffuse increase in the density of the mesenteric fat with poor definition of the segmental mesenteric vessels. A small amount of lesser sac ascites is also present. Stomach (St); tail of pancreas (P). **B:** Rescan after 1-hr delay shows progressive hemorrhagic mesenteric edema and development of a hemorrhagic effusion (H) within the lesser sac surrounding the obstructed small bowel loops.

may result from irregular clot resorption or intermittent bleeding (220). In most cases, intraperitoneal blood contains focal areas of clot that are higher in attenuation than the free intraperitoneal blood. These localized clots are helpful in determining the bleeding site, as they usually form adjacent to the organ from which the hemorrhage originated (50). Occasionally, fresh blood within a hematoma or confined within a peritoneal space may show a "hematocrit effect" with sedimented erythrocytes producing a dependent layer of high attenuation (Fig. 43). The most common site of blood accumulation on CT scans after upper abdominal trauma is Morison's pouch (50,120). The right paracolic gutter is another common site of blood collection, even in cases of splenic trauma. With extensive hemorrhage, large collections of blood may fill the pelvis with little blood in upper abdominal sites. Therefore, it is important to include the pelvis in any CT examination performed for suspected intraabdominal hemorrhage, particularly in patients who have sustained blunt abdominal trauma (50). Before beginning the examination, adequate oral contrast material should be administered to opacify all abdominal and pelvic bowel loops.

If a CT examination without intravenous contrast material has been obtained, viewing the images with a narrow window width is helpful to accentuate the density difference between the fresh blood and the adjacent soft tissues. However, in most cases a precontrast CT examination is unnecessary and one can begin the study with intravenous contrast material administered as a bolus. The contrast enhancement helps to demonstrate injuries to the liver, spleen, and kidneys and makes intraperitoneal fluid collections more apparent by increasing the density of the surrounding tissues. Extravasation of intravenous contrast material, resulting in an area of fluid whose attenuation is higher than the remainder of the acute hemoperitoneum, is an indicator of significant active bleeding (193).

Magnetic resonance imaging also can be used to demonstrate intraperitoneal hemorrhage. However, many patients referred for suspected intraabdominal hemorrhage are unstable and require extensive monitoring and supportive equipment, making MRI less practical. A hematoma <48 hours old may have a nonspecific signal intensity (204). Intraabdominal hematoma >3 weeks old can have a specific appearance referred to as the concentric ring sign, in which a thin peripheral rim that is dark on all sequences surrounds a bright inner ring that is most distinctive on T1-weighted images (69).

Intraperitoneal bile accumulation (biloma) is caused by iatrogenic, traumatic, or spontaneous rupture of the biliary tree (210). The bile elicits a low-grade inflammatory response that generally walls off the collection by the formation of a thin capsule or inflammatory adhesions within the mesentery and omentum (114,210). Most bilomas appear round or oval and have attenuation values of <20 HU. Those complicated by hemorrhage or infection may be higher in density. Bilomas are usually confined to the upper abdomen. Although most are located in the right upper quadrant, left upper quadrant bilomas are not uncommon, occurring in approximately 30% of cases (141,210) (see Fig. 34). Because the CT appearance is not specific, biloma cannot be distinguished from other abdominal fluid collections and either needle aspiration or hepatobiliary scintigraphy is usually required to establish the diagnosis. Most bilomas can be treated successfully with percutaneous catheter drainage (141,210).

Intraabdominal collections of urine may result from urinary tract obstruction or from surgery or trauma involving the kidney, ureter, or bladder. Free intraperitoneal urine usually results from traumatic rupture of the bladder dome. Computed tomographic examination of patients with intraperitoneal bladder rupture performed after cystography or intravenous contrast material administration will show high-density fluid freely filling the peritoneal spaces. Although localized collections of urine (urinomas) usually occur within the retroperitoneal space, an intraperitoneal urinoma can occur if the anatomic boundaries of the retroperitoneum have been disrupted by trauma or prior surgery (77). On CT images obtained without intravenous contrast material, the attenuation value of a urinoma is <20 HU. After administration of intravenous contrast medium, however, the attenuation value can increase due to accumulation of opacified urine in the fluid collection. Thus, delayed CT imaging may be helpful in establishing the diagnosis of urinoma.

Lymphoceles are abnormal accumulations of lymphatic fluid usually resulting from operative disruption of lymphatic vessels. The most common procedures to cause lymphoceles are renal transplantation and retroperitoneal

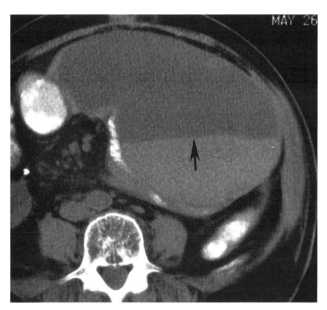

FIG. 43. Intraperitoneal hematoma in an anticoagulated patient. Unenhanced CT examination demonstrates a large fluid collection containing a hematocrit level (*arrow*) with higher attenuation erythrocytes layering dependently.

lymph node dissection. Although most lymphoceles are confined to the retroperitoneum, intraperitoneal lymphoceles do occur. The more common manifestation of intraperitoneal lymph leakage is chylous ascites, usually resulting from lymphatic obstruction by tumor (165). A lymphocele has a nonspecific appearance and cannot be distinguished from other abdominal fluid collections by its CT or MRI features alone. The diagnosis can be established by percutaneous aspiration (165,215). Chylous ascites usually is indistinguishable from other types of ascitic fluid. Occasionally, however, the diagnosis may be suggested if negative Hounsfield numbers, due to the high fat content of lymph, are detected. The rare finding of a fat–fluid level in ascitic fluid is pathognomonic of chylous ascites (79).

The Mesentery

Normal Anatomy

The small bowel mesentery is a broad, fan-shaped fold of peritoneum that connects the jejunum and ileum to the posterior abdominal wall (64). It originates at the duodenojejunal flexure just to the left of the spine and extends obliquely to the ileocecal junction. Within its two fused layers are contained the intestinal branches of the superior mesenteric artery and vein, lymphatic vessels, lymph nodes, nerves, and variable amounts of fat. On CT, the mesentery appears as a fat-containing area central to the small bowel loops within which the jejunal and ileal vessels can be identified as distinct, round, or linear densities (191) (Fig. 44). Normal lymph nodes <1 cm in diameter are occasionally identified. The normal mesenteric fat is similar in attenuation to the subcutaneous fat (-100 to -160 HU) (190). In patients with a large amount of ascites, the pleated nature of the mesentery can be appreciated as fluid outlines the mesenteric folds (Fig. 45).

The transverse mesocolon, which extends from the anterior surface of the pancreas to the transverse colon, contains the middle colic arteries and veins (Fig. 46). On the right, the root of the mesocolon is continuous with the duodenocolic ligament and thus the posterior aspect of the hepatic flexure. Medially it crosses the descending duodenum and head of pancreas extending along the lower anterior edge of the body and tail of the pancreas. On the left it is continuous with the phrenicocolic and splenorenal ligaments (134). In most patients, the transverse mesocolon is readily identified on CT as a fat-containing area extending from the pancreas, particularly at the level of the uncinate process, to the margin of the colonic wall (90). In thin patients, the transverse mesocolon may be difficult to identify due to lack of mesenteric fat and the steeply oblique orientation of the mesentery in such patients. Nevertheless, the middle colic branches of the transverse mesocolon can be identified in nearly all patients (191). The root of the small bowel mesentery at its origin near the duodenojejunal flexure is continuous with the root of the transverse mesocolon (131). The sigmoid mesocolon, extending from the posterior pelvic wall and containing the sigmoid and hemorrhoidal vessels, can usually be identified deep within the pelvis (Fig. 47).

Pathologic Conditions Involving the Mesentery and Peritoneum

Mesenteric abnormalities are readily identified on CT in all but the leanest patients because of the abundance of fat present within the normal mesentery. Various pathologic processes, both benign and malignant, may infiltrate the mesentery causing an increase in attenuation

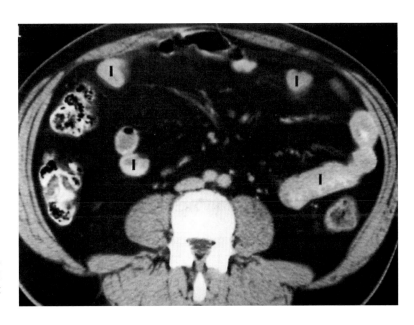

FIG. 44. Normal small bowel mesentery. The jejunal and ileal vessels appear as round and curvilinear densities within the mesenteric fat central to the small intestinal loops (I).

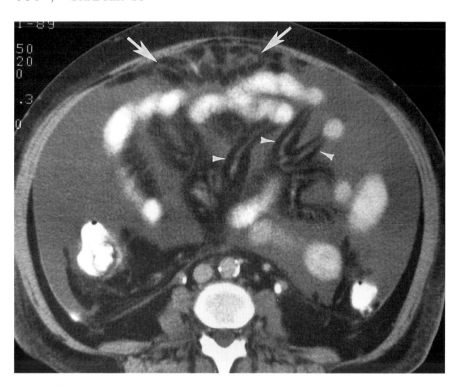

FIG. 45. Massive ascites. Low attenuation ascites outlines the greater omentum (*arrows*) and the leaves of the small bowel mesentery (*arrowheads*). The jejunal vessels are easily identified within the mesenteric fat.

of the mesenteric fat, distortion of the mesenteric architecture, and loss of definition of the mesenteric vessels. Some of these processes may also cause thickening of the peritoneal lining. Detection of mesenteric abnormalities requires rigorous attention to CT technique. It is particularly important to opacify the GI tract with oral contrast material so that unopacifed bowel is not mistaken for a mesenteric mass. Conversely, a small mesenteric mass can be obscured if surrounded by unopacified bowel loops. Approximately 500 ml of an oral contrast agent should be given at least 1 hr prior to the examination in order to opacify the distal small bowel. Another 500 ml of contrast material should be given 15 min before the examination to opacify the stomach and proximal small bowel. If bowel cannot confidently be distinguished from a mesenteric mass, additional contiguous scans through the suspicious area can be obtained after additional oral contrast material has been administered or after delay allows transit of more proximal contrast material. Occasionally, it is helpful to opacify the colon per rectum with a dilute contrast solution or air in order to differentiate a redundant sigmoid colon from a pelvic mass.

Magnetic resonance imaging is not as valuable as CT for detecting, characterizing, and delineating mesenteric abnormalities. Peristaltic and respiratory motion artifacts can degrade MR images and limit spatial resolution in the region of the mesentery. In addition, lack of a reliable oral contrast agent for MRI makes it difficult to differentiate mesenteric masses from bowel loops in many cases. The MRI appearance of nodular or thickened, enhancing peritoneum is a nonspecific finding, with considerable overlap between benign and malignant causes (15,73,97).

Edema

Diffuse mesenteric edema is most commonly the result of hypoalbuminemia, usually caused by either cirrhosis or the nephrotic syndrome. Mesenteric ischemia and mesenteric venous or lymphatic obstruction are less common causes. The CT findings characteristic of mesenteric edema include increased density of the mesenteric fat, poor definition of segmental mesenteric vessels, relative sparing of the retroperitoneal fat, and association with subcutaneous edema (190). Bowel wall thickening also is present in some patients. When this pattern is identified, careful evaluation of the root of the mesentery should be made to exclude a focal tumor mass obstructing mesenteric vessels and creating secondary edema (190). Although diffuse infiltration of the mesentery by metastatic tumor may have an appearance similar to that of mesenteric edema, it can sometimes be distinguished from edema by the rigidity of the mesenteric leaves. Lateral decubitus or prone scans may be helpful in demonstrating the mesenteric fixation.

Pancreatitis

Computed tomography has established roles in the initial diagnosis, assessment of prognosis, evaluation of

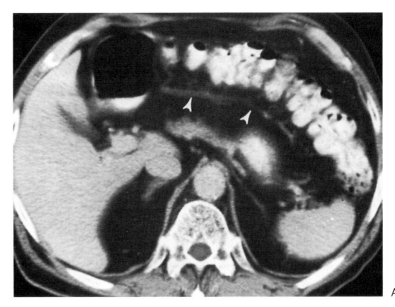

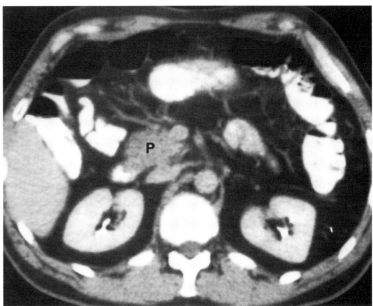

FIG. 46. Normal transverse mesocolon. **A:** The middle colic vessels (*arrowheads*) are easily identifiable within the fat posterior to the transverse colon. **B:** The fat and vessels within the transverse mesocolon are often easiest to identify at the level of the uncinate process of the pancreas (P).

complications, direction of image-guided intervention, and follow-up of pancreatitis (8,9).

The transverse mesocolon is affected by dissection of pancreatic enzymes in a small percentage of patients with acute pancreatitis (126,192). In patients with fulminant pancreatitis, the mesocolon is involved approximately one third of the time (90). The small bowel mesentery is involved much less commonly. The main CT finding in patients with mesenteric inflammation related to pancreatitis is streaky or confluent increased density of the mesenteric fat (Fig. 48). Dissection by pancreatic enzymes along the mesenteric leaves can result in formation of abscesses, pseudocysts, hemorrhage, enteric fistulae, and late bowel stenoses (90). The presence of air bubbles in a mesenteric fluid collection may be due to an abscess, necrosis without infection, or communication with the GI tract. Patients with mesenteric involvement demonstrated by CT have a higher morbidity and mortality than patients without CT evidence of mesenteric spread (90).

Crohn Disease

Crohn disease is a chronic granulomatous disease of the alimentary tract that most commonly involves the small intestine or colon. The major benefit of CT scanning in patients with Crohn disease is to identify and characterize the extramucosal abnormalities, many of which cause separation of bowel loops on barium studies (59). Most importantly, CT is helpful in differentiating mesenteric abscess from fibrofatty proliferation or diffuse inflammatory reaction of the mesentery (Fig. 49). Bowel wall thickening and mes-

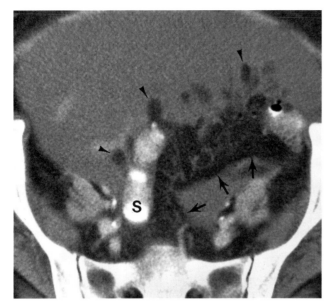

FIG. 47. The sigmoid mesocolon (*arrow*) is well demonstrated in this patient with a large amount of ascites. Sigmoid colon(s); appendices epiploicae (*arrowheads*).

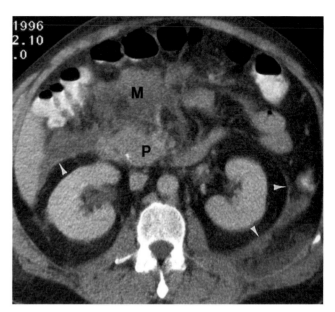

FIG. 48. Acute pancreatitis. The transverse mesocolon (M) is diffusely increased in density by extension of peripancreatic fluid and inflammation. Fluid is also present in the retroperitoneal interfascial planes (*arrowheads*). Head of pancreas (P).

enteric adenopathy are also well demonstrated (116,142). Fibrofatty mesenteric proliferation, the most common cause of bowel loop separation, is characterized by increased density of the fat between the separated loops (−70 to −90 HU) and lack of a soft tissue mass or fluid collection in the affected region (52,59). Diffuse inflammatory reaction of the mesentery produces a similar increase in density of the mesenteric fat but has no clearly defined borders. An abscess can be confidently diagnosed when a well-marginated near-water density mass is identified. Occasionally the mass may contain air and oral contrast material, indicating communica-

tion with bowel (59,96). Computed tomography can also be helpful in identifying and defining the extent of sinus tracts and fistulae. In cases in which a mesenteric mass has an attenuation value near that of soft tissue, it may be difficult to differentiate an abscess from an inflammatory mass (96). Occasionally, the identification of fibrofatty proliferation of the mesentery on CT can be helpful in establishing a diagnosis of Crohn disease when a patient's inflammatory bowel disease is difficult to classify clinically, as mesenteric fat

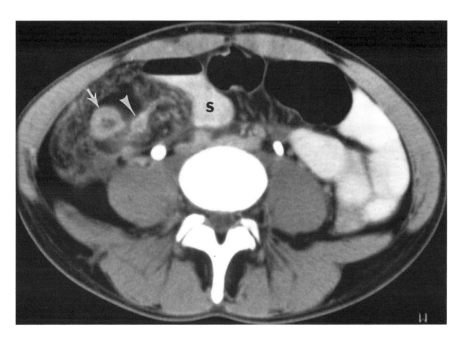

FIG. 49. Crohn disease. The mesenteric fat surrounding the thickened ascending colon (*arrow*) and terminal ileum (*arrowhead*) is diffusely inflamed and edematous, producing mass effect on adjacent dilated small bowel loops (s).

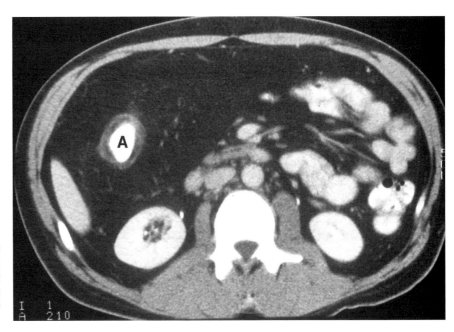

FIG. 50. Fibrofatty proliferation of mesenteric fat in a patient with Crohn disease. Marked proliferation of fat within the mesentery of the ascending colon (A) displaces small bowel loops to the left side of the abdomen.

proliferation does not appear to be a feature of ulcerative colitis (63) (Fig. 50). Fibrofatty proliferation and increased blood flow are responsible for the CT appearance of vascular dilatation and tortuosity, as well as wide spacing and prominence of the vasa recta ("comb sign") seen in association with affected bowel segments (132) (Fig. 51).

Diverticulitis

Although the barium enema examination has long served as the primary imaging test for diagnosing diverticulitis, it does not delineate the extracolonic extent of dis-

ease. The advantage of CT is that it clearly delineates the extracolonic extent of disease, while not requiring direct distention of the colon with contrast material.

The most common CT finding in patients with diverticulitis is inflammation of the pericolonic fat, characterized by poorly defined soft tissue density and fine linear strands in the fat adjacent to the involved colon (81,113) (Fig. 52). Other CT findings include colon wall thickening, intramural sinus tracts, mural or extramural abscesses (Fig. 53), fistulae, and peritonitis (189,199). In addition, because CT images the entire abdomen, it is useful in demonstrating other complications of diverticulitis such as bladder involvement, ureteral obstruction, and distant abscesses. The sensitivity of

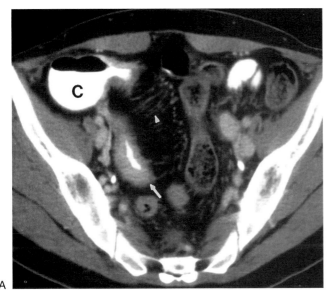

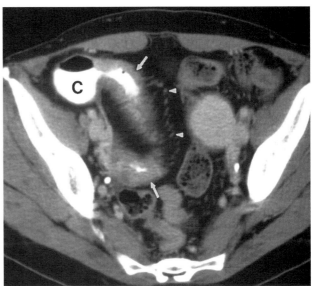

A   B

FIG. 51. Comb sign in patient with Crohn disease. **A, B:** Two contiguous CT images demonstrate prominent vasa recta (*arrowheads*) coursing through proliferative mesenteric fat to supply inflamed thick-walled terminal ileum (*arrows*). Cecum (C).

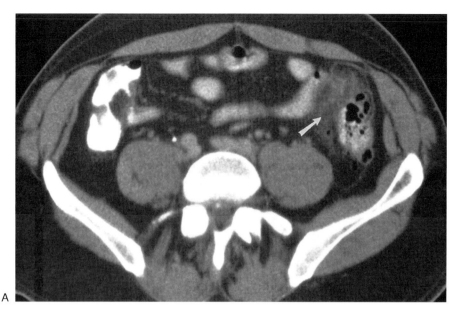

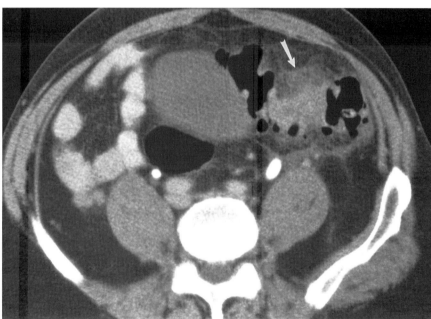

FIG. 52. Diverticulitis. Increased density in the mesenteric fat (*arrows*) adjacent to the descending (**A**) and sigmoid colon (**B**). Multiple air-filled diverticula can be identified along the wall of the colon.

CT for the diagnosis of diverticulitis has been reported to be higher than that of contrast enema (93% versus 80%) (31). In one study, CT demonstrated the extracolonic extent and complications of diverticulitis more accurately than contrast enema examination in 41% of cases (81). The association of colonic wall thickening and pericolonic inflammatory changes is not pathognomonic for diverticulitis and can be mimicked by perforated colon carcinoma, pelvic inflammatory disease, appendicitis, endometriosis, Crohn disease, and other forms of colitis.

Peritonitis

Peritonitis is an inflammation of the peritoneum that can result from numerous causes and can be either local-ized or diffuse. The major types of peritonitis include bacterial, granulomatous, and chemical (164). Although bacterial peritonitis is sometimes primary, it usually results secondarily from perforation of an abdominal viscus. Common etiologies include appendicitis, diverticulitis, perforated ulcer, perforated carcinoma, acute cholecystitis, pancreatitis, salpingoopheritis, and abdominal surgery (164). With diffuse peritonitis, the CT findings consist of thickening of the peritoneum and mesentery, increased density of the mesenteric fat, and ascites (216) (Fig. 54). This CT appearance is nonspecific and can also be seen in patients with metastatic cancer or peritoneal mesothelioma.

Tuberculous peritonitis has become a relatively uncommon disease. It is believed to occur by direct extension

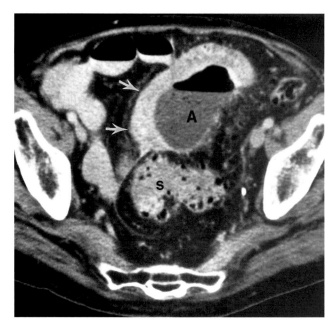

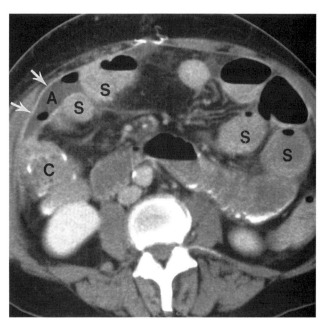

FIG. 53. Diverticulitis with a pericolonic abscess. A near-water-density fluid collection (A) with air–fluid level and enhancing wall displaces an adjacent small bowel loop (*arrows*). The sigmoid colon (S) contains many diverticula.

FIG. 54. Peritonitis secondary to perforated Crohn disease. Contrast-enhanced CT demonstrates thickened, enhancing peritoneum (*arrows*) and an adjacent air-containing fluid collection (A). Ascending colon (C); small bowel loops (S).

(ruptured lymph nodes or perforation of a tuberculous lesion in the GI or genitourinary tract) or by lymphatic or hematogenous spread (203). The CT appearance of tuberculous peritonitis is varied. The most common CT feature is lymphadenopathy, predominantly in the mesenteric and peripancreatic areas (82) (Fig. 55). Central low density within the enlarged lymph nodes, presumably due

to caseation necrosis, is seen in approximately 40% of patients (47,82). Disseminated mycobacterium tuberculosis infection is found in approximately three fourths of HIV-infected patients who have enlarged low-attenuation lymph nodes, whereas *Mycobacterium avium-intracellulare* (MAI) infection more often results in soft tissue attenuation lymphadenopathy (167). High-density ascites (20 to

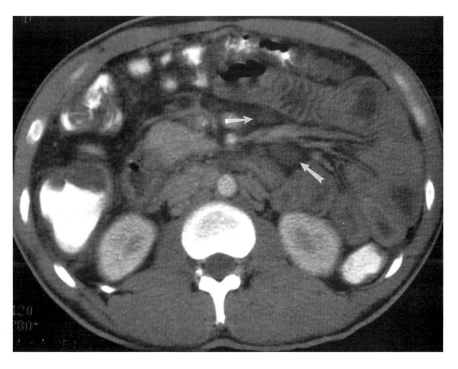

FIG. 55. Tuberculosis. Low-density mesenteric lymphadenopathy (*arrows*).

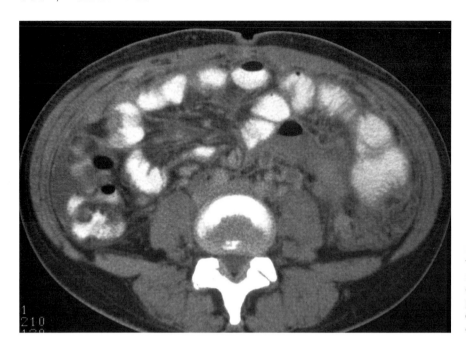

FIG. 56. Tuberculous peritonitis. Diffuse omental, mesenteric and peritoneal thickening with a small amount of high-density ascites in the right paracolic gutter. The appearance is indistinguishable from that of peritoneal carcinomatosis.

45 HU) is another characteristic feature of tuberculous peritonitis, the increased density being related to the high protein content of the fluid (40,47,75,82). Additional CT findings include thickening and nodularity of peritoneal surfaces, mesentery, and omentum (40,47,82) (Fig. 56). Although these CT features are highly suggestive of tuberculous peritonitis, they are not pathognomonic, and other diseases, such as nontuberculous peritonitis, lymphoma, metastatic carcinoma, peritoneal mesothelioma, and pseudomyxoma peritonei, should be included in the differential diagnosis. The presence of mesenteric changes, soft tissue nodules with a diameter of at least 5 mm, and peritoneal masses with low-attenuation center favors tuberculous peritonitis over metastatic carcinoma, which more commonly has more prominent omental involvement (67).

A rare condition, peritoneal *Echinococcus multilocularis* infection, results in multiple low-attenuation, thin-walled, cystic lesions on peritoneal and omental surfaces (198). As with many of the entities discussed above, the appearance is nonspecific.

Mesenteric Panniculitis

Mesenteric panniculitis, mesenteric lipodystrophy, and idiopathic retractile mesenteritis are descriptive terms used to characterize different stages of a pathologic process that results in fibrofatty thickening of the mesentery. In each, inflammation (panniculitis), fatty degeneration (lipodystrophy), or fibrosis (retractile) predominates (102,121). The association of fat necrosis and acute pancreatitis is well recognized (54). Fat necrosis, which can affect the mesentery, omentum, or retroperitoneum, can

also be caused by infection, recent surgery, or a foreign body (94). The CT appearance varies from soft tissue attenuation mesenteric infiltration (Fig. 57) to nodular masses with soft tissue and/or fat attenuation (102,121) (Fig. 58). Calcification in the necrotic central portion may also be detected (76). Cystic components may be seen, representing dilated lymphatics due to lymphatic and/or venous obstruction (95). In some cases, when fat attenuation is present, the CT appearance may not be distinguishable from that of a liposarcoma or a fat-containing teratoma (Fig. 58). When soft tissue attenuation nodules are present, differential diagnostic considerations include carcinoid, desmoid tumor, mesenteric lymphoma, and metastatic carcinoma. The MRI appearance varies, with signal characteristics suggesting fluid or inflammation (low on T1, high on T2), fat (high on T1, low on T2), or fibrosis (low on T1 and T2) (102).

Segmental omental infarction can result in CT findings in the omentum similar to those described above in the mesentery (10,166). Omental infarction can be idiopathic or associated with adhesions, prior surgery, trauma, or omental torsion (10,27). Torsion of the greater omentum sometimes results in a characteristic CT appearance consisting of fibrous and fatty folds in a converging radial pattern (27).

Mesenteric Cysts

A large variety of benign and malignant entities can present as cystic mesenteric or omental masses. These include lymphangioma, enteric duplication cyst, mesothelial cyst, ovarian cyst, non-pancreatic pseudocyst, cystic mesothelioma, cystic mesenchymal tumor, and cystic ter-

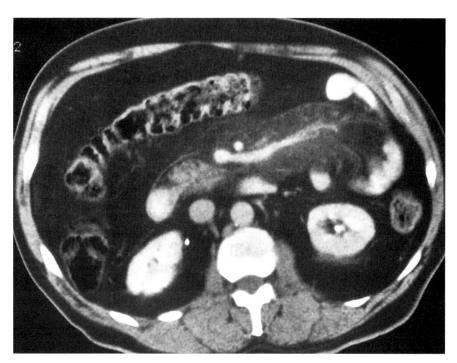

FIG. 57. Mesenteric panniculitis. The fat of the small bowel mesentery is diffusely increased in density with loss of definition of segmental mesenteric vessels.

atoma. Although CT findings may suggest a specific diagnosis in some cases, histologic diagnosis is often needed (173, 196).

Mesenteric cysts appear on CT as well-defined, near-water-density, abdominal masses that sometimes contain thin higher density septa (74). In some cases a thin wall can be identified peripherally. Mesenteric cysts are benign masses containing either serous or chylous fluid (205). Chylous cysts occasionally have a pathognomonic fat–fluid layer, demonstrable with CT, MRI, or ultrasound.

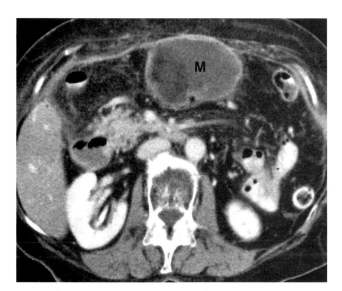

FIG. 58. Fat necrosis. A large, well-defined mass (M) contains mixed soft tissue and fat attenuation components. The mass arose within the transverse mesocolon after partial pancreatectomy for pancreatic cancer.

The etiology of these cysts is poorly understood. They usually present as an asymptomatic abdominal mass but can cause chronic abdominal pain or acute pain secondary to a complication such as torsion, rupture, hemorrhage, or GI obstruction. The most common location of a mesenteric cyst is in the small bowel mesentery, with the mesocolon and omentum being less common sites of origin (74,184). The cysts are usually single, but can be multiple and vary widely in size. In children the cysts may fill most of the abdomen (74). Although the cyst content is usually water density, cysts containing mucinous fluid or hemorrhage can have higher CT numbers (216). Lymphangioma is usually multilocular with an imperceptible wall. CT attenuation values and MRI signal intensity may indicate the presence of fat (196).

Other Nonneoplastic Processes Involving the Mesentery

Mesenteric hemorrhage, similar to hemorrhage elsewhere in the peritoneum, has a varied appearance depending on the age and extent of the bleeding. Acute mesenteric hemorrhage may produce localized, well-defined, soft tissue masses adjacent to bowel loops or larger "cake-like" masses that displace the bowel loops (216). When presenting as a focal mass, mesenteric hematoma can be mistaken for a primary or metastatic mesenteric tumor, an exophytic tumor of the bowel, or a mesenteric cyst with hemorrhage (168). With diffuse involvement the mesenteric fat is obliterated. The attenuation of the hematoma is initially high with a gradual decrease in attenuation over a period of weeks followed by

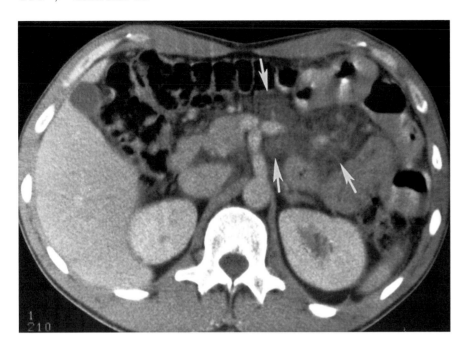

FIG. 59. Whipple disease. The small bowel mesentery contains multiple confluent low attenuation lymph node masses (*arrows*).

gradual resorption of the remaining seroma. After complete resorption, the mesentery may appear to return to normal or may contain residual fibrosis (216).

Pseudotumoral lipomatosis of the mesentery refers to the excessive proliferation of normal mesenteric fat. This benign condition can be idiopathic or can be seen in association with obesity, Cushing syndrome, or steroid therapy (111). On contrast studies of the GI tract, mesenteric lipomatosis may displace bowel loops, simulating an abdominal mass or ascites. Computed tomography can exclude the presence of neoplasm by showing that the displacement is due to either diffuse or focal accumulation of normal fat (34,111,188).

Systemic amyloidosis is characterized by diffuse extracellular tissue deposition of an amorphous eosinophilic protein-polysaccharide complex (38). Amyloidosis can occur as a primary process or in association with chronic inflammatory disease or multiple myeloma. Involvement of the mesentery, when extensive, is easily demonstrated by CT (2). The CT appearance, consisting of increased density of mesenteric fat with encasement of mesenteric vessels, is indistinguishable from other disease processes causing diffuse mesenteric infiltration including peritonitis, metastatic carcinoma, and peritoneal mesothelioma.

The most commonly recognized radiographic manifestation of Whipple disease is thickening of the valvulae conniventes of the small bowel. However, CT is capable of demonstrating some of the less well-recognized extraintestinal manifestations of the disease including lowdensity retroperitoneal and mesenteric lymphadenopathy, and sacroiliitis (112,171) (Fig. 59). The enlarged lymph nodes in Whipple disease may be low in attenuation secondary to deposition of neutral fat and fatty acids within the nodes (112).

Mesenteric venous thrombosis is responsible for 5% to 15% of cases of intestinal ischemia (65). The superior mesenteric vein (SMV), which is involved in 95% of these cases, is easily imaged by CT. The typical appearance of chronic SMV thrombosis consists of enlargement of the vein with central low density surrounded by a higher density wall (174) (Fig. 60). The wall of the vein enhances after administration of intravenous contrast material, possibly due to enhancement of the arterially supplied vasa vasorum (226). The thrombus may be higher in attenuation than soft tissue when SMV thrombosis is acute. Associated portal venous or splenic venous thrombosis may be seen (174). In some cases, mesenteric venous thrombosis is associated with increased density of the mesenteric fat and poor definition of segmental mesenteric vessels, due to mesenteric edema (190). Thickening of the bowel wall may also be present. If the mesenteric ischemia is severe enough to cause bowel infarction, intramural, portal vein, or mesenteric vein gas may also be identified (49). These associated findings are usually absent when the thrombus is non-occlusive (Fig. 61).

Endometriosis can diffusely involve the peritoneum with cystic, solid, or mixed masses throughout the omentum, mesentery, and peritoneal surfaces (Fig. 62). High-attenuation ascites may also be present. Although the CT appearance is nonspecific, this diagnosis should be considered in women of childbearing age. Differential diagnostic considerations include peritoneal carcinomatosis, pseudomyxoma peritonei, lymphoma, and tuberculous peritonitis.

Castleman disease is an idiopathic, benign entity characterized by proliferation of lymphoid tissue into tumoral masses. It is most often seen as a solitary mediastinal mass but can occur as solitary or widespread mesenteric

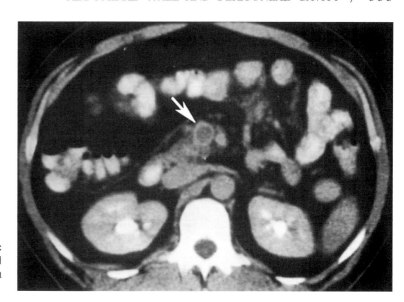

FIG. 60. Thrombosis of the superior mesenteric vein (SMV). The SMV (*arrow*) is enlarged and contains central low density surrounded by a higher density wall.

disease (51,53). Classically, marked enhancement is seen on CT (51,53).

Primary Neoplasms

Primary neoplasms of the peritoneum are rare and are generally of mesenchymal origin. The mesenteric desmoid tumor is a non-encapsulated, locally invasive form of fibromatosis (143). It occurs predominantly in patients with Gardner's syndrome who have undergone abdominal surgery, although it occasionally occurs as an isolated abnormality (13,118,143). On CT, a desmoid tumor appears as a soft tissue mass displacing adjacent visceral structures (13) (Figs. 63 and 64). Although the mass may appear well circumscribed, it often has irregular margins reflecting its infiltrative nature (Figs. 63 and 64). Attenuation values range from 40 to 60 HU (13,118). Other neoplasms such as mesenteric metastases and lymphoma can present a similar CT appearance. On MRI a desmoid tumor appears low in signal intensity on T1-weighted images and remains relatively low in intensity on T2-weighted images, reflecting its largely fibrous composition (Fig. 64).

Lipomatous tumors, which occur predominantly in the retroperitoneum, rarely involve the peritoneal cavity. Benign lipomas (Fig. 65) consist predominantly of fat, which is reflected in their CT attenuation and MR signal characteristics. Multiple histologic subtypes of liposarcoma exist, each with corresponding CT and MR characteristics. Well-differentiated liposarcoma can be of lipomatous or sclerosing type, with CT and MR appearance of fat or muscle, respectively. Myxoid liposarcoma has an appearance on unenhanced CT that is similar to water, with reticular enhancement after administration of intravenous contrast material. Round cell and pleiomorphic liposarcomas are nonfatty tumors with nonspecific soft tissue appearance on CT and MRI (97).

Benign or malignant primary peritoneal tumors other than desmoid and lipomatous tumors are extremely rare but can arise from any of the mesenchymal tissue elements (73,105,124) (Figs. 66 and 67). Primary mesenteric and omental teratomas have also been reported (73,214).

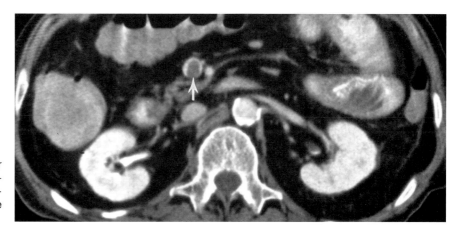

FIG. 61. Thrombosis of the superior mesenteric vein (SMV). Contrast material flows around the periphery of a nonocclusive thrombus (*arrow*) within the SMV.

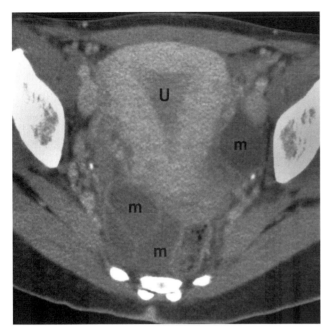

FIG. 62. Endometriosis. Multiple homogenous near-water attenuation cystic masses (m) occupy the adnexal regions of the pelvis. Uterus (U).

Because both benign and malignant primary peritoneal tumors may demonstrate cystic, solid, and complex features, histologic diagnosis is usually required.

Mesothelioma is a rare malignant neoplasm arising from the serosal lining of the pleura, peritoneum, and pericardium. Peritoneal involvement may occur, either alone or in combination with pleural involvement. Computed tomographic findings in patients with peritoneal mesothelioma include peritoneal thickening that may appear irregular or nodular, omental and mesenteric thickening, and ascites (66,170, 218) (Fig. 68). It can also appear as a multilocular cystic mass (151) (Fig. 69). The mesenteric involvement may produce a "stellate" appearance due to thickening of the perivascular bundles by tumor (218). The CT appearance of peritoneal mesothelioma may be indistinguishable from peritoneal carcinomatosis, lymphoma, and benign disease processes such as tuberculous peritonitis. The amount of ascites relative to the soft tissue component of mesothelioma may be disproportionately small as compared with peritoneal carcinomatosis in which ascites is usually a prominent feature (170).

Secondary Neoplasms

The most common malignant neoplasms involving the peritoneum are metastatic carcinoma and lymphoma. Metastases usually arise from the stomach, colon, or ovary; and less commonly from the pancreas, biliary tract, or uterus (1,41). Renal cell carcinoma and transitional cell

carcinoma of the bladder are reported as rare sites of origin (163,200). Prior to the availability of CT, peritoneal metastases were not detectable radiographically until they were large enough to displace adjacent organs or cause intestinal obstruction. Now with the use of CT, peritoneal metastases less than 1 cm in diameter can be detected before they are large enough to cause symptoms. Rigorous attention to technique is important in detecting small mesenteric and omental tumor implants. Intraperitoneal air or iodinated contrast material may improve the detection of implants in some intraperitoneal compartments (26,72). Although CT remains the imaging method of choice for detecting peritoneal and mesenteric implants, newer MRI techniques, including breath-hold gradient echo imaging with fat suppression and gadolinium enhancement, show promise for demonstrating peritoneal tumors (115,182) (Fig. 70). However, non-breath-hold MRI techniques suffer from image degradation due to motion artifact from respiration, cardiac activity, and bowel peristalsis, and from lack of a satisfactory GI contrast agent. Detection of implants by MRI is improved in the presence of ascites, with greatest contrast achieved on T1-weighted images obtained with fat suppression and gadolinium enhancement.

In patients with a large amount of ascites, ultrasound is capable of demonstrating superficial peritoneal and omental tumor nodules as small as 2 to 3 mm because of the acoustic window provided by the peritoneal fluid (223). However, it is difficult to detect peritoneal masses with ultrasound in patients with little or no ascites. Furthermore, centrally located tumors are poorly imaged by

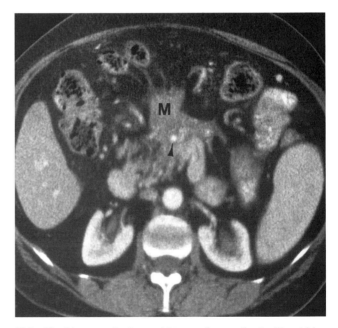

FIG. 63. Mesenteric desmoid tumor in a patient without history of Gardner syndrome. Enhancing soft tissue attenuation mass with irregular margins (M) encases the superior mesenteric artery (*arrowhead*).

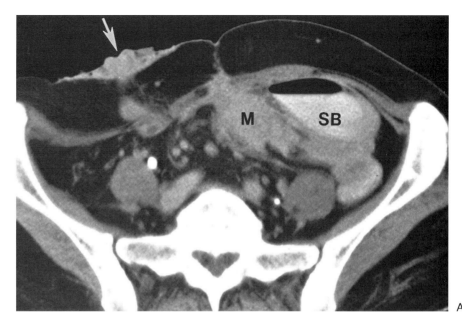

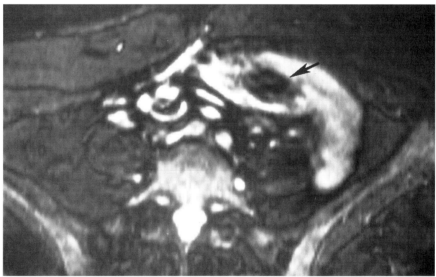

FIG. 64. Mesenteric desmoid tumors in two patients with Gardner syndrome. **A:** CT demonstrates a soft tissue attenuation mass (M) adjacent to an obstructed gas and oral contrast-filled small bowel loop (SB) in this patient who has had a total colectomy and ileostomy (arrow). **B:** T2-weighted MR image with fat suppression shows that the mass (*arrow*) is low in signal intensity.

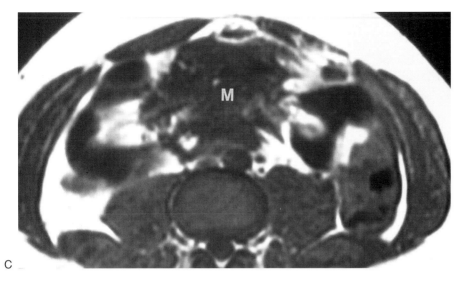

C

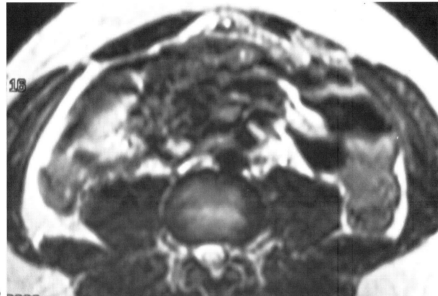

D

FIG. 64. (*Continued.*) In another patient, T1- (C) and T2-weighted (D) MR images show a large mesenteric mass with irregular margins. The signal intensity of the mass is low on both sequences due to its fibrous composition. (Courtesy of Rodney H. Reznek, M.D., St. Bartholomew's Hospital, London, England.)

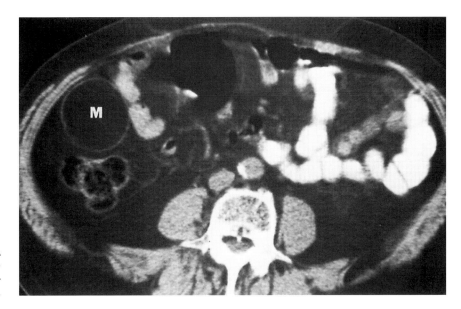

FIG. 65. Benign mesenteric lipoma. A well-defined mass (M) of homogeneous fat density is present in the mesentery anterior to the ascending colon.

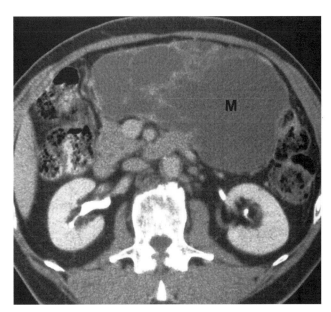

FIG. 66. Primary angiosarcoma of the omentum. Large mass (M) in the greater omentum containing near-water attenuation and enhancing soft tissue attenuation components.

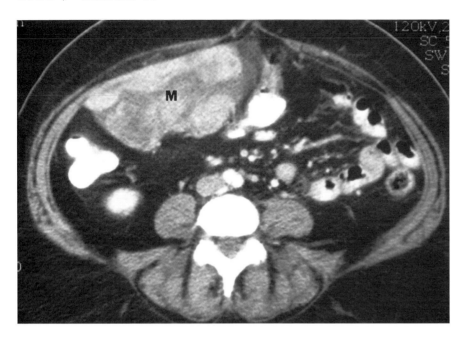

FIG. 67. Spindle cell sarcoma of the omentum. Large heterogeneously enhancing, vascular mass (M) in the greater omentum displaces adjacent bowel.

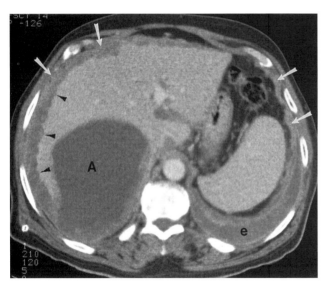

FIG. 68. Peritoneal and pleural mesothelioma. Contrast-enhanced CT demonstrates nodular thickening of the peritoneum (*arrows*) and of the serosal surface of the liver (*arrowheads*). A loculated collection of malignant ascites (A) indents the right lobe of the liver from the subhepatic space. Note the high-attenuation left pleural effusion (e) and pleural thickening.

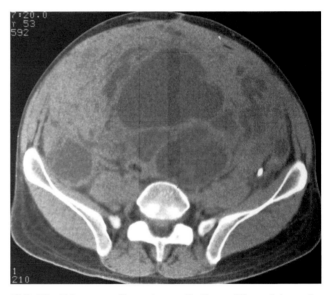

FIG. 69. Primary peritoneal mesothelioma. The pelvic cavity is replaced by a large heterogeneous peritoneal mass containing soft tissue attenuation solid and low-attenuation cystic components.

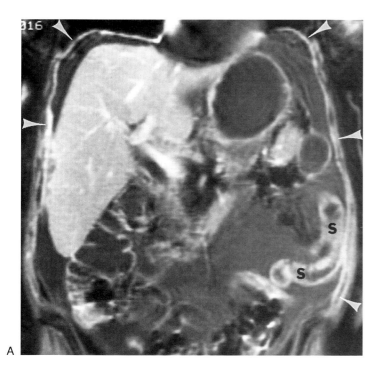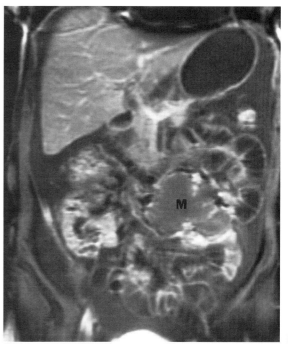

A   B

FIG. 70. Metastatic ovarian carcinoma demonstrated by MRI in two patients. T1-weighted spoiled gradient echo images with fat suppression acquired after i.v. administration of gadolinium and oral administration of dilute barium (Courtesy of Russell N. Low, M.D., Sharp and Children's MRI Center, San Diego, California). **A:** Coronal image demonstrates diffuse peritoneal thickening and enhancement (*arrowheads*). Thickening and enhancement of small bowel loop (S) indicates serosal involvement. Ascites is present. **B:** Coronal image shows ascites and a mesenteric metastasis (M).

ultrasound due to the acoustic impedance of bowel gas and mesenteric fat (21).

Metastatic neoplasm can disseminate through the peritoneal cavity by four pathways: direct spread along mesenteric and ligamentous attachments, intraperitoneal seeding, lymphatic extension, and embolic hematogenous dissemination (133). Many neoplasms metastasize predominantly by one particular route producing characteristic CT findings (107).

Direct Spread Along Peritoneal Surfaces

Malignant neoplasms of the stomach, colon, pancreas, and ovary that have penetrated beyond the borders of these organs can spread directly along the adjacent visceral peritoneal surfaces to involve other peritoneal structures. Neoplastic spread along peritoneal pathways can also involve bowel at some distance from the primary tumor. The transverse mesocolon serves as a major route of spread from the stomach, colon, and pancreas. The gastrocolic ligament (greater omentum) is another important pathway between stomach and colon. Gastric malignancies can also extend along the gastrosplenic ligament to the spleen, whereas neoplasms in the tail of the pancreas may spread via the phrenicocolic ligament to involve the anatomic splenic flexure of the colon (134). Biliary neoplasms often spread along the gastrohe-

patic and hepatoduodenal ligaments. Ovarian carcinoma spreads diffusely along all adjacent mesothelial surfaces. The CT appearance of direct peritoneal extension of tumor depends on the degree of spread. Early peritoneal infiltration produces an increase in the density of the fat adjacent to the neoplasm. More advanced spread results in a mass that is contiguous with the primary neoplasm and often extends along the expected course of the ligamentous attachment to involve adjacent organs (153) (Fig. 71). Because of their continuity with the retroperitoneum, the peritoneal ligaments, in addition to serving as the avenues of intraperitoneal tumor spread, also serve as conduits of disease spread between the peritoneum and retroperitoneum (134) (Fig. 71).

Neoplastic infiltration of the greater omentum can produce a distinctive CT appearance ranging from small nodules or strands of soft tissue that increase the density of the fat anterior to the colon or small intestine (Fig. 72) to large masses that separate the colon or small intestine from the anterior abdominal wall (''omental cakes'') (36,109) (Figs. 73 and 74). Extensive neoplastic infiltration of the omentum is produced most frequently by metastatic ovarian carcinoma but can occur with other neoplasms. Occasionally omental or other peritoneal metastases from ovarian carcinoma calcify (Fig. 75). This is most commonly seen with serous papillary cystadenocarcinoma in which psammomatous calcifications are seen

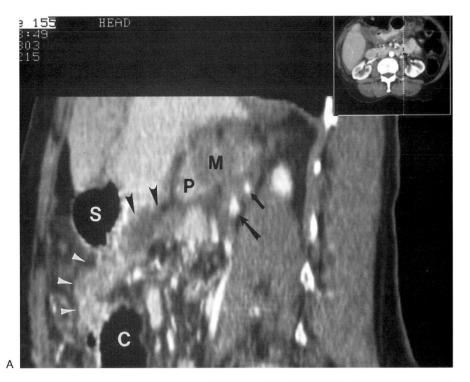

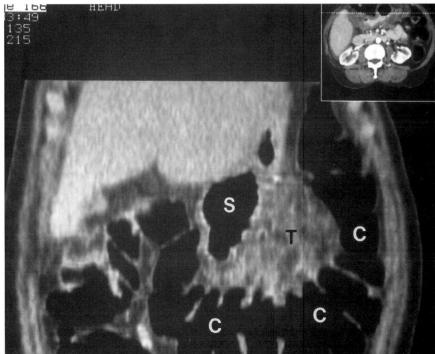

FIG. 71. Pancreatic adenocarcinoma extending to gastrocolic ligament. **A:** Left-sided sagittal reformatted image shows spread of tumor along the transverse mesocolon (*black arrowheads*) to the gastrocolic ligament (*white arrowheads*). The renal artery (*small arrow*) and ovarian vein (*large arrow*) are encased by the tumor. Transverse colon (C); pancreatic mass (M); normal pancreas (P); stomach (S). **B:** Coronal reconstructed image shows extensive tumor involvement of the gastrocolic ligament (T). Transverse colon (C); stomach (S). (Reprinted with permission from Heiken JP, Brink JA, Vannier MW. Spiral (helical) CT. *Radiology* 1993;189:647–656.)

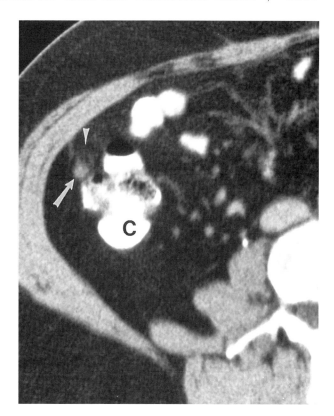

FIG. 72. Omental metastasis from colon adenocarcinoma. Small soft tissue nodule (*arrow*) and minimal soft tissue density strands (*arrowhead*) are present in the omental fat adjacent to the right colon (C).

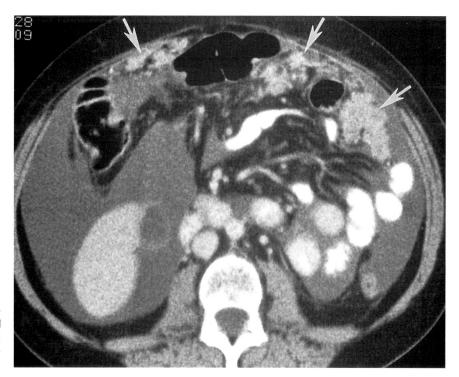

FIG. 73. Metastatic ovarian carcinoma. The omental fat is replaced by multiple soft tissue attenuation masses (*arrows*). A large amount of ascites is also present.

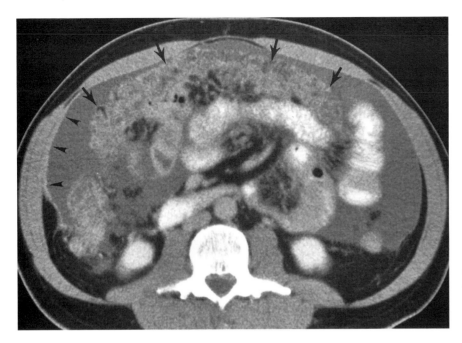

FIG. 74. Metastatic colon carcinoma. Confluent soft tissue masses ("omental cake") (*arrows*) separate the colon and small bowel from the anterior abdominal wall. Peritoneal thickening and enhancement (*arrowheads*) and a large amount of ascites are also evident.

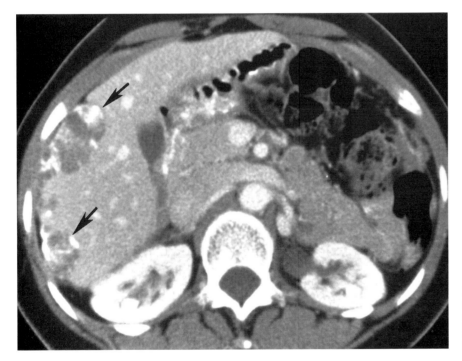

FIG. 75. Calcified peritoneal metastases from ovarian carcinoma. Metastatic implants on the surface of the liver (*arrows*) contain irregular high-attenuation foci of calcification.

histologically (136). Inflammatory thickening of the omentum, such as that produced by peritonitis, may be indistinguishable from neoplastic infiltration of the omentum (36) (Fig. 56).

Involvement of the small bowel mesentery by carcinoid tumor often produces a characteristic CT appearance. The triad of calcification within a mesenteric mass, radiating soft tissue strands due to reactive desmoplasia around the mass, and mural thickening of an adjacent bowel loop is highly suggestive of this diagnosis (159,222) (Fig. 76). Calcification may be detected in up to 70% of cases (159) (Fig. 77). Many patients have liver metastases at the time of diagnosis.

Intraperitoneal Seeding

Intraperitoneal seeding of neoplasm depends on the natural flow of fluid within the peritoneal cavity, which is governed by the compartmentalization of the peritoneal spaces in combination with the effects of gravity and changes in intraabdominal pressure caused by respiration (103). The most common sites of pooling of ascites and subsequent fixation and growth of peritoneal metastases are the pouch of Douglas (Fig. 78), the lower small bowel mesentery near the ileocecal junction (Fig. 79), the sigmoid mesocolon, and the right paracolic gutter (129). The primary neoplasms that most commonly spread by this

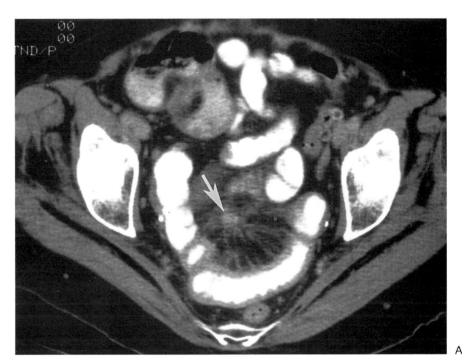

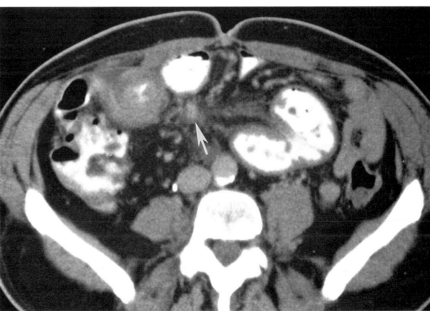

FIG. 76. Carcinoid tumor. **A, B:** In each of two patients, a small mesenteric soft tissue mass (*arrow*) is surrounded by radiating soft tissue attenuation strands extending to an adjacent loop of thick-walled small bowel.

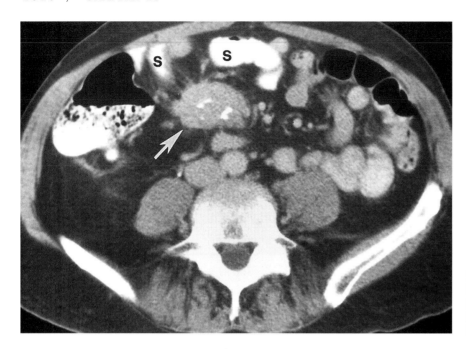

FIG. 77. Carcinoid tumor. Calcifications are present in this mesenteric soft tissue mass (*arrow*). Radiating soft tissue strands extend to an adjacent small bowel loop (s).

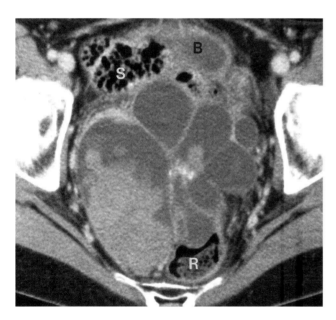

FIG. 78. Metastatic ovarian carcinoma. Large peritoneal implant in the pouch of Douglas. The mass contains cystic and solid components with a central area of calcification. Rectum (R); sigmoid colon (S); urinary bladder (B).

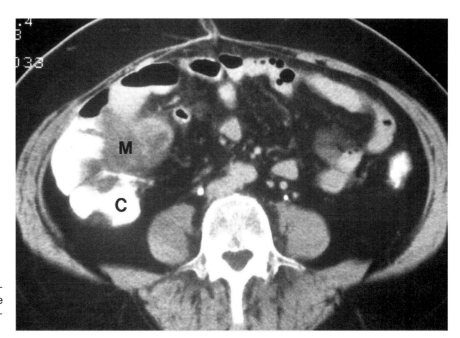

FIG. 79. Metastatic ovarian carcinoma. Heterogeneous mass (M) in the small bowel mesentery near the ileocecal valve. Cecum (C).

route are adenocarcinoma of the ovary, colon, stomach, and pancreas. On CT scans, seeded metastases appear as soft tissue masses, frequently associated with ascites, at one or more of the sites of normal pooling (88). In some cases the peritoneum is diffusely thickened (Fig. 80). If a moderate amount of ascites is present, peritoneal implants less than 1 cm in diameter can be identified. If the metastases are very small, ascites may be the only sign of intraperitoneal seeding. When little or no ascites is present, the only CT manifestation of intraabdominal carcinomatosis may be replacement of the normal mesenteric fat density with soft tissue density.

The small bowel mesentery and the greater omentum are frequently involved by intraperitoneally disseminated tumor. Four general CT patterns of mesenteric involvement have been described: rounded masses, cake-like masses, ill-defined masses, and a stellate pattern (217). Rounded masses are seen most commonly with non-Hodgkin lymphoma (due primarily to lymphadenopathy rather than intraperitoneal seeding) (18, 217) (Fig. 81) but can also be seen with other metastatic tumors (Fig. 82). Irregular ill-defined and cake-like masses are seen most often with ovarian carcinoma, although non-Hodgkin lymphoma (Fig. 83) and metastatic carcinoma sometimes produce a similar appearance. Cystic mesenteric masses are an occasional mani-

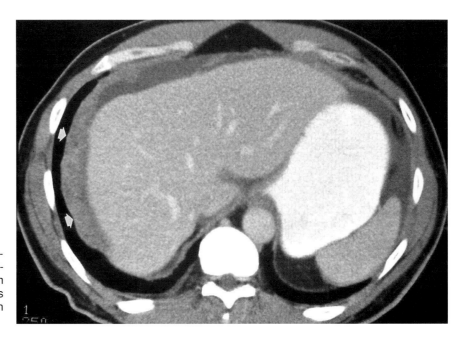

FIG. 80. Peritoneal metastases. Contrast-enhanced CT demonstrates diffuse thickening of the peritoneum (*arrows*) and a small amount of ascites in a patient with metastatic colon carcinoma.

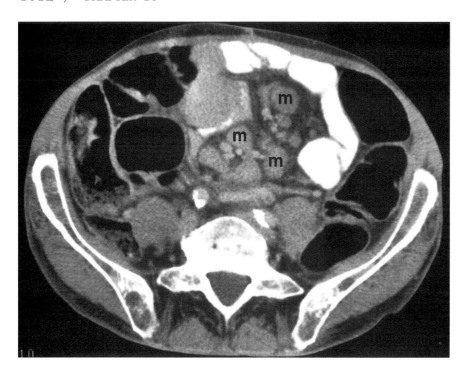

FIG. 81. Mesenteric lymphadenopathy in a patient with lymphoma. Multiple small and moderate-sized mesenteric masses (m) are present within the mesentery.

festation of ovarian carcinoma (Fig. 84). The stellate pattern, consisting of a radiating pattern of the mesenteric leaves, can be produced by a number of metastatic carcinomas, including ovarian, pancreatic, colonic, and breast (Fig. 85). This pattern results from diffuse mesenteric tumor infiltration causing thickening and rigidity of the perivascular bundles (109). These mesenteric patterns, although characteristic of metastatic involvement, are by no means specific and can be mimicked by primary peritoneal neoplasms such as mesothelioma

and by inflammatory processes such as pancreatitis and tuberculous peritonitis (see Fig. 48).

A distinctive CT appearance is produced by pseudomyxoma peritonei in which the peritoneal surfaces become diffusely involved with large amounts of mucinous material. This condition results from rupture of a mucinous cystadenocarcinoma or cystadenoma, usually of the ovary or appendix. Computed tomographic findings include low-attenuation masses that may be surrounded by discrete walls (Fig. 86) or diffuse intraperitoneal low-attenuation material that may contain septations and often

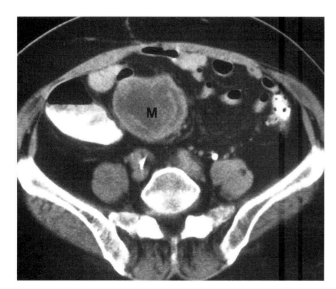

FIG. 82. Metastatic leiomyosarcoma. Large, heterogeneous mass (M) with central low attenuation involves the small bowel mesentery.

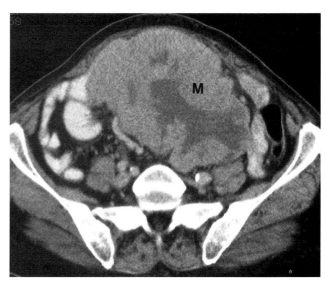

FIG. 83. Non-Hodgkin lymphoma. Large, irregular, mesenteric mass (M) displaces adjacent bowel loops.

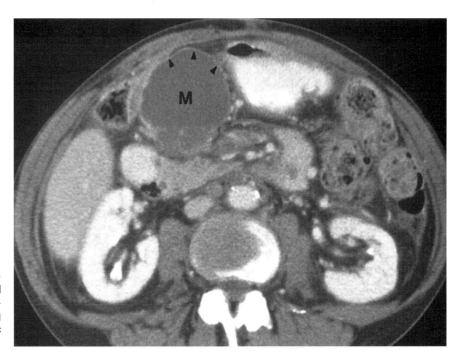

FIG. 84. Cystic metastasis from ovarian carcinoma. Contrast-enhanced CT demonstrates a near-water attenuation mass (M) with a thin enhancing rim (*arrowheads*) in the gastrocolic ligament.

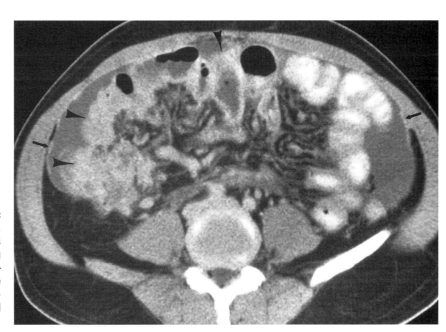

FIG. 85. Peritoneal and mesenteric metastases from colon carcinoma. Contrast-enhanced CT demonstrates ascites with diffuse peritoneal thickening (*arrows*), omental implants (*arrowheads*), and mesenteric infiltration. The mesenteric vascular bundles are thickened, and the mesentery has a rigid appearance.

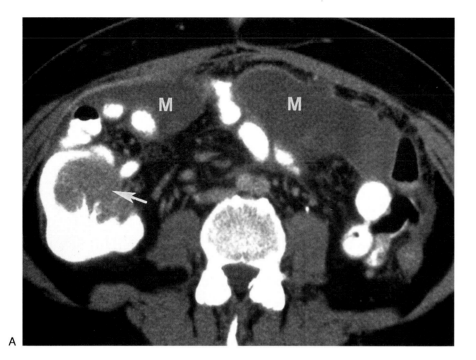

A

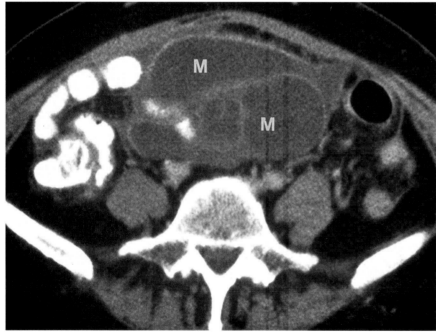

B

FIG. 86. Pseudomyxoma peritonei. **A,B:** Multiple near-water attenuation masses (M) with discrete enhancing walls are distributed throughout the peritoneal cavity. The primary tumor responsible for the peritoneal disease was a mucinous adenocarcinoma of the cecum (*arrow*).

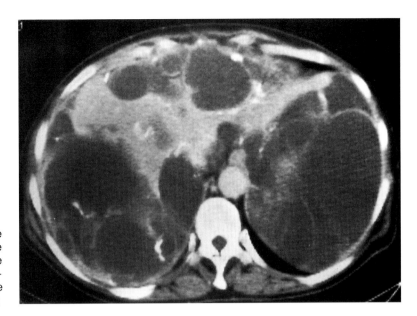

FIG. 87. Pseudomyxoma peritonei. Multiple low-attenuation intraperitoneal masses cause scalloping of the liver margin. Many of the masses contain septations and mural calcification. (Courtesy of Mark E. Baker, M.D., The Cleveland Clinic Foundation, Cleveland, Ohio.)

causes scalloping of the liver margin (39,122,147, 183,225) (Fig. 87). Occasionally the walls or septations contain calcification (122). If the walls of the cystic masses are thin, the CT appearance may be similar to that produced by loculated ascites. Scalloping of the liver margin by extrinsic pressure of the gelatinous masses and failure of bowel loops to float up toward the anterior abdominal wall may be useful in differentiating pseudomyxoma peritonei from ascites (183).

Lymphatic Dissemination

Lymphatic extension plays a minor role in the intraperitoneal dissemination of metastatic carcinoma (130) but is the primary mode of spread of lymphoma to mesenteric lymph nodes. At the time of presentation, approximately 50% of patients with non-Hodgkin lymphoma have mesenteric lymph node involvement, whereas only 5% of patients with Hodgkin disease have mesenteric disease at presentation (58). Identification of mesenteric lymph node disease is extremely important as it almost always indicates the need for chemotherapy, sometimes in combination with radiation therapy (107). American Burkitt lymphoma is a B-cell lymphoma, primarily affecting children and young adults, that usually produces bulky extranodal tumors in the abdomen (61).

On CT the appearance of mesenteric lymph node involvement by lymphoma ranges from small round or oval masses within the mesenteric fat (see Fig. 81) to large confluent masses displacing adjacent bowel loops (18,109,217) (see Fig. 83). Large confluent masses of lymphomatous nodes may surround the superior mesenteric artery and veins, producing a "sandwich-like"

appearance (139) (Fig. 88). Occasionally, the earliest CT sign of mesenteric lymphoma is an increased number of normal size (<1 cm) lymph nodes within the mesentery. However, mild mesenteric lymphadenopathy is a nonspecific finding and does not always represent lymphoma. Non-neoplastic causes of mesenteric lymphadenopathy include infiltrative and inflammatory disease such as Crohn disease (43), sarcoidosis, Whipple disease (112,171), sprue (93), giardiasis, tuberculous peritonitis (82), MAI (Fig. 89), mastocytosis (43), and acquired immune deficiency syndrome (AIDS) (138,149). After radiation or combined radiation and chemotherapy treatment of non-Hodgkin lymphoma, peripheral curvilinear calcifications may be seen in the mesenteric masses (30). Occasionally, enlarged mesenteric vessels oriented perpendicular to the plane of the CT section may simulate mesenteric lymphadenopathy. Enhancement of mesenteric vessels after intravenous contrast material administration easily distinguishes them from lymph nodes. Alternatively, MRI can distinguish vessels with flowing blood from lymph nodes by virtue of the signal void on spin-echo sequences or high signal intensity on flow-sensitive gradient echo sequences. When lymphoma disseminates to peritoneal surfaces other than the mesentery (peritoneal lymphomatosis), the CT appearance may be indistinguishable from that of metastatic carcinoma (107) (Fig. 90). Patients with AIDS-related lymphoma often present with more advanced disease (150).

Embolic Metastases

Tumor emboli may be spread via the mesenteric arteries to the antimesenteric border of bowel where the cells

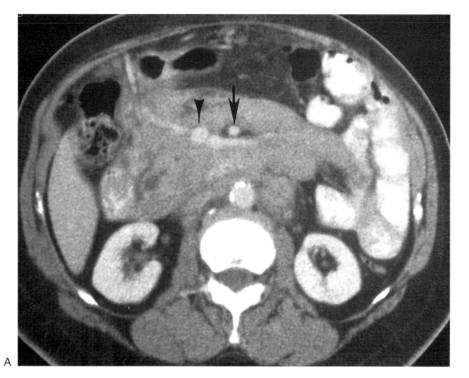

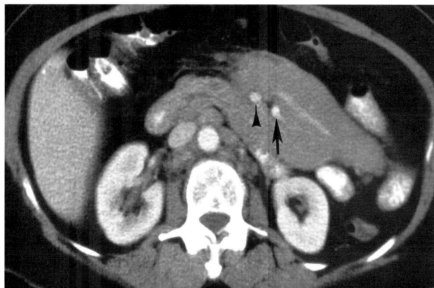

FIG. 88. Confluent mesenteric lymphadenopathy. **A, B:** In each of two patients with non-Hodgkin lymphoma, large confluent masses of involved lymph nodes surround the superior mesenteric artery (*arrow*) and vein (*arrowhead*), producing a sandwich-like appearance.

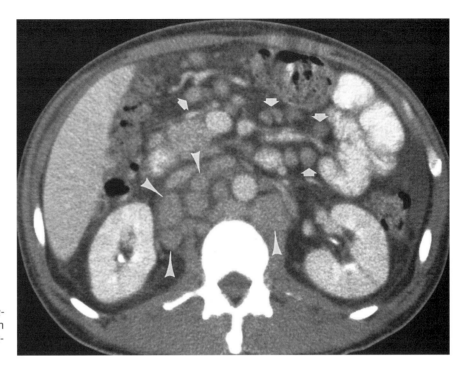

FIG. 89. *Mycobacterium avium-intracellulare* (MAI) infection resulting in mesenteric (*arrows*) and retroperitoneal (*arrowheads*) lymphadenopathy.

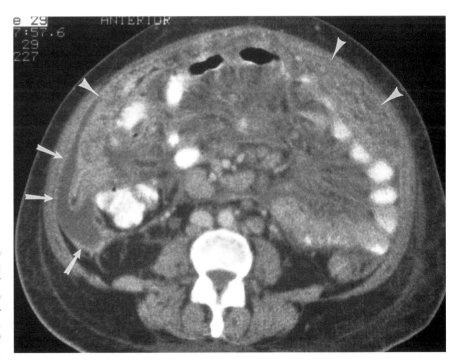

FIG. 90. Peritoneal dissemination of non-Hodgkin lymphoma (peritoneal lymphomatosis). Midabdominal CT image shows ascites and diffuse peritoneal (*arrows*), omental (*arrowheads*), and mesenteric thickening. The appearance is indistinguishable from that of peritoneal carcinomatosis.

implant and subsequently grow into intramural tumor nodules (133). On CT, these embolic metastases may produce thickening of the mesenteric leaves or focal bowel wall thickening, occasionally with recognizable ulceration. The most common neoplasms to spread in this manner are melanoma and carcinoma of the breast or lung.

REFERENCES

1. Ackerman LV. *Atlas of tumor pathology. Fascicles 23 and 24: Tumors of the retroperitoneum mesentery and omentum.* Washington, DC: Armed Forces Institute of Pathology, 1954.
2. Allen HA, Vick CW, Messmer JM, Parker GA. Diffuse mesenteric amyloidosis: CT, sonographic, and pathologic findings. *J Comput Assist Tomogr* 1985;9:196–198.
3. Altemeier WA, Culbertson WR, Fullen WD, Shook CD. Intraabdominal abscess. *Am J Surg* 1973;125:70–79.
4. Arenas AP, Sanchez LV, Albillos JM, Borruel SN, Roldan JR, Lozano FO. Direct dissemination of pathologic abdominal processes through perihepatic ligaments: identification with CT. *RadioGraphics* 1994;14:515–527.
5. Aronberg DJ, Stanley RJ, Levitt RG, Sagel SS. Evaluation of abdominal abscess with computed tomography. *J Comput Assist Tomogr* 1978;2:384–387.
6. Auh YH, Lim JH, Kim KW, Lee DH, M.-G. L, Cho KS. Loculated fluid collections in hepatic fissures and recesses: CT appearance and potential pitfalls. *RadioGraphics* 1994;14:529–540.
7. Baker ME, Weinerth JL, Andriani RT, Cohan RH, Dunnick NR. Lumbar hernia: diagnosis by CT. *AJR* 1987;148:565–567.
8. Balthazar EJ. CT diagnosis and staging of acute pancreatitis. *Radiol Clin North Am* 1989;27:19–37.
9. Balthazar EJ, Freeny PC, vanSonnenberg E. Imaging and intervention in acute pancreatitis. *Radiology* 1994;193:297–306.
10. Balthazar EJ, Lefkowitz RA. Left-sided omental infarction with associated omental abscess: CT diagnosis. *J Comput Assist Tomogr* 1993;17:379–381.
11. Balthazar EJ, Subramanyam BR, Megibow AJ. Spigelian hernia: CT and ultrasonography diagnosis. *Gastrointest Radiol* 1984;9:81–84.
12. Barakos JA, Jeffrey RB, Federle MP, Wing VW, Laing FC, Hightower DR. CT in the management of periappendiceal abscess. *AJR* 1986;146:1161–1164.
13. Baron RL, Lee JKT. Mesenteric desmoid tumors. *Radiology* 1981;140:777–779.
14. Becker G, Hess CF, Grund KE, Hoffmann W, Bamberg M. Abdominal wall metastasis following percutaneous endoscopic gastrostomy. *Support Care Cancer* 1995;3:316–316.
15. Bennett HF, Balfe DM. MR imaging of the peritoneum and abdominal wall. *MRI Clin North Am* 1995;3:99–120.
16. Bergstrom M, Erickson K, Levander B, Svendsen P, Larsson S. Variation with time of the attenuation values of intracranial hematomas. *J Comput Assist Tomogr* 1977;1:57–63.
17. Berna JD, Garcia-Medina V, Guirao J, Garcia-Medina J. Rectus sheath hematoma: diagnostic classification by CT. *Abdom Imag* 1996;21:62–64.
18. Bernardino ME, Jing BS, Wallace S. Computed tomography diagnosis of mesenteric masses. *AJR* 1979;132:33–36.
19. Bradley WG, Schmidt PG. Effect of methemoglobin formation on the MR appearance of subarachnoid hemorrhage. *Radiology* 1985;156:99–103.
20. Brasfield RD, Das Gupta TK. Desmoid tumors of the anterior abdominal wall. *Surgery* 1969;65:241–246.
21. Bree RL, Schwab RE. Contribution of mesenteric fat to unsatisfactory abdominal and pelvic ultrasonography. *Radiology* 1981;140:773–776.
22. Brown JJ, van Sonnenberg E, Gerber KH, Strich G, Wittich GR, Slutsky RA. Magnetic resonance relaxation times of percutaneously obtained normal and abnormal body fluids. *Radiology* 1985;154:727–731.
23. Buhr J, Hurtgen M, Heinrichs CM, Graf M, Padberg WM. Implantation metastases following laparoscopic cholecystectomy in gallbladder carcinoma. *Deutsche Medizinische Wochenschrift* 1996;121:57–61.
24. Bydder GM, Kreel L. Attenuation values of fluid collections within the abdomen. *J Comput Assist Tomogr* 1980;4:145–150.
25. Callen PW. Computed tomographic evaluation of abdominal and pelvic abscesses. *Radiology* 1979;131:171–175.
26. Caseiro-Alves F, Goncalo M, Abraul E, Pinto E, Oliveira C, Ramos V. Induced pneumoperitoneum in CT evaluation of peritoneal carcinomatosis. *Abdom Imag* 1995;20:52–55.
27. Ceuterick L, Baert AL, Marchal G, Kerremans R, Geboes K. CT diagnosis of primary torsion of greater omentum. *J Comput Assist Tomogr* 1987;11:1083–1084.
28. Charnsangavej C, DuBrow RA, Varma DG, Herron DH, Robinson TJ, Whitley NO. CT of the mesocolon - Part 1. Anatomic considerations. *RadioGraphics* 1993;13:1035–1045.
29. Charnsangavej C, DuBrow RA, Varma DG, Herron DH, Robinson TJ, Whitley NO. CT of the mesocolon - Part 2. Pathologic considerations. *RadioGraphics* 1993;13:1309–1322.
30. Cheng J, Castellino. Post-treatment calcification of mesenteric non-Hodgkin lymphoma: CT findings. *J Comput Assist Tomogr* 1989;13:64–66.
31. Cho KC, Morehouse HT, Alterman DD, Thurhill BA. Sigmoid diverticulitis; diagnostic role of CT comparison with barium enema studies. *Radiology* 1990;176:111–115.
32. Cirocco WC, Schwartzman A, Golub RW. Abdominal wall recurrence after laparoscopic colectomy for colon cancer. *Surgery* 1994;116:842–846.
33. Cohen JM, Weinreb JC, Maravilla KR. Fluid collections in the intraperitoneal and extraperitoneal spaces: comparison of MR and CT. *Radiology* 1985;155:705–708.
34. Cohen WN, Seidelmann FE, Bryan PJ. Computed tomography of localized adipose deposits presenting as tumor masses. *AJR* 1977;128:1007–1011.
35. Coode PE, McGuinness FE, Rawas MM, Griffith GG. Diffuse lipomatosis involving the thoracic and abdominal wall: CT features. *J Comput Assist Tomogr* 1991;15:341–343.
36. Cooper C, Jeffrey RB, Silverman PM, Federle MP, Chun GH. Computed tomography of omental pathology. *J Comput Assist Tomogr* 1986;10:62–66.
37. Cooper C, Silverman PM, Davros WJ, Zeman RK. Delayed contrast enhancement of ascitic fluid on CT: frequency and significance. *AJR* 1993;161:787–790.
38. Cryer PE, Kissane J. Infiltrative gastrointestinal disease. *Am J Med* 1974;57:127–134.
39. Dachman AH, Lichtenstein JE, Friedman AC. Mucocele of the appendix and pseudomyxoma peritonei. *AJR* 1985;144:923–929.
40. Dahlene DH, Stanley RJ, Koehler RE, Shin MS, Tishler JMA. Abdominal tuberculosis: CT findings. *J Comput Assist Tomogr* 1984;8:443–445.
41. Daniel O. The differential diagnosis of malignant disease of the peritoneum. *Br J Surg* 1951;39:147–156.
42. DeMeo JH, Fulcher AS, Austin RF. Anatomic CT demonstration of the peritoneal spaces, ligaments, and mesenteries: normal and pathologic proceses. *RadioGraphics* 1995;15:755–770.
43. Deutsch SJ, Sandler MA, Alpern MB. Abdominal lymphadenopathy in benign disease: CT detection. *Radiology* 1987;163:335–338.
44. Dobrin PB, Gully PH, Greenlee HB, et al. Radiologic diagnosis of an intra-abdominal abscess. *Arch Surg* 1986;121:41–46.
45. Dodds WJ, Foley WD, Lawson TL, Stewart ET, Taylor A. Anatomy and imaging of the lesser peritoneal sac. *AJR* 1985;144:567–575.
46. Dooms GC, Fisher MR, Hricak H, Higgins CB. MR of intramuscular hemorrhage. *J Comput Assist Tomogr* 1985;9:908–913.
47. Epstein BM, Mann JH. CT of abdominal tuberculosis. *AJR* 1982;139:861–866.
48. Faxon HH. Subphrenic abscess. *N Engl J Med* 1940;222:289–299.
49. Federle MP, Chun G, Jeffrey RB, Raynor R. Computed tomographic findings in bowel infarction. *AJR* 1984;142:91–95.
50. Federle MP, Jeffrey RB Jr. Hemoperitoneum studied by computed tomography. *Radiology* 1983;148:187–192.

51. Ferreiros J, Leon NG, Mata MI, Casanova R, Pedrosa CS, Cuevas A. Computed tomography in abdominal Castleman's disease. *J Comput Assist Tomogr* 1989;13:433–436.
52. Frager DH, Goldman M, Beneventano TC. Computed tomography in Crohn disease. *J Comput Assist Tomogr* 1983;7:819–824.
53. Garber SJ, Shaw DG. Case report: the ultrasound and computed tomography appearance of mesentric Castleman disease. *Clin Radiol* 1991;43:429–430.
54. Gedgaudas RK, Rice RP. Radiologic evaluation of complicated pancreatitis. *CRC Crit Rev Diagn Imag* 1981;15:319–367.
55. Gerzof SG, Johonson WC, Robbins AH, Nabseth DC. Expanded criteria for percutaneous abscess drainage. *Arch Surg* 1985;120:227–232.
56. Ghahremani GG, Jiminez MA, Rosenfeld M, Rochester D. CT diagnosis of occult incisional hernias. *AJR* 1987;148:139–142.
57. Gleeson NC, Nicosia SV, Mark JE, Hoffman MS, Cavanagh D. Abdominal wall metastases from ovarian cancer after laparoscopy. *Am J Obstet Gynecol* 1993;169:522–523.
58. Goffinet DR, Castellino RA, Kim H, et al. Staging laparotomies in unselected previously untreated patients with non-Hodgkin's lymphoma. *Cancer* 1973;32:672–681.
59. Goldberg HI, Gore RM, Margulis AR, Moss AA, Baker EL. Computed tomography in the evaluation of Crohn disease. *AJR* 1983;140:277–282.
60. Gomori JM, Grossman RI, Goldberg HI, Zimmerman RA, Bilaniuk LT. Intracranial hematomas: imaging by high-field MR. *Radiology* 1985;157:87–93.
61. Goodman P, Raval B. CT of the abdominal wall. *AJR* 1990;154:1207–1211.
62. Gore RM, Callen PW, Filly RA. Lesser sac fluid in predicting the etiology of ascites: CT findings. *AJR* 1982;139:71–74.
63. Gore RM, Marn CS, Kirby DF, Vogelzang RL, Neiman HL. CT findings in ulcerative, granulomatous and indeterminate colitis. *AJR* 1984;143:279–284.
64. Goss CM. *Gray's anatomy of the human body,* 29th American edition. Goss CM, ed. Philadelphia: Lea and Febiger, 1973.
65. Grendell JH, Ockner RK. Mesenteric venous thrombosis. *Gastroenterology* 1982;82:358–372.
66. Guest PJ, Reznek RH, Selleslage D, Geraghty R, Slevin M. Peritoneal mesothelioma: the role of computed tomography in diagnosis and follow up. *Clin Radiol* 1992;45:79–84.
67. Ha HK, Jung JI, Lee MS, et al. CT differentiation of tuberculous peritonitis and peritoneal carcinomatosis. *AJR* 1996;167:743–748.
68. Haaga JR, Alfidi RJ, Havrilla TR, et al. CT detection and aspiration of abdominal abscesses. *AJR* 1977;128:465–474.
69. Hahn PF, Saini S, Stark DD, Papanicolaou N, Ferrucci JT Jr. Intraabdominal hematoma: the concentric-ring sign in MR imaging. *AJR* 1987;148:115–119.
70. Halber MD, Daffner RH, Morgan CL, et al. Intraabdominal abscess: current concepts in radiologic evaluation. *AJR* 1979;133:9–13.
71. Halliday P, Halliday H. Subphrenic abscess: a study of 241 patients at the Royal Prince Edward Hospital. *Br J Surg* 1976;63:352.
72. Halvorsen RA, Panushka C, Oakley GJ, Letourneau JG, Adcock LL. Intraperitoneal contrast material improves the CT detection of peritoneal metastases. *AJR* 1991;157:37–40.
73. Hamrick-Turner JE, Chiechi MV, Abbitt PL, Ros PR. Neoplastic and inflammatory processes of the peritoneum, omentum, and mesentery: diagnosis with CT. *RadioGraphics* 1992;12:1051–1068.
74. Haney PJ, Whitley NO. CT of benign cystic abdominal masses in children. *AJR* 1984;142:1279–1281.
75. Hanson RD, Hunter. Tuberculous peritonitis: CT appearance. *AJR* 1985;144:931–932.
76. Hayashi S, Oyama K, Hirkawa K, Oda M, Kogure T. Mesenteric panniculitis — case report and its radiolgoical diagnosis including CT. *Rinsho Hoshasen* 1982;27:143–146.
77. Healy ME, Teng SS, Moss AA. Uriniferous pseudocyst: computed tomographic findings. *Radiology* 1984;153:757–762.
78. Heiken JP, Brink JA, Sagel SS. Helical CT: abdominal applications. *RadioGraphics* 1994;14:919–924.
79. Hibbeln JF, Wehmueller MD, Wilbur AC. Chylous ascites: CT and ultrasound appearance. *Abdom Imag* 1995;20:138–140.
80. Hudson TM, Vandergriend RA, Springfield DS, et al. Aggressive fibromatosis: evaluation by computed tomography and angiography. *Radiology* 1984;150:495–501.
81. Hulnick DH, Megibow AJ, Balthazar EJ, Naidich DP, Bosniak MA. Computed tomography in the evaluation of diverticulitis. *Radiology* 1984;152:491–495.
82. Hulnick DH, Megibow AJ, Naidich DP, Hilton S, Cho KC, Balthazar EJ. Abdominal tuberculosis: CT evaluation. *Radiology* 1985;157:199–204.
83. Ichikawa T, Koyama A, Fujimoto H, et al. Abdominal wall desmoid mimicking intra-abdominal mass: MR features. *Magn Reson Imag* 1994;12:541–544.
84. Jacobs JE, Birnbaum BA, Siegelman ES. Heterotopic ossification of midline abdominal incisions: CT and MR imaging findings. *AJR* 1996;166:579–584.
85. Jacquet P, Averbach AM, Jacquet N. Abdominal wall metastasis and peritoneal carcinomatosis after laparoscopic-assisted colectomy for colon cancer. *Eur J Surg Oncol* 1995;21:568–570.
86. Jaques P, Mauro M, Safrit H, Yankaskas B, Piggott B. CT features of intraabdominal abscesses: prediction of successful percutaneous drainage. *AJR* 1986;146:1041–1045.
87. Jatzko G, Lisborg P, Horn M, Dinges HP. Abdominal wall implantation metastasis 2 years after apparently uneventful laparoscopic cholecystectomy. *Chirurg* 1994;65:812–814.
88. Jeffrey RB. CT demonstration of peritoneal implants. *AJR* 1980;135:323–326.
89. Jeffrey RB. Computed tomography of the peritoneal cavity and mesentery. In: Moss AA, Gamsu G, Genant HK, eds. *Computed tomography of the body.* Philadelphia: WB Saunders, 1983.
90. Jeffrey RB, Federle MP, Laing BC. Computed tomography of mesenteric involvement in fulminant pancreatitis. *Radiology* 1983;147:185–188.
91. Jeffrey RB, Tolentino CS, Federle MP, Laing FC. Percutaneous drainage of periappendiceal abscess: review of 20 patients. *AJR* 1987;149:59–62.
92. Jolles H, Coulam CM. CT of ascities: differential diagnosis. *AJR* 1980;135:315–322.
93. Jones B, Bayless TM, Fishman EK, Siegelman SS. Lymphadenopathy in celiac disease: computed tomographic observations. *AJR* 1984;142:1127–1132.
94. Katz ME, Heiken JP, Glazer HS, Lee JKT. Intraabdominal panniculitis: clinical, radiographic, and CT features. *AJR* 1985;145:293–296.
95. Kawashima A, Fishman EK, Hruban RH, Kuhlman JE, Lee RP. Mesenteric panniculitis presenting as a multilocular cystic mesenteric mass: CT and MR evaluation. *Clin Imag* 1993;17:112–116.
96. Kerber GW, Greenberg M, Rubin JM. Computed tomography evaluation of local and extraintestinal complications of Crohn's disease. *Gastrointest Radiol* 1984;9:143–148.
97. Kim T, Murakami T, Oi H, et al. CT and MR imaging of abdominal liposarcoma. *AJR* 1996;166:829–833.
98. Knochel JQ, Koehler PR, Lee TG, Welch DM. Diagnosis of abdominal abscesses with computed tomography, ultrasound and 111In leukocyte scans. *Radiology* 1980;137:425–432.
99. Koehler PR, Moss AA. Diagnosis of intra-abdominal and pelvic abscesses by computerized tomography. *JAMA* 1980;244:49–52.
100. Korobkin M, Callen PW, Filly RA, Hoffer PB, Shimshak RR, Kressel HY. Comparison of computed tomography, ultrasonography, and gallium-67 scanning in the evaluation of suspected abdominal abscess. *Radiology* 1978;129:89–93.
101. Korobkin M, Moss AA, Callen PW, DeMartini WJ, Kaiser JA. Computed tomography of subcapsular splenic hematoma: clinical and experimental studies. *Radiology* 1978;129:441–445.
102. Kronthal AJ, Kang YS, Fishman EK, Jones B, Kuhlman JE, C. TCM. MR imaging in sclerosing mesenteritis. *AJR* 1991;156:517–519.
103. Lawdahl RB, Moss CN, VanDyke JA. Inferior lumbar (Petit's) hernia. *AJR* 1986;147:744–745.
104. Lee G-HM, Cohen AJ. CT imaging of abdominal hernias. *AJR* 1993;161(March):1209–1213.
105. Lee JT, Kim MJ, Yoo HS, Suh JH, Jeong HJ. Primary leiomyosarcoma of the greater omentum: CT findings. *J Comput Assist Tomogr* 1991;15:92–94.
106. Levine CD, Patel UJ, Silverman PM, Wachsberg RH. Low attenua-

tion of acute traumatic hemoperitoneum on CT scans. *AJR* 1996; 166:1089–1093.

107. Levitt RG. Abdominal wall and peritoneal cavity. In: Sagel SS, Stanely RJ, eds. *Computed body tomography.* New York: Raven Press, 1983.

108. Levitt RG, Biello DR, Sagel SS, et al. Computed tomography and 67Ga citrate radionuclide imaging for evaluating suspected abdominal abscess. *AJR* 1979;132:529–534.

109. Levitt RG, Sagel SS, Stanley RJ. Detection of neoplastic involvement of the mesentery and omentum by computed tomography. *AJR* 1978;131:835–838.

110. Lewin JR, Patterson EA. CT recognition of spontaneous intraperitoneal hemorrhage complicating anticoagulant therapy. *AJR* 1980; 134:1271–1272.

111. Lewis VL, Shaffer HA, Williamson BRJ. Pseudotumoral lipomatosis of the abdomen. *J Comput Assist Tomogr* 1982;6:79–82.

112. Li DKB, Rennie CS. Abdominal computed tomography in Whipple's disease. *J Comput Assist Tomogr* 1981;5:249–252.

113. Lieberman JM, Haaga JR. Computed tomography of diverticulitis. *J Comput Assist Tomogr* 1983;7:431–433.

114. Lorenz R, Beyer D, Peters PE. Detection of intraperitoneal bile accumulations: significance of ultrasonography, CT, and cholescintigraphy. *Gastrointest Radiol* 1984;9:213–217.

115. Low RN, Alzate GD, Sigeti JS, Sebrechts CP, Barone R, Lacey C. Double-contrast MR imaging of peritoneal tumors with dilute barium oral contrast, intravenous gadolinium, and breath-hold FMPSPGR imaging. *Radiology* 1996;201(P):252.

116. Lubat E, Balthazar EJ. The current role of computerized tomography in inflammatory disease of the bowel. *Am J Gastroenterol* 1988;83:107–113.

117. Lundstedt C, Hederstrom E, Holmin T, Lunderquist A, Navne T, Owman T. Radiologic diagnosis in proven intra-abdominal abscess formation. *Gastrointest Radiol* 1983;8:261–266.

118. Magid D, Fishman EK, Jones B, Hoover HC, Feinstein R, Siegleman SS. Desmoid tumors in Gardner syndrome: use of computed tomography. *AJR* 1984;142:1141–1145.

119. Maklad NF, Doust BD, Baum JK. Ultrasonic diagnosis of postoperative intra-abdominal abscess. *Radiology* 1974;113:417–422.

120. Mall JC, Kaiser JA. CT diagnosis of splenic laceration. *AJR* 1980; 134:265–269.

121. Mata JM, Inaraja L, Martin J, Olazabal A, Castilla MT. CT features of mesenteric panniculitis. *J Comput Assist Tomogr* 1987;11: 1021–1023.

122. Mayes GB, Chuang VP, Fisher RG. CT of pseudomyxoma peritonei. *AJR* 1981;136:807–808.

123. McAfee JG, Samin A. In-111 labeled leukocytes: a review of problems in image interpretation. *Radiology* 1985;155:221–229.

124. McDonnell CH, McLeod M, Baker ME. Primary peritoneal neuroblastoma: computed tomography findings. *Clin Imag* 1990;14:41–43.

125. McDougall IR, Baumert JE, Lantiere RL. Evaluation of 111In leukocyte whole body scanning. *AJR* 1979;133:849–854.

126. Mendez G, Isikoff MB, Hill MC. CT of acute pancreatitis: interim assessment. *AJR* 1980;135:463–469.

127. Meyers MA. Roentgen significance of the phrenicocolic ligament. *Radiology* 1970;95:539–545.

128. Meyers MA. The spread and localization of acute intraperitoneal effusions. *Radiology* 1970;95:547–554.

129. Meyers MA. Distribution of intra-abdominal malignancy seeding: dependency on dynamics of flow of ascitic fluid. *AJR* 1973;119: 198–206.

130. Meyers MA. *Dynamic radiology of the abdomen: normal and pathologic anatomy,* 2nd ed. New York: Springer–Verlag, 1982.

131. Meyers MA, Evans JA. Effects of pancreatitis on the small bowel and colon: spread along mesenteric planes. *AJR* 1973;119:151–165.

132. Meyers MA, McGuire PV. Spiral CT demonstration of hypervascularity in Crohn disease: vascular jejunization of the ileum or the comb sign. *Abdom Imag* 1995;20:327–332.

133. Meyers MA, McSweeney J. Secondary neoplasm of bowel. *Radiology* 1972;105:1–11.

134. Meyers MA, Oliphant M, Berne AS, Feldberg MAM. The peritoneal ligaments and mesenteries: pathways of intraabdominal spread of disease. *Radiology* 1987;163:593–604.

135. Meziane MA, Fishman EK, Siegelman SS. Computed tomographic diagnosis of obturator foramen hernia. *Gastrointest Radiol* 1983; 8:375–377.

136. Mitchell DG, Hill MC, Hill S, Zaloudek C. Serous carcinoma of the ovary: CT identification of metastatic calcified implants. *Radiology* 1986;158:649–652.

137. Molmenti EP, Balfe DM, Kanterman RY, Bennett HF. Anatomy of the retroperitoneum: observations of the distribution of pathologic fluid collections. *Radiology* 1996;200:95–103.

138. Moon KL, Federle MP, Abrams DI, Volberding P, Lewis BJ. Kaposi sarcoma and lymphadenopathy syndrome: limitations of abdominal CT in acquired immnunodeficiency syndrome. *Radiology* 1984;150:479–483.

139. Mueller PR, Ferrucci JT Jr, Harbin WP, Kirkpatrick RH, Simeone JF, Wittenberg J. Appearance of lymphomatous involvement of the mesentery by ultrasonography and body computed tomography: the sandwich sign. *Radiology* 1980;134:467–473.

140. Mueller PR, Ferrucci JT Jr, Simeone JF, et al. Lesser sac abscesses and fluid collections: drainage by transhepatic approach. *Radiology* 1985;155:615–618.

141. Mueller PR, Ferrucci JT Jr, Simeone JF, et al. Detection and drainage of bilomas: special considerations. *AJR* 1983;140:715–720.

142. Nanakawa S, Takahashi M, Takagi K, Takano M. The role of computed tomography in management of patients with Crohn disease. *Clin Imag* 1993;17:193–198.

143. Naylor EW, Gardner EJ, Richards RC. Desmoid tumors and mesenteric fibromatosis in Gardner's syndrome. *Arch Surg* 1979;114: 1181–1185.

144. Neff CC, vanSonnenberg E, Casola G, et al. Diverticular abscesses: percutaneous drainage. *Radiology* 1987;163:15–18.

145. New PFJ, Aronow S. Attenuation measurements of whole blood and blood fractions in computed tomography. *Radiology* 1976; 121:635–640.

146. Norman D, Price D, Boyd D, Fishman R, Newton TH. Quantitative aspects of computed tomography of the blood and cerebrospinal fluid. *Radiology* 1977;123:335–338.

147. Novetsky GJ, Berlin L, Epstein AJ, Lobo N, Miller SH. Pseudomyxoma peritonei. *J Comput Assist Tomogr* 1982;6:398–399.

148. Nunez D, Huber JS, Yrizarry JM, Mendez G, Russell E. Nonsurgical drainage of appendiceal abscess. *AJR* 1986;146:587–589.

149. Nyberg DA, Federle MP, Jeffrey RB, Bottles K, Wofsy CB. Abdominal CT findings of disseminated mycobacterium avium-intracellulare in AIDS. *AJR* 1985;145:297–299.

150. Nyberg DA, Jeffrey RB Jr, Federle MP, Bottles K, Abrams DI. AIDS-related lymphomas: evelution by abdominal CT. *Radiology* 1986;159:59–63.

151. O'Neil JD, Ros PR, Storm BL, Buck JL, Wilkinson EJ. Cystic mesothelioma of the peritoneum. *Radiology* 1989;170:333–337.

152. Ochsner A, Graves AM. Subphrenic abscess: an analysis of 3372 collected and personal cases. *Ann Surg* 1933;98:961–990.

153. Oliphant M, Berne AS. Computed tomography of the subperitoneal space: demonstration of direct spread of intraabdominal disease. *J Comput Assist Tomogr* 1982;6:1127–1137.

154. Oliphant M, Berne AS, Meyers MA. Imaging the direct bidirectional spread of disease between the abdomen and the female pelvis via the subperitoneal space. *Gastrointest Radiol* 1988;13: 285–298.

155. Oliphant M, Berne AS, Meyers MA. Bidirectional spread of disease via the subperitoneal space: the lower abdomen and left pelvis. *Abdom Imag* 1993;18:117–125.

156. Oliphant M, Berne AS, Meyers MA. Spread of disease via the subperitoneal space: the small bowel mesentery. *Abdom Imag* 1993;18:109–116.

157. Oliphant M, Berne AS, Meyers MA. Direct spread of subperitoneal disease into solid organs: radiologic diagnosis. *Abdom Imag* 1995; 20:141–147.

158. Pandolfo I, Blandino A, Gaeta M, Racchiusa S, Chirico G. CT findings in palpable lesions of the anterior abdominal wall. *J Comput Assist Tomogr* 1986;10:629–633.

159. Pantongrag-Brown L, Buetow PC, Carr NJ, Lichtenstein JE, Buck JL. Calcification and fibrosis in mesenteric carcinoid tumor: CT findings and pathologic correlation. *AJR* 1995;164:387–391.

160. Pastakia B, Horvath K, Kurtz D, Udelsman R, Doppman JL. Giant

rectus sheath hematomas of the pelvis complicating anticoagulant therapy: CT findings. *J Comput Assist Tomogr* 1984;8:1120–1123.

161. Patten RM, Shuman WP, Teefey S. Subcutaneous metastases from malignant melanoma: prevalence and findings on CT. *AJR* 1989;152:1009–1012.

162. Peters JC, Reinertson JS, Polansky SM, Lamont BM, Fortune JB. CT demonstration of traumatic ventral hernia. *J Comput Assist Tomogr* 1988;12:710–711.

163. Pevarski DJ, Mergo PJ, Ros PR. Peritoneal carcinomatosis due to transitional cell carcinoma of the bladder: CT findings in two patients. *AJR* 1995;164:929–930.

164. Pitt HA. Peritonitis, intraabdominal abscess, and retroperitoneal abscess. 5. In: Shackelford RT, Zuidema GD, eds. *Surgery of the alimentary tract,* 2nd ed. Philadelphia: WB Saunders, 1986.

165. Press OW, Press NO, Kaufman SD. Evaluation and management of chylous ascites. *Ann Intern Med* 1982;96:358–364.

166. Puylaert JBCM. Right-sided segmental infarction of the omentum: clinical, US and CT findings. *Radiology* 1992;185:169–172.

167. Radin R. HIV infection: analysis in 259 consecutive patients with abnormal abdominal CT findings. *Radiology* 1995;197:712–722.

168. Raghavendra BN, Grieco AJ, Balthazar EJ, Megibow AJ, Subramanyam BR. Diagnostic utility of sonography and computed tomography in spontaneous mesenteric hematoma. *Am J Gastroenterol* 1982;77:570–573.

169. Ray CE Jr, Wilbur AC. CT diagnosis of concurrent hematomas of the psoas muscle and rectus sheath: case reports and review of anatomy, pathogenesis, and imaging. *Clin Imag* 1993;17:22–26.

170. Reuter K, Raptopoulos V, Reale F, et al. Diagnosis of peritoneal mesothelioma: computed tomography, sonography, and fine-needle aspiration biopsy. *AJR* 1983;140:1189–1194.

171. Rijke AM, Falke THM, de Vries RRP. Computed tomography in whipple disease. *J Comput Assist Tomogr* 1983;7:1101–1102.

172. Rodrigues A, Whitten CG. Roentgenologic clinical pathologic case. *Invest Radiol* 1993;28:260–262.

173. Ros PR, Olmsted WW, Moser RP, Dachman AH, Hjermstad BH, Sobin LH. Mesenteric and omental cysts: histologic classification with imaging correlation. *Radiology* 1987;164:327–332.

174. Rosen A, Korobkin M, Silverman PM, Dunnick NR, Kelvin FM. Mesenteric vein thrombosis: CT identification. *AJR* 1984;143:83–86.

175. Rubin JI, Gomori JM, Grossman RI, Gefter WB, Kressel HY. High-field MR imaging of extracranial hematomas. *AJR* 1987;148:813–817.

176. Rust RJ, Kopecky KK, Holden RW. The triangle sign: a CT sign of intraperitoneal fluid. *Gastrointest Radiol* 1984;9:107–113.

177. Safrit HD, Mauro MA, Jaques PF. Percutaneous abscess drainage in Crohn's disease. *AJR* 1987;148:859–862.

178. Sanders RC. The changing epidemiology of subphrenic abscess and its clinical and radiological consequences. *Br J Surg* 1970;57:449–455.

179. Schechter S, Eisenstat TE, Oliver GC, Rubin RJ, Salvati EP. Computerized tomographic scan-guided drainage of intra-abdominal abscesses. *Dis Colon Rectum* 1994;37:984–988.

180. Schneekloth G, Terrier F, Fuchs WA. Computed tomography of intraperitoneal abscesses. *Gastrointest Radiol* 1982;7:35–41.

181. Seabold JE, Wilson DG, Lieberman LM, Boyd CM. Unsuspected extra-abdominal sites of infection: scintigraphic detection with indium-111-labeled leukocytes. *Radiology* 1984;151:213–217.

182. Semelka RC, Lawrence PH, Shoenut JP, Heywood M, Kroeker MA, Lotocki R. Primary ovarian cancer: prospective comparison of contrast-enhanced CT and pre- and postcontrast, fat-suppressed MR imaging, with histologic correlation. *J Magn Reson Imag* 1993;3:99–106.

183. Seshul MB, Coulam CM. Pseudomyxoma peritonei: computed tomography and sonography. *AJR* 1981;136:803–806.

184. Shackelford GD, McAlister WH. Cysts of the omentum. *Pediatr Radiol* 1975;3:152–155.

185. Shackelford RT, Grose WE. Groin hernia. 5. In: Shackelford RT, Zuidema GD, eds. *Surgery of the Alimentary tract,* 2nd ed. Philadelphia: WB Saunders, 1986.

186. Sharif HS, Clark DC, Aabed MY, Aideyan OA, Haddad MC, Mattsson TA. MR imaging of thoracic and abdominal wall infec-

tions: comparison with other imaging procedures. *AJR* 1990;154:989–995.

187. Sherman JJ, Davis JR, Jeseph JE. Subphrenic abscess: a continuing hazard. *Am J Surg* 1969;117:117–123.

188. Shin MS, Ferrucci JT, Wittenberg J. Computed tomographic diagnosis of pseudoascites (floating viscera syndrome). *J Comput Assist Tomogr* 1978;2:594–597.

189. Siewert B, Raptopoulos V. CT of the acute abdomen: findings and impact on diagnosis and treatment. *AJR* 1994;163:1317–1324.

190. Silverman PM, Baker ME, Cooper C, Kelvin F. CT appearance of diffuse mesenteric edema. *J Comput Assist Tomogr* 1986;10:67–70.

191. Silverman PM, Kelvin FM, Korobkin M, Dunnick NR. Computed tomography of the normal mesentery. *AJR* 1984;143:953–957.

192. Silverstein W, Isikoff MB, Hill MC, Barkin J. Diagnostic imaging of acute pancreatitis: prospective study using CT and sonography. *AJR* 1981;137:497–502.

193. Sivit CJ, Peclet MH, Taylor GA. Life-threatening intraperitoneal bleeding: demonstration with CT. *Radiology* 1989;171:430.

194. Sones PJ. Percutaneous drainage of abdominal abscesses. *AJR* 1984;142:35–39.

195. Steck CW, Helwig EB. Cutaneous endometriosis. *Clin Obstet Gynecol* 1966;9:373–383.

196. Stoupis C, Ros PR, Abbitt PL, Burton SS, Gauger J. Bubbles in the belly: imaging of cystic mesenteric or omental masses. *RadioGraphics* 1994;14:729–737.

197. Swensen SJ, McLeod RA, Stephens DH. CT of extracranial hemorrhage and hematomas. *AJR* 1984;143:907–912.

198. Taneja K, Gothi R, Kumar K, Jain S, Mani RK. Peritoneal echinococcus multilocularis infection: CT appearance. *J Comput Assist Tomogr* 1990;14:493–494.

199. Taourel P, Pradel J, Fabre JM, Cover S, Seneterre E, Bruel JM. Role of CT in the acute nontraumatic abdomen. *Semin Ultrasound CT MRI* 1995;16:151–164.

200. Tartar VM, Heiken JP, McClennan BL. Renal cell carcinoma presenting with diffuse peritoneal metastases: CT findings. *J Comput Assist Tomogr* 1991;15:450–453.

201. Taylor KJW, Sullivan DC, Wasson JF, Rosenfield AT. Ultrasound and gallium for the diagnosis of abdominal and pelvic abscesses. *Gastrointest Radiol* 1978;3:281–286.

202. Terrier F, Revel D, Pajannen H, Richardson M, Hricak H, Higgins CB. MR imaging of body fluid collections. *J Comput Assist Tomogr* 1986;10:953–962.

203. Thoeni RF, Margulis AR. Gastrointestinal tuberculosis. *Semin Roentgenol* 1979;14:283–294.

204. Unger EC, Glazer HS, Lee JKT, Ling D. MRI of extracranial hematomas: preliminary observations. *AJR* 1986;146:403–407.

205. Vanek VW, Phillips AK. Retroperitoneal, mesenteric, and omental cysts. *Arch Surg* 1984;119:838–842.

206. vanSonnenberg E, D Agostino HB, Casola G, Halasz NA, Sanchez RB, Goodacre BW. Percutaneous abscess drainage: current concepts. *Radiology* 1991;181:617–626.

207. vanSonnenberg E, Mueller PR, Ferrucci JT Jr. Percutaneous drainage of 250 abdominal abscesses and fluid collections. *Radiology* 1984;151:337–341.

208. vanSonnenberg E, Mueller PR, Wittenberg J, et al. Comparative utility of ultrasound and computed tomography in suspected abdominal abscesses. In 66th Scientific Assembly and Annual Meeting of the Radiological Society of North America, 1980, Dallas, Texas.

209. vanSonnenberg E, Wittich GR, Casola G, et al. Periappendiceal abscesses: percutaneous drainage. *Radiology* 1987;163:23–26.

210. Vazquez JL, Thorsen MK, Dodds WJ, et al. Evaluation and treatment of intraabdominal bilomas. *AJR* 1985;144:933–938.

211. Vincent LM, Mauro MA, Mittelstaedt CA. The lesser sac and gastrohepatic recess: sonographic appearance and differentiation of fluid collections. *Radiology* 1984;150:515–519.

212. Wall SD, Hricak H, Bailey GD, Kerlan RK, Goldberg HI, Higgins CB. MR of pathologic abdominal fluid collections. *J Comput Assist Tomogr* 1986;10:746–750.

213. Wang SM, Wilson SE. Subphrenic abscess: the new epidemiology. *Arch Surg* 1977;112:934–936.

214. Whang SH, Lee KS, Kim PN, Bae WK, Lee BH. Omental teratoma in an adult: a case report. *Gastrointest Radiol* 1990;15:301–302.

215. White M, Mueller PR, Ferrucci JT Jr, et al. Percutaneous drainage of postoperative abdominal and pelvic lymphoceles. *Am J Gastroenterol* 1985;145:1065–1069.
216. Whitley NO. Mesenteric disease. In: Meyers MA, ed. *Computed tomography of the gastrointestinal tract.* New York: Springer–Verlag, 1986.
217. Whitley NO, Bohlman ME, Baker LP. CT patterns of mesenteric disease. *J Comput Assist Tomogr* 1982;6:490–496.
218. Whitley NO, Brenner DE, Antman KH, Grant D, Aisner J. CT of peritoneal mesothelioma: analysis of eight cases. *AJR* 1982;138: 531–535.
219. Wolf GC, Kopecky KK. MR imaging of endometriosis arising in cesarean section scar. *J Comput Assist Tomogr* 1989;13:150–152.
220. Wolverson MK, Crepps LF, Sundaram M, Heiberg E, Vas WG, Shields JB. Hyperdensity of recent hemorrhage at body computed tomography: incidence and morphologic variation. *Radiology* 1983;148:779–784.
221. Wolverson MK, Jagannadharao B, Sundaram M, Joyce PF, Riaz MA, Shields JB. CT as a primary diagnostic method in evaluating intraabdominal abscess. *AJR* 1979;133:1089–1095.
222. Woodard PK, Feldman JM, Paine SS, Baker ME. Midgut carcinoid tumors: CT findings and biochemical profiles. *J Comput Assist Tomogr* 1995;19:400–405.
223. Yeh H-C. Ultrasonography of peritoneal tumors. *Radiology* 1979; 133:419–424.
224. Yeh H-C, Rabinowitz JG. Ultrasonography and computed tomography in inflammatory abdominal wall lesions. *Radiology* 1982; 144:859–863.
225. Yeh H-C, Shafir MK, Slater G, Meyer RJ, Cohen BA, Geller SA. Ultrasonography and computed tomography in pseudomyxoma peritonei. *Radiology* 1984;153:507–510.
226. Zerhouni EA, Barth KA, Siegelmann SS. Demonstration of venous thrombosis by computed tomography. *AJR* 1980;134:753–758.

CHAPTER 17

Retroperitoneum

Joseph K. T. Lee, James N. Hiken, and Richard C. Semelka

The retroperitoneum, bounded anteriorly by the parietal peritoneum and posteriorly by the transversalis fascia, extends from the diaphragm superiorly to the level of pelvic viscera inferiorly. At the level of the kidneys, the retroperitoneal space is divided into three compartments—the perirenal space, surrounded by the anterior and posterior pararenal spaces. Two types of viscera exist in the retroperitoneal space: the true embryonic retroperitoneal organs (i.e., adrenal glands, kidneys, ureters, and gonads), and those structures closely attached to the posterior abdominal wall and only partly covered by the peritoneum (i.e., aorta, inferior vena cava, pancreas, portions of the duodenum, colon, lymph nodes, and nerves).

The diagnosis of retroperitoneal pathology has historically presented a challenge to physicians. The signs and symptoms of retroperitoneal diseases are myriad and often subtle. Because computed tomography (CT) and magnetic resonance imaging (MRI) allow direct, noninvasive demonstration of normal and pathologic retroperitoneal anatomy with a high level of clarity, both methods have had a major impact on the evaluation of retroperitoneal diseases (137,238). With current technology, diagnostic images can be obtained even in very emaciated patients (Fig. 1). In this chapter, discussion will be limited to diseases involving the great vessels, lymph nodes, and psoas muscle, as well as primary retroperitoneal neoplasms. Diseases related to other solid retroperitoneal organs, such as the kidneys, the adrenals, and the pancreas, are covered in other chapters.

TECHNIQUES

Computed Tomography

As in other parts of the body, careful patient preparation and attention to technical details are essential to obtain an optimal CT evaluation of the retroperitoneum. A survey examination of the retroperitoneum is routinely performed with contiguous 5- to 10-mm slice using either a dynamic incremental technique or a helical technique. Except in emergency situations in which the CT examination must be performed without delay (e.g., in patients with suspected ruptured abdominal aortic aneurysms), retroperitoneal CT should be done only after the patient has ingested oral contrast media. Approximately 1,000 ml of oral contrast material (dilute barium suspension or iodinated water-soluble contrast material) is given to the patient at least 1 hour before the examination to opacify the colon and distal small bowel loops. An additional 300 to 500 ml of contrast is given approximately 15 minutes before the study to opacify the stomach and proximal small bowel loops. If the pelvis is to be included, a contrast material enema (200 ml) occasionally may be necessary to expedite opacification of rectosigmoid and descending colon. Although the retroperitoneum can be adequately studied without the use of intravenous contrast material, most retroperitoneal CT studies are now performed with intravenous contrast material to allow distinction between vascular and nonvascular structures, to determine the vascularity of a retroperitoneal mass and its effect on the urinary tract, and to maximize detection of focal lesions in solid abdominal organs. One hundred fifty to 200 ml of a 60% iodine solution are administered intravenously via a power injector as either a uniphasic (e.g., 2 to 3 ml/sec) or biphasic (e.g., 2 to 3 ml/sec for the initial 50 ml, followed by 1 ml/sec for the remainder) injection. Images are obtained 30 to 45 seconds after the initiation of contrast delivery. Thorough bowel opacification, coupled with optimal delivery of intravenous contrast material, allows detection of retroperitoneal abnormalities even in the leanest patient (Fig. 1). The

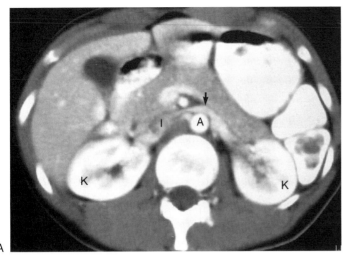

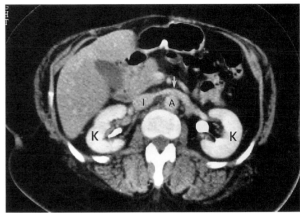

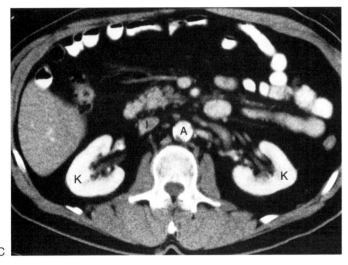

FIG. 1. Computed tomography images of the normal retroperitoneum in patients with variations in body habitus. **A:** Thin patient with little body fat. **B:** Relative paucity of retroperitoneal and mesenteric fat compared with subcutaneous fat, a pattern common in women. **C:** Relative prominence of retroperitoneal and mesenteric fat compared with subcutaneous fat, a pattern common in men. A, aorta; I, IVC; K, kidney; *arrow,* left renal vein.

introduction of helical CT has allowed production of detailed three-dimensional displays of retroperitoneal vascular structures including the renal arteries (221). Because multiple scans can be obtained in a single breath-hold, the resulting three-dimensional image reformations in these areas are not degraded by the respiratory misregistration that limits such images derived from standard CT scans. Furthermore, the shorter imaging time of helical CT allows more uniform and intense vascular enhancement during the entire scan. Optimal results can be achieved by delivering contrast material at a rate of 3 to 5 ml/sec (220), coupled with thinner collimation (e.g., 3 mm) and matched table speed (pitch = 1.0). However, use of thin collimation with matched table speed results in coverage of a small volume. Use of a higher pitch (up to 2.0) allows greater cephalocaudal coverage with only a minimal loss of longitudinal resolution. Another approach to increasing the volume of coverage is to use variable-collimation and overlapping reconstructions, which provides thin sections through the renal arteries as well as adequate cephalocaudal coverage (278). Using the latter technique, two consecutive helical acquisitions are obtained: the first with

3-mm collimation to cover the superior mesenteric artery and the renal arteries, followed by 7-mm collimation to reach the aortic bifurcation. Images are reconstructed with overlap: the 7-mm collimated scans are reconstructed at 4-mm intervals, and the 3-mm scans at 2-mm intervals.

Although a scan delay of 25 seconds works well for most patients, circulation time in some patients with abdominal aortic aneurysms is prolonged. Therefore, scan timing for helical CT angiography of the aorta generally is determined with a low volume intravenous contrast material test injection. In these instances, 18 ml of contrast material is injected at the rate to be used for the study (i.e., 3 to 5 ml/sec). Beginning 14 seconds and ending 32 seconds after the start of the bolus, single-level scans are acquired every 2 seconds at the top of the volume to be imaged. A time–density curve of aortic attenuation values is then generated from the test injection data. Alternatively, aortic attenuation value measurements from each scan can be recorded manually. The scan delay is then set at 2 seconds before peak aortic enhancement.

Magnetic Resonance Imaging

The retroperitoneum can likewise be successfully examined with MRI. Transverse images are obtained in all patients, usually with 8- to 10-mm collimation at 10- to 12-mm intervals. In addition, coronal and sagittal images often are performed to better define abnormalities of the aorta, inferior vena cava, and psoas muscle. The use of a 2-mm interslice gap reduces "cross talk" between consecutive sections.

As in the case of CT, an MR oral contrast agent can aid in the differentiation of bowel from other normal or pathologic tissue. Although perflubron (perfluorooctyl-bromide, or PFOB, Imagent, Alliance Pharmaceutical, San Diego, California), which causes darkening of the bowel lumen, has received FDA approval, it has not achieved widespread clinical acceptance because of its high cost. This agent appears as a signal void on T1- and T2-weighted images because it lacks mobile protons. PFOB is dense and has a low surface tension, progressing rapidly through the small bowel to reach the colon in 30 minutes. It has a short-lived oily taste and may leak inadvertently through the rectum in the first 3 hours after oral administration (195). Oral magnetic particles (OMP, Nycomed, Oslo, Norway), another darkening agent, has also received FDA approval. This agent is low in signal on T1-and T2-weighted images because of the magnetic susceptibility effects of iron. OMP is generally well tolerated: side effects are mostly mild, consisting of nausea, vomiting, and diarrhea in approximately 5% of patients. It is effective with all pulse sequences, except for gradient refocused echo (GRE) sequences, which demonstrate an undesirable amount of magnetic susceptibility (195).

Both T1- and T2-weighted sequences are required for lesion detection and characterization. T1-weighted imaging can be achieved with either a breath-hold GRE sequence (for example, FLASH, or spoiled GRASS) or a conventional spin-echo (SE) sequence (TR 300 to 1,000 msec, TE as short as possible). Although an SE sequence is less affected by magnetic susceptibility artifact, we prefer GRE for the T1-weighted sequence because it allows multiple sections to be obtained within a single breath-hold, resulting in high-quality images without respiratory-related artifacts and with minimal artifacts from bowel peristalsis. At 1.5T, with a TR of 130 msec, TE 4 msec, flip angle 80°, and one excitation, a total of 14 sections can be obtained in 19 seconds. The short acquisition time of a GRE sequence allows serial dynamic imaging after intravenous administration of a gadolinium (Gd) contrast agent. T2-weighted imaging (TR, >1,500 msec; TE, >70 msec) can be achieved with a conventional SE or a rapid SE (e.g. fast SE or turbo-spin echo) technique. Fat suppression can be applied to both techniques. The advantage of rapid SE over conventional SE sequences is a substantial reduction in data acquisition time. The reduced acquisition time can be used to improve

spatial resolution (by increasing imaging matrix elements) or to obtain stronger T2 weighting (by increasing TR and obtaining later echoes) without significantly prolonging the total imaging time. Although rapid SE provides better image quality and contrast-to-noise ratio for cystic abdominal lesions than does conventional SE, the qualitative conspicuousness and contrast-to-noise ratio of solid abdominal lesions are decreased (39). T2-weighted rapid SE technique combined with fat saturation reduces ghosting artifact and increases the contrast range of nonfatty tissues.

To assess the vascular system, various MR angiographic (MRA) methods have been employed. Data are acquired using a GRE sequence or its variant (e.g., turbo GRE) based on either time of flight (TOF) or phase contrast (PC) technique. Dynamic arterial phase Gd-enhanced GRE also may be used as an angiographic technique (62,206). Although two-dimensional (2-D) TOF technique is relatively accurate and requires less time, in-plane flow saturation of tortuous vessels and vessels with slow flow often leads to suboptimal images. Although the PC method is more sensitive to slow flow, it is more time consuming. In practice, 2-D or three-dimensional (3-D) TOF GRE technique is used to evaluate the abdominal aorta, whereas 2-D TOF turbo-FLASH or 2-D cine PC technique is better suited to assessing the iliac arteries (67,243,274). Magnetic resonance angiograms reconstructed with maximum intensity projection (MIP) rendering technique allow display of the entire retroperitoneal arterial and venous system in multiple projections (67).

AORTA

Normal Anatomy

Computed Tomography

The abdominal aorta begins at the hiatus of the diaphragm and usually extends along the ventral aspect of the lumbar spine to the level of the fourth lumbar vertebra, where it divides into the two common iliac arteries. On CT scans, the aorta appears as a circular soft-tissue density in a prevertebral location. The caliber of the abdominal aorta decreases as it progresses distally towards the bifurcation. Men usually have larger diameter vessels than age-matched women, and aortic diameter gradually increases with age in both sexes (113). Computed tomographic measurements of the normal aortic diameter at the level of the renal hila vary from a mean of 1.53 cm in women in their fourth decade, to 2.10 cm in men in their eighth decade. Normal infrarenal aortic dimensions (just proximal to the bifurcation) are smaller, averaging 1.43 cm and 1.96 cm, respectively, in these two groups of patients. Aortic diameter less than 12 mm at the level of

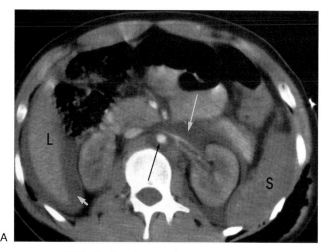 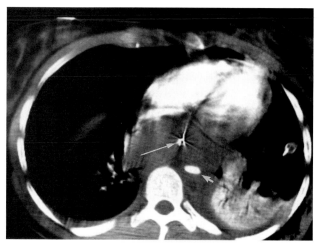

FIG. 2. Small aorta in a 17-year-old woman in shock after a motor vehicle accident. **A:** Contrast-enhanced CT scan shows a 7-mm-diameter aorta *(long black arrow)* associated with intraperitoneal *(short white arrow)* and retroperitoneal *(long white arrow)* hemorrhage. **B:** At 7 cm superiorly, there is a large mediastinal hematoma surrounding the aorta *(short arrow)* and esophagus *(long arrow)* which has artifact from a nasogastric tube. At surgery, thoracic aortic transection was found with dissection of hemorrhage into the retroperitoneum and peritoneal cavity. L, liver; S, spleen.

renal arteries should raise the possibility of hypovolemic shock (231) (Fig. 2).

The major branches arising from the abdominal aorta that can be seen on both conventional CT scans and projectional helical CT angiograms include the celiac trunk, the superior mesentery artery, the renal arteries, and the inferior mesenteric artery. Small accessory renal arteries likewise can be demonstrated on projectional helical CT angiograms when data are acquired with 3-mm collimation and reconstructed at 1.5-mm intervals (201).

The noncalcified aortic wall cannot be distinguished from its intraluminal blood on precontrast scans except in anemic patients. Whereas the attenuation value of the blood in the aortic lumen ranges from 50 to 70 Hounsfield units (HU) in normal subjects, it is considerably less in patients with a markedly reduced hematocrit. Thus, a visible, noncalcified aortic wall is a clue to the presence of anemia. After bolus intravenous administration of water-soluble iodinated contrast medium, the attenuation value of the aortic lumen can rise to as high as +400 HU.

Magnetic Resonance Imaging

Flowing blood has an appearance on MR images that is distinct from that of stationary tissue. Depending on the imaging technique used, blood may be bright or dark. In general, blood flowing at normal velocities (faster than 10 cm/sec) usually produces no signal on SE sequences (especially at long TEs) and bright signal on GRE sequences (especially at short TEs) because of the TOF phenomenon. Therefore, the aorta and its major branches appear as areas of signal void (111) on SE images, but as bright foci on GRE images. With either technique,

these arteries can be distinguished easily from the surrounding retroperitoneal structures (Fig. 3). However, the thin wall of the normal aorta usually is not clearly identified as a separate structure on either SE or GRE images. When transaxial images are obtained with a multislice SE technique, the aorta often demonstrates signal in the most cranial slice of the imaged volume as a result of a flow-related enhancement effect (22). Placement of a presaturation band above the imaging volume eliminates this effect and ensures that flowing blood remains black (67).

By means of GRE sequences triggered with electrocardiography, blood flow in the abdominal aorta and renal arteries can be quantified by measuring the flow-induced phase shift (167,269). Measurements thus obtained agree closely with those obtained by either Doppler ultrasound or clearance of *p*-aminohippurate.

Pathologic Conditions

Atherosclerosis

Computed Tomography

Atherosclerotic changes of the aorta can be detected on CT scans. These include calcification in the wall, mild ectasia, and tortuosity. Although the aorta usually is located in a prevertebral position, it may either be parallel to the spine or even lie to the right of the vertebral column in patients with severe atherosclerosis. Atheromatous plaque and chronic mural thrombus may be lower in attenuation value than the flowing blood; they are best appreciated on postcontrast scans (Fig. 4). Occlusion of a vessel likewise can be demonstrated on postcontrast scans (Fig. 5).

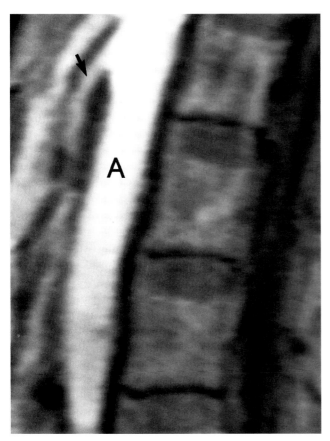

FIG. 3. MR of normal abdominal aorta. Sagittal post-Gd T1-weighted FLASH image (140/4/80°) shows enhancement of normal aorta (A) and proximal superior mesenteric artery *(arrow)*.

Luminal narrowing of renal and mesenteric arteries can be seen on helical CT angiograms using MIP rendering technique (220,222). In one study (220), computed tomographic angiography depicted all main and accessory renal arteries that were seen at conventional arteriography. Computed tomograpic angiography was 92% sensitive and 83% specific for the detection of grade 2 to 3 renal artery stenosis (≥70% stenosis).

Magnetic Resonance Imaging

Atherosclerotic changes of the aorta also can be seen on MR images. Calcification of the aortic wall appears as an arc or circumferential rim of low signal intensity. On SE images, atheromatous plaques and thrombus produce intraluminal signals of various intensities (7,109,151). Whereas organized thrombi have low signal intensity on both T1- and T2-weighted SE images, fresh unorganized thrombi have high signal intensity on T1- and T2-weighted images (37). Atheromatous plaques and thrombi can be differentiated easily from the aortic lumen, which usually appears as an area of signal void. However, slow blood flow may result in intraluminal signal. The signal

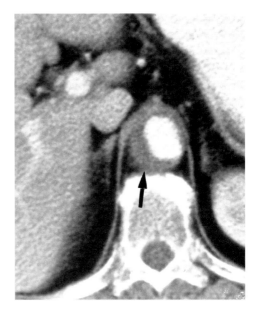

FIG. 4. Atheromatous plaque in a normal-size aorta. The atheroma *(arrow)* has a lower attenuation value and is clearly differentiated from the aortic lumen on this postcontrast CT image.

from slow flow can be distinguished from that of atheromatous plaques and thrombus by comparing the signal intensities on first and second echo images. Slow flow may show an increase in the absolute signal intensity on the second or even echo, whereas the signal produced by thrombus and the atheromatous plaque decreases in intensity on the second echo (Fig. 6). This increase in signal strength in blood vessels with slow flow has been described as an even-echo rephasing effect (22).

On GRE images, atheromatous plaque and thrombi usually are less intense than flowing blood. The signal differ-

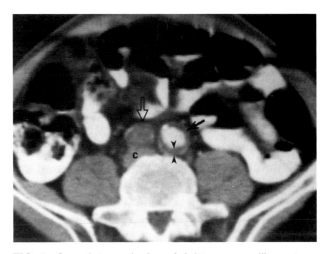

FIG. 5. Complete occlusion of right common iliac artery. Postcontrast CT image demonstrates an enhanced, ectatic left common iliac artery *(arrow)*. There is no enhancement of right common iliac artery *(open arrow)*. C, inferior vena cava; *arrowheads,* atheromatous plaque.

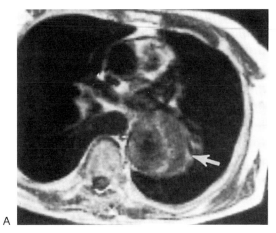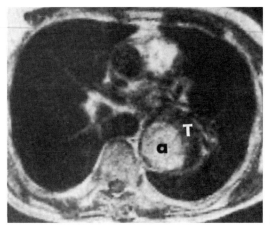

A

B

FIG. 6. Differentiation between slow flow and atheromatous thrombus in a descending thoracic aneurysm. **A:** Transverse MR image (500/30) shows an aneurysmal descending aorta *(arrow)*. The lumen size cannot be accurately discerned on this image. **B:** On second-echo image (500/60), there is an increase in signal intensity in the aortic lumen (a) that is related to slow flow. The thrombus (T), which shows decrease in signal intensity, can therefore be easily distinguished from the aortic lumen. (From ref. 93.)

ence between atheromatous plaque or thrombus and flowing blood can be accentuated on post-Gd GRE images.

Several studies have shown that stenosis (50% or greater) of the aorta and the renal arteries can be depicted on either noncontrast or Gd-enhanced MRA with a high degree of accuracy (134,163,205,234). Stenosis in the proximal 3 cm of renal artery is more accurately demonstrated than stenosis more than 3 cm from the origin. Although the sensitivity of detecting vessel stenosis was 100% in some studies, overgrading of luminal narrowing occurred in up to 40% of cases, with severe stenosis misconstrued as vessel occlusion (234). A higher specificity was achieved when MRA was obtained during intravenous infusion of gadolinium (205).

Aortic Aneurysms

The abdominal aorta must exceed 3 cm in diameter in an elderly patient to be considered aneurysmally dilated (113). In patients less than 50 years old, however, the normal abdominal aorta should not measure more than 2 cm in diameter.

In the United States, abdominal aortic aneurysms (AAAs) are mostly due to atherosclerosis. Infectious (mycotic, syphilitic) or traumatic causes are uncommon. Approximately 90% of the AAAs are infrarenal because the applied pressure load at this location is highest as a result of reflected pressure waves from the aortic bifurcation (56). Larger aneurysms tend to grow at a more rapid rate than smaller ones. In one study (161), the annual growth rate for aneurysms less than 4 cm, between 4 and 5 cm, and greater than 5 cm in diameter were 5.3 mm, 6.9 mm, and 7.4 mm, respectively. The incidence of rupture varies with the size of the aneurysm. Whereas the risk of rupture

approaches zero for aneurysms less than 3.5 cm in diameter, the risk exceeds 20% for aneurysms larger than 5 cm in diameter (161,188). Accepted indications for surgical repair of AAA include size greater than 4 cm, rapid rate of aneurysm expansion (increase of 5 mm or more in 6 months), known mycotic aneurysm, pain, concomitant occlusive disease, iliac or femoral artery aneurysms, or peripheral emboli (28,131).

The surgical approach to repair of AAA depends on whether the aneurysm involves the renal arteries. Infrarenal aneurysms can be approached via a routine transab-

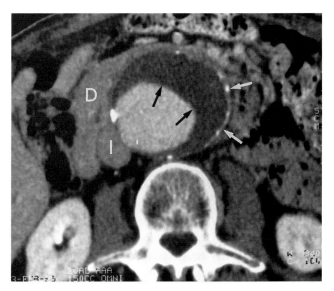

FIG. 7. Abdominal aortic aneurysm. Contrast-enhanced CT scan shows a 7-cm-diameter, fusiform, infrarenal abdominal aortic aneurysm. Note the rim of intimal calcification *(white arrows)* and the crescentic mural thrombus *(black arrows)*. I, IVC; D, duodenum.

dominal incision with the aorta clamped proximally below the renal arteries. Juxtarenal aneurysms (originating within 1 to 2 cm of the main renal arteries) can be approached either in the same fashion or through a retroperitoneal incision with the aorta usually clamped above the renal arteries (3). Suprarenal extension of an aneurysm requires a suprarenal or occasionally even a supraceliac proximal aortic clamp and concomitant renal revascularization via either a retroperitoneal or thoracoabdominal approach (3).

An alternative approach to surgical repair of AAA is the use of endovascular stented graft. The device consists of either a Dacron or an autogenous vein graft sutured to a balloon-expandable stent. The stented graft is placed through a remote arteriotomy site, advanced under fluoroscopic guidance to its predetermined location, and secured into position. Early results have been promising (20,194).

Computed Tomography

Abdominal aortic aneurysms can be detected and differentiated from a tortuous aorta by CT regardless of the presence or absence of aortic wall calcification. Although calcification is most commonly mural, it also may be present within a thrombus. Measurements of aortic diameter obtained on CT correlate precisely with those found at surgery (8,14, 98,192,197). The lumen can be differentiated from the adjacent atheroma/thrombus following intravenous injection of contrast agents (166) (Fig. 7). The origin and the length of an aneurysm, as well as its relationship to renal and iliac arteries, can be traced on both serial axial scans (Fig. 8) and projectional CT angiograms (Fig. 9). With 5-mm collimated sections, the overall accuracy of CT in predicting aneurysmal location with respect to the renal arteries exceeds 95% (97). However, the positive predictive value of nonhelical CT in determining renal artery involvement (the frequency with which the renal arteries are correctly predicted to be involved) has been low (262). Volume averaging of a tortuous juxtarenal aneurysm may produce an appearance suggesting involvement of the main renal arteries when, in fact, these vessels are actually immediately cephalad to the aneurysm. The ability to depict the proximal extent of the juxta- and suprarenal aneurysms and to identify renal artery stenosis of greater than 70% has improved significantly with the use of 2-mm-collimation helical CT technique (257).

Because less than one third of patients with ruptured

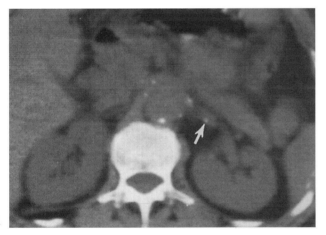

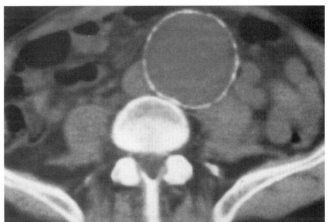

FIG. 8. Infrarenal aortic aneurysm with involvement of both iliac arteries. **A:** The aorta is normal in size at the level of the left renal artery *(arrow).* **B:** At 5 cm caudal to (A), the aorta is calcified and markedly dilated. **C:** Scan obtained 2 cm caudal to (B) shows dilation of both proximal common iliac arteries (IA).

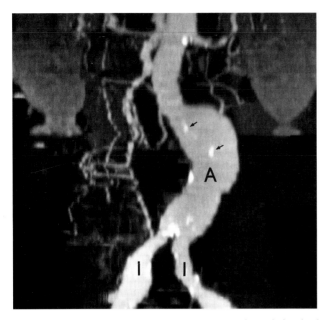

FIG. 9. Computed tomographic angiogram of an abdominal aortic aneurysm. Maximum intensity projection (MIP) image from a CT arteriogram (spiral technique: 3-mm collimation, 6-mm/sec table speed, 1-mm reconstruction intervals) shows a 5-cm infrarenal aortic aneurysm (A) extending into the common iliac arteries (I). The central calcifications *(arrowheads)* represent intimal calcifications in the anterior and posterior aortic walls projected onto the lumen by the 3-D rendering and do not suggest dissection. (Courtesy of Jay Heiken, M.D., St. Louis, Missouri.)

AAA present with the classic triad of abdominal pain, hypotension, and a pulsatile mass (172), and because more than 40% of normotensive patients with known or suspected AAAs and abdominal pain do not have a ruptured aneurysm (141,164), CT is an effective imaging study for evaluating hemodynamically stable patients with suspected leaking AAAs. In the latter group of patients, the delay imposed by obtaining a preoperative CT study usually does not adversely affect patient outcome, and the information obtained from the CT study can aid substantially in both preoperative and intraoperative management (141).

The CT diagnosis of ruptured AAA is based on demonstration of obscuration or anterior displacement of the aneurysm by an irregular, high-density (approximately +70 HU on noncontrast scans) mass or collection, which extends into one or both perirenal spaces and, less commonly, pararenal spaces (Fig. 10). Although intravenous contrast material is not required for the diagnosis of ruptured AAA, contrast-enhanced dynamic CT may document active arterial extravasation either as a focal high-density area (attenuation values of 80 to 130 HU) surrounded by a large hematoma, or as a diffuse area of high density (122). Additional findings include anterior displacement of the kidney by the hematoma and enlargement or obscuration of the psoas muscle. A focally indistinct aortic margin on contrast-enhanced scans, and focal discontinuity of a calcified rim, may indicate the site of rupture, but neither sign is specific (86,214). A finding that is frequently associated with AAA rupture is a

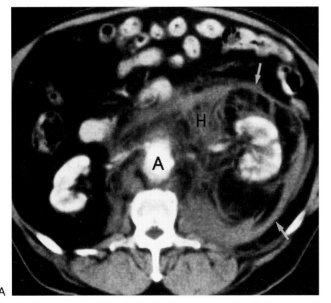

A

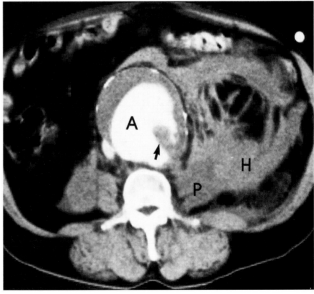

B

FIG. 10. Ruptured abdominal aortic aneurysm. **A:** Contrast-enhanced CT scan shows irregular soft-tissue strands representing acute hemorrhage (H) extending from the aneurysm (A) into the left perirenal space. Note the thickened perirenal fascia *(arrows)*. **B:** At 5 cm caudad, acute hemorrhage (H) is hyperdense compared with psoas muscle (P). Note the irregular intraluminal thrombus *(arrow)* within the aorta.

crescent-shaped area of high attenuation within the wall or mural thrombus of the aneurysm. Furthermore, in the absence of signs of active AAA rupture, the identification of a high-attenuation crescent sign should raise the suspicion of impending rupture (177,200) (Fig. 11). Although a variety of retroperitoneal masses, such as lymphadenopathy, perianeurysmal fibrosis, and masses in the psoas muscle, are occasionally present in patients with AAAs and may conceivably be confused with areas of rupture (232), false positive CT diagnoses of ruptured AAAs are extremely rare. False negative CT diagnoses are equally uncommon.

In comparison to acute rupture, a chronic pseudoaneurysm (false aneurysm) appears as a well-defined, usually round mass with an attenuation value similar to or lower than that of the native aorta on noncontrast scans. On postcontrast scans, the lumen of the aneurysm, as well as its communication with the aorta, may enhance (Fig. 12). A mycotic aneurysm usually has a saccular, irregular contour, and it contains little or no mural calcification. It enhances to a degree similar to the adjacent normal-appearing aorta (Fig. 13). The diagnosis can be confidently made based on CT findings if gas is seen within the wall of the aorta (261). Additional features that often aid in the diagnosis include splenic infarcts, lack of atherosclerotic changes in the other vessels, and the rapidity of its appearance. A nonenhancing periaortic mass representing inflammatory tissue and blood from a contained aortic rupture may be present (100). In chronic forms, erosion of the adjacent vertebral body and a paravertebral soft-tissue mass may be identified (11). An infected atherosclerotic aortic aneurysm, likewise, can be demonstrated on CT (Fig. 14).

A rare complication of AAA is the development of an aortocaval fistula. The CT findings that suggest this diagnosis include early equivalent enhancement of the inferior vena cava and aorta; enlarged, poorly functioning kidneys; and perirenal "cobwebs" (138).

Dissection of the aorta usually originates in the thorax but sometimes extends into the abdomen. Its diagnosis is based on demonstration of an intimal flap with enhancement of both the true and false lumina after intravenous administration of contrast medium (68,101,102,145) (Fig. 15). Aortic cobwebs, most likely representing residual ribbons of media that have been incompletely sheared from the aortic wall during the dissection process, are occasionally seen; they can serve as an anatomic marker of the false lumen (268). When the false lumen does not fill with contrast medium, a CT diagnosis of aortic dissection still may be suggested if inward displacement of intimal calcification is present (Fig. 15). However, caution must be taken not to confuse thrombus calcification with displaced calcified intima, as the two may appear similar (251) (Fig. 16). Although hyperdensity of the aortic wall at multiple levels has been reported to be specific for acute aortic dissection (108), 40% of patients without dissection in one series demonstrated this finding on noncontrast scans (142). Nevertheless, a hyperdense aortic wall tends to be uniformly thick throughout the vessel circumference in patients without dissection, whereas hyperdense thickening usually is eccentric in the uncommon form of dissection that occurs when intramural hematoma develops without intimal rupture (272).

Magnetic Resonance Imaging

Magnetic resonance imaging is an accurate method for demonstrating AAAs (7,74,81,151). It can accurately depict the size of an aneurysm, its relationship to the origin of the renal arteries, and the status of the iliac arteries in all patients (Fig. 17). Although only transaxial images are needed to determine the presence and size of an AAA, sagittal sections more directly display the cephalocaudad extent of the aneurysm and its relationship to the visceral arteries (Fig. 18). Coronal images are of limited value for demonstrating cephalocaudal extent, as usually only a portion of the aorta is seen on any one section because of the tortuosity of the aorta and the normal lordosis of most patients (151). However, coronal images are of greatest value in demonstrating the renal arteries. Accessory renal arteries and renal artery stenosis are poorly depicted on conventional SE images; they are much better shown on dynamic contrast-enhanced 3-D TOF MR angiograms. However, because of limited spatial resolution, grading of stenosis remains difficult even with MRA

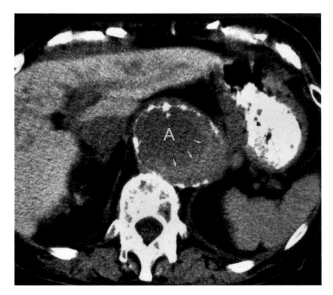

FIG. 11. High-attenuating crescent in early rupture of an aortic aneurysm. Noncontrast CT scan shows an abdominal aortic aneurysm (A) with a high-attenuating crescent *(arrowheads)* posterolaterally. Emergent surgery in this 82-year-old female with back pain disclosed very early aneurysm rupture at this site. (Courtesy of Jay Heiken, M.D., St. Louis, Missouri.)

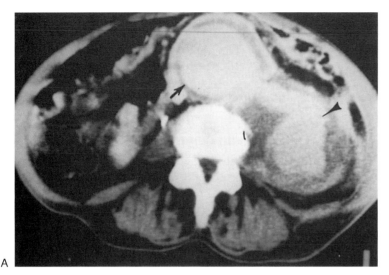

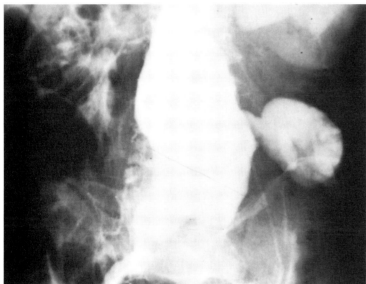

FIG. 12. Aortic aneurysm and associated chronic pseudoaneurysm. **A:** Postcontrast CT image demonstrates a large abdominal aortic aneurysm extending posterolaterally into the left paravertebral area. Note the centrally enhanced lumen in both the true *(arrow)* and the false *(arrowhead)* aneurysms. The lower-density periphery represents either an atheroma or a thrombus. The left psoas muscle is obscured by the pseudoaneurysm. **B:** The abdominal arteriogram shows findings similar to those of the CT study.

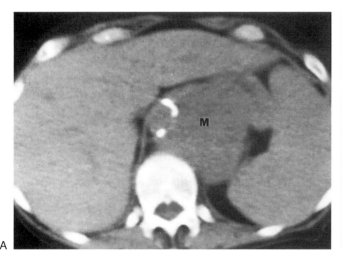

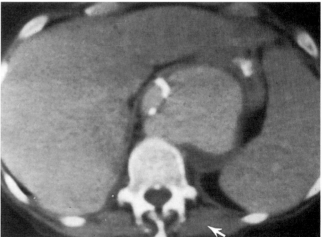

FIG. 13. Mycotic aortic aneurysm. **A:** Non-contrast-enhanced CT image shows a large soft-tissue mass (M) adjacent to the calcified descending aorta. This could be confused with lymphadenopathy. **B:** Postcontrast image demonstrates enhancement of this mass to the same degree as the aorta, thus establishing its vascular nature.

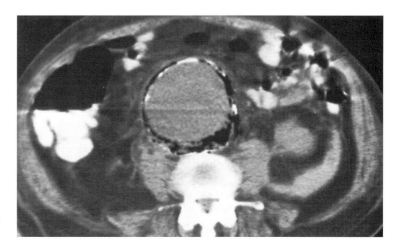

FIG. 14. Infected atherosclerotic aortic aneurysm. Numerous air bubbles are seen within the wall of this fusiform aneurysm.

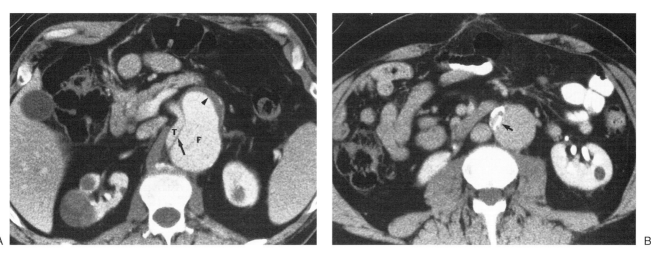

A

B

FIG. 15. Aortic dissection in a preexisting saccular abdominal aortic aneurysm. **A:** Contrast-enhanced CT scan demonstrates a saccular outpouching of an aortic aneurysm with a crescent of hypodense mural thrombus *(arrowhead)*. There is associated dissection with visible intimal flap *(arrow)* and enhancement of both true (T) and false (F) lumens. Incidentally noted are bilateral renal cell carcinomas. **B:** AT 2 cm caudad, there is inward displacement of intimal calcification *(arrow)*.

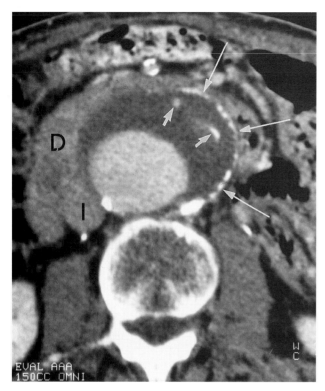

FIG. 16. Mural thrombus with calcification in an abdominal aortic aneurysm. Contrast-enhanced CT scan shows a 7-cm-diameter abdominal aortic aneurysm. Within the mural thrombus, there are calcifications *(short arrows)* that are distinct from the intact rim of intimal calcification *(long arrows)*. This is in contrast to the displaced intimal calcification that may be seen in aortic dissection, in which case the peripheral rim of intimal calcification is disrupted or distorted. I, IVC; D, duodenum.

(132). Because of its ability to detect blood flow without the use of intravenous contrast medium, MR also can be used to diagnose mycotic aortic aneurysms (183).

Because of its relatively long imaging time and the difficulty in monitoring critically ill patients, MRI has not been used to evaluate patients with suspected rupture of AAAs. Furthermore, MRI cannot distinguish acute hematoma from other fluid collections because of their similar signal intensities.

Magnetic resonance imaging is as accurate as CT and arteriography in the detection of aortic dissection (6,55,89,93,133). The MR diagnosis of an aortic dissection requires the demonstration of an intimal flap, which can be easily identified when both the true and false lumina appear as signal void areas on SE images (Fig. 19). On occasion, intraluminal signal may appear in the false channel as a result of slow blood flow or thrombus. As stated previously, slow flow can be differentiated from thrombus by comparing the signal intensity on the first and second echo image. They also can be differentiated on flow-sensitive GRE or phase images. In general, the false channel is more likely than the true channel to show evidence of slow blood flow and thrombus.

The inability of MRI to consistently demonstrate small calcification is not of clinical significance in most patients. However, in the rare case of complete thrombosis of the false channel, the detection of an intimal flap by MRI may not be possible. In these patients, CT can more easily diagnose an aortic dissection if inward displacement of intimal calcification can be demonstrated.

On rare occasions, concentric or eccentric aortic wall thickening may be the only sign of acute dissection (270). The wall thickening may be homogeneous and isointense,

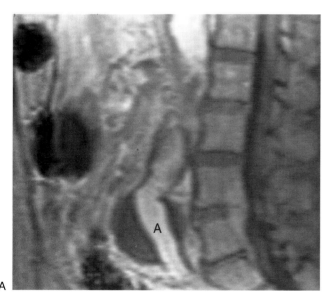

A

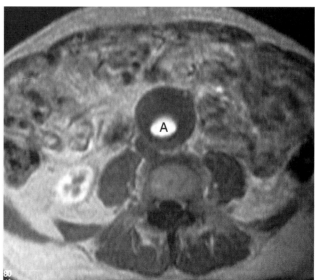

B

FIG. 17. Infrarenal aortic aneurysm. Sagittal **(A)** and transaxial **(B)** post-Gd, T1-weighted FLASH images (140/4/80°) show a 5-cm infrarenal aortic aneurysm. The aortic lumen (A) can be easily separated from hypointense mural thrombus.

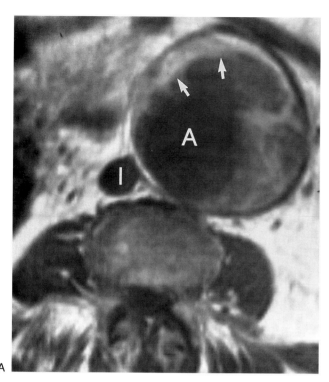
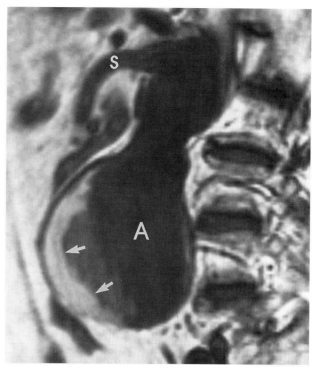

A

B

FIG. 18. Abdominal aortic aneurysm. Transaxial **(A)** and sagittal **(B)** gated T1-weighted SE images (501/15) show fusiform dilation of the infrarenal aorta measuring 5 cm at its widest diameter. The central lumen retains its flow void (A), whereas the peripheral high signal represents mural thrombus *(arrows)*. Note the superior mesenteric artery (S) arises from a slightly ectatic aortic segment. I, IVC.

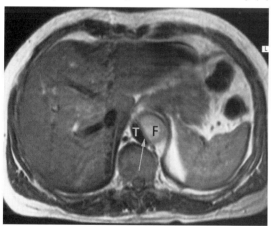
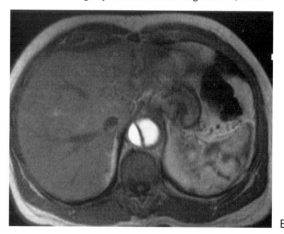

A

B

FIG. 19. Aortic dissection. **A:** Transaxial gated T1-weighted SE image (1219/25) shows an intimal flap *(arrow)*. Flow void in the true lumen (T) is a result of high velocity flow, whereas signal in the false lumen (F) is a result of slow flow or thrombosis. **B:** Post-Gd T1-weighted FLASH image (140/4/80°) at the same level shows enhancement of both lumens with better delineation of the intimal flap. **C:** Image obtained at the level of the superior mesenteric artery take-off demonstrates poor enhancement of the left kidney resulting from renal artery involvement.

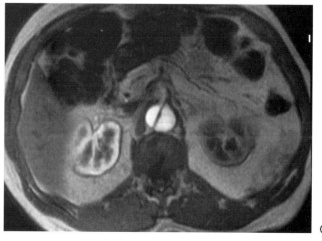

C

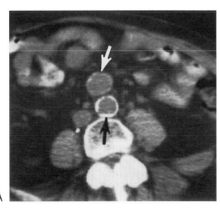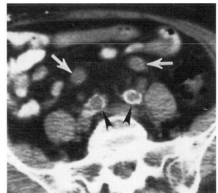

FIG. 20. CT appearance of normal aortoiliac graft with end-to-side anastomosis. **A:** The aortic graft *(white arrow)* lies anterior to the native, calcified aorta *(black arrow)*. **B:** The iliac artery grafts *(arrows)* lie several centimeters anterior to the native vessels *(arrowheads)*.

although it often contains hyperintense foci on the T1-weighted images.

Aortic dissection can likewise be diagnosed on GRE sequence (Fig. 19), which requires a much shorter imaging time than SE sequence. Imaging of the entire aorta can be completed with a GRE sequence within a few minutes. Gadolinium-enhanced GRE is an effective means of demonstrating blood flow in the aorta (Fig. 19), and, in patients with diminished renal function, the lack of nephrotoxicity of gadolinium may be advantageous. Limitations of GRE imaging include increased magnetic susceptibility artifact and, if gadolinium is not administered, its inability to distinguish subacute hematoma in the aortic wall from flowing blood.

Postoperative Complications

Computed Tomography. Aortic grafts are performed for replacing aneurysms and bypassing occlusive vascular disease. The CT appearance of aortic grafts depends on the type of surgery performed (128,169). There are three common configurations for the proximal anastomosis in these grafts: (a) end-to-side anastomosis; (b) end-to-end anastomosis; and (c) end-to-end anastomosis within the sac of an aneurysm.

Postoperative aortas can be distinguished from native atherosclerotic aortas because the graft is of slightly higher attenuation than unenhanced blood on noncontrast CT scans and its lumen is perfectly round and smooth, whereas the patent lumen of an atherosclerosis aorta is usually slightly irregular. In the case of an end-to-side anastomosis, the graft is seen ventral to the native aorta (Fig. 20). The iliac branches of the graft are seen as two dense circular structures anterior to the calcified native iliac arteries, which are commonly thrombosed. The bifurcation of the graft is usually located 2 to 3 cm cephalad to the native aortic bifurcation. The CT appearance of end-to-end anastomosis differs from that of end-to-side

anastomosis in its complete interruption of the native aorta at the anastomotic site. Therefore, the distal native aorta is not opacified on postcontrast scans. In patients who have an end-to-end anastomosis within the sac of an aneurysm (endoaneurysmorrhaphy), the aneurysm sac is wrapped around the graft to provide an additional layer between the graft and duodenum to reduce the risk of aortoduodenal fistula formation. A collection of serous fluid, or soft-tissue attenuation, often can be identified between the synthetic graft and the native aortic wrap (Fig. 21). This collection usually resolves within 3 months (165) (Fig. 22).

Postoperative complications of abdominal aortic graft surgery that can be diagnosed by CT include hemorrhage and false aneurysm formation, major vessel or graft limb occlusion, infection, and aortoenteric fistula (AEF) (52,103,112,124,128,165,168). When acute hemorrhage is suspected, a noncontrast CT scan is often helpful to

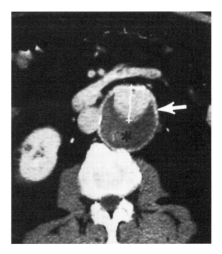

FIG. 21. CT appearance of normal aortoiliac graft: end-to-end anastomosis within an aneurysmal sac. A layer of fluid (*) with near water density is present between the native aortic wall *(arrow)* and the synthetic graft *(measuring cursor)*.

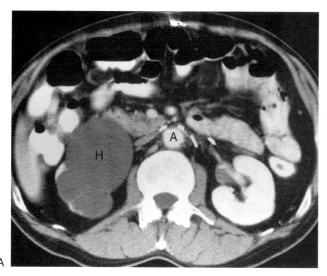
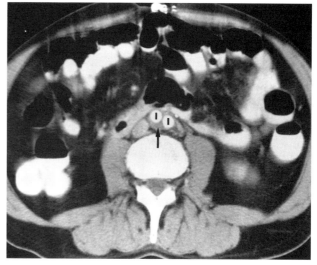

A   B

FIG. 22. Computed tomographic appearance of a normal aortobifemoral graft. **A:** Surgical clips mark the level of the end-to-end aortic anastomosis (A). Chronic right hydronephrosis (H) is a result of congenital ureteropelvic junction obstruction. **B:** Inferiorly, the iliac limbs (I) of the graft lie within the wrap of the native aortic wall. A small hypodense collection *(arrow)* is commonly seen between the graft and the aortic wrap, representing serous fluid or organized hemorrhage.

identify the increased attenuation of fresh blood. False aneurysms occur at the suture line and are more common in the femoral area than in the region of the aortoiliac system. They appear as paragraft fluid collections, which may enhance to the same degree as the native aorta or graft on postcontrast scans (Figs. 23,24).

The diagnosis of graft occlusion is based on the demonstration of a low-density lumen representing thrombus with lack of enhancement after administration of contrast medium. When a graft becomes infected, an irregular collection of fluid and soft-tissue attenuation is often present around the prosthesis, sometimes associated with small pockets of gas (165) (Fig. 25). These gas collections usually are multiple in number and posterior in location, and most often they occur more than 10 days after the initial surgery (104). This is in contradistinction to a "normal" gas collection seen in the immediate postoperative period, which usually is solitary and anterior in location (Fig. 26). Because gas occurs only in a small percentage of perigraft infections and because gas may be a normal finding in the immediate postoperative period, needle aspiration of a suspicious perigraft fluid collection is advised in any patient with suspected infection.

Computed tomography features of AEF are similar to those of graft infection and include paragraft fluid and extraluminal air (165). Although not specific, thickening

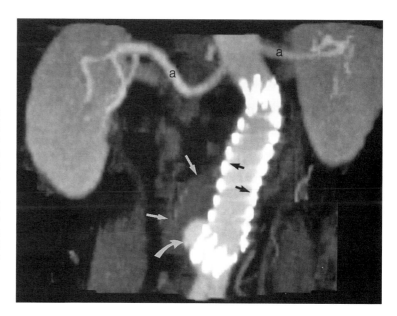

FIG. 23. Computed tomographic angiogram of an abdominal aortic aneurysm treated with an internal stent and complicated by pseudoaneurysm formation. Maximum intensity projection (MIP) image from a CT angiogram (spiral technique: 3-mm collimation, 5-mm/sec table speed, 2-mm reconstruction intervals) shows the metallic surface of an expandable intraluminal aortic stent *(arrows)*. Note the relatively normal diameter of the enhancing aortic lumen. At the inferior edge of the stent, there is a pseudoaneurysm *(white arrows)* with a large amount of thrombus and a relatively small enhancing patent lumen *(curved white arrow)*. a, renal arteries. (Courtesy of Jay Heiken, M.D., St. Louis, Missouri.)

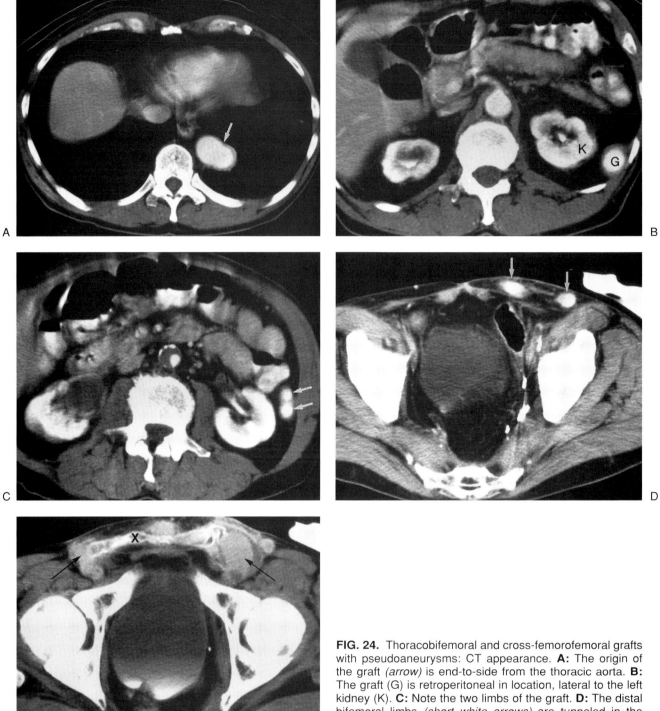

FIG. 24. Thoracobifemoral and cross-femorofemoral grafts with pseudoaneurysms: CT appearance. **A:** The origin of the graft *(arrow)* is end-to-side from the thoracic aorta. **B:** The graft (G) is retroperitoneal in location, lateral to the left kidney (K). **C:** Note the two limbs of the graft. **D:** The distal bifemoral limbs *(short white arrows)* are tunneled in the subcutaneous tissues. **E:** The original cross-femorofemoral graft (X) has become occluded. Pseudoaneurysms *(long black arrows)* are present as enhancing dilations at the bilateral distal anastomoses of the thoracobifemoral graft.

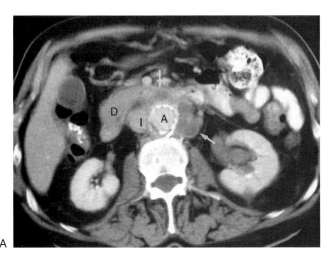 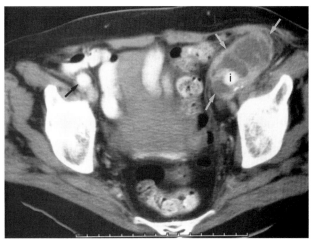

FIG. 25. Infected aortobifemoral graft. **A:** Contrast-enhanced CT image at the level of the proximal end-to-end anastomosis demonstrates a complex fluid collection with enhancing walls *(arrows)* surrounding the aortic graft (A). I, IVC; D, duodenum. **B:** The left iliac limb (i) is surrounded by a large abscess *(white arrows)*. The right iliac limb *(black arrow)* is normal.

of the small bowel, especially the third portion of the duodenum, adjacent to paragraft fluid, is highly suggestive of an AEF. Additional findings, such as extravasation of oral contrast material around the graft, intravasation of intravenous contrast material into unopacified small bowel, or small bowel hematomas, are rare (140,162,279).

In patients in whom endovascular stented grafts have been placed to treat AAAs, helical CT is a sensitive means of assessing the status of the grafts (218). Decreased or stable size of the aneurysmal sac without perigraft channels on the follow-up CT study obtained several months

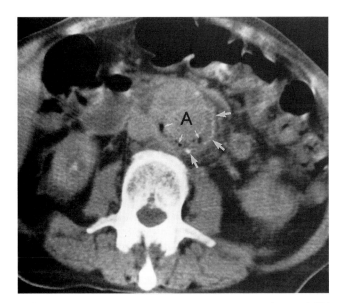

FIG. 26. Infected aortic graft. Poorly contrast-enhanced CT scan shows multiple gas foci *(small arrows)* present between the aortic graft (A) and the calcified intima *(large arrows)* of the overlying native aortic wrap. Benign postoperative gas is typically solitary and anterior in location.

after the procedure signifies technical success. Persistence or recurrence of perigraft channels is the most likely cause of later enlargement of an aneurysm and suggests procedure failure.

Magnetic Resonance Imaging. Magnetic resonance imaging also can be used to evaluate abdominal aortic grafts. Graft complications, such as infections, pseudoaneurysms, limb occlusions, and bleeding, all have been demonstrated by MRI (12,13,103,126). The prosthetic graft itself does not produce any signal and, therefore, cannot be delineated as a separate structure if blood flow within the graft is rapid enough to produce a signal void on SE images (126). In patients who have an end-to-end anastomosis within the sac of an aneurysm, a collection of fluid that shows relatively low signal intensity on T1-weighted images and a high signal intensity on T2-weighted images, is routinely seen on MRI studies obtained up to 6 weeks after surgery (Fig. 27). After 3 months, a perigraft collar of low signal intensity is often seen on T1- and T2-weighted images and likely represents fibrosis or the wall of the native aorta adherent to the graft (graft incorporation) (13). A perigraft fluid collection that increases in size or persists beyond 3 months should cause concern about infection.

On MRI, perigraft abscesses appear as fluid collections that have low to medium signal intensity (iso- or hyperintense to muscle) on T1-weighted images and high intensity on T2-weighted images (iso- or hyperintense to fat). Inflammation in surrounding tissues, characterized by a nonhomogeneously increased signal intensity of the psoas muscles adjacent to the graft, also can be seen. Gadolinium-enhanced T1-weighted fat-suppressed imaging accentuates the contrast difference between nonenhancing low signal abscess fluid and adjacent enhancing inflammatory tissue. However, the infected nature of the

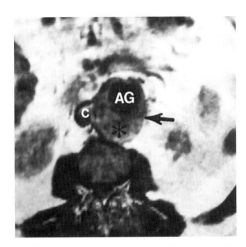

FIG. 27. MRI appearance of a normal aortic graft: end-to-end anastomosis within an aneurysmal sac. Note the presence of a large fluid collection (*) between the native aortic wall *(arrow)* and the synthetic graft (AG). c, inferior vena cava.

fluid cannot be ascertained on the basis of MR signal intensities alone. A significant limitation of MRI is its inability to detect small collections of gas. In addition, MRI cannot reliably differentiate between a collection of gas and a small cluster of calcifications.

Clinical Applications

Although both CT and MRI can detect the presence and the size of aortic aneurysms and their internal character with a high degree of accuracy (7,14,98,151,197), ultrasound remains the procedure of choice in patients with suspected AAA because of its ease of performance, lack of ionizing radiation, lower cost, and portability. In patients who have had an unsuccessful or equivocal sonographic examination as a result of postsurgical scar tissue, obesity, or abundant bowel gas, either a CT or an MRI study may be performed. However, in most cases, we prefer CT to MRI. On some occasions, optimal CT evaluation of the abdominal aorta requires the intravenous administration of contrast material, for example to differentiate a pseudoaneurysm from periaortic lymphadenopathy. Thus, in patients who have a contraindication to the use of iodinated contrast material, it is advantageous to perform MRI rather than a CT examination.

Although both CTA and MRA are capable of demonstrating vascular stenosis, they are not accurate enough to replace conventional angiography or digital subtraction arteriography for preoperative evaluation of all patients with AAAs (129,163). Before elective AAA repair, arteriography is still performed in most patients with thoracoabdominal, juxtarenal, or suprarenal aneurysms, suspected renal artery stenosis, aortoiliac occlusive disease, and mesenteric or peripheral arterial insufficiency (250).

In our experience, CT is superior to ultrasound and

MRI in detecting infected aortic grafts and leaking AAAs because of its superior ability to demonstrate small collections of air, its proven ability to diagnose recent hemorrhage, and the ease with which patients can be monitored during the study.

Although not universally accepted, MRI can be performed as the initial imaging study in a clinically stable patient who is suspected of having a dissecting aortic aneurysm (198). Magnetic resonance imaging can accurately detect aortic dissections and define their superior and inferior extents. Although CT is also highly accurate in the diagnosis of an aortic dissection (249), the CT diagnosis of a dissection usually requires the administration of iodinated contrast material, which is clinically important if additional angiographic studies are contemplated. If MRI or CT shows a type A dissection, angiography may be needed to evaluate the status of the coronary arteries and aortic valve.

INFERIOR VENA CAVA AND ITS TRIBUTARIES

Normal Anatomy

Computed Tomography

The inferior vena cava (IVC) is formed by the confluence of the two common iliac veins at the level of the fifth lumbar vertebra. From this point, it ascends along the vertebral column on the right of the aorta to the level of the diaphragm and enters the chest, terminating in the right atrium. Although it is in close proximity to the lumbar vertebral bodies in its most caudal position, it assumes a more ventral position at its cephalic end.

The shape, which may be round or flat, and the size of the inferior vena cava vary from patient to patient and even in the same patient at different levels. Performance of a Valsalva maneuver usually results in more distension of the IVC in normal subjects. In patients undergoing CT for abdominal trauma, a flat IVC at multiple levels may be an important sign of hypovolemia resulting from major hemorrhage. In some cases, the demonstration of the collapsed IVC may precede the clinical detection of shock (123). The renal veins, which are located ventral to the renal arteries, often can be seen in their entirety entering the vena cava. The left renal vein usually is longer than the right and passes across the midline between the abdominal aorta and the superior mesenteric artery. The main hepatic veins and their tributaries converge into the vena cava near the diaphragm. A small, oval collection of fat that lies medial to the IVC, at or above the level of confluence of the hepatic veins and the IVC, may be seen in some normal patients. This collection is contiguous to the fat around the subdiaphragmatic portion of the esophagus, and its presence or absence is not related to obesity (180).

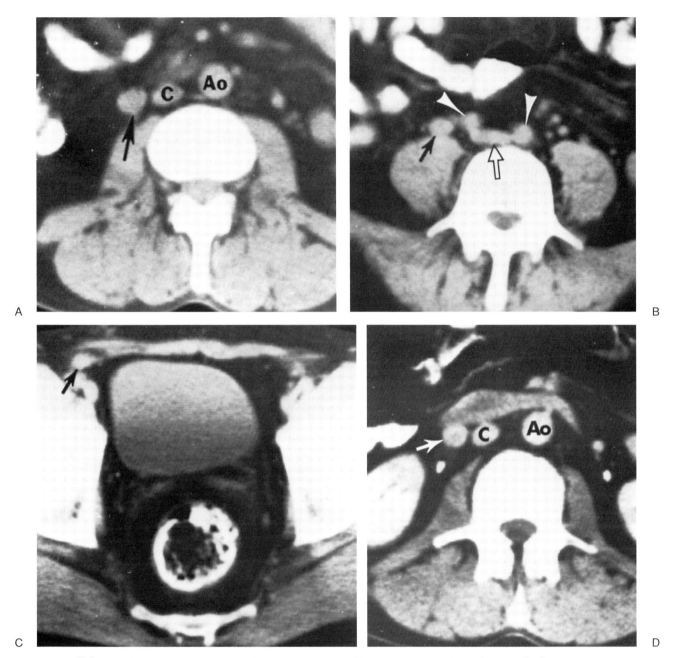

FIG. 28. An enlarged right gonadal vein in a man with an asymptomatic varicocele. **A:** Precontrast CT image just below both kidneys shows an oval soft-tissue density *(arrow)* lateral to the inferior vena cava (c). **B:** At the level of the common iliac artery *(arrowheads)*, an extra soft-tissue density *(arrow)* lies anterior to the psoas muscle and lateral to the iliac artery. *Open arrow,* confluence of the common iliac vein. **C:** At the level of the acetabulum, the soft-tissue density *(arrow)* is seen near the internal (deep) inguinal ring. The presence of such a soft-tissue density over several images indicates that this is a tubular structure. **D:** Postcontrast image at a level slightly above (A) demonstrates the previously noted soft-tissue structure *(arrow)* to enhance to a similar degree as the adjacent inferior vena cava (c), thus documenting its vascular nature. Scrutiny of sequential images and intravenous administration of contrast material often are needed to clarify such complex venous anomalies. Ao, aorta; c, inferior vena cava.

The IVC, the iliac veins, and the renal veins can be easily seen even on noncontrast CT scans. The main hepatic veins and their tributaries also can be seen on noncontrast scans because they have a slightly lower attenuation than the normal hepatic parenchyma. At least a portion of normal-caliber gonadal vein can be traced on consecutive contrast-enhanced scans in a majority of patients. Whereas the right gonadal vein drains directly into the IVC, approximately 4 cm below the junction of the right renal vein and the IVC (211), the left gonadal vein usually drains into the left renal vein. Below the left renal vein, the left gonadal vein is often seen posterior to the inferior mesenteric vein and anterior to the left psoas muscle. The gonadal veins may be enlarged in multiparous women and in men with varicoceles (Fig. 28).

The attenuation value of the lumen of the IVC is similar to that of the abdominal aorta and thus varies with the hematocrit of the patient. However, in comparison to the aortic wall, the wall of the IVC is thin and rarely visible as a discrete structure even in severely anemic patients.

Magnetic Resonance Imaging

The IVC and its tributaries are well delineated by MRI because of the excellent contrast between vascular struc-

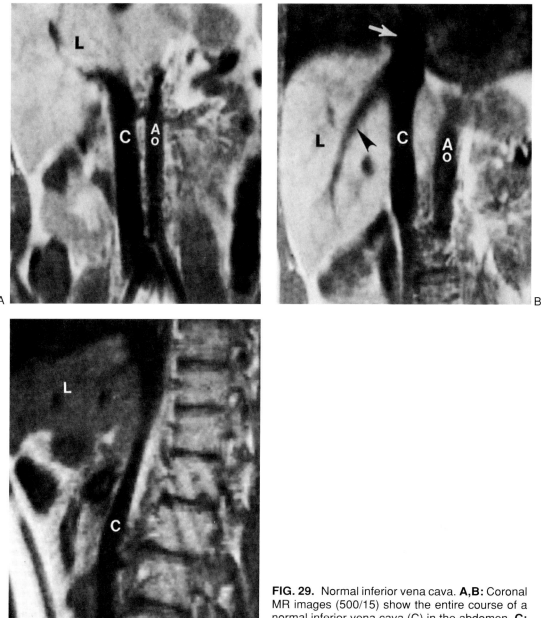

FIG. 29. Normal inferior vena cava. **A,B:** Coronal MR images (500/15) show the entire course of a normal inferior vena cava (C) in the abdomen. **C:** Sagittal MR image (500/30) in another patient. L, liver; *arrowhead*, right hepatic vein; *arrow*, junction between inferior vena cava and right atrium. Ao, abdominal aorta.

tures with flowing blood and adjacent soft tissue. The normal IVC demonstrates no intraluminal signal on SE images (Fig. 29) but appears as a high-signal-intensity structure on GRE sequences. As in the aorta, flow-related enhancement effect (also called slice-entry phenomenon) can produce a signal in the IVC when transverse SE images are obtained. Unlike the aorta, the flow-related signal is observed on the most caudal slice of the imaged volume because of the opposite direction of the flow of blood.

Normal Variations (Congenital Anomalies)

Knowledge of the various developmental anomalies of the venous system and recognition of their CT/MRI appearances are critical for proper image interpretation. Misinterpretation of venous anomalies as pathology may lead to unnecessary surgical evaluation.

The IVC is formed by the successive development and regression of three paired veins (43,44,217) (Fig. 30). Early in embryogenesis, the posterior supracardinal and more anterior subcardinal veins are formed. Later, the most caudal segment of the right supracardinal vein becomes the infrarenal vena cava. The middle segment joins with part of the right subcardinal vein to form the renal portion of the IVC. The cephalic portion of the IVC is formed from the efferent veins of the liver. The portion of the right supracardinal vein cephalad to the kidneys becomes the azygos vein; similarly, that portion on the left forms the hemiazygos system. The rest of the left cardinal system undergoes involution.

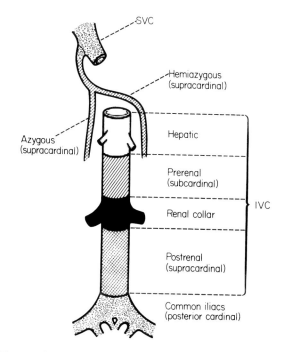

FIG. 30. Schematic diagram showing the precursors of different segments of the inferior vena cava.

Interruption of normal regression of any of these venous structures results in different anomalies. Azygos vein continuation is an anomaly of the suprarenal segment. Circumaortic venous rings and retroaortic left renal vein involve the renal segment. Circumcaval ureter, transposition, and duplication of the IVC involve the infrarenal segment. Schematic representations of these various anomalies are shown in Figure 31. Most of these venous anomalies can be confidently diagnosed on noncontrast CT scans by tracing their course on contiguous slices. If confusion persists on noncontrast CT scans, the vascular nature of these structures can be proven by intravenous contrast material administration.

Congenital anomalies of the IVC likewise can be demonstrated by MRI (47,80,82,228). The venous channels are readily differentiated from retroperitoneal fat, muscle, and enlarged lymph nodes without the use of intravenous contrast medium. Whereas contiguous transverse CT or MR images are adequate for defining the anomalous venous anatomy, the entire system can be displayed more elegantly by axial CT or MRA.

Interrupted Inferior Vena Cava with Azygos/Hemiazygos Continuation

When the subcardinal vein fails to connect with the hepatic veins during the 6th fetal week, blood returns to the heart from the postrenal segment through the azygos/hemiazygos system, and the hepatic veins drain directly into the right atrium (24,43,44,90). Rare variations include portal and hemiazygos continuation of the IVC (82) and hemiazygos continuation of a left IVC (186). This anomaly usually occurs as an isolated lesion but occasionally can be associated with cardiac abnormalities or other visceral anomalies such as the asplenia and polysplenia syndromes.

On transverse CT or MRI study, a normal IVC is seen from the confluence of common iliac veins to the level of both kidneys. An intrahepatic segment of the IVC, which lies anterior to the right diaphragmatic crus and posterior to the caudate lobe of the liver, is absent. However, an enlarged azygos vein, and often a hemiazygos vein as well, can be seen in the retrocrural space on both sides of the aorta. The azygos vein can be further traced on more cephalic scans to the level where it arches anteriorly to join the superior vena cava or just below the level of the aortic arch (Figs. 32,33).

Circumaortic Left Renal Vein

There is a true vascular ring about the aorta in this anomaly. The preaortic left renal vein crosses from the left kidney to the IVC at the expected level of the renal veins. The additional retroaortic left renal vein (or veins) connects to the IVC by descending caudally and crossing

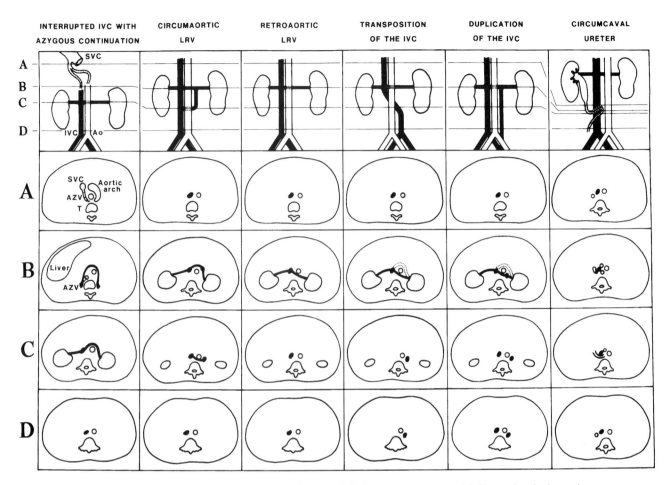

FIG. 31. Diagram showing relationships of aorta, inferior vena cava, and left renal vein in various congenital venous anomalies. (Adapted from ref. 217.)

the spine behind the aorta, usually one to two vertebrae below the level of the preaortic left renal vein (217). On a CT or an MRI study, a normal, albeit somewhat diminutive, left renal vein can be seen in its preaortic position. The anomalous retroaortic left renal vein is identified in a more caudal position.

Retroaortic Left Renal Vein

In this anomaly, the anterior subcardinal veins regress completely and only the retroaortic supracardinal veins remain to connect the left kidney to the IVC (217,252). The retroaortic left renal vein can be seen either at the same level as a normal left renal vein or in a more caudal position, sometimes as low as the confluence of iliac veins.

Transposition of the Inferior Vena Cava

Anomalous regression of the right cardinal veins and persistence of the left cardinal system result in transposition of the IVC (43,217). In this entity, a single IVC ascends on the left side of the spine and crosses either anterior or posterior to the aorta at the level of the renal veins to ascend further to the right atrium on the right side of the spine (Fig. 34). The characteristic appearance on CT or transverse MRI examination is a single IVC to the right of the aorta at levels above the renal vein, a vascular structure either crossing anterior or posterior to the aorta at the level of the renal veins, and a large, single IVC to the left of the spine at levels below the renal veins.

Duplication of the Inferior Vena Cava

In duplication of the IVC, there is an IVC, albeit smaller than usual in size, along the right side of the spine (43,75,217). In addition, a left-sided IVC ascends to the level of the renal veins to join the right-sided IVC through a vascular structure that may pass either anterior or posterior to the aorta at the level of the renal veins. Either vena cava can be the predominant vessel, or they can be of equal size. On a CT or an MRI study, a single right-sided IVC is seen at levels above the renal veins. A vascular

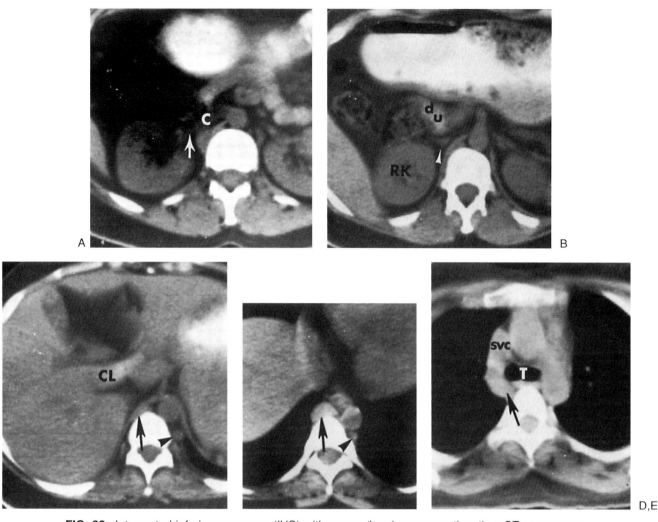

FIG. 32. Interrupted inferior vena cava (IVC) with azygos/hemiazygos continuation: CT appearance. **A:** At the level of renal hilum, the right renal vein *(white arrow)* drains into the IVC (C). **B:** Image through the upper pole of the right kidney (RK) shows absence of an IVC. Note that the right adrenal gland *(white arrowhead)* lies directly posterior to the descending duodenum (du). **C:** At the level of the hepatic hilus, enlarged azygos *(arrow)* and hemiazygos *(arrowhead)* veins can be seen in the retrocrural space. An intrahepatic segment of the IVC, which normally is situated posterior to the caudate lobe of the liver (CL), is not present in this case. **D:** A more cephalic image, again demonstrating abnormally enlarged azygos *(arrow)* and hemiazygos *(arrowhead)* veins. **E:** At the level of tracheal bifurcation (T), the enlarged azygos vein *(arrow)* drains into the superior vena cava (svc).

structure crossing either anterior or posterior to the aorta is seen at the level of the renal veins, and two vena cavae, one on each side of the aorta, are present below the level of the renal veins (Fig. 35). A duplicated left IVC can be differentiated from a dilated left gonadal vein by following its course to the more caudal scans. Whereas a duplicated left IVC ends at the level of common iliac veins, a dilated left gonadal vein can be traced further inferiorly to the level of the inguinal canal (217).

Circumcaval Ureter

Embryologically, a circumcaval ureter results from anomalous regression of the most caudal segment of the supracardinal vein and the persistence of the subcardinal vein. Consequently, the ureter passes behind and around the medial aspect of the IVC as it courses to the bladder. Although more commonly described on the right, a left retrocaval ureter associated with a left IVC also has been described (199). As in other types of vena caval anomalies, circumcaval ureter may be discovered as an incidental radiographic finding. However, patients with this condition sometimes present with signs and symptoms related to right ureteral obstruction. Whereas asymptomatic patients or patients with minimal caliectasis require only occasional follow-up, patients with significant renal obstruction often require surgical correction.

Inasmuch as circumcaval ureter has a characteristic appearance on excretory urography (medial deviation of the

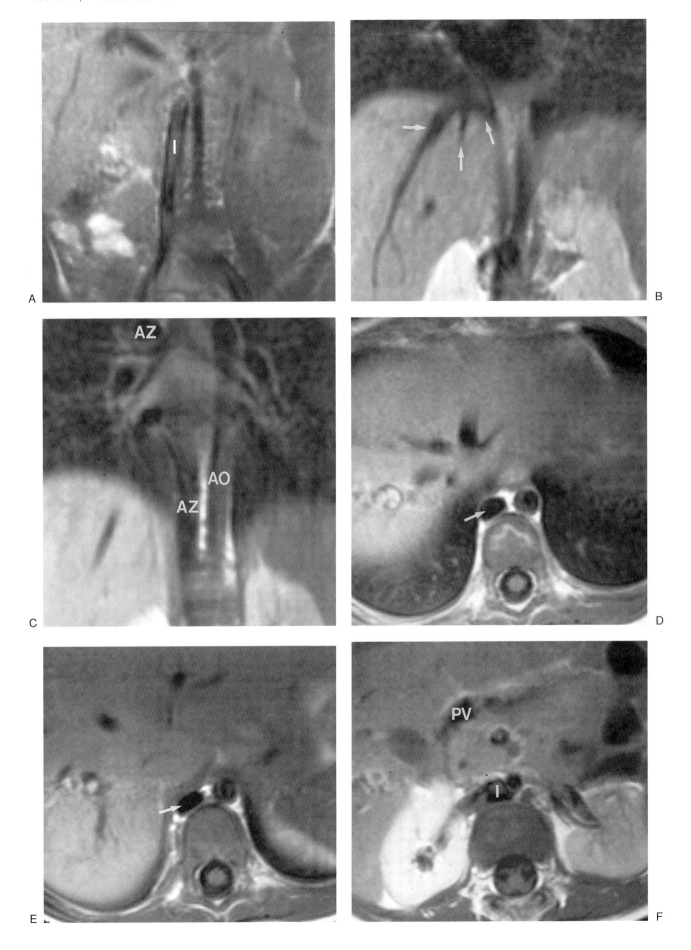

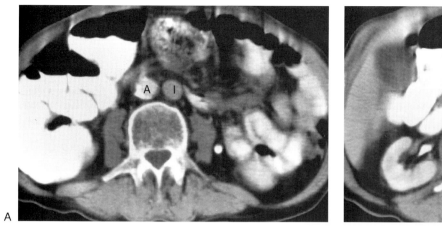

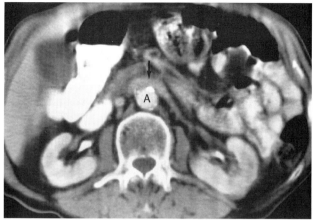

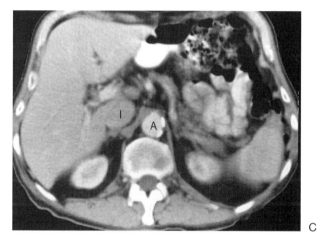

FIG. 34. Transposition of the IVC. **A:** Contrast-enhanced CT shows the anomalous infrarenal IVC (I) to the left of the calcified aorta (A). No right-sided IVC is present. **B:** Superiorly, the left IVC crosses the aorta anteriorly via the left renal vein *(arrow)*. **C:** The suprarenal IVC (I) is in its normal location.

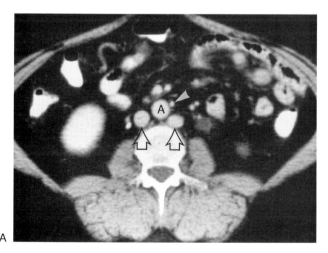

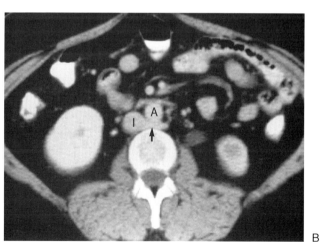

FIG. 35. Duplication of the IVC with retroaortic left renal vein. **A:** Contrast-enhanced CT image through the origin of the inferior mesenteric artery *(arrowhead)* shows two inferior vena cavae *(open arrow)*. A, aorta. **B:** Superiorly, the left IVC drains into the right IVC via a retroaortic left renal vein *(arrow)*. Above this level, only one IVC (I) is seen on the right.

FIG. 33. Interruption of the IVC with azygos continuation. **A,B,C:** Coronal MR images show a normal infrarenal IVC (I) and hepatic veins *(arrows)*. There is no intrahepatic IVC. Posteriorly, the azygos vein (AZ) is enlarged to the size of the aorta (AO). **D,E,F:** Transaxial MR images also show absence of the intrahepatic IVC and an enlarged azygos vein *(arrow)*. The infrarenal IVC (I) is normal. Note the decreased enhancement of the left kidney in this patient with acute pyelonephritis. PV, portal vein.

upper one third of the ureter with sharp turn toward the pedicle of the third or fourth lumbar vertebra producing a "reverse J" configuration), a definitive diagnosis by conventional imaging methods often requires concomitant opacification of the ureter and IVC (i.e., inferior vena cavography in conjunction with retrograde ureteral pyelography). Computed tomography can eliminate the need for vena cavography in corroborating the diagnosis, should this be considered necessary. With CT, the proximal right ureter can be seen coursing medially behind and then anteriorly around the IVC so as to encircle it partially (Fig. 36). The distal ureter may be better distended and delineated with the aid of a lower abdominal compression device (87).

Pathologic Conditions

Venous Thrombosis

Computed Tomography

Tumoral and nontumoral thromboses of the IVC can be identified but not differentiated from each other on CT scans, unless hypervascularity is shown in the tumoral thrombus by bolus dynamic CT (54,112,130,170,236, 256,266). Most of the tumoral thrombus in the IVC and renal veins arise from a primary renal or adrenal neoplasm, although extension from a uterine myoma (intravenous leiomyomatosis) may also occur (130,216). In cases of catheter-induced septic thrombosis, gas bubbles have been identified within the thrombi. In addition, inflammatory changes also can be observed surrounding the occluded vein (182) (Fig. 37). Thrombosis of the renal and gonadal veins has been similarly documented (92,230). Because the right renal vein is shorter and more obliquely oriented than the longer, more horizontal left renal vein, direct demonstration of thrombus is achieved less frequently on the right than on the left (Fig. 38). However, the use of thinner sections (e.g., 5 mm) coupled with dynamic incremental technique improves visualization of both renal veins (277). The involved segment of the vein can be either normal in caliber or substantially enlarged. Enlargement of the cava (or the renal vein) secondary to a thrombus can be strongly suggested on non-contrast-enhanced scans alone because dilatation is often more focal in cases of thrombosis in comparison to the more generalized dilatation seen secondary to increased blood

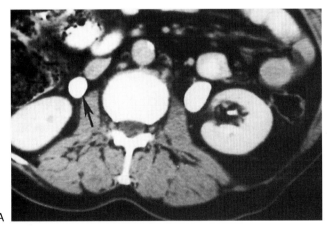

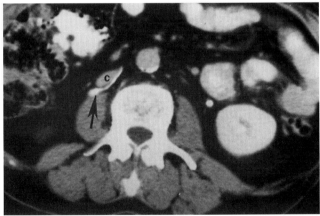

FIG. 36. Circumcaval ureter. **A:** Postcontrast CT image demonstrates a dilated proximal right ureter *(arrow)*. **B:** At 1 cm caudal to (A), the right ureter *(arrow)* passes behind the inferior vena cava (c). **C:** At 1 cm caudal to (B), the right ureter *(arrow)* lies anterior to the inferior vena cava (c). This is in contrast to the normal left ureter *(arrowhead)*, which lies along the anterolateral aspect of the psoas muscle.

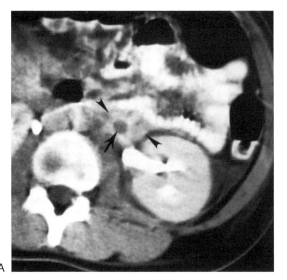
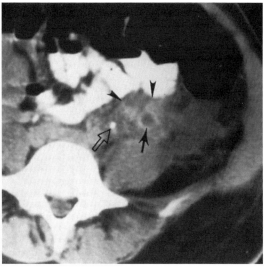

FIG. 37. Postpartum septic thrombosis of the left ovarian vein. Sequential postcontrast CT images demonstrate a thrombosed left ovarian vein *(arrow)* and its surrounding inflammatory changes *(arrowheads). Open arrow,* left ureter.

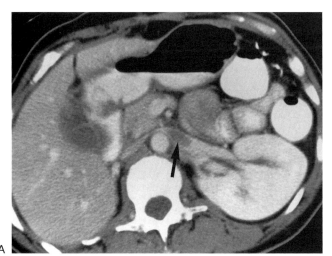
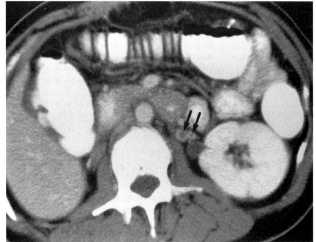
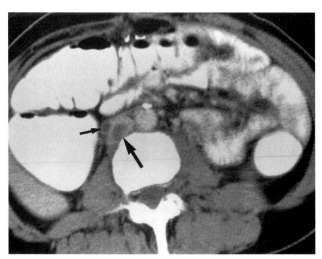

FIG. 38. Thrombosis of multiple vessels in a patient with ovarian cancer: CT appearance. Contrast-enhanced CT scan shows intraluminal hypodense filling defects representing thrombi within the opacified lumens of the left renal vein **(A)** *(arrow)*, left gonadal veins **(B)** *(arrows)*, and right gonadal vein *(small arrow)* and IVC *(large arrow)* **(C)**.

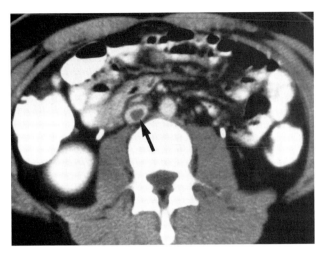

FIG. 39. Thrombus within the IVC. Contrast-enhanced CT shows a hypodense filling defect within the opacified lumen of the IVC *(arrow)*.

flow or increased vascular resistance at the level of the diaphragm and right atrium. In cases of complete caval obstruction, extensive venous collaterals may also be identified by CT (190). These include the paravertebral venous system and its communications with the ascending lumbar veins and the azygos/hemiazygos system; gonadal, periureteric, and other retroperitoneal veins; abdominal wall veins; hemorrhoidal venous plexus; and the portal venous system.

The definitive diagnosis of venous thrombosis by CT depends on demonstration of an intraluminal thrombus (Fig. 39). Whereas a fresh thrombus has a density similar to or higher than that of circulating blood, an old thrombus is of lower density than the surrounding blood on noncontrast scans. When the occlusion is complete, the involved segment remains unenhanced on postcontrast scans. In the case of chronic occlusion, the IVC may become atrophic and calcified (Fig. 40). In cases in which the venous occlusion is partial, the thrombus appears as a low-density filling defect surrounded by iodine-containing blood. However, caution must be taken not to confuse true intraluminal defects with those caused by laminar flow phenomenon; in the latter, the slower-flowing enhanced blood staying close to the wall and unopacified blood flowing centrally suggest a luminal thrombus (15,91). This "defect" is commonly seen in the IVC at the end of a bolus injection when a foot vein is used. At present, there are probably few if any indications for administering contrast media via a foot vein injection. Bolus injection of contrast material through an arm vein followed by serial dynamic scans is the preferred method for examining the patency of the venous system.

A "pseudothrombus" artifact also may occur in the suprarenal vena cava with a bolus injection or rapid infusion even when an arm vein is used (260). This defect is most pronounced just at and cephalad to the renal vein origins, although it can be seen as high as the intrahepatic vena cava (Fig. 41). It is caused by the poor mixing between the densely opacified renal venous effluent and the less densely opacified infrarenal caval blood. This artifact can be differentiated from a true thrombus by its unsharp border, a higher attenuation, and the use of delayed scans.

Thrombosis of the ovarian vein, classically associated with postpartum (puerperal) endometritis, pelvic inflammatory disease, and gynecologic surgery (226,230), also can occur in patients with malignant tumors, particularly those undergoing chemotherapy (119) (see Fig. 38). On CT, puerperal ovarian vein thrombosis appear as a well-defined tubular retroperitoneal mass extending from the pelvis to the infrarenal IVC. The mass corresponds to the dilated gonadal vein and usually contains a central low-attenuation region representing thrombus (226). Other common CT findings include a nonhomogeneously enhancing pelvic mass, and fluid in an enlarged uterus. Inflammatory changes also may be seen around the occluded vein (see Fig. 37).

Magnetic Resonance Imaging

On SE images, venous thrombus produces an intraluminal signal and can be differentiated from slow flow by comparing the signal intensities on the first and second

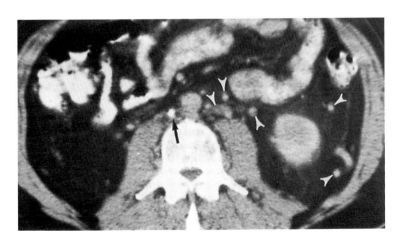

FIG. 40. Chronic vena caval thrombosis. Postcontrast CT image demonstrates a calcified, atrophic inferior vena cava *(arrow)*. Note multiple enhancing collateral vessels in the retroperitoneum *(arrowheads)*.

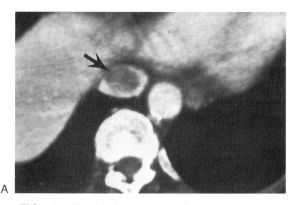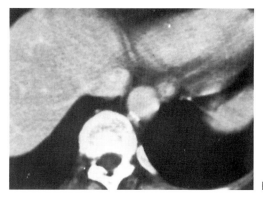

A   B

FIG. 41. Pseudothrombus in the inferior vena cava. **A:** CT image at the level of the diaphragm obtained 1 min after a bolus intravenous injection of contrast material into an arm vein shows a central, hypodense defect within the IVC *(arrow).* **B:** Repeat image at the same level several minutes later demonstrates uniform enhancement of the IVC, without evidence of a thrombus.

echoes or by using a phase-sensitive imaging sequence (73,78,114,115). Additional MR manifestations of caval thrombosis include focal dilation of the vena cava and the presence of venous collateral vessels that appear as tubular structures emitting little or no signal. Magnetic resonance imaging may distinguish tumor thrombus from bland thrombus on the basis of their signal characteristics. Magnetic resonance imaging features of tumor thrombus include isointensity with the primary neoplasm and loss of definition of the vena caval wall. High signal intensity on first and second echo images is indicative of a bland thrombus. Lack of enhancement after intravenous administration of gadolinium also favors a bland thrombus (88) (Fig. 42). Thrombi of intermediate signal intensity can be seen in both entities. The reliability of MRI in differentiating between bland and tumor thrombi is yet to be determined in a large group of patients.

Transverse views are often sufficient for the diagnosis of caval thrombosis; sagittal and coronal sections more directly display the cephalocaudal extent of the thrombus. The latter information is particularly important for the planning of resection of tumor thrombus (Fig. 42).

In contradistinction to SE images, venous thrombus appears as an area of lower signal on GRE images. Because GRE takes less time than SE, the former is the preferred technique. MRA based on the GRE sequence is especially effective in demonstrating the entire venous system. However, false positive diagnosis may occur at the confluence of vessels where mixing of blood may reduce the signal of flowing blood, simulating a thrombus. Likewise, subacute thrombus, which is often hyperintense, may be confused with flowing blood and lead to a false negative diagnosis. Both of these potential problems can be resolved by repeating the GRE sequence after intravenous administration of Gd compound. In one study (10), a combination of SE and GRE images significantly increased the accuracy of diagnosis of abdominal venous thrombosis.

Membranous Obstruction

Membranous or segmental obstruction of the IVC is a common cause of chronic Budd-Chiari syndrome in Asia and South Africa. Although patients usually present in adulthood, many regard this condition as a congenital anomaly (273). In membranous obstruction of the IVC, the hepatic segment of the IVC is obstructed by a fibromuscular membrane or replaced by a cordlike fibrous tissue. In the former, the IVC usually appears normal and the membrane is rarely seen on CT scans, unless it is calcified (136). In the latter, the IVC is narrowed and obliterated segmentally. In both situations (160), CT also may show obliteration of hepatic veins, systemic collaterals (such as enlarged azygos vein), cirrhosis, portal hypertension, hepatic neoplasms, and ascites.

Primary Neoplasm

Leiomyosarcoma originating from the wall of the IVC is a rare retroperitoneal neoplasm that occurs most commonly in older women (26). Leiomyosarcomas most frequently are located between the diaphragm and the renal veins. Although they can be purely extrinsic or intrinsic (intramural or intraluminal), most commonly they have both an extrinsic and an intraluminal component. Contrast-enhanced CT or MR often shows a heterogeneously enhancing, well-circumscribed, right-sided retroperitoneal mass inseparable from the IVC, with displacement of adjacent organs such as the right kidney, pancreas, duodenum, and aorta (254) (Figs. 43,44). In upper IVC leiomyosarcomas, differentiation from a primary right adrenal carcinoma with venous extension may be difficult.

Intracaval Filters

Computed tomography is a simple noninvasive method for evaluating the position of the IVC filters and its rela-

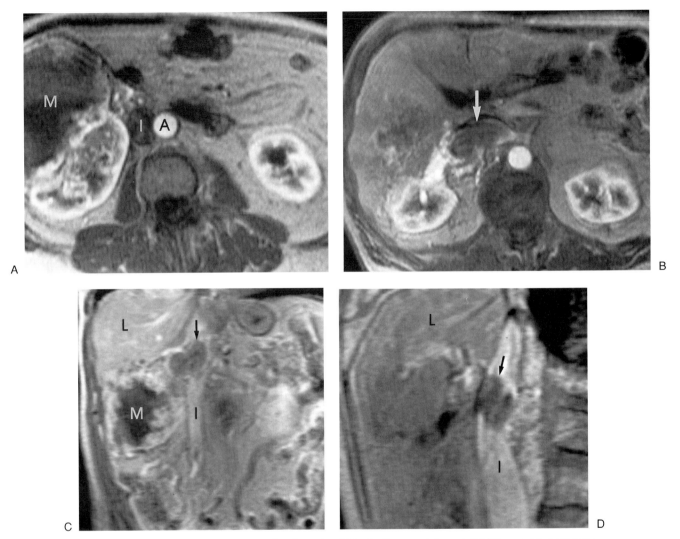

FIG. 42. Renal cell carcinoma extending into the IVC. **A:** Transaxial post-Gd T1-weighted FLASH image (140/4/80°) shows a large necrotic right renal mass (M). A, aorta; I, IVC. **B:** Superiorly, enhancing tumor thrombus *(arrow)* is present within the dilated IVC. Coronal **(C)** and sagittal **(D)** images clearly demonstrate the cephalic extent of the tumor thrombus *(arrow)* within the infrahepatic IVC (I). L, liver.

tion to the renal veins. It can reveal filter perforation and retroperitoneal hematoma (179). Likewise, patency of the IVC, filter position, trapped thrombi, and the presence of vascular obstruction and turbulence can be evaluated with MRI in patients with certain low-artifact caval filters (246,247). Spin echo and GRE images play complementary roles in such an evaluation. In our experience, caval filters often yield fewer artifacts on MR images than CT scans.

Clinical Application

Ultrasound is a well-established technique for evaluating the IVC (193,229). Ultrasound is superior to CT for identifying the echogenic membrane or the fibrous cord

in the IVC (160). It also can detect caval thrombus from the level of the renal veins to the right atrium in most patients. However, the inability of ultrasound to clearly demonstrate the rest of the IVC because of overlying bowel gas has limited its use (127).

Although there are no data comparing the accuracy of CT and venography in detecting nontumoral thrombosis of the IVC and its major branches, CT is reported to have a similar overall accuracy in the detection of IVC and main renal vein invasion by renal cell carcinoma. In one study (266), the overall accuracy of CT was 93% in detecting inferior vena caval invasion and 82% in detecting main renal vein invasion. It is often harder to be certain of tumor thrombus in the right renal vein, which is shorter than its counterpart on the left. Computed tomography is not able to detect tumor

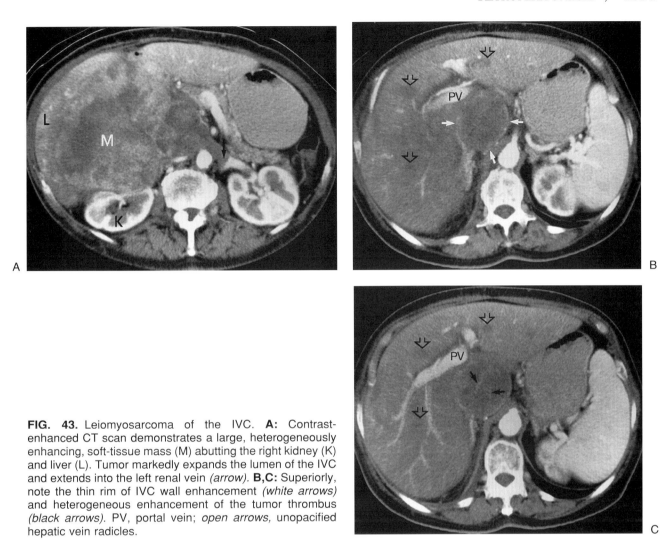

FIG. 43. Leiomyosarcoma of the IVC. **A:** Contrast-enhanced CT scan demonstrates a large, heterogeneously enhancing, soft-tissue mass (M) abutting the right kidney (K) and liver (L). Tumor markedly expands the lumen of the IVC and extends into the left renal vein *(arrow).* **B,C:** Superiorly, note the thin rim of IVC wall enhancement *(white arrows)* and heterogeneous enhancement of the tumor thrombus *(black arrows).* PV, portal vein; *open arrows,* unopacified hepatic vein radicles.

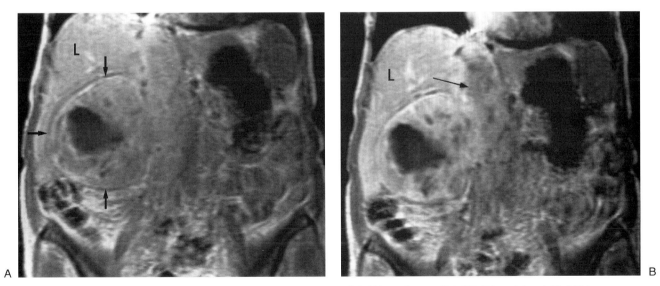

FIG. 44. Leiomyosarcoma of the IVC. Coronal pre-Gd **(A)** and post-Gd **(B)** T1-weighted FLASH images (140/4/80°) show a large retroperitoneal mass *(short arrows)* with peripheral enhancement. Central hypointensity results from tissue necrosis or cystic degeneration, commonly seen in leiomyosarcomas. Heterogeneously enhancing tumor extends into a dilated IVC *(long arrow).* L, liver.

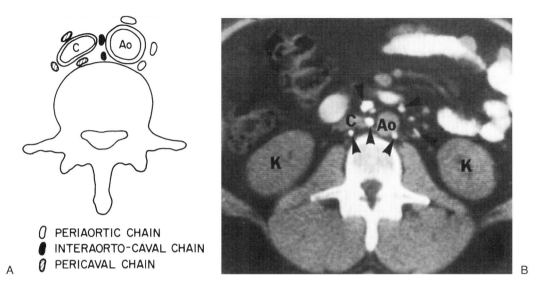

FIG. 45. A: Schematic drawing denoting distribution of periaortic and pericaval lymph nodes. **B:** CT image in a patient after lymphangiography, showing normal distribution of retroperitoneal lymph nodes *(arrowheads)*. Ao, aorta; C, inferior vena cava; K, kidney.

thrombus in intrarenal venous branches; however, this is of limited clinical significance, as the presence of only intrarenal vein invasion by tumor does not alter surgical management (266).

Although earlier studies indicate that MRI and CT are equally accurate in demonstrating vena caval thrombus (78,114), a more recent study has shown that MRI is equal to venocavography but more sensitive than CT and ultrasound for detecting tumor thrombus in the main renal vein and the IVC in 431 patients with surgically staged renal cell carcinoma (127). The ability to evaluate the IVC without iodinated contrast material and the ability to display the entire venous system using projectional MRA should make MRI the ideal technique for evaluating patients with suspected venous pathology. In spite of this, because of the limited availability of MR imagers and because of the ease and speed with which CT can survey the entire retroperitoneum, CT remains the screening procedure of choice in most institutions. Furthermore, many of the venous abnormalities are detected incidentally on CT studies performed for other unrelated indications. Magnetic resonance imaging, nevertheless, should be performed in patients who have a contraindication to iodinated contrast material or in patients in whom the prior CT findings are equivocal.

LYMPH NODES

Normal Anatomy

Normal unopacified lymph nodes are routinely seen as small, flat, soft tissue densities on CT scans ranging from 3 to 10 mm in size (258). Short-axis measurements should be used to minimize errors caused by node orientation.

In the retroperitoneum, lymph nodes can be found adjacent to the anterior, posterior, medial, and lateral walls of the IVC and aorta (Fig. 45). Lymph nodes also can be seen as nonenhancing soft-tissue densities in the root of the mesentery and along the course of the major venous structures draining to the IVC and portal vein (233). In the pelvis, lymph nodes can be identified in close proximity with the iliac vessels. Although less commonly seen, lymph nodes also can be found anterior to the psoas muscle and adjacent to the posterior iliac crest (35,267). Although the internal architecture of a lymph node generally is not discernible on CT, benign fibrolipomatous changes have been shown on CT scans on rare occasions (Fig. 46).

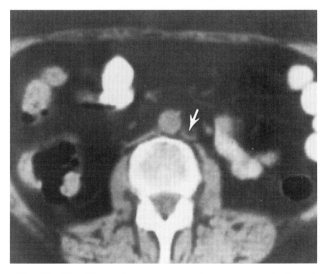

FIG. 46. Fibrolipomatous changes in a para-aortic lymph node. Note that the central portion *(arrow)* of this lymph node has an attenuation value similar to that of retroperitoneal fat.

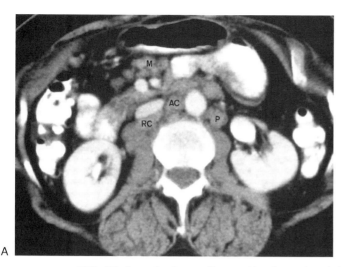 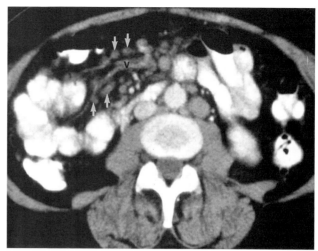

FIG. 47. Lymphadenopathy resulting from chronic lymphocytic leukemia: CT appearance. **A:** Enlarged nodes are present in para-aortic (P), interaortocaval (AC), retrocaval (RC), and mesenteric (M) regions. **B:** Small nodes *(arrows)* extend along mesenteric veins (V).

Normal abdominal and pelvic lymph nodes can likewise be seen on MRI (58,281). However, because of their small size and the poorer spatial resolution of MRI, normal nodes are seen less frequently on MRI studies than on CT scans. Furthermore, lymph nodes opacified by lymphographic contrast cannot be distinguished from retroperitoneal fat because of the similar relaxation times between fat and lymphographic contrast material (30). As with CT, the internal architecture of a normal lymph node generally cannot be evaluated with MRI. The signal intensity of normal nodes usually is similar to that of pathologically enlarged lymph nodes.

Pathologic Conditions

Computed Tomography

The diagnosis of retroperitoneal lymphadenopathy by CT is based upon recognition of nodal enlargement, sometimes concomitant with displacement or obscuration of normal structures in far advanced disease (2,18,25, 71,139,147,212,227). Except in unusually lean or cachetic patients, enlarged lymph nodes generally are well profiled by surrounding fat. Retrocrural and portahepatis nodes should not exceed 6 mm, whereas the upper limit of normal for gastrohepatic ligament nodes is 8 mm (33,61). Retroperitoneal, celiac axis, mesenteric, and pelvic nodes greater than 10 mm in size are considered abnormal (Figs. 47,48), but multiple, slightly smaller (8- to 10-mm) nodes in these regions should be viewed with suspicion. A CT-guided percutaneous needle biopsy or a follow-up study may be indicated in such problem cases.

The CT presentation of malignant lymphadenopathy may vary from (a) one or several discrete enlarged lymph nodes, to (b) a more conglomerate group of contiguous enlarged nodes similar in size to the aorta or IVC, to (c) a large homogeneous mass, in which individual nodes are no longer recognizable, obscuring the contours of normal surrounding structures (Fig. 49). Massive enlargement of retroaortic and retrocaval nodes may cause anterior displacement of these vessels.

Because intranodal architecture is not discernible on CT, lymph nodes that are normal in size but infiltrated with neoplastic cells cannot be distinguished as abnormal by CT. Furthermore, CT usually cannot differentiate between benign and malignant causes of lymph node enlargement. Diffuse lymph node enlargement secondary to

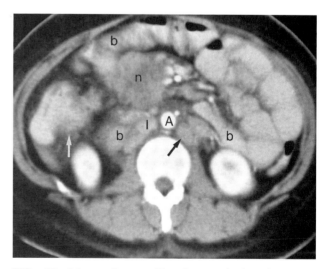

FIG. 48. Adenopathy resulting from colonic adenocarcinoma. Contrast-enhanced CT scan shows left para-aortic *(black arrow)* and mesenteric adenopathy (n), as well as an ulcerating mass *(white arrow)* in the ascending colon. Note the slight hyperdensity of bowel (b) distinguishing it from adenopathy. A, aorta; I, IVC.

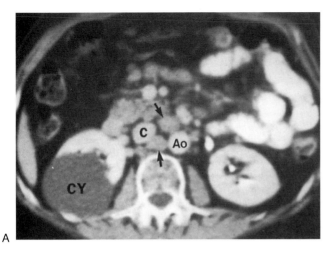

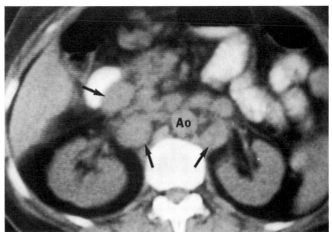

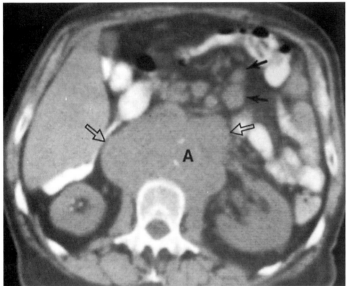

FIG. 49. Retroperitoneal lymphadenopathy in three different patients with lymphoma. **A:** Mild lymph node enlargement. Postcontrast CT image shows that individual lymph nodes (arrows) are enlarged, but their discrete outlines have been maintained. Ao, aorta; C, inferior vena cava; CY, renal cyst. **B:** Moderate lymph node enlargement. Enlarged lymph nodes have coalesced to form soft-tissue masses (arrows), each of which is slightly larger than the adjacent aorta (Ao). **C:** Homogeneous soft-tissue mass (open arrows), resulting in obscuration of retroperitoneal vascular structure. Note that the location of the aorta (A) is identified by virtue of its mural calcification. Arrows, enlarged mesenteric nodes.

viral or granulomatous disease cannot be differentiated from lymphoma or metastases based on CT findings alone (153), although the massive type of conglomeration described almost never is seen with the benign conditions. The inability of CT to distinguish benign from malignant causes of lymphadenopathy poses a problem for patients with AIDS-related disease, because benign nodal hyperplasia, mycobacterial infections, lymphoma, and metastases from Kaposi sarcoma (KS) occur with equal frequency in these patients (181). Although 80% of hyperdense (relative to iliopsoas muscle) lymph nodes seen on dynamic sequential bolus CT scans in patients with AIDS are caused by the epidemic form of KS, hyperdense lymphadenopathy can occur in other AIDS-related diseases as well (110). Percutaneous needle biopsy of the enlarged nodes under CT guidance is often needed to establish a histologic diagnosis.

A definite CT diagnosis may be possible in Whipple disease. In this disease, the attenuation value of the enlarged lymph nodes often is quite low, ranging from +10 HU to +30 HU (157) (Fig. 50). This relatively low density most likely is caused by the deposition of fat and fatty acids in the lymph nodes. Enlarged, low-density lymph nodes also may be seen in patients with *Mycobacterium* infection (more common with *M. tuberculosis* than with *M. avium-intracellulare*), histoplasmosis, testicular neoplasms, particularly teratocarcinoma, epidermoid carcinoma of the genitourinary tract, and rarely in patients with lymphoma (207,208) (Fig. 51). Usually, this is the result of necrosis or liquefaction within the neoplasm. Calcified enlarged nodes may be postinflammatory or can be seen in mucinous carcinoma, sarcomas, and treated lymphomas. Rarely, calcifications may be seen even in untreated lymphomas (Fig. 52).

Benign and malignant lymphadenopathy may exhibit mild (mean, +6 HU) to pronounced (mean, +61 HU) enhancement after intravenous administration of iodinated contrast material with maximal enhancement occurring 1 to 2 minutes after injection (118,202,203) (Fig. 53). Contrast enhancement may be homogeneous,

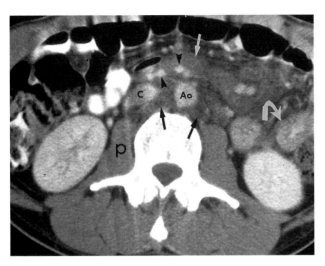

FIG. 50. Whipple disease. Enlarged retroperitoneal *(black arrows)* and mesenteric *(white arrow)* lymph nodes are present. Note that the attenuation value of the lymph nodes is lower than that of psoas muscle (p). Ao, aorta; c, inferior vena cava; *black arrowhead,* superior mesenteric vessels; *curved white arrow,* thickened jejuneum.

nonhomogeneous, or peripheral. Lymph nodes that have a low attenuation value (<30 HU) on noncontrast scans and exhibit peripheral enhancement are suggestive of *M. tuberculosis* infection (203).

Other entities, such as retroperitoneal fibrosis, perianeurysmal fibrosis, and false aortic aneurysm (see Fig. 23) also may exhibit findings on CT resembling malignant lymphadenopathy (1,18,239). However, the soft-tissue mass seen in idiopathic retroperitoneal fibrosis or perianeurysmal fibrosis usually has a more regular border than that seen with malignant lymphadenopathy. False aortic aneurysms usually can be distinguished from lymphadenopathy on postcontrast scans. Although the inferior extent of the right crus of the diaphragm or vascular abnormalities and anomalies—such as an enlarged gonadal vein (see Fig. 28), a duplicated IVC, and a dilated azygos or hemiazygos vein—could conceivably be confused with an enlarged lymph node, careful examination of multiple contiguous scans and concomitant use of intravenous iodinated contrast medium can separate these entities from lymphadenopathy.

Magnetic Resonance Imaging

Abnormal retroperitoneal lymph nodes are identified on the basis of nodal enlargement rather than by any characteristic signal intensity (149). Although in vitro study has shown that lymph nodes containing metastases have a significantly longer T2 than normal and hyperplastic nodes (264), in vivo tissue characterization based on relaxation times or signal intensities has not been possible (59,149). Enlarged lymph nodes resulting from malignant

disease cannot be distinguished from those resulting from benign processes. Furthermore, lymph nodes that are of normal size but are partially or totally replaced with a neoplasm will not be identified as abnormal by MRI.

Abnormal lymph nodes usually have a homogeneous MRI appearance, but they may appear nonhomogeneous as a result of calcification or necrosis. In one study, more than 60% of high-grade non-Hodgkin lymphoma (NHL) nodes had a nonhomogeneous MR appearance (corresponding to necrosis) on T2-weighted images in contrast to low-grade NHL nodes, which were mostly homogeneous. Furthermore, patients with high-grade NHL and a homogeneous signal intensity pattern had a better survival rate than those with a nonhomogeneous pattern (213).

On T1-weighted images, the signal intensity of lymph nodes is slightly higher than that of iliopsoas muscle and diaphragmatic crura and is much lower than the signal intensity of fat (Fig. 54). On rare occasions, lymph nodes may be nearly isointense to fat on T1-weighted images because of hemorrhage or melanin (Fig. 55). On images obtained with longer repetition times or longer echo delay times, the contrast between lymph nodes and muscle increases, and that between nodes and fat decreases. Thus, on T2-weighted images, lymph nodes are easily distinguished from muscle and diaphragmatic crura but may be difficult to differentiate from surrounding retroperitoneal fat because of their similar signal intensities (58,149). In general, abnormal lymph nodes are better demonstrated on the T1-weighted and proton-density-weighted images. Fat-suppression techniques such as excitation-spoiling T2-weighted SE or short tau inversion recovery (STIR) are useful at demonstrating lymph nodes in the upper abdomen in emaciated patients, as lymph nodes have higher signal intensity than surrounding tissue (106). The multiplanar capability of MRI has not facilitated the detection of lymphadenopathy. Images obtained in the sagittal or coronal planes usually do not contribute additional clinically useful information.

Lymph nodes are easily separated from blood vessels on either SE or GRE images without the use of intravenous contrast medium. As a result, displacement or encasement of blood vessels by lymphadenopathy is well demonstrated by MRI (Figs. 54,56). However, oral contrast medium should be used to facilitate differentiation of bowel loops and lymph nodes by MRI. This is especially important in patients with sparse retroperitoneal fat in whom such a distinction is often difficult.

Clinical Applications

Lymphoma

The accuracy of CT in detecting intra-abdominal and pelvic lymphadenopathy in patients with lymphoma has been studied by several groups of investigators. Results

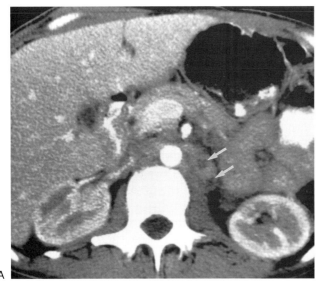

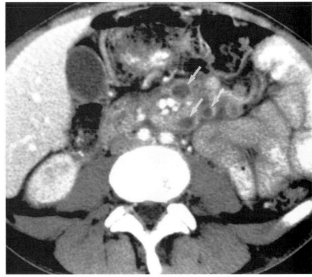

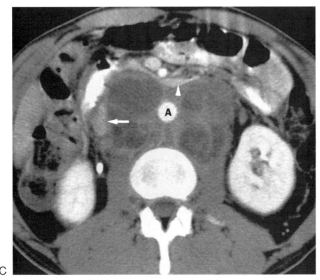

FIG. 51. Low-density lymph nodes. In a patient with AIDS, contrast-enhanced CT scans show hypodense, enlarged nodes *(arrows)* in the para-aortic region **(A)** and small bowel mesentery **(B)** from culture-proven *Mycobacteria avium-intracellulare* (MAI). In another patient with metastatic seminoma **(C)**, contrast-enhanced CT scan shows hypodense adenopathy surrounding the aorta. Note the elevation of the aorta (A), lateral displacement of the IVC *(arrow)*, and anterior displacement of the left renal vein *(arrowhead)*.

from these studies are generally influenced by the types of CT scanners used, expertise of the interpreters, and types of patients selected. The reported accuracy has ranged from 68% to 100%, with a false positive rate varying from 0% to 25% (2,18,19,25,34,65,153,171, 212,276). False positive cases largely result from confusion with unopacified bowel loops or normal vascular structures, a problem that is easily resolved by rigorous attention to technique. False positive diagnoses also can result from misinterpretation of lymphadenopathy secondary to benign inflammatory disease, as malignant. False negative interpretations almost always are secondary to the inability to recognize replaced but normal-sized or minimally enlarged lymph nodes as abnormal. Even with increasing experience in scan interpretation, coupled with meticulous scanning techniques, this limitation remains a problem for CT and accounts for most of the false negative interpretations.

Bipedal lymphangiography (LAG) has been the tech-

nique employed in the past to investigate possible retroperitoneal lymph node abnormalities. However, the method is time consuming, occasionally difficult to perform, and uncomfortable for the patient. In patients with severe cardiopulmonary disease, LAG may be medically contraindicated. The introduction of CT has provided a method for easy assessment of the retroperitoneal lymph nodes and for simultaneous evaluation of lymph nodes and organs elsewhere in the abdomen. Efforts have been made by several investigators to compare the clinical efficacy of LAG with that of CT. Although most investigators, including ourselves, found CT to have an accuracy comparable to LAG in detecting retroperitoneal and pelvic lymph node involvement by lymphoma (18,19,65,69,240,276), others (34) showed LAG to be a slightly more accurate test in evaluating patients with clinically early-stage Hodgkin disease. However, all groups found CT capable of detecting lymph nodes in areas where the lymphographic contrast

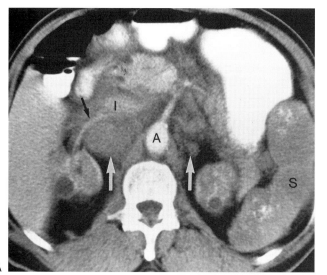
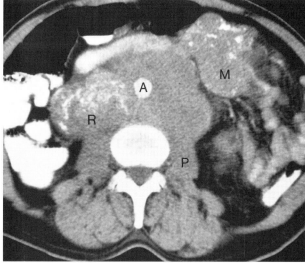

FIG. 52. Calcified lymphoma before treatment. **A:** Contrast-enhanced CT scan through the origin of the superior mesenteric artery demonstrates enlarged retrocaval and para-aortic nodes *(arrows).* Amorphous calcifications are noted in focal splenic lesions. Small renal cysts are present in both kidneys. S, spleen; *black arrow,* encased right renal artery. **B:** CT scan obtained 7 cm caudad shows calcified mesenteric (M) and retrocaval lymphadenopathy (R), an extremely atypical feature for untreated lymphoma. The rest of the retroperitoneal adenopathy is of soft-tissue density. Note anterior displacement of the aorta (A) and obscuration of the psoas (P) margin.

medium does not reach, such as nodes around the celiac axis, retrocrural space, renal hilus, and splenic and hepatic hila, as well as in the mesentery (Fig. 57). Lymphomatous infiltration of various intra-abdominal organs, such as the liver, the spleen, the kidneys, and the gastrointestinal tract, also can be seen on CT scans (Figs. 58–61), although the sensitivity of CT in detecting early or minimal parenchymal lymphoma is low (2,34,176,240). Such nodal and extranodal areas fre-

quently are involved at presentation with NHL. Demonstration of lymphomatous involvement of iliopsoas muscle, adrenal glands, gynecologic organs, and pancreas by CT also has been reported (94). Computed tomography also may be superior to LAG in delineating the exact extent of intra-abdominal nodal involvement because lymph nodes totally replaced by lymphoma are not opacified at all by LAG.

There is nearly unanimous agreement (36,48,147,187)

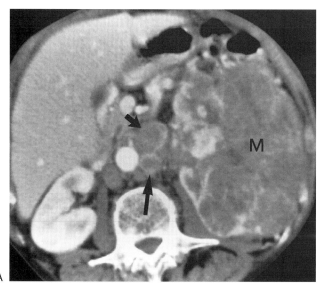
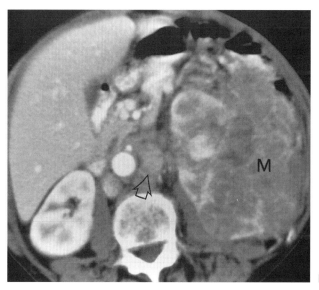

FIG. 53. Enhancing adenopathy resulting from metastatic renal cell carcinoma. Contrast-enhanced CT scans show para-aortic adenopathy demonstrating **(A)** heterogeneous *(short arrow),* rim *(long arrow),* and **(B)** homogeneous *(open arrow)* enhancement. Note the large renal mass (M).

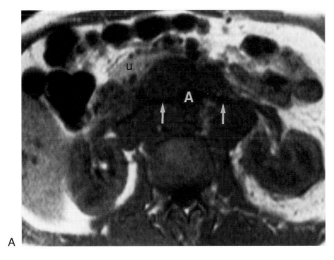

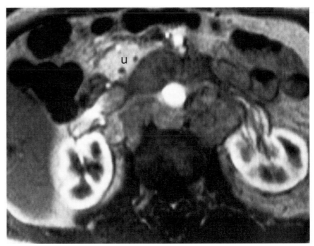

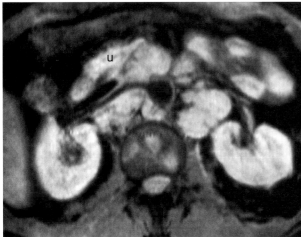

FIG. 54. Extensive adenopathy resulting from metastatic prostate adenocarcinoma. **A:** Transaxial T1-weighted FLASH image (140/4/80°) shows lobulated circumaortic (A) tissue encasing the renal arteries *(arrows).* **B:** Transaxial post-Gd T1-weighted FLASH image (140/4/80°) shows significant nodal enhancement. Note the anterior displacement of the aorta, a feature commonly seen with lymphadenopathy but not in retroperitoneal fibrosis. **C:** Transaxial post-Gd FATSAT proton density-weighted SE image (2400/15) shows the increased sensitivity to contrast enhancement using this sequence. U, uncinate process.

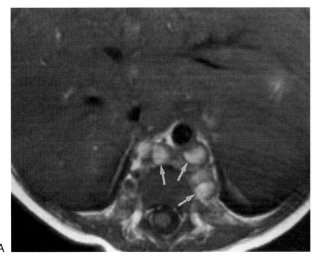

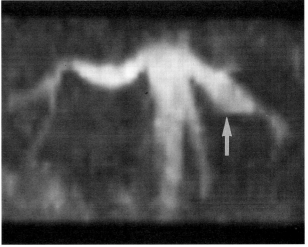

FIG. 55. Hemorrhagic adenopathy in a patient with Kawasaki disease. **A:** Transaxial gated T1-weighted SE image (729/15) shows multiple hyperintense enlarged retrocrural nodes *(arrows)* reflecting hemorrhagic contents. **B:** Maximum intensity projection (MIP) image of an MR angiogram (3D-FISP, 30/7/25°) shows a fusiform left renal artery aneurysm *(arrow).*

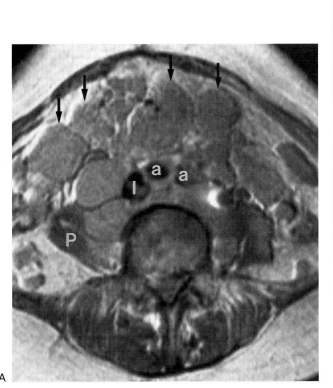

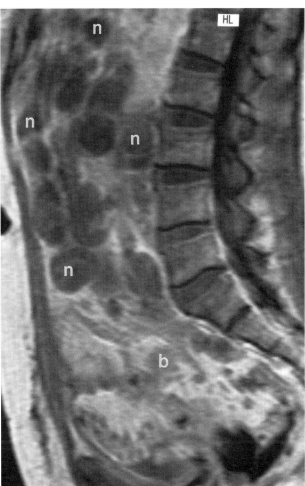

A

B

FIG. 56. Lymphoma. **A:** Transaxial proton-density-weighted fast spin echo (FSE) image (3500/19) shows enlarged paracaval, common iliac, and mesenteric *(arrows)* nodes slightly hyperintense to muscle. Note the anterolateral displacement of the right psoas muscle (P). a, common iliac arteries; I, IVC. **B:** Sagittal T1-weighted FLASH image (140/4/80°) better demonstrates the cephalocaudad extent of the mesenteric adenopathy (n). Note the nodes are hypointense to bowel (B).

that CT should assume the primary radiologic role in staging patients with NHL because of the tendency of this disease to exhibit bulky lymphadenopathy in multiple sites and because of the high incidence of mesenteric lymph node involvement (>50%). Lymphangiography is rarely needed in this group of patients. In one study (204), clinical stage would have been incorrect in 5% and initial management incorrect in 3% of patients with NHL if LAG had been omitted entirely from diagnostic evaluation. Other radiologic studies such as upper gastrointestinal series and barium enema are necessary only when specific symptoms of a patient suggest involvement of these organs.

Controversy regarding whether CT or LAG should be used for the initial staging of Hodgkin disease has become less heated in recent years. Although some centers continue to use LAG as a primary imaging method and use CT only as a complementary tool in a few selected cases,

others, including ourselves, have replaced LAG with CT as the primary imaging method. A positive CT scan eliminates the need for a lymphangiogram. A negative CT scan can exclude nodal disease with a high degree of confidence. Lymphangiography certainly is valuable when the CT scans are equivocal, and, after a negative CT scan, it can be reassuring. Moreover, in some instances, it may detect replaced but normal-sized lymph nodes. Staging laparotomy is still required for many patients at the time of initial presentation because of the inability of CT to detect microscopic disease in both lymph nodes and the spleen.

In addition to being used as an initial staging procedure, CT also has been used to follow response to various methods of treatment. In institutions where both CT and LAG are used for the initial staging of patients with newly diagnosed lymphomas, post-LAG plain radiographs rather than CT are obtained serially to monitor

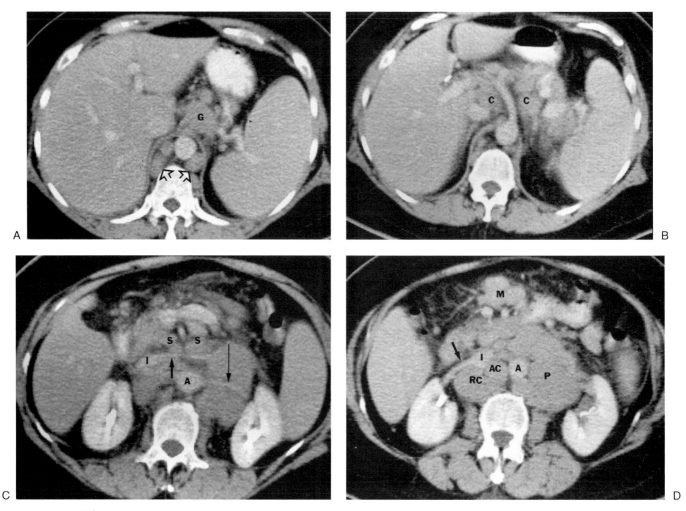

FIG. 57. Adenopathy in a patient with lymphoma. **A–D:** Contrast-enhanced CT scans demonstrate extensive adenopathy involving the retrocrural *(open arrow)*, gastrohepatic ligament (G), celiac axis (C) superior mesenteric artery axis (S), para-aortic (P), interaortocaval (AC), retrocaval (RC), and mesenteric (M) regions. Note the encasement of the left renal artery *(long arrow)* and both renal veins *(short arrows)* as well as the splenomegaly. A, aorta; I, IVC.

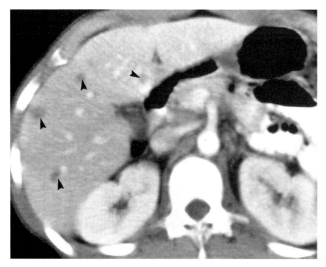

FIG. 58. Hepatic lymphoma. Multiple hypodense lesions *(arrowheads)* representing lymphoma are present in both lobes of the liver.

posttreatment response because of the lower cost. A repeat CT study is performed only when progression of disease is detected on surveillance radiographs (196). It should be emphasized that in patients with massive lymphadenopathy on the initial study, the follow-up scans may not always revert to normal even when patients are in complete clinical remission. Fibrotic changes secondary to prior radiation or chemotherapy may appear either as discrete, albeit smaller, soft-tissue masses or as a thin sheath causing obscuration of the discrete outlines of the aorta and IVC (Fig. 62). Unfortunately, CT is incapable of differentiating between viable residual neoplasm and such fibrotic changes caused by chemotherapy or radiotherapy. Additional follow-up study, or surgical or percutaneous biopsy, is often necessary for such a differentiation. Despite this limitation, CT provides a more accurate delineation of progression or regression of the disease process than any other radiologic procedure (150).

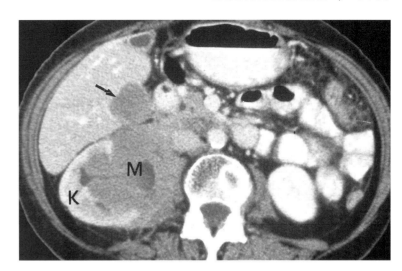

FIG. 59. Renal lymphoma. Postcontrast CT image demonstrates a large, irregular hypodense mass (M) infiltrating the right kidney (K). Note the obscuration of the right psoas muscle. *Arrow,* Hepatic lymphoma.

Testicular Neoplasms

Testicular neoplasms are the most common solid cancers in male patients 15 to 34 years old, accounting for a significant percentage of all cancer deaths in this group. Histologically, the germ cell testicular tumors are composed of different cell types. For therapeutic purposes, they are classified into seminomatous and nonseminomatous categories. Although most seminomas are treated by radiation therapy, most nonseminomatous (and some seminomatous) tumors are treated by retroperitoneal lymphadenectomy or chemotherapy (38). Accurate preoperative determination of tumor extent helps in the design of radiation ports for seminomas and in the choice of initial mode of treatment (surgery versus chemotherapy) in the nonseminomatous group. Testicular tumors tend to metastasize via the lymphatic system. A thorough understanding of the distribution and pattern of lymphatic spread by testicular cancer is helpful in interpreting CT findings. In general, the testicular lymphatics, which fol-low the course of the testicular arteries and veins, drain directly into the lymph nodes in or near the renal hilus (Fig. 63). These lymph nodes (sentinel nodes) lie lateral to the lumbar nodes and are usually not opacified by bipedal LAG (40). After involvement of these sentinel nodes, the lumbar para-aortic nodes become involved (unilaterally or bilaterally), followed by spread to the mediastinal and supraclavicular nodes or hematogenous dissemination to the lungs, liver, and brain.

Data from a large surgical series showed nodal metastases from the right testis tend to be midline, with primary zones of involvement being the interaortocaval, precaval and preaortic lymph node groups (57) (Fig. 64). Although previous studies showed that the lymphatic drainage from the right testis not infrequently "crosses over" to the left side without involving the ipsilateral side, involvement of the contralateral left para-aortic node (or nodes) without concomitant involvement of interaortocaval nodes in pa-

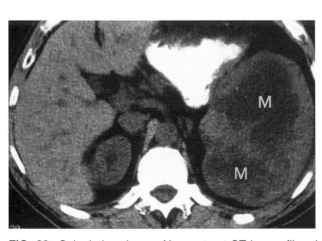

FIG. 60. Splenic lymphoma. Noncontrast CT image filmed at narrow windows shows multiple ill-defined hypodense splenic masses (M).

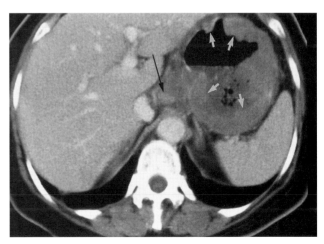

FIG. 61. Gastric lymphoma. Contrast-enhanced CT scan demonstrates lobulated gastric wall thickening *(white arrows)* and an enlarged gastrohepatic ligament lymph node *(black arrow).*

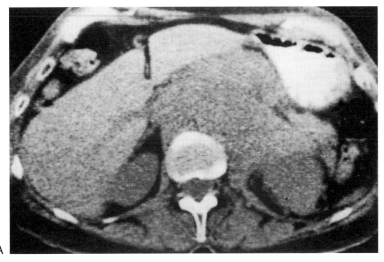

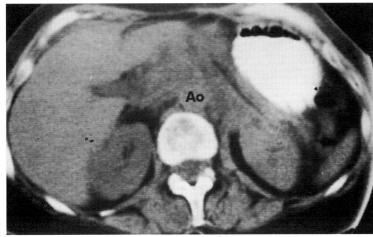

FIG. 62. Residual fibrosis after chemotherapy. **A:** Initial image in this patient with Hodgkin disease shows massive retroperitoneal lymphadenopathy obscuring the aorta and IVC. The patient was started on chemotherapy, and serial CT images documented gradual improvement. **B:** A follow-up study 2 years after (A) demonstrates persistent residual soft-tissue density partially obscuring the aorta (Ao). Surgical biopsy of this area showed only residual fibrosis.

tients with a right-sided testicular tumor was not found. If lymph nodes in the right renal hilar region are normal in size, then lymph nodes in the right suprahilar area are always uninvolved.

Nodal metastases from the left testis show a predilection for left para-aortic nodal groups, followed by preaortic and interaortocaval nodal groups (Fig. 65). In contradistinction to right-sided testicular drainage, left suprahilar nodes have been found to be involved even when renal hilar nodal groups are grossly normal. However, contralateral hilar nodes are always free of disease if the ipsilateral lymph nodes are not involved.

Although both testes have lymphatic channels to the ipsilateral external iliac nodes, isolated involvement of the external iliac, inguinal, and femoral nodes is most common when the primary drainage routes have been altered by previous inguinal surgery. Also, if the tumor locally involves the epididymis, it may spread via lymphatic routes to the distal aortic or proximal common iliac group.

The overall accuracy achieved by CT examinations compares very favorably with that of bipedal LAG

(31,64,69,152,159,223,248). The reported accuracy of CT is in the range of 70% to 90%, with a sensitivity of 40% to 60% and a specificity approaching 100% (32,49). In general, CT has a higher specificity but a lower sensitivity than LAG (32) because of its inability to detect metastasis in a normal-sized lymph node. Although lowering the size criteria for a normal lymph node from 15 mm to 5 mm increases the sensitivity of CT, it is associated with a concomitant decrease in the specificity of the exam without significant change in its overall accuracy (241). Computed tomography does have a theoretical advantage over LAG in detecting early metastases to renal hilar nodes, a nodal group not normally opacified with bipedal LAG. Furthermore, CT is superior to LAG in delineating the exact extent of the tumor mass, knowledge important in the planning of radiation therapy (Fig. 66). Computed tomography also can be used to detect metastases to extralymphatic organs such as the liver and the lung.

Computed tomography is the preferred method in staging patients with known testicular neoplasms. Lymphangiography should be reserved for cases in which the CT scans are equivocal or negative. Because over 90% of

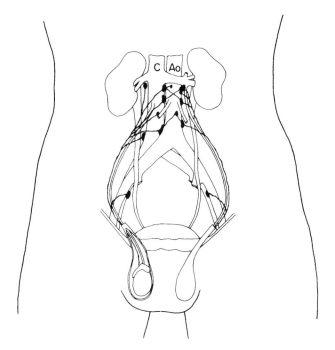

FIG. 63. Schematic diagram showing lymphatic drainage from the testis and epididymis. The testis drains primarily into lymph nodes at or below the level of the renal hilum, whereas the epididymis drains into the distal aortic or proximal iliac nodal group.

the nonseminomatous testicular tumors produce alpha-fetoprotein (AFP) or the beta subunit of human chorionic gonadotropin (β-HCG), serial determination of the serum level of these tumor markers is an extremely accurate method to follow therapeutic response and to detect possible recurrence (120,144). In one study, 82% of enlarging masses in patients with negative serum tumor markers after chemotherapy for nonseminomatous germ cell tumors represented mature teratomas (191). Computed tomography can be used to confirm a recurrence anatomically when serum markers become positive. Because the great majority of pure seminomas do not produce either HCG or AFP, CT has become the procedure of choice for following the response to chemotherapy and radiation therapy in this group of patients (120,152). As with substantial lymphomatous lymph node involvement, residual retroperitoneal masses may remain on CT scans even after successful treatment of metastatic testicular carcinoma. Such masses may represent posttreatment fibrosis or teratoma (usually in nonseminomatous germ cell tumor); they cannot be distinguished reliably from residual viable neoplasm by CT (235,242).

Other Metastatic Diseases

Nodal metastases from other primary tumors likewise can be detected on CT scans when the involved lymph nodes are enlarged (see Figs. 48,54). Because of its ability to evaluate the liver, adrenals, and abdominal lymph nodes simultaneously, CT has been used as part of an abdominal oncologic survey in patients with known malignant neoplasms with a propensity for metastases to these areas, such as melanoma and colon carcinoma. Computed tomography is also used to document suspected recurrence or follow response to various treatments in these patients.

In contradistinction to lymphoma, nodal metastases from primary epithelial cancer of the genitourinary tract frequently cause replacement without enlarging the lymph node, a condition not discernible on CT scans (154). Furthermore, metastases to the pelvic lymph nodes usually antedate involvement of retroperitoneal lymph nodes in these cases. The role of CT in primary epithelial carcinoma of the genitourinary tract is covered in Chapter 20, Pelvis.

Role of Other Noninvasive Imaging Methods

Besides LAG and CT, other noninvasive diagnostic tests (i.e., ultrasound and gallium scintigraphy) also have been reported to be of some value in the detection of abdominal lymphadenopathy. Ultrasound has been quite accurate in detecting retroperitoneal adenopathy (23,31,49); however, it is often difficult to obtain adequate scans of the lower abdomen because of bowel gas. In obese patients, examination of the retroperitoneal area by ultrasound also is difficult because of marked attenuation of the sound beam by the abundant subcutaneous and mesenteric fat. The use of gallium-67 (Ga-67) imaging in detecting intra-abdominal nodal involvement by malignant lymphoma has been generally disappointing. In a

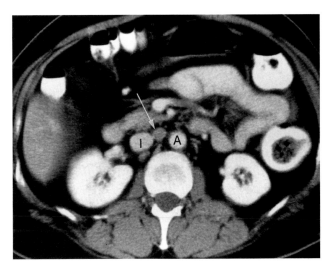

FIG. 64. Interaortocaval adenopathy. This nodal region *(arrow)*, between the aorta (A) and IVC (I), can be the first site of nodal metastasis from ovarian and testicular neoplasms, typically right-sided primaries.

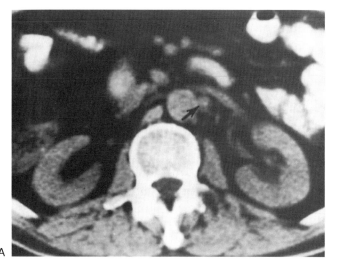

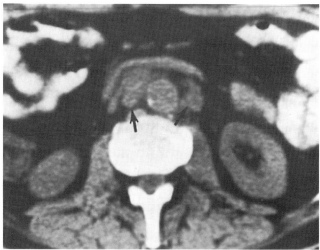

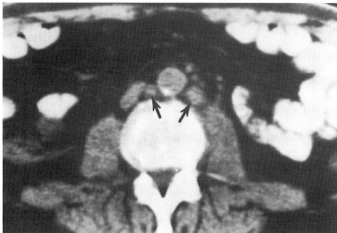

FIG. 65. Nodal metastases from embryonal cell carcinoma of left testis. Enlarged lymph nodes *(arrows)* are noted in the left para-aortic and interaortocaval chains at several levels. **A:** CT image through renal hilus. **B:** CT image through lower poles of both kidneys. **C:** CT image below both kidneys.

large cooperative study (125), the true positive rate for detecting intra-abdominal disease was 48%. However, Ga-67 SPECT (single photon emission computed tomography) has been shown to be valuable after treatment in excluding disease in patients with residual masses at CT (84,85).

Magnetic resonance imaging is comparable to CT in the detection of retroperitoneal lymphadenopathy in adults (58,72,149). In one study of infradiaphragmatic lymphadenopathy in children and adolescents with Hodgkin disease, MRI using a STIR (short tau inversion recovery) sequence showed more abnormal nodes than CT and LAG in the upper abdomen, but it was equal to LAG and superior to CT in the lower abdomen and pelvis (106). Magnetic resonance imaging has several advantages with respect to CT. One advantage is its ability to distinguish vascular structures from soft-tissue structures without the use of iodinated contrast material. In particular, mildly enlarged pelvic lymph nodes may be difficult to detect by CT because of the great variability in location, diameter, and orientation of the pelvic arteries and veins. This is especially true in patients in whom adequate opacifica-

tion of both the arteries and veins is not achieved because of technical reasons. Even with the administration of intravenous contrast material, mildly enlarged pelvic nodes still may be confused with pelvic vessels because both will enhance (118). In these instances, pelvic lymphadenopathy is more easily demonstrated by MRI. Venous anomalies, prominent gonadal veins, and collateral vessels all may mimic retroperitoneal lymphadenopathy on noncontrast CT studies, but they are easily shown to be vascular structures by MRI.

Another advantage of MRI is in the evaluation of some postsurgical patients. On CT scans, metallic clips and prostheses produce streak artifacts that can obscure significant regions of interest. However, the surgical clips most commonly used at our institutions for abdominal surgical procedures are made of tantalum or other material that produces minimal artifacts and does not degrade the MR studies (59,72,174). Large metallic objects, such as hip prostheses, produce a focal loss of signal but otherwise do not interfere with MRI of the pelvis.

Magnetic resonance imaging does have several limitations compared with CT. With optimal opacification of

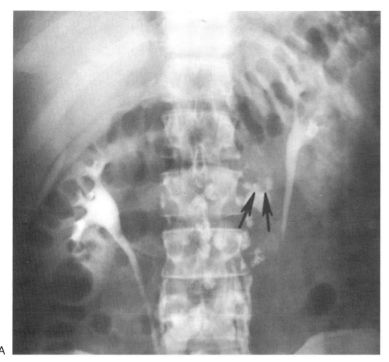
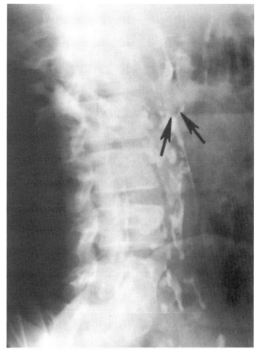
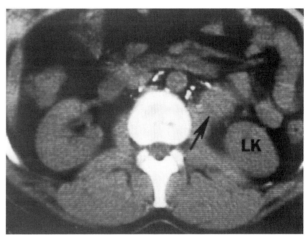

FIG. 66. Metastatic retroperitoneal lymphadenopathy in a patient with left testicular seminoma. Anteroposterior **(A)** and left posterior oblique **(B)** views of the abdomen from a bipedal lymphangiogram show a well-defined peripheral filling defect involving at least one left para-aortic lymph node *(arrows)* at the level of the second lumbar vertebra, compatible with nodal metastases. **C:** CT image demonstrates a large metastatic mass *(arrow)* not appreciated on the preceding lymphangiogram. LK, left kidney.

bowel loops, CT can more easily detect lymphadenopathy in patients who have little retroperitoneal fat, and in patients in whom the retroperitoneal tissue planes have been altered by surgery. Because of the poorer spatial resolution of MRI, a cluster of normal-sized lymph nodes could appear as a single enlarged node on the MRI study. Finally, MRI is unable to detect small calcifications in lymph nodes, a limitation that is of greater significance in the evaluation of the mediastinum than in the retroperitoneum and pelvis.

Although a survey MRI examination of the abdomen and pelvis can be completed by T1-weighted GRE sequence in less than a minute, a thorough MR examination that consists of both T1- and T2-weighted sequences still takes more time than a comparable CT study. Furthermore, CT is less expensive and is more available than

MRI. Therefore, in most institutions, CT remains the imaging procedure of choice for screening the retroperitoneum for evidence of lymphadenopathy. If the CT findings are equivocal, an MRI study should be performed. Magnetic resonance imaging should be considered the primary imaging technique in those patients whose exposure to ionizing radiation should be limited. This includes pediatric patients, especially if multiple follow-up examinations are anticipated, and pregnant patients in their second and third trimesters.

An important application of MRI is in the evaluation of patients who have undergone radiation therapy or chemotherapy and have a residual retroperitoneal mass. As mentioned previously, CT is frequently unable to distinguish residual fibrotic changes from viable neoplasms (156,158). Several investigators have shown that MRI

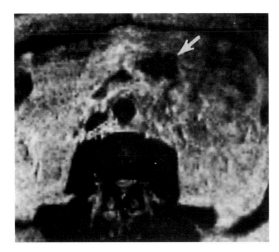

FIG. 67. Fibrosis after successful treatment of non-Hodgkin lymphoma. T2-weighted MR image (2100/90) shows a low-intensity mass *(arrow)* in the mesentery, representing residual fibrosis. Lymphadenopathy would have a signal intensity similar to that of fat on this sequence.

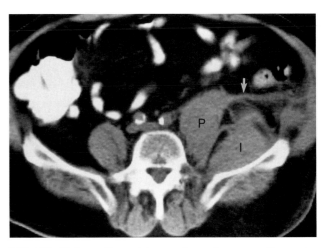

FIG. 68. Retroperitoneal hemorrhage in over-anticoagulation. Isodense hemorrhage enlarges the left psoas (P) and iliacus (I) muscles with ill-defined strands *(arrow)* extending into the pararenal spaces.

may be able to distinguish posttreatment fibrosis from residual or recurrent tumor (66,95,209). Demonstration of uniform low signal intensity (similar to that of muscle) on T1- and T2-weighted images suggests that the soft-tissue mass represents fibrosis (Fig. 67). However, regions of intermediate to high signal intensity on T2-weighted images may represent not only viable tumor but benign processes such as necrosis or inflammation. This is especially true in the first 6 months after initiation of therapy. Caution is necessary as MR signal intensities reflect only gross histologic characteristics and cannot exclude microscopic foci of residual disease. Serial MRI studies may be of greater value than any one isolated examination in monitoring patients who have responded poorly to therapy.

RETROPERITONEAL HEMORRHAGE

Retroperitoneal hemorrhage occurs most commonly in patients on anticoagulant therapy (Figs. 68,69), following trauma, or as a complication of an aortic aneurysm (Fig. 70) or a retroperitoneal tumor. Bleeding into the retroperitoneum has been reported to occur in a high percentage of patients after translumbar aortography (17,42) and percutaneous renal biopsy (215). It also may occur in patients with a bleeding diathesis or vasculitis (224).

Although acute onset of abdominal pain and development of an abdominal mass in association with a decreasing hematocrit are suggestive of retroperitoneal hemorrhage, clinical signs and symptoms may be ambiguous, delayed, or misleading. The diagnosis of retroperitoneal hemorrhage by plain abdominal radiographs lacks both sensitivity and specificity.

Computed Tomography

Computed tomography is an accurate noninvasive imaging method for detecting retroperitoneal hemorrhage (63,77,224). On CT scans, it appears as an abnormal soft-tissue density, either well localized or diffusely expanding the retroperitoneum (224) (Figs. 68–70). Its location and attenuation characteristics depend on the source and duration of the hemorrhage.

Hemorrhage resulting from renal biopsy is centered around the traumatized kidney, whereas that associated with a leaking abdominal aortic aneurysm (Fig. 70) or

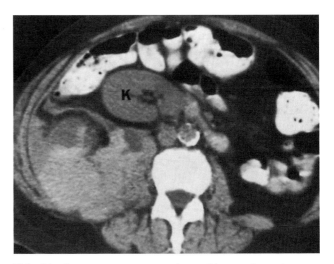

FIG. 69. Spontaneous retroperitoneal hemorrhage in a patient on anticoagulant therapy. Non-contrast-enhanced CT image shows a mixed-attenuation mass involving right perirenal and posterior pararenal spaces. Some areas of this mass have relatively high attenuation values, compatible with acute hemorrhage. Note anteromedial displacement of the right kidney (K).

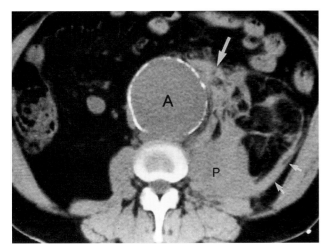

FIG. 70. Noncontrast CT scan shows enlargement of the left psoas muscle (P) due to isodense hemorrhage from a ruptured abdominal aortic aneurysm (A). Note the strands of hemorrhage *(long arrow)* extending into the left perirenal space, and the thickening of the Zuckerkandl fascia *(short arrow)*.

translumbar aortography generally surrounds the aorta before extending into the adjacent retroperitoneum. An acute hematoma (+70 to +90 HU) has a higher attenuation value than circulating blood because clot formation and retraction cause greater concentration of red blood cells (245,271). As stated previously, contrast-enhanced dynamic CT may document active arterial extravasation either as a focal high-density area surrounded by a large hematoma or as a diffuse area of high density (122). A subacute hematoma often has a lucent halo and a soft-tissue density center. A chronic hematoma appears as a low density mass (+20 to +40 HU) with a thick, dense rim (189,245). Peripheral calcification also may be present. Although hyperdensity is quite specific for acute hematoma, the appearance of retroperitoneal hemorrhage on CT is by no means pathognomonic. A subacute hematoma can be confused with a retroperitoneal tumor; a chronic hematoma may have an appearance similar to that of an abscess, a lymphocele, a cyst, or a urinoma. Differentiation among these entities often requires correlation with the patient's clinical history. Decreasing size and attenuation value of the retroperitoneal mass, seen with serial scanning, are reassuring signs that a diagnosis of hematoma is correct in cases in which the clinical features are equivocal (45).

Magnetic Resonance Imaging

The MRI appearance of retroperitoneal hemorrhage depends not only on the age of the hematoma but also on the magnetic field strength. The signal intensity of an acute hematoma imaged at low magnetic field (0.15 to 0.5 tesla) is less than that of muscle on T1-weighted images and slightly higher than that of muscle on T2-weighted images (244). On the other hand, acute hematoma examined at high magnetic field (1.5 T) has a signal intensity similar to that of muscle on T1-weighted images, and marked hypointensity on T2-weighted images (99,280). Marked hypointensity on T2-weighted images is attributed to the presence of intracellular deoxyhemoglobin, which causes T2 shortening. This effect is more pronounced on GRE images than on SE images. A fluid–fluid level with greater signal in the dependent layer on T1-weighted images also has been described in large, acute hematomas (105).

As the hematoma ages, it assumes a more characteristic MRI appearance. On T1-weighted images, a subacute hematoma often has three distinct layers of signal: a low-intensity rim corresponding to the hemosiderin-laden fibrous capsule, a high-intensity (similar to fat) peripheral zone, and a medium-intensity central core (slightly greater than muscle) (105,222,253). On T2-weighted images, the signal intensity of the central core increases relative to that of the peripheral zone, whereas the rim remains low in intensity. With further maturation of the hematoma, the central core, which represents the retracted clot, continues to diminish in size, and the entire hematoma eventually becomes a homogeneous, high-signal intensity mass surrounded by a low-intensity rim on both T1- and T2-weighted images. Progressive increase in signal intensity of a hematoma parallels the formation of methemoglobin (21).

Although hematoma may have a characteristic MRI appearance, the specificity of this appearance is yet unknown. Hemorrhage into a tumor may be indistinguishable from a bland hematoma, and fluid containing a high protein content may have a similar appearance. Furthermore, fluid–fluid levels resulting from settling of debris within an abscess may simulate the appearance of sedimented blood. Because of the limited availability of MR imagers and because of the ease with which the diagnosis of acute hematoma can be made on CT, CT will remain the procedure of choice in imaging patients with suspected acute retroperitoneal hemorrhage (i.e., of less than 2 weeks' duration). However, MRI may provide a more specific diagnosis than CT in less acute cases in which CT findings are nonspecific.

RETROPERITONEAL FIBROSIS

Retroperitoneal fibrosis, a disease process often insidious in its clinical presentation, is characterized pathologically by fibrous tissue proliferation along the posterior aspect of the retroperitoneal cavity, causing encasement of blood vessels and ureters. The process may extend into the pelvis, resulting in narrowing of the rectosigmoid colon (117). The histologic features range from an active inflammatory process to a more acellular, hyalinized reac-

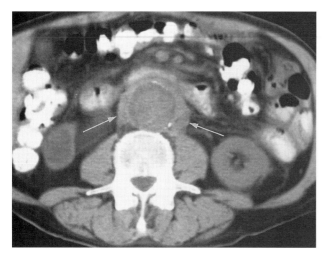

FIG. 71. Perianeurysmal fibrosis. Noncontrast CT scan shows an infrarenal abdominal aortic aneurysm associated with a sharply marginated rind of fibrotic soft tissue *(arrows)*.

tion (76). Although most of the reported cases are idiopathic, certain drugs such as methysergide, primary or metastatic tumors, aneurysms, and aneurysm surgery have all been associated with similar pathologic alterations in the retroperitoneum (1,175,259). In cases in which retroperitoneal fibrosis is associated with an aortic aneurysm (Fig. 71), a heterogeneous population of leukocytes (i.e., polymorphonuclear leukocytes, lymphocytes, and plasma cells) can be found within the perianeurysmal tissues. Therefore, it has been suggested that perianeurysmal fibrosis may be the end result of an exaggerated inflammatory response to luminal thrombi or their breakdown products permeating the aortic wall (1). The lack of any hemosiderin-laden macrophages in the periaortic tissue negates the possibility of prior dissection or rupture (175). The development of an inflammatory abdominal aortic

aneurysm from an uncomplicated aneurysm over a period of 6.5 months has been documented by CT (146).

The CT appearance of retroperitoneal fibrosis is quite variable. Although some have no detectable abnormality, others present as a well-marginated sheath of soft-tissue density with obscuration of the aorta and IVC (29,76) (Fig. 72). On rare occasion, retroperitoneal fibrosis may even present as single or multiple soft tissue masses with irregular borders, an appearance quite similar to that of primary retroperitoneal tumor or malignant lymphadenopathy. Although slight anterior displacement of the aorta may occur on rare occasions (27), marked anterior displacement of the great vessels is not seen in idiopathic retroperitoneal fibrosis, and this may serve as a useful sign in differentiating it from primary retroperitoneal tumor or malignant lymphadenopathy (53).

On noncontrast CT scans, retroperitoneal fibrosis usually has an attenuation value similar to that of muscle, although focal or uniform hyperdensity also has been reported (219). On postcontrast scans, it may exhibit exuberant enhancement (1,219,259). Whereas the precontrast hyperdensity of retroperitoneal fibrosis has been attributed to the high physical density of collagen within these tissues, contrast enhancement is said to be in part a result of the abundant capillary network (219) (Fig. 72). Malignant causes of retroperitoneal fibrosis cannot be differentiated from nonmalignant causes based on CT findings (219) (Fig. 73).

In view of the spectrum of histologic findings, a variable MR appearance for retroperitoneal fibrosis would be expected. Although nonmalignant retroperitoneal fibrosis often has homogeneous low signal intensity similar to that of psoas muscle on both T1- and T2-weighted images (Fig. 74), it also may have heterogeneous medium signal intensity on T2-weighted images, being hyperintense to muscle but slightly hypointense to fat (9,116,151,185,

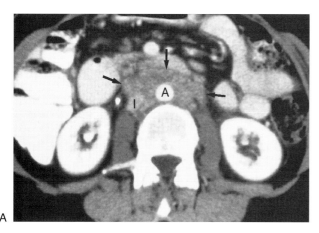
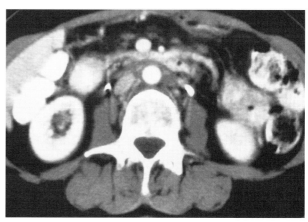

A   B

FIG. 72. Idiopathic retroperitoneal fibrosis. **A:** Contrast-enhanced CT scan shows mildly enhancing circumferential para-aortic soft tissue *(arrows)* encasing the IVC (I) and left ureter. Enhancement suggests an acute process or a malignant etiology. **B:** A follow-up study shows reduction of the para-aortic soft tissue after treatment with tamoxifen. Lack of enhancement is now consistent with chronic fibrosis.

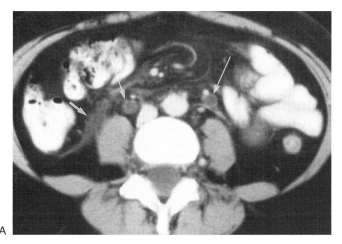
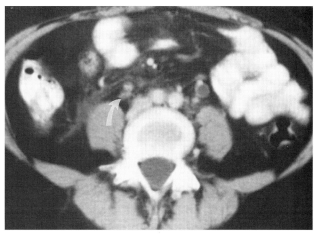

FIG. 73. Malignant retroperitoneal fibrosis due to metastatic breast cancer. **A:** Contrast-enhanced CT scan shows bilateral obstructive hydroureter *(long white arrows)* with a sheet of abnormal retroperitoneal soft tissue *(short white arrow).* **B:** Inferiorly, tissue extends to the right ureter with abnormal enhancement *(curved white arrow)* at the site of obstruction.

275). The former appearance probably reflects a more mature and quiescent stage of the disease and can be distinguished from malignant retroperitoneal fibrosis, which has heterogeneous signal intensity, similar to or slightly lower than fat on T2-weighted images (9). Except when the disease has reached a quiescent stage (Fig. 74), both benign and malignant retroperitoneal fibroses usually enhance after intravenous administration of gadolinium (Figs. 75,76). If malignant retroperitoneal fibrosis is suspected based on imaging findings, it is recommended that multiple, deep tissue samples be acquired at biopsy, because relatively few malignant cells may be admixed with inflammatory cells of the collagen network (5).

Magnetic resonance imaging can demonstrate encasement of retroperitoneal vessels by retroperitoneal fibrosis without the use of iodinated contrast material. Gradient echo imaging and MRA techniques are effective methods for evaluating the extent of vascular involvement and collateral vessel formation.

PRIMARY RETROPERITONEAL TUMORS

Primary retroperitoneal neoplasms comprise a rare and diverse group of tumors. The vast majority are malignant and of mesodermal origin. They tend to be large at initial presentation because they generally must reach a large size to compress adjacent structures sufficiently to produce symptoms (Fig. 77). Malignant fibrous histiocytoma, liposarcoma, leiomyosarcoma, fibrosarcoma, and malignant germ cell tumor are the tumor types most frequently encountered. Benign retroperitoneal neoplasms are uncommon and include lipomas, paragangliomas, neurogenic tumors, hemangiomas, lymphangiomas, and mature

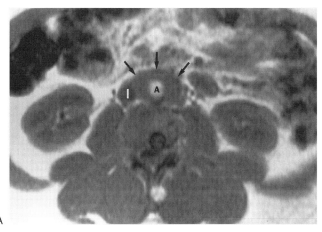
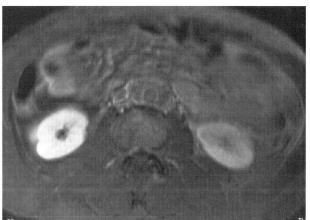

FIG. 74. Chronic retroperitoneal fibrosis. **A:** Transaxial T1-weighted FLASH image (140/4/80°) shows sharply defined hypointense tissue *(arrows)* encasing the aorta (A). I, IVC. **B:** Post-Gd FATSAT T1-weighted SE image (600/15) shows no enhancement of circumaortic tissue.

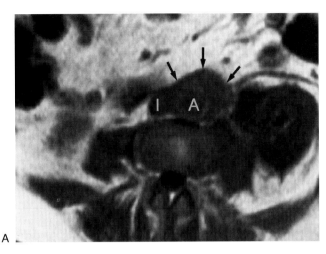

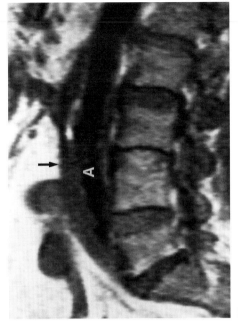

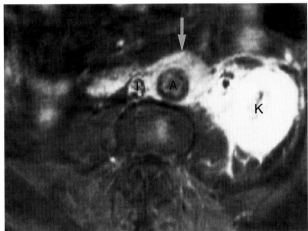

FIG. 75. Acute retroperitoneal fibrosis. Transaxial **(A)** and sagittal **(B)** T1-weighted SE images (600/15) show a hypointense rind of tissue *(arrows)* surrounding the aorta (A). I, IVC. **C:** Transaxial post-Gd FATSAT T1-weighted SE image (600/15) shows significant tissue enhancement *(arrows)* reflecting the extensive capillary network present before fibrosis becomes chronic. At this stage, this entity cannot be distinguished from metastatic disease. K, kidney.

teratomas. The diagnosis of tumors arising from the retroperitoneal tissues is readily accomplished with CT even when they are relatively small (237,238). Such neoplasms, usually sarcomas, appear on CT generally as soft-tissue-density masses that displace, compress, or obscure the normal retroperitoneal structures. Computed tomography can usually differentiate primary retroperitoneal neoplasms from retroperitoneal lymphomas. Whereas the former tend to be heterogeneous on CT, lymphomas are usually homogeneous (46). Provided that some perivisceral fat is present, CT can accurately define the size, extent, and composition of the tumors as well as their effect on neighboring structures. Adjacent organs may be invaded, but clear planes of separation cannot always be seen. Predictions as to definite invasion of normal structures, with implications toward surgical resectability, should be offered with caution.

Although most solid retroperitoneal tumors have attenuation values similar to that of muscle tissue, a specific histologic diagnosis occasionally can be suggested based on unique CT findings. Lipomas appear as sharply marginated, homogeneous masses with CT densities equal to that of normal fat. A lymphangioma with high lipid content can simulate a lipoma on CT scans (51,83).

With the exception of exceedingly rare, very well differentiated liposarcomas, which are difficult to distinguish from lipomas even at surgery and on pathologic examination, most malignant liposarcomas can be distinguished from benign lipomas by CT (83,263). Liposarcomas usually are inhomogeneous, poorly marginated, or infiltrative, and they have CT numbers greater than those of the patient's normal fat (see Fig. 68). They also may exhibit contrast enhancement. Three distinct CT patterns have been described that reflect the amount and distribution of fat within the liposarcomas (83). The solid pattern has CT numbers greater than +20 HU; the mixed pattern has discrete fatty areas less than −20 HU and other areas greater than +20 HU; and a pseudocystic pattern has a

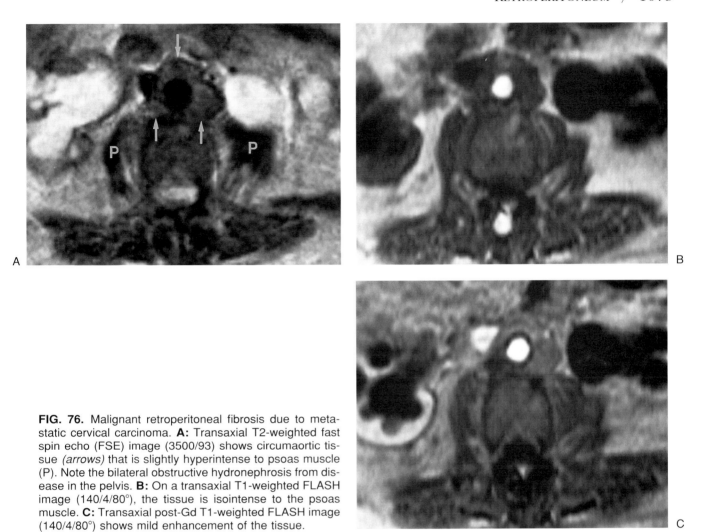

FIG. 76. Malignant retroperitoneal fibrosis due to metastatic cervical carcinoma. **A:** Transaxial T2-weighted fast spin echo (FSE) image (3500/93) shows circumaortic tissue *(arrows)* that is slightly hyperintense to psoas muscle (P). Note the bilateral obstructive hydronephrosis from disease in the pelvis. **B:** On a transaxial T1-weighted FLASH image (140/4/80°), the tissue is isointense to the psoas muscle. **C:** Transaxial post-Gd T1-weighted FLASH image (140/4/80°) shows mild enhancement of the tissue.

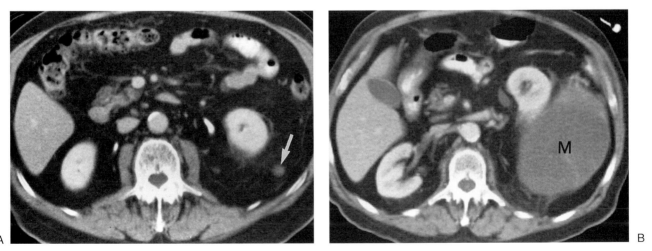

FIG. 77. Retroperitoneal liposarcoma. **A:** Contrast-enhanced CT scan performed for unrelated reasons shows an incidental 1-cm soft-tissue nodule *(arrow)* within the left perirenal space. **B:** Follow-up study 1 year later shows a large perirenal soft-tissue density mass (M) displacing the left kidney anteriorly.

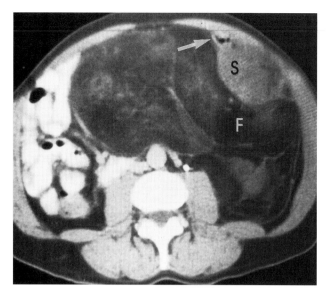

FIG. 78. Retroperitoneal liposarcoma. Contrast-enhanced CT scan shows a large retroperitoneal mass of mixed fat (F) and soft-tissue (S) attenuation. The descending colon *(arrow)* is displaced anteromedially, indicating the retroperitoneal location of the tumor.

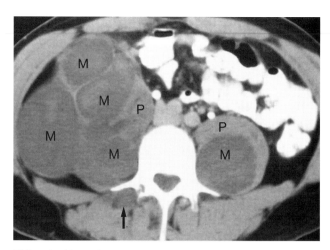

FIG. 79. Neurofibromatosis with neurofibrosarcoma. Contrast-enhanced CT scan demonstrates two slightly enhancing, hypodense masses (M) extending along the course of the lumbar nerves and displacing the psoas muscles (P) anteriorly. The location is typical for a neurogenic tumor and the gross asymmetry should raise suspicion for sarcomatous degeneration. A smaller neurofibroma lies posterior to the right transverse process *(arrow)*.

homogeneous density between +20 HU and −20 HU. The well-differentiated liposarcoma with abundant mature fat generally still has a mixed pattern (Fig. 78); poorly differentiated tumors with little fat, and liposarcomas with round-cell or pleomorphic histology are seen as solid pattern and are indistinguishable on CT scans from other soft-tissue-density neoplasms (Fig. 77) (135). The pseudocystic pattern results from averaging of a homogeneous mixture of fat and solid connective tissue and may simulate a cystic lymphangioma (225).

Although a mature teratoma of the retroperitoneum also may contain foci of mature fat, it usually can be differentiated from other fat-containing neoplasms by the presence of fluid density, a fat−fluid level, and calcifications (50). Benign neurogenic neoplasms such as a neurofibroma often have a homogeneous low attenuation value, equal to or slightly higher than water but much lower than paraspinal muscle. A plexiform neurofibroma is an interdigitating network of fingerlike bands of tumor occurring along a nerve and its branches. Retroperitoneal plexiform neurofibromas can be recognized because they are typically bilaterally symmetrical and situated in a parapsoas or presacral location. Asymmetry in size and attenuation of a larger mass suggests the possibility of a malignant tumor of the nerve sheath (16) (Fig. 79).

Tissue necrosis and cystic degeneration within a solid neoplasm also may result in areas of lower attenuation (less than muscle). This is particularly common in leiomyosarcomas (173) (Fig. 80). Although malignant fibrohistiocytoma and hemangiopericytoma may have CT features similar to leiomyosarcoma (4,96,143), they more commonly contain amorphous and dystrophic calcifica-

tions. Furthermore, hemangiopericytoma may exhibit exuberant contrast enhancement similar to that of hemangioma as a result of its hypervascularity (143).

Although extra-adrenal retroperitoneal paragangliomas have no unique CT feature, the diagnosis may be suggested if a soft-tissue mass is seen along the abdominal aorta. Determination of serum catecholamine is helpful in establishing the diagnosis, as a significant percentage of patients with this neoplasm have an elevated level (107).

Like CT, MRI cannot provide a specific histologic diagnosis in most cases. The only tumors that can be diagnosed on the basis of their MRI appearance are mature teratomas,

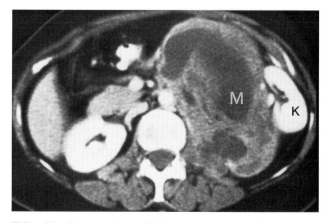

FIG. 80. Retroperitoneal leiomyosarcoma. Contrast-enhanced CT scan demonstrates a large, heterogeneously enhancing mass (M) displacing the left kidney (K) laterally. Irregular hypodense regions represent tissue necrosis and cystic degeneration commonly seen in leiomyosarcoma.

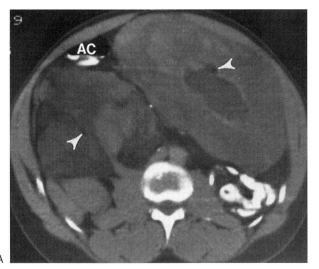
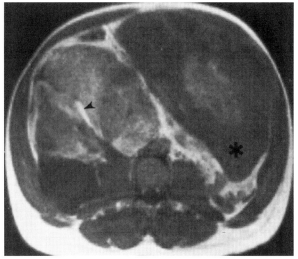

FIG. 81. Retroperitoneal liposarcoma. **A:** CT image demonstrates a large mixed-density occupying nearly the entire abdomen. The mass has only a few foci of fat density *(arrowheads)*. AC, ascending colon. **B:** Tl-weighted MR image (500/15) at a level similar to that of (A). Note that the tumor has heterogeneous signal intensities. Whereas some areas are isointense to muscle (*), other areas are isointense to fat *(arrowhead)*.

lipomas, and possibly liposarcomas (41,60). Unlike lipomas, which are homogeneous and have the same signal intensity as fat on all pulse sequences, liposarcomas are usually inhomogeneous and may not have any areas of fatlike signal intensity (Fig. 81). As with CT, MRI features of a liposarcoma depend on the relative amounts of intracellular lipid and mucin, and the degree of cellularity (263).

Computed tomography should be the procedure of choice in screening patients with possible retroperitoneal tumors suspected on the basis of either abnormal findings on physical examination or other radiologic studies; its accuracy is exceedingly high, quite comparable to that in patients with retroperitoneal lymphoma or metastatic testicular cancer. The inability of CT to differentiate among most cell types is not critical because surgery is performed in all patients with primary retroperitoneal neoplasm, regardless of the histology. Furthermore, if histologic characterization is required before surgery, this can be achieved easily by performing a CT-guided percutaneous biopsy. In patients with known primary retroperitoneal tumors, CT can be used to assess response to treatment and to document possible recurrence. Although the superior soft-tissue contrast resolution of MRI and its multiplanar imaging capability allow accurate localization of retroperitoneal masses and assessment of their relationship to adjacent organs and vessels, insufficient additional information is provided by MRI, compared to CT, to warrant its routine use.

PSOAS

Normal Anatomy

Computed Tomography

The psoas major, psoas minor, and iliacus muscles are a group of muscles that function as flexors of the thigh and trunk. The psoas major muscle originates from fibers arising from the transverse processes of the 12th thoracic vertebra as well as all lumbar vertebrae. The muscle fibers fuse and pass inferiorly in a paraspinal location. As it exits from the pelvis, the psoas major assumes a more anterior location, merging with the iliacus to become the iliopsoas muscle. The iliopsoas passes beneath the inguinal ligament to insert on the lesser trochanter of the femur. At its superior attachment, the psoas muscle passes beneath the arcuate ligament of the diaphragm. The psoas muscle is in a fascial plane that directly extends from the mediastinum to the thigh.

The psoas minor is a long, slender muscle, located immediately anterior to the psoas major. When present, it arises from the sides of the body of the 12th thoracic and first lumbar vertebrae, and from the fibrocartilage between them. It ends in the long flat tendon, which inserts on the iliopectineal eminence of the innominate bone.

On CT scans, the normal psoas major muscles are delineated clearly in almost every patient as paired paraspinal structures. The proximal portion of the psoas muscle is triangular in shape, whereas the distal end has a more rounded appearance. The size of the psoas major muscle increases in a cephalocaudad direction. When visible, especially in young, muscular individuals, the psoas minor appears as a small, rounded, soft-tissue mass anterior to the psoas major (Fig. 82). Caution must be taken not to confuse this muscle with an enlarged lymph node. The sympathetic trunk as well as the lumbar veins and arteries are sometimes seen as small soft-tissue densities located just medial to the psoas muscles and lateral to the lumbar spine. However, differentiation between an artery,

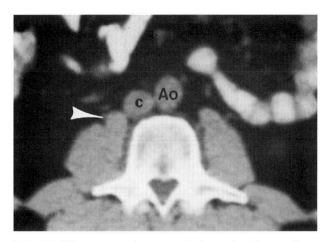

FIG. 82. The psoas minor muscle *(arrowhead)*, prominent in some muscular individuals on CT, should not be confused with an enlarged lymph node. Ao, aorta; c, IVC.

a vein, and a nerve in this location is not possible on noncontrast scans.

Magnetic Resonance Imaging

The psoas muscle has a low signal intensity on both T1- and T2-weighted images. A T1-weighted pulse sequence provides the best contrast between the muscle and adjacent retroperitoneal fat; both T2-weighted and post-Gd, T1-weighted, fat-suppressed sequences can clearly differentiate normal from the abnormal psoas (148,265). To evaluate the psoas muscle, images in the transaxial plane should be obtained. If an abnormality is noted in the muscle, additional coronal or sagittal views may help delineate the extent of disease and determine if there is involvement of the spine (265).

Pathology

Neoplasm

Neoplastic disease can involve the psoas muscle by one of three mechanisms: (a) total replacement, (b) medial displacement, and (c) lateral displacement (148). In the case of lateral displacement, a paraspinal mass, which often represents enlargement of lymph nodes, is present between the spine and psoas muscle.

On CT, lymphomas and other malignant retroperitoneal neoplasms can result in enlargement or obscuration of the psoas muscle, regardless of the underlying mechanism. The involved muscle most often has an attenuation value similar to that of the normal one, although areas of low attenuation also may be present (Figs. 83,84).

On MRI, the abnormal muscle has a signal intensity higher than that of the normal psoas on both T1- and T2-weighted images. On T1-weighted images, the signal intensity of the diseased muscle is less than that of fat unless hemorrhage has occurred, in which case high intensity signal may be observed in the abnormal region. Because of its superior contrast sensitivity, MRI is superior to CT in separating normal from abnormal psoas muscle (Figs. 85,86). We have encountered cases in which the CT study showed apparent enlargement of the psoas muscle, but subsequent MRI examination demonstrated that the psoas muscle was compressed and displaced laterally by a mass. However, neither examination can reliably differentiate mere contiguity from superficial invasion.

Inflammatory Lesions

Infection within the psoas muscle is commonly a result of direct extension from contiguous structures such as the spine, kidney, bowel loops, and pancreas. With the

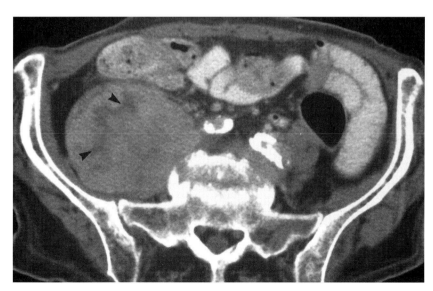

FIG. 83. Non-Hodgkin lymphoma involving the right psoas muscle. CT image demonstrates a markedly enlarged right psoas muscle, with areas of lower attenuation value *(arrowheads)*. The CT findings are nonspecific and can be confused with hemorrhage or infection involving the psoas muscle.

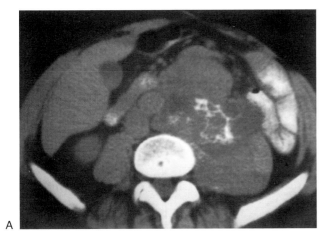
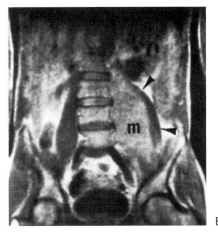

FIG. 84. Apparent psoas enlargement due to metastatic colon carcinoma. **A:** CT image demonstrates a large retroperitoneal mass, with amorphous calcifications obscuring the contour of the left psoas muscle. **B:** Coronal MR image (900/30) shows a large medium-intensity paraspinal mass (m) displacing a relatively normal left psoas *(arrowheads)* laterally. The paraspinal mass most likely represents nodal metastases. Calcification is not seen on this MR image. (From ref. 148.)

decreasing incidence of tuberculous involvement of the spine, the majority of psoas abscesses now encountered are of pyogenic origin. On CT scans, the involved psoas muscle is often diffusely enlarged, usually with central areas of lower density (0 to 30 HU) (79,121,178,210). The size and extent of the abscess usually can easily be delineated; visualization of the abscess frequently can be improved on the scans by intravenous administration of iodinated contrast material (Fig. 87). Uniform enlargement of a psoas muscle with areas of lower density is not specific for an inflammatory process. With the exception

of a single case report in which gas within the psoas muscle resulted from an intravertebral vacuum cleft, a benign manifestation of vertebral body necrosis (255), demonstration of gas bubbles within the psoas muscle is virtually pathognomonic of an abscess (Fig. 88). In cases in which the CT findings are nonspecific, CT can be used to guide percutaneous needle aspiration of the observed abnormality to obtain tissue for histologic examination and bacteriologic culture. In cases in which the diagnosis of psoas abscess is certain, CT can be used to guide percutaneous drainage (184).

Psoas abscess can likewise be detected by MRI. Abscesses have a signal intensity equal to or greater than

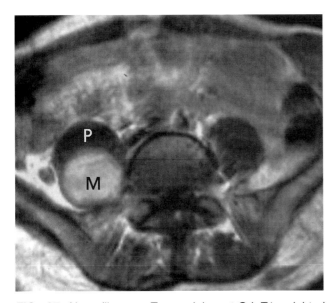

FIG. 85. Neurofibroma. Transaxial post-Gd T1-weighted FLASH image (140/4/80°) shows a homogeneously enhancing, sharply margined mass (M) along the course of a lumbar nerve. Note the characteristic anterior displacement of the psoas muscle (P).

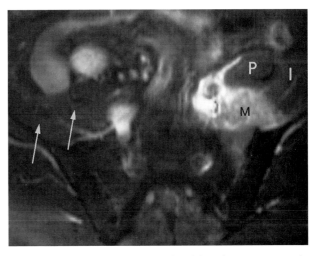

FIG. 86. Melanoma metastasis involving the psoas muscle. Transaxial post-Gd FATSAT T1-weighted SE image (600/15) shows an enhancing mass (M) displacing the psoas (P) and iliacus (I) muscles anterolaterally. *Arrows,* normal right iliopsoas muscle.

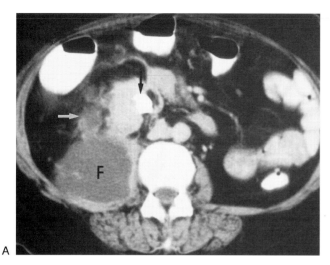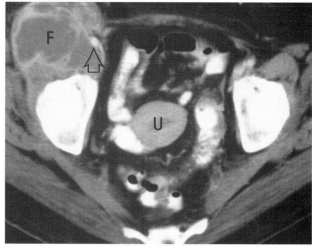

A   B

FIG. 87. Psoas abscess from an infected urinoma. **A:** Contrast-enhanced CT scan shows a fluid collection (F) tracking within the right psoas muscle. Note the obstructing renal calculus *(black arrow)* and the communication of the psoas collection with the right perinephric space *(white arrow)*. **B:** CT scan at the level of the acetabulum demonstrates the inferior extent of this fluid collection to be located at the site of the right psoas muscle attachment. Note the enhancement of its wall and septations. Culture grew *E. coli.* U, uterus. *Open arrow,* external iliac artery.

that of normal muscle on T1-weighted images, and a high signal intensity on T2-weighted images (148,265). Because of the similarity in signal characteristics, psoas inflammation or abscess cannot be differentiated by MRI from psoas involvement by neoplastic disease. A major limitation of MRI is its inability to consistently detect small collections of air that may be present within the abscess. If detected, a collection of air would appear as a focal region of signal void on both T1- and T2-weighted images. However, a focal calcification in the muscle could have a similar appearance.

Other Conditions

Although the psoas may undergo spontaneous hemorrhage as a result of over-anticoagulation (see Fig. 68), a hematoma involving this muscle also can result from a leaking aortic aneurysm (see Fig. 70). As mentioned previously, the CT attenuation value of a hematoma varies from about +20 to +90 HU, depending on its age. Hematoma, abscess, and neoplasm, with or without central necrosis, all can have identical CT appearances (155).

The MRI appearance of intramuscular hemorrhage also

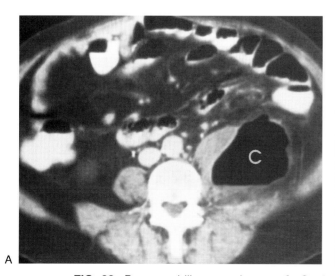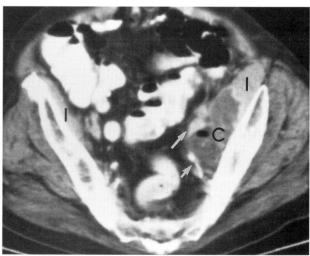

A   B

FIG. 88. Psoas and iliopsoas abscess. **A:** Contrast-enhanced CT scan shows a large collection of gas and fluid (C) within the left psoas muscle. **B:** Inferiorly, the collection tracks within the psoas and iliacus muscles. Note the medial displacement of both external (long arrow) and internal (short arrow) iliac vessels, confirming the retroperitoneal location of the abscess. I, iliopsoas muscles.

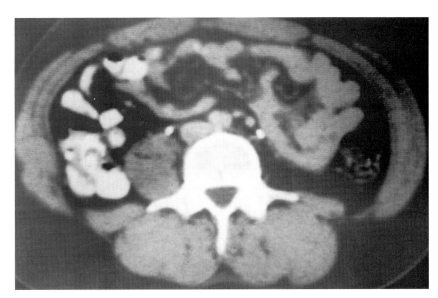

FIG. 89. Psoas atrophy. Note absence of left psoas muscle in this patient with a history of polio. The right psoas is normal.

depends upon the age of the hematoma (253). As stated previously, acute hematoma may have a nonspecific MRI appearance, whereas subacute and chronic hematomas often have more characteristic features.

Atrophy of the psoas muscle secondary to neuromuscular disorders is similarly easily identified, because a uniform decrease in the size of the muscle bulk on the involved side is seen (Fig. 89). On occasion, the involved muscles have a low density on CT as a result of partial fatty replacement.

Clinical Application

The plain radiograph is neither sensitive nor specific in assessment of disease processes involving the psoas muscle. Both psoas margins may be poorly visualized, or not visualized, in a substantial number of normal subjects (70). Furthermore, pathologic conditions involving the medial aspect of the psoas muscle cannot be initially identified on plain radiographs. Although ultrasound is also capable of demonstrating the normal and abnormal psoas muscle, this examination is often difficult or incomplete because of overlying bowel gas. In addition, sonography may be difficult to perform successfully in obese patients.

Although MRI can clearly depict psoas disease and provide better contrast between normal and abnormal psoas muscle than CT, it does not appear to offer any advantage over CT in terms of either sensitivity or specificity for routine use. Furthermore, most patients with an abnormality of the psoas muscle may not present with a specific sign and symptom that would enable the clinician to limit diagnosis of the lesion to the psoas compartment. In most instances, the psoas is mentioned only as one of many possible areas affected. At present, CT is still a better screening procedure in these situations, because it requires a shorter imaging time and is more readily avail-

able (148). An MRI study should be performed if the CT findings are equivocal or negative in patients with persistent symptoms referable to the psoas compartment. In these instances, MRI may detect a subtle abnormality and help facilitate the planning of any additional diagnostic or therapeutic procedures.

REFERENCES

1. Aiello MR, Cohen WM. Inflammatory aneurysms of the abdominal aorta. *J Comput Assist Tomogr* 1980;4:265–267.
2. Alcorn FS, Mategrano VC, Petasnick JP, Clark JW. Contributions of computed tomography in the staging and management of malignant lymphoma. *Radiology* 1977;125:717–723.
3. Allen BT, Anderson CB, Rubin BG, Flye MW, Baumann DS, Sicard GA. Preservation of renal function in juxtarenal and suprarenal abdominal aortic aneurysm repair. *J Vasc Surg* 1993;17:948–959.
4. Alpern MB, Thorsen MK, Kellman GM, Pojunas K, Lawson TL. CT appearance of hemangiopericytoma. *J Comput Assist Tomogr* 1986;10:264–267.
5. Amis ES. Retroperitoneal fibrosis. *AJR* 1991;157:321–329.
6. Amparo EG, Higgins CB, Hricak H, Sollitto R. Aortic dissection: magnetic resonance imaging. *Radiology* 1985;155:399–406.
7. Amparo EG, Hoddick WK, Hricak H, Sollitto R, Justich E, Filly RA, Higgins CB. Comparison of magnetic resonance imaging and ultrasonography in the evaluation of abdominal aortic aneurysms. *Radiology* 1985;154:451–456.
8. Andersen PE Jr, Lorentzen JE. Comparison of computed tomography and aortography in abdominal aortic aneurysms. *J Comput Assist Tomogr* 1983;7:670–673.
9. Arrive L, Hricak H, Tavares NJ, Miller TR. Malignant versus nonmalignant retroperitoneal fibrosis: differentiation with MR imaging. *Radiology* 1989;172:139–143.
10. Arrive L, Menu Y, Dessarts I, Dubray B, Vullierme MP, Vilgrain V, Najmark D, Nahum H. Diagnosis of abdominal venous thrombosis by means of spin-echo and gradient-echo MR imaging: analysis with receiver operating characteristic curves. *Radiology* 1991;181:661–668.
11. Atlas SW, Vogelzang RL, Bressler EL, Gore RM, Bergan JJ. CT diagnosis of a mycotic aneurysm of the thoracoabdominal aorta. *J Comput Assist Tomogr* 1984;8:1211–1212.
12. Auffermann W, Olofsson P, Stoney R, Higgins CB. MR imaging

of complications of aortic surgery. *J Comput Assist Tomogr* 1987; 11:982–989.

13. Auffermann W, Olofsson PA, Rabahie GN, Tavares NJ, Stoney RJ, Higgins CB. Incorporation versus infection of retroperitoneal aortic grafts: MR imaging features. *Radiology* 1989; 172:359–362.

14. Axelbaum SP, Schellinger D, Gomes NM, Ferris RA, Hakkal HG. Computed tomographic evaluation of aortic aneurysms. *AJR* 1976; 125:75–78.

15. Barnes PA, Bernardino ME, Thomas JL. Flow phenomenon mimicking thrombus: a possible pitfall of the pedal infusion technique. *J Comput Assist Tomogr* 1982; 6:304–306.

16. Bass JC, Korobkin M, Francis IR, Ellis JH, Cohan RH. Retroperitoneal plexiform neurofibromas: CT findings. *AJR* 1994; 163:617–620.

17. Bergman AB, Neiman HL. Computed tomography in the detection of retroperitoneal hemorrhage after translumbar aortography. *AJR* 1978; 131:831–833.

18. Best JJK, Blackledge G, Forbes WStC, Todd IDH, Eddleston B, Crowther D, Isherwood I. Computed tomography of abdomen in staging and clinical management of lymphoma. *Br Med J* 1978; 2:1675–1677.

19. Blackledge G, Best JJK, Crowther D, Isherwood I. Computed tomography in the staging of patients with Hodgkin's disease: a report on 136 patients. *Clin Radiol* 1980; 31:143–148.

20. Blum U, Langer M, Spillner G, Mialhe C, Beyersdorf F, Buitrago-Tellez C, Voshage G, Duber C, Schlosser V, Cragg AH. Abdominal aortic aneurysms: preliminary technical and clinical results with transfemoral placement of endovascular self-expanding stent-grafts. *Radiology* 1996; 198:25–31.

21. Bradley WG Jr, Schmidt PG. Effect of methemoglobin formation on the MR appearance of subarachnoid hemorrhage. *Radiology* 1985; 156:99–103.

22. Bradley WG Jr, Waluch V. Blood flow: magnetic resonance imaging. *Radiology* 1985; 154:443–450.

23. Brascho DJ, Durant JR, Green LE. The accuracy of retroperitoneal ultrasonography in Hodgkin's disease and non-Hodgkin's lymphoma. *Radiology* 1977; 125:485–487.

24. Breckenridge JW, Kinlaw WB. Azygos continuation of inferior vena cava: CT appearance. *J Comput Assist Tomogr* 1980; 4:392–397.

25. Breiman RS, Castellino RA, Harell GS, Marshall WH, Glatstein E, Kaplan HS. CT-pathologic correlations in Hodgkin's disease and non-Hodgkin's lymphoma. *Radiology* 1978; 126:159–166.

26. Brewster DC, Athanasoulis CA, Darling RC. Leiomyosarcoma of the inferior vena cava: diagnosis and surgical management. *Arch Surg* 1976; 111:1081–1085.

27. Brooks AP, Reznek RH, Webb JAW. Aortic displacement on computed tomography of idiopathic retroperitoneal fibrosis. *Clin Radiol* 1989; 40(1):51–52.

28. Brown PM, Pattenden R, Gutelius JR. The selective management of small abdominal aortic aneurysms: the Kingston study. *J Vasc Surg* 1992; 125:21–27.

29. Brun B, Laursen K, Sorensen IN, Lorentzen JE, Kristensen JK. CT in retroperitoneal fibrosis. *AJR* 1981; 137:535–538.

30. Buckwalter KA, Ellis JH, Baker DE, Borello JA, Glazer GM. Pitfall in MR imaging of lymphadenopathy after lymphangiography. *Radiology* 1986; 161(3):831–832.

31. Burney BT, Klatte EC. Ultrasound and computed tomography of the abdomen in the staging and management of testicular carcinoma. *Radiology* 1979; 132:415–419.

32. Bussar-Maatz R, Weissbach L. Retroperitoneal lymph node staging of testicular tumours: TNM study group. *Br J Urol* 1993; 72(2):234–240.

33. Callen PW, Korobkin M, Isherwood I. Computed tomographic evaluation of the retrocrural prevertebral space. *AJR* 1977; 129:907–910.

34. Castellino RA, Hoppe RT, Blank N, Young SW, Neumann C, Rosenberg SA, Kaplan HS. Computed tomography, lymphography, and staging laparotomy: correlations in initial staging of Hodgkin disease. *AJR* 1984; 143:37–41.

35. Castellino RA. Lymph nodes of the posterior iliac crest: CT and lymphographic observations. *Radiology* 1990; 175:687–689.

36. Castellino RA, Marglin S, Blank N. Hodgkin disease, the non-Hodgkin lymphomas, and the leukemias in the retroperitoneum. *Semin Roentgenol* 1980; 15:288–301.

37. Castrucci M, Mellone R, Vanzulli A, De Gaspari A, Castellano R, Astore D, Chiesa R, Grossi A, Del Maschio A. Mural thrombi in abdominal aortic aneurysms: MR imaging characterization—useful before endovascular treatment? *Radiology* 1995; 197:135–139.

38. Catalona WJ. Current management of testicular tumors. *Surg Clin North Am* 1982; 62:1119–1127.

39. Catasca JV, Mirowitz SA. T2-Weighted MR imaging of the abdomen: fast spin-echo vs conventional spin-echo sequences. *AJR* 1994; 162:61–67.

40. Chiappa S, Uslenghi C, Bonadonna G, et al. Combined testicular and foot lymphangiography in testicular carcinomas. *Surg Gynecol Obstet* 1966; 123:10–14.

41. Choi BI, Chi JG, Kim SH, Chang KH, Han MC. MR imaging of retroperitoneal teratoma: correlation with CT and pathology. *J Comput Assist Tomogr* 1989; 13(6):1083–1086.

42. Chuang VP, Fried AM, Chen CQ. Computed tomographic evaluation of para-aortic hematoma following translumbar aortography. *Radiology* 1979; 130:711–712.

43. Chuang VP, Mera CE, Hoskins PA. Congenital anomalies of the inferior vena cava. Review of embryogenesis and presentation of a simplified classification. *Br J Radiol* 1974; 47:206–213.

44. Churchill RJ, Wesby G III, Marsan RE, Moncada R, Reynes CJ, Love L. Computed tomographic demonstration of anomalous inferior vena cava with azygous continuation. *J Comput Assist Tomogr* 1980; 4:398–402.

45. Cisternino SJ, Neiman HL, Malave SR Jr. Diagnosis of retroperitoneal hemorrhage by serial computed tomography. *J Comput Assist Tomogr* 1979; 3:686–688.

46. Cohan RH, Baker ME, Cooper C, Moore JO, Saeed M, Dunnick NR. Computed tomography of primary retroperitoneal malignancies. *J Comput Assist Tomogr* 1988; 12(5):804–810.

47. Cory DA, Ellis JH, Bies JR, Olson EW. Retroaortic left renal vein demonstrated by nuclear magnetic resonance imaging. *J Comput Assist Tomogr* 1984; 8:339–340.

48. Crowther D, Blackledge G, Best JJK. The role of computed tomography of the abdomen in the diagnosis and staging of patients with lymphoma. *Clin Hematol* 1979; 83:567–591.

49. Damgaard-Pedersen K, von der Maase H. Ultrasound and ultrasound guided biopsy, CT and lymphography in the diagnosis of retroperitoneal metastases in testicular cancer. *Scand J Urol Nephrol* 1991; 137:139–144.

50. Davidson AJ, Hartman DS. Lymphangioma of the retroperitoneum: CT and sonographic characteristics. *Radiology* 1990; 175:507–510.

51. Davidson AJ, Hartman DS, Goldman SM. Mature teratoma of the retroperitoneum: radiologic, pathologic, and clinical correlation. *Radiology* 1989; 172:421–425.

52. Davis JH. Complications of surgery of the abdominal aorta. *Am J Surg* 1975; 130:523–527.

53. Degesys GE, Dunnick NR, Silverman PM, Cohan RH, Illescas FF, Castagno A. Retroperitoneal fibrosis: use of CT in distinguishing among possible causes. *AJR* 1986; 146:57–60.

54. Didier D, Racle A, Etievent JP, Weill F. Tumor thrombus of the inferior vena cava secondary to malignant abdominal neoplasms: US and CT evaluation. *Radiology* 1987; 162:83–89.

55. Dinsmore RE, Wedeen VJ, Miller SW, Rosen BR, Fifer M, Vlahakes GJ, Edelman RR, Brady TJ. MRI of dissection of the aorta: recognition of the intimal tear and differential flow velocites. *AJR* 1986; 146:1286–1288.

56. Dobrin PB. Pathophysiology and pathogenesis of aortic aneurysms: current concepts. *Surg Clin North Am* 1989; 69:687–703.

57. Donohue JP, Zachary JM, Maynard B. Distribution of nodal metastases in non-seminomatous testis cancer. *J Urol* 1982; 128:315–320.

58. Dooms GC, Hricak H, Crooks LE, Higgins CB. Magnetic resonance imaging of the lymph nodes: comparison with CT. *Radiology* 1984; 153:719–728.

59. Dooms GC, Hricak H, Moseley ME, Bottles K, Fisher M, Higgins CB. Characterization of lymphadenopathy by magnetic resonance relaxation times: preliminary results. *Radiology* 1985; 155:691–697.

60. Dooms GC, Hricak H, Sollitto RA, Higgins CB. Lipomatous tumors and tumors with fatty component: MR imaging potential and comparison of MR and CT results. *Radiology* 1985;157:479–483.

61. Dorfman RE, Alpern MB, Gross BH, Sandler MA. Upper abdominal lymph nodes: criteria for normal size determined with CT. *Radiology* 1991;180(2):319–322.

62. Douek PC, Revel D, Chazel S, Falise B, Villard J, Amiel M. Fast MR angiography of the aortoiliac arteries and arteries of the lower extremity: value of bolus-enhanced, whole-volume subtraction technique. *AJR* 1995;165:431–437.

63. Druy ME, Rubin BE. Computed tomography in the evaluation of abdominal trauma. *J Comput Assist Tomogr* 1979;3:40–44.

64. Dunnick NR, Javadpour N. Value of CT and lymphography: distinguishing retroperitoneal metastases from non-seminomatous testicular tumors. *AJR* 1981;136:1093–1099.

65. Earl HM, Sutcliffe SBJ, Fry IK, Tucker AK, Young J, Husband J, Wrigley PFM, Malpas JS. Computerised tomography (CT) abdominal scanning in Hodgkin's disease. *Clin Radiol* 1980;31:149–153.

66. Ebner F, Kressel HY, Mintz MC, et al. Tumor recurrent versus fibrosis in the female pelvis: differentiation with MR at 1.5T. *Radiology* 1988;166:333–340.

67. Edelman RR. MR angiography: present and future. *AJR* 1993;161:1–11.

68. Egan TJ, Neiman HL, Herman RJ, Malave SR, Sanders JH. Computed tomography in the diagnosis of aortic aneurysm dissection or traumatic injury. *Radiology* 1980;136:141–146.

69. Ehrlichman RJ, Kaufman SL, Siegelman SS, Trump DL, Walsh PC. Computerized tomography and lymphangiography in staging testis tumors. *J Urol* 1980;126:179–181.

70. Elkin M, Cohen G. Diagnostic value of the psoas shadow. *Clin Radiol* 1962;13:210–217.

71. Ellert J, Kreel L. The role of computed tomography in the initial staging and subsequent management of the lymphomas. *J Comput Assist Tomogr* 1980;4:368–391.

72. Ellis JH, Bies JR, Kopecky KK, Klatte EC, Rowland RG, Donohue JP. Comparison of NMR and CT imaging in the evaluation of metastatic retroperitoneal lymphadenopathy from testicular carcinoma. *J Comput Assist Tomogr* 1984;8:709–719.

73. Erdman WA, Weinreb JC, Cohen JM, Buja LM, Chaney C, Peshock RM. Venous thrombosis: clinical and experimental MR imaging. *Radiology* 1986;161:233–238.

74. Evancho AM, Osbakken M, Weidner W. Comparison of NMR imaging and aortography for preoperative evaluation of abdominal aortic aneurysm. *Magn Reson Med* 1985;2:41–55.

75. Faer MJ, Lynch RD, Evans HO, Chin FK. Inferior vena cava duplication: demonstration by computed tomography. *Radiology* 1979;130:707–709.

76. Fagan CJ, Larrieu AJ, Amparo EG. Retroperitoneal fibrosis: ultrasound and CT features. *AJR* 1979;133:239–243.

77. Federle MP, Goldberg HI, Kaiser JA, Moss AA, Jeffrey RB, Mall JC. Evaluation of abdominal trauma by computed tomography. *Radiology* 1981;138:637–644.

78. Fein AB, Lee JKT, Balfe DM, Heiken JP, Ling D, Glazer HS, McClennan BL. Diagnosis and staging of renal cell carcinoma: a comparison of MR imaging and CT. *AJR* 1987;148:749–753.

79. Feldberg MAM, Koehler PR, van Waes PFGM. Psoas compartment disease studied by computed tomography. *Radiology* 1983;148:505–512.

80. Fisher MR, Hricak H, Higgins CB. Magnetic resonance imaging of developmental venous anomalies. *AJR* 1985;145:705–709.

81. Flak B, Li DKB, Ho BYB, Knickerbocker WJ, Fache S, Mayo J, Chung W. Magnetic resonance imaging of aneurysms of the abdominal aorta. *AJR* 1985;144:991–996.

82. Friedland GW, deVries PA, Nino-Murcia M, King BF, Leder RA, Stevens S. Congenital anomalies of the inferior vena cava: embryogenesis and MR features. *Urol Radiol* 1992;13:237–248.

83. Friedman AC, Hartman DS, Sherman J, Lautin EM, Goldman M. Computed tomography of abdominal fatty masses. *Radiology* 1981;139:415–429.

84. Front D, Ben-Haim S, Israel O, Epelbaum R, Haim N, Even-Sapir E, Kolodny GM, Robinson E. Lymphoma: predictive value of Ga-67 scintigraphy after treatment. *Radiology* 1992;182:359–363.

85. Front D, Israel O, Epelbaum R, Haim SB, Sapir EE, Jerushalmi J, Kolodny GM, Robinson E. Ga-67 SPECT before and after treatment of lymphoma. *Radiology* 1990;175:515–519.

86. Gale ME, Johnson WC, Gerzof SG, Robbins AH. Problems in CT diagnosis of ruptured abdominal aortic aneurysms. *J Comput Assist Tomogr* 1986;10:637–641.

87. Gefter WB, Arger PH, Mulhern CB, Pollack HM, Wein AJ. Computed tomography of circumcaval ureter. *AJR* 1978;131:1086–1087.

88. Gehl HB, Bohndorf K, Klose KC. Inferior vena cava tumor thrombus: demonstration by Gd-DTPA enhanced MR. *J Comput Assist Tomogr* 1990;14(3):479–481.

89. Geisinger MA, Risius B, O'Donnell JA, Zelch MG, Moodie DS, Graor RA, George CR. Thoracic aortic dissection: magnetic resonance imaging. *Radiology* 1985;155:407–412.

90. Ginaldi S, Chuang VP, Wallace S. Absence of hepatic segment of the inferior vena cava with azygous continuation. *J Comput Assist Tomogr* 1980;4:112–114.

91. Glazer GM, Callen PW, Parker JJ. CT diagnosis of tumor thrombus in the inferior vena cava: avoiding the false-positive diagnosis. *AJR* 1981;137:1265–1267.

92. Glazer GM, Francis IR, Gross BH, Amendola MA. Computed tomography of renal vein thrombosis. *J Comput Assist Tomogr* 1984;8:288–293.

93. Glazer HS, Gutierrez F, Levitt RG, Lee JKT, Murphy WA. The thoracic aorta studied by MR imaging. *Radiology* 1985;157:149–156.

94. Glazer HS, Lee JKT, Balfe DM, Mauro M, Griffith RC, Sagel SS. Unusual CT manifestations of non-Hodgkin's lymphoma. *Radiology* 1983;149:211–217.

95. Glazer HS, Lee JKT, Levitt RG, Heiken JP, Ling D, Totty WG, Balfe DM, Emami B, Wasserman T, Murphy WA. Radiation fibrosis: differentiation from recurrent tumor by MR imaging. *Radiology* 1985;156:721–726.

96. Goldman SM, Davidson AJ, Neal J. Retroperitoneal and pelvic hemangiopericytomas: clinical, radiologic, and pathologic correlation. *Radiology* 1988;168:13–17.

97. Gomes MN, Choyke PL. Improved identification of renal arteries in patients with aortic aneurysms by means of high-resolution computed tomography. *J Vasc Surg* 1987;6:262–268.

98. Gomes NM, Hufnagel CA. CT scanning: a new method for the diagnosis of abdominal aortic aneurysms. *J Cardiovasc Surg* 1979;20:511–515.

99. Gomori JM, Grossman RI, Goldberg HI, Zimmerman RA, Bilaniuk LT. Intracranial hematomas: imaging by high-field MR. *Radiology* 1985;157:87–93.

100. Gonda RL Jr, Gutierrez OH, Azodo MVU. Mycotic aneurysms of the aorta: radiologic features. *Radiology* 1988;168:343–346.

101. Goodwin JD, Herfkens RL, Skioldebrand CG, Federle MP, Lipton MJ. Evaluation of dissections and aneurysms of the thoracic aorta by conventional and dynamic CT scanning. *Radiology* 1980;136:125–133.

102. Gross SC, Barr I, Eyler WR, Khaja F, Goldstein S. Computed tomography in dissection of the thoracic aorta. *Radiology* 1980;136:135–139.

103. Guinet C, Buy JN, Ghossain MA, Mark AS, Jardin M, Fourmestraux J, Dimaria G, Vadrot D. Aortic anastomotic pseudoaneurysms: US, CT, MR, and angiography. *J Comput Assist Tomogr* 1992;162(2):182–188.

104. Haaga JR, Baldwin N, Reich NE, Beven E, Kramer A, Weinstein A, Havrilla TR, Seidelmann FE, Namba AH, Parrish CM. CT detection of infected synthetic grafts: preliminary report of a new sign. *AJR* 1978;131:317–320.

105. Hahn PF, Saini S, Stark DD, Papanicolaou N, Ferrucci JT Jr. Intraabdominal hematoma: the concentric-ring sign in MR imaging. *AJR* 1987;148:115–119.

106. Hanna SL, Fletcher BD, Boulden TF, Hudson MM, Greenwald CA, Kun LE. MR imaging of infradiaphragmatic lymphadenopathy in children and adolescents with Hodgkin disease: comparison with lymphography and CT. *J Magn Reson Imaging* 1993;3(3):461–470.

107. Hayes WS, Davidson AJ, Grimley PM, Hartman DS. Extraadrenal retroperitoneal paraganglioma: clinical, pathologic, and CT findings. *AJR* 1990;155(6):1247–1250.

108. Heiberg E, Wolverson MK, Sundaram M, Shields JB. CT charac-

teristics of aortic atherosclerotic aneurysm versus aortic dissection. *J Comput Assist Tomogr* 1985;9:78–83.

109. Herfkens RJ, Higgins CB, Hricak H, Lipton MJ, Crooks LE, Sheldon DE, Kaufman L. Nuclear magnetic resonance imaging of atherosclerotic disease. *Radiology* 1983;148:161–166.

110. Herts BR, Megibow AJ, Birnbaum BA, Kanzer GK, Noz ME. High-attenuation lymphadenopathy in AIDS patients: significance of findings at CT. *Radiology* 1992;185:777–781.

111. Higgins CB, Goldberg H, Hricak H, Crooks LE, Kaufman L, Brasch R. Nuclear magnetic resonance imaging of vasculature of abdominal viscera: normal and pathologic features. *AJR* 1983;140: 1217–1225.

112. Hilton S, Megibow AJ, Naidich DP, Bosniak MA. Computed tomography of the postoperative abdominal aorta. *Radiology* 1982; 145:403–407.

113. Horejs D, Gilbert PM, Burstein S, Vogelzang RL. Normal aortoiliac diameters by CT. *J Comput Assist Tomogr* 1988;12(4):602–603.

114. Hricak H, Amparo E, Fisher MR, Crooks L, Higgins CB. Abdominal venous system: assessment using MR. *Radiology* 1985;156: 415–422.

115. Hricak H, Demas BE, Williams RD, McNamara MT, Hedgecock MW, Amparo EG, Tanagho EA. Magnetic resonance imaging in the diagnosis and staging of renal and perirenal neoplasms. *Radiology* 1985;154:709–715.

116. Hricak H, Higgins CB, Williams RD. Nuclear magnetic resonance imaging in retroperitoneal fibrosis. *AJR* 1983;141:35–38.

117. Hulnick DH, Chatson GP, Megibow AJ, Bosniak MA, Ruoff M. Retroperitoneal fibrosis presenting as colonic dysfunction: CT diagnosis. *J Comput Assist Tomogr* 1988;12(1):159–161.

118. Husband JE, Robinson L, Thomas G. Contrast enhancing lymph nodes in bladder cancer: a potential pitfall on CT. *Clin Radiol* 1992;45(6):395–398.

119. Jacoby WT, Cohan RH, Baker ME, Leder RA, Nadel SN, Dunnick NR. Ovarian vein thrombosis in oncology patients: CT detection and clinical significance. *AJR* 1990;155:291–294.

120. Javadpour N, Doppman JL, Bergman SM, Anderson T. Correlation of computed tomography and serum tumor markers in metastatic retroperitoneal testicular tumor. *J Comput Assist Tomogr* 1978;2: 176–180.

121. Jeffrey RB Jr, Callen PW, Federle MP. Computed tomography of psoas abscesses. *J Comput Assist Tomogr* 1980;4:639–641.

122. Jeffrey RB Jr, Cardoza JD, Olcott EW. Detection of active intraabdominal arterial hemorrhage: value of dynamic contrast-enhanced CT. *AJR* 1991;156:725–729.

123. Jeffrey RB Jr, Federle MP. The collapsed inferior vena cava: CT evidence of hypovolemia. *AJR* 1988;150:431–432.

124. Johnson KK, Russ PD, Bair JH, Friefeld GD. Diagnosis of synthetic vascular graft infection: comparison of CT and gallium scans. *AJR* 1990;154(2):405–409.

125. Johnston GS, Go MF, Benna RS, Larson SM, Andrews GA, Hubner KF. Gallium-67 citrate imaging in Hodgkin's disease: final report of cooperative group. *J Nucl Med* 1977;18:692–698.

126. Justich E, Amparo EG, Hricak H, Higgins CB. Infected aortoiliofemoral grafts: magnetic resonance imaging. *Radiology* 1985;154: 133–136.

127. Kallman DA, King BF, Hattery RR, Charboneau JW, Ehman RL, Guthman DA, Blute ML. Renal vein and inferior vena cava tumor thrombus in renal cell carcinoma: CT, US, MRI and venacavography. *J Comput Assist Tomogr* 1992;16(2):240–247.

128. Kam J, Patel S, Ward RE. Computed tomography of aortic and aortoiliofemoral grafts. *J Comput Assist Tomogr* 1982;6:298–303.

129. Kandarpa K, Piwnica-Worms D, Chopra PS, Adams DF, Hunink MG, Donaldson MC, Whittemore AD, Mannick JA, Harrington DP. Prospective double-blinded comparison of MR imaging and aortography in the preoperative evaluation of abdominal aortic aneurysms. *J Vasc Interv Radiol* 1992;3:83–89.

130. Kaszar-Seibert DJ, Gauvin GP, Rogoff PA, Vittimberga FJ, Margolis S, Hilgenberg AD, Saal DK, Goldsmith GO. Intracardiac extension of intravenous leiomyomatosis. *Radiology* 1988;168: 409–410.

131. Katz DA, Littenberg B, Cronenwett JL. Management of small abdominal aortic aneurysms. *JAMA* 1992;268:2678–2686.

132. Kaufman JA, Geller SC, Peterson MJ, Cambria RP, Prince MR,

Waltman AC. MR imaging (including MR angiography) of abdominal aortic aneurysms: comparison with conventional angiography. *AJR* 1994;163:203–210.

133. Kersting-Sommerhoff BA, Higgins DB, White RD, Sommerhoff CP, Lipton MJ. Aortic dissection: sensitivity and specificity of MR imaging. *Radiology* 1988;166:651–655.

134. Kim D, Edelman RR, Kent KC, Porter DH, Skillman JJ. Abdominal aorta and renal artery stenosis: evaluation with MR angiography. *Radiology* 1990;174:727–731.

135. Kim T, Murakami T, Oi H, Tsuda K, Matsushita M, Tomoda K, Fukuda H, Nakamura H. CT and MR imaging of abdominal liposarcoma. *AJR* 1996;166:829–833.

136. Kobayashi A, Matsui O, Takashima T, Ueno T, Kawahara E, Sugihara M, Kurosaki M, Notsumata K, Takayanagi N. Calcification in caval membrane causing primary Budd-Chiari syndrome: CT demonstration. *J Comput Assist Tomogr* 1988;12(3):401–404.

137. Korobkin M, Callen PW, Fisch AE. Computed tomography of the pelvis and retroperitoneum. *Radiol Clin North Am* 1979;17:301–318.

138. Koslin DB, Kenney PJ, Stanley RJ, Van Dyke JA. Aortocaval fistula: CT appearance with angiographic correlation. *J Comput Assist Tomogr* 1987;11(2):348–350.

139. Kreel L. The EMI whole body scanner in the demonstration of lymph node enlargement. *Clin Radiol* 1976;27:421–429.

140. Kukora JS, Rushton FW, Cranston PE. New computed tomographic signs of aortoenteric fistula. *Arch Surg* 1984;119:1073–1075.

141. Kvilekval KHV, Best IM, Mason RA, Newton GB, Giron F. The value of computed tomography in the management of symptomatic abdominal aortic aneurysms. *J Vasc Surg* 1990;12:28–33.

142. Landay MJ, Virolainen H. ''Hyperdense'' aortic wall: potential pitfall in CT screening for aortic dissection. *J Comput Assist Tomogr* 1991;15(4):561–564.

143. Lane RH, Stephens DH, Reiman HM. Primary retroperitoneal neoplasms: CT findings in 90 cases with clinical and pathologic correlation. *AJR* 1989;152:83–89.

144. Lange PH, Fraley EE. Serum alpha-fetoprotein and human chorionic gonadotropin in the treatment of patients with testicular tumors. *Urol Clin North Am* 1977;4:383–406.

145. Larde D, Belloir C, Vasile N, Frija J, Ferrane J. Computed tomography of aortic dissection. *Radiology* 1980;136:147–151.

146. Latifi HR, Heiken JP. CT of inflammatory abdominal aortic aneurysm: development from an uncomplicated atherosclerotic aneurysm. *J Comput Assist Tomogr* 1992;16(3):484–486.

147. Lee JKT, Balfe DM. Computed tomographic evaluation of lymphoma patients. *CRC Crit Rev Diagn Imaging* 1981;18:1–28.

148. Lee JKT, Glazer HS. Psoas muscle disorders: MR imaging. *Radiology* 1986;160:683–687.

149. Lee JKT, Heiken JP, Ling D, Glazer HS, Balfe DM, Levitt RG, Dixon WT, Murphy WA. Magnetic resonance imaging of abdominal and pelvic lymphadenopathy. *Radiology* 1984;153:181–188.

150. Lee JKT, Levitt RG, Stanley RJ, Sagel SS. Utility of body computed tomography in the clinical follow-up of abdominal masses. *J Comput Assist Tomogr* 1978;2:607–611.

151. Lee JKT, Ling D, Heiken JP, Glazer HS, Sicard GA, Totty WG, Levitt RG, Murphy WA. Magnetic resonance imaging of abdominal aortic aneurysms. *Radiology* 1984;143:1197–1202.

152. Lee JKT, McClennan BL, Stanley RJ, Sagel SS. Computed tomography in the staging of testicular neoplasms. *Radiology* 1978;130: 387–390.

153. Lee JKT, Stanley RJ, Sagel SS, Levitt RG. Accuracy of computed tomography in detecting intraabdominal and pelvic adenopathy in lymphoma. *AJR* 1978;131:311–315.

154. Lee JKT, Stanley RJ, Sagel SS, McClennan BL. Accuracy of CT in detecting intraabdominal and pelvic lymph node metastases from pelvic cancers. *AJR* 1978;131:675–679.

155. Lenchik L, Dovgan DJ, Kier R. CT of the iliopsoas compartment: value in differentiating tumor, abscess, and hematoma. *AJR* 1994; 162:83–86.

156. Lewis E, Bernardino ME, Salvador PG, Cabanillas FF, Barnes PA, Thomas JL. Post-therapy CT-detected mass in lymphoma patients: is it viable tissue? *J Comput Assist Tomogr* 1982;6:792–795.

157. Li DKB, Rennie CS. Abdominal computed tomography in Whipple's disease. *J Comput Assist Tomogr* 1981;5:249–252.

158. Libshitz HI, Jing BS, Wallace S, Logothetis CJ. Sterilized metastases: a diagnostic and therapeutic dilemma. *AJR* 1983;140:15–19.

159. Lien HH, Kolbenstvedt A, Talle K, Fossa SD, Klepp O, Ous S. Comparison of computed tomography, lymphography, and phlebography in 200 consecutive patients with regard to retroperitoneal metastases from testicular tumor. *Radiology* 1983;146:129–132.

160. Lim JH, Park JH, Auh YH. Membranous obstruction of the inferior vena cava: comparison of findings at sonography, CT, and venography. *AJR* 1992;159:515–520.

161. Limet R, Sakalihassan N, Albert A. Determination of the expansion rate and incidence of rupture of abdominal aortic aneurysm. *J Vasc Surg* 1991;14:540–548.

162. Lineaweaver WC, Clore F, Alexander RH. Computed tomography diagnosis of acute aortoiliac catastrophes. *Arch Surg* 1982;117:1095–1097.

163. Loubeyre P, Revel D, Garcia P, Delignette A, Canet E, Chirossel P, Genin G, Amiel M. Screening patients for renal artery stenosis: value of three-dimensional time-of-flight MR angiography. *AJR* 1994;162:847–852.

164. Louridas G, Gaylis H. Management of tender abdominal aortic aneurysm. *S Afr Med J* 1988;74:165–167.

165. Low RN, Wall SD, Jeffrey RB Jr, Sollitto RA, Reilly LM, Tierney LM Jr. Aortoenteric fistula and perigraft infection: evaluation with CT. *Radiology* 1990;175:157–162.

166. Machida K, Tasaka A. CT patterns of mural thrombus in aortic aneurysms. *J Comput Assist Tomogr* 1980;4:840–842.

167. Maier SE, Maier D, Boesiger P, Moser UT, Vieli A. Human abdominal aorta: comparative measurements of blood flow with MR imaging and multigated Doppler US. *Radiology* 1989;171:487–492.

168. Mark AS, McCarthy SM, Moss AA, Price D. Detection of abdominal aortic graft infection: comparison of CT and In-labeled white blood cell scans. *AJR* 1985;144:315–318.

169. Mark AS, Moss AA, Lusby R, Kaiser JA. CT evaluation of complications of abdominal aortic surgery. *Radiology* 1982;145:409–414.

170. Marks WM, Korobkin M, Callen PW, Kaiser JA. CT diagnosis of tumor thrombosis in the renal vein and inferior vena cava. *AJR* 1978;131:843–846.

171. Marshall WH, Breiman RS, Harell GS, Glatstein E, Kaplan HS. Computed tomography of abdominal paraaortic lymph node disease: preliminary observations with a 6 second scanner. *AJR* 1977;128:759–764.

172. Marston WA, Ahlquist R, Johnson G, Meyer AA. Misdiagnosis of ruptured abdominal aortic aneurysms. *J Vasc Surg* 1992;16:17–22.

173. McLeod AJ, Zornoza J, Shirkhoda A. Leiomyosarcoma: computed tomographic findings. *Radiology* 1984;152:133–136.

174. Mechlin M, Thickman D, Kressel HY, Gefter W, Joseph P. Magnetic resonance imaging of postoperative patients with metallic implants. *AJR* 1984;143:1281–1284.

175. Megibow AJ, Ambos MA, Bosniak MA. Computed tomographic diagnosis of ureteral obstruction secondary to aneurysmal disease. *Urol Radiol* 1980;1:211–215.

176. Megibow AJ, Balthazar EJ, Nadich DP, Bosniak MA. Computed tomography of gastrointestinal lymphoma. *AJR* 1983;141:541–547.

177. Mehard WB, Heiken JP, Sicard GA. High-attenuation crescent in abdominal aortic aneurysm wall at CT: sign of acute or impending rupture *(abstr)*. *Radiology* 1994;192:359–362.

178. Mendez G, Isikoff MB, Hill MC. Retroperitoneal processes involving the psoas demonstrated by computed tomography. *J Comput Assist Tomogr* 1980;4:78–82.

179. Miller CL, Wechsler RJ. CT evaluation of Kimray-Greenfield filter complications. *AJR* 1986;147(1):45–50.

180. Miyake H, Suzuki K, Ueda S, Yamada Y, Takeda H, Mori H. Localized fat collection adjacent to the intrahepatic portion of the inferior vena cava: a normal variant on CT. *AJR* 1992;158:423–425.

181. Moon KL, Federle MP, Abrams DI, Volberding P, Lewis BJ. Kaposi sarcoma and lymphadenopathy syndrome: limitations of abdominal CT in acquired immunodeficiency syndrome. *Radiology* 1984;150:479–483.

182. Mori H, Fukuda T, Isomoto I, Maeda H, Hayashi K. CT diagnosis of catheter-induced septic thrombus of vena cava. *J Comput Assist Tomogr* 1990;14(2):236–238.

183. Moriarty JA, Edelman RR, Tumeh SS. CT and MRI of mycotic aneurysms of the abdominal aorta. *J Comput Assist Tomogr* 1992;16(6):941–943.

184. Mueller PR, Ferrucci JT Jr, Wittenberg J, Simeone JF, Butch RJ. Iliopsoas abscess: treatment by CT-guided percutaneous catheter drainage. *AJR* 1984;142:359–362.

185. Mulligan SA, Holley HC, Koehler RE, Koslin DB, Rubin E, Berland LL, Kenney PJ. CT and MR imaging in the evaluation of retroperitoneal fibrosis. *J Comput Assist Tomogr* 1989;13(2):277–281.

186. Munechika H, Cohan RH, Baker ME, Cooper CJ, Dunnick NR. Hemiazgos continuation of a left inferior vena cava: CT appearance. *J Comput Assist Tomogr* 1988;12(2):328–330.

187. Neumann CH, Robert NJ, Canellos G, Rosenthal D. Computed tomography of the abdomen and pelvis in non-Hodgkin lymphoma. *J Comput Assist Tomogr* 1983;7:846–850.

188. Nevitt MP, Ballard DJ, Hallett JW. Prognosis of abdominal aortic aneurysms: a population-based study. *N Engl J Med* 1989;321:1009–1014.

189. New PFJ, Aronow S. Attenuation measurements of whole blood and blood fractions in computed tomography. *Radiology* 1976;121:635–640.

190. Pagani JJ, Thomas JL, Bernardino ME. Computed tomographic manifestations of abdominal and pelvic venous collaterals. *Radiology* 1982;142:415–419.

191. Panicek DM, Toner GC, Heelan RT, Bosl GJ. Nonseminomatous germ cell tumors: enlarging masses despite chemotherapy. *Radiology* 1990;175:499–502.

192. Papanicolaou N, Wittenberg J, Ferrucci JT Jr, Stauffer AE, Waltman AC, Simeone JF, Mueller PR, Brewster DC, Darling RC. Preoperative evaluation of abdominal aortic aneurysms by computed tomography. *AJR* 1986;146:711–715.

193. Park JH, Lee JB, Han MC, Choi BI, Im CK, Chang KH, Yeon KM, Kim CW. Sonographic evaluation of inferior vena caval obstruction: correlative study with vena cavography. *AJR* 1985;145:757–762.

194. Parodi JC. Endovascular repair of abdominal aortic aneurysms and other arterial lesions. *J Vasc Surg* 1995;21:549–557.

195. Pels Rijcken TH, Davis MA, Ros PB. Intraluminal contrast agents for MR imaging of the abdomen and pelvis. *J Magn Reson Imaging* 1994;4:291–300.

196. Pera A, Cepek M, Shirkhoda A. Lymphangiography and CT in the follow-up of patients with lymphoma. *Radiology* 1987;164(3):631–633.

197. Perrett LV, Sage MR. Computed tomography of abdominal aortic aneurysms. *J Surg* 1978;48:275–277.

198. Petasnick JP. Radiologic evaluation of aortic dissection. *Radiology* 1991;180(2):297–305.

199. Pierro JA, Soleimanpour M, Bory JL. Left retrocaval ureter associated with left inferior vena cava. *AJR* 1990;155:545–546.

200. Pillari G, Chang JB, Zito J, et al. Computed tomography of abdominal aortic aneurysm: an in vivo pathological report with a note on dynamic predictors. *Arch Surg* 1988;123:727–732.

201. Platt JF, Ellis JH, Korobkin M, Reige KA, Konnak JW, Leichtman AB. Potential renal donors: comparison of conventional imaging with helical CT. *Radiology* 1996;198:419–423.

202. Pombo F, Rodriquez E, Caruncho MV, Villalva C, Crespo C. CT attenuation values and enhancing characteristics of thoracoabdominal lymphomatous adenopathies. *J Comput Assist Tomogr* 1994;18(1):59–62.

203. Pombo F, Rodriquez E, Mato J, Perez-Fontan J, Rivera E, Valvuena L. Patterns of contrast enhancement of tuberculous lymph nodes demonstrated by computed tomography. *Clin Radiol* 1992;46(1):13–17.

204. Pond GD, Castellino RA, Horning S, Hoppe RT. Non-Hodgkin lymphoma: influence of lymphography, CT, and bone marrow biopsy on staging and management. *Radiology* 1989;170:159–164.

205. Prince MR. Gadolinium-enhanced MR aortography. *Radiology* 1994;191:155–164.
206. Prince MR, Narasimham DL, Stanley JC, Chenevert TL, Williams DM, Marx MV, Cho KJ. Breath-hold gadolinium-enhanced MR angiography of the abdominal aorta and its major branches. *Radiology* 1995;197:785–792.
207. Radin DR. Disseminated histoplasmosis: abdominal CT findings in 16 patients. *AJR* 1991;157(5):955–958.
208. Radin DR. Intraabdominal *Mycobacterium tuberculosis* vs *Mycobacterium avium-intracellulare* infections in patients with AIDS: distinction based on CT findings. *AJR* 1991;156(3):487–491.
209. Rahmouni A, Tempany C, Jones R, Mann R, Yang A, Zerhouni E. Lymphoma: monitoring tumor size and signal intensity with MR imaging. *Radiology* 1993;188:455–451.
210. Ralls PW, Boswell W, Henderson R, Rogers W, Boger D, Halls J. CT of inflammatory disease of the psoas muscle. *AJR* 1980;134:767–770.
211. Rebner M, Gross BH, Korobkin M, Ruiz J. CT appearance of right gonadal vein. *J Comput Assist Tomogr* 1989;13(3):460–462.
212. Redman HC, Glatstein E, Castellino RA, Federal WA. Computed tomography as an adjunct in the staging of Hodgkin's disease and non-Hodgkin's lymphomas. *Radiology* 1977;124:381–385.
213. Rehn SM, Nyman RS, Glimelius BLG, Hagberg HE, Sundstrom JC. Non-Hodgkin lymphoma: predicting prognostic grade with MR imaging. *Radiology* 1990;176:249–253.
214. Rosen A, Korobkin M, Silverman PM, Moore AV Jr, Dunnick NR. CT diagnosis of ruptured abdominal aortic aneurysm. *AJR* 1984;143:265–268.
215. Rosenbaum R, Hoffsten PE, Stanley RJ, Klahr S. Use of computerized tomography to diagnose complications of percutaneous renal biopsy. *Kidney Int* 1978;14:87–92.
216. Rotter AJ, Lundell CJ. MR of intravenous leiomyomatosis of the uterus extending into the inferior vena cava. *J Comput Assist Tomogr* 1991;15(4):690–693.
217. Royal SA, Callen PW. CT evaluation of anomalies of the inferior vena cava and left renal vein. *AJR* 1979;132:759–763.
218. Rozenblit A, Marin ML, Veith FJ, Cynamon J, Wahl SI, Bakal SW. Endovascular repair of abdominal aortic aneurysm: value of postoperative follow-up with helical CT. *AJR* 1995;165:1473–1479.
219. Rubenstein WA, Gray G, Auh YH, Honig CL, Thorbjarnarson B, Williams JJ, Haimes AB, Zirinsky K, Kazam E. CT of fibrous tissues and tumors with sonographic correlation. *AJR* 1986;147:1067–1074.
220. Rubin GD, Dake MD, Napel S, Jeffrey RB, McDonnell CH, Sommer FG, Wexler L, Williams DM. Spiral CT of renal artery stenosis: comparison of three-dimensional rendering techniques. *Radiology* 1994;190:181–189.
221. Rubin GD, Walker PJ, Dake MD, Napel S, Jeffrey RB, McDonnel CH, Mitchell RS, Miller DC. Three-dimensional spiral computed tomographic angiography: an alternative imaging modality for the abdominal aorta and its branches. *J Vasc Surg* 1993;18(4):656–664.
222. Rubin JI, Gomori JM, Grossman RI, Gefter WB, Kressel HY. High-field MR imaging of extracranial hematomas. *AJR* 1987;148:813–817.
223. Safer ML, Green JP, Crews QE Jr, Hill DR. Lymphangiographic accuracy in the staging of testicular tumors. *Cancer* 1975;35:1603–1605.
224. Sagel SS, Siegel MJ, Stanley RJ, Jost RG. Detection of retroperitoneal hemorrhage by computed tomography. *AJR* 1977;129:403–407.
225. Sarno RC, Carter BL, Bankoff MS. Cystic lymphangiomas: CT diagnosis and thin needle aspiration. *Br J Radiol* 1984;57:424–426.
226. Savader SJ, Otero RR, Savader BL. Puerperal ovarian vein thrombosis: evaluation with CT, US, and MR imaging. *Radiology* 1988;167:637–639.
227. Schaner EG, Head GL, Doppman JL, Young RC. Computed tomography in the diagnosis, staging, and management of abdominal lymphoma. *J Comput Assist Tomogr* 1977;1:176–180.
228. Schultz CL, Morrison S, Bryan PJ. Azygous continuation of the inferior vena cava: demonstration by NMR imaging. *J Comput Assist Tomogr* 1984;8:774–776.
229. Schwerk WB, Schwerk WN, Rodeck G. Venous renal tumor extension: a prospective US evaluation. *Radiology* 1985;156:491–495.
230. Shaffer PB, Johnson JC, Bryan D, Fabri PJ. Diagnosis of ovarian vein thrombophlebitis by computed tomography. *J Comput Assist Tomogr* 1981;5:436–439.
231. Shin MS, Berland LL, Ho KJ. Small aorta: CT detection and clinical significance. *J Comput Assist Tomogr* 1990;14(1):102–103.
232. Siegel CL, Cohan RH. CT of abdominal aortic aneurysms. *AJR* 1994;163:17–29.
233. Silverman PM, Kelvin FM, Korobkin M, Dunnick NR. Computed tomogrqaphy of the normal mesentery. *AJR* 1984;143:953–957.
234. Sivananthan UM, Ridgway JP, Bann K, Verma SP, Cullingworth J, Ward J, Rees MR. Fast magnetic resonance angiography using turbo-FLASH sequences in advanced aortoiliac disease. *Br J Radiol* 1993;66(792):1103–1110.
235. Soo CS, Bernardino ME, Chuang VP, Ordonez N. Pitfalls of CT findings in post-therapy testicular carcinoma. *J Comput Assist Tomogr* 1981;5:39–41.
236. Steele JR, Sones PJ, Heffner LT Jr. The detection of inferior vena cava thrombosis with computed tomography. *Radiology* 1978;128:385–386.
237. Stephens DH, Sheedy PF, Hattery RR, Williams B. Diagnosis and evaluation of retroperitoneal tumors by computed tomography. *AJR* 1977;129:395–402.
238. Stephens DH, Williamson B Jr, Sheedy PF II, Hattery RR, Miller WE. Computed tomography of the retroperitoneal space. *Radiol Clin North Am* 1977;15:377–390.
239. Sterzer SK, Herr HW, Mintz I. Idiopathic retroperitoneal fibrosis misinterpreted as lymphoma by computed tomography. *J Urol* 1979;122:405–406.
240. Stomper PC, Cholewinski SP, Park J, Bakshi SP, Barcos MP. Abdominal staging of thoracic Hodgkin disease: CT-lymphangiography-Ga-67 scanning correlation. *Radiology* 1993;187(2):381–386.
241. Stomper PC, Fung CY, Socinski MA, Jochelson MS, Garnick MB, Ritchie JP. Detection of retroperitoneal metastases in early-stage nonseminomatous testicular cancer: analysis of different CT criteria. *AJR* 1987;149(6):1187–1190.
242. Stomper PC, Kalish LA, Garnick MB, Richie JP, Kantoff PW. CT and pathologic predictive features of residual mass histologic findings after chemotherapy for nonseminomatous germ cell tumors: can residual malignancy or teratoma be excluded? *Radiology* 1991;180:711–714.
243. Swan JS, Grist TM, Weber DM, Sproat IA, Wojtowycz MM. MR angiography of the pelvis with variable velocity encoding and a phased-array coil. *Radiology* 1994;190:363–369.
244. Swensen SJ, Keller PL, Berquist TH, McLeod RA, Stephens DH. Magnetic resonance imaging of hemorrhage. *AJR* 1985;145:921–927.
245. Swensen SJ, McLeod RA, Stephens DH. CT of extracranial hemorrhage and hematomas. *AJR* 1984;143:907–912.
246. Teitelbaum GP, Ortega HV, Vinitski S, Clark RA, Watanabe AT, Matsumoto AH, Rifkin MD, Barth KH. Optimatization of gradient-echo imaging parameters for intracaval filters and trapped thromboemboli. *Radiology* 1990;174:1013–1019.
247. Teitelbaum GP, Ortega HV, Vinitski S, Stern H, Tsuruda JS, Mitchell DG, Rifkin MD, Bradley WG Jr. Low-artifact intravascular devices: MR imaging evaluation. *Radiology* 1988;168:713–719.
248. Thomas JL, Bernardino ME, Bracken RB. Staging of testicular carcinoma: comparison of CT and lymphangiography. *AJR* 1981;137:991–996.
249. Thorsen MK, San Dretto MA, Lawson TL, Foley WD, Smith DF, Berland LL. Dissecting aortic aneurysms: accuracy of computed tomographic diagnosis. *Radiology* 1983;148:773–777.
250. Todd GJ, Nowygrod R, Benvenisty A, Buda J, Reemtsma K. The accuracy of CT scanning in the diagnosis of abdominal and thoracoabdominal aortic aneurysms. *J Vasc Sury* 1991;13:302–309.
251. Torres WE, Maurer DE, Steinberg HV, Robbins S, Bernardino ME. CT of aortic aneurysms: the distinction between mural and thrombus calcification. *AJR* 1988;150:1317–1319.
252. Turner RJ, Young SW, Castellino RA. Dynamic continous com-

puted tomography: study of retroaortic left renal vein. *J Comput Assist Tomogr* 1980;4:109–111.

253. Unger EC, Glazer HS, Lee JKT, Ling D. MRI of extracranial hematomas: preliminary observations. *Radiology* 1986;146:403–407.

254. van Rooij WJJ, Martens F, Verbeeten B Jr, Dijkstra J. CT and MR imaging of leiomyosarcoma of the inferior vena cava. *J Comput Assist Tomogr* 1988;12(3):415–419.

255. Van Bockel SR, Mindelzun RE. Gas in the psoas muscle secondary to an intravertebral vacuum cleft: CT characteristics. *J Comput Assist Tomogr* 1987;11(5):913–915.

256. VanBreda A, Rubin BE, Druy EM. Detection of inferior vena cava abnormalities by computed tomography. *J Comput Assist Tomogr* 1979;3:164–169.

257. Van Hoe L, Baert AL, Gryspeerdt S, Marchal G, Lacroix H, Wilms G, Mertens L. Supra- and juxtarenal aneurysms of aorta: preoperative assessment with thin-section spiral CT. *Radiology* 1996;198:443–448.

258. Vinnicombe SJ, Norman AR, Nicholson V, Husband JE. Normal pelvic lymph nodes: evaluation with CT after bipedal lymphangiography. *Radiology* 1995;194:349–355.

259. Vint VC, Usselman JA, Warmath MA, Dilley RB. Aortic perianeurysmal fibrosis: CT density enhancement and ureteral obstruction. *AJR* 1980;134:577–580.

260. Vogelzang RL, Gore RM, Neiman HL, Smith SJ, Deschler TW, Vrla RF. Inferior vena cava CT pseudothrombus produced by rapid arm-vein contrast infusion. *AJR* 1985;144:843–846.

261. Vogelzang RL, Sohaey R. Infected aortic aneurysms: CT appearance. *J Comput Assist Tomogr* 1988;12(1):109–112.

262. Vowden P, Wilkinson D, Ausobsky JR, Kester RC. A comparison of three imaging techniques in the assessment of an abdominal aortic aneurysm. *J Cardiovasc Surg* 1989;30:891–896.

263. Waligore MP, Stephens DH, Soule EH, McLeod RA. Lipomatous tumors of the abdominal cavity: CT appearance and pathologic conditions. *AJR* 1981;137:539–545.

264. Weiner JI, Chako AC, Merten CW, Gross S, Coffey EL, Stein HL. Breast and axillary tissue MR imaging: corelation of signal intensities and relaxation times with pathologic findings. *Radiology* 1986;160:299–305.

265. Weinreb JC, Cohen JM, Maravilla KR. Iliopsoas muscles: MR study of normal anatomy and disease. *Radiology* 1985;156:435–440.

266. Weyman PJ, McClennan BL, Stanley RJ, Levitt RG, Sagel SS. Comparison of computed tomography and angiography in the evaluation of renal cell carcinoma. *Radiology* 1980;137:417–424.

267. William MP, Cook JV, Duchesne GM. Psoas nodes—an overlooked site of metastasis from testicular tumours. *Clin Radiol* 1989;40:607–609.

268. Williams DM, Joshi A, Dake MD, Deeb GM, Miller DC, Abrams GD. Aortic cobwebs: an anatomic marker identifying the false lumen in aortic dissection—imaging and pathologic correlation. *Radiology* 1994;190:167–174.

269. Wolf RL, King BF, Torres VE, Wilson DM, Ehman RL. Measurement of normal renal artery blood flow: cine phase-contrast MR imaging vs clearance of *p*-aminohippurate. *AJR* 1993;161(5):995–1002.

270. Wolff KA, Herold CJ, Tempany CM, Parravano JG, Zerhouni EA. Aortic dissection: atypical patterns seen at MR imaging. *Radiology* 1991;181:489–495.

271. Wolverson MK, Crepps LF, Sundaram M, Heiberg E, Vas WG, Shields JB. Hyperdensity of recent hemorrhage at body computed tomography: incidence and morphologic variation. *Radiology* 1983;148:779–784.

272. Yamada T, Tada S, Harada J. Aortic dissection without intimal rupture: diagnosis with MR imaging and CT. *Radiology* 1988;168:347–352.

273. Yamamoto S, Yokoyama T, Takeshige K, Iwatsuki S. Budd-Chiari syndrome with obstruction of inferior vena cava. *Gastroenterology* 1968;54:1070–1084.

274. Yucel EK, Silver MS, Carter AP. MR angiography of normal pelvic arteries: comparison of signal intensity and contrast-to-noise ratio for three different inflow techniques. *AJR* 1994;163:197–201.

275. Yuh WTC, Barloon TJ, Sickels WJ, et al. Magnetic resonance imaging in the diagnosis and followup of idiopathic retroperitoneal fibrosis. *J Urol* 1989;141:602–605.

276. Zelch MG, Haaga JR. Clinical comparison of computed tomography and lymphangiography for detection of retroperitoneal lymphadenopathy. *Radiol Clin North Am* 1979;17:157–168.

277. Zeman RK, Cronan JJ, Rosenfield AT, Lynch JH, Jaffe MH, Clark LR. Renal cell carcinoma: dynamic thin-section CT assessment of vascular invasion and tumor vascularity. *Radiology* 1988;167:393–396.

278. Zeman RK, Silverman PM, Berman PM, Weltman DI, Davros WJ, Gomes MN. Abdominal aortic aneurysms: evaluation of variable-collimation helical CT and overlapping reconstruction. *Radiology* 1994;193:555–560.

279. Zeppa MA, Forrest JV. Aortoenteric fistula manifested as an intramural duodenal hematoma. *AJR* 1991;157:47–48.

280. Zimmerman RD, Deck MDI. Intracranial hematomas: imaging by high-field MR. *Radiology* 1986;159:565–566.

281. Zirinsky K, Auh YH, Rubenstein WA, Kneeland JB, Whalen JP, Kazam E. The portacaval space: CT with MR correlation. *Radiology* 1985;156:453–460.

CHAPTER 18

The Kidney

Philip J. Kenney and Bruce L. McClennan

Computed tomography (CT) has had a profound impact on diagnostic uroradiology. It has proven useful for imaging the complete spectrum of renal and ureteral disorders (260). Despite the continued availability of less expensive imaging methods, and despite advances in sonography and magnetic resonance imaging (MRI), CT has continued to play a major role in diagnosis, management, and follow-up of patients with urologic disease. CT should be used in many areas for definitive evaluation of lesions suspected from other studies, such as intravenous urography or sonography, but for many disorders, the diagnostic power of CT is so definitive that its use as the primary diagnostic imaging procedure is justified, and other studies are not required (Table 1).

To a large degree, the power of CT lies in its ability to display the entire urinary tract in cross section. Normal and abnormal structures are directly shown, without the potential confusion of overlying structures, as may occur with urography, and without the potential for obscuration by bowel gas or bone, as may occur with sonography. Structures that previously were barely visible or only inferred, such as the retroperitoneal fascia, are clearly and reproducibly seen (164,222). Because of its much higher contrast sensitivity, CT allows differentiation of tissues with much less density difference than could be identified by plain radiography; thus, there is greater sensitivity to detection of calcification, faint or limited contrast excretion, and "radiolucent" calculi (e.g., urate). Computed tomography can image the urinary tract even without contrast media, so that useful information can be derived in patients with renal failure or other contraindications to the use of intravenous contrast. Additionally, CT can display enhancement or excretion patterns, extremely valuable diagnostic criteria for many diseases, which is not possible with sonography.

The technologic evolution of CT has further enhanced its valuable diagnostic role for urologic disease. CT provides better spatial resolution and signal-to-noise ratio than MRI. Rapid scan times (less than 2 seconds per slice) avoid respiratory motion artifact. Current scanners allow imaging with both rapid acquisition and thin slices, so that images of high quality can be obtained during the optimal time of enhancement after intravenous contrast administration. CT can be performed quickly and with reproducible technique, which is particularly important in very sick patients. Computed tomography is a noninvasive study, although the patient is exposed to X-rays and, when needed, intravenous contrast medium.

TABLE 1. *Indications for renal CT and/or MRI*

Renal masses: cyst, tumor, pseudotumor, calcification, AVM
    Evaluate lesions that are indeterminate on US, IVU; stage solid masses
Oncologic management
    Tumor detection (unknown primary), metastasis search
    Renal involvement in lymphoma, treatment planning, follow-up
Infection: acute, chronic, abscess, XGP, TB
Trauma
    Exclude or detect and characterize renal injury, follow-up for complications
Calculus disease
    Distinguish between radiolucent calculi and TCCA
Renal failure: hydronephrosis, parenchymal disease
Miscellaneous: congenital anomalies, vascular disease (renal ischemia, venous thrombosis, arterial stenosis), transplants

AVM, arteriovenous malformation; US, ultrasound; IVU, intravenous urography; XGP, xanthogranulomatous pyelonephritis; TB, tuberculosis; TCCA, transitional cell carcinoma.

Although many renal abnormalities are evident on post-contrast CT images, complete evaluation of the kidney by CT requires both pre- and postcontrast images (Fig. 1). Calculi may be obscured by contrast medium excretion, and diagnosis of masses requires assessment of enhancement, which is only accurate if pre- and postcontrast attenuation can be compared. Thus, for evaluation of known or suspected renal masses, or for evaluation of hematuria, both pre- and postcontrast images should be obtained. Five-millimeter collimation is usually sufficient, but thinner sections may be useful for small masses. A sufficient dose of intravenous contrast medium must be used, but smaller doses of nonionic contrast (150 ml) provide comparable image quality to higher doses of ionic contrast media (180 ml). Helical CT offers significant advantages for urinary tract CT. It allows collection of a set of images from a volume of tissue during a single suspended respiration, allowing truly contiguous slices to be obtained (161). Slice misregistration between pre- and postcontrast images is avoided. Images of the kidney (the cortical enhancement phase) can be acquired during the earliest nephrographic phase on spiral CT (Fig. 2). Some lesions, however, may be more conspicuous after some delay (47). Helical CT provides superior reformatted images, and it may improve diagnosis of renal vascular dis-eases. Although it has been shown that helical CT better displays fine anatomic details of the kidney, particularly the renal arteries and veins (340), there are few scientific studies comparing transaxial and helical CT for specific urinary tract diagnoses other than renal masses.

High-quality renal CT can be accomplished with either dynamic incremental or helical technique. Precontrast scans are obtained with 5-mm slice collimation at 5-mm increments through the kidneys. Iodinated contrast medium (180 ml of ionic contrast or 150 ml of nonionic contrast) is administered intravenously via a power injector at 3 ml/sec. With dynamic incremental technique, a 2-sec scan time and a 4-sec interscan pause [120 to 140 kV(p) (kilovolt peak), 140 to 170 mAs (milliampere second)] are used. Scans are obtained 60 sec after the initiation of contrast administration, from the diaphragm to the top of either kidney, using 5-mm slice collimation at 10-mm slice intervals. Contiguous 5-mm scans then are obtained through both kidneys. In helical mode, scanning is begun 70 sec after the initiation of contrast administration, using 1 sec scan time at 1:1 pitch. One to two groups of helical sets (7 by 7 mm through the liver, 5 by 5 mm though the kidneys) are obtained with 7- to 10-sec intergroup pause.

Computed tomography is a valuable tool in evaluation of many suspected urinary tract disorders (Table 1). The

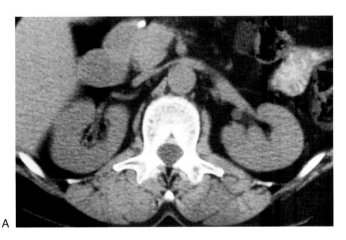

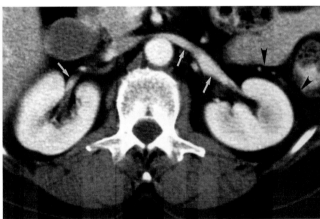

FIG. 1. Normal renal CT. **A:** The kidneys are isodense with muscle on this noncontrast CT image. **B:** The renal parenchyma and renal veins *(arrows)* enhance brightly after intravenous contrast; note anterior renal fascia *(arrowheads)*. **C:** Postcontrast CT shows opacified renal pelvis *(arrow)* and renal vein branches *(arrowheads)* coursing anteromedially through renal sinus fat.

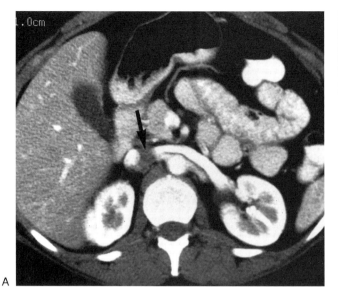

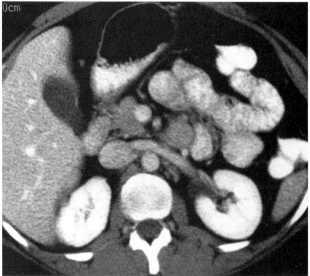

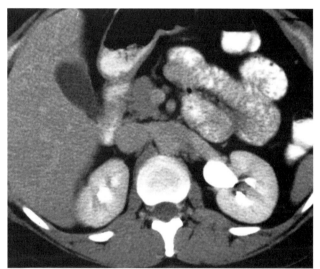

FIG. 2. Renal enhancement patterns. **A:** At 70 sec after rapid bolus injection of 125 cc of Ioversol, there is very dense opacification of renal cortex and veins. Note streaming effect in inferior vena cava *(arrow)*. **B:** At 130 sec after injection, the medulla has also become brightly enhanced; the renal pelvis is not yet opacified, but the renal vein is less well opacified than in (A). **C:** At 10 min after injection, the pelvis is well filled, with renal parenchyma washing out, and the renal vein is poorly opacified.

exact role of CT in relation to other diagnostic tools continues to evolve. Contrast-enhanced CT can distinguish a benign cyst from a solid renal neoplasm and is the preferred imaging method for suspected renal masses. Staging and follow-up of renal neoplasms, evaluation of renal infection and trauma, and investigation of a kidney that is nonvisualized by sonography or urography are all commonly accomplished with CT.

The capability of MRI for evaluation of urinary tract disorders has improved dramatically (133,220,269). A variety of techniques can be used to produce images with good spatial resolution, virtually free of motion and other artifacts (Figs. 3,4,5). Respiratory and flow compensation have markedly improved spin echo images, but T1-weighted gradient recalled echo (GRE) sequences performed during suspended respiration are the preferred method. Faster techniques for obtaining heavily T2-weighted images are also useful. Flow-sensitive methods allow very high accuracy in evaluation of the renal vascu-

lature (66,255). The greatest advance has been the use of MRI contrast agents that are excreted by the kidney (36) (Figs. 4,5). The use of gadolinium (Gd)-containing agents in conjunction with breath-hold GRE sequences allows performance of pre- and postcontrast MRI in a fashion analogous to CT, with similar or higher accuracy for detection and diagnosis of renal masses (269). Fat-sensitive methods, including radiofrequency selective fat-suppression and phase-sensitive methods, can be used to document the presence of fat in a lesion, or to make enhancement or local tumor extension more visible by eliminating potentially obscuring fat signal. The insensitivity of MRI to calcification is a limitation for urologic diagnosis.

Despite the marked advances in MRI technology, the high cost and more limited availability has restricted its use to a largely adjunctive imaging role at present. MRI is most useful in evaluating renal masses in patients with contraindication to the use of intravenous contrast, or in whom contrast-enhanced CT has been inadequate for di-

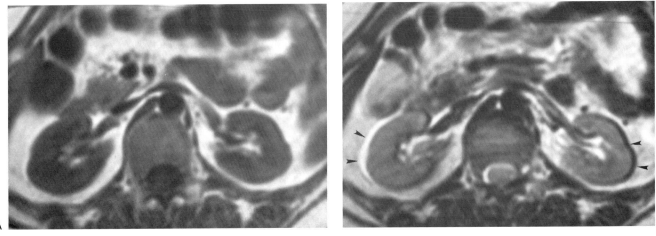

A

B

FIG. 3. Normal renal MRI. **A:** T1-weighted SE image (500/11) shows the renal medulla has lower signal than cortex; blood vessels show signal void. **B:** T2-weighted fast SE image (2400/85) shows renal parenchyma diffusely more intense than muscle, slightly less intense than fat; note chemical shift artifact *(arrowheads).*

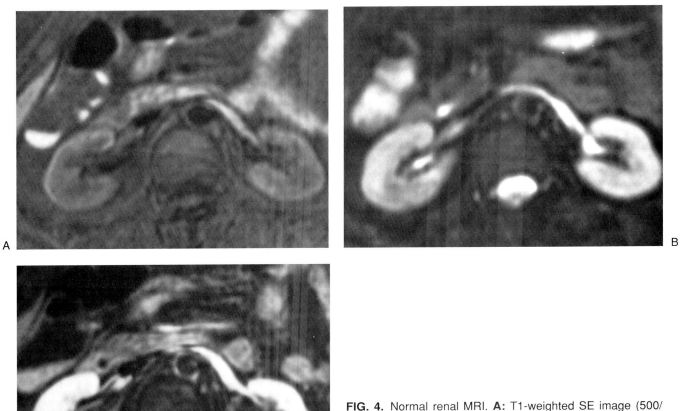

A

B

C

FIG. 4. Normal renal MRI. **A:** T1-weighted SE image (500/11) with fat suppression shows corticomedullary differentiation well. **B:** T2-weighted fast SE image with fat suppression shows better contrast between renal parenchyma and the suppressed fat, with no chemical shift artifact. Compare to Fig. 3B. **C:** Fat-suppressed T1-weighted SE image (400/11) after Gd-DTPA shows marked increase in signal of the renal parenchyma. Compare to (A).

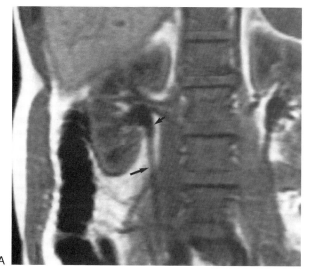

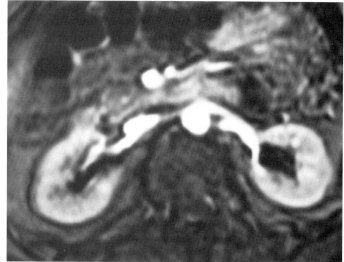

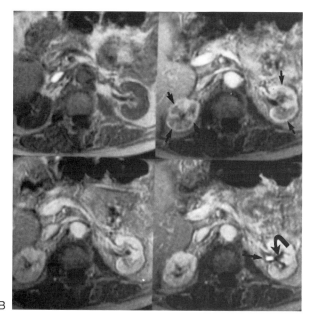

FIG. 5. Normal renal MRI. **A:** Coronal T1-weighted GRE image (2-D FLASH 140/4/70°) done during suspended respiration shows good corticomedullary differentiation with no motion artifact; note bright fat in the renal sinus with low signal pelvis and ureter *(arrows)*. **B:** serial GRE images (FMPSPGR 125/4) before and after Gd-DTPA show early cortical enhancement *(arrows)* within the first minute after contrast, followed by diffuse parenchymal enhancement; note high *(arrow)* and low signal *(curved arrow)* portions of collecting system on 5-min image). **C:** Transaxial GRE image after Gd-DTPA (SPGR 18/8/30°) shows normal high signal in blood vessels and diffusely enhanced renal parenchyma.

agnosis or staging. However, MRI is useful for renal vascular disorders. Initial enthusiasm for the use of MRI in evaluation of renal transplants has waned; the role of newer methods, including contrast excretion, flow assessment, or spectroscopy, has yet to be defined. Although MRI may be capable of demonstrating the site and cause of obstructive uropathy, its role for this is limited by cost factors (115).

Magnetic resonance imaging of the kidney has routinely been performed with T1- and T2-weighted images (Fig. 3). Transaxial images are standard; images acquired in the coronal or sagittal plane may be useful, especially for evaluation of upper or lower pole masses. T1-weighted images are excellent for depiction of anatomy of the kidneys and adjacent organs, and for evaluation of signal characteristics of renal masses. Both spin echo (SE) and GRE methods are effective, but GRE images during suspended respiration are preferred (Fig. 5). Contrast-en-

hanced [e.g., Gd-DTPA (diethylene-triamine penta-acetic acid)] images are mandatory for evaluation of a renal mass. Fat-suppressed T1 sequences are helpful for assessing contrast enhancement, as they accentuate the signal difference between the high-signal renal parenchyma and the normally high-signal fat (Fig. 4). The same type of images should be obtained before and after Gd-DTPA. It has not been established whether rapid-sequence dynamic studies are more diagnostic than a single contrast-enhanced sequence. Fat-suppressed T1-weighted images are also useful to detect the presence of fat in a mass.

Although T2-weighted images have traditionally been done, they yield little information about renal lesions. Enhancement characteristics are more important, as T2-weighted characteristics of both benign and malignant lesions are variable. T2-weighted images are most useful to screen for metastatic disease to liver or bone. If done, T2-weighted images are improved by fat suppression, as this makes the interface of the kidney or a mass more distinct against the retroperitoneal fat and reduces artifact (Fig. 4). It is unproven whether standard or fast SE images are preferable. When staging a renal mass, scanning should extend from the right atrium to the lower pole of the kidney; a flow-sensitive GRE sequence should be used, as it has been shown to be most accurate for detecting renal invasion by tumors.

When done with SE techniques and multiple sequences, MRI is a lengthy procedure. However, if GRE sequences are used and SE T2-weighted sequences deleted, MRI can be accomplished in nearly the same overall time as CT.

NORMAL ANATOMY

Computed Tomography

The cross-sectional anatomy of the normal kidney is clearly demonstrated by CT. The low-attenuation fat in the renal sinus outlines the collecting system and blood vessels, which course anteromedially. The perinephric fat outlines the surface of the kidney, which is usually smooth and curved, except where there is fetal lobation. There may be a deep indentation, commonly on the anterior surface just superior to the renal sinus (the interreticular cleft) (Fig. 6). The renal capsule cannot be visualized as separate from the renal parenchyma, as it is extremely closely applied. The perirenal fascia and bridging renorenal septa, however, are commonly seen as linear soft-tissue-density structures (164,222). These septa extend between the kidney and the anterior or posterior renal fascia, or from the anterior to the posterior surface of the kidney. The anterior renal fascia is often seen on the left, less often on the right, as a thin line separating the kidney

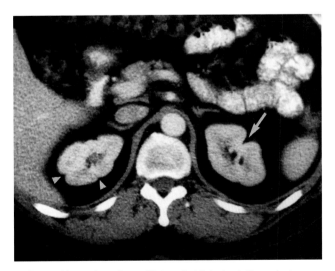

FIG. 6. Normal variant. Note slight indentations between renal lobes *(arrowheads)* and interrenicular defect *(arrow)*.

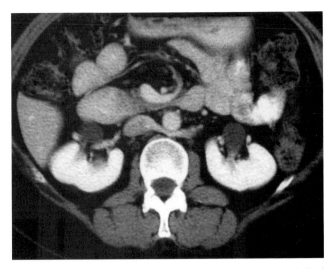

FIG. 7. Malrotation. Both renal pelves are directed anteriorly.

from the pancreas and other structures of the anterior pararenal space (see Fig. 1). The posterior renal fascia is commonly seen posterior to both kidneys. This fascia is multilayered, and it may thicken or separate because of infiltration of fluid collections in various disorders (240).

On noncontrast images, the renal parenchyma is of homogeneous soft-tissue density [30 to 60 Hounsfield units (HU)] (see Fig. 1). The pelvis and portions of the collecting system may be seen as water-density structures, but the calyces can rarely be seen without contrast excretion. Immediately after intravenous administration of iodinated contrast medium, the renal vasculature and the renal cortex enhance brightly. There is sharp distinction between the cortex and the medulla within the first 60 seconds after contrast medium administration, but both cortex and medulla attain moderate enhancement rapidly. On delayed images (about 2 minutes), the medulla may be somewhat brighter than the cortex (see Fig. 2B). The collecting system fills with very densely enhanced urine in patients with normal renal function; with thin sections, the calyceal anatomy may be seen. The ureter can be seen exiting the renal sinus and coursing anteroinferiorly over the psoas muscle. The renal vessels can be clearly seen, with the larger renal vein anterior to the renal artery. The left renal vein is easily seen as it passes anterior to the aorta and posterior to the superior mesenteric artery to enter the inferior vena cava. The right renal vein has a short, oblique superior course and can be difficult to visualize. With malrotation, the renal hila face directly anteriorly (Fig. 7).

Magnetic Resonance Imaging

Detailed anatomy of the kidney can be shown with current MRI techniques. The appearance of specific structures varies with the imaging sequence. Because of greater water content, the medulla has somewhat longer

T1 and T2 values (163). Thus, on T1-weighted SE or GRE images, the normal kidney shows distinct corticomedullary differentiation (14) (Figs. 3,5). The normal cortex is of medium signal (similar to liver) and the medulla is of lower signal. Urine has very low signal intensity, and fat in the renal sinus or perinephric space is very intense (Fig. 5A). On the moderately T2-weighted images typically used in clinical practice, corticomedullary differentiation is usually not seen, with both cortex and medulla having similar hyperintensity (often nearly isointense with retroperitoneal fat). However, on very heavily T2-weighted images, the medulla is slightly more intense than cortex. Urine is more intense than fat on T2-weighted images. Both the imaging technique and flow will affect the appearance of the normal renal arteries and veins. On most SE sequences, there should be a signal void in patent vessels; however, slow flow can result in spurious signal that can be misconstrued as thrombus. Gradient recalled echo techniques with inflow phenomena and flow compensation display patent vessels as very bright.

T1-weighted images performed after intravenous administration of Gd-DTPA shows striking enhancement of the kidney (Figs. 4,5). On Gd-enhanced T1-weighted SE images, the renal parenchyma appears uniformly hyperintense, nearly isointense to fat, in patients with normal renal function. Complex patterns may be seen, with rapid sequential GRE imaging, resulting in part from the nonlinear relationship of signal intensity to Gd concentration (with very high concentration resulting in low signal) (Fig. 5B). There is brighter enhancement of the cortex than of the medulla in the first minute or two after Gd-DTPA; although rarely seen clinically, there may be a phase with a drop in signal in the medulla because of hyperconcentration, followed by equilibration between medulla and cortex in 3 to 5 minutes (40,267). Sometimes the urine displays low signal intensity because of highly concentrated Gd-DTPA, but this is more often seen in the renal pelvis or bladder than the parenchyma.

Several studies have documented that Gd-DTPA, which is excreted by glomerular filtration, is well tolerated, with no evidence of toxicity even in patients with renal failure (40,116,249). The clearance of the agent will be delayed, however, in patients with severe renal failure (265). In part, the excellent patient tolerance may be related to the significantly lower volume used compared with that of iodinated contrast medium used in CT (306).

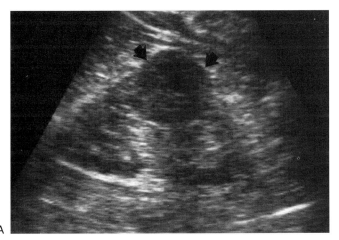

A

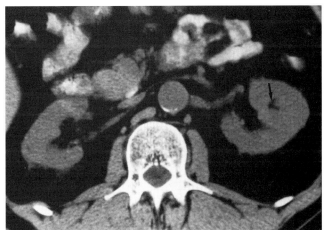

B

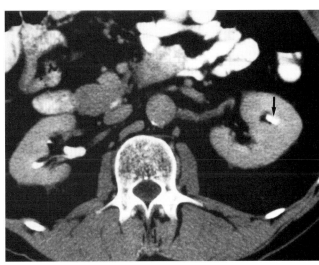

C

FIG. 8. Pseudotumor. **A:** Sonogram shows an apparent solid mass *(arrows)*. **B:** Precontrast CT image shows corresponding isodense area of thickening with central fat-attenuation focus *(arrow)*. **C:** Contrast-enhanced CT image shows isodense enhancement, with filling of a calyx *(arrow)*.

NORMAL VARIANTS AND CONGENITAL ANOMALIES

A number of variations can occur during the embryological development of the kidney. Recognition of these normal variants is needed to avoid misinterpreting them as pathologic. The kidney is formed by the fusion of several (approximately 14) reniculi, each of which consists of a central pyramid surrounded by cortical tissue. These give rise to the renal lobes. Depending on the pattern of fusion, the kidney parenchyma may be of uniform thickness with a smooth surface, or it may have seemingly thickened portions with surface irregularities (333) (Fig. 6). A variety of pseudotumors may occur, including the so-called column of Bertin (junctional parenchyma), dromedary hump, and hilar lip. These may simulate masses, particularly on sonography (Fig. 8). However, these pseudotumors can be distinguished from pathologic masses by both CT and MRI. On CT, they will show isodensity with renal parenchyma on both pre- and postcontrast images; they will be isointense with renal paren-

chyma on all MRI sequences, including postcontrast images. Compensatory hypertrophy, especially if focal due to segmental disease such as atrophic chronic pyelonephritis, may also simulate a mass, but it should show tissue characteristics identical to those of normal renal parenchyma.

An extrarenal pelvis may be incorrectly taken as evidence of obstruction. A search for secondary signs can avoid misdiagnosis. If the ureter is well filled with contrast and of normal caliber, if the excretion pattern is symmetric with the contralateral kidney, if parenchymal thickness is preserved, and if there is no calyceal dilation (better shown with thin section, helical CT), then significant obstruction can be excluded. Venous anomalies, such as retroaortic or circumaortic renal veins or persistent left-sided or duplicated inferior vena cava, are easily recognized on CT.

Malpositioned and anomalous kidneys are readily evaluated by CT or MRI. Displacement of the kidney by enlarged spleen or liver or by abnormal masses will be evident, because both the malposition and the causative

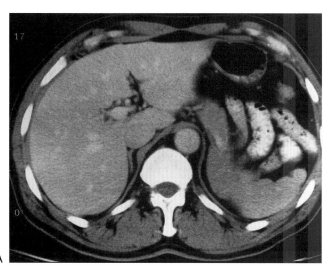

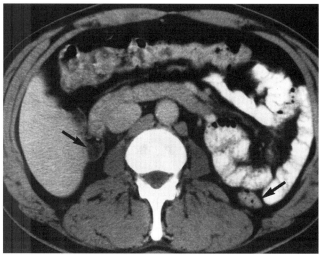

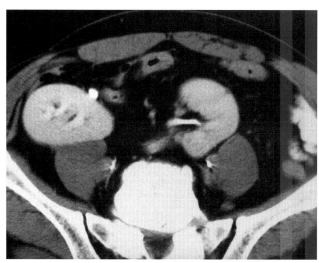

FIG. 9. Bilateral pelvic kidneys. **A:** The spleen and tail of pancreas are medially located. **B:** The colon *(arrows)* is located medially on both sides. **C:** Both kidneys lie in the pelvis.

agent are shown. Congenital malposition, including ectopy and malrotation, are readily diagnosed, and fusion anomalies such as horseshoe kidney and cross-fused ectopy are evident from the position and uniformity of the parenchyma and contour (Figs. 9–11). Other anomalies such as ectopic, malrotated, and atrophic kidneys have characteristic appearances. Frequently, kidneys in anomalous locations have somewhat distorted architecture. There may be minimal renal sinus fat, as the calyces are near the surface with an extrarenal pelvis (73). Although a peculiar-appearing mass may result on noncontrast images, postcontrast CT allows recognition that there is an anomalous kidney. Renal agenesis is inferred from absence of a kidney, compensatory hypertrophy of the remaining kidney, and the expected pattern of organ displacement. Absence of the left kidney from the renal fossa is accompanied by medial displacement of the splenic flexure of the colon, medial angulation of the pancreatic tail, and a flat, disc-like adrenal gland (152) (Figs. 9,11). On the right, the duodenum, proximal small bowel, or hepatic flexure may fill the corresponding space (Fig. 9). With any renal anomaly, one must look for associated genital anomalies. Computed tomography is highly accurate in distinguishing true congenital agenesis from atrophic, nonfunctioning kidneys.

Duplication anomalies can be well demonstrated by CT. With nonobstructed ureteral duplication, the two ureters can be followed on sequential contrast-enhanced images as they exit the renal sinus and extend to join each other or the bladder (Fig. 12). With obstructed systems, the hydronephrotic segment of the kidney and the nonenhancing dilated ureter can be followed to its point of termination, whether ectopic or not (Fig. 13). Duplications with obstruction, including ectopic ureterocele and other forms of ectopic insertion, are well demonstrated

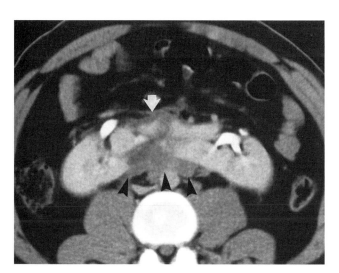

FIG. 10. Horseshoe kidney. On a CT image done to evaluate hematuria after a motor vehicle accident, there is a laceration *(arrow)* of the isthmus of a horseshoe kidney with hematoma posteriorly *(arrowheads).*

with MRI, because the ectopic insertion in various pelvic locations (such as the vagina, perineum, seminal vesicle, and urethra) can be graphically displayed because of the direct coronal or sagittal capability. Nevertheless, in many patients, and especially in children, sonography will be sufficient for diagnosis.

Abnormalities of the renal sinus rarely cause diagnostic problems on CT or MRI. Renal sinus lipomatosis is seen in about 1% of the adult population (105), often resulting from loss of volume from the kidney with aging. In nearly all cases, the expanded renal sinus will be filled with fat density (although, rarely, an admixture of fibrous tissue may raise the attenuation value to near-water range). On MRI, fat is recognizable, as it is hyperintense on both T1- and T2-weighted images.

CONTRAST MEDIA IN RENAL COMPUTED TOMOGRAPHY

Radiopaque intravenous contrast material is essential for the optimal performance of renal CT. The detection and definition of pathologic conditions depends on optimal contrast enhancement. Following intravenous administration of contrast media, there is rapid diffusion into the extracellular space and extravascular compartments. Immediately after this, plasma reentry occurs and renal excretion ensues. Contrast-assisted renal CT, using dynamic imaging techniques including helical acquisitions, depends on the physiologic properties of contrast material to provide information on the enhancement characteristics of normal and pathologic tissues (34,137). Functional assessment of the kidney can be achieved relying on the basic principles of vascular opacification and contrast material excretion by the kidney (142,198,199). Quantitative information is available from perfusion imaging (198,199). Planimetric calculations using contrast-enhanced renal CT can also be used to estimate differential renal function (15,199). The transit time of a bolus of contrast material has been studied in animals and humans (199,232). Contrast material clearance can be calculated using regional tracer clearance techniques, which are common practice for single photon emission computed tomography (SPECT) and positron emission tomography (PET) imaging. Dividing the maximum gradient of a time–density curve by the aortic contrast peak can provide tissue perfusion values (i.e., 4.7 ml/min/ml of renal tissue for renal cortex perfusion) (198,199).

Dynamic contrast-enhanced renal CT depends on the same urographic principles as those that account for the appearance and quality of the nephrogram and pyelogram during intravenous urography. Radiopaque contrast media can be imaged, particularly using fast CT techniques (i.e., helical and/or electron beam), in the three renal compartments: (a) vascular, (b) interstitium (the renal interstitial space is extremely small), and (c) tubules. Both functional

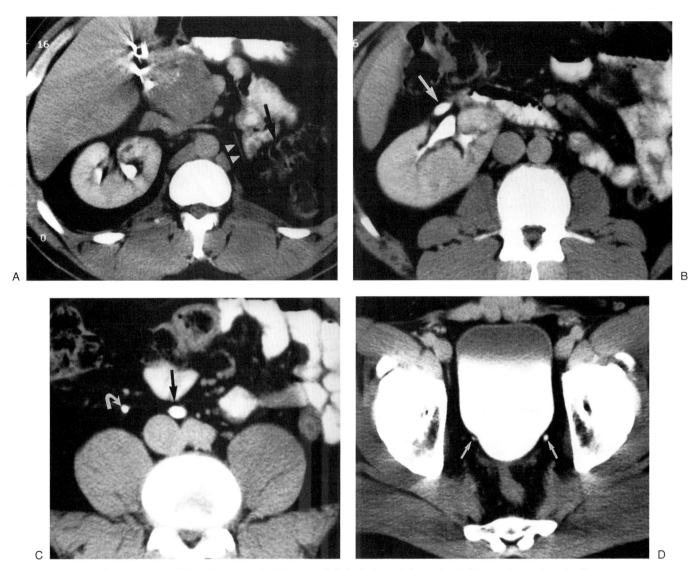

FIG. 11. Crossed fused ectopy. **A:** Note medial deviation of the splenic flexure *(arrow)* and a linear left adrenal *(arrowheads)*. **B:** Note a second ureter *(arrow)* in front of the pelvis. **C:** The left ureter *(arrow)* passes anterior to the inferior vena cava. Note right ureter *(curved arrow)*. **D:** Both ureters *(arrows)* enter the bladder in normal position.

and morphologic information may help determine the status of the vascular supply to an ischemic or traumatized kidney (96,118,137,188). Renal CT may be diagnostic in these two conditions, using computed tomography angiography (CTA) with helical acquisition and reconstruction techniques (278). The salvageability of an obstructed system may be determined by the amount of residual functional parenchyma present and the quantitative information available from functional imaging (198,199). A contrast-enhanced CT renogram similar to the radioisotope renogram can be used to assess the presence and significance of renal obstruction (63,64). The glomerular filtration rate can be estimated using contrast-enhanced CT techniques (2), and Gd-based MRI contrast media may give similar information (94).

Methods for delivery of contrast for renal CT are typi-

cally intravenous bolus or infusion methods, or some combination of each, utilizing a peripheral vein (34). Hand or mechanical power injection techniques yield suitable opacification if a large peripheral vein is used and there is an adequate amount and flow rate of contrast media. Power injectors have become the preferred method for delivering ionic or nonionic contrast media for renal CT. Intra-arterial injections, small peripheral hand or foot vein infusions, or injection of central lines may be required. Small bore, peripheral access, central venous catheters should not be injected with a power injector, and the same is true for subcutaneously placed Infusaport or Port-a-cath devices. It is essential to check for back flow prior to injection of central venous catheters.

Rapid injections (i.e., 3 to 5 ml/sec) will lead to rapid peak plasma levels and ideally a "square wave" form

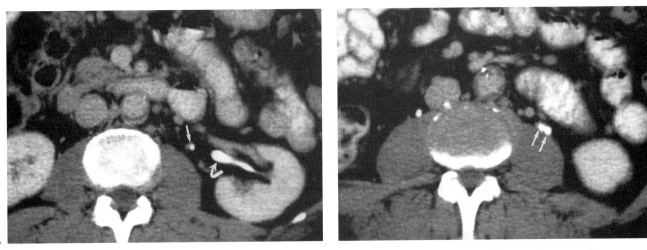

FIG. 12. Ureteral duplication. **A:** Note upper pole segment ureter *(arrow)* at level of lower pole segment pelvis *(curved arrow)* **B:** The twin ureters *(arrows)* course along the psoas; the ureters joined proximal to the ureterovesical junction.

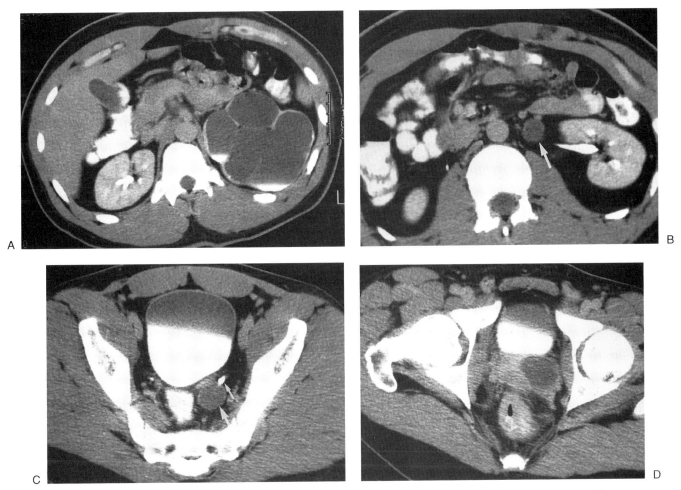

FIG. 13. Ureteral duplication, obstructed ectopic ureter. **A:** On CT done to evaluate a left upper pole mass discovered on urogram, the left upper pole is hydronephrotic. **B:** At a more caudal level, note the unopacified dilated upper pole ureter *(arrow)* passing the normal lower pole collecting system. **C:** Both ureters *(arrows)* course in close proximity through the pelvis. **D:** The upper pole ureter inserts ectopically in the prostate (note there is no ureterocele).

to the plasma concentration curve (2,45,64). Mechanical injectors can satisfactorily accomplish this task with programmed injection rates. Increasing the injection speed from 5 ml/min to 8 to 10 ml/min will enhance opacification, but these rates are rarely necessary for renal CT (45).

For a given injection rate, the time of the peak plasma level is directly related to the volume of contrast material given and inversely related to the patient's blood volume (33). It is also dependent on cardiac output, renal blood flow, and the type (osmolality) of contrast material chosen (33). Time–density curves, serial densitimetric measurements, and tissue perfusion values can all be calculated with existing software programs (20,335).

Prolonged administration using a drip infusion of contrast material or slow power injection is rarely required today with modern sub-5-second CT scanning systems and in particular with helical CT. Total doses of between 20 and 50 g of iodine per patient are common for renal CT, but smaller intravenous injections of 10 to 30 cc of a 32% to 66% solution of contrast material are usually sufficient for evaluation of renal masses. Because of the beam-hardening artifacts occasionally seen with high concentrations of contrast material in the renal collecting system or parenchyma, evaluations of subtle renal pathology (e.g., invasion from transitional cell carcinoma) may require smaller intravenous injections [i.e., 10 to 20 cc of a 30% to 35% solution (wt/vol)] of contrast material. There is no dominant influence from any of the physical, chemical, or molecular structural features of modern water-soluble contrast agents that might effect the choice of one agent over another for renal CT. Selection may reasonably be based on the concentration desired, cost, patient tolerance, and safety.

With contrast-enhanced renal CT, there is a linear relationship between the iodine concentration and the CT number, or Hounsfield unit (30). Hounsfield units may reflect the blood or tissue concentration of contrast material, but they may vary due to beam hardening, scanner geometry, and volume averaging. An increase in the plasma concentration of contrast material will increase the HU of renal parenchyma. A high peak plasma level, and therefore a higher cortical CT number on the order of 80 to 100 HU, is achieved after a bolus injection of contrast material. The peak plasma concentration and renal cortical CT number achieved after a slower injection or infusion of contrast material are therefore lower than after bolus injections, but the peak achieved will be maintained longer (34). Peak tissue perfusion values for the cortex are always greater than the medullary portion of the kidney by a ratio of between 2:1 and 4:1 (198). Imaging during the early or very early contrast enhancement phase (vascular nephrogram), particularly with helical CT, may actually obscure pathology, because the normal medulla may be difficult to separate from a mass or other pathologic condition. Therefore, later phase CT images

(i.e., corticomedullary junction phase or tubular nephrogram and pyelogram phase) are all important. The stages of dynamic contrast-enhanced renal CT have been described as triphasic: (a) major vascular opacification (arteries and veins), early vascular nephrogram phase, (b) nephrogram, combination vascular and tubular nephrogram phase, and (c) pyelogram (calyceal filling) phase. Some authors refer to these phases as the bolus phase, the nonequilibrium phase, and the equilibrium phases, respectively (33,65,242). With serial dynamic imaging after an intravenous bolus injection, the aorta, the main renal arteries, and the renal veins are initially opacified, followed immediately by an intense vascular nephrogram defining the corticomedullary junction. Interstitial perfusion is not an important consideration, as it might be in other organs, because the interstitial space of the kidney is so small and because of the excretory nature of the kidney. Time–density curves for each renal artery should closely parallel the aorta in the absence of significant renal artery stenosis or increased intrarenal vascular resistance (160,242). The attenuation value of normal renal parenchyma will increase to 80 to 120 HU after standard contrast material injections. The appearance time of the corticomedullary junction and the degree of opacity will depend on the patient's renal function, cardiac output, and body habitus, and the method and amount of contrast material delivery (160). The arteriovenous difference measured during the second (nonequilibrium) phase is in the range of 10 to 30 HU. As contrast material reaches the renal tubules, medullary opacification begins. Typically, this is between 1 and 3 minutes after the start of the injection. During this time, the medulla may appear denser than the cortex. The third or last (equilibrium) phase occurs at approximately 2 minutes after injection and progresses rapidly within 3 to 4 minutes to the pyelogram phase where calyceal and pelvic filling is observed. Degree of distention is proportional to the dose and type of contrast material used, and ionic contrast media are associated with greater osmotic diuresis.

PATHOLOGIC CONDITIONS

Renal Masses

Initial evaluation of patients with hematuria or other signs suggestive of a renal mass is best done by intravenous urography or, increasingly, sonography. However, CT is the standard method for definitive investigation unless a mass is clearly a cyst, using strict sonographic criteria. Patients with a malignancy that commonly metastasizes to the kidney, or who have a palpable mass in the region of the kidney, may have CT as a first study. A CT is indicated in patients with persistent upper tract hematuria, even if intravenous urography or sonography has been negative.

When performed before and after intravenous contrast, CT is clearly more sensitive for detection of renal masses than sonography or urography (3,315). It also more easily allows the exclusion of pathology as well as the rendering of a specific diagnosis. For example, many renal pseudotumors will not be distinguishable from true renal neoplasms by sonography, but they are distinguishable on CT (Fig. 8).

Computed tomography has, in fact, had a major impact on the mode of presentation of renal masses. A very large number of renal masses are now initially detected as unsuspected, incidental findings on CT scans done for other reasons (5,56). Many others are incidental findings on sonography. Because of the widespread use of sonography and CT and their ability to define extremely small lesions, management of the small, incidentally detected renal mass has become a challenge (56). Although most small solid renal masses are renal carcinomas (53, 177,219), it is controversial whether a small neoplasm requires radical nephrectomy. It is even unclear whether removal of a tiny, low-grade renal neoplasm is likely to lengthen the survival of a patient, particularly if the patient is elderly or has other significant disease. However, vigorous imaging evaluation and follow-up of such indeterminate renal masses results in significant cost.

Recent advances in MRI have made it an even more powerful tool, both for diagnosis and staging of renal carcinoma. With state-of-the-art technique, including pre- and postcontrast (Gd-DTPA)-enhanced scans, MRI is at least as accurate as CT for diagnosis of renal masses. It is

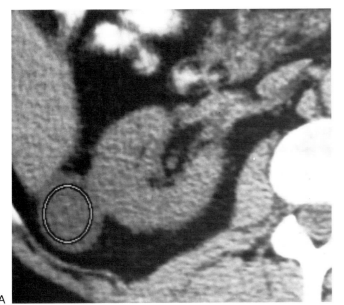

A

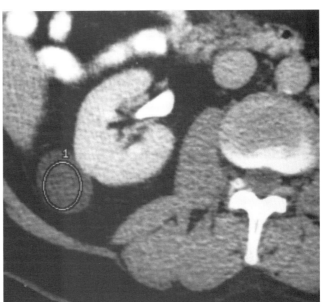

B

	104	105	106	107	108	109	110	111	112	113	114
350	8	15	21	28	32	-4	-27	14	12	-20	-2
351	22	26	5	-2	36	42	1	22	67	39	13
352	7	6	-14	-24	-2	12	-7	-19	10	17	29
353	0	22	13	-18	9	28	32	20	-10	2	8
354	-18	-3	29	11	20	29	22	50	38	10	3
355	1	0	-10	-17	-20	-12	-2	-21	1	2	21
356	28	11	4	-2	10	3	-2	6	-8	-41	-11
357	0	7	-12	10	36	23	1	13	27	-4	-37
358	11	37	0	-23	-10	-2	18	47	53	6	-9
359	4	28	27	28	24	4	-14	1	20	36	20
360	-23	-15	6	10	14	1	-6	28	37	43	22

C

FIG. 14. Simple cyst. **A:** Precontrast CT image shows homogeneous mass that had mean attenuation of 1 HU. **B:** Postcontrast CT image shows no enhancement; the attenuation measured 5 HU. **C:** Note on pixel report a few negative pixel readings, but there are no clusters of 3 to 6 contiguous negative pixels.

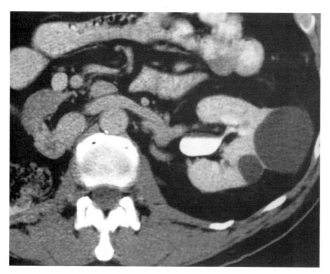

FIG. 15. Pseudoseptate cyst. Two simple cysts compress normal renal parenchyma between them.

clearly indicated in patients who cannot tolerate iodinated contrast (249,269). For these patients, MRI should replace CT for evaluation of a sonographically detected indeterminate mass (56).

Cysts

The most common renal mass in the adult is a cyst. Simple renal cysts arise from the cortex. If a lesion fulfills all the strict criteria for a cyst on sonography, no further imaging evaluation is needed. Diagnostic features of simple cysts on CT are (a) smooth, round shape; (b) homogeneous water-attenuation fluid content; (c) smooth, sharp interface with adjacent renal parenchyma; (d) imperceptible cyst wall (Fig. 14). Sometimes on transaxial CT, a thin rim of renal parenchyma may surround the cyst (especially polar cysts); also, two adjacent cysts may compress renal parenchyma between them (Fig. 15). Occasionally, a beak of renal parenchyma may be produced at the margin between cyst and kidney (266). If such masses otherwise fulfill CT criteria for a cyst, they should not be pursued aggressively. Although a variety of technical factors affects CT attenuation numbers, the latter can nevertheless be very useful in the diagnosis of renal masses. Simple

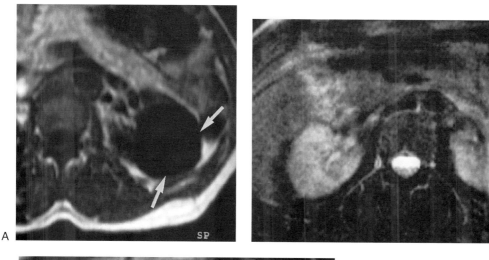

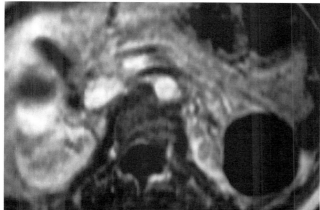

FIG. 16. Simple cyst, MRI. **A:** Axial T1-weighted GRE (FLASH 140/6/70°) image shows a large, homogeneous, very low signal mass *(arrows)*. **B:** On fast SE T2-weighted image (4000/90), the mass is homogeneous and very hyperintense. **C:** After intravenous Gd-DTPA, the mass remains low signal, but the kidney parenchyma enhances. Compare with (A).

cysts will have homogeneous density in the water range and should not have a density over 20 HU. There should be no significant increase in the attenuation after contrast. However, because of various factors, including volume averaging and beam hardening (by the iodine concentrated in the adjacent renal parenchyma), an increase of less than 10 HU should not be considered definite enhancement (24). The cyst contents should also remain homogeneous after contrast. Accurate assessment of enhancement requires appropriate section thickness—the slice thickness should be no more than half the diameter of the mass. Volume averaging may result in spurious ''enhancement'' when the slice includes part of the cyst and part of the renal parenchyma, because the CT attenuation value is an average of marked increase in attenuation of a small portion of renal parenchyma, and the unenhancing cyst contents.

Cysts may be solitary or multiple, and they can arise anywhere in the kidney. They tend to increase in size and number with age (60). Although growth is slow, when followed for years, increase in size will be seen. Cysts are usually asymptomatic. However, they may cause hematuria, and, if large, they may cause compressive mass effect, which can lead to hypertension or obstruction of the collecting system. In such circumstances, cyst aspiration and sclerosis is justified.

Although simple cortical cysts have a quite distinctive appearance on MRI, it is not necessary in general to evaluate simple cysts (149,191). Simple cysts have the same morphologic features on MRI as on CT: they are round and homogeneous, with a smooth, sharp interface with renal parenchyma and an imperceptible wall. Their signal mirrors that of water (or cerebral spinal fluid), they are very hypointense on T1-weighted images, and they are very hyperintense (brighter than fat) on T2-weighted images (Fig. 16). No enhancement will occur after intravenous Gd-DTPA (although volume averaging also occurs with MRI, and signal intensity numbers are not standardized, so no accurate numerical criteria can be used).

Calyceal diverticula may be discovered on CT as incidental findings, and on occasion they are imaged after sonography, because these lesions may appear complicated, with calculi, debris, or milk of calcium within the diverticulum. These cystic spaces are lined by transitional epithelium and communicate with the collecting system through a narrow opening. They are commonly small and intrarenal, but they may be large and extend to the surface of the kidney (Fig. 17). They are of water density on precontrast images unless calculi or milk of calcium is present. The latter is seen as a layered high density, which will shift with change in patient position (295). Most calyceal diverticula will show some filling with contrast, but this may occur only on delayed scans; if no delayed images are obtained, such lesions may be misdiagnosed as complicated cysts.

A variety of complex or complicated cystic masses occurs (Figs. 18–22), most of which are benign and of no clinical consequence. Nonetheless, they must be distinguished from renal malignancy (51,53). Computed tomography and MRI are very useful for this purpose, with CT playing the primary imaging role. A simple cyst may become complicated as a result of hemorrhage, infection, or other processes that thicken some or all of the wall and may increase the density of the contents (24,113,252). Calcification within the wall or a septum may occur (Figs. 18,20) (53). Acute bleeding into a cyst may present with pain, and a fluid level may be seen within an acutely hemorrhagic cyst. The cyst may show increase in size on serial studies.

Hyperdense cysts have an attenuation value greater than renal parenchyma on precontrast CT images, commonly measuring 40 to 90 HU (Fig. 19) (24,48, 50,114,342). This may be a result of bleeding into the cyst, with concentration of the protein components of blood. Some of these cysts contain a material as thick and dark as crankcase oil, and others contain inspissated white material (similar to milk of calcium), but some have clear amber fluid with a high protein content (84,294). Most hyperdense cysts are solitary, but they may be multiple; they are quite common in autosomal dominant polycystic disease (175). Hyperdense cysts may appear sonolucent, but in many cases sonography shows internal echoes because of the thick nature of the contents. If the lesion is small (most are less than 3 cm), homogeneous, and shows no enhancement on postcontrast images, and if it has no other complicating factor (such as calcification), diagnosis of benign hyperdense cyst can be made. If a hyperdense lesion is first detected by CT, sonography may be helpful, because it may confirm the cystic nature. Follow-up of hyperdense cysts (with the exception of those in polycystic disease) is prudent to confirm their benign nature, because, rarely, renal carcinoma may have the appearance of a hyperdense cyst (76,114).

Several other findings may occur in cystic lesions that raise the level of suspicion for carcinoma. Thickening or irregularity of the wall, heterogeneity of the contents, calcification in the wall, and multilocularity or septation are all findings that may be seen in benign cystic lesions but also can be found in cystic forms of renal neoplasms, including renal cell carcinoma, Wilms tumor, and others (51,112,113,252). Bosniak has described a classification of renal cystic masses that is useful in clarifying the risk of malignancy and aids in the management of complicated cystic lesions (24). This classification is largely based on CT findings, but it utilizes information from sonography, MRI, and follow-up. A type 1 lesion fulfills all the strict criteria for a simple cyst and no further workup or treatment is needed. A type 2 lesion contains features that raise concern, such as thin septation, minimal mural calcification, and high-density contents without other disturbing features. Type 2 lesions have minimal risk of

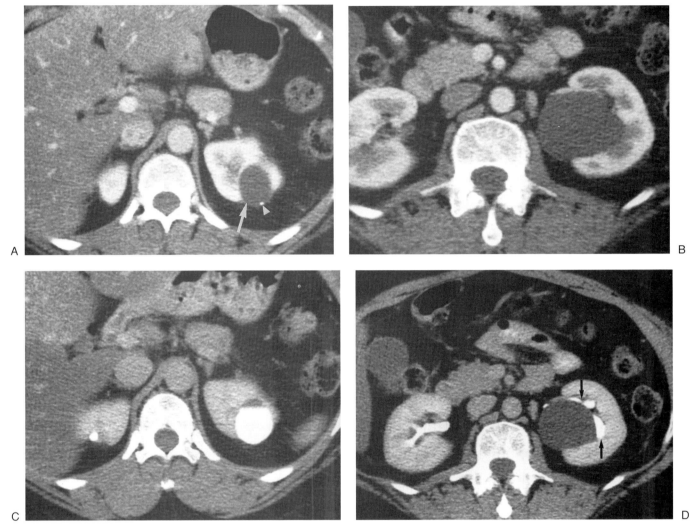

FIG. 17. Calyceal diverticulum and parapelvic cyst. **A:** Early postcontrast CT image shows a water-attenuation lesion *(arrow)* with a fleck of calcification *(arrowhead)*. **B:** Another water-attenuation structure is seen at the hilum. **C:** The 5-min delayed image shows contrast layering in the upper pole lesion, confirming it is a calyceal diverticulum. **D:** Delayed image shows collecting system *(arrows)* compressed by the other lesion, a parapelvic cyst.

malignancy (4). Type 3 lesions are those with one or more features suggestive of malignancy, but without definitive signs of malignancy (i.e., soft-tissue components with definite enhancement after contrast by either CT or MRI). Thick or nodular septations, thick or irregular calcification, nodularity or thickening of the wall, or heterogeneous density are all features of type 3 lesions. A lesion with a question of enhancement (increase in attenuation value of less than 10 HU) may be put in this category. In one study, type 3 lesions had an approximately 50% rate of malignancy. They thus should be followed very closely or treated surgically, with the realization, however, that half will be benign. A type 4 lesion contains some definitely enhancing area, and, thus, it is a cystic neoplasm. A further refinement of this system has been proposed to categorize lesions as ''type 2F'' if they have several of the features

of a type 2 lesion or some features of type 3. This group requires close, careful follow-up with CT, but not immediate surgery (26).

Magnetic resonance imaging can be useful in evaluating complicated renal masses. The same morphologic criteria (e.g., homogeneity, sharp margination, thickness of wall, and septa) can be used as with CT. In addition, the great sensitivity of MRI to tissue characteristics can be useful because hemorrhage or other alteration of the cyst contents will be reflected by heterogeneity and change in the signal characteristics. Complicated cysts have higher signal intensity than water on T1-weighted images, and they are variably intense on T2-weighted images (Figs. 21,22). If MRI shows a typical simple cyst (homogeneous low signal on T1 and high signal on T2), neoplasm is effectively excluded (191). However, when using only unenhanced T1- and

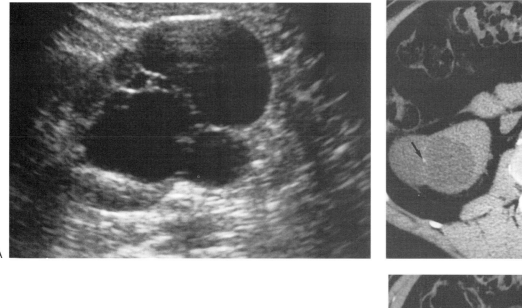

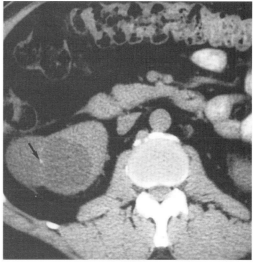

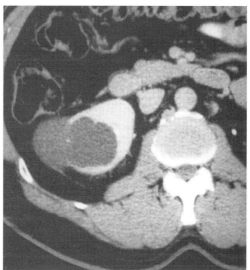

FIG. 18. Septate cyst. **A:** Sonogram shows complex, septated cyst arising from the right lower pole. **B:** On precontrast CT, there is a small fleck of calcification *(arrow)* on a septum; all components measured water attenuation. **C:** Postcontrast image shows no enhancement.

T2-weighted images, complicated cysts cannot be reliably distinguished from renal neoplasms (130,191). The availability of MRI contrast agents provides the opportunity to determine enhancement. As with CT, cysts do not enhance, but both benign and malignant neoplasms exhibit enhancement on post-Gd studies. MRI is equivalent to CT for distinction of cysts from neoplasms (250,269), and currently it is the preferred procedure to evaluate complicated cysts in patients who cannot tolerate iodinated contrast. To clearly recognize enhancement, however, careful comparison of the appearance of the mass on the same type of sequence before and after Gd-DTPA is needed, because complicated cysts are typically hyperintense on T1-weighted images. Otherwise, such hyperintensity may be misconstrued as enhancement (268). As stated previously, it is easier to appreciate subtle contrast enhancement on fat-suppressed images than on non-fat-suppressed images.

Parapelvic Cysts

Noncortical cysts occur adjacent to the renal parenchyma. Most cysts seen in the renal hilar region are believed to be of lymphatic origin and are usually called parapelvic cysts because of their location. These may be solitary but frequently are multiple. Etiology is obscure, but no hereditary pattern is known. Such cysts typically replace the renal sinus fat and displace or compress adjacent structures, including renal parenchyma, pelvis, and hilar vessels. When solitary, these cysts are larger, often several centimeters in size, and round or oval (see Fig. 17). When multiple, they are usually smaller, and they may be ovoid or lobulated (Fig. 23). They are most often of water density but may be somewhat higher attenuation. There is neither enhancement nor communication with the collecting system after contrast medium administration (although increase in attenuation after retrograde pyelography has been reported, presumably due to extravasation

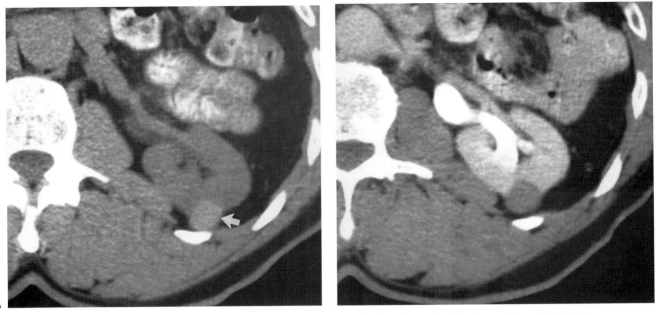

FIG. 19. Hyperdense cyst. **A:** A 1.8-cm homogeneous lesion *(arrow)* with attenuation of 72 HU is shown on precontrast CT. **B:** Postcontrast, the attenuation is 74 HU; the lesion has shown no change on follow-up.

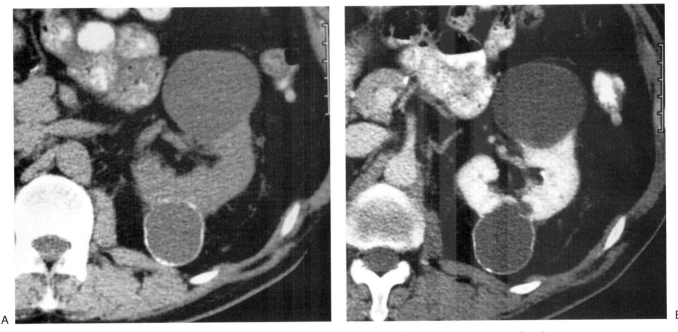

FIG. 20. Calcified cyst. **A:** On noncontrast CT image, note two homogeneous water-density masses; the anterior lesion has an imperceptible wall; calcification is evident in the wall of the posterior lesion. **B:** There is no enhancement of either cyst postcontrast.

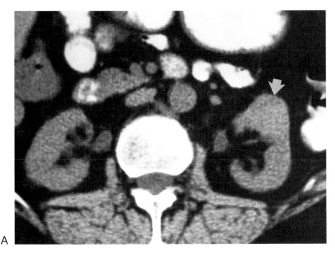

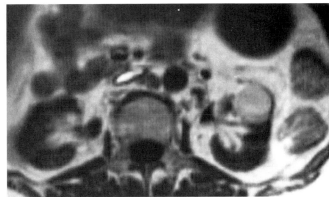

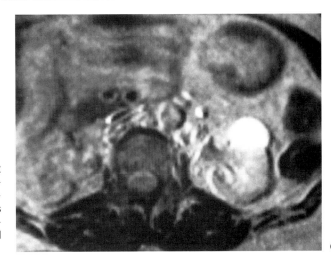

FIG. 21. Complicated cyst. **A:** Noncontrast CT on a patient with renal failure shows an isodense bulge *(arrow)*. **B:** On T1-weighted SE image (400/20), the mass is homogeneously hyperintense. **C:** On T2-weighted SE image (1500/80), the mass is homogeneous and more intense than fat; there was no enhancement and no change on follow-up. Findings are typical of a hemorrhagic cyst.

and communication) (193). On unenhanced CT images (as well as sonography and MRI), they may simulate hydronephrosis. However, their true nature is obvious on contrast-enhanced CT, as the contrast-filled infundibula are seen, effaced or compressed by the parapelvic cyst(s) (Fig. 23). These lesions are of no clinical significance unless they enlarge enough to cause obstructive uropathy. Some of these cysts are thought to develop as a result of prior obstruction with resultant urine extravasation, the so-called parapelvic uriniferous pseudocysts (119,205).

Cystic Diseases

Autosomal Dominant Polycystic Kidney Disease

ADPCKD (autosomal dominant polycystic kidney disease) is a hereditary disorder affecting multiple organ systems; it has 100% penetrance but variable expressivity. In most patients, the disease results from a genetic lesion on the short arm of chromosome 16 (221). Renal disease is the predominant clinical feature, with between 5% and 10% of all end-stage renal disease resulting from ADPCKD, but the process affects many other organ sys-

tems. Hypertension is very common even before the onset of renal failure. Cerebral aneurysms occur in 5% to 10% (with cerebral hemorrhage occurring in about 8%), and aortic aneurysm, aortic dissection, and valvular heart disease are much more common than in the general population (125). Cysts are found not only in the kidneys, but also in the liver in up to 50%, in the pancreas in about 7%, and in the spleen in less than 5% of patients (125). Hepatic function is not impaired, however, even when the liver is diffusely involved.

Autosomal dominant polycystic kidney disease presents in several ways. The average age of onset of renal failure is in the sixth decade (125,221). Often the diagnosis is made because of screening, usually by sonography, of the offspring of an affected individual. Virtually all patients with the disease have sonographically detectable cysts by age 30 (221). Patients may present with a palpable mass, because the kidneys become enlarged with increasing number and size of cysts. Not infrequently, patients present with complications of the renal disease, including flank pain, hematuria, or urinary tract infection. Nephrolithiasis (usually uric acid calculi) has been reported in up to 36% of cases (179).

Although CT and MRI are not usually indicated for

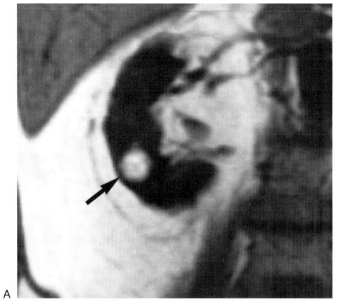

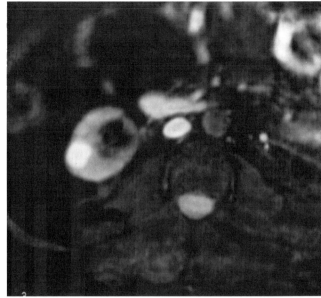

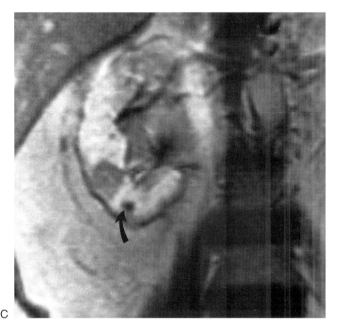

FIG. 22. Complicated cyst. **A:** Coronal T1-weighted GRE image (FLASH 130/4/80°) shows hyperintense lesion *(arrow)*. **B:** The lesion is markedly hyperintense on transaxial fat-suppressed, T2-weighted SE image (2500/90). **C:** There is no enhancement after intravenous administration of Gd-DTPA (coronal FLASH 130/4/80°). Note the additional small simple cyst *(curved arrow)* seen only on postcontrast image.

screening of suspected subjects, they can be useful for evaluation of complications, and they both show typical patterns that are virtually diagnostic of the disorder. Multiple macroscopic cysts ranging from a few millimeters to several centimeters are seen throughout the full thickness of the renal parenchyma (Fig. 24) (167). Early in life, or in poorly penetrant forms, only a few cysts may be seen in the kidneys, overlapping with the appearance of multiple sporadic simple cysts. Detection of cysts in other organs will be a useful clue to the diagnosis. With progression, the kidneys gradually enlarge as the cysts become more numerous, become larger, and replace the renal parenchyma (Fig. 24B,C). Bilateral involvement is usual, but sometimes the disease is quite asymmetric, and, rarely, only one kidney shows significant disease (Fig. 24D) (55,167,169,176). Although the cysts

may have the typical appearance of simple cysts on CT, high-density cysts are common, resulting from the frequency of hemorrhage into the cysts (175). Only 31% of patients in one study had no hyperdense cysts (175). Calcification of the cyst walls is also common, again most likely resulting from old hemorrhage. About 50% of ADPCKD patients have calcifications on CT, including calcified cysts and renal calculi (179). Calcification in these cysts does not carry the same degree of concern for renal carcinoma as it does in the general population. Although there is some controversy, there have been no publications convincingly establishing an increased incidence of renal cell carcinoma (RCC) in ADPCKD. Nevertheless, RCC does occur in these patients, and the same diagnostic criteria are used on CT. Thus it is very important to assess enhancement with pre- and

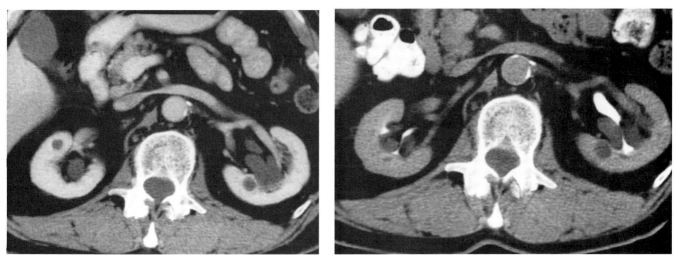

FIG. 23. Parapelvic cysts. **A:** Early postcontrast CT image shows several water-attenuation structures in both renal hila. **B:** Delayed image shows the collecting system passing between several parapelvic cysts.

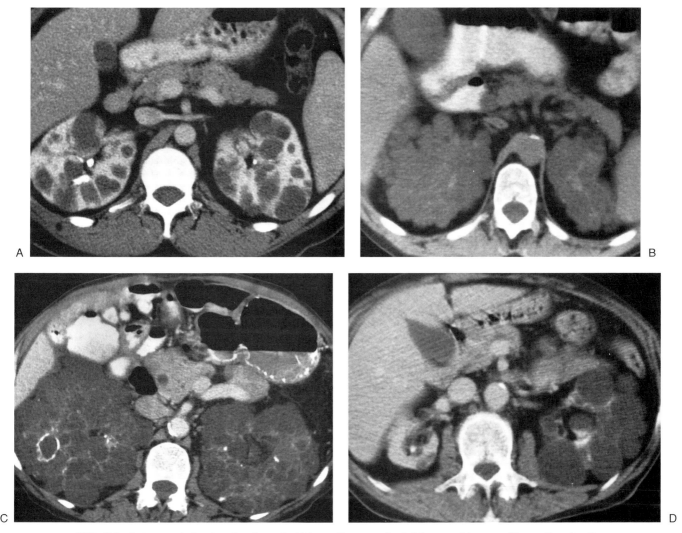

FIG. 24. Autosomal dominant polycystic kidney disease. **A:** A 30-year-old man with positive family history, but no renal failure, shows numerous cysts throughout the parenchyma. **B:** Initial noncontrast CT in another patient shows polycystic kidneys. **C:** After 6 years, there is progression, with larger kidneys, more numerous cysts, and increased calcification. **D:** In a different patient, there is marked asymmetry in involvement.

postcontrast scans. Magnetic resonance imaging may be used as an alternative if there is a concern over the nephrotoxicity of iodinated contrast. Computed tomography is very useful in evaluating hematuria in patients with ADPCKD because it can detect cyst hemorrhage, can distinguish calculi from cyst calcification, and can diagnose renal neoplasms with higher accuracy than sonography.

Magnetic resonance imaging may reveal a characteristic pattern in patients with ADPCKD. In addition to enlargement of the kidneys and the presence of multiple cysts scattered throughout the parenchyma, there almost invariably are cysts of varying signal intensity on both T1- and T2-weighted images (Fig. 25) (126). This is a result of hemorrhage of varying age within the cysts, so that some cysts are low signal on T1-weighted images and high on T2-weighted images, whereas others have high signal on T1-weighted images, but remain low signal on T2-weighted

images. The effect of hemorrhage into cysts is complex, but it may produce shortening of both T1 and T2 values, so there may be increased signal on T1, but decreased on T2, compared to simple cysts (126). Heterogeneity and layering may be seen, even in some cysts that are homogeneous on CT. Hemorrhagic cysts often show layering, with the dependent layer hyperintense on T1-weighted images but hypointense on T2-weighted images, and with the nondependent layer showing the reverse pattern (Fig. 25) (256). Renal carcinoma can be detected on MRI in these patients as the tumor enhances with intravenous Gd-DTPA.

Acquired Cystic Disease of the Kidney

Nonhereditary cystic disease of the kidney is common in any form of end-stage renal disease, but is particularly

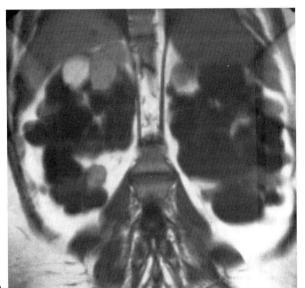

A

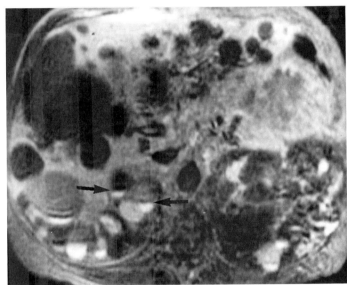

B

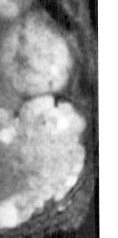

C

FIG. 25. Autosomal dominant polycystic kidney disease, MRI. **A:** Coronal T1-weighted (400/20) image shows multiple cysts with signal intensity ranging from low to very high intensity. **B:** In another patient, transaxial T1-weighted SE image (500/15) shows multiple renal and hepatic cysts; note some cysts have fluid—fluid levels with the dependent portion being hyperintense *(arrows).* **C:** On fat-suppressed T2-weighted SE image (2000/60), some of the dependent material is now hypointense *(arrow).*

common in patients on chronic dialysis, whether hemo- or peritoneal dialysis (192). Incidence ranges from 47% to 87% (37,138,173), depending on the duration of dialysis, with an 80% incidence reported after the third year (138). The exact etiology is not certain, and ischemia, fibrosis, unknown metabolites, and inadequate control of renal disease have been postulated as causes. Hyperplasia of tubular epithelium occurs, which results in blockage and dilatation of nephrons, leading to cyst formation. There is a definite increase in renal carcinoma, with incidences between 5% and 19% reported (37,93,135, 138,173). Thus, follow-up of patients on dialysis longer than 3 years may be indicated.

Early in the disease process, the kidneys are small with only a few cysts. The renal contour often is preserved, with most of the cysts small (<0.5 cm) and completely intrarenal. Although renal size may continue to decrease the first few years on dialysis, eventually the renal size begins to increase, as the cysts become more numerous and larger (2 to 3 cm). In a longitudinal CT study, 57% had some cysts at the beginning of dialysis; 87% did after 7 years. The kidney volume increased from 79 to 150 cc (178). Hemorrhage can occur both into the cyst and into the subcapsular or perinephric space. This can cause increased attenuation, heterogeneity, thickening, and calcification of the cyst walls. Eventually, after many years of dialysis, the kidneys may achieve an appearance nearly indistinguishable from that in ADPCKD (Fig. 26), even with calcifications. However, cysts do not occur in other organs.

As with ADPCKD, CT is superior to sonography for detection of complications, particularly RCC (302). Intravenous contrast medium can usually be used, if the patients already are on dialysis, but MRI is also an effective method for diagnosis of RCC. Detection of an enhancing lesion on either CT or MRI is presumptive evidence of RCC (Fig. 26). Although a renal adenoma may be suggested if the lesion is less than 3 cm, nevertheless nephrectomy should be seriously considered, because it is not possible to accurately differentiate a small renal carcinoma from an adenoma without surgery.

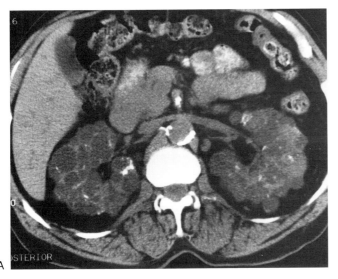

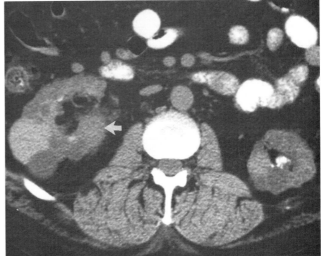

FIG. 26. Acquired cystic disease. **A:** Multiple cysts and calcifications are noted on noncontrast CT image in this patient who has been on hemodialysis for 16 years. **B:** In another chronic dialysis patient, multiple cysts are shown on precontrast CT image; note high-attenuation medial lesion *(arrow).* **C:** Postcontrast CT image shows enhancement of the medial lesion *(arrow)*; a renal carcinoma was resected.

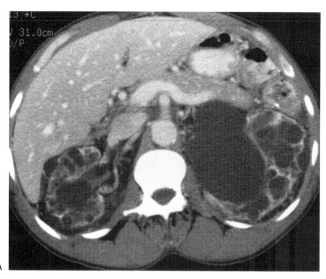

A   B

FIG. 27. Tuberous sclerosis. **A:** Both kidneys contain many cysts. **B:** More inferiorly, an angiomyolipoma is also present *(arrow).*

Although acquired cystic disease due to dialysis has been reported to regress after successful renal transplantation (138), it has also been reported that renal carcinoma may occur in native kidneys after transplantation (180). The premalignant potential of the cyst may remain for some time, and investigation of the native kidneys may be indicated in transplant patients with hematuria.

Tuberous Sclerosis

Tuberous sclerosis (TS) is an autosomal dominant hereditary disorder resulting from a defect on chromosome 9 (35). It has somewhat variable presentation, and, although the usual clinical features are seizure disorder, mental retardation, and cutaneous lesions, patients may not be recognized to have the disease until adulthood. Several renal lesions have been associated with TS, although the association with angiomyolipomas is best known (104,258). Cysts are seen in about 15%. Occasionally, numerous cysts are present in a pattern similar to that in ADPCKD (Fig. 27) (35,202). Renal failure may occur, although this is uncommon. These cysts have a hyperplastic epithelial lining, as in acquired cystic disease. There may in fact be an increased incidence of RCC in TS patients, with an incidence of 1% reported (104,299).

Angiomyolipomas (AMLs) occur in 40% to 80% of patients with TS (310). Commonly, these are numerous, bilateral, and small (Fig. 28). However, they may be solitary or there may be only a few. Recent longitudinal studies have also shown that there is a propensity for AMLs in TS to grow and to hemorrhage, requiring angioembolization or surgery (310). The diagnosis of AML can be made if the presence of fat is documented by CT or MRI. Hyperechogenicity on sonography is not adequate, because small RCCs may also be hyperechoic.

The rarest renal manifestation of TS is lymphangioleiomyomatosis. The process, most commonly seen in the chest, apparently results from smooth muscle proliferation that obstructs lymphatic channels, resulting in development of cystic lesions. Fluid-density masses may be seen in the perinephric space in such cases (141).

Von Hippel-Lindau Disease

Another autosomal dominant hereditary disorder that may affect the kidney is von Hippel-Lindau (VHL) disease (41). The causative defect has been localized to the short arm of chromosome 3 (43,171,172). Several phenotypes exist. The commonest includes presentation with retinal and CNS hemangioblastomas, renal cysts and cancers, and pancreatic cysts, but not pheochromocytoma. The next commonest pattern includes hemangioblastomas, pheo-

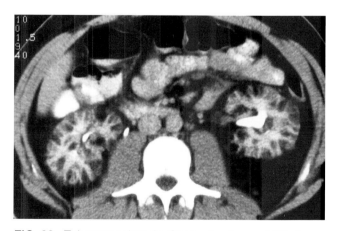

FIG. 28. Tuberous sclerosis. Contrast-enhanced CT shows numerous small, fat-attenuation lesions scattered throughout both kidneys, all angiomyolipomas.

chromocytoma, and islet cell tumors of the pancreas, but not pancreatic or renal cysts, or renal cancers. In the least common form, hemangioblastomas, pheochromocytoma, and renal and pancreatic disease are found (43). Renal cysts are found in 60%; they are usually bilateral and may mimic ADPCKD, especially because pancreatic cysts may be seen (Fig. 29) (172). Seventy-four percent of renal masses in VHL patients are cystic (42). RCC can be expected to develop in up to 45% of patients, and, historically, one third of the deaths have been caused by RCC (43). Although it is uncommon for a cyst to degenerate into a tumor, many of the RCCs in VHL are partly cystic (Fig. 29). Angiography has been shown to have a sensitivity of only 35% for diagnosing RCC in VHL (200). Because the RCCs in these patients are commonly small when initially detected, CT is probably preferable to MRI, but no comparative study has yet been reported. Small tumors may be missed on initial CT, but with careful follow-up, enlarging lesions should be detected. Removal of lesions that reach 3 cm in diameter is recommended, with an attempt at renal-conserving surgery rather than radical nephrectomy,

because it is likely RCC will eventually develop in the contralateral kidney (43).

Other Cystic Diseases

Multilocular cystic nephroma is a localized cystic disease of the kidney believed by many to represent a benign neoplasm (11,113,187,223). It is uncommon, of unknown etiology, and has no hereditary pattern. It is seen most often in two groups: young boys (3 months to 4 years of age), and adult women (over 30 years of age) (113,223). The pathologic characteristics are (a) it is unilateral and solitary, (b) it consists of multiple noncommunicating epithelial-lined cysts separated by fibrous septa that contain no renal parenchyma, (c) a well-defined capsule is common, (d) the uninvolved kidney tissue is normal, and (e) the cysts do not communicate with the collecting system, but, not uncommonly, a portion of the mass may herniate into the renal pelvis. Primitive blastema cells may be found in the septa (146). The usual multilocular

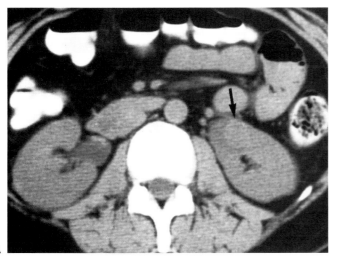

A

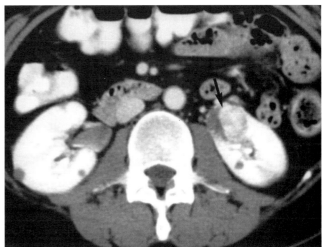

B

FIG. 29. Von Hippel-Lindau disease. Noncontrast CT **(A)** and postcontrast CT **(B)** at same the level show an enhancing mass (arrow) within a cyst. **C:** More superiorly, another enhancing mass (curved arrow) and multiple cysts are present, as well as pancreatic cysts (arrows). Two renal carcinomas were removed.

C

cystic nephroma has no malignant potential and is often an incidental finding, but it may cause symptoms when large. On CT, a multiloculated cystic mass ranging from a few centimeters to over 10 cm is shown (Fig. 30). The cysts have water-attenuation value or slightly higher. The septa are usually thin with no enhancement (59). Septal calcification is seen in about 10%, and often it is curvilinear (187). High density or other signs of hemorrhage are rarely seen in multilocular cystic nephroma. In general, these lesions are in the Bosniak type 3 category, and they can be difficult to discriminate from cystic renal carcinoma (82,111–113,223,225,252,324). If CT or MRI shows thick or nodular enhancing septa, the mass must be considered renal carcinoma until proven otherwise, usually by resection. If there are no enhancing compo-

nents, benign multiloculated cyst is likely, and the lesion may be followed if it is not so large as to cause symptoms (59).

Multicystic dysplastic kidney is usually encountered in neonates or infants, either as a finding on prenatal sonogram or as a palpable mass after birth. These can persist into adult life, but they are small masses in adults as they do not grow from childhood, and they often regress completely (289,314). The CT appearance is characteristic: a small to moderate-sized cystic mass with peripheral calcification, occupying the expected location of a kidney (Fig. 31) (298). The lesion may be uni- or multiloculated, and no contrast excretion occurs. The contralateral kidney often is hypertrophied, and may have ureteropelvic junction disproportion or partial obstruction.

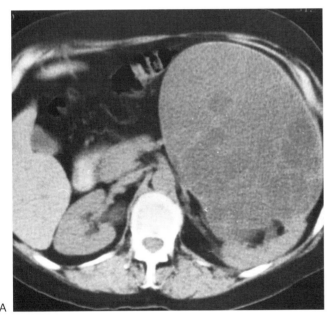

A

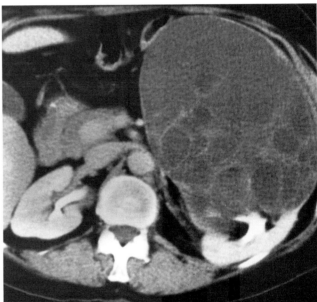

B

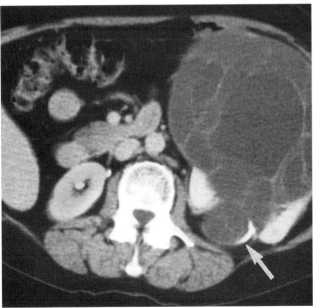

C

FIG. 30. Multilocular cystic nephroma. **A:** A palpable mass was found in this otherwise healthy 50-year-old woman; noncontrast CT shows a large complex mass. **B:** The mass contains multiple septations on postcontrast CT image. **C:** The mass bulges into the distorted collecting system *(arrow).*

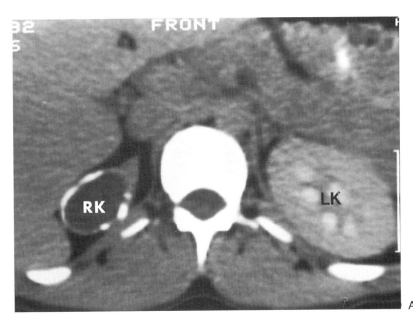

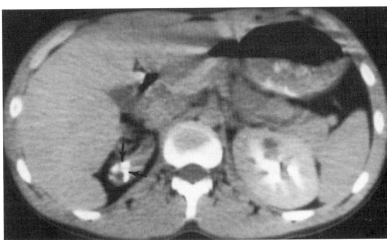

FIG. 31. Adult multicystic dysplastic kidney. **A:** Postcontrast CT image shows enlarged left kidney (LK) and the calcified cystic remnant of the right kidney (RK). **B:** Cephalad by 1 cm, clumps of calcification *(arrows)* are noted within the posterior aspect of the dysplastic right kidney.

MALIGNANT RENAL NEOPLASMS

Renal Cell Carcinoma

Renal cell carcinoma (RCC) is the most common primary malignant tumor of the kidney and accounts for 3% of all malignancies (194). In 1995, 28,800 new cases were expected, with 11,700 cancer deaths resulting from RCC, up from 22,500 and 9,600, respectively, in 1988 (277,327). It is, in fact, the commonest solid tumor of the kidney, and the focus of evaluation of renal masses is to distinguish the commonest benign mass, a cyst, from RCC. The cells of origin are tubular cells, and RCC is typically an adenocarcinoma, with several histologic variations. Clear cell type is commonest, but cystic variants, granular cell, sarcomatoid, and papillary RCC also occur.

There has been a major change in the presentation of RCC, with many small carcinomas now detected as serendipitous findings on CT done for unrelated reasons (56).

The overall 5-year survival has improved from 51% in 1977 to 1979, to 56% in 1983 to 1989 (327). To some degree, this is a result of detection of RCC at an earlier stage in the disease, when the tumor is smaller and of lower stage and is more likely to be cured by surgical resection, which is still the only effective treatment. The widespread use of both sonography and CT have improved the ability to detect small tumors in patients with signs such as hematuria and in asymptomatic individuals. The sensitivity of CT in detecting lesions 3 cm or less is much higher (94%) than that of sonography (79%) or intravenous urography (67%) (3,315). In one study, 48% of RCCs were incidentally detected, compared to 13% from the era before ultrasound and CT (159). In a survey of Japanese hospitals, the number of incidental cases rose from 20 in 1980 to 338 in 1988 (5). These incidentally discovered tumors are typically smaller (25% smaller than 3 cm, versus only 5% smaller than 3 cm in the pre-CT era) (280) and of lower stage, with a better prognosis (76.5% 5-year survival) (5).

TABLE 2. *Indications for CT for renal neoplasms*

Urogram suspicious for renal mass
Sonogram suspicious for renal mass other than benign cyst
Normal findings on urography/sonography, but suspicious signs or symptoms (e.g., persistent hematuria)
Metastases from unknown primary
Paraneoplastic syndromes
Syndromes with high incidence of renal neoplasms, including von Hippel-Lindau disease, acquired renal cystic disease
Previous treatment for renal cell carcinoma

Computed tomography is currently the method of choice for evaluation of suspected renal neoplasms and for staging of a neoplasm detected by other means (Table 2) (174,341). Proper technique must be used to achieve high accuracy (26). Both pre- and postcontrast images are mandatory. Section thickness must be appropriate to the size of the lesions. For lesions less than 2 cm in diameter, 3- to 5-mm contiguous sections should be used. At least 30 to 40 g of iodine (150 to 180 ml) should be injected as a rapid bolus. Attenuation measurements must increase by at least 10 HU to be certain of enhancement. These methods will help avoid potential pitfalls, such as volume averaging, which can cause both spurious elevations in attenuation values and failure to detect enhancement.

Using the above principles, accurate diagnoses of renal masses can be made with dynamic incremental (nonhelical) CT. Helical CT offers several potential advantages (279). A volume of tissue can be imaged during a single suspended respiration. If the volume is selected appropriately, and consistently for pre- and postcontrast images, the entire mass will be imaged, and pre- and postcontrast images will be comparable. This avoids the problem of respiratory misregistration,

which may result in a nondiagnostic study. Helical CT allows for very rapid imaging, so that images of the renal vein can be done during peak enhancement, improving detectability of tumor thrombus. However, if images of the kidney are done only in the very early postcontrast period (corticomedullary phase), small lesions may be less detectable (Fig. 32). Lesions that lie in the more central portion of the kidney may be difficult to distinguish from the normal medullary parenchyma, which is not yet enhanced. In one study, only 25 centrally located lesions were detected on helical CT corticomedullary phase images, but 111 were present on nephrographic phase images (47). Both false positive and false negative misdiagnoses can result. Greater diagnostic accuracy may be achieved by allowing a greater postinjection delay to obtain nephrographic phase images, or by obtaining both early corticomedullary images and then re-scanning the kidney to get nephrographic images.

The diagnosis of RCC by CT or MRI is based on recognition of the altered renal contour, parenchyma, collecting system, and renal sinus fat, as well as the characteristics of the mass lesion itself. Diagnostic criteria include the following:

1. A mass that bulges the renal contour (Figs. 33,34). Because RCC arises from the cortex, it is usually peripheral, and 94% to 96% are exophytic (128,336). If arising from cortex near the hilum, it may bulge into the renal sinus.

2. Attenuation value or signal intensity characteristics of the mass differ from normal renal parenchyma. On precontrast CT, most RCCs are nearly isodense with renal parenchyma, and somewhat heterogeneous; small tumors often are homogeneously isodense (Fig. 35), whereas large masses typically are hypodense and heterogeneous

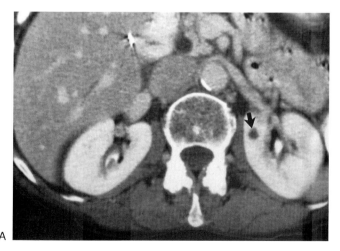
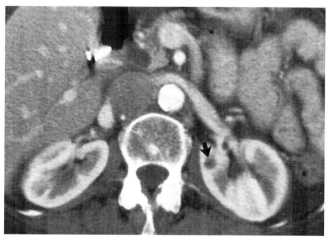

FIG. 32. Effect of CT technique on lesion conspicuity. **A:** CT image done 160 sec after intravenous contrast injection with 5 mm nonhelical scan shows a small renal cyst *(arrow)*. **B:** On follow-up CT, done with helical technique, 5-mm slice obtained during the corticomedullary phase shows the lesion *(arrow)* to be more subtle.

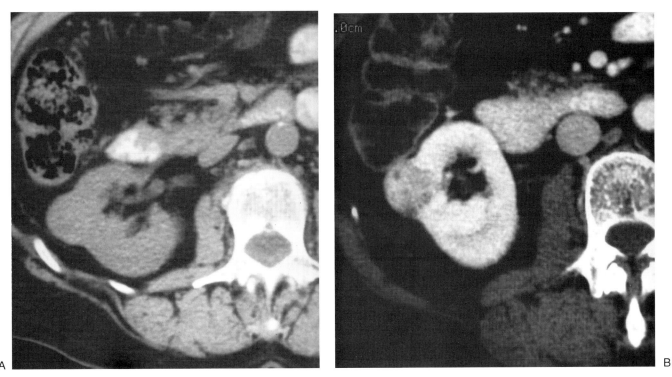

FIG. 33. Renal carcinoma, incidental. **A:** Noncontrast CT (done to evaluate a solid mass detected incidentally at sonography) shows a 2.6-cm mass measuring 26 HU. **B:** Postcontrast, the density is 160 HU; a stage I renal carcinoma was enucleated.

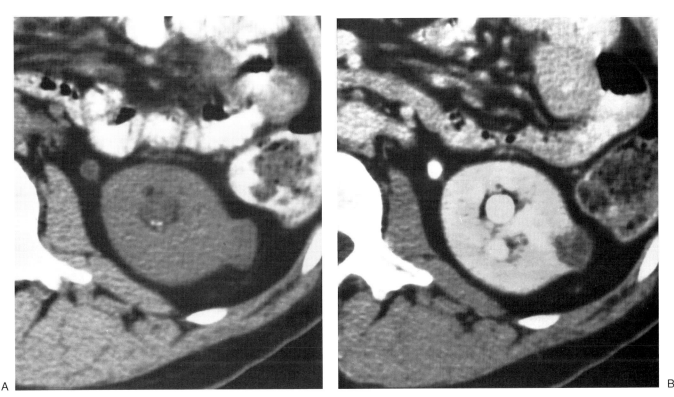

FIG. 34. Cystic renal carcinoma, incidental. **A:** Precontrast CT shows a 15-mm lesion measuring 15 HU. **B:** Postcontrast, the lesion is heterogeneous; attenuation measured 37 HU. A cystic renal carcinoma, stage I, was enucleated.

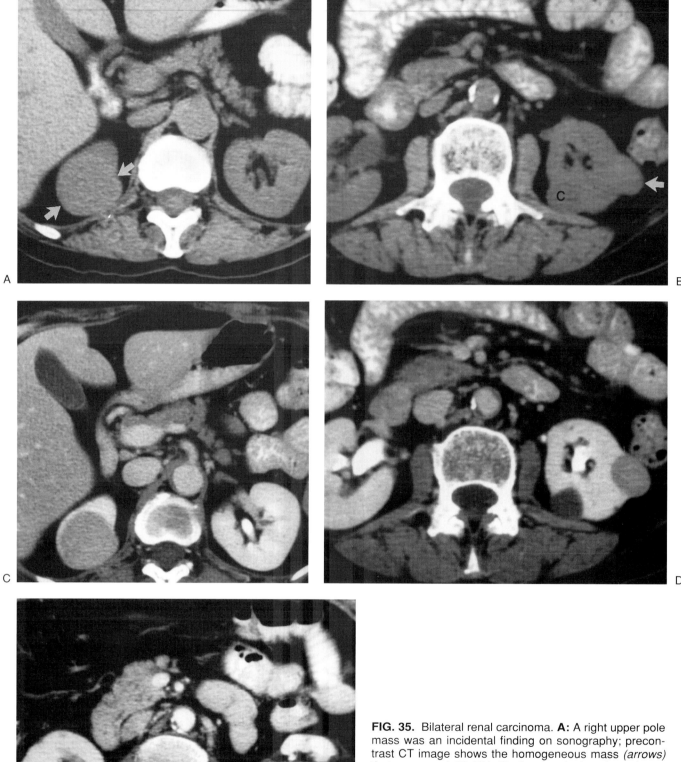

FIG. 35. Bilateral renal carcinoma. **A:** A right upper pole mass was an incidental finding on sonography; precontrast CT image shows the homogeneous mass *(arrows)* that measured 28 HU. **B:** Another lesion *(arrow)* protrudes from the left kidney (37 HU); note cyst (C). **C:** Postcontrast, the right mass is homogeneous and sharply marginated, measuring 3.5 cm and 114 HU. **D:** The left lesion is sharply marginated, measuring 2 cm and 105 HU; bilateral enucleations were done revealing low grade renal carcinomas. **D:** Follow-up CT shows a surgical defect, but no recurrent tumor.

as a result of central necrosis (Figs. 36–39). Hemorrhagic tumors are hyperdense (332). Calcification is common in RCC, demonstrated on CT in about 25% to 30% (19,336). The likelihood of calcification increases with size: only 3% of a series of RCCs less than 3 cm in diameter showed calcification (332), whereas in another study, 33% of RCCs over 3 cm contained calcification on CT (19). On unenhanced MRI, RCC is commonly intermediate in signal intensity between cortex and medulla on T1-weighted images, and usually somewhat hyperintense to parenchyma on T2-weighted images (81) (Figs. 40,41). Small RCCs are difficult to diagnose on both CT and MRI performed without contrast medium (130,133).

3. Enhancement that differs from normal renal parenchyma (Figs. 33–35,40). Virtually all RCCs show some enhancement, but less than that of renal parenchyma, on CT or MRI (26,77,268,336). Patterns of enhancement are variable. Small, well-differentiated tumors tend to show homogeneous enhancement (Fig. 35); moderate-sized tumors usually show some heterogeneity, and they commonly appear more heterogeneous after contrast medium administration than before (Figs. 38,39) (336). Large tumors may be mostly necrotic with a central low-density, nonenhancing area; a thick or nodular enhancing wall can be seen in nearly all cases (Figs. 37A, 39C). MRI is also a very sensitive detector of enhancement, with patterns similar to those on CT (Fig. 40) (250,269).

4. An unsharp margin between the mass and renal parenchyma is very suggestive of malignancy (Fig. 39). This, however, is common only in larger tumors, with over 80% of small RCC being well marginated (Figs. 33–35) (19,332). Pseudoencapsulation (a thin, low-attenuation or low signal intensity border) also may be seen in RCC, both on CT and MRI.

5. When present, the wall of a predominantly cystic RCC is perceptibly thick and usually irregular (59); there may be multiple thick septations with enhancement (Figs. 36,37).

6. Secondary signs, when present, such as venous extension, metastases, lymphadenopathy or adjacent organ invasion, are indicative of malignancy (Figs. 39,42,43).

Nearly all RCCs show some of these criteria, such that very few renal masses remain indeterminate today. In several studies, CT has a diagnostic accuracy of over 95% (51,320). With helical CT, accuracy may be even higher. Nevertheless, with small renal masses diagnosis can be difficult. A 17% false positive diagnosis of RCC was reported, even with helical CT (278). Follow-up of indeterminate masses can be helpful, because RCCs will grow (mean rate, 0.5 cm/year) more rapidly than benign lesions (18).

If MRI is done without intravenous Gd-DTPA, its sensitivity for small renal tumors is much less than that of contrast-enhanced CT. A large percentage of small RCCs are isointense on both T1- and T2-weighted images (237). Based on T1- and T2-weighted images alone, 24% of renal masses remain indeterminate (130). However, when Gd-DTPA is used, MRI is equivalent in accuracy to CT for detection and diagnosis of RCC (77,269). All RCCs

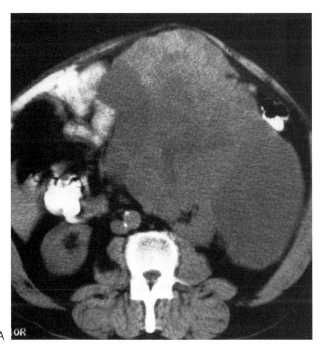
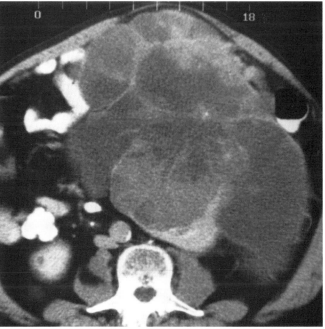

FIG. 36. Cystic renal carcinoma. **A:** Precontrast CT image shows a huge multiloculated cystic mass arising from the left kidney. **B:** Postcontrast, there are areas of enhancement; a stage I cystic renal carcinoma was resected.

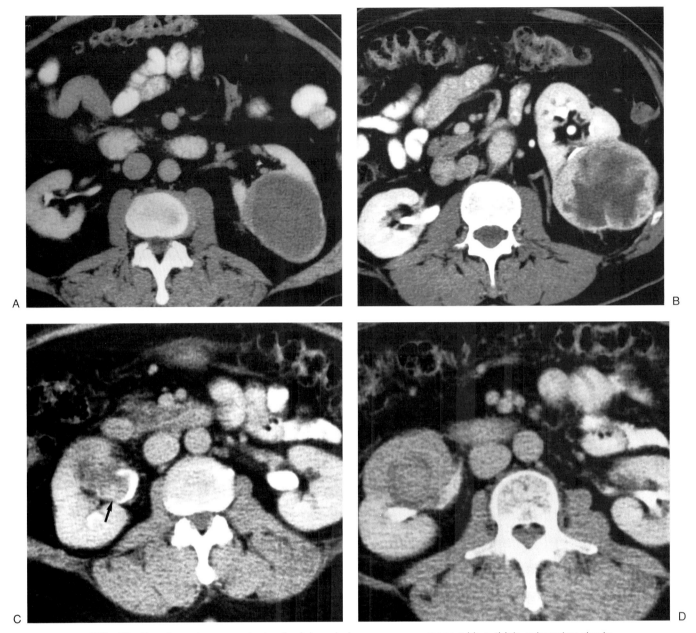

FIG. 37. Renal carcinoma variants. **A:** A largely homogeneous mass with a thick enhancing rim is shown; a papillary adenocarcinoma with extensive central necrosis was resected. **B:** In a different patient who presented with pulmonary metastases, there is a very heterogeneous mass; biopsy revealed a rhabdoid variant renal carcinoma. **C:** A pelvic filling defect was seen on a urogram in this patient with hematuria; postcontrast CT shows a mass protruding into the pelvis *(arrow)*. **D:** More inferiorly, the mass involves the lower pole parenchyma; a renal carcinoma was resected.

were detected by both CT and MRI in one large study (269). Although it is almost always possible to distinguish cyst from tumor, in some cases it is difficult to differentiate RCCs from other solid renal neoplasms, including oncocytoma, metastasis, lymphoma, and renal sarcoma. Whereas histologic type cannot be reliably predicted, papillary carcinomas often display calcification, diminished enhancement, central cystic or necrotic change, and low stage (235).

Knowledge of the staging of RCC is important, so that appropriate information is provided to determine resectability and prognosis. The Robson system (247) is still used by most urologists, but the TNM system is also used, especially in Europe (Table 3). Although most small RCCs are of low stage, some small tumors may metastasize (280) (Fig. 42B); conversely, some massive tumors are low stage (Fig. 36). Thus, it is critical to apply specific staging criteria using CT or MRI. It may be difficult to distinguish stage I (confined within the renal capsule) from stage II (extending into the perinephric fat but not

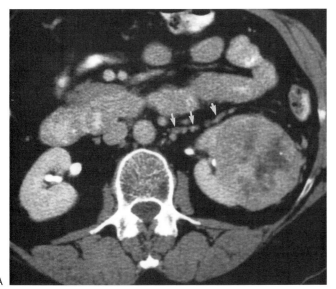

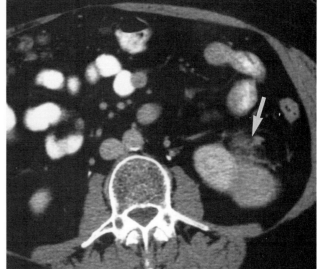

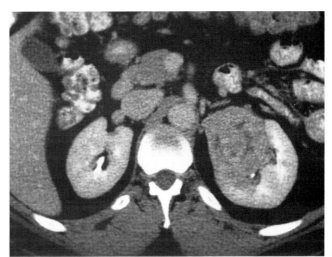

FIG. 38. Renal carcinoma stage II. **A:** A 7.2-cm poorly marginated, heterogeneously enhancing mass is present; note the enlarged vessels in the perinephric space *(arrows)*. **B:** More inferiorly, there is extension of tumor into the perinephric fat *(arrow)*, confirmed surgically. **C:** In another patient, this 6-cm renal carcinoma was found to be stage II pathologically, but shows it has a smooth outer margin on CT.

TABLE 3. *Staging renal cell carcinoma: Robson's classification versus TNM*

Robson	Disease extent	TNM
I	Tumor confined to kidney (small, intrarenal)	T1
	Tumor confined to kidney (large)	T2
II	Tumor spread to perinephric fat, but within Gerota's fascia	T3a
IIIA	Tumor spread to renal vein or cava	T3b
IIIB	Tumor spread to local lymph nodes (LN)	N1–N3
IIIC	Tumor spread to local vessels and LN	T3b, N1–N3
IVA	Tumor spread to adjacent organs (excluding ipsilateral adrenal)	T4
IVB	Distant metastasis	M1a–d, N4

beyond Gerota's fascia) tumors by either CT (145) or MRI (Fig. 38) (81,269,320). Demonstration of thickening of the renal fascia, including the bridging septa, and of dilated, tortuous vessels coursing through the perinephric space are not reliable signs of tumor extension. They most often are the result of edema, inflammation, or engorgement of vessels because of the increased blood flow through a vascular tumor, rather than the result of direct tumor spread (Fig. 38). However, distinction between stage I and II tumors is not critical, because both are resectable and both have good prognoses.

The presence of lymph node metastases in the renal hilum or retroperitoneum indicates stage III and confers a poorer prognosis (Figs. 39,43) (194). There is a high association of local recurrence in patients with lymph node involvement at presentation. Lymph nodes larger than 1 cm (short axis diameter) are considered abnormal on both CT and MRI. The sensitivity of CT for detection of adenopathy resulting from RCC has been reported to be over 95% (291). Nodes larger than 2 cm are almost

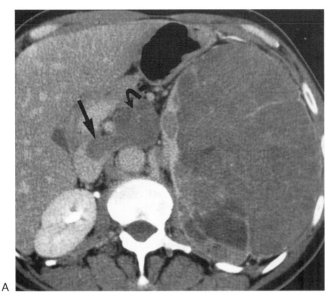

A

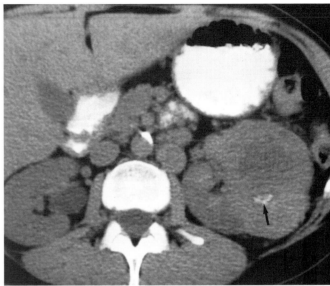

B

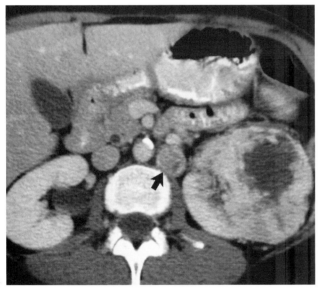

C

FIG. 39. Renal carcinoma, stage III. **A:** A large heterogeneous mass with extension into the vena cava *(arrow)* and lymphadenopathy *(curved arrow)* is seen on postcontrast CT. **B:** Precontrast CT in another patient shows a heterogeneous mass with some calcification *(arrow).* **C:** On postcontrast CT, the mass demonstrates heterogeneous enhancement and poor margination; note the lymphadenopathy *(arrow),* confirmed pathologically. The renal vein was uninvolved.

always involved with tumor. Unfortunately, not all enlarged nodes harbor tumor, as some are enlarged because of reactive hyperplasia (291). Thus, nephrectomy is often done despite enlarged nodes. Although adenopathy can usually be recognized on contrast-enhanced CT, nodes can be more easily distinguished from vessels on MRI (because of the signal void phenomenon on SE images) (Fig. 43), and MRI is slightly more accurate in the diagnosis of nodal disease (81,131). However, MRI also relies on enlargement of nodes for diagnosis, because signal intensity of hyperplastic nodes is similar to that of lymph node metastases. Also, care must be taken not to misinterpret adenopathy on MRI by measuring the craniocaudal length on sagittal or coronal views, because normal nodes are longer in that dimension.

Adrenal gland involvement by RCC is found in less than 10% of cases, and it is more frequent in large tumors

replacing much of the kidney, or upper pole tumors (95). Contralateral adrenal metastases are very rare. CT has been shown to be very accurate with no false positive CT diagnoses reported in one study (95). CT is also very accurate at detecting abnormally enlarged adrenals; however, incidental nonhyperfunctioning adenomas may simulate metastases (95).

Stage III is also indicated by extension of tumor into the renal vein or inferior vena cava (Figs. 39,43,44). This is very uncommon with small tumors; in a study of over 400 cases of RCC, none with venous extension were smaller than 4.5 cm (148). Surgical planning depends on the exact extent of the thrombus. Although prognosis is poorer than stage II, maximum survival rates are achieved by surgical resection if the entire tumor and thrombus can be successfully removed. Increased caliber of the renal vein is suggestive of thrombus, but this is a nonspe-

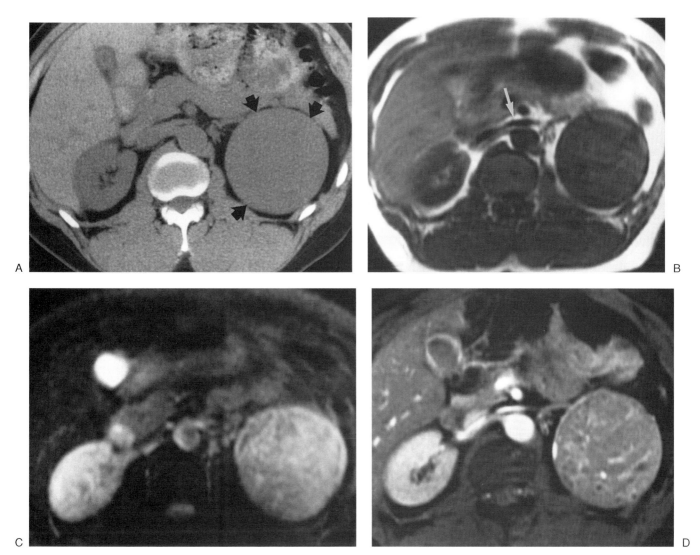

FIG. 40. MRI, renal carcinoma. **A:** Noncontrast CT in this patient with renal failure shows enlargement of the left upper pole *(arrows)*. **B:** T1-weighted SE image (400/12) shows the mass to be slightly heterogeneous, nearly isointense with the normal right renal parenchyma; note the left renal vein is patent *(arrow)*. **C:** On fat-suppressed, T2-weighted SE image (2500/70), the mass is well marginated, slightly heterogeneous, and nearly isointense with the normal right renal parenchyma. **D:** On Gd-DTPA-enhanced breath-hold GRE image (SPGR 52/12/45°), heterogeneous enhancement of the mass is shown; a stage I renal carcinoma was resected.

cific sign, as the renal vein may be dilated because of increased flow from a very vascular tumor. Contrast-enhanced scans are needed for accurate diagnosis. The tumor thrombus is usually detectable as a filling defect outlined by the brightly enhanced flowing blood (Fig. 39), especially when the vessel is only partly filled with tumor thrombus (190,285,339). Care must be taken not to over-diagnose thrombus in the inferior vena cava (IVC) based on streaming of unopacified blood returning from the lower extremities (see Fig. 2A) (285). If the vessel is completely occluded, enlarged paravertebral collaterals may be seen (83). Tumor thrombus is more readily detected in the left renal vein (because of its longer, transverse course) than the right (which has a short, oblique

course). Tumor within the IVC usually can be recognized because of increased diameter of the vessel and lack of the usual dense enhancement. On delayed or poorly enhanced scans, the tumor thrombus may be isodense with venous blood and difficult to recognize (Fig. 44). Overall, CT has an approximate sensitivity of 80% and specificity of 96% for the diagnosis of venous invasion (145,148).

Magnetic resonance imaging can be even more accurate for detection of venous invasion. In several studies, MRI has had a sensitivity between 80% and 100% for detection of IVC tumor thrombus, superior to that of CT, and equivalent to venacavography (129,147,148,239). Tumor thrombus produces a filling defect, replacing the expected signal void in flowing vessels on SE images (Fig. 43).

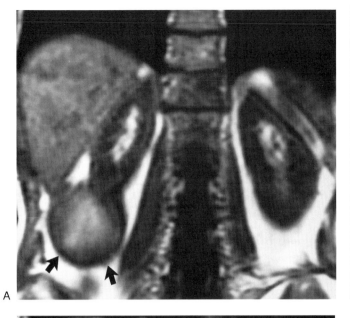

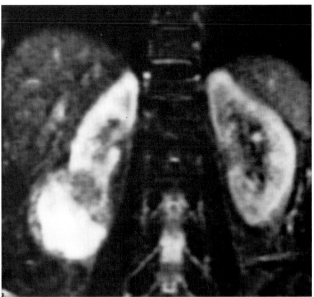

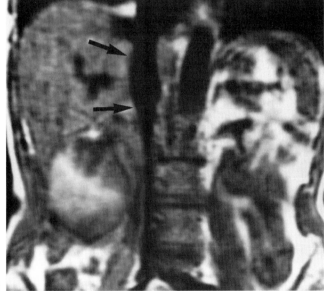

FIG. 41. MRI, renal carcinoma. **A:** Coronal T1-weighted SE image (500/15) shows a large mass *(arrows)* extending from the right lower pole with a hyperintense center. **B:** The inferior vena cava *(arrows)* is normal. **C:** A fat-suppressed, coronal, T2-weighted SE image (2000/90) shows the mass has a very hyperintense center and is well marginated; the mass showed enhancement after Gd-DTPA injection; a stage I renal carcinoma with central hemorrhagic necrosis was resected.

However, slow or turbulent flow may also produce apparent filling defects. Gradient echo sequences with flow compensation that makes flowing blood appear very bright make tumor thrombus readily recognizable as a filling defect (Fig. 44). In a comparison of SE and GRE methods, the GRE method was clearly superior, with 100% sensitivity for IVC tumor and 88% for renal veins (255). The multiplanar imaging capacity of MRI aids in accurate demonstration of the extent of the tumor thrombus (Fig. 44). MRI may be capable in some cases of distinguishing bland thrombus from tumor thrombus, as only the latter will enhance with Gd-DTPA.

Direct spread to contiguous organs indicates stage IV and a very poor prognosis (Fig. 42A). Such patients are not surgical candidates. This is an uncommon cir-

cumstance today. In many instances, direct tumor spread is detectable on CT, as the tumor crosses and obliterates the normal tissue planes between the kidney and adjacent organs, such as the liver, pancreas, spleen, or psoas muscle. However, a diagnosis based only on the loss of tissue planes may lead to false positive diagnoses, because in many cases, the tumor abuts, but has not invaded, the organ. Invasion of the liver also may be falsely suggested because of volume averaging of an oblique interface in the transverse plane. Local extension can be more accurately detected by MRI, because the most appropriate imaging plane can be selected to avoid volume averaging (147). Also, tumor has distinctly different signal (hyperintense) on T2-weighted images than psoas muscle and liver (hypoin-

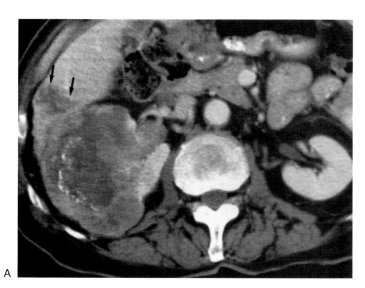
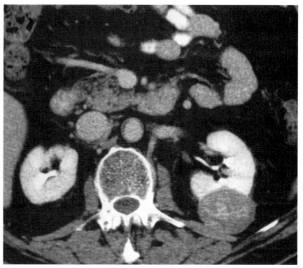

A

B

FIG. 42. Renal carcinoma, stage IV. **A:** This large, calcified renal carcinoma extends directly into the liver *(arrows)*; omental disease was also present (not shown). **B:** In a different patient, who presented with pulmonary metastases, a 3.5 × 4 cm renal carcinoma is shown on postcontrast CT.

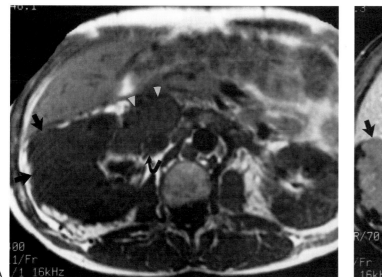
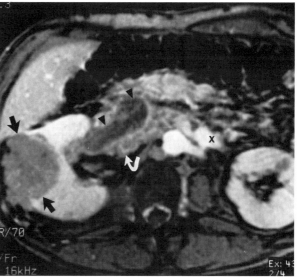

A

B

FIG. 43. MRI, stage III renal carcinoma. **A:** T1-weighted SE image (400/11) shows a right renal mass *(arrows)*, retroperitoneal adenopathy *(curved arrows)*, and enlargement of the renal vein with loss of signal void *(arrowheads)*. **B:** Gd-DTPA-enhanced, T1-weighted GRE image (SPGR 116/2.7/70°) shows enhancement of the mass *(arrows)* and the tumor thrombus *(arrowheads)* is seen as a defect, rather than the expected high signal of flowing blood [compare with left renal vein (X)]; note adenopathy *(curved arrows)*.

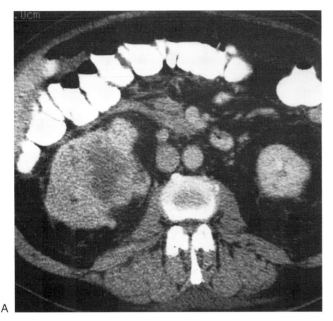

A

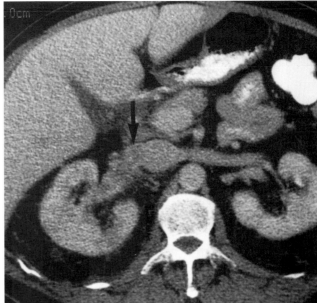

B

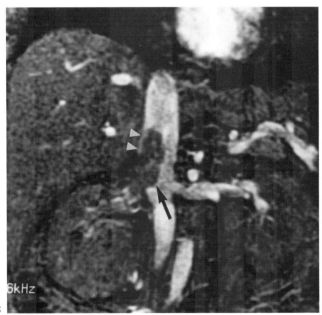

C

FIG. 44. MRI, stage III renal carcinoma. **A:** A right lower pole tumor is evident on postcontrast CT. **B:** Because of poor enhancement, it is unclear whether the renal vein is invaded *(arrow)*. **C:** Coronal GRE image (SPGR 34/13/35°) shows tumor thrombus extending into the inferior vena cava *(arrow)*; note the lateral wall is not involved *(arrowheads)*; the tumor was extracted successfully.

tense), so that invasion can usually be clearly seen or excluded (147) (Fig. 41).

Metastases to distant organs also confer stage IV and a very poor long-term prognosis. As a general rule, the extent and number of metastases relate to tumor size and vascularity (194). On rare occasions, however, renal carcinoma may present with distant metastases even when the primary tumor is less than 3 cm (51,53). The lung, mediastinum, skeleton, brain, and liver are the commonest sites. Renal carcinoma may present with a metastasis (particularly skeletal) before the primary tumor has become symptomatic. Because about 5% of RCCs are bilateral, very careful examination of the contralateral kidney is mandatory in every case.

Angiography and Biopsy

With CT and MRI, accurate detection, diagnosis, and staging is possible in nearly all cases of renal mass. The few indeterminate lesions are usually very small. The role for angiography is limited, primarily because nearly all questions can be answered by less invasive and less expensive methods (320). Angiography is useful if angioembolization is needed, usually for palliation of symptoms or bleeding in nonsurgical cases. Angiography also may be useful in surgical planning of nephron-sparing resection. Contrast venacavography also has been almost entirely replaced by CT and MRI. Percutaneous renal biopsy is rarely indicated, not because it is inaccurate, but because in most instances it is superfluous. Most cases of RCC are definitively diagnosed by their CT or MRI appearance, and they require surgical removal. The few very small or complex lesions that are indeterminate are those that are particularly difficult to diagnose by biopsy or angiography as well. Biopsy, however, may be useful in cases of unresectable, apparently malignant tumor of uncertain histology (e.g., metastasis or lymphoma versus RCC), where treatment may be altered by knowledge of the cell type. In such a population, a sensitivity of 80% and a specificity of 100% with minimal complications have been reported. In that study, all of the patients with RCC with metastases at the time of presentation died within 1 year (211).

Treatment and Follow-Up

In addition to the initial diagnosis and staging of RCC, CT and MRI play an important role in the follow-up of patients treated with surgery, angioinfarction, or chemother-apy (17). Those who are at the highest risk for having persistent or recurrent disease are those with bulky tumors; venous, nodal, or adrenal involvement; and incomplete resection (194). Because the recurrence rate of stage I or II tumors after radical nephrectomy is so low, routine follow-up may not be justified, although CT should be done if there are any signs or symptoms suggestive of a recurrence. Follow-up of stage III tumors that have been successfully resected is justified because of the greater incidence of recurrence; this should be concentrated in the first 2 years after surgery. Baseline and follow-up CT in the first 2 years after nephron-sparing surgery is also reasonable, especially because of concern about unrecognized multicentricity (214). Because most recurrences occur in the abdomen, follow-up studies should scrutinize the renal bed, liver, remaining kidney, adrenals, and retroperitoneum. A tumor recurrence is indicated by a soft-tissue mass in the renal fossa, local organ abnormalities, and sometimes by asymmetric focal enlargement of the psoas muscle (Fig. 45). Abscess, seroma, or lymphocele should not be confused with recurrence, as they are largely water attenuation.

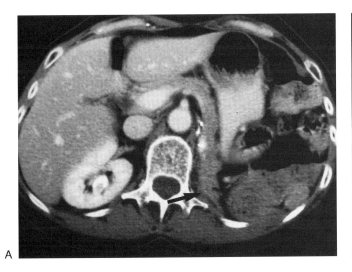

A

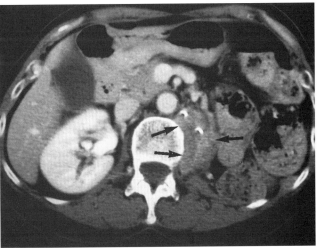

B

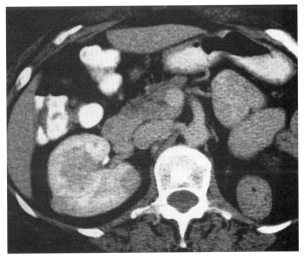

C

FIG. 45. Follow-up of renal carcinoma. **A:** This patient complained of new onset of back pain 3 years after left radical nephrectomy for renal carcinoma; note the pancreatic tail is now lying adjacent to the spine *(arrow)*. **B:** At a more caudal level, there is a heterogeneous mass *(arrows)* in the region of surgical clips, indicative of recurrence. **C:** In a different patient, CT done because of new onset of hypertension 8 years after resection of a stage I renal carcinoma shows several enhancing masses in the remaining right kidney; nephrectomy was done and confirmed multiple RCCs.

Nephron-sparing surgery is increasing in frequency, because excellent results have been reported with small, low stage RCC (181,204). Because of this, the postoperative appearance of the surgically altered kidney must be recognized. Postoperative fluid collections, including hematoma and abscess, are not uncommon, but they are seen in the early postoperative period and resolve within weeks to months. Wedge-shaped or concave defects are usually detectable in the region of the removed tumor (150) (Fig. 35E). There should be no abnormally enhancing tissue present and identification of such is suggestive of recurrence (150). A baseline postoperative CT is very useful to aid detection of recurrences. Because of the possibility of multifocal disease, the remaining kidney must be very carefully searched for additional lesions that may have been too small to recognize at initial presentation.

Urothelial Carcinoma

The second commonest primary malignancy of the kidney arises from the urothelium (12). Of these, 85% to 95% are transitional cell carcinoma (TCCA), about 10% are squamous cell carcinoma (SCCA), and less than 1% are adenocarcinomas (91). Overall, these tumors are about one fifth as common as RCC (168). Hematuria, either gross or microscopic, is the commonest sign, with flank pain or weight loss as the presenting symptom in less than one fourth. Because the signs and symptoms are so

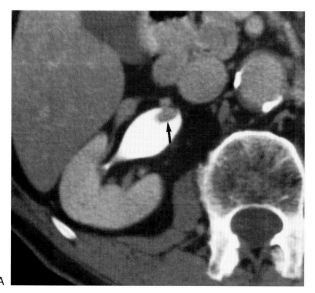

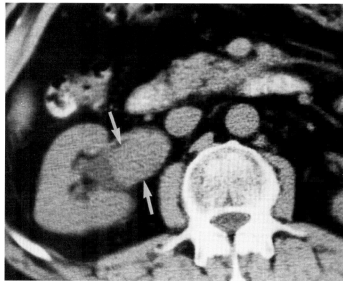

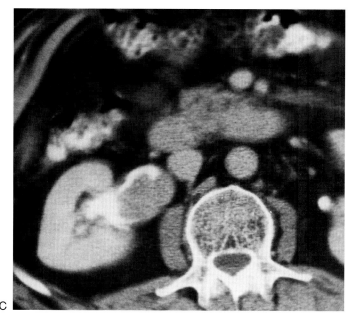

FIG. 46. Transitional cell carcinoma. **A:** Postcontrast CT image shows a soft-tissue filling defect *(arrow)*. **B:** Precontrast CT image in another patient shows a soft-tissue mass *(arrows)* in the fluid-filled right pelvis. **C:** Postcontrast image shows the mass as a filling defect.

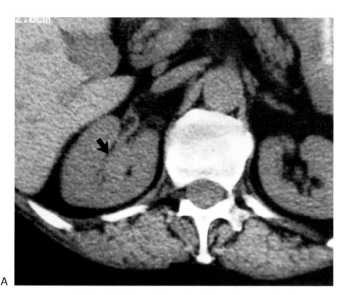
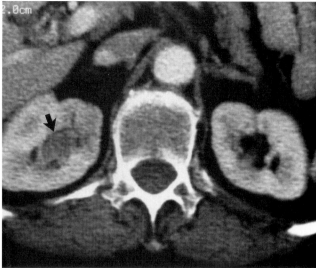

A   B

FIG. 47. Transitional cell carcinoma. **A:** Precontrast CT image shows a lesion that measured 24 HU in the right upper pole calyx *(arrow)*. **B:** On helical CT image 90 sec after injection of contrast, the lesion measured 45 HU; note the collecting system is not yet well opacified. Note obliteration of the right renal sinus fat compared to the normal left upper pole.

nonspecific, imaging is crucial in the diagnosis. Urography, sonography, or retrograde pyelography is often the initial study for suspected upper tract urothelial tumors. Cytology may be diagnostic, although it does not localize the lesion, and cytology is often falsely negative with upper tract TCCA. Computed tomography is often done as a staging procedure, but it has particular advantages for diagnosing uroepithelial tumors when there has been loss of function of the kidney resulting from chronic obstruction, and when there is need to distinguish carcinoma from other causes of radiolucent filling defects (12,38, 153,228).

Computed tomography can determine the nature of a radiolucent filling defect in the intrarenal collecting system or ureter. Noncontrast CT images show TCCA as a soft-tissue-density filling defect (10 to 40 HU) (91,216,224), whereas calculi range from 75 to over 500 HU (Fig. 46). Thus, even "radiolucent" urate calculi will be separable from TCCA by CT. Blood clot usually measures about 50 to 60 HU precontrast, although acute blood may measure up to 80 HU. After intravenous contrast medium administration, TCCA enhances a little (Figs. 47,48) (an increase of 10 to 30 HU) (91,216,224). Thus, CT can distinguish TCCA from calculus, clot, dilated pelvis, and parapelvic cyst. Although most patients with calculus disease can be managed without CT, CT can be very accurate in detecting

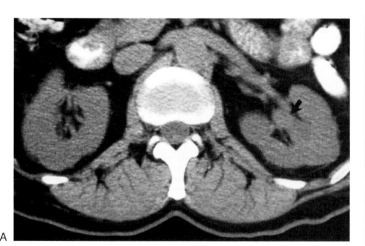
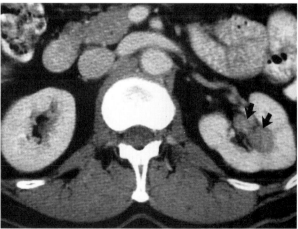

A   B

FIG. 48. Transitional cell carcinoma. **A:** Precontrast CT shows soft-tissue filling collecting system *(arrow)* in region where irregular narrowing of the infundibulum was seen on urography. **B:** An enhancing soft-tissue mass is seen in the collecting system *(arrows)* at the same level on postcontrast image.

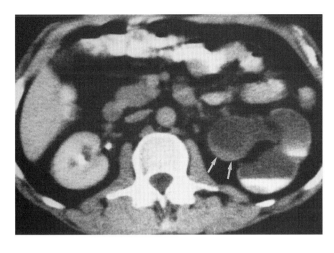

FIG. 49. Transitional cell carcinoma. Urography showed a nonfunctioning left kidney; hydronephrosis is shown on postcontrast CT; note the crescentic thickening of the pelvis *(arrows)*. Transitional cell carcinoma was confirmed at surgery.

stones not only in patients with radiolucent filling defects but also in patients with hematuria and nondiagnostic prior studies. However, precontrast as well as postcontrast images are critical (because calculi may be obscured by the contrast); thin contiguous or overlapping sections in the area of interest also may be needed.

A variety of patterns on CT may be caused by TCCA of the kidney (Figs. 46–50). Most often, there is an intraluminal soft-tissue mass in the pelvis, calyces, or ureter (12,91,216). This is usually isodense with renal parenchyma precontrast, and enhances less than renal parenchyma (12,216). The tumor may be outlined by contrast in the pelvis (Fig. 46), or the tumor may infiltrate some or all of the renal sinus. Calcification can occur in TCCA, usually appearing as stippled calcification on the surface of a soft-tissue mass (71). Transitional cell carcinoma may merely cause thickening or irregularity of the wall of the calyces, pelvis, or ureter (12,216) (Fig. 49). This can be seen as concentric or eccentric thickening of the pelvis or ureter (Figs. 49,51) (12). Dilatation of the col-

lecting system above a subtle soft-tissue mass may be seen (91,216). If the tumor arises from a calyx, a centrally located renal mass will result (12,168). The soft-tissue mass is often ill defined and grows centrifugally, expanding the kidney without deforming the surface, such that the reniform shape is largely preserved (Fig. 50). Focal alteration of the nephrogram may be seen, especially with peripheral tumors (28). There may be early delay in nephrogram, with a late persistent dense nephrogram (28,91). Transitional cell carcinoma may be highly invasive, infiltrating the renal parenchyma, and it may produce massive, necrotic tumors sometimes replacing the entire kidney (29). Although rare, renal vein and vena cava invasion have been reported. In most instances, the appearance is distinct from that of RCC or other tumors such as lymphoma, but occasionally a precise histologic diagnosis may not be possible. In some rare cases, RCC may invade the pelvis, simulating a urothelial primary (Fig. 37) (208). Percutaneous biopsy may be done, but only as a last resort, because of the possibility of needle tract seeding (probably more common with TCCA than other tumors). Frozen sections may be done at the time of surgical removal. However, direct endoscopic biopsy is a preferred method for establishing the diagnosis preoperatively.

Although the diagnosis may be clear from other studies, CT is the most accurate imaging procedure available for detection and staging of urothelial tumors. Recent reports indicate detection of 86% of TCCAs by CT (216). Staging is important to plan therapy, as stage III and IV tumors have poor a prognosis (Table 4) (284). CT is not capable of distinguishing tumors that are superficial from those that deeply invade the muscle layers (12,195). However, it is accurate (85%) at detecting invasion beyond the pelvic wall or metastatic disease (216). Local extension or distant metastases preclude nephroureterectomy, the surgical procedure of choice for confined tumors (49).

Squamous carcinoma of the renal pelvis is associated with chronic inflammation, resulting from calculus disease, urinary stasis, and chronic infection (313,325). It is more aggressive

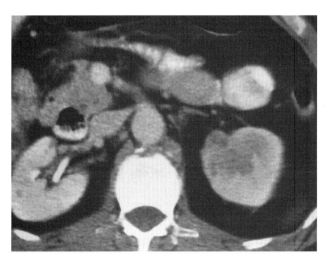

FIG. 50. Infiltrative transitional cell carcinoma. Note the poorly marginated lower attenuation region that involves the left upper pole without altering the contour; transitional cell carcinoma was confirmed at nephrectomy.

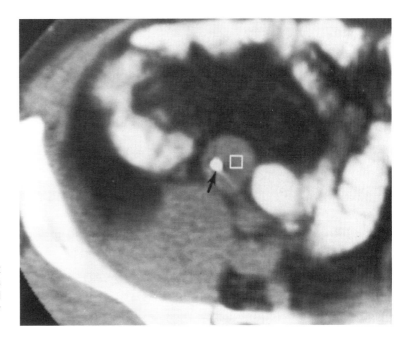

FIG. 51. Transitional cell carcinoma of the right ureter; note semilunar pattern. The cursor is placed over an eccentric portion of the thickened ureteral wall. The *arrow* points to the eccentrically situated ureteral stent. (From ref. 12.)

and carries a worse prognosis than TCCA. On CT, SCCA rarely appears as a discrete intraluminal filling defect but is more often an ill-defined (sometimes circumferential) thickening of the pelvic wall, or an infiltrating mass with a tendency to grow extraluminally (210). Invasion of renal parenchyma or adjacent organs is often seen (210). Adenocarcinoma, cholesteatoma, and metastases to the urothelium are rare causes of masses that simulate TCCA on CT (8,12).

Little has been reported on the utility of MRI in upper tract urothelial tumors. MRI is capable of demonstrating large TCCA, especially with the use of Gd-DTPA to enhance the collecting system. Unless iodinated contrast medium cannot be used, there is no advantage of MRI over CT.

Renal Sarcoma

Sarcomas arising in the kidney itself are rare, accounting for about 1% of renal malignancies (274). These are

TABLE 4. *Staging classification of upper tract urothelial tumors*

Finding	Grabstad Cummings	UICC
Carcinoma in situ	I	Tis
Limited to mucosa	I	Ta
Tumor involves submucosa	II	T1
Muscle invasive tumor	III	T2
Tumor invades parenchyma	III	T3
Tumor invades peripelvic or periureteral tissue	III	T3
Invasion of contiguous organs	IV	T4
Lymph node metastases	IV	N1–N3
Distant metastases	IV	M1

From refs. 49, 284.
UICC, International Union against Cancer.

highly malignant tumors. Leiomyosarcoma is the commonest primary renal sarcoma. It is believed to arise from the renal capsule or from the wall of an intrarenal vessel walls. Fibrosarcoma, liposarcoma, osteosarcoma, rhabdomyosarcoma, clear cell sarcoma, and others also occur (229,274). On CT and MRI, its appearance is similar to that of RCC. Typically, renal sarcomas are very large at presentation. Detection of a very large, malignant-appearing tumor arising in the kidney suggests sarcoma. Large, poorly marginated, irregularly-shaped, focal masses that are heterogeneous with low-attenuation areas (central necrosis) precontrast, and show heterogeneous enhancement after contrast, are typical. Calcification occurs in 10% (274). Some have a very peripheral location, probably resulting from origination from the renal capsule (Fig. 52). Lymphadenopathy, extension to involve adjacent organs, and metastases to lung, liver, and bone are common. It is not possible in most cases to diagnose the type of sarcoma based on CT appearances, but the presence of fat suggests liposarcoma, and the presence of dense calcification, osteosarcoma. On MRI, renal sarcomas appear similar to large RCCs, with heterogeneous low signal on T1-weighted images, heterogeneous high signal on T2-weighted images, and irregular enhancement after intravenous administration of Gd-DTPA. Because of the size and the possibility of local extension, MRI can be useful for diagnosis and staging. Renal sarcoma may be detected as an incidental tumor at a lower stage (Fig. 53). Although it is often difficult to distinguish renal sarcoma from RCC, treatment principles are the same.

Metastases and Lymphoma

Metastases to the kidneys are not rare, although they are usually asymptomatic. Autopsy series report an incidence

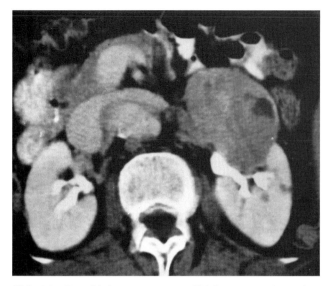

FIG. 52. Renal leiomyosarcoma. CT done to evaluate hematuria in this 74-year-old woman reveals a heterogeneous mass arising from the periphery of the left kidney.

between 2% and 20% (39). Primary sources include bronchogenic carcinoma, colorectal, breast, melanoma, testes, and gynecologic malignancies, and a variety of others (39,128). In most instances, renal metastases are found in patients with known malignancies, usually in association with other metastatic disease (Fig. 54). In such cases, there is no diagnostic dilemma. It is uncommon for a metastasis to present as a solitary renal mass in a patient with no history of malignancy. However, a primary renal carcinoma may develop in a patient with another malignancy. In some circumstances, such as a case of a solitary renal mass in a patient with a remote history of a malignancy, or in a case of a patient presenting with a new malignancy that rarely metastasizes to the kidney, metastases must be distinguished from primary renal carci-

noma. Recognition of the CT imaging features can be useful, but sometimes percutaneous biopsy is needed.

Computed tomography is the most cost-efficient screening method for renal metastases, and it is the standard imaging tool for evaluation of oncologic patients. It is more sensitive than sonography and less costly than MRI (which is probably equivalent in sensitivity, although no large comparative studies have been published). Most metastases are small (<3 cm), multiple (>50%), and noncontour deforming (39,128) (Fig. 55). They may be wedge-shaped or appear infiltrating (Figs. 55,56) (128). On precontrast CT images, metastases are commonly isodense with renal parenchyma, and they enhance less than renal parenchyma after intravenous contrast medium administration. When large, they may be heterogeneous because of central necrosis (Fig. 54).

Renal metastases are typically associated with metastases elsewhere; renal vein invasion is rare. Thus, renal metastases are usually distinctive compared to RCC, which is solitary in 96% of cases, and more typically exophytic, bulging the renal contour (128). Perirenal metastases may occur, seen as soft-tissue nodules in the perinephric fat; these may or may not be associated with renal lesions (Fig. 55). Melanoma, bronchogenic carcinoma, and lymphoma are the commonest sources of perirenal metastases (322).

Approximately 5% of patients with lymphoma will have renal involvement during their disease course (120). Up to 50% have renal involvement at autopsy. Renal lymphoma is usually not clinically evident, and it is most often detected by imaging evaluation of patients presenting with, or being followed for, lymphoma. Non-Hodgkin lymphoma is considerably more common than Hodgkin disease (92% versus 8%) (244), although the imaging appearances are similar. Primary renal lymphoma is very rare, as there is no lymphatic tissue normally residing in the kidney. Involvement of the kidney may be by hematogenous seeding or direct contiguous spread. In about

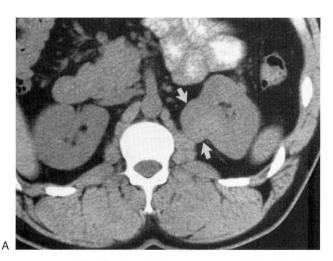

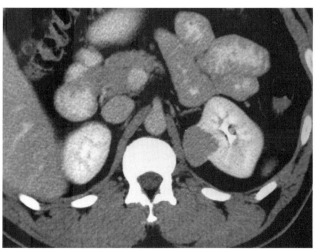

A   B

FIG. 53. Renal leiomyosarcoma. **A:** In this 39-year-old man, precontrast CT shows an isodense 3.5-cm lesion *(arrows).* **B:** After contrast, there is homogeneous enhancement.

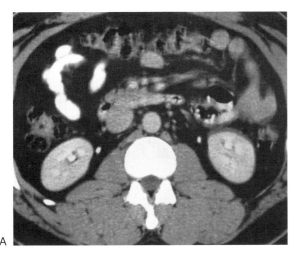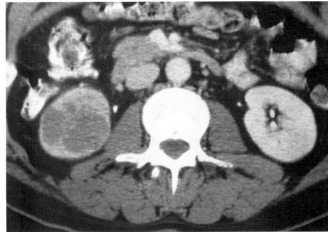

FIG. 54. Renal metastases. **A:** Baseline CT in this patient with lung cancer shows the lower poles to be normal. **B:** After 10 months, a large mass is shown in the right lower pole; there were also new skeletal metastases.

half of cases, renal lymphoma represents a relapse in patients previously treated for lymphoma.

CT has been shown to be superior to sonography for detection of lymphoma in the kidney (319), and it is the standard method for evaluation and follow-up of abdominal lymphoma in general. Incidence of renal involvement on CT scans of lymphoma patients is between 2.7 and 6% (261). Several different patterns (110,120) may be seen:

1. Most commonly, there is direct contiguous spread of a typical retroperitoneal lymphomatous mass into the renal sinus or parenchyma (Fig. 57).
2. Multifocal masses (31%)
3. A solitary mass (23%)

4. There may be diffuse enlargement of both kidneys without discrete masses, but this pattern is not commonly seen with contrast-enhanced CT (12%) (244).

Discrete solid masses are common (244) (Figs. 58,59). These masses are usually homogeneous and isodense with renal parenchyma on precontrast images, although occasionally they may be of slightly lower or higher density. Following contrast injection, homogeneous enhancement (10 to 30 HU) that is significantly less than renal parenchyma is typical (110,120). Heterogeneous enhancement may be seen with larger, necrotic lesions (Figs. 58,59). Enhancement may be patchy or wedge shaped. Necrosis or calcification may be seen after treatment.

Extension into the perirenal space occurs in 40% of

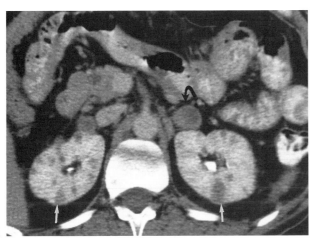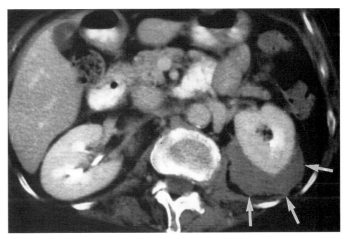

FIG. 55. Renal metastases. **A:** Contrast-enhanced CT images show numerous bilateral small, round, and some wedge-shaped *(arrows)* lesions in the kidneys of this patient with melanoma. Adrenal metastases are also present *(curved arrow)*. **B:** In a different patient with widespread metastatic melanoma, a large perirenal mass is present *(arrows)*.

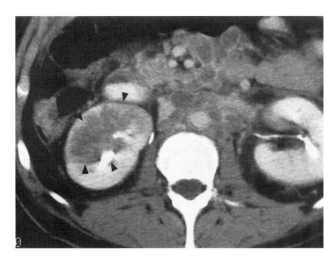

FIG. 56. Renal metastases. A lung cancer had been resected 1 year previously; contrast-enhanced CT shows an infiltrative lesion of the right kidney *(arrowheads)* and retroperitoneal adenopathy. Percutaneous biopsy revealed metastatic lung cancer.

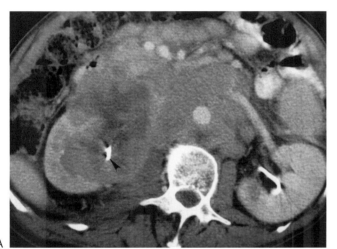

A

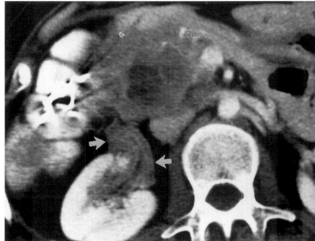

B

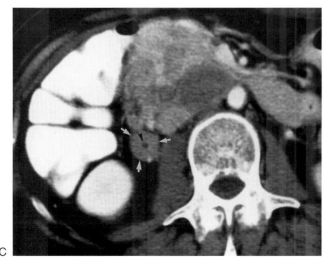

C

FIG. 57. Renal lymphoma. **A:** Extensive retroperitoneal adenopathy with direct extension into the right kidney is evident in this patient with recurrent non-Hodgkin lymphoma; note stent previously placed in right ureter *(arrowhead)*. **B:** In another patient with non-Hodgkin lymphoma, tumor infiltrates the renal sinus *(arrows)*, narrowing the pelvis. **C:** More caudally, the lymphoma encases the ureter *(arrows)*.

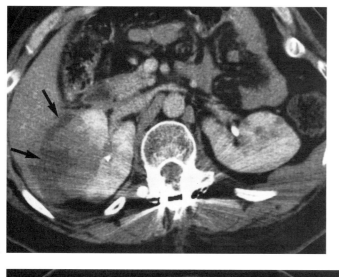

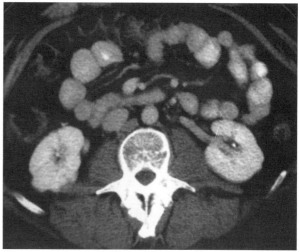

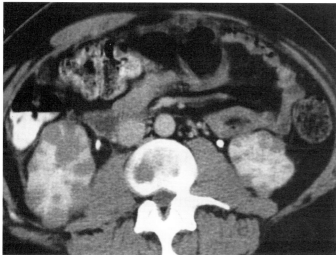

FIG. 58. Renal lymphoma. **A:** In this patient who had presented with lymphoma in the spine, follow-up CT shows a large right renal mass *(arrows)*. **B:** More caudally, multiple smaller homogeneous lesions are present. **C:** After chemotherapy, the lymphomatous deposits have resolved, with some residual scarring.

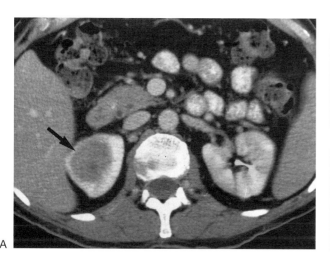

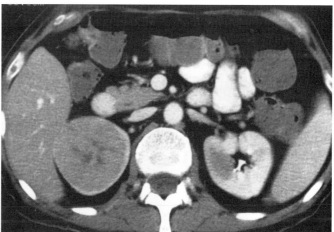

FIG. 59. Renal lymphoma in an AIDS patient, whose CT 3 months earlier had been normal. **A:** Postcontrast CT image shows a 4-cm mass *(arrow)*. **B:** After 3 months, the right upper pole mass is 6.5 cm and more heterogeneous; note the new left upper pole mass. Growth this rapid is more typical of lymphoma than of renal carcinoma.

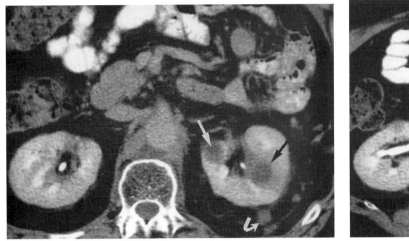
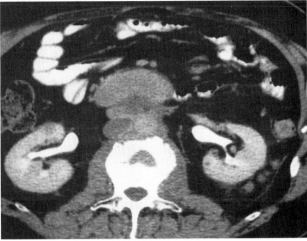

FIG. 60. Renal lymphoma. **A:** Note intrarenal *(arrows)* and perirenal lesions *(curved arrow).* **B:** More caudally, retroperitoneal lymphadenopathy and perirenal nodules are shown.

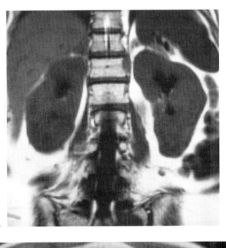
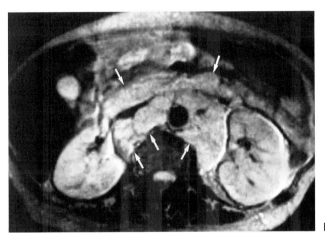

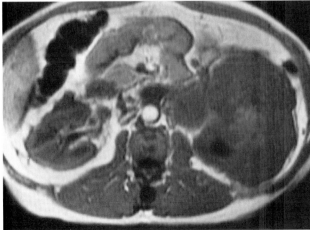
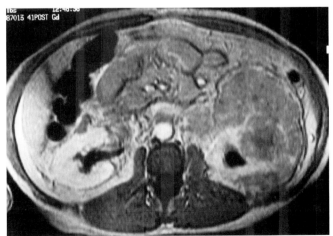

FIG. 61. MRI of renal lymphoma. **A:** Coronal T1-weighted SE image (400/16) shows the kidneys are enlarged with loss of corticomedullary differentiation due to infiltration by lymphoma. **B:** Transaxial T2-weighted SE image (1600/80) shows retroperitoneal adenopathy *(arrows)* and infiltration of the kidneys with lesions isointense to fat. **C:** In another patient, T1-weighted GRE image (FLASH 154/6/75°) shows a large heterogeneous left renal mass. **D:** Following intravenous Gd-DTPA, the mass shows heterogeneous enhancement that is less than that of renal parenchyma.

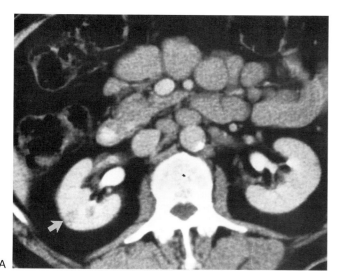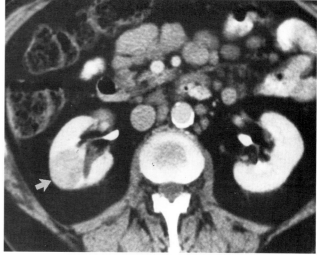

FIG. 62. Renal carcinoma in lymphoma patient. **A:** A small renal lesion *(arrow)* was presumed to be lymphoma in this patient being treated for non-Hodgkin lymphoma. **B:** After 4 years, the lymphoma has regressed somewhat, but the renal mass is larger; a stage I renal carcinoma was resected.

patients with renal lymphoma, sometimes being the only disease manifestation (196,244). This may be in the form of multiple discrete nodules in the perirenal fat (Fig. 60). Conversely, there may be sheetlike or diffuse infiltration of the perirenal space with low-density material replacing the retroperitoneal fat, often with little displacement of organs. The only other disease that causes this pattern of spread with any frequency is melanoma.

Experience with MRI for renal lymphoma is limited, and no large comparative series with CT have been published. In general, lymphoma in the kidney produces focal lesions, causing some mass effect and disruption of corticomedullary architecture normally seen on T1-weighted images by one or more multiple low signal intensity masses. The lesions are hyperintense on T2-weighted images (Fig. 61) (110). Enhancement after Gd-DTPA will occur (Fig. 61). It must always be kept in mind, especially with long-term follow-up of lymphoma or other oncology patients, that a second primary RCC may occur (Fig. 62).

BENIGN RENAL TUMORS

Adenoma and Oncocytoma

There is presently much controversy concerning the renal adenoma. Although this is defined as a benign neoplasm of renal tubule cell origin, it is debated whether this is a distinct benign lesion or whether it is merely a premalignant lesion that eventually becomes a renal carcinoma (236). It is also increasingly uncertain whether there is any criterion useful for making a distinction between adenoma and carcinoma by imaging. In the past, a well-encapsulated solid neoplasm of the renal cortex less than 3 cm in diameter, with no metastases and no necrosis, hemorrhage, mitoses, or atypia histologically,

was considered an adenoma. However, most small, solid, renal cortical neoplasms currently detected are renal carcinomas, and they have identical appearances on CT and on MRI. Although patients at high risk for developing renal neoplasia (such as those with end-stage renal disease, and especially those on dialysis) may be considered to have adenomas when small, slow-growing, solid masses are identified, neither size nor imaging appearance is capable of excluding renal carcinoma. All such patients should be followed closely.

Oncocytomas are a type of renal adenoma with a distinctive histologic appearance, including large, polysomal, eosinophilic epithelial cells with mitochondria-rich cytoplasm arranged in solid trabecular or tubular patterns (10, 46,166,236). Mitotic activity is absent and there is no hemorrhage or necrosis. Although most often solitary, multiple and bilateral oncocytomas do occur. They range in size from less than 1 to over 20 cm (mean, 6.7 cm), and patient age ranges from 26 to 94 years (207). About 4% of renal tumors are oncocytomas (207). These are well-circumscribed lesions on CT. When small, they typically are round or ovoid and isodense with renal parenchyma before contrast, and they show homogeneous enhancement after intravenous contrast (Fig. 63), a pattern not distinct from that of a small renal carcinoma (see Fig. 35) (143). When larger, a central stellate scar may be seen (Fig. 64) (10). This is a branching, low-attenuation (10 to 20 HU) (236), nonenhancing area. When a scar is present, the remainder of the lesion enhances homogeneously. However, a scar is rarely seen in oncocytomas less than 5 cm in size. More problematic is the fact that central necrosis in a renal carcinoma can appear very similar to this central stellate scar (46). Thus, whatever the size, oncocytoma cannot be reliably differentiated from renal carcinoma by CT (62). In a large comparison of oncocytoma to renal carcinoma,

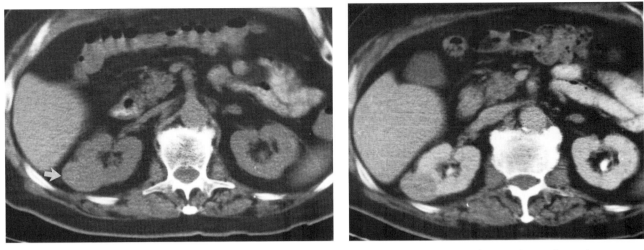

FIG. 63. Oncocytoma. **A:** Precontrast CT shows a 3.5-cm mass isodense to renal parenchyma *(arrow)*. **B:** Contrast-enhanced CT shows the lesion is homogeneous, well circumscribed, and enhances less than renal parenchyma.

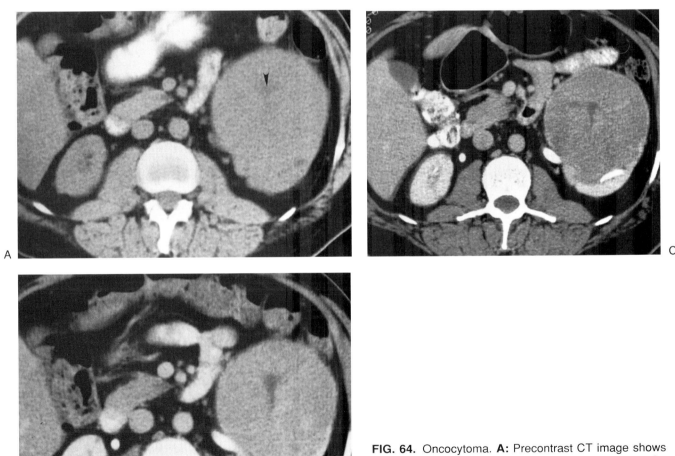

FIG. 64. Oncocytoma. **A:** Precontrast CT image shows a 10-cm mass isodense to renal parenchyma except for a central low-attenuation region *(arrowhead)*. **B:** After contrast, there is homogeneous enhancement except for the central scar; note rim of normal kidney *(curved arrow)*. **C:** Follow-up CT 2 years later shows no change.

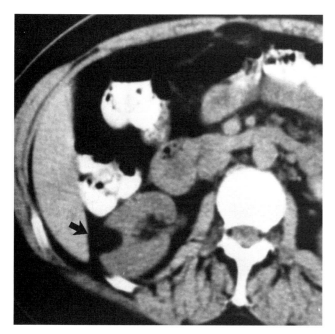

FIG. 65. Angiomyolipoma. Noncontrast CT shows a homogeneous fat density (−68 HU) lesion *(arrow)*.

82% of oncocytomas less than 3 cm were homogeneous. However, 42% of the renal carcinomas less than 3 cm were also homogeneous. Conversely, in 33% of oncocytomas over 3 cm, the central low-attenuation area appeared indistinguishable from a necrotic center, and thus these were indistinguishable from RCC as well (62).

Reports on the MRI appearance of oncocytomas indicate they are of low to moderate signal on T1- and hyperintense on T2-weighted images. If present, the central scar is seen as a lower signal area on T1- but may be of very intense signal on T2-weighted images. Homogeneous enhancement (except the central scar) can be expected after intravenous Gd-DTPA. However, the MRI appearance is not distinct from that of RCC (10,69, 243,281). It is also now believed that no angiographic pattern is pathognomonic of oncocytoma. Thus, any lesion over 3 cm, even if suspected of being an oncocytoma, should be removed, although a nephron-sparing approach would be preferred.

Several other unusual renal tumors may be found that do not have distinctive appearances on CT and MRI, including fibroma, leiomyoma, and extramedullary hematopoiesis. The great majority of fibrous histiocytomas are malignant, although a few benign ones occur.

A

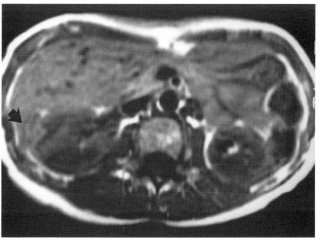

B

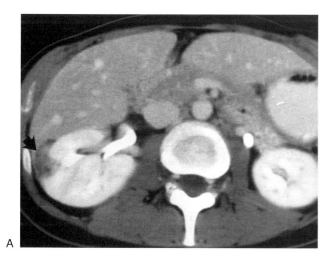

C

FIG. 66. Angiomyolipoma. **A:** CT after contrast shows a heterogeneous mass *(arrow)* with a few small low-attenuation areas; convincing fat attenuation could not be measured. **B:** On T1-weighted SE image (300/15), the lesion has high signal *(arrow)*; high signal was also present on T2-weighted images. **C:** The lesion retains high signal on water suppressed T1 SE weighted (300/15) sequence, documenting the presence of fat.

One of the rarest of all renal lesions is the capillary or cavernous hemangioma. This neoplasm is composed of blood-filled epithelial spaces (venous lakes) that crowd into the medullary portion of the kidney. Angiography shows a hypovascular mass with bowed, pruned-appearing intrarenal arteries. The lesion appears as a well-defined central (medullary) mass with diminished contrast-material enhancement at CT. A history of intermittent gross hematuria over several years in a teenager or young adult may provide an important clue to the existence of such a rare benign tumor.

Lymphangiomyoma may present as a cystic, multiloculated renal mass (141). Juxtaglomerular cell tumors are rare, but they have a typical presentation. Patients are usually young (third decade), severely hypertensive with hypokalemia and hyperaldosteronism. A solitary solid homogeneous renal mass, commonly about 2 cm in size, is

seen. These are typically peripheral, lying just below the renal capsule, and they enhance poorly. High density may be seen because of hemorrhage (75,309).

Angiomyolipoma

Angiomyolipomas (AMLs) are benign renal neoplasms that consist of varying amounts of mature adipose tissue, smooth muscle, and thick-walled blood vessels (22, 109,308). Although they can spread locally and may rarely involve local lymph nodes, the clinical course is benign, with no distant metastases (109,300,308). The term *hamartoma* (a benign mass composed of disorganized tissues normally found in an organ) is sometimes used, but *choristoma* (a benign mass composed of disorganized tissues not normally found in the organ) is a more

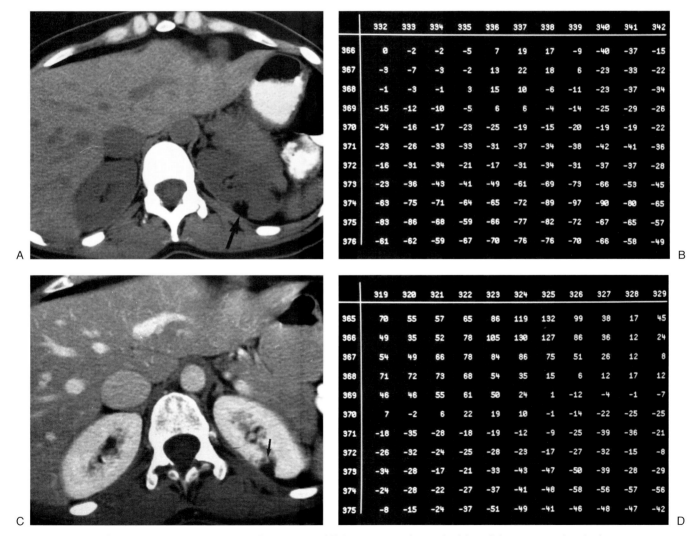

FIG. 67. Angiomyolipoma. **A:** Precontrast CT image reveals an incidental low-attenuation lesion *(arrow)*. **B:** Average attenuation was −33 HU; note on pixel report clusters of pixels with negative numbers. **C:** Contrast-enhanced CT shows small areas of bright enhancement *(arrow)*. **D:** Average postcontrast density was 12 HU; note on pixel report some negative numbers and some areas with high positive numbers.

appropriate term because smooth muscle is not normally found in renal parenchyma. About 80% of patients with TS have AMLs, and in these patients, multiplicity is the rule. Numerous bilateral small AMLs are typical of TS patients (see Fig. 28) and about 30% of TS patients have cysts (310). However, large or solitary AMLs can be seen in TS. Conversely, about 80% of cases of AML occur in patients without TS; in these patients, typically middle-aged women, solitary lesions are the rule. Multiple AMLs in non-TS patients do occur sporadically (31,264). Whether sporadic or associated with TS, two basic tenets remain the same: diagnosis is made by documentation of fat in the lesion, and management is guided by the size of the mass.

Angiomyolipomas range from being nearly completely fatty (Fig. 65) to being nearly all soft tissue (Fig. 66). They may be small and completely intrarenal, but often they are exophytic, especially as they enlarge. When small, they usually are asymptomatic, but when large they may cause significant displacement of organs by mass effect or hemorrhage. In about 40% of cases, signs or symptoms include pain, palpable mass, hemorrhage, and hematuria (288). Accurate diagnosis of AML can be made in virtually all cases using CT, which is very sensitive to the low attenuation of fat (22). Thin sections (3 to 5 mm) and small region-of-interest (ROI) measurements may be needed in small lesions or those with only tiny amounts of fat (25). Measurement of densities on precontrast images is preferable, since the enhancement of the blood vessels coursing through the fat may increase the average density of the lesion to the water or soft tissue range (Fig. 67). In lesions with very small amounts of fat, analysis of the individual pixel CT numbers can be diagnostic (297). However, care must be taken when using pixel reports. One can diagnose fat only if several (at least 3 to 6) contiguous pixels have fat attenuation values (<-20), because individual pixels in cysts may have low numbers (see Figs. 14,67). With careful technique, an area measuring less than -20 HU will usually be seen; in a few cases, especially when only postcontrast images, thick slices, or large ROIs are measured, density readings may be somewhat higher (-15 to -10 HU).

Computed tomography is the preferred diagnostic tool for AML. Although most AMLs are hyperechoic on sonography, other renal tumors, including RCC, may be very echogenic as well (87). Computed tomography must be done to document the presence of fat. Although MRI may be even more sensitive to the presence of fat and may be diagnostic of AML, its role is limited because noncontrast CT will suffice in most instances. If MRI is used, AML will usually appear as a complex lesion with at least some area that is hyperintense on both T1- and T2-weighted images. Because other substances, particularly old hemorrhage, can be hyperintense on T1-weighted and T2-weighted images (256), chemical shift methods should be used for clarification. Fat-containing

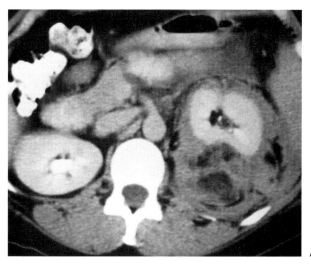

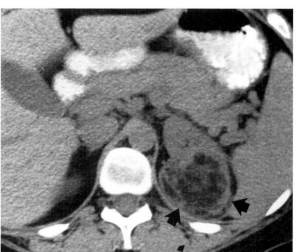

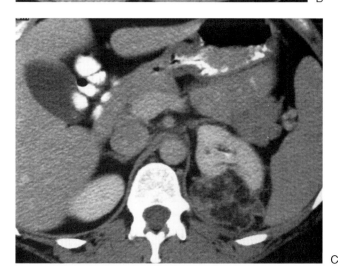

FIG. 68. Angiomyolipoma with hemorrhage. A: Contrast-enhanced CT was done to evaluate acute left flank pain in this 40-year-old woman; perirenal hemorrhage is present. B: Follow-up CT 6 weeks later shows resolution of the hematoma and a fat-containing mass *(arrows)* on precontrast CT. C: The mass shows enhancement of the vascular component; segmental resection was performed.

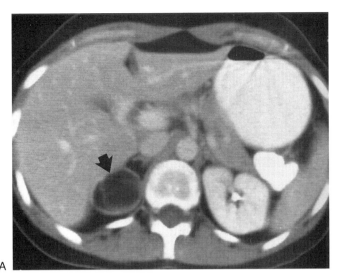
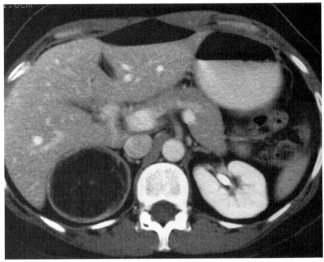

FIG. 69. Angiomyolipoma, growth. **A:** A 2.9-cm angiomyolipoma *(arrow)* was incidentally discovered in this 56-year-old asymptomatic woman. **B:** The lesion has grown to 6.5 cm, 7 years later, and the patient has intermittent flank pain; segmental resection was performed.

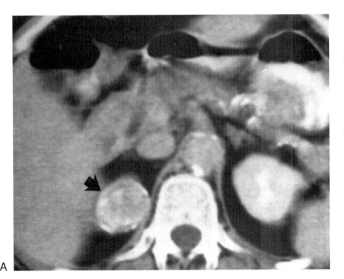
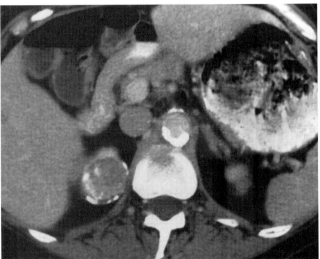

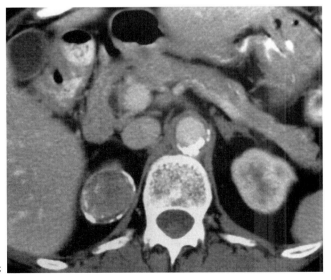

FIG. 70. Indeterminate renal mass. **A:** Contrast-enhanced CT shows a hyperdense renal mass *(arrow)* as an incidental finding in this 60-year-old woman with severe cardiac disease. **B:** Follow-up noncontrast CT 6 months later yielded central density of 72 HU; there is central calcification however. Postcontrast CT showed no definite enhancement; because of the heart disease, the patient was followed. **C:** CT 1 year later shows no change.

areas will show loss of signal with radiofrequency fat suppression, or retention of signal with water suppression. This may prove the presence of even tiny amounts of fat when this cannot be documented by CT (Fig. 66). Although the use of GRE images with opposed phase technique [echo time (TE) selected so that water and fat protons have opposite phase, resulting in phase cancellation and loss of signal compared to in-phase TE image] can be useful to document the presence of fat, if a lesion is nearly all fat there may not be significant phase cancellation and, thus, no recognizable loss of signal. There usually is enhancement of AMLs after administration of intravenous Gd-DTPA.

Several longitudinal studies have investigated the longterm outcome of AMLs (21,151,217,288,310). It is now clear that surgical intervention is required in only a minority of cases. If a patient has had a significant hemorrhage, surgical removal (preferably by a nephron-sparing method) is indicated (Fig. 68), although good results have also been achieved with angioembolization (151). Up to 36% of AMLs will increase in size; growth is more likely in lesions over 4 cm (288). Thus, asymptomatic patients with AML over 4 cm do not require urgent intervention but do merit relatively close follow-up (yearly CT or sonography) (Fig. 69). Although there seems to be even greater predilection for growth in TS patients (217,288), the management principles are the same.

In general, the detection of fat within a renal mass allows diagnosis of AML. Nevertheless, rare instances have been reported of masses other than AML that contained, or appeared to contain (290), fat. In some, a large tumor (RCC

and oncocytoma) engulfed perinephric or renal sinus fat as it grew (54,233). Some rare teratoid Wilms tumors have been reported to contain fat (227,323). Fat has been reported within renal carcinoma in two cases with osseous metaplasia (122,290) and in one in a tumor thrombus (238). In these cases, some features atypical for AML were present (calcification, renal vein extension). Perspective must be maintained; fat in a malignant renal tumor is extraordinarily rare. When fat is detected in a renal mass, the diagnosis should be AML unless there are atypical features. In any case, because of the possibility of growth, follow-up should be done.

INDETERMINATE MASSES

With careful technique and use of the diagnostic criteria previously described, as well as pertinent history and laboratory findings, very few renal masses are indeterminate today (9,51). Broad categories of CT-indeterminate masses include the following: (a) technically indeterminate CT images; (b) cystlike masses; (c) tumorlike masses with problematic features.

Technically indeterminate CT images are often a result of a scan done for unrelated purposes, not a directed renal mass evaluation. If only postcontrast images were obtained, there can be no certainty of enhancement. Thus, a hyperdense cyst (or hyperintense lesion on MRI) may be thought to be an enhancing lesion. Thick or noncontiguous slices, motion artifact, data-poor images in very large patients, incorrect field of view, inadequate dose of

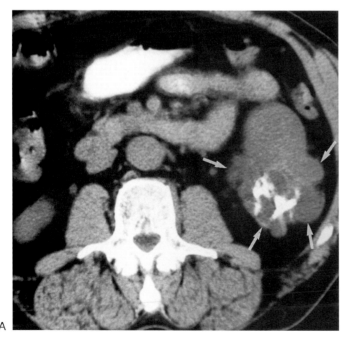
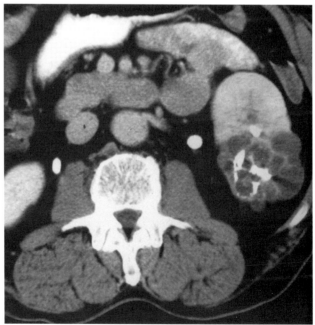

A   B

FIG. 71. Calcified renal cell carcinoma. **A:** Precontrast CT image shows dense calcifications in a lobulated mass *(arrows)*. **B:** On postcontrast CT image, the mass is multiseptated with slightly thick enhancing septa; a cystic renal carcinoma was resected.

contrast, long delay after contrast injection, and other factors can produce either nondiagnostic images or spurious density readings. In most such cases, repeat CT, directed for evaluation of the suspected mass, with pre- and postcontrast images and appropriately thin sections in the region of the mass, will provide definitive information (Fig. 70). Helical CT may be particularly advantageous. MRI also may help diagnose a lesion indeterminate on CT (191).

Cystic masses in the Bosniak type 3 category may be considered indeterminate, because they have about a 50% chance of malignancy (Fig. 71). The criteria for type 3 cystic lesions have been discussed. In such cases, clinical factors, including age and intercurrent illness, will direct management toward either close follow-up or surgery. Rarely do other diagnostic procedures aid in assessment of lesions that are type 3 by CT and MRI (51). Type 2F lesions (those with some disturbing findings but not quite type 3) should be followed closely.

Some renal masses closely resemble solid neoplasms but exhibit confusing CT features. This category includes very small lesions that are truly difficult to characterize because even with thin sections, accurate assessment of enhancement is difficult (Fig. 72). There is an overlap of the appearance of hemorrhagic and hyperdense cysts and renal carcinoma (76,114) (Figs.

19,73–5). Angiomyolipomas with little or no fat, and lesions suspected of being oncocytoma, fall into this category. So do neoplasms that may or may not be renal in origin (such as adrenal tumors, retroperitoneal sarcomas, and metastases) (248). Also, ill-defined masses involving the kidney, with diffuse enlargement, and perhaps with extrarenal spread, may be inflammatory, such as xanthogranulomatous pyelonephritis (XGP). For very small lesions (<1.5 cm), close follow-up is usually the best approach. Even a very small RCC is unlikely to grow or metastasize very rapidly; if followed with CT every 6 months for up to 2 years, growth should be detected, indicating whether surgery is needed. Conversely, for very large masses, percutaneous biopsy or surgery will usually be needed more urgently.

CALCIFIED RENAL MASSES

Calcifications may occur in both benign and malignant renal masses (184,321). In the past, calcification alone was considered a feature suggesting malignancy, because RCC is the commonest calcified renal mass (61). About 25% of RCCs contain calcification on CT (336); less than 1% of cysts are calcified on radiography (61). However, the exact location of the calcification and other features

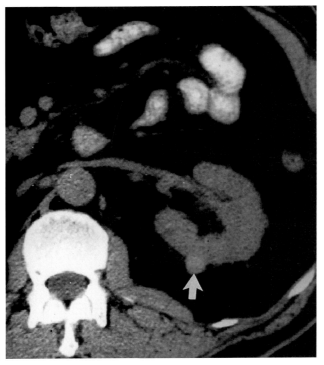

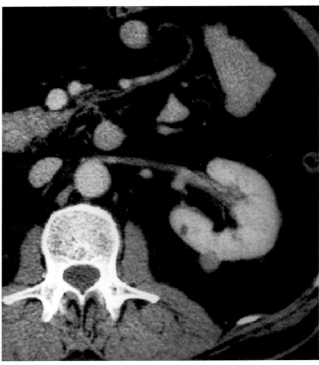

A   B

FIG. 72. Indeterminate renal mass. **A:** A 1 cm homogeneous high density (72 HU) lesion *(arrow)* was an incidental finding on this noncontrast CT. **B:** Contrast-enhanced CT (5 mm section thickness) measured 83 HU. Considerations are hyperdense cyst or renal carcinoma. Local resection revealed hemorrhagic cyst.

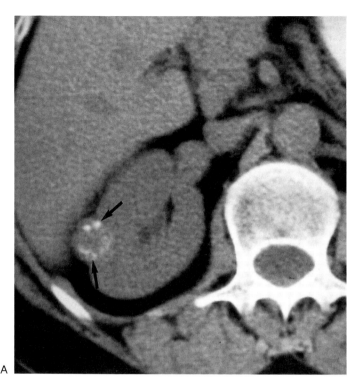
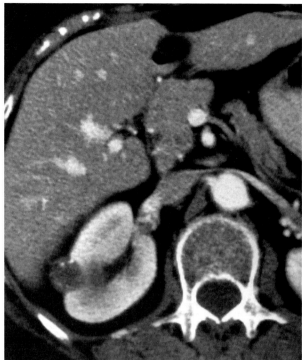

FIG. 73. Hemorrhagic cyst. **A:** Precontrast CT image shows a thick calcified wall *(arrows)*; the 2-cm mass measured 42 HU centrally. **B:** After contrast, the lesion measured 54 HU. Because of pain and patient anxiety, the lesion was removed surgically.

of the mass can be shown by CT, so that in many cases a definitive diagnosis can be made (157,321). Whereas MRI may help to evaluate such masses, it cannot demonstrate the calcification well. Calcified renal masses fall into three groups: (a) soft-tissue masses containing calcification; (b) predominantly cystic masses with focal, mural, or septal calcification; and (c) indeterminate masses. Diagnosis of a calcified tumor can be made in two situations: if the calcification is within the substance of the mass, not truly peripheral (Figs. 39B,76A), or if there is peripheral calcification but also an enhancing area of soft tissue within the mass (Fig. 76B). A variety of patterns of calcification are found in RCC, including punctate, amorphous, linear, and curvilinear, peripheral calcification. Renal neoplasms that are calcified may have a better prognosis (157,321). Other renal tumors that are rarely calcified include Wilms tumor, TCCA, SCCA, and metastases (6,111,162).

If CT shows the calcification to be limited to the wall or septa of a cystic mass, and the mass otherwise fulfills criteria for a cyst (homogeneous water-density contents, no enhancing solid component, or thick walls), a benign calcified cyst can be diagnosed with confidence (see Fig. 20). If the calcification is very dense or thick, follow-up is suggested. Although sonography is rarely useful in evaluating calcified cysts, MRI may be used to assess disturbing features, particularly enhancement. Indeterminate calcified lesions are those in which there is some

other disturbing feature in addition to calcification—such as high density or heterogeneous contents, thick walls or septations, or questionable enhancement (see Fig. 71). Such lesions are in the Bosniak type 3 category and should at least be followed very closely.

Inflammatory masses and hematomas also may calcify. Hydatid cysts of the kidney often are calcified, and these may raise suspicion of RCC because hydatid disease is uncommon in the United States. Detection of daughter cysts suggests the diagnosis, because calcified RCC rarely is multilocular (59). Arteriovenous malformations, aneurysms, and even AML may present as a calcified mass, but, with typical features on CT and MRI, a diagnosis can usually be made.

INFECTION

Acute Infection

In most cases, clinical signs such as fever, chills, flank pain or tenderness, and laboratory results such as leukocytosis (80%), pyuria, and bacteriuria will indicate presence of acute urinary tract infection. Urine cultures are positive in 75% and blood cultures in 50% (27). In many cases, no imaging is needed if there is prompt clinical response to appropriate antibiotics. If clinical signs and symptoms are unclear, or if response to treatment is poor, imaging

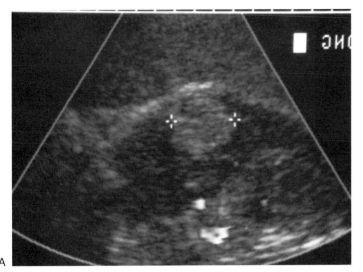

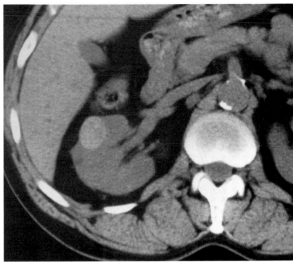

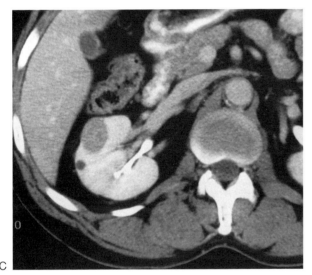

FIG. 74. Hyperdense renal carcinoma. **A:** Sonogram reveals a hyperechoic mass *(between cursors)* in this 60-year-old man with microscopic hematuria. **B:** Precontrast CT shows the mass is hyperdense (60 HU). **C:** Following intravenous contrast administration, the mass enhances (88 HU) and is slightly more heterogeneous.

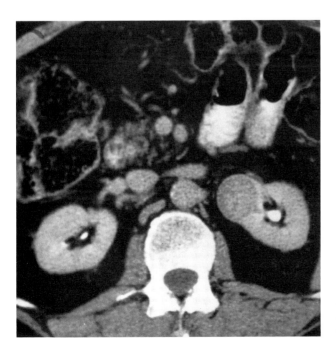

FIG. 75. Renal carcinoma in melanoma patient. A 3-cm solid mass was the only abnormality in this patient being followed for melanoma; biopsy revealed renal carcinoma.

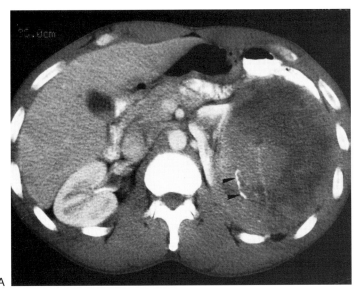

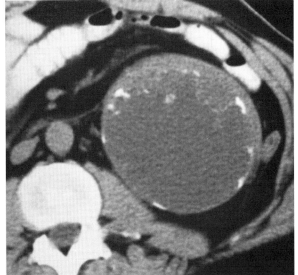

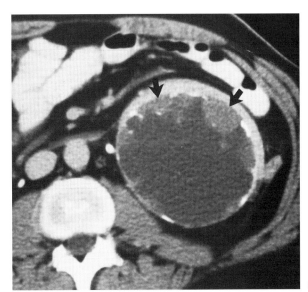

FIG. 76. Calcified renal carcinomas. **A:** Curvilinear calcification and a left upper pole mass were seen on urography; contrast-enhanced CT shows the calcification *(arrowheads)* lies within a heterogeneously enhancing mass. A renal cell carcinoma was resected. **B:** In a different patient, precontrast CT image shows a predominantly cystic mass with peripheral calcification. **C:** Post-contrast image shows enhancing mural nodules *(arrows)*; a renal carcinoma was resected.

is often performed to detect potential complications. It is less important to document acute pyelonephritis, which almost invariably responds to antibiotics, than to identify complicating factors such as hydronephrosis, calculi, and abscess. Intravenous urography is rarely used for serious infections, as it often fails to show any abnormality in cases of acute pyelonephritis or small renal abscesses; conversely several different processes can result in nonvisualization, such as severe pyelonephritis, or pyonephrosis (102,307). Although sonography can detect hydronephrosis, calculi, and some abscesses, it is much less revealing than CT (27,102,282). In many cases of acute pyelonephritis, sonography will be normal although CT shows definite abnormalities (301). Although radionuclide scintigrams are very sensitive to renal changes resulting from infection, in adults they do not distinguish the various pathologic processes. CT is the most revealing imaging procedure for renal infections.

A variety of terms have been promulgated for acute bacterial infection of the kidney, but *acute pyelonephritis* is the preferred term (170,301,317,338). Others terms (such as *acute focal bacterial nephritis* and *lobar nephronia*) have enjoyed popular usage (301); however, neither pathology nor treatment is different than for what is classically called acute pyelonephritis. The CT features of acute pyelonephritis are: (a) renal swelling, producing enlargement of the affected kidney; (b) focal hypoattenuation; and (c) mass effect. There are round or wedge-shaped areas in the parenchyma whose attenuation is either normal, decreased (because of edema or necrosis), or occasionally increased (because of hemorrhage) (246) on precontrast images. After contrast, these areas show diminished enhancement compared to normal parenchyma on early images (Figs. 77–79) (27,102,282). The wedge-shaped areas in fact do enhance, but much less than normal parenchyma, as a result of edema or vaso-

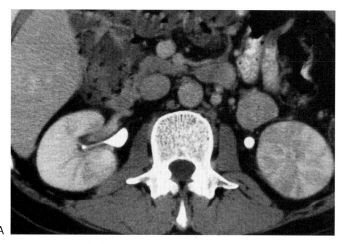 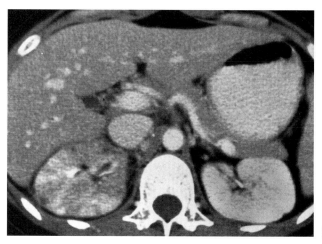

A   B

FIG. 77. Acute pyelonephritis. **A:** Contrast-enhanced CT reveals numerous low-attenuation wedges and streaks in both kidneys. **B:** Patchy low attenuation of much of the right kidney is shown on contrast-enhanced CT, in a different patient.

spasm caused by the infection. On delayed images up to 24 hours, there may be increased density in, or on the periphery of, these areas (140).

In some cases, one or more focal areas of the kidney are severely involved, with sparing of other regions (98,102,282). There may be a single masslike region as a result of swelling due to edema (this is focal pyelonephritis, formerly called acute focal bacterial nephritis to distinguish it from neoplasm) (Fig. 78) (170). Patchy decreased enhancement may be limited to this focal mass. A very frequent (77%) finding in acute infections is thickening of the renal fascia and thickening of the septa in the perinephric space, a result of hyperemia and inflammatory edema (Fig. 78) (282).

Despite treatment with adequate antibiotics, CT abnor-

malities may persist for several weeks to months (283). Persistence of a focal mass may increase the suspicion of tumor, but it must be recognized as an acceptable sequela until followed for up to 6 months (283). With the severe parenchymal infection that causes focal CT abnormalities, scar formation is not uncommon, and polar or global atrophy may be seen (Fig. 79) (283).

Emphysematous pyelonephritis is a severe, gas-forming infection of the renal substance, usually due to *Escherichia coli* or other gram-negative organisms. This process is nearly always seen in diabetics (134,218,253,312). Because of the impaired vascular supply and the diminished host immunity in such patients, *E. coli* and other gram-negative bacteria (that are facultative anaerobes) proliferate in an anaerobic environment, producing CO_2

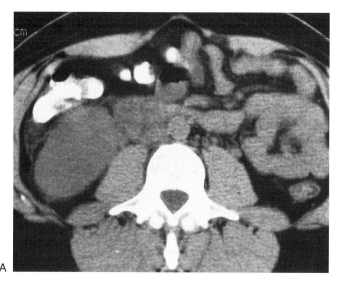 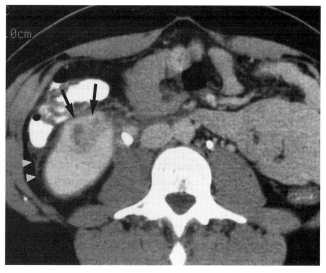

A   B

FIG. 78. Focal acute pyelonephritis. **A:** Precontrast CT image shows swelling of the right lower pole. **B:** After contrast, a focal, heterogeneous, mixed-attenuation lesion is evident *(arrows)*; note thickening of the fascia *(arrowheads)*.

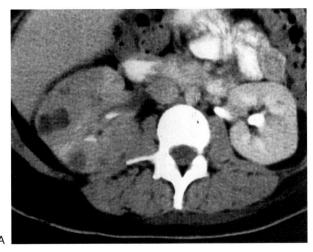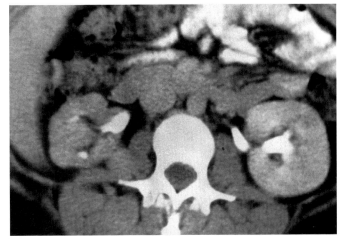

A

B

FIG. 79. Acute pyelonephritis with scarring. **A:** Note the swelling, poor excretion, and patchy low attenuation of the right kidney in this young female patient with acute *E. coli* pyelonephritis. **B:** Follow-up CT 10 months later shows irregular scarring of the right kidney.

from the necrotic tissue (197). Patients may present with signs of acute infection, but often they are found comatose from diabetic ketoacidosis. Although plain radiographs or sonography may suggest the presence of gas in the kidney, CT is most informative, showing the precise localization of the gas. In emphysematous pyelonephritis, gas is seen in the renal parenchyma itself, not merely in the collecting system (as may be the case with reflux of air from the bladder, or gas due to fistulae) (Figs. 80,81). Gas may extend to the subcapsular, perinephric, and para-renal spaces and may cross to the contralateral retroperito-neal spaces, even when the other kidney is not infected (Fig. 80). Although nephrectomy is the treatment of choice for severely involved kidneys, medical treatment

combined with percutaneous drainage has been successful in mild cases. Since CO_2 is rapidly absorbed, there should be rapid decrease in the gas if there is a good response to medical therapy, and persistent gas on follow-up CT indicates ongoing infection (197).

Pyonephrosis results from infection of a hydronephrotic kidney. This may present either as an acute or chronic infection with up to 15% of patients being afebrile (334). Thus, this entity must be distinguished from acute pyelonephritis, renal abscess, and XGP. Urography is of little use, because the kidney is usually nonfunctioning. Sonography is usually diagnostic and can guide percutaneous aspiration and nephrostomy placement. However, CT is often used in such a setting. CT will show dilation of the

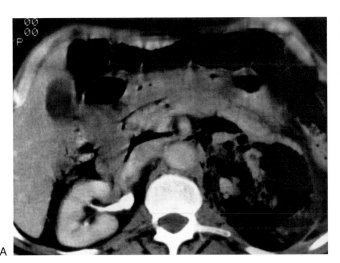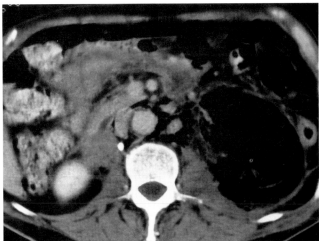

A

B

FIG. 80. Emphysematous pyelonephritis. **A:** This diabetic was found comatose; extensive gas throughout the left renal parenchyma with extension into the perinephric space and crossing over into the right anterior pararenal space is shown on this contrast-enhanced CT image. There is no involve-ment of the right kidney. **B:** More inferiorly, retroperitoneal gas is evident. Left nephrectomy was performed.

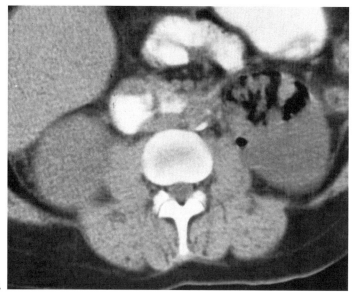

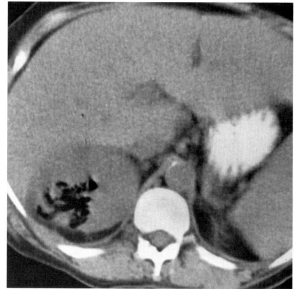

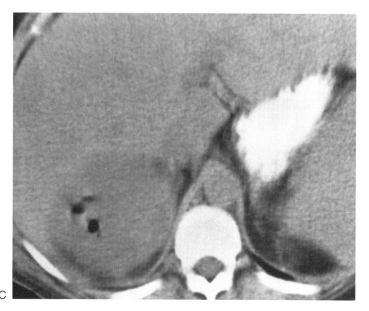

FIG. 81. Bilateral emphysematous pyelonephritis. **A:** Noncontrast CT image demonstrates gas in the left renal parenchyma. **B:** A focus of gas in the right upper pole is also evident. **C:** Left nephrectomy was performed and antibiotics given; follow-up CT 5 days later shows decrease in gas on the right.

collecting system and poor excretion. Thickening of the pelvic wall and of Gerota's fascia are common (90); increased density or heterogeneity of the pelvic contents may be seen but is rare. CT also can show the cause of the obstruction.

The role of MRI in evaluation of acute renal infection is limited to patients who either cannot undergo a contrast-enhanced CT study or have an equivocal CT exam. It is more difficult to produce good MRI images of very ill patients. Little experience exists with MRI in the diagnosis of urinary tract infections. Although changes resulting from renal infections are not specific on noncontrast or delayed contrast-enhanced SE images (low signal on T1-, high signal on T2-weighted images: variable enhancement, similar to that in neoplasms), and no advantage of MRI over CT has been reported (107) using SE sequences, dynamic contrast-enhanced MRI performed with breath-held T1-weighted GRE sequence allows detection of changes (e.g., striated nephrogram, patchy nonenhancing areas) previously possible only with contrast-enhanced CT.

Renal Abscess

Renal abscess is increasingly uncommon, largely because most acute infections are effectively treated. Most renal abscesses currently are a result of an ascending infection and are usually due to gram-negative urinary pathogens, particularly *E. coli* (36%) (27,88). Less than 10% result from hematogenous seeding, usually caused by *Staphylococcus* (27,88). Renal abscesses also may be a complication of trauma, surgery, contiguous spread from other organs, or lymphatic spread (27,165). In most cases today, a renal abscess results from breakdown and coalescence of microabscesses due to acute pyelonephritis that is inadequately treated. An abscess is a necrotic, devascularized cavity, often filled with pus. Although many present with acute infection, sometimes the diagnosis is obscure because the patient has only vague symptoms such as flank pain, weakness, and weight loss (27,88,271). Fever is absent in a third, a normal urinalysis is found in 25%, and positive urine cultures are found in only a third of patients (206). Thus, renal abscess must be distinguished both from acute pyelonephritis and from renal tumors. Computed tomography is the best procedure for this evaluation, identifying 96% of abscesses in two large series (88,282). Although sonography will identify an abnormality, it is less sensitive than CT (88,282), and the appearance may not be distinguishable from a renal neoplasm (Fig. 82).

In many cases of renal abscess (50%), the entire kidney is enlarged (282). In some, a focal mass bulges the renal contour. Inflammatory changes in the perinephric space and thickening of Gerota's fascia are common (77% and 42%, respectively) (282). A focal low-attenuation area (near water density) is seen on precontrast images; there will be no enhancement in the center of the lesion (Figs. 82,83). Commonly there is a thick, slightly irregular and ill-defined rind of enhancing tissue surrounding the abscess cavity. There may be septations in the abscess (Fig. 82). The remainder of the kidney may be normal, or it may show changes of pyelonephritis. The presence of gas in the lesion is pathognomonic of abscess, but it is unusual.

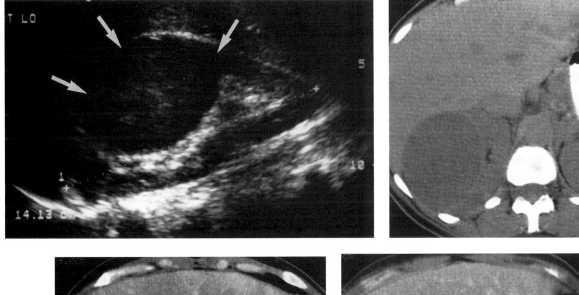

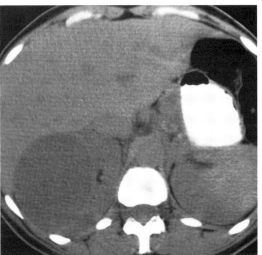

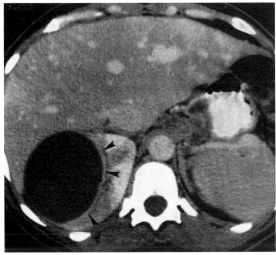

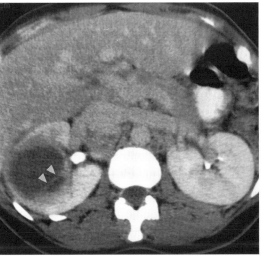

FIG. 82. Renal abscess. A: Sonogram reveals a large mass *(arrows)* with internal echoes in the right kidney in this febrile 38-year-old female patient; retroperitoneal lymphadenopathy was also present. B: On precontrast CT image, the mass is of low attenuation (10 HU). C: The mass does not enhance after intravenous contrast, but there is an enhancing rim *(arrowheads)*. D: More caudally, a septum is evident *(arrowheads)*; percutaneous aspiration yielded pus and a drain was placed. *E. coli* was cultured.

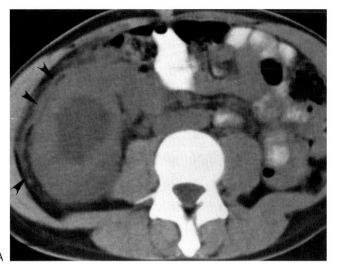
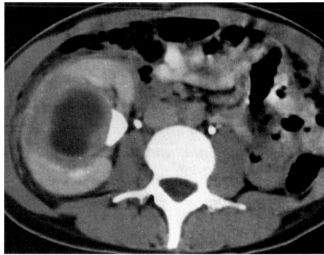

A

B

FIG. 83. Renal abscess. **A:** noncontrast CT reveals enlargement of the right kidney with a central low attenuation (14 HU) area; note the thickened renal fascia *(arrowheads)*. **B:** Contrast-enhanced CT shows a thick enhancing rim but a nonenhancing center; percutaneous aspiration yielded pus.

It is sometimes difficult to distinguish an indolent abscess from a necrotic renal tumor (57). In such a case, percutaneous needle biopsy may be required. In general, once an abscess is identified, needle aspiration should be done for definitive diagnosis, for culture, and for placement of drains, which has been shown to improve outcome (165). CT will show sequelae of renal abscesses for weeks to months, especially if treated without drainage. Focal scarring often results (283).

Chronic Renal Infections

The characteristic changes of chronic pyelonephritis seen with urography are also readily identified with CT.

A focal parenchymal scar overlying a blunted calyx indicates the diagnosis, whether single or multiple areas are involved. This is distinct from an infarct scar, wherein the calyx is not blunted.

Xanthogranulomatous pyelonephritis is an uncommon chronic infection that has a specific pathology, typically occurring in an obstructed kidney. There is accumulation of lipid-laden macrophages (xanthoma cells) and a granulomatous infiltrate because of the failure of local immunity (117). In 85%, the entire kidney is involved, but the disease may be focal. Computed tomography is very useful, because the findings on sonography and occasionally urography are nonspecific (99,117,124,226,311). On CT, XGP is associated with: (a) a large central calculus,

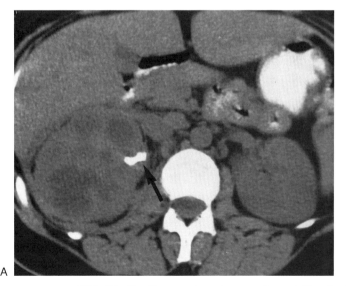
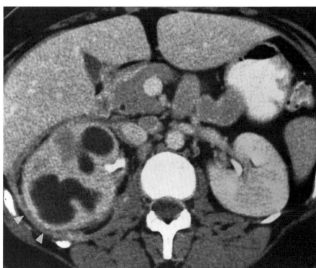

A

B

FIG. 84. Xanthogranulomatous pyelonephritis. **A:** A calculus in the renal pelvis *(arrow)* and low-attenuation areas in the parenchyma are noted on precontrast CT in this 41-year-old female patient with right flank pain and low grade fever for months. **B:** No excretion occurs from the right kidney on postcontrast image, but there is enhancement of the rims of the low-attenuation xanthoma collections; note the fascial thickening *(arrowheads)*. Nephrectomy was performed.

often a staghorn; (b) enlargement of the kidney (or of a segment); (c) poor or no excretion of contrast into the collecting system; and (d) multiple focal low-attenuation (−10 to +30 HU) masses scattered throughout the involved portions of the kidney (Fig. 84). The low-attenuation collections represent dilated, debris-filled calyces and xanthoma collections. The collections themselves do not enhance, and there is no excretion of contrast, but there is bright enhancement of the rims of the collections, because of inflammatory hypervascularity. Although XGP is usually found in the setting of chronic obstruction, often the renal pelvis is less dilated than might be expected for high grade chronic obstruction. Also, the renal sinus fat is often obliterated by inflammation (226) (Fig. 84). Perinephric extension occurs in about 14% and is well shown on CT (44,99,124,311), fistulae may develop (296), and gas may rarely be seen. Some variations occur: the kidney may be small, and calculi may be absent, making it difficult to distinguish XGP from other infections or neoplasm. Nephrectomy is indicated in any case, but partial nephrectomy can be done for the focal form.

Renal tuberculosis (TB) is uncommon, but the frequency has recently been increasing because of resistant organisms and the increase in patients with acquired immune deficiency syndrome (AIDS). A variety of renal abnormalities may result from TB, depending on the stage of the process at the time of presentation. The early calyceal changes cannot be seen using CT, but parenchymal scars, calcification (usually parenchymal, within tuberculomas), and low-attenuation parenchymal masses (granulomas) are common (58,100,234). In many cases, parenchymal changes predominate; in others obstruction resulting from infundibular, pelvic, or ureteral strictures is the predominant finding; renal calculi also occur. In later cases, CT shows a small hydronephrotic shell; the diagnosis of TB is suggested by stricturing of the pelvis or ureter (Fig. 85). Marked thickening of the wall of the ureter or pelvis may be seen on CT. Computed tomography also is excellent at demonstrating perirenal ex-

tension or fistulae to adjacent organs, such as the colon or duodenum.

Fungal infections in the kidney also are on the rise with the increasing population of immune-compromised patients, including transplant recipients, patients with malignancies, and AIDS patients (329). Fungi can cause pyelonephritis and renal abscess with the same CT appearance as bacterial infections (57,85). Fungal infection is suggested when multiple microabscesses are seen, in the kidney or in the spleen or liver (273). Slough of urothelium, inflammatory cells, and mycelia into the collecting system can form a fungus ball. Such patients often have poor renal function, and careful attention to the density of the pelvic contents is required to recognize a fungus ball on noncontrast CT. The pelvis will be dilated but filled with material of soft-tissue attenuation, rather than water attenuation.

Malacoplakia is a very uncommon chronic infection that can affect the kidney, although it is more commonly found in other organs, particularly the bladder. Renal malacoplakia is much more common in women than in men, and patients are usually debilitated or immune suppressed. It can occur in renal transplants. It results when a bacterial infection, most often E. coli, cannot be eradicated because of a local immune failure, and a chronic granulomatous inflammatory process develops. In about 75%, the process is multifocal, and it may be bilateral. Multiple soft-tissue masses of varying size may be seen on CT (136). These lesions enhance less than normal renal parenchyma after intravenous contrast, but they do enhance because of the inflammatory vascularity. Hydronephrosis and nephrolithiasis are not seen, and the masses do not calcify. There may be perinephric extension however. If unifocal, the lesion may mimic RCC; when multiple, metastases or lymphoma may be considered. Pathologic examination is often needed for diagnosis; large histiocytes (von Hanseman cells) and basophilic intracytoplasmic inclusions (Michaelis-Gutmann bodies) are pathognomonic (136).

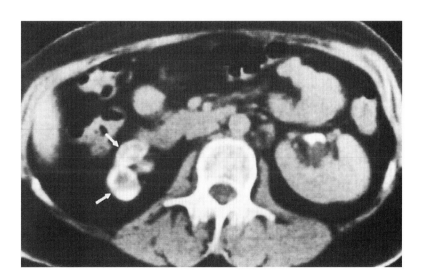

FIG. 85. End-stage renal tuberculosis. Post-contrast CT image shows a small, nonfunctioning right kidney with rim calcifications *(arrows)*. Diagnosis. autonephrectomy (putty kidney).

Hydatid disease is very uncommon in North America, but is endemic in parts of the world and may be seen in immigrants or travelers. The kidneys are involved in only about 2% to 3% (1). The disease results from infestation by the larval form of the tapeworm *Echinococcus granulosus*. Signs and symptoms are nonspecific, including flank mass, hematuria, dysuria, fever, and hypertension. The cysts may rupture into the collecting system, and renal colic may be a presenting symptom due to hydatiduria (1). The CT appearance may be characteristic, usually showing a multilocular cystic mass with mural calcification (Fig. 86). There may be enhancement of the thick walls. The presence of small, daughter cysts within

the main cyst is characteristic, and it is different from the usual appearance of a calcified RCC. However, occasionally there may be a noncalcified unilocular cyst that may be difficult to distinguish from an infected simple cyst (1).

A number of pathologic conditions affect the kidneys of patients with AIDS, and CT may be useful in demonstrating these. Kaposi sarcoma, lymphoma, or RCC may produce renal masses in AIDS patients (201) (see Fig. 59). All types of renal infections, including pyelonephritis, abscess, fungal infections, and TB, are more common in AIDS patients. Opportunistic infectious agents, such as *Pneumocystis carinii, Mycobacterium avium-intracellu-*

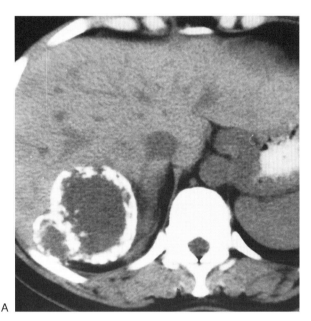

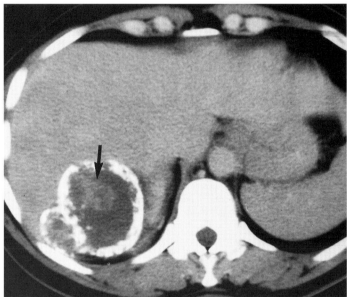

FIG. 86. Renal hydatid disease. **A:** Precontrast CT shows a multiloculated calcified mass in this patient who had traveled in South America. **B:** Postcontrast CT image shows area of enhancement within the mass *(arrow).* **C:** A more caudal image shows the mass arises from the right kidney.

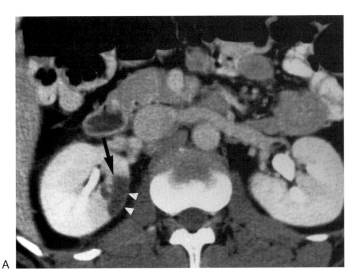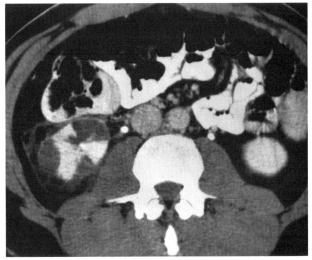

FIG. 87. Renal infarcts. **A:** Contrast-enhanced CT was done to investigate acute back pain, leukocytosis, and fever; a focal nonenhancing area is present *(arrow)*; note a thin enhancing capsular rim *(arrowheads).* **B:** Several more infarcts are present in the lower pole; angiography revealed a dissection of the right renal artery.

lare, and cytomegalovirus, can involve the kidney; all of these can produce multiple, small calcifications scattered throughout the kidneys (201). Human immunodeficiency virus (HIV)-associated nephropathy is most often seen in HIV patients who are young, black men with a history of intravenous drug abuse. On CT, the kidneys are normal to large in size; there may be a striated nephrogram after intravenous contrast (201).

Renal replacement lipomatosis is a quite unusual process that produces a striking CT appearance (127,212). It is associated with chronic infection and calculi, commonly central, often obstructing (105,292,305). The kidney may be large or small but is usually nonfunctioning. Most of the renal parenchyma has been replaced by fat,

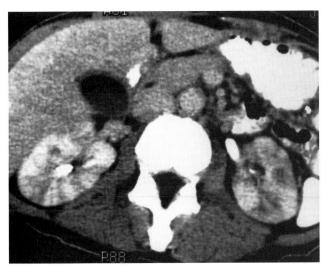

FIG. 88. Polyarteritis. Contrast-enhanced CT demonstrates diffuse, patchy, low-attenuation areas; angiogram revealed typical changes of polyarteritis nodosum.

in many cases leaving only a ghost of a kidney containing calculi. Pararenal fascia are thickened, and there may be fistulae. A fatty mass causing displacement of adjacent structures, suggestive of liposarcoma, can also be seen (212).

RENAL VASCULAR DISEASES

Although sonography and radionuclide techniques are often considered the primary procedures, and although arteriography remains the gold standard, CT and to a lesser degree MRI can be either suggestive or diagnostic of a variety of vascular disorders of the kidney. Infarction of the kidney, often due to embolic phenomena, may present with nonspecific acute symptoms. Contrast-enhanced CT can distinguish renal infarction from other acute abdominal disorders (331). The renal parenchyma will show total lack of enhancement, despite normal size and shape. There may be a thin peripheral rim of enhancement as a result of capsular vessels (96), and there may be central medullary enhancement, probably from ureteral or other collaterals (188). A segmental infarct will show a sharply demarcated nonenhancing area (Fig. 87). Follow-up studies show atrophy of the infarcted area. However, persistent wedge-shaped cortical defects have been described in a number of conditions other than ischemia, including renal contusion, infection, and collagen vascular disease (96). MRI also may show distinctive changes. Corticomedulary differentiation is lost in an infarcted region. The infarcted area may be lower signal than normal on T1- and T2-weighted images, or it may be higher signal because of hemorrhage. There is no change in signal after Gd-DTPA administration (156). Although usually not diagnostic, CT can show striking

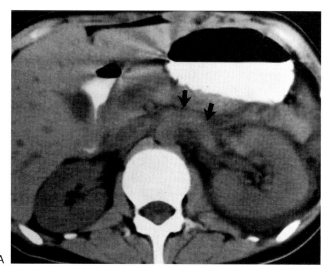
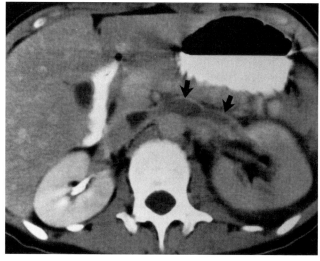

FIG. 89. Renal vein thrombosis. **A:** Precontrast CT in this patient with nephrotic syndrome shows high density in the left renal vein *(arrows)*. **B:** After contrast administration, a filling defect is evident in the left renal vein *(arrows)*. Note the left kidney is swollen and excreting poorly.

findings in cases of vasculitis, with either multiple small infarcts, or multiple patchy or wedge-shaped areas of altered perfusion in a pattern similar to acute pyelonephritis (231) (Fig. 88).

In addition to tumor thrombus, thrombosis of the renal vein may occur as a result of trauma or hypercoagulable states, and it is quite common (up to 33%) in patients with nephrotic syndrome (303,318). Computed tomography can be diagnostic, but it requires careful technique with precontrast localization of the renal veins, rapid bolus of an adequate amount of iodinated contrast, and imaging during maximum vascular enhancement phase. With this technique, CT has been reported to have 92%

sensitivity and 100% specificity (318). Thrombus is seen as a low-attenuation filling defect in the renal vein, which may have increased or decreased caliber (Figs. 89,90) (97,318). There may also be engorged perirenal collaterals if the process is chronic (326). The kidney may be enlarged with prolonged visualization of the corticomedullary junction on contrast-enhanced CT images (97). Magnetic resonance imaging is also quite accurate in detecting renal vein thrombus and avoids the use of iodinated contrast. The combination of SE and gradient echo sequences resulted in only one false negative and one false positive in a series of 41 patients (303).

Computed tomography can detect renal artery aneu-

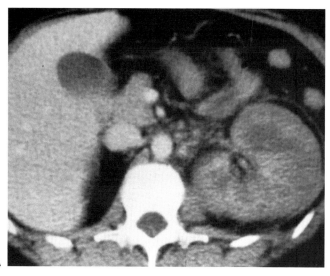
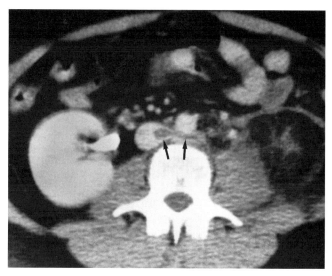

FIG. 90. Renal vein thrombosis. **A:** Contrast-enhanced CT image shows a swollen, poorly excreting left kidney; note lack of a normal renal vein in the expected location. **B:** More caudal image shows thrombus in a retroaortic left renal vein *(arrows)* just extending into the inferior vena cava. (Courtesy of Howard Holley, M.D.)

rysms, arteriovenous malformations (AVMs) (Fig. 91), and arteriovenous fistulas (AVFs) unless they are very small. These may be clinically unsuspected, or present with a bruit, hematuria, or subjective symptoms, and they can be distinguished from nonvascular masses because they enhance as much as other vascular structures, such as the aorta and IVC. Imaging early during the maximum vascular enhancement phase is crucial, as on noncontrast or delayed images the lesion may be nearly isodense with renal parenchyma and can simulate a mass. Renal artery aneurysms are usually round with peripheral calcification and lie in the renal sinus, adjacent to the main or proximal branches of the renal artery. AVMs and AVFs are variable in size and location and also may be calcified. When there is a large shunt, dilatation of the renal vein and collaterals is a suggestive sign. MRI also can demonstrate these lesions with recognition of their vascular nature because of either signal void on SE, or bright signal on GRE images (Fig. 91).

Although renal artery stenosis accounts for perhaps 1% of all hypertension, it is an important process to recognize, because it can be cured by percutaneous angioplasty or surgery. Although other methods are currently used for screening, considerable investigation of CT and MRI has been stimulated by the search for a noninvasive tool that could replace arteriography, which still remains the gold standard. Computed tomography can show calcified plaques of the renal artery and its origin; however, although this is correlated with stenosis, the predictive value of this finding alone is poor (275). With the advent of helical CT technology, rapid acquisition of data from a volume of tissue during suspended respiration can be done, so that true contiguous images can be reconstructed. When done with 30 to 40 contiguous 1-sec tube rotations and continuous table incrementation following a 30-sec bolus of a high volume of contrast, 3-D reconstructions can be done to produce a CT angiogram (70,257). High-quality images have been produced with such techniques, with reliable visualization of both main and accessory renal vessels (70,257). With a maximum intensity projection (MIP) method, a sensitivity of 92%, and specificity of 83% has been reported (257). However, the method does require the use of a large amount of iodinated contrast and a relatively long breath hold. The time of peak enhancement varies, especially in those with cardiovascular disease, and may need to be determined in each patient (257). Because of tube heat limits, CT angiography of obese patients may be limited. The technique also has a tendency to overestimate the degree of stenosis (257).

Magnetic resonance imaging also may be used to produce reconstructed angiogram-like images, usually with gradient echo techniques in which flowing blood is high signal, and with maximum intensity projection and 3-D reconstruction (Fig. 92). A variety of methods have been investigated, including 2-D and 3-D time-of-flight and phase contrast. Some have used suspended respiration and/or cardiac gating, and some have not. Although several studies have demonstrated that the main renal artery can be reliably seen, detection of accessory vessels is poor (40%) (67). Vessels less than 2 mm in diameter are hard to image (183). Only the proximal 3.5 cm of the main renal artery is reliably well seen, with unreliable visualization of intrarenal branches. However, results have been promising, with 80% to 100% sensitivity and 76% to 91% specificity reported (66,183). One comparative study suggests coronal 2-D phase contrast methods are best, but this technique continues to evolve. Magnetic resonance angiography (MRA) also has a tendency to overestimate degree of stenosis (183). Phase contrast MRI techniques also offer the ability to quantitate the renal artery blood flow. Good correlation with blood flow measurement by p-aminohippurate has been shown both in flow phantoms and in vivo (68,330). This may aid in assessing the significance of stenoses, and it may be useful in renal transplant evaluation (209). Renal MRA is limited by relatively long imaging times, by artifacts related to respiratory and other motion, and by spatial resolution and signal-to-noise ratios that result from attempting to image the small renal vascular structures with the large standard body coil. Nevertheless, improvements in MRI technology, including stronger and faster gradients, phased array body coils, and faster imaging sequences, are likely to increase the utility of MRA.

RENAL FAILURE

Computed tomography and MRI play a limited but sometimes very useful role in evaluation of renal failure. Sonography and radionuclide studies are usually sufficient to distinguish obstructive from other causes of renal failure (316). However, CT can determine the presence, size, shape, location, number, and appearance (including hydronephrosis and calcification) of kidneys in all azotemic patients even without i.v. contrast medium, and CT can be used in those in whom sonography is inadequate (Fig. 93) (86). Not only the presence of hydronephrosis, but also the thickness of cortex (which may help in determining salvageability of the kidney) can be well shown with CT. Often CT can demonstrate the etiology of the obstruction, even without contrast (Fig. 94) (23,155). If contrast can be tolerated, even a reduced amount can help in this assessment, but delayed views are often needed (Fig. 94) to prove or rule out obstruction. Pitfalls on CT include parapelvic cysts on noncontrast scans, and extrarenal pelves or dilated calyces due to pyelonephritis or postobstructive atrophy. Computed tomography is more sensitive than urography to subtle changes in excretion caused by obstruction, but it is not as quantitative as is diuresis scintigraphy. Asymmetric excretion with delayed calyceal filling and persistent nephrogram is an indication of acute obstruction. However, such changes also can

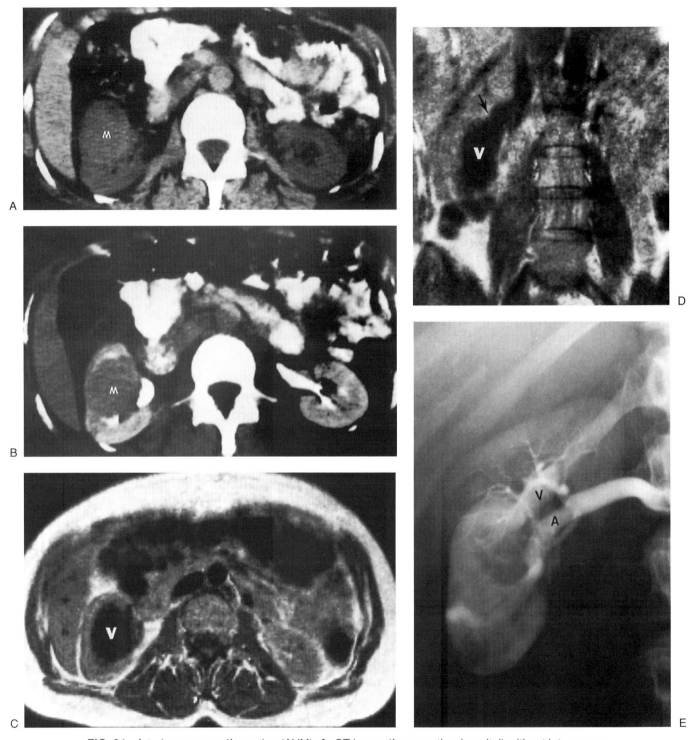

FIG. 91. Arteriovenous malformation (AVM). **A:** CT image (from another hospital) without intravenous contrast material shows a mass (M) with higher attenuation than the normal renal parenchyma in the right kidney. **B:** A delayed, nondynamic, postcontrast CT image shows that the mass (M) is now lower in attenuation than the renal parenchyma. **C:** Transaxial SE image (1500/35) shows a large signal void (V) area in the right renal hilum compatible with a vascular malformation. **D:** Coronal proton-density-weighted SE image (1500/35) demonstrates a large vein *(arrow)* draining from the malformation (V) into the IVC. **E:** Angiogram demonstrates that there is a large AVM. The draining vein (V) and feeding artery (A) are well seen.

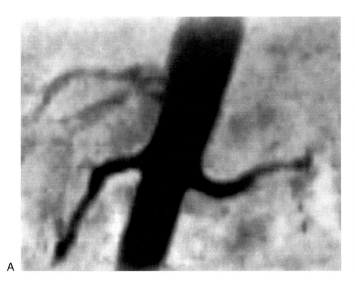

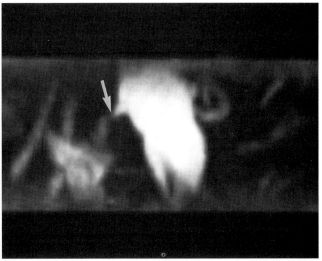

A

B

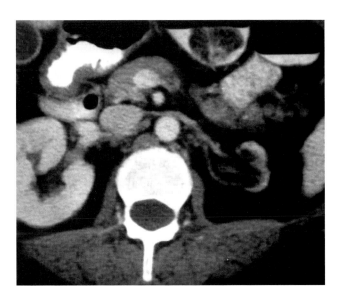

C

FIG. 92. Magnetic resonance angiography. **A:** MIP reconstruction of a normal volunteer (3-D time of flight 33/8/20°) shows normal main renal arteries; note intrarenal vessels are not shown. **B:** Right renal artery stenosis *(arrow)* and left renal artery occlusion are demonstrated on this magnetic resonance angiogram (cardiac gaged 3-D time of flight with selective inversion recovery 13/6/20°/TI 300). **C:** Digital subtraction contrast angiogram confirms the MRA findings.

FIG. 93. Atrophic kidney. note hypertrophy of the right and marked atrophy of the left kidney, but absence of hydronephrosis.

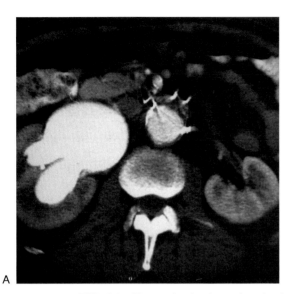
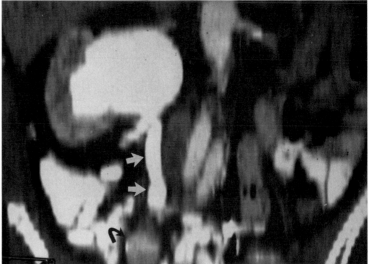

A   B

FIG. 94. Obstructive hydronephrosis. **A:** Delayed images after contrast show marked right hydrone-phrosis (note aneurysm repair). **B:** The dilated opacified ureter can be easily followed on coronal reconstruction. The ureter *(arrows)* is obstructed by an iliac artery aneurysm *(curved arrow).*

result from vascular disease, acute tubular necrosis (ATN), infection, trauma, acute glomerulonephritis, and others (189). Prolonged or diffusely dense CT nephrograms may occur in patients with glomerular nephritis, acute tubular necrosis, leukemia, urate nephropathy, myoglobulinuria, obstruction, and contrast-induced nephrotoxicity (7,98,139).

In addition to hydronephrosis, CT can demonstrate typical patterns in other renal diseases that may lead to renal failure. Chronic pyelonephritis results in an irregular renal contour with focal cortical scarring and calyceal blunting, whereas renal ischemia leads to small, smooth kidneys. Acquired cystic disease, ADPCKD, and renal TB have been discussed. Chronic glomerulonephritis leads to small kidneys with poor excretion; cortical calcification is rarely seen. Acute renal disorders typically show enlarged, poorly excreting kidneys (Fig. 95). Calcification may be focal, diffuse, medullary, or cortical in cases of oxalosis and acute cortical necrosis. Medullary nephrocalcinosis can be recognized as multiple, small, medullary calcifications, but it requires precontrast images and may be difficult to distinguish from nephrolithiasis (Fig. 96) (241,293). Multiple, tiny, focal calcifications scattered through the parenchyma can result from *Pneumocystis carinii, Mycobacterium avium-intracellulare* or cytomegalovirus infection in AIDS patients (201). On CT, HIV-associated nephropathy typically shows nephromegaly and poor excretion in a setting of severe renal failure and nephrotic syndrome (201). In patients with no history of preexisting renal failure, CT demonstration of persistent increased density in the renal parenchyma 24 to 48 hours or more after intravenous contrast is suggestive of contrast-associated nephrotoxicity (Fig. 97) (185). Vicarious excretion into the gallbladder may also be seen. Al-

though an attenuation value of over 140 HU is strongly indicative of acute nephrotoxicity, values of 55 to 110 HU have been suggested as an indication to avoid further insult, by avoiding additional intravenous contrast or other nephrotoxic drugs (185).

Magnetic resonance imaging can demonstrate many abnormalities related to renal function. It can readily demonstrate dilated ureters and aid in diagnosis of obstructive uropathy, which may be very useful when using MRI to stage gynecologic, prostatic, and bladder malignancies. Calculi are not well shown on MRI, because they produce no signal; however, when they are large enough, a low

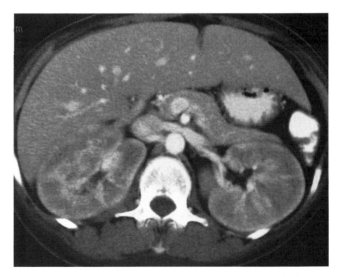

FIG. 95. Lupus nephritis. This patient with systemic lupus erythematosus had recently begun dialysis for acute renal failure; on contrast-enhanced CT, both kidneys are swollen with poorly enhancing pyramids.

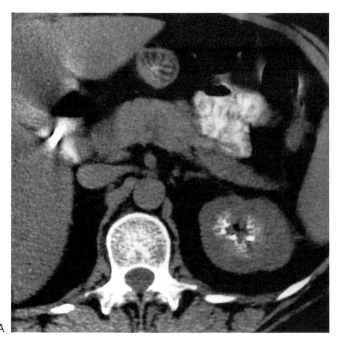
A

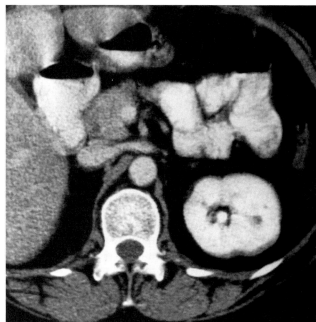
B

FIG. 96. Nephrocalcinosis. A: Precontrast CT image shows calcification limited to the medullary pyramids. B: Contrast-enhanced CT shows no abnormalities.

signal filling defect may be seen. The normal corticomedullary distinction (CMD) seen on T1-weighted images is lost in a variety of acute and chronic renal diseases. In one study, this correlated with serum creatinine over 3.0 mg/dl; loss of CMD after Gd-DTPA correlated with serum creatinine over 10.0 mg/dl (270). These changes are not specific for any particular disease, however. Obstruc-

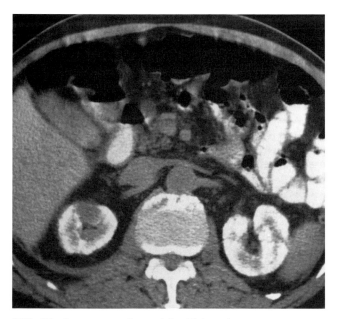

FIG. 97. Contrast nephrotoxicity. This patient's serum creatinine increased from 3.0 to 8.0 mg/dl in the 8 days following coronary angiogram; note the persistent dense nephrograms and gallbladder opacification (arrow).

tion also causes an alteration in the normal excretion pattern of Gd-DTPA (267).

One MRI method that has some potential for evaluation of obstructive uropathy is RARE (rapid acquisition with relaxation enhancement) urography (123). In this modification of an old method, heavily T2-weighted images in the coronal plane, with fat suppression result in dramatic images of dilated urinary systems. This can document the dilatation, show a point of obstruction, and perhaps show an obstructing lesion, such as intraluminal neoplasm (254). Nonobstructive dilatations and obstruction from an extrinsic mass can be suggested by the appearance of the ureter. However, it is as yet unclear what the role of such methods will be. Cost effectiveness is an undefined issue. The inability to clearly detect calcifications, the limited spatial resolution, and the difficulty in detecting low-grade, partial obstruction may limit the usefulness (115).

RENAL TRANSPLANTS

Most renal transplant complications are adequately evaluated using a combination of radionuclide procedures and sonography (especially with color and power Doppler). Distinction between acute rejection, ATN, and obstruction and detection of fluid collections is usually accomplished expeditiously (287). Computed tomography can be used as an adjunctive tool, especially in patients with infected or open surgical wounds or with suspicion of intra-abdominal abscess (52,89,158). Fluid collections can be readily detected by CT, which may aid in distinction of hematoma, abscess, lympho-

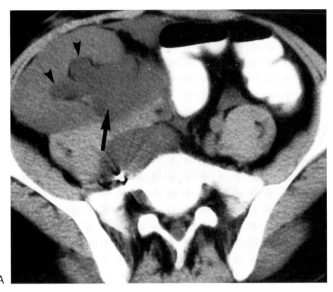
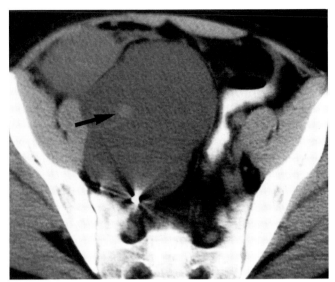

FIG. 98. Lymphocele following renal transplant. **A:** Recent decline in function of the renal transplant noted in this patient; noncontrast CT image shows dilated collecting system *(arrowheads)* and a fluid collection medial to the pelvis *(arrow)*. **B:** The large fluid collection is well shown with the external iliac vessels *(arrow)* coursing through it.

cele, or urinoma (Fig. 98) (215). Tumors can arise in transplants, and CT or MRI can be useful for detection and staging; MRI may be preferred to avoid iodinated contrast.

Considerable initial enthusiasm was expressed for the potential use of MRI in evaluating transplant complications (13,106,132,304). There is loss of CMD in cases of acute rejection, probably as a result of edema. There also may be loss of CMD in chronic rejection, resulting from interstitial fibrosis (144). However, although loss of CMD was found in one study in 73% of cases of rejection, it was also found in 71% with ATN (182). It also may result from cyclosporine toxicity, infection, and obstruction (182,328). Thus, MRI findings are too insensitive and nonspecific to justify the cost (182,328). MRI is, however, very capable of demonstrating fluid collections and hydronephrosis. New techniques with gadolinium enhancement (108,121), quantitative flow evaluation (209), and even spectroscopy (103) offer promise. If MRI can allow evaluation of both morphologic changes and function, it may find a role, but much further investigation is needed.

RENAL TRAUMA

Renal injuries occur in about 10% of trauma victims. Most result from blunt injuries, particularly motor vehicle accidents, but penetrating injuries are increasing. The majority (75% to 85%) are minor and do not require treatment, but some are life threatening. Computed tomography can play a very important role in detecting and categorizing renal injuries (78,80,213,245). It has been shown to be more accurate than other imaging methods

for classification of renal injuries (32,230). Computed tomography also offers the great advantages of noninvasiveness, ease of performance, and ability to evaluate all organ systems. Thus, CT is a primary method for evaluation of severely traumatized patients with suspected multisystem injury, and it should be used when significant renal injuries are suspected, either because of gross hematuria (especially with hematuria after penetrating injury) or findings on other studies. Other procedures, primarily intravenous urography, may be used in stable patients when severe injury is unlikely, such as a patient with microscopic hematuria and no alteration of vital signs (213). Computed tomography also should be avoided if the patient is very unstable, unless a CT suite is located in close proximity to the emergency department.

When evaluating for renal trauma, CT should be done with both oral and intravenous contrast; precontrast images usually are unnecessary; delayed images may be needed if there is a fluid collection to detect extravasation. The whole range of renal injuries can be demonstrated with CT with accurate determination of the size and location of hematomas (79). Renal contusion is shown as a focal area of diminished enhancement; an intrarenal hematoma is similar but shows no enhancement. A focal infarct is also nonenhancing but has sharp margins and a wedge shape. A superficial parenchymal laceration is seen as an ill-defined defect in the cortex; a deep laceration extends into the collecting system and commonly will be associated with extravasation into the perinephric space. Lacerations often are associated with hematomas (see Fig. 10). Subcapsular hematomas are fluid collections (often hyperdense when acute) delimited by the renal capsule;

when large, they are lenticular and compress the kidney. Perinephric hematoma fills the entire perinephric space and does not compress the kidney, although it may displace it (Fig. 99). A renal fracture should be diagnosed when a single plane of disruption divides the kidney into two major fragments; extravasation is often seen. A shattered kidney is divided into multiple fragments; the capsule may be intact or ruptured also, and massive hemorrhage is frequent. Renal artery occlusion usually is a result of intimal disruption and acute thrombosis, and such a kidney shows no enhancement (although a cortical rim may be seen) (186,286). There usually is no significant hematoma. With true renal artery avulsion, severe retroperitoneal bleeding occurs as well as renal nonfunction. Such patients have very high mortality, and rarely reach the CT suite. Ureteropelvic junction avulsion is indicated by extravasation in the region of the renal sinus with intact parenchyma (154). Computed tomography also can be very useful in follow-up of trauma patients, for assessment of continued extravasation or bleeding in patients treated conservatively, or for detection of abscess or rebleeding in those treated surgically. Magnetic resonance imaging, however, is rarely used in a trauma setting.

PERINEPHRIC PROCESSES

Many of the disease processes that involve the perirenal areas begin as primary renal processes, but some begin in other adjacent organs. CT often can reveal the origin and nature of these processes and fully define their extent. The anatomy of the retroperitoneum has been previously described. Processes that frequently affect the extraperitoneal pararenal spaces are hemorrhage, urine or lymph extravasation, pancreatic effusions, and either primary or metastatic tumors.

Hemorrhage

Hemorrhage into the perirenal or posterior pararenal spaces may be extensive without showing any significant change on plain abdominal radiographs or urography; sonography is also less capable of demonstrating retroperitoneal hemorrhage than CT (16,92,259). Even when done without intravenous contrast, CT is the best procedure for evaluation of suspected retroperitoneal hemorrhage. Acute hemorrhage typically measures 60 to 80 HU whereas chronic hematomas measure 10 to 40 HU. Hematomas have a variable appearance on MRI depending on age. Whereas a hematoma may be confined to the subcapsular, perinephric, or pararenal space, large hemorrhages commonly occupy several spaces. Hemorrhages may be seen on CT as either discrete fluid collections, or thick strands of material tracking along the bridging septa or fascial planes, which may serve as the barriers to the spread of the hematoma (Fig. 99).

Trauma, either blunt or penetrating, is the most common cause of hemorrhage in the retroperitoneum. This may be isolated or associated with renal injury. Iatrogenic injuries, including renal biopsy, nephrostomy placement, and extracorporeal shock wave lithotripsy (ESWL), as well as angiographic procedures (including bleeding extending proximally from a femoral puncture) are important causes (251). Subcapsular hematomas are less commonly seen with penetrating trauma than with blunt;

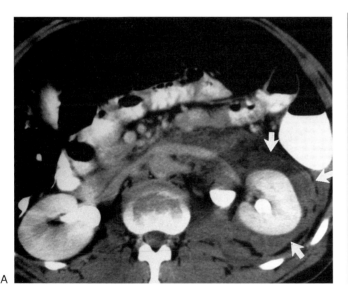
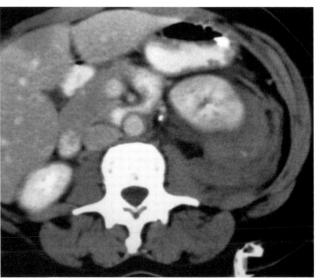

A   B

FIG. 99. Perinephric hemorrhage. **A:** In this patient with von Willebrand disease and evidence of a recent hemorrhage, contrast-enhanced CT shows extensive hematoma filling the perinephric space *(arrows).* **B:** This patient was stabbed in the back (note drain in wound; perinephric hematoma displaces the kidney anteriorly but there is no parenchymal laceration.

they can result from ESWL. Spontaneous renal or perirenal hemorrhage (with no antecedent trauma) and hemorrhage in patients on anticoagulants merit evaluation because the incidence of underlying pathology is very high, including RCC (60%) and AML (17%) (16). Computed tomography is the best procedure to demonstrate the hematoma and identify the etiology (16). In cases of spontaneous hemorrhage in which initial CT is negative, arteriography may be done. However, in a stable patient, repeat CT after the hematoma resolves is often diagnostic of a tumor originally obscured by the hematoma (see Fig. 68).

Other causes of perirenal hemorrhage include arteritis, interstitial nephritis, excessive anticoagulation, bleeding diathesis, polycystic disease, and bleeding aneurysms. Although most abdominal aortic aneurysms rupture into the perirenal spaces or psoas compartment, blood may dissect into the anterior pararenal space or within the layers of the anterior pararenal fascia (262).

Urinoma

Urine extravasation into the perirenal spaces can occur spontaneously but is usually secondary to urinary tract obstruction or trauma, including iatrogenic injury from percutaneous or ureteroscopic manipulation and ESWL (203). Computed tomography is superior to urography or sonography for detecting urine extravasation and defining the extent and etiology (74,203). However, in an acute setting, urography may be the initial study. With acute urinary extravasation, the contrast-enhanced urine can be seen to extravasate, although delayed views may be needed. With time, the kidney may become nonfunctional and contrast extravasation is not seen. A chronic urinoma can result from extravasation

in the face of chronic obstruction. Urinomas are usually of low attenuation value (−10 to +20 HU). They have low intensity on T1- and high on T2-weighted MR images. Chronic urinomas typically have well-defined walls, which are occasionally calcified, mimicking a chronic hematoma, seroma, abscess, retroperitoneal cyst, or lymphocele.

Abscess

A number of conditions predispose to perinephric inflammatory disease, but most are extensions of preexisting renal inflammatory disease (206,271). Although usually confined within Gerota's fascia, aggressive infections may break down existing barriers and involve contiguous spaces and organs. Patients with diabetes mellitus, calculi, renal obstruction, congenital anomalies, and polycystic disease are prone to perinephric abscess, usually with a concomitant renal abscess. E. coli and Proteus are the commonest organisms, with Staphylococcus seen in a few (271). Other local inflammatory conditions such as diverticulitis, Crohn disease, or appendicitis may spread to the perinephric space (Fig. 100). Hematogenous spread to the perinephric space from a remote site of infection rarely occurs. Pancreatic abscesses or pseudocysts may extend into the perinephric space, and they commonly will produce thickening of the posterior pararenal fascia (Fig. 101) (240,276). Computed tomography is the best procedure for demonstrating perinephric abscess (271).

Although MRI is capable of displaying these lesions, it has disadvantages: its long imaging time in very ill patients and the insensitivity to calcification and gas. The CT and MRI appearance of perinephric abscesses is similar to that of renal or other abscess, with localization of

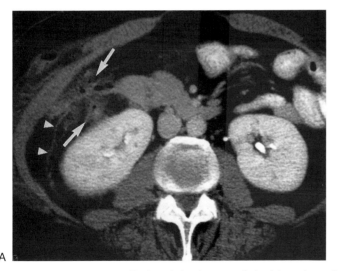
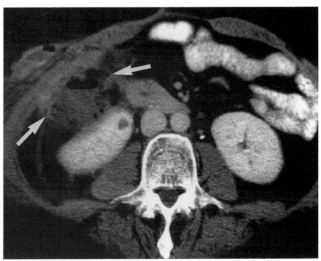

A   B

FIG. 100. Perinephric abscess. **A:** In this patient with Crohn disease, there is thickening of the anterior renal fascia *(arrowheads)* with gas bubbles in perinephric and anterior pararenal spaces *(arrows).* **B:** More caudally, an abscess *(arrows)* is shown in the perinephric space with extension into the abdominal wall.

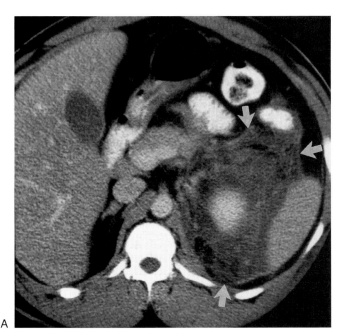
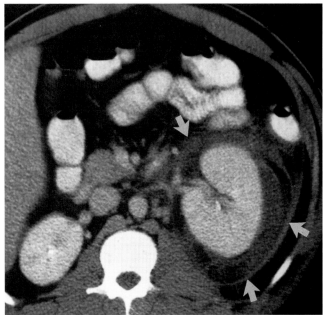

FIG. 101. Pancreatitis. **A:** Severe phlegmonous pancreatitis extends from the tail of the pancreas to surround the left upper pole *(arrows)*. **B:** The fluid collection extends more inferiorly in the perinephric space *(arrows)*.

a discrete fluid collection within the perirenal space itself. The lesion often insinuates itself throughout the perinephric space and can extend inferiorly as far as the femoral region and superiorly into the chest. Thick enhancing walls and gas bubbles or gas–fluid levels may be seen. Thickening of Gerota's fascia and perinephric stranding is common (Fig. 100) (271). It may be difficult in some cases to exclude necrotic neoplasm, but percutaneous aspiration should be diagnostic. Either percutaneous or surgical drainage is needed. Rapid diagnosis using CT, and early drainage have resulted in low mortality and high cure rates (165,271).

Neoplasms

A variety of uncommon tumors can arise in or invade the perinephric spaces. These can be clearly demonstrated with CT and MRI, but they may present diagnostic difficulties as they may resemble aggressive adrenal or renal carcinomas, renal sarcoma, lymphoma, or metastases (272). Liposarcoma is the most common capsular or perinephric mesenchymal neoplasm (72). Malignant fibrous histiocytoma also may arise in the perirenal region (Fig. 102) (101).

Typical CT and MRI features of juxtarenal mesenchymal sarcomas include: (a) inward displacement of renal parenchyma, with smooth interfaces; (b) enlarged capsular collateral vessels; (c) little or no contrast enhancement (except in very poorly differentiated tumors); and (d) very large tumors that displace rather than invade local struc-

tures. As these tumors tend to be very large, the interfaces often are better shown on coronal or sagittal MRI images than transaxial CT. The CT and MRI characteristics of many such tumors are similar to those of malignant tumors elsewhere. Liposarcomas usually contain at least some recognizable fat, usually mixed with some ill-defined soft-tissue component (72). Some may, however,

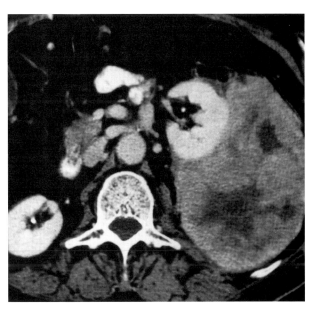

FIG. 102. Malignant fibrous histiocytoma. Contrast-enhanced CT was done to evaluate a palpable mass; note the left kidney is displaced forward by a large heterogeneous mass, but the renal surface is intact; an MFH was resected.

be nearly all mature fat. T1-weighted fat-suppressed MRI images, before and after gadolinium, can be very helpful, because demonstration of enhancing, non-fatty components is indicative of liposarcoma, not lipoma. MRI may be more sensitive for this than CT, but no comparative study has been published. Both CT and MRI can usually suggest the primary extrarenal source of the mass (Fig. 102).

REFERENCES

1. Afsar H, Yagci F, Meto S, Aybasti N. Hydatid disease of the kidney: evaluation and features of diagnostic procedures. *J Urol* 1994;151:567–570.
2. Almen T, Bergquist D, Frennby B, et al. Use of urographic contrast media to determine glomerular filtration rate (GFR). *Invest Radiol* 1991;26:S72–74.
3. Amendola MA, Bree RL, Pollack H, et al. Small renal cell carcinomas: resolving a diagnostic dilemma. *Radiology* 1988;166:637–641.
4. Aronson S, Frazier HA, Galuch JD, Hartman DS, Christenson PJ. Cystic renal masses: usefulness of the Bosniak classification. *Urol Radiol* 1991;13:83–90.
5. Aso Y, Homma Y. A survey on incidental renal cell carcinoma in Japan. *J Urol* 1992;147:340–343.
6. Ayers R, Curry NS, Gordon L, Bradford BF. Renal metastases from osteogenic sarcoma. *Urol Radiol* 1985;7:39–41.
7. Badiola-Varela CM. Acute renal cortical necrosis: contrast-enhanced CT and pathologic correlation. *Urol Radiol* 1992;14:159–160.
8. Balfe DM, McClennan BL, AufderHeide J. Multimodal imaging in evaluation of two cases of adenocarcinoma of the renal pelvis. *Urol Radiol* 1981;3:19–23.
9. Balfe DM, McClennan BL, Stanley RJ, Weyman PJ, Sagel SS. Evaluation of renal masses considered indeterminate on computed tomography. *Radiology* 1982;142:421–428.
10. Ball DS, Friedman AC, Hartman DS, Radecki PD, Caroline DF. Scar sign of renal oncocytoma: magnetic resonance imaging appearance and lack of specificity. *Urol Radiol* 1986;8:46–48.
11. Banner MP, Pollack HM, Chatten J, Witzleben C. Multilocular renal cysts; radiologic-pathologic correlation *AJR* 1981;136:239–247.
12. Baron RL, McClennan BL, Lee JKT, Lawson TL. Computed tomography of transitional-cell carcinoma of the renal pelvis and ureter. *Radiology* 1982;144:125–130.
13. Baumgartner BR, Nelson RC, Ball TI, et al. MR imaging of renal transplants. *AJR* 1986;147:949–953.
14. Baumgartner BR, Nelson RC, Torres WE, Malko JA, Peterson JE, Bernardino ME. Renal corticomedullary junction. Performance of T$_1$-weighted MR pulse sequences. *Invest Radiol* 1989;24:884–887.
15. Bellin MF, Richard F, Gobin P, et al. CT renal planimetry: effectiveness in the evaluation of individual renal function. *Urol Radiol* 1992;14:168–171.
16. Belville JS, Morgentaler A, Loughlin KR, Tumeh SS. Spontaneous perinephric and subcapsular renal hemorrhage: evaluation with CT, US, and angiography. *Radiology* 1989;172:733–738.
17. Bernardino ME, deSantos LA, Johnson DE, Bracken RB. Computed tomography in the evaluation of post-nephrectomy patients. *Radiology* 1979;130:183–187.
18. Birnbaum BA, Bosniak MA, Megibow AJ, Lubat E, Gordon RB. Observations on the growth of renal neoplasms. *Radiology* 1990;176:695–701.
19. Birnbaum BA, Bosniak MA, Krinsky GA, Cheng D, Waisman J, Ambrosino MM. Renal cell carcinoma: correlation of CT findings with nuclear morphologic grading in 100 tumors. *Abdom Imaging* 1994;19:262–266.
20. Blomley MJK, Coulden R, Bufkin C, Lipton MJ, Dawson P. Contrast bolus dynamic CT for the measurement of solid organ perfusion. *Invest Radiol* 1993;28(suppl 5):S72–97.

21. Blute ML, Malek RS, Segura JW. Angiomyolipoma: clinical metamorphosis and concepts for management. *J Urol* 1988;139:20–24.
22. Bosniak MA. Angiomyolipoma (harmatoma) of the kidney; a preoperative diagnosis is possible in virtually every case. *Urol Radiol* 1981;3:135–142.
23. Bosniak MA, Megibow AJ, Ambos MA, Mitnick JS, Lefleur RS, Gordon R. Computed tomography and ureteral obstruction. *AJR* 1982;138:1107–1114.
24. Bosniak MA. The current radiological approach to renal cysts. *Radiology* 1986;158:1–10.
25. Bosniak MA, Megibow AJ, Hulnick DH, Horii S, Raghavendra BN. CT diagnosis of renal angiomyolipoma: the importance of detecting small amounts of fat. *AJR* 1988;151:497–501.
26. Bosniak MA. The small (≤3.0 cm) renal parenchymal tumor: detection, diagnosis, and controversies. *Radiology* 1991;179:307–317.
27. Bova JG, Potter JL, Arevalos E, Hopens T, Goldstein HM, Radwin HM. Renal and perirenal infection: the role of computerized tomography. *Urology* 1985;133:375–378.
28. Breatnach ES, Stanley RJ, Lloyd K. Focal obstructive nephrogram: an unusual CT appearance of a transitional cell carcinoma. *J Comput Assist Tomogr* 1984;8:1019–1022.
29. Bree RL, Schultz SR, Hayes R. Large infiltrating renal transitional cell carcinomas: CT and ultrasound features. *J Comput Assist Tomogr* 1990;14:381–385.
30. Brennan RE, Curtis JA, Pollack HM, Weinberg I. Sequential changes in the CT numbers of the normal canine kidney following intravenous contrast administration. I. The renal cortex. *Invest Radiol* 1979;14:141–148.
31. Bret PM, Bretagnolle M, Gaillard D, et al. Small, asymptomatic angiomyolipomas of the kidney. *Radiology* 1985;154:7–10.
32. Bretan PN, McAninch JW, Federle MP, Jeffrey RB. Computerized tomographic staging of renal trauma: 85 consecutive cases. *J Urol* 1986;136:561–565.
33. Burbank FH. Determinants of contrast enhancement of intravenous digital subtraction angiography. *Invest Radiol* 1983;18:308–316.
34. Burgener FA, Hamlin DJ. Contrast enhancement in abdominal CT: bolus vs. infusion. *AJR* 1981;137:351–358.
35. Campos A, Figueroa ET, Gunasekaran S, Garin EH. Early presentation of tuberous sclerosis as bilateral renal cysts. *J Urol* 1993;149:1077–1079.
36. Carr DH, Brown J, Bydder GM, et al. Gadolinium-DTPA as a contrast agent in MRI: initial clinical experience in 20 patients. *AJR* 1984;143:215–224.
37. Cho C, Friedland GW, Swenson RS. Acquired renal cystic disease and renal neoplasms in hemodialysis patients. *Urol Radiol* 1984;6:153–157.
38. Cholankeril JV, Freundlich R, Ketyer S, Spirito AL, Napolitano J. Computed tomography in urothelial tumors of renal pelvis and related filling defects. *J Comput Assist Tomogr* 1986;10:263–272.
39. Choyke PL, White EM, Zeman RK, Jaffe MH, Clark LR. Renal metastases: clinicopathologic and radiologic correlation. *Radiology* 1987;162:359–363.
40. Choyke PL, Frank JA, Girton ME, et al. Dynamic Gd-DTPA-enhanced MR imaging of the kidney: experimental results. *Radiology* 1989;170:713–720.
41. Choyke PL, Filling-Katz MR, Shawker TH, et al. von Hippel-Lindau disease: radiologic screening for visceral manifestations. *Radiology* 1990;174:815–820.
42. Choyke PL, Glenn GM, Walther MM, et al. The natural history of renal lesions in von Hippel-Lindau disease: a serial CT study in 28 patients. *AJR* 1992;159:1229–1234.
43. Choyke PL, Glenn GM, Walther MM, Patronas NJ, Linehan WM, Zbar B. Von Hippel-Lindau disease: genetic, clinical, and imaging features. *Radiology* 1995;194:629–642.
44. Chuang C-K, Lai M-K, Chang P-L, et al. Xanthogranulomatous pyelonephritis: experience in 36 cases. *J Urol* 1992;147:333–336.
45. Claussen CD, Banzer D, Pfretzschner C, Kalender WA, Schorner W. Bolus geometry and dynamics after intravenous contrast medium injection. *Radiology* 1984;153:365–368.
46. Cohan RH, Dunnick NR, Degesys GE, Korobkin M. Computed tomography of renal oncocytoma. *J Comput Assist Tomogr* 1984;8:284–287.

47. Cohan RH, Sherman LS, Korobkin M, Bass JC, Francis IR. Helical CT of renal masses: assessment of corticomedullary and nephrographic phase images. *Radiology* 1995;196:445–450.

48. Coleman BG, Arger PH, Mintz MC, Pollack HM, Banner MP. Hyperdense renal masses. A computed tomography dilemma. *AJR* 1983;143:291–294.

49. Cummings KB. Nephroureterectomy: rationale in the management of transitional cell carcinoma of the upper urinary tract. *Urol Clin North Am* 1980;7:569–578.

50. Curry NS, Brock JG, Metcalf JS, Sens MA. Hyperdense renal mass: unusual CT appearance of a benign renal cyst. *Urol Radiol* 1982;4:33–36.

51. Curry NS, Reinig J, Schabel SI, Ross P, Vujic I, Gobien RP. An evaluation of the effectiveness of CT vs. other imaging modalities in the diagnosis of atypical renal masses. *Invest Radiol* 1984;19:447–452.

52. Curry NS, Frangos DN, Tague DF. Computed tomography of end-stage renal transplant rejection. *J Comput Assist Tomogr* 1986;10:51–53.

53. Curry NS, Schabel SI, Betsill WL Jr. Small renal neoplasms: diagnostic imaging, pathologic features, and clinical course. *Radiology* 1986;158:113–117.

54. Curry NS, Schabel SI, Garvin AJ, Fiol G. Intra-tumoral fat in a renal oncocytoma mimicking angiomyolipoma. *AJR* 1990;154:307–308.

55. Curry NS, Chung CJ, Gordon B. Unilateral renal cystic disease in an adult. *Abdom Imaging* 1994;19:366–368.

56. Curry NS. Small renal masses (lesions smaller than 3 cm): imaging evaluation and management. *AJR* 1995;164:355–362.

57. Cyran KM, Kenney PJ. Asymptomatic renal abscess: evaluation with gadolinium DTPA-enhanced MRI. *Abdom Imaging* 1994;19:267–269.

58. Dahlene DH, Stanley RJ, Koehler RE, Shin MS, Tishler JM. Abdominal tuberculosis: CT findings. *J Comput Assist Tomogr* 1984;8:443–445.

59. Dalla-Palma L, Pozzi-Mucelli F, di Donna A. Cystic renal tumors: US and CT findings. *Urol Radiol* 1990;12:67–73.

60. Dalton D, Neiman H, Grayhack JT. The natural history of simple renal cysts: a preliminary study. *J Urol* 1986;135:905–908.

61. Daniel WW, Hartman GW, Witten DM, Farrow GM, Kelalis PP. Calcified renal masses. *Radiology* 1972;103:503–508.

62. Davidson AJ, Hayes WS, Hartman DS, McCarthy WF, Davis CJ. Renal oncocytoma and carcinoma: failure of differentiation with CT. *Radiology* 1993;186:693–696.

63. Dawson RH, Dunnick NR, Leder RA, Baker ME. Extravasation of nonionic radiologic contrast medium: efficacy of conservative treatment. *Radiology* 1990;176:65–69.

64. Dawson P, Peters AM. Dynamic contrast bolus computed tomography for the assessment of renal function. *Invest Radiol* 1993;28:1039–1042.

65. Dean PB, Kivisaari L, Kormano M. Contrast enhancement pharmacokinetics of six ionic and nonionic contrast media. *Invest Radiol* 1983;18:368–374.

66. Debatin JF, Spritzer CE, Grist TM, et al. Imaging of the renal arteries: value of MR angiography. *AJR* 1991;157:981–990.

67. Debatin JF, Sostman HD, Knelson M, Argabright M, Spritzer CE. Renal magnetic resonance angiography in the preoperative detection of supernumerary renal arteries in potential kidney donors. *Invest Radiol* 1993;28:882–889.

68. Debatin JF, Ting RH, Wegmüller H, et al. Renal artery blood flow: quantitation with phase-contrast MR imaging with and without breath holding. *Radiology* 1994;190:371–378.

69. Defossez SM, Yoder IC, Papanicolaou N, Rosen BR, McGovern F. Nonspecific magnetic resonance appearance of renal oncocytoma: report of 3 cases and review of the literature. *J Urol* 1991;145:552–554.

70. Dillon EH, van Leeuwen MS, Fernandez MA, Mali WPTM. Spiral CT angiography. *AJR* 1993;160:1273–1278.

71. Dinsmore BJ, Pollack HM, Banner MP. Calcified transitional cell carcinoma of the renal pelvis. *Radiology* 1988;167:401–404.

72. Dooms GC, Hricak H, Sollitto RA, Higgins CB. Lipomatous tumors and tumors with fatty component: MR imaging potential and comparison of MR and CT results. *Radiology* 1985;157:479–483.

73. Dretler SP, Pfister R, Hendren WH. Extrarenal calyces in the ectopic kidney. *J Urol* 1970;103:406–410.

74. Dunnick NR, Long JA, Javadpour N. Perirenal extravasation of urographic contrast medium demonstrated by computed tomography. *J Comput Assist Tomogr* 1980;4:538–539.

75. Dunnick NR, Hartman DS, Ford KK, Davis CJ Jr, Amis ES Jr. The radiology of juxtaglomerular tumors. *Radiology* 1983;147:321–326.

76. Dunnick NR, Korobkin M, Clark WM. CT demonstration of hyperdense renal carcinoma. *J Comput Assist Tomogr* 1984;8:1023–1024.

77. Eilenberg SS, Lee JKT, Brown JJ, Morowitz SA, Tartar VM. Renal masses: evaluation with gradient-echo Gd-DTPA-enhanced dynamic MR imaging. *Radiology* 1990;176:333–338.

78. Erturk E, Sheinfeld J, DiMarco PL, Cockett ATK. Renal trauma: evaluation by computerized tomography. *J Urol* 1985;133:946–949.

79. Fanney DR, Casillas J, Murphy BJ. CT in the diagnosis of renal trauma. *Radiographics* 1990;10:29–40.

80. Federle MP, Goldberg HI, Kaiser JA, Moss AA, Jeffrey RB, Mall JC. Evaluation of abdominal trauma by computed tomography. *Radiology* 1981;138:637–644.

81. Fein AB, Lee JKT, Balfe DM, et al. Diagnosis and staging of renal cell carcinoma: a comparison of MR imaging and CT. *AJR* 1987;148:749–753.

82. Feldberg MAM, vanWaes PFGM. Multilocular cystic renal cell carcinoma. *AJR* 1982;138:953–955.

83. Ferris RA, Kirschner LP, Mero JH, McCabe DJ, Moss ML. Computed tomography in the evaluation of inferior vena caval obstruction. *Radiology* 1979;130:7–10.

84. Fishman MC, Pollack HM, Arger PH, Banner MD. High protein content: another cause of CT hyperdense benign renal cysts. *J Comput Assist Tomogr* 1983;7:1103–1106.

85. Flechner SM, McAninch JW. Aspergillosis of the urinary tract: ascending route of infection and evolving patterns of disease. *J Urol* 1981;125:598–601.

86. Forbes WSSC, Isherwood I, Fawcitt RA. Computed tomography in the evaluation of the solitary or unilateral nonfunctioning kidney. *J Comput Assist Tomogr* 1987;2:389–394.

87. Forman HP, Middleton WD, Melson GL, McClennan BL. Hyperechoic renal cell carcinomas: increase in detection at US. *Radiology* 1993;188:431–434.

88. Fowler JE, Perkins T. Presentation, diagnosis and treatment of renal abscesses: 1972–1988. *J Urol* 1994;151:847–851.

89. Fuld IL, Matalon TA, Vogelzang RL, et al. Dynamic CT in the evaluation of physiologic status of renal transplants. *AJR* 1984;142:1157–1160.

90. Fultz PJ, Hampton WR, Totterman SMS. Computed tomography of pyonephrosis. *Abdom Imaging* 1993;18:82–87.

91. Gatewood OMB, Goldman SM, Marshall FF, Siegelman SS. Computerized tomography in the diagnosis of transitional cell carcinoma of the kidney. *J Urol* 1982;127:876–887.

92. Gebel M, Kuhn K, Dohring W, Freise J. Ultrasonography and computed axial tomography in the detection and monitoring of renal hematomas following ultrasonically guided percutaneous renal biopsy. *Radiology* 1985;28:25–27.

93. Gehrig JJ, Gottheiner TI, Swensen RS. Acquired cystic disease of the end-stage kidney. *Am J Med* 1985;79:609–620.

94. Gibson RJ, Meanock CI, Torrie EPH, Walker TM. An assessment of Gd-DTPA as a CT contrast agent in the renal tract. *Clin Radiol* 1993;47:278–279.

95. Gill IS, McClennan BL, Kerbl K, Carbone JM, Wick M, Clayman RV. Adrenal involvement from renal cell carcinoma: predictive value of computerized tomography. *J Urol* 1994;152:1082–1085.

96. Glazer GM, Francis IR, Brady TM, Teng SS. Computed tomography of renal infarction: clinical and experimental observations. *AJR* 1983;140:721–727.

97. Glazer GM, Francis IR, Gross BH, Amendola MA. Computed tomography of renal vein thrombosis. *J Comput Assist Tomogr* 1984;8:288–293.

98. Gold RP, McClennan BL, Rottenberg RR. CT appearance of acute inflammatory disease of the renal interstitium. *AJR* 1983;141:343–349.

99. Goldman SM, Hartman DS, Fishman EK, Finizio JP, Gatewood

OM, Siegelman SS. CT of xanthogranulomatous pyelonephritis: radiologic–pathologic correlation. *AJR* 1984;142:963–969.

100. Goldman SM, Fishman EK, Hartman DS, Kim YC, Siegelman SS. Computed tomography of renal tuberculosis and its pathological correlates. *J Comput Assist Tomogr* 1985;9:771–776.

101. Goldman SM, Hartman DS, Weiss SW. The varied radiographic manifestation of retroperitoneal malignant fibrous histiocytoma revealed through 27 cases. *J Urol* 1986;135:33–38.

102. Goldman SM, Fishman EK. Upper urinary tract infection: the current role of CT, ultrasound, and MRI. *Semin Ultrasound CT MR* 1991;12:335–360.

103. Grist TM, Charles HC, Sostman HD. Renal transplant rejection: diagnosis with ^{31}P MR spectroscopy. *AJR* 1991;156:105–112.

104. Gutierrez OH, Burgener FA, Schwartz S. Coincident renal cell carcinoma and renal angiomyolipoma in tuberous sclerosis. *AJR* 1979;132:848–850.

105. Hadar H, Meiraz D. Renal sinus lipomatosis. Differentiation from space-occupying lesion with aid of computed tomography. *Urology* 1980;15:86–90.

106. Halasz NA. Differential diagnosis of renal transplant rejection: Is MR imaging the answer? *AJR* 1986;147:954–955.

107. Hamlin DJ, Kaude NAJV, Fitzsimmons JR, Gaskin JM. Magnetic resonance imaging of renal abscess in an experimental animal model. *Acta Radiol Diagn* 1985;26:315–319.

108. Hanna S, Helenon O, Legendre C, et al. MR imaging of renal transplant rejection. *Acta Radiol* 1991;32:42–46.

109. Hartman DS, Goldman SM, Friedman AC, David CJ, Madewell JE, Sherman JL. Angiomyolipoma: ultrasonic-pathologic correlation. *Radiology* 1981;139:451–458.

110. Hartman DS, Davis CJ Jr, Goldman SM, Friedman AC, Fritzsche P. Renal lymphoma: radiologic–pathologic correlation of 21 cases. *Radiology* 1982;144:759–766.

111. Hartman DS, Davis CJ Jr, Madewell JE, Friedman AC. Primary malignant renal tumors in the second decade of life: Wilms tumor versus renal cell carcinoma. *J Urol* 1982;127:888–891.

112. Hartman DS, Davis CJ, Johns T, Goldman SM. Cystic renal cell carcinoma. *Urology* 1986;28:145–153.

113. Hartman DS, Davis CJ, Sanders RC, Johns TT, Smirniotopoulos J, Goldman SM. The multiloculated renal mass: considerations and differential features. *Radiographics* 1987;7:29–52.

114. Hartman DS, Weatherby E III, Laskin WB, Brody JM, Corse W, Baluch JD. Cystic renal cell carcinoma: CT findings simulating a benign hyperdense cyst. *AJR* 1992;159:1235–1237.

115. Hattery RR, King BF. Tecnique and application of MR urography. *Radiology* 1995;194:25–27.

116. Haustein J, Niendorf HP, Krestin G, et al. Renal tolerance of gadolinium-DTPA/dimeglumine in patients with chronic renal failure. *Invest Radiol* 1992;27:153–156.

117. Hayes WS, Hartman DS, Sesterhenn IA. From the archives of the AFIP. Xanthogranulomatous pyelonephritis. *Radiographics* 1991;11:485–498.

118. Haynes JW, Walsh JW, Brewer WH, Vick CW, Allen HA. Traumatic renal artery occlusion: CT diagnosis with angiographic correlation. *J Comput Assist Tomogr* 1984;8:731–733.

119. Healy ME, Teng SS, Moss AA. Uriniferous pseudocyst: computed tomographic findings. *Radiology* 1984;153:757–762.

120. Heiken JP, McClennan BL, Gold RP. Renal lymphomas. *Semin Ultrasound CT MR* 1986;7:58–66.

121. Hélénon O, Attlan E, Legendre C, et al. Gd-DOTA-enhanced MR imaging and color Doppler US of renal allograft necrosis. *Radiographics* 1992;12:21–33.

122. Hélénon O, Chrétien Y, Paraf F, Melki P, Denys A, Moreau JF. Renal cell carcinoma containing fat: demonstration with CT. *Radiology* 1993;188:429–430.

123. Hennig J, Friedburg H, Ströbel B. Rapid nontomographic approach to MR myelography without contrast agents. *J Comput Assist Tomogr* 1986;10:375–378.

124. Hertle L, Becht E, Klose K, Rumpelt HJ. Computed tomography in xanthogranulomatous pyelonephritis. *Eur Urol* 1984;10:385–386.

125. Higashihara E, Aso Y, Shimazaki J, Ito H, Koiso K, Sakai O. Clinical aspects of polycystic kidney disease. *J Urol* 1992;147:329–332.

126. Hilpert PL, Friedman AC, Radecki PD, et al. MRI of hemorrhagic renal cysts in polycystic kidney disease. *AJR* 1986;146:1167–1172.

127. Honda H, McGuire CW, Barloon TJ, Hashimoto K. Replacement lipomatosis of the kidney: CT features. *J Comput Assist Tomogr* 1990;14:229–231.

128. Honda H, Coffman CE, Berbaum KS, Barloon TJ, Masuda K. CT analysis of metastatic neoplasms of the kidney. *Acta Radiol* 1992;33:39–44.

129. Horan JJ, Robertson CN, Choyke PL, et al. The detection of renal carcinoma extension into the renal vein and inferior vena cava: a prospective comparison of venacavography and magnetic resonance imaging. *J Urol* 1989;142:943–948.

130. Hovsepian DM, Levy H, Amis ES, Newhouse JH. MR evaluation of renal space-occupying lesions: diagnostic criteria. *Urol Radiol* 1990;12:74–79.

131. Hricak H, Demas BE, Williams RD, et al. Magnetic resonance imaging in the diagnosis and staging of renal and perirenal neoplasms. *Radiology* 1985;154:709–715.

132. Hricak H, Terrier F, Marotti M, et al. Post-transplant renal rejection: comparison of quantitative scintigraphy, US and MR imaging. *Radiology* 1987;162:685–688.

133. Hricak H, Thoeni RF, Carroll PR, Demas BE, Marotti M, Tanagho EA. Detection and staging of renal neoplasms: a reassessment of MR imaging. *Radiology* 1988;166:643–649.

134. Hudson MA, Weyman PJ, van der Vliet AH, Catalona WJ. Emphysematous pyelonephritis: successful management by percutaneous drainage. *J Urol* 1986;136:884–886.

135. Hughson MD, Hennigar GR, McManus JFA. Atypical cysts, acquired renal cystic disease and renal cell tumors in end-stage dialysis kidneys. *Lab Invest* 1980;42:475–480.

136. Hurwitz G, Reimund E, Moparty KR, Hellstrom WJG. Bilateral renal parenchymal malacoplakia: a case report. *J Urol* 1992;147:115–117.

137. Ishikawa I, Onouchi Z, Saito Y, et al. Renal cortex visualization and analysis of dynamic CT curves of the kidney. *J Comput Assist Tomogr* 1981;5:695–701.

138. Ishikawa I. Uremic acquired cystic disease of kidney. *Urology* 1985;26:101–107.

139. Ishikawa I, Saito Y, Onouchi Z, et al. Delayed contrast enhancement in acute focal bacterial nephritis: CT features. *J Comput Assist Tomogr* 1985;9:894–897.

140. Ishikawa I, Tateishi K, Onouchi Z, et al. Persistent wedge-shaped contrast enhancement of the kidney. *Urol Radiol* 1985;7:45–47

141. Jacobs JE, Sussman SK, Glickstein MF. Renal lymphangiomyoma—A rare cause of a multiloculated renal mass. *AJR* 1989;152:307–308.

142. Jakobsen JA, Lundby B, Kristoffersen DT, Borch KW, Hald JK, Berg KJ. Evaluation of renal function with delayed CT after injection of nonionic monomeric and dimeric contrast media in healthy volunteers. *Radiology* 1992;182:419–424.

143. Jasinski RW, Amendola MA, Glazer GM, Bree RL, Gikas PW. Computed tomography of renal oncocytoma. *Comput Radiol* 1985;9:307–314.

144. Jennerholm S, Backman U, Bohman SO, Hemmingsson A, Nyman R. Magnetic resonance imaging of the transplanted kidney. Correlation to function and histopathology. *Acta Radiol* 1990;31:499–503.

145. Johnson CD, Dunnick NR, Cohan RH, Illescas FF. Renal adenocarcinoma: CT staging of 100 tumors. *AJR* 1987;148:59–63.

146. Joshi VV, Beckwith JB. Multilocular cyst of the kidney (cystic nephroma) and cystic, partially differentiated nephroblastoma. *Cancer* 1989;64:466–479.

147. Kabala JE, Gillatt DA, Persad RA, Penry JB, Gingell JC, Chadwick D. Magnetic resonance imaging in the staging of renal cell carcinoma. *Br J Radiol* 1991;64:683–689.

148. Kallman DA, King BF, Hattery RR, Charboneau JW, Ehman RL, Guthman DA, Blute ML. Renal vein and inferior vena cava tumor thrombus in renal cell carcinoma: CT, US, MRI, and venacavography. *J Comput Assist Tomogr* 1992;16:240–247.

149. Karstaedt N, McCullough DL, Wolfman NT. Magnetic resonance imaging of the renal mass. *J Urol* 1986;136:566–570.

150. Kauczor H-U, Schadmand-Fischer S, Filipas D, Schwickert HC, Steinbach F, Schild HH, Thelen M. CT after enucleation of renal cell carcinoma. *Abdom Imaging* 1994;19:361–365.

151. Kennelly MJ, Grossman HB, Cho KJ. Outcome analysis of 42 cases of renal angiomyolipoma. *J Urol* 1994;152:1988–1991.

152. Kenney PJ, Robbins GL, Ellis DA, Spirt BA. Adrenal glands in patients with congenital renal anomalies: CT appearance. *Radiology* 1985;155:181–182.

153. Kenney PJ, Stanley RJ. Computed tomography of ureteral tumors. *J Comput Assist Tomogr* 1987;11:102–107.

154. Kenney PJ, Panicek DM, Witanowski LS. Computed tomography of ureteral disruption. *J Comput Assist Tomogr* 1987;11:480–484.

155. Kenney PJ. CT and MRI of upper urinary tract obstruction. In: Goldman SM, Gatewood WMB, eds. *CT and MRI of the genitourinary tract*. New York: Churchill Livingston, 1990;117–148.

156. Kim SH, Park JH, Han JK, Han MC, Kim S, Lee JS. Infarction of the kidney: role of contrast enhanced MRI. *J Comput Assist Tomogr* 1992;16:924–928.

157. Kim WS, Goldman SM, Gatewood OMB, et al. Computed tomography in calcified renal masses. *J Comput Assist Tomogr* 1981;5:855–860.

158. Kittredge RD, Brensilver J, Pierce JC. Computed tomography in renal transplant problems. *Radiology* 1978;127:165–169.

159. Konnak JW, Grossman HB. Renal cell carcinoma as an incidental finding. *J Urol* 1985;134:1094–1096.

160. Kormano M, Partaren K, Soimakallio S, Kivimaki T. Dynamic contrast enhancement of the upper abdomen and effect of contrast medium and body weight. *Invest Radiol* 1983;18:364–367.

161. Korobkin M. 1993 plenary session: imaging symposium. *Radiographics* 1994;14:885–886.

162. Kumar R, Amparo EG, David R, Fagan CJ, Morettin LB. Adult Wilms' tumor: clinical and radiographic features. *Urol Radiol* 1984;6:164–169.

163. Kundel HL, Schlakman B, Joseph PM, Fishman JE, Summers R. Water content and NMR relaxation time gradients in the rabbit kidney. *Invest Radiol* 1986;21:12–17.

164. Kunin M. Bridging septa of the perinephric space: anatomic, pathologic and diagnostic consideration. *Radiology* 1986;158:361–365.

165. Lang EK. Renal, perirenal, and pararenal abscesses: percutaneous drainage. *Radiology* 1990;174:109–113.

166. Lautin EM, Gordon PM, Friedman AC, et al. Radionuclide imaging and computed tomography in renal oncocytoma. *Radiology* 1981;138:185–190.

167. Lawson TL, McClennan BL, Shirkhoda A. Adult polycystic kidney disease: ultrasonographic and computed tomographic appearance. *J Clin Ultrasound* 1981;6:295–302.

168. Leder RA, Dunnick NR. Transitional cell carcinoma of the pelvicalices and ureter. *AJR* 1990;155:713–722.

169. Lee JKT, McClennan BL, Kissane JM. Unilateral polycystic kidney disease. *AJR* 1978;130:1165–1167.

170. Lee JKT, McClennan BL, Melson GL, Stanley RJ. Acute focal bacterial nephritis: emphasis on gray scale sonography and computed tomography. *AJR* 1980;135:87–92.

171. Levine E, Lee KR, Weigel JW, Farber B. Computed tomography in the diagnosis of renal carcinoma complicating Hippel-Lindau syndrome. *Radiology* 1979;130:703–706.

172. Levine E, Collins DL, Horton WA, Schmenke RN. CT screening of the abdomen in von Hippel-Lindau disease. *AJR* 1982;139:505–510.

173. Levine E, Grantham JJ, Slusher SL, Greathouse JL, Krohn BP. CT of acquired cystic kidney disease and renal tumors in long-term dialysis patients. *AJR* 1984;142:125–131.

174. Levine E. CRC diagnosis: computed tomography of renal masses. *Crit Rev Diagn Imaging* 1985;24:91–200.

175. Levine E, Grantham JJ. High-density renal cysts in autosomal dominant polycystic kidney disease demonstrated by CT. *Radiology* 1985;154:477–482.

176. Levine E, Huntrakoon M. Unilateral renal cystic disease: CT findings. *J Comput Assist Tomogr* 1989;13:273–276.

177. Levine E, Huntrakoon M, Wetzel LH. Small renal neoplasms: clinical, pathologic, and imaging features. *AJR* 1989;153:69–73.

178. Levine E, Slusher SL, Grantham JJ, Wetzel LH. Natural history of acquired renal cystic disease in dialysis patients: a prospective longitudinal CT study. *AJR* 1991;156:501–506.

179. Levine E, Grantham JJ. Calcified renal stones and cyst calcifica-

180. Levine LA, Gburek BM. Acquired cystic disease and renal adenocarcinoma following renal transplantation. *J Urol* 1994;151:129–132.

181. Licht MR, Novick AC, Goormastic M. Nephron sparing surgery in incidental versus suspected renal cell carcinoma. *J Urol* 1994;152:39–42.

182. Liou JTS, Lee JKT, Heiken JP, Totty WG, Molina PL, Flye WM. Renal transplants: Can acute rejection and acute tubular necrosis be differentiated with MR imaging? *Radiology* 1991;179:61–65.

183. Loubeyre P, Revel D, Garcia P, et al. Screening patients for renal artery stenosis: value of three-dimensional time-of-flight MR angiography. *AJR* 1994;162:847–852.

184. Love L, Yedicka J. Computed tomography of internally calcified renal cysts. *AJR* 1985;145:1225–1227.

185. Love L, Lind JA Jr, Olson MC. Persistent CT nephrogram: significance in the diagnosis of contrast nephropathy. *Radiology* 1989;172:125–129.

186. Lupetin AR, Mainwaring BL, Daffner RH. CT diagnosis of renal artery injury caused by blunt abdominal trauma. *AJR* 1989;153:1065–1089.

187. Madewell JE, Goldman SM, Davis CJ Jr, Hartman DS, Feigin DS, Lichtenstein JE. Multilocular cystic nephroma: a radiographic–pathologic correlation of 58 patients. *Radiology* 1983;146:309–321.

188. Malmed AS, Love L, Jeffrey RB. Medullary CT enhancement in acute renal artery occlusion. *J Comput Assist Tomogr* 1992;16:107–109.

189. Mangano FA, Zaontz M, Pahira JJ, et al. Computed tomography of acute renal failure secondary to rhabdomyolysis. *J Comput Assist Tomogr* 1985;9:777–779.

190. Marks WM, Korobkin M, Callen PW, Kaiser JA. CT diagnosis of tumor thrombosis of the renal vein and inferior vena cava. *AJR* 1978;131:843–846.

191. Marotti M, Hricak H, Fritzsche P, Crooks LE, Hedgcock MW, Tanagho EA. Complex and simple renal cysts: comparative evaluation with MR imaging. *Radiology* 1987;162:679–684.

192. Matson MA, Cohen EP. Acquired cystic kidney disease: occurrence, prevalence, and renal cancers. *Medicine* 1990;69:217–226.

193. Mayer DP, Baron RL, Pollack HM. Increase in CT attenuation values of parapelvic renal cysts after retrograde pyelography. *AJR* 1982;139:991–993.

194. McClennan BL. Computed tomography in the diagnosis and staging of renal cell carcinoma. *Semin Urol* 1985;3:111–131.

195. McCoy JG, Honda H, Reznicek M, Williams RD. Computerized tomography for detection and staging of localized and pathologically defined upper tract urothelial tumors. *J Urol* 1991;146:1500–1503.

196. McMillin KI, Gross BH. CT demonstration of peripelvic and periureteral non-Hodgkin lymphoma. *AJR* 1985;144:945–946.

197. Michaeli J, Mogle P, Perlberg S, Heiman S, Caine M. Emphysematous pyelonephritis. *J Urol* 1984;131:203–208.

198. Miles KA. Measurement of tissue perfusion by dynamic computed tomography. *Br J Radiol* 1991;64:409–412.

199. Miles KA, Hayball MP, Dixon AK. Functional imaging of changes in human intrarenal perfusion using quantitative dynamic computed tomorlraphy. *Invest Radiol* 1994;29:911–914.

200. Miller DL, Choyke PL, Walther MM, Doppman JL, Kragel PJ, Weiss GH, Linehan WM. Von Hippel-Lindau disease: inadequacy of angiography for identification of renal cancers. *Radiology* 1991;179:833–836.

201. Miller FH, Parikh S, Gore RM, Nemcek AA Jr, Fitzgerald SW, Vogelzang RL. Renal manifestations of AIDS. *Radiographics* 1993;13:587–596.

202. Mitnick JS, Bosniak MA, Mitton S, Raghavendra BN, Subramanyam BR, Genieser NB. Cystic renal disease in tuberous sclerosis. *Radiology* 1983;147:85–87.

203. Mitty HA. CT for diagnosis and management of urinary extravasation. *AJR* 1980;134:497–501.

204. Moll V, Becht E, Ziegler M. Kidney preserving surgery in renal cell tumors: indications, techniques and results in 152 patients. *J Urol* 1993;150:319–323.

205. Morag B, Rubenstein ZJ, Hertz M, Solomon A. Computed tomog-

raphy in the diagnosis of renal parapelvic cysts. *J Comput Assist Tomogr* 1983;7:833–836.
206. Morgan WR, Nyberg LM Jr. Perinephric and intrarenal abscesses. *Urology* 1985;26:529–536.
207. Morra MN, Das S. Renal oncocytoma: a review of histogenesis, histopathology, diagnosis and treatment. *J Urol* 1993;150:295–302.
208. Munechika H, Kushihashi T, Gokan T, Hasimoto T, Higaki Y, Ogawa Y. A renal cell carcinoma extending into the renal pelvis simulating transitional cell carcinoma. *Urol Radiol* 1990;12:11–14.
209. Myers BD, Sommer FG, Li K, et al. Determination of blood flow to the transplanted kidney. *Transplantation* 1994;57:1445–1450.
210. Narumi Y, Sato T, Hori S, et al. Squamous cell carcinoma of the uroepithelium: CT evaluation. *Radiology* 1989;173:853–856.
211. Niceforo JR, Coughlin GF. Diagnosis of renal cell carcinoma: value of fine-needle aspiration cytology in patients with metastases or contraindications to nephrectomy. *AJR* 1993;161:1303–1305.
212. Nicholson DA. Case report: replacement lipomatosis of the kidney—Unusual CT features. *Clin Radiol* 1992;45:42–43.
213. Nicolaisen GS, McAninch JW, Marshall GA, Bluth RF, Carroll PR. Renal trauma: re-evaluation of the indications for radiographic assessment. *J Urol* 1985;133:183–187.
214. Nissenkorn I, Bernheim J. Multicentricity in renal cell carcinoma. *J Urol* 1995;153:620–622.
215. Novick AC, Irish C, Steinmuller D, Buonocore E, Cohen C. The role of computerized tomography in renal transplant patients. *J Urol* 1981;125:15–18.
216. Nyman U, Oldbring J, Aspelin P. CT of carcinoma of the renal pelvis. *Acta Radiol* 1992;33:31–38.
217. Oesterling JE, Fishman EK, Goldman SM, Marshall FF. The management of renal angiomyolipoma. *J Urol* 1986;135;1121–1124.
218. Olazabal A, Velasco M, Martinez A, Villavicencio H, Codina M. Emphysematous pyelonephritis. *Urology* 1987;29:95–98.
219. Ozen H, Colowick A, Freiha FS. Incidentally discovered solid renal masses: What are they? *Br J Urol* 1993;72:274–276.
220. Papanicolaou N, Hahn PF, Edeman RR, et al. Magnetic resonance imaging of the kidney. *Urol Radiol* 1986;8:139–150.
221. Parfrey PS, Bear JC, Morgan J, et al. The diagnosis and prognosis of autosomal dominant polycystic kidney disease. *N Engl J Med* 1990;323:1085–1090.
222. Parienty RA, Pradel J, Picard JD, Ducellier R, Lubrano JM, Smolarski N. Visibility and thickening of the renal fascia on computed tomograms. *Radiology* 1981;139:119–124.
223. Parienty RA, Pradel J, Imbert MC, Picard JD, Savant P. Computed tomography of multilocular cystic nephroma. *Radiology* 1981;140:135–139.
224. Parienty RA, Ducellier R, Pradel J, Lubrano J-M, Francois C, Francois R. Diagnostic value of CT numbers in pelvocalyceal filling defects. *Radiology* 1982;145:743–747.
225. Parienty RA, Pradel J, Parienty I. Cystic renal cancer: CT characteristics. *Radiology* 1985;157:741–744.
226. Parker MD, Clark RL. Evolving concepts in the diagnosis of xanthogranulomatous pyelonephritis. *Urol Radiol* 1989;11:7–15.
227. Parvey LS, Warner RM, Callihan TR, Magill HS. CT demonstration of fat tissue in malignant renal neoplasms: atypical Wilms' tumor. *J Comput Assist Tomogr* 1981;5:851–854.
228. Pollack HM, Arger PH, Banner MP, Mulhern CB, Coleman BG. Computed tomography of renal pelvic filling defects. *Radiology* 1981;138:645–651.
229. Pollack HM, Banner MP, Amendola MA. Other malignant neoplasms of the renal parenchyma. *Semin Roentgenol* 1987;22:260–274.
230. Pollack HM, Wein AJ. Imaging of renal trauma. *Radiology* 1989;172:297–308.
231. Pope TL, Buschi AJ, Moore TS, Williamson BRJ, Brenbridge ANAG. CT features of renal polyarteritis nodosa. *AJR* 1981;136:986–987.
232. Potts DG, Brody AS, Shafik IM, et al. Demonstration of renal tubular flow by selective angiographic computed tomography. *Can Assoc Rad* 1993;44:364–370.
233. Prando A. Letters: intratumoral fat in a renal cell carcinoma. *AJR* 1991;156:871.

234. Premkumar A, Lattimer J, Newhouse JH. CT and sonography of advanced urinary tract tuberculosis. *AJR* 1987;148:65–69.
235. Press GA, McClennan BL, Melson GL, Weyman PJ, Mauro MA, Lee JKT. Papillary renal cell carcinoma: CT and sonographic evaluation. *AJR* 1984;143:1005–1010.
236. Quinn MJ, Hartman DS, Friedman AC, et al. Renal oncocytoma: new observations. *Radiology* 1984;153:49–53.
237. Quint LE, Glazer GM, Chenevert TL, et al. In vivo and in vitro MR imaging of renal tumors: histopathologic correlation and pulse sequence optimization. *Radiology* 1988;169:359–362.
238. Radin DR, Chandrasoma P. CT demonstration of fat density in renal cell carcinoma. *Acta Radiol* 1992;33:365–367.
239. Rahmouni A, Mathieu D, Berger J-F, Montazel J-L, Chopin DK, Vasile N. Fast magnetic resonance imaging in the evaluation of tumoral obstructions of the inferior vena cava. *J Urol* 1992;148:14–17.
240. Raptopoulous V, Kleinman PK, Marks S, Snyder M, Silverman PM. Renal fascial pathway: posterior extension of pancreatic effusions within the anterior pararenal space. *Radiology* 1986;158:367–374.
241. Rausch HP, Hanefeld F, Kaufman HJ. Medullary nephrocalcinosis and pancreatic calcifications demonstrated by ultrasound and CT in infants after treatment with ACTH. *Radiology* 1984;153:105–107.
242. Reiser UJ. Study of bolus geometry after after intravenous contrast medium injection: dynamic quantitative measurement (chronogram) using an x-ray CT device. *J Comput Assist Tomogr* 1984;8:251–262.
243. Remark RR, Berquist TH, Lieber MM, Charboneau JW, Hartman GW. Magnetic resonance imaging of renal oncocytoma. *Urology* 1988;31:176–179.
244. Reznek RH, Mootoosamy I, Webb JAW, Richards MA. CT in renal and perirenal lymphoma: a further look. *Clin Radiol* 1990;42:233–238.
245. Rhyner P, Federle MP, Jeffrey RB. CT of trauma to the abnormal kidney. *AJR* 1984;142:747–750.
246. Rigsby CM, Rosenfield AT, Glickman MG, Hodson J. Hemorrhagic focal bacterial nephritis: findings on gray-scale sonography and CT. *AJR* 1986;146:1173–1177.
247. Robson CJ. The results of radical nephrectomy for renal cell carcinoma. *J Urol* 1969;101:297–301.
248. Rofsky NM, Bosniak MA, Weinreb JC, Coppa GF. Giant renal cell carcinoma: CT and MR characteristics. *J Comput Assist Tomogr* 1989;13:1078–1080.
249. Rofsky NM, Weinreb JC, Bosniak MA, Libes RB, Birnbaum BA. Renal lesion characterization with gadolinium-enhanced MR imaging: efficacy and safety in patients with renal insufficiency. *Radiology* 1991;180:85–89.
250. Rominger MB, Kenney PJ, Morgan DE, Bernreuter WK, Listinsky JJ. Gadolinium-enhanced MR imaging of renal masses. *Radiographics* 1992;12:1097–1116.
251. Rosenbaum R, Hoffsten PE, Stanley RJ, Klahr S. Use of computerized tomography to diagnose complications of percutaneous renal biopsy. *Kidney Int* 1978;14;87–92.
252. Rosenberg ER, Korobkin M, Foster W, Silverman PM, Bowie JD, Dunnick NR. The significance of septations in a renal cyst. *AJR* 1985;144:593–595.
253. Rosi P, Selli C, Carini M, Rosi MF, Mottola A. Xanthogranulomatous pyelonephritis: clinical experience with 62 cases. *Eur Urol* 1986;12:96–100.
254. Rothpearl A, Frager D, Subramanian A, et al. MR urography: technique and application. *Radiology* 1995;194:125–130.
255. Roubidoux MA, Dunnick NR, Sostman HD, Leder RA. Renal carcinoma: detection of venous extension with gradient-echo MR imaging. *Radiology* 1992;182:269–272.
256. Roubidoux MA. MR imaging of hemorrhage and iron deposition in the kidney. *Radiographics* 1994;14:1033–1044.
257. Rubin GD, Dake MD, Napel S, et al. Spiral CT of renal artery stenosis: comparison of three-dimensional rendering techniques. *Radiology* 1994;190:181–189.
258. Rumancik WM, Bosniak MA, Rosen RJ, Hulnich D. Atypical renal and pararenal hamartoma associated with lymphangiomatosis. *AJR* 1984;142:971–972.
259. Sagel SS, Siegel MJ, Stanley RJ, Jost RG. Detection of retroperito-

neal hemorrhage by computed tomography. *AJR* 1977;129:403–407.

260. Sagel SS, Stanley RJ, Levitt RJ, Geisse G. Computed tomography of the kidney. *Radiology* 1977;124:359–370.

261. Salem YH, Miller HC. Lymphoma of genitourinary tract. *J Urol* 1994;151:1162–1170.

262. Sandler CM, Jackson H, Kaminsky RI. Right perirenal hematoma secondary to a leaking abdominal aortic aneurysm. *J Comput Assist Tomogr* 1981;5:264–266.

263. Sandler CM, Raval B, David CR. Computed tomography of the kidney. *Urol Clin North Am* 1985;12:657–665.

264. Sant GR, Ucci AA Jr, Meres EM Jr. Multicentric angiomyolipoma: renal and lymph node involvement. *Urology* 1986;28:111–113.

265. Schuhmann-Giampieri G, Krestin G. Pharmacokinetics of Gd-DTPA in patients with chronic renal failure. *Invest Radiol* 1991;26:975–979.

266. Segal AJ, Spitzer RM. Pseudo thick-walled renal cyst by CT. *AJR* 1979;132:827–828.

267. Semelka RC, Hricak H, Tomei E, Floth A, Stoller M. Obstructive nephropathy: evaluation with dynamic Gd-DTPA-enhanced MR imaging. *Radiology* 1990;175:797–803.

268. Semelka RC, Hricak H, Stevens SK, Finegold R, Tomei E, Carroll PR. Combined gadolinium-enhanced and fat-saturation MR imaging of renal masses. *Radiology* 1991;178:803–809.

269. Semelka RC, Shoenut JP, Kroeker MA, MacMahon RG, Greenberg HM. Renal lesions: controlled comparison between CT and 1. 5-T MR imaging with nonenhanced and gadolinium-enhanced fat-suppressed spin-echo and breath-hold FLASH techniques. *Radiology* 1992;182:425–430.

270. Semelka RC, Corrigan K, Ascher SM, Brown JJ, Colindres RE. Renal corticomedullary differentiation: observation in patients with differing serum creatinine levels. *Radiology* 1994;190:149–152.

271. Sheinfeld J, Erturk E, Spataro RF, Cockett ATK. Perinephric abscess: current concepts. *J Urol* 1987;237:191–194.

272. Shirkhoda A. Computed tomography of perirenal metastases. *J Comput Assist Tomogr* 1986;10:435–438.

273. Shirkhoda A. CT findings in hepatosplenic and renal candidiasis. *J Comput Assist Tomogr* 1987;11:795–798.

274. Shirkhoda A, Lewis E. Renal sarcoma and sarcomatoid renal cell carcinoma: CT and angiographic features. *Radiology* 1987;162:353–357.

275. Siegel CL, Ellis JH, Korobkin M, Dunnick NR. CT detected renal arterial calcification: correlation with renal artery stenosis on angiography. *AJR* 1994;163:867–872.

276. Siegelman SS, Copeland BE, Saba GP, Cameron JL, Sanders RC, Zerhouni EA. CT of fluid collections associated with pancreatitis. *AJR* 1980;134:1121–1132.

277. Silverberg E, Lubera JA. Cancer Statistics 1988. *CA Cancer J Clin* 1988;380:5–22.

278. Silverman PM, Cooper CJ, Weltman DI, Zeman RK. Helical CT: practical considerations and potential pitfalls. *Radiographics* 1995;15:25–36.

279. Silverman SG, Lee BY, Seltzer SE, Bloom DA, Corless CL, Adams DF. Small (≤3 cm) renal masses: correlation of spiral CT features and pathologic findings. *AJR* 1994;163:597–605.

280. Smith SJ, Bosniak MA, Megibow AJ, Hulnick DH, Horii SC, Raghavendra BN. Renal cell carcinoma: earlier discovery and increased detection. *Radiology* 1989;170:699–703.

281. Sohn HK, Kim SY, Seo HS. MR imaging of a renal oncocytoma. *J Comput Assist Tomogr* 1987;11:1085–1087.

282. Soulen MC, Fishman EK, Goldman SM, Gatewood OMB. Bacterial renal infection: role of CT. *Radiology* 1989;171:703–707.

283. Soulen MC, Fishman EK, Goldman SM. Sequelae of acute renal infections: CT evaluation. *Radiology* 1989;173:423–426.

284. Spiessl B, Beahrs OH, Hermanek P, et al. Renal pelvis and ureter. In: Spiessl B, Beahrs OH, Hermanek P, Hutter RVP, Scheibe O, Sobin LH, Wagner G, eds. *UICC-TNM atlas: illustrated guide to the TNM/pTNM-classification of malignant tumours.* Berlin: Springer-Verlag, 1989;260.

285. Steele JR, Soes PJ, Heffner LT. The detection of inferior vena caval thrombosis with computed tomography. *Radiology* 1978;128:385–386.

286. Steinberg DL, Jeffrey RB, Federle MP, McAninch JW. The com-

287. puterized tomography appearance of renal pedicle injury. *J Urol* 1984;132:1163–1164.

287. Steinberg HV, Nelson RC, Murphy FB, et al. Renal allograft rejection: evaluation by Doppler US and MR imaging. *Radiology* 1987;162:237–242.

288. Steiner MS, Goldman SM, Fishman EK, Marshall FF. The natural history of renal angiomyolipoma. *J Urol* 1993;150:1782–1786.

289. Strife JL, Souza AS, Kirks DR, Strife CF, Gelfand MJ, Wacksman J. Multicystic dysplastic kidney in children: US follow-up. *Radiology* 1993;186:785–788.

290. Strotzer M, Lehner KB, Becker K. Detection of fat in a renal cell carcinoma mimicking angiomyolipoma. *Radiology* 1993;188:427–428.

291. Studer UE, Scherz S, Scheidegger J, Kraft R, Sonntag R, Ackermann D, Zingg EJ. Enlargement of regional lymph nodes in renal cell carcinoma is often not due to metastases. *J Urol* 1990;144:243–245.

292. Subramanyam BR, Bosniak MA, Horii SC, Megibow AJ, Balthazar EJ. Replacement lipomatosis of the kidney: diagnosis by computed tomography and sonography. *Radiology* 1983;148:791–792.

293. Sumner RE, Volberg FM, Karstaedt N, Ward CF, Lorentz WB. Hypophosphatasia and nephrocalcinosis demonstrated by ultrasound and CT. *Clin Nephrol* 1984;22:317–319.

294. Sussman S, Cochran ST, Pagani JJ, et al. Hyperdense renal masses: a CT manifestation of hemorrhagic renal cysts. *Radiology* 1984;150:207–211.

295. Sussman SK, Goldberg RP, Griscom HT. Milk of calcium hydronephrosis in patients with paraplegia and urinary-enteric diversion: CT demonstration. *J Comput Assist Tomogr* 1986;10:257–259.

296. Sussman SK, Gallmann WH, Cohan RH, Saeed M, Lawton JS. CT findings in xanthogranulomatous pyelonephritis with coexistent renocolic fistula. *J Comput Assist Tomogr* 1987;11:1188–1090.

297. Takahashi K, Honda M, Okubo RS, Hyodo H, Takakusaki H, Yokoyama H, Ohsawa T. CT pixel mapping in the diagnosis of small angiomyolipomas of the kidneys. *J Comput Assist Tomogr* 1993;17:98–101.

298. Takao R, Amamoto Y, Matsunaga N, et al. Computed tomography of multicystic kidney. *J Comput Assist Tomogr* 1980;4:548–549.

299. Takeyama M, Arima M, Sagawa S, Sonoda T. Preoperative diagnosis of coincident renal cell carcinoma and renal angiomyolipoma in nontuberous sclerosis. *J Urol* 1982;128:579–581.

300. Tallarigo C, Baldassarre R, Bianchi G, et al. Diagnostic and therapeutic problems in multicentric renal angiomyolipoma. *J Urol* 1992;148:1880–1884.

301. Talner LB, Davidson AJ, Lebowitz RL, Dalla-Palma L, Goodman SM. Acute pyelonephritis: Can we agree on terminology? *Radiology* 1994;192:297–305.

302. Taylor AJ, Cohen EP, Erickson SJ, Olson DL, Foley WD. Renal imaging in long-term dialysis patients: a comparison of CT and sonography. *AJR* 1989;153:765–767.

303. Tempany CMC, Morton RA, Marshall FF. MRI of the renal veins: assessment of nonneoplastic venous thrombosis. *J Comput Assist Tomogr* 1992;16:929–934.

304. Terrier F, Hricak H, Revel D, et al. Magnetic resonance imaging in the diagnosis of acute renal allograft rejection and its differentiation from acute tubular necrosis. Experimental study in the dog. *Invest Radiol* 1985;20:617–625.

305. Thierman D, Haaga JR, Anton P, LiPuma JP. Renal replacement lipomatosis. *J Comput Assist Tomogr* 1983;7:341–343.

306. Thomsen HS, Dorph S, Larsen S, et al. Urine profiles and kidney histology after intravenous injection of ionic and nonionic radiologic and magnetic resonance contrast media in normal rats. *Acta Radiol* 1994;1:128–135.

307. Thornbury JR. Acute renal infections. *Urol Radiol* 1991;12:209–213.

308. Totty WG, McClennan BL, Melson GL, Patel R. Relative value of computed tomography and ultrasonography in the assessment of renal angiomyolipoma. *J Comput Assist Tomogr* 1981;5:173–177.

309. Van den Berg JC, Hermus ARMM, Rosenbusch GR. Juxtaglomerular cell tumour of the kidney as cause of hypertension: a case report. *Br J Radiol* 1992;65:542–545.

310. Van Baal JG, Smits NJ, Keeman JN, Lindhout D, Verhoef S.

The evolution of renal angiomyolipomas in patients with tuberous sclerosis. *J Urol* 1994;152:35–38.

311. Varma DG, Rojo JR, Thomas R, Walker PD. Computed tomography of xanthogranulomatous pyelonephritis. *J Comput Assist Tomogr* 1985;9:241–247.

312. Vas W, Carlin B, Salimi Z, Tang-Barton P, Tucker D. CT diagnosis of emphysematous pyelonephritis. *Comput Radiol* 1985;9:37–39.

313. Vas W, Salimi Z, Tang-Barton P, Vargas F, Sidarthan AS. Computed tomography and ultrasound demonstration of squamous cell carcinoma. *Comput Tomogr* 1985;9:87–89.

314. Wacksman J, Phipps L. Report of the multicystic kidney registry: preliminary findings. *J Urol* 1993;150:1870–1872.

315. Warshauer DM, McCarthy SM, Street L, et al. Detection of renal masses: sensitivities and specificities of excretory urography/linear tomography, US, and CT. *Radiology* 1988;169:363–365.

316. Webb JAW, Reznek RH, White FE, Cattell WR, Fry IK, Baker LRI. Can ultrasound and computed tomography replace high-dose urography in patients with impaired renal function? *Q J Med* (new series 53) 1984;211:411–425.

317. Wegenke JD, Malek GH, Alter AJ, Olson JG. Acute lobular nephronia. *J Urol* 1986;135:343–345.

318. Wei LQ, Rong ZK, Gui L, Shan RD. CT Diagnosis of renal vein thrombosis in nephrotic syndrome. *J Comput Assist Tomogr* 1991;15:454–457.

319. Weinberger E, Rosenbaum DM, Pendergrass TW. Renal involvement in children with lymphomas: comparison of CT with sonography. *AJR* 1990;155:347–349.

320. Weyman PJ, McClennan BL, Stanley RJ, Levitt RG, Sagel S. Comparison of computed tomography and angiography in the evaluation of renal cell carcinoma. *Radiology* 1980;137:417–424.

321. Weyman PJ, McClennan BL, Lee JKT, Stanley RJ. CT of calcified renal masses. *AJR* 1982;138:1095–1099.

322. Wilbur AC, Turk JN, Capek V. Perirenal metastases from lung cancer: CT diagnosis. *J Comput Assist Tomogr* 1992;16:589–591.

323. Williams MA, Schropp KP, Noe HN. Fat containing renal mass in childhood: a case report of teratoid Wilms tumor. *J Urol* 1994;151:1662–1663.

324. Wills JS. Cystic adenocarcinoma of the kidney mimicking multilocular renal cyst. *Urol Radiol* 1983;5:51–53.

325. Wimbish JK, Sanders MM, Samuels BI, Francis IR. Squamous cell carcinoma of the renal pelvis: case report. *Urol Radiol* 1983;5:267–269.

326. Winfield AC, Gerlock AJ, Shaff MI. Perirenal cobwebs: a CT sign of renal vein thrombosis. *J Comput Assist Tomogr.* 1981;5:705–708.

327. Wingo PA, Tong T, Bolder S. Cancer Statistics 1995. *CA Cancer J Clin* 1995;45:8–30.

328. Winsett MZ, Amparo EG, Fawcett HD, Kumar R, Johnson RF Jr, Bedi DG, Winsett OE. Renal transplant dysfunction: MR evaluation. *AJR* 1988;150:319–323.

329. Wise GJ, Silver DA. Fungal infections of the genitourinary system. *J Urol* 1993;149:1377–1388.

330. Wolf RL, King BF, Torres VE, Wilson DM, Ehman RL. Measurement of normal renal artery blood flow: cine phase-contrast MR imaging vs clearance of *p*-aminohippurate. *AJR* 1993;161:995–1002.

331. Wong WS, Moss AA, Federle MP, Cochran ST, London SS. Renal infarction: CT diagnosis and correlation between CT findings and etiologies. *Radiology* 1984;150:201–205.

332. Yamashita Y, Takahashi M, Watanabe O, et al. Small renal cell carcinoma: pathologic and radiologic correlation. *Radiology* 1992;184:493–498.

333. Yeh HC, Halton KP, Shapiro RS, Rabinowitz JG, Mitty HA. Junctional parenchyma: revised definition of hypertrophic column of Bertin. *Radiology* 1992;185:725–732.

334. Yoder IC, Pfister RC, Lindfors KK, Newhouse JH. Pyonephrosis: imaging and intervention. *AJR* 1983;141:735–740.

335. Young SW, Noon LMA, Marincek B. Dynamic computed tomographic-density study of normal human tissue after intravenous contrast administration. *Invest Radiol* 1980;16:36–39.

336. Zagoria RJ, Wolfman NT, Karstaedt N, Hinn GC, Dyer RB, Chen YM. CT features of renal cell carcinoma with emphasis on relation to tumor size. *Invest Radiol* 1990;25:261–266.

337. Zagoria RJ, Bechtold RE, Dyer RB. Staging of renal adenocarcinoma: role of various imaging procedures. *AJR* 1995;164:363–370.

338. Zaontz MR, Pahira JJ, Wolfman M, Gargurevich AJ, Zeman RK. Acute focal bacterial nephritis: a systematic approach to diagnosis and treatment. *J Urol* 1985;133:752–757.

339. Zeman RK, Cronan JJ, Rosenfield AT, Lynch JH, Jaffe MH, Clark LR. Renal cell carcinoma: dynamic thin-section CT assessment of vascular invasion and tumor vascularity. *Radiology* 1988;167:393–396.

340. Zeman RK, Zeiberg AS, Davros WJ, et al. Routine helical CT of the abdomen: image quality considerations. *Radiology* 1993;189:395–400.

341. Zimmer WD, Williamson B Jr, Hartman GW, Hattery RR, O'Brien PC. Changing patterns in the evaluation of renal masses: economic implications. *AJR* 1984;143:285–289.

342. Zirinsky K, Auh YH, Rubenstein WA, Williams JJ, Pasmantier MW, Kazam E. CT of hyperdense renal cyst: sonographic correlation. *AJR* 1984;143:151–156.

CHAPTER 19

The Adrenals

Philip J. Kenney and Joseph K. T. Lee

Computed tomography (CT) is the primary diagnostic imaging method for evaluation of adrenal disorders. When optimal CT scanning technique is used, the normal or pathologic adrenal glands can be well visualized in virtually 100% of patients (1,73,101,158). Large and small masses and hyperplasia can be readily detected when present. With modern CT scanners, imaging of the adrenals can be achieved even in the most emaciated patients, and in patients who are unable to suspend respiration.

The adrenals can be well imaged with axial slices. Most adrenal masses can be detected with rapid scanning with 8 to 10 mm contiguous slice technique. However, thinner slices (3 to 5 mm, contiguous) should be made if small lesions are suspected or if initial screening is negative in a patient strongly suspected of having adrenal disease (Fig. 1). Both helical CT and contiguous thin slices allow better reformatted images (in sagittal or coronal plane), which sometimes can be useful in determining whether a mass arises from the adrenal, liver, or kidney. Helical CT also will avoid the potential problem of slice misregistration resulting from erratic breathing by the patient. However, helical CT images have slightly less edge sharpness (15). Whether this has any effect on diagnostic accuracy in detecting small lesions has not been established.

The normal adrenal glands and most masses can usually be detected without the use of intravenous iodinated contrast material. However, intravenous contrast may be useful to characterize the enhancement pattern of masses, improving the ability to make a specific diagnosis. Whereas general screening can be adequately done with postcontrast scans only, performance of pre- and postcontrast scans can be useful for the most accurate differential diagnosis of a mass (e.g., for distinguishing adenoma, myelolipoma, and malignancy). Rapid sequential imaging of the adrenal region after bolus injection of contrast is also helpful in distinguishing adrenal masses from adjacent vascular structures and other organs, such as the kidney, liver, and pancreas (9,12,99). Oral contrast should be used routinely as it helps delineate the gastrointestinal structures of the upper abdomen, and it helps avoid mistaking a bowel structure for an adrenal mass (9,133,134).

Great strides have been made in magnetic resonance imaging (MRI) of the abdomen; and with current techniques, the adrenals also can be delineated in nearly all patients with MRI (21,42,102,105,132). Patients who are claustrophobic, are unstable or erratic breathers, exceed the size limits, or have pacemakers cannot be evaluated with MRI. State-of-the-art MRI scanners now produce thin sections (5 to 8 mm) with good spatial resolution and signal-to-noise ratio. The use of respiratory compensation techniques, or rapid imaging sequences that can be performed during suspended respiration, produce images without significant motion artifacts. Fat-suppression methods allow avoidance of chemical shift artifact that can obscure fine detail on T2-weighted images. Fat suppression also makes normal adrenals very conspicuous on T2-weighted images: they are bright, in contrast to surrounding retroperitoneal fat. Intravenous contrast agents are now available for MRI, and they provide information about enhancement patterns of masses that is similar to that obtained with contrast-enhanced CT. Techniques sensitive to the presence of lipid (such as phase contrast or the Dixon method, STIR (short inversion time inversion recovery sequence), and radiofrequency-selective fat suppression) are most useful in differentiating between subacute hemorrhage and fat-containing adrenal masses, both of which can appear as high signal lesions on T1-weighted spin echo images.

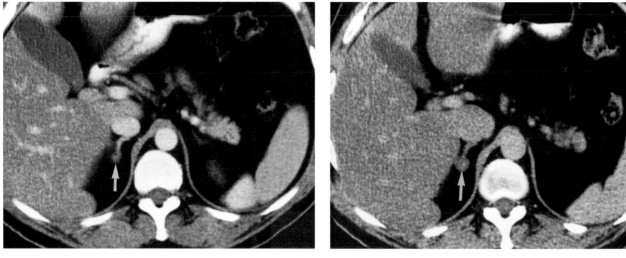

FIG. 1. Use of thinner collimation. **A:** CT with 10-mm contiguous sections demonstrates an equivocal right adrenal nodule *(arrow)*. **B:** Repeat with contiguous 3-mm sections clearly shows a small nodule *(arrow)*.

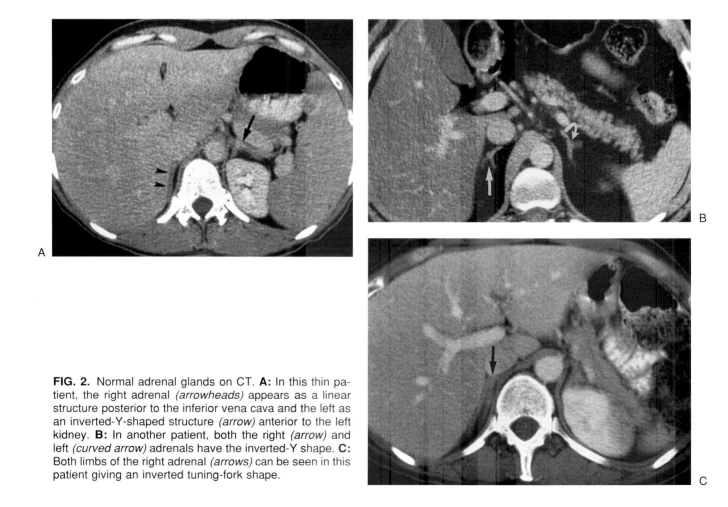

FIG. 2. Normal adrenal glands on CT. **A:** In this thin patient, the right adrenal *(arrowheads)* appears as a linear structure posterior to the inferior vena cava and the left as an inverted-Y-shaped structure *(arrow)* anterior to the left kidney. **B:** In another patient, both the right *(arrow)* and left *(curved arrow)* adrenals have the inverted-Y shape. **C:** Both limbs of the right adrenal *(arrows)* can be seen in this patient giving an inverted tuning-fork shape.

An MRI evaluation of the adrenals should usually consist of both T1- and T2-weighted images. Either spin echo or gradient refocused echo (GRE) T1-weighted images are acceptable, with rapid GRE T1-weighted images during a breath-hold preferred, as they take less time and provide sharper images. T2-weighted images done with fat suppression also provide better margination of the adrenals and masses. Whether standard or fast spin echo sequences are better for detection and characterization of adrenal lesions has not been clearly determined, but fast imaging sequences can result in good quality images in less time. T1-weighted GRE images performed with an echo time (TE) at which lipid and water protons are in opposed phases are useful, because loss of signal documents the presence of lipid (97,145). Dynamic serial T1-weighted images obtained after intravenous administration of gadolinium diethylene-triamine penta-acetic acid (Gd-DTPA) are used to show enhancement patterns of adrenal masses (84). Whereas axial images are standard, coronal and sagittal images may be useful for displaying anatomic relationships of large adrenal masses, and for detecting the organ of origin of a large mass. Despite the many improvements in MRI that allow more rapid data acquisition, an MRI examination of the adrenals is still a relatively lengthy procedure compared to CT, because several different imaging sequences must be performed.

NORMAL ANATOMY

The adrenal glands are paired retroperitoneal organs that lie in a suprarenal location and are enclosed within the perinephric fascia. They are surrounded by a variable amount of retroperitoneal fat. The right adrenal is usually seen directly superior to the upper pole of the right kidney (Figs. 2,3), with its most caudal portion just anterior to the upper pole. The right adrenal is directly posterior to the inferior vena cava and insinuates between the right lobe

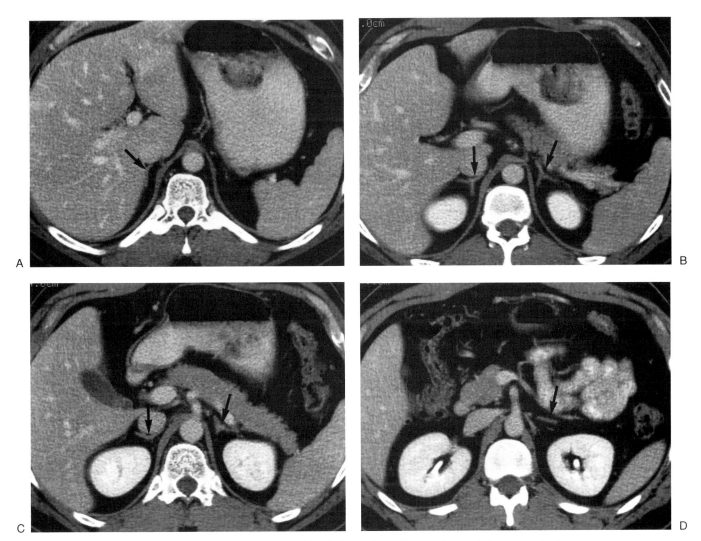

FIG. 3. Normal adrenal glands on CT. **A,B,C:** Note the different shape of the adrenals *(arrows)* on each sequential section. **D:** The left adrenal ends at the level of the left renal vein.

of the liver and the right crus of the diaphragm. If there is a paucity of retroperitoneal fat, the right adrenal can be difficult to visualize, but with state-of-the-art CT it is usually recognizable (Fig. 2). The left adrenal may be seen at the same level as the right, but often it is slightly more caudal. It is anteromedial to the upper pole of the left kidney and is usually seen on CT in the same slice as the left kidney. The left adrenal lies lateral to the aorta and the left diaphragmatic crus, and superior to the left renal vein. A portion of the pancreas or the splenic vessels may be immediately anterior to the left adrenal. When performing a dedicated (thin section) CT of the adrenals, it is important to obtain a sufficient number of images, because the adrenals each extend about 2 to 4 cm in craniocaudal direction, and because masses may protrude superiorly or inferiorly, with other slices showing apparently normal adrenal morphology.

The adrenals have a complex three-dimensional shape; this results in a variety of appearances on cross-sectional images. Both glands anatomically have a medial and a lateral limb extending posteriorly from a central ridge. The right adrenal may appear as a linear structure paralleling the diaphragmatic crus (Fig. 2). This appearance is a result of visualization of the medial limb, without recognition of the lateral limb, which is often closely apposed to the liver. With excellent technique, both limbs of the right adrenal can be seen, resulting in an inverted tuning fork shape (Fig. 2). Inverted V, Y, L, and other configurations may be seen (101,158). The left adrenal most often has an inverted V or Y shape, but it may be triangular or have other shapes (101,158) (Fig. 2). Commonly, the adrenals in an individual have a slightly different configuration on each slice (Fig. 3). The most caudal portions of both adrenals may appear as horizontal linear structures. The adrenals have the same shape on axial MRI as on CT (Figs. 4,5). On coronal views, the adrenals usually

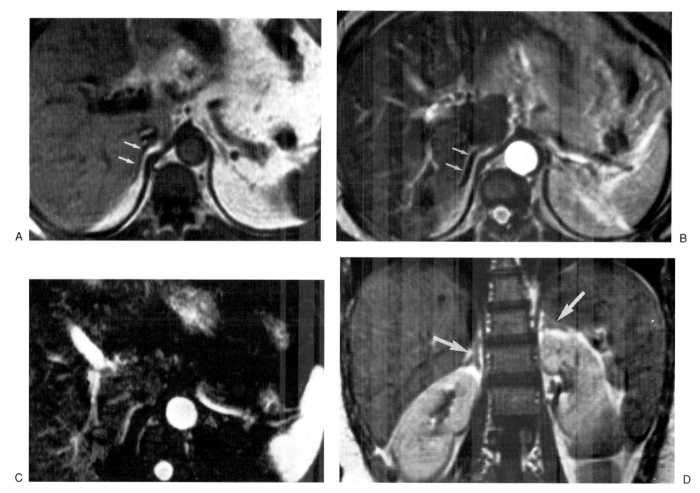

FIG. 4. Normal adrenal glands on MRI. **A:** The linear-appearing normal right adrenal *(arrows)* is clearly seen with lower signal than the liver on this T1-weighted GRE scan (2-D FLASH) (130/4/80°) done during suspended respiration. **B:** On heavily T2-weighted spin echo image (2300/90), the right adrenal *(arrows)* appears nearly isointense with liver. **C:** On fat-suppressed T2-weighted image (2300/90), the adrenal is seen free of chemical shift artifact, but the gland now appears hyperintense to liver. **D:** Coronal T1-weighted spin echo image (500/15) after gadolinium DTPA shows the adrenals *(arrows)* remain nearly isointense with the liver, whereas the kidneys are brightly enhanced.

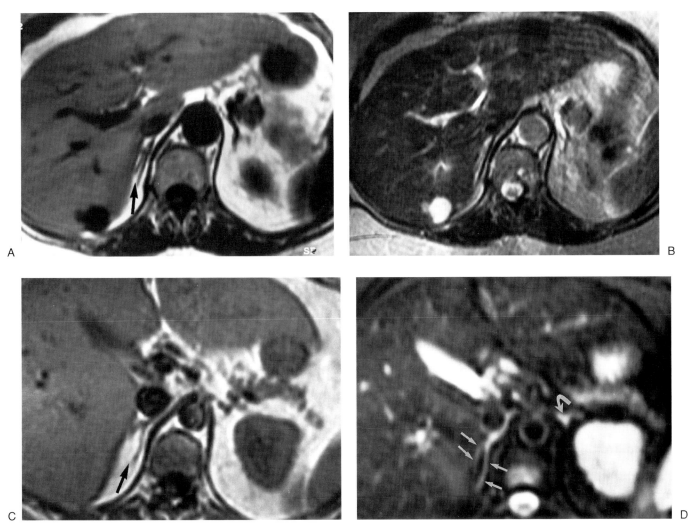

FIG. 5. Normal adrenal glands on MRI. **A,C:** In these two different patients, T1-weighted spin echo images (TR 500 ms, TE 15 ms) show the right adrenals as bilimbed structures *(arrows)*. **B:** On standard T2-weighted image (TR 2000 ms, TE 80 ms), both adrenals are not as clearly defined as in A because of chemical shift artifact. **D:** With the use of fat suppression (TR 1800 ms, TE 80 ms), both limbs of the right adrenal *(arrows)* as well as the left adrenal are more clearly defined (compare with C).

are seen as inverted V- or Y-shaped structures just superior to the upper poles of the kidneys (Fig. 4).

On precontrast CT, the adrenals have a soft-tissue density similar to that of the liver. If very early postcontrast scans are obtained, there is considerable enhancement, which fades quickly to moderate enhancement—slightly less than that of liver (Fig. 6). The adrenal cortex and medulla cannot be reliably distinguished by either CT or MRI. On T1-weighted MRI images, the adrenals have a medium signal intensity, similar to that of the liver, somewhat greater than the diaphragmatic crus but much less than the surrounding fat (21,25). On standard T2-weighted images, the adrenals are hypointense to fat and isointense to liver, but they are hyperintense to the crus (Fig. 4). There is less difference between adrenal and fat signal intensities on T2-weighted images, and significant chemical shift artifact may obscure details of

the normal adrenals (Fig. 5). On fat-suppressed T2-weighted images, however, the normal adrenals appear somewhat brighter than liver, and are much brighter than the suppressed fat (Fig. 5). Thus, normal adrenals and small masses are best seen on T1-weighted or fat-suppressed T2-weighted images. The normal adrenals do not demonstrate marked enhancement after intravenous administration of gadolinium compounds. The adrenals can be clearly separated from adjacent vessels because of the signal void phenomenon on spin echo images or flow enhancement on GRE images.

There are no standardized measurements of normal adrenal size, and there is considerable variability in the lengths of the limbs. However, the surface of the adrenals should be quite smooth, without protruding nodules, and the limbs should have uniform thickness. Although no strict measurements have been standardized, any area

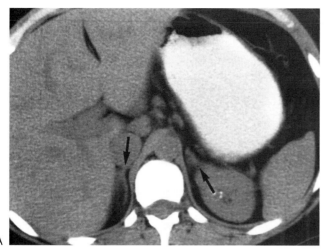

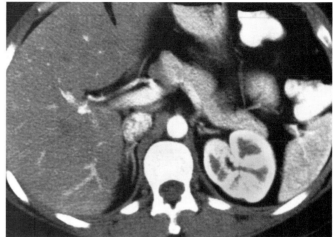

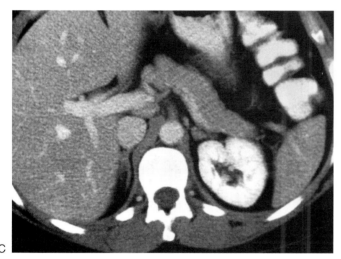

FIG. 6. Normal adrenal glands: enhancement pattern on helical CT. **A:** Precontrast CT image shows both right and left adrenal glands *(arrows)* have attenuation similar to the diaphragmatic crura. **B:** Immediately following rapid bolus intravenous injection of 125 ml of nonionic iodinated contrast, both adrenals show bright enhancement, brighter than liver or crura. **C:** At 90 seconds after contrast, the enhancement is similar to that of the liver.

thicker than 10 mm is probably abnormal (73,101). It must be recognized that in the face of stress (as may be seen in severely ill patients), the adrenals may become enlarged in response to physiologically high circulating adrenocorticotropic hormone (ACTH) levels (Fig. 7).

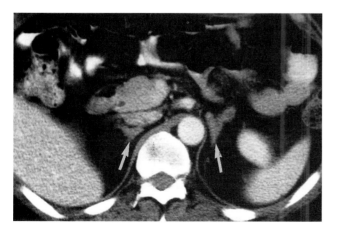

FIG. 7. Stress-induced adrenal hyperplasia. Both adrenals *(arrows)* show smooth thickening in this patient undergoing treatment for staphylococcal sepsis.

Congenital absence of the adrenal glands is quite rare (119). The vast majority of patients with renal agenesis or ectopy do have an ipsilateral adrenal gland (75,119). However, in such patients the adrenal is in the shape of a flat disc parallel to the spine. On cross-sectional images with CT or MRI, these glands will be seen as linear structures (Fig. 8), either in the expected location or slightly more caudal. In contrast, patients who have had simple nephrectomy, or who have undergone severe renal atrophy, the adrenals have a normal shape (75). There may be greater difficulty evaluating the adrenals in such patients, because removal of the perinephric fascia and the kidneys allows other organs to move adjacent to the adrenals—bowel loops on the right; medial movement of the tail of the pancreas; and bowel loops, splenic vessels, or spleen on the left.

PSEUDOTUMORS

A variety of normal structures may simulate an adrenal mass if meticulous technique is not used (9). The routine use of oral contrast and rapid scanning after bolus intrave-

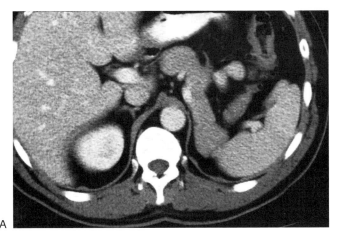 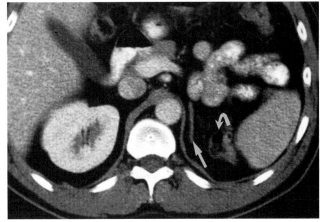

FIG. 8. Anomalous adrenal in patient with renal agenesis. **A:** Note the normal right adrenal, and the posteromedial placement of the tail of the pancreas. **B:** More inferiorly, the left adrenal *(arrow)* is seen with a linear configuration; note the medially placed splenic flexure of the colon *(curved arrow).*

nous contrast will usually allow these pseudotumors to be distinguished from true adrenal masses. Pseudotumors are less common on the right, because there are fewer adjacent organs. Rarely, the duodenum or colon may produce a mass-like appearance (134). Either an accessory spleen or the presence of the pancreatic tail in an unusual location may produce a rounded structure in the region of the left adrenal (Fig. 9). Most often, a splenic lobulation can be seen to connect with the spleen if contiguous slices are done, and both splenic lobulations and accessory spleens will have the same attenuation value as the spleen on pre- and postcontrast scans. Either tortuous or dilated splenic arteries and veins can simulate a left adrenal mass (9,12,99). This is particularly common when there is portal hypertension; the left inferior phrenic vein that passes

immediately anterior to the left adrenal may dilate as a collateral pathway from the splenic vein to the left renal vein (12). These vascular pseudotumors can be identified by their tubular nature, which can be recognized on sequential contiguous slices as well as by their bright enhancement after intravenous administration of iodinated contrast medium. Adjacent bowel, particularly a gastric diverticulum (133,138) or redundant gastric fundus (Fig. 10), and occasionally a small bowel loop, may be misconstrued as a left adrenal mass if there is not adequate oral contrast.

Pseudotumors present less of a difficulty to MRI, partly because of the multiplanar imaging capability and partly because of the ease with which pathologic masses, which have moderate signal intensity, can be distinguished from

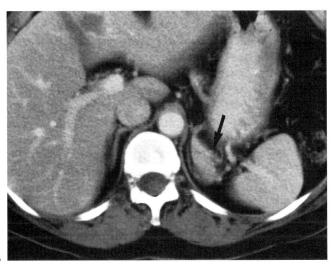 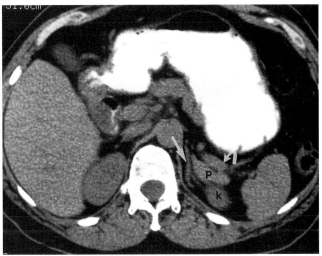

FIG. 9. Adrenal pseudotumor. **A:** Routine CT done with 10-mm contiguous slice technique shows a possible left adrenal mass *(arrow).* **B:** Repeat CT with contiguous 3-mm slices shows the normal left adrenal *(arrow);* volume averaging of the tail of the pancreas accounted for the adrenal pseudotumor (P, pancreas; k, upper pole of left kidney; *curved arrow,* splenic vein).

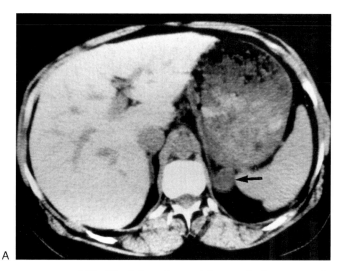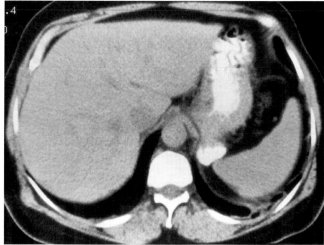

A

B

FIG. 10. Adrenal pseudotumor. **A:** An apparent mass is seen in the region of the left adrenal *(arrow)* on this CT done without oral contrast. **B:** Following oral contrast administration, CT shows the apparent mass was a gastric diverticulum. The normal left adrenal was seen more inferiorly.

vessels, which either have signal void on spin echo images or very bright signal on GRE sequences.

PATHOLOGY

A variety of pathologic processes can affect the adrenal glands. Some cause endocrine disorders (functional diseases), either hyperfunction or adrenal insufficiency, and some do not produce biochemical abnormalities. Although both CT and MRI provide accurate depiction of the adrenal morphology, both functional and nonfunctional disorders may produce similar appearances, so correlation of imaging findings with the endocrine status is usually necessary for diagnosis. In patients with biochemical evidence of adrenal hyperfunction, a CT examination is valuable because of its ability to differentiate between a focal mass, hyperplastic glands, and normal adrenals. A pathologic diagnosis can usually be made based on the imaging appearance of an adrenal mass and the clinical history, even when there is no adrenal dysfunction. Thus, other diagnostic studies can be avoided. MRI has diagnostic capabilities equivalent to those of CT. Detection of small masses and documentation of normal adrenal morphology can probably be better done with CT, because of its better spatial resolution. However, MRI has better tissue characterization capabilities, which may be useful in certain circumstances.

The accuracy of CT for diagnosis of adrenal masses has been reported as being better than 90% (1,39,83). With proper technique, masses smaller than 5 mm can be detected. A normal appearance of the adrenal effectively excludes the presence of an adrenal tumor. Because many small adrenal masses are isodense with adrenal tissue, they are detected as focal bulges on the otherwise smooth adrenal surface. Focal enlargement is

a more important finding than any measurement. Some small masses have only a minimal attachment to the adrenal, whereas large masses may obliterate the adrenal glands. Inability to visualize a normal adrenal is suggestive of adrenal origin, but extra-adrenal malignant masses can engulf or invade the adrenal. If an adrenal mass becomes very large, its exact site of origin can be difficult to determine, especially on CT. Large hepatic, renal, or retroperitoneal tumors may simulate an adrenal mass. In these cases, demonstration of a normal adrenal gland essentially excludes the possibility that the mass is adrenal in origin. Conversely, the presence of adrenal hyperfunction confirms an adrenal origin. The pattern of displacement of organs likewise may be helpful in determining the center of origin, because most tumors grow centrifugally. Right adrenal masses typically displace the kidney inferiorly, and the inferior vena cava anteriorly, whereas hepatic masses rarely displace the vena cava anteriorly. Computed reconstructions along other orthogonal planes may help in recognizing the origin of such a large mass. On MRI, with multiplanar imaging and better tissue contrast, it is often easier to determine the organ of origin of an upper abdominal mass. The distinction between an adrenal and a renal mass can be achieved by MRI if the upper pole renal cortex is shown to be intact.

Adrenal hyperplasia may result in diffuse thickening of the adrenal glands, but retention of the normal shape. This enlargement is usually smooth, but there may be nodularity. However, bilateral enlargement, whether smooth or nodular, is indicative of hyperplasia. A significant number of patients with clinical and biochemical evidence of hyperplasia will have normal adrenals with CT (63,117). In part, this is because there may be significant hyperfunction of the adrenal cortex before enough thickening has occurred to be recognizable. Thus, a normal appearance of the adrenals does not exclude hyperplasia. With current CT technique, focal nodules are frequently noted in hyperplastic glands. These are usually smaller than 5 mm, but they can be several centimeters in size (35,142). Adrenal hyperplasia can be diagnosed when there are bilateral nodules or when there is nodularity associated with bilateral adrenal thickening. With primary functional adrenal tumors, the ipsilateral remaining adrenal tissue and contralateral adrenal gland should be normal or atrophic. However, it is not always possible to distinguish an adenoma from a solitary hyperplastic nodule by CT.

Detection of hyperplasia is important in evaluation of patients with functional disorders. Although both MRI and CT can show markedly enlarged glands, CT is preferable because it is better able to detect subtle alterations of adrenal morphology. On MRI, hyperplastic adrenals can be seen to be enlarged, but the signal intensity of the tissue is similar to that of normal adrenal gland. On occasion, the adrenals are found to be enlarged in patients with no evidence of adrenal dysfunction. These findings are not clinically significant. A number of conditions have been associated with such nonspecific hyperplasia, including acromegaly (100%), hyperthyroidism (40%), hypertension with arteriosclerosis (16%), diabetes mellitus (3%), and a variety of malignancies (142). In some cases, this adrenal enlargement is a response to physiologic stress (Fig. 7). On imaging, the appearance is indistinguishable from hyperplasia producing adrenal hyperfunction.

Magnetic resonance imaging has several advantages in evaluating adrenal pathology. In addition to depicting the morphology of the adrenal, MRI can show the signal intensity of various types of masses on different imaging sequences, which may allow more specific characterization. Whereas the magnetic susceptibility effect of acute hemorrhage is best demonstrated on GRE images, subacute hematoma can be best seen on T1-weighted GRE or spin echo sequences. Although mature fat can be identified on T1-weighted or fat-suppressed images, other lipid-containing structures are discernible by using opposed phase imaging. Benign tissues, such as hyperplasia and adenoma, are rather similar in signal intensity to normal adrenal tissue, whereas malignancy is typically heterogeneously hyperintense on T2-weighted images. The local extent of malignant disease may show up well, especially with fat-suppressed T2-weighted images and multiplanar scanning. MRI has been shown to be comparable to CT in detection of adrenal masses.

CUSHING SYNDROME

Cushing syndrome results from excess production of cortisol by the adrenal cortex. In about 85% of cases, this is a result of excess ACTH production (an ACTH-dependent disorder) resulting from a pituitary adenoma or hyperplasia (80%), or coming from an ectopic source (71). The dexamethasone suppression test can aid in distinguishing pituitary from ectopic sources of elevated ACTH, because urinary cortisol secretion is not suppressed in cases of ectopic ACTH (71). About 15% of cases of Cushing syndrome are ACTH independent, usually due to a cortical adenoma or adrenal carcinoma, rarely secondary to primary nodular hyperplasia (71,116). Adrenal CT is performed in patients with Cushing syndrome to distinguish ACTH-dependent (hyperplasia) from ACTH-independent (focal mass) disorders, and to determine the location of the focal mass in the latter. In patients with an adenoma or a carcinoma, the remaining ipsilateral and the contralateral adrenals are normal or atrophic. Surgical removal of an adenoma (or of a resectable carcinoma) is curative. Biochemical testing can be extremely useful.

Computed tomography is virtually 100% accurate for detection of adrenal adenomas resulting in hypercortisolism (36,39,63). These adenomas are almost always over 2 cm at the time of presentation, are usually in the range 2 to 5 cm (32), and are readily seen on CT, especially because these patients have abundant retroperitoneal fat (Figs. 11,12). The masses are smooth, round or oval, and relatively homogeneous, with little enhancement after intravenous contrast. Most often they have a soft-tissue-attenuation value, but they may be near water attenuation because of relatively high lipid content (100,130). Calcification can be found in adenomas, although it is rare (76). The contralateral adrenal is commonly visibly thinner than normal, indicating atrophy from ACTH suppression (Fig. 12). With these findings, and in the proper clinical setting, no further investigation is needed. It should be noted that the CT appearances of different types of adenomas are indistin-

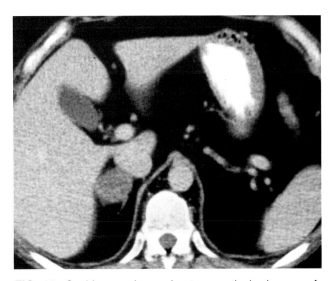

FIG. 11. Cushing syndrome due to a cortical adenoma. A round, 2.9-cm mass is seen in the right adrenal; the left was normal. Surgery confirmed a cortical adenoma.

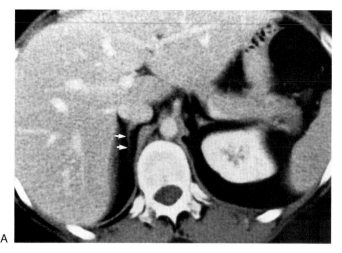 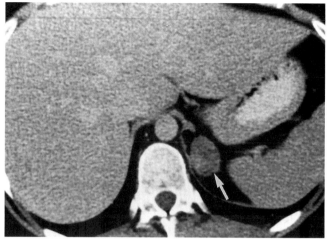

A   B

FIG. 12. Cushing syndrome due to a cortical adenoma. **A:** The right adrenal *(arrows)* is atrophic in this patient with hypercortisolism. **B:** More superiorly, there is a 2.5 × 3 cm left adrenal mass *(arrow).*

guishable, whether they produce excess cortisol or aldosterone, or they are not hyperfunctioning (125).

Magnetic resonance imaging is equally accurate in patients with such adenomas, because of their size (116). Typically, the signal intensity of the adenomas is similar to that of liver on T1-weighted images, and similar or only slightly greater on T2-weighted images (Fig. 13) (42,124). After intravenous administration of gadolinium compounds, enhancement is only moderate, it is relatively

homogeneous, and it shows significant washout in 10 minutes in most cases (92). The presence of intracellular lipid can be documented by the phase-contrast method (97). Although adrenal adenomas and cysts may have similar attenuation values on CT, they are readily distinguished on MRI, because cysts are very hyperintense on T2-weighted images and do not enhance.

A normal CT or MRI appearance does not exclude hyperplasia (117). In fact, in the absence of a focal mass,

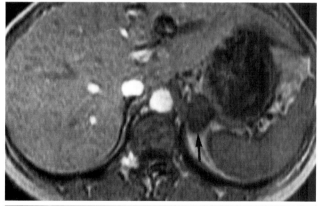 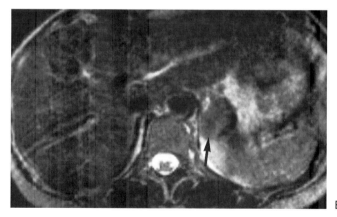

A   B

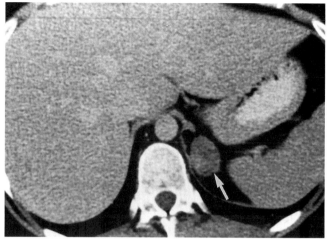

C

FIG. 13. Cushing syndrome due to a cortical adenoma. **A:** T1-weighted GRE (144/6/75°) image done during suspended respiration shows a homogeneous 2.2 × 3.2 cm mass in the left adrenal *(arrow)* with signal intensity slightly less than that of liver. **B:** On T2-weighted image (2000/90), the mass *(arrow)* is lower signal than fat, similar to liver. **C:** Following intravenous administration of gadolinium DTPA. T1-weighted GRE scan (144/6/75°) shows only mild enhancement, which rapidly washed out. Surgery confirmed the lesion was a cortical adenoma.

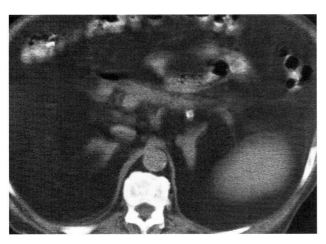

FIG. 14. Adrenal hyperplasia due to ectopic ACTH. This patient with carcinoma of the lung developed hypercortisolism. CT shows increased retroperitoneal fat and marked smooth thickening of both adrenals.

a patient with biochemical evidence of hypercortisolism and normal adrenals can confidently be given the diagnosis of hyperplasia as long as exogenous steroid use is excluded. Most often, both adrenals become smoothly thickened due to excess ACTH. The thickening may become massive, especially with ectopic ACTH production (32) (Fig. 14). Adrenal nodules ranging from 6 mm to 7 cm may be seen in 12% to 15% of patients with ACTH-dependent Cushing syndrome (32) (Fig. 15). Although usually bilateral, such nodules may be unilateral (117). Careful examination will usually show some evidence of bilateral enlargement. Primary pigmented nodular adrenocortical disease is a rare disorder producing Cushing syn-

drome. It tends to present in younger patients than the other types of Cushing syndrome. Elevated cortisol is found, with very low ACTH levels. On CT, multiple bilateral nodules up to 3 cm are typical. Unlike macronodular hyperplasia due to excess ACTH, the cortex between the nodules is atrophic (33,34). On MRI, the nodules are relatively low signal on both T1- and T2-weighted images.

PRIMARY ALDOSTERONISM

Primary aldosteronism (Conn syndrome) results from excess adrenal production of the mineralocorticoid aldosterone. It is characterized by reduced plasma renin levels, hypokalemia, and hypertension. Biochemical tests for the disorder indicate the inability to suppress aldosterone excretion with normal saline infusion, and the lack of change in serum aldosterone levels with postural change (13). As many as 95% of cases result from an autonomous cortical adenoma (aldosteronoma); most of the remaining cases result from primary idiopathic bilateral hyperplasia (121). A few rare cases have been reported to have resulted from bilateral adenomas, unilateral hyperplasia, and adrenal carcinoma (54,143). Correct diagnosis is important, because surgical removal of an aldosteronoma is curative (121), but partial and even bilateral total adrenalectomy commonly fails to cure hypertension in patients with hyperplasia (57).

On CT, aldosteronomas appear as round or oval lesions, similar to other adenomas, but typically smaller than cortisol-producing adenomas (38,49,121,157) (Fig. 16). They are rarely over 3 cm, and usually in the range 5 to 35 mm, with a median size of 16 to 17 mm (38,121). Because of a relatively high lipid content, they often

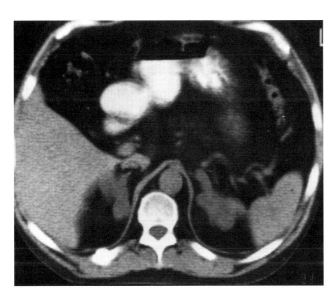

FIG. 15. Cushing's syndrome due to massive nodular hyperplasia. CT reveals marked enlargement of both adrenals with multiple large nodules. Patient underwent adrenalectomy, confirming nodular adrenal hyperplasia.

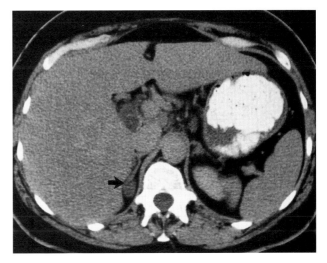

FIG. 16. Aldosteronoma. CT image shows a 1-cm mass in the medial limb of the left adrenal *(arrow)*. The mass has an attenuation value slightly lower than that of adjacent normal adrenal tissue.

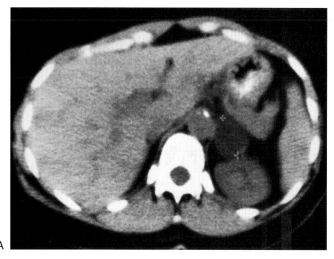 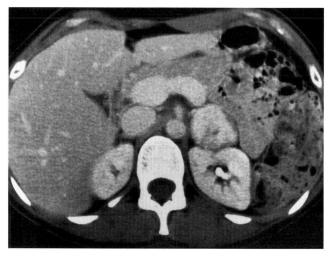

A   B

FIG. 17. Aldosteronomas. **A:** CT without intravenous contrast in this patient with hyperaldosteronism shows a low-attenuation (−14 HU) mass arising in the left adrenal; although the homogeneous low attenuation simulates a cyst, a 3-cm solid aldosteronoma (with a large lipid component) was resected. **B:** A 4-cm left adrenal mass with marked heterogeneous enhancement is shown in this patient with hyperaldosteronism; surgical resection confirmed aldosteronoma.

(50%) have an attenuation value similar to that of water (−10 to +10) (38,100) (Fig. 17). This propensity for low attenuation should be recognized, so that a low-attenuation mass discovered in a patient with documented hyperaldosteronism is not misdiagnosed as a cyst.

Because aldosteronomas are typically small, they present a greater challenge than cortisol-producing adenomas. Early publications reported a sensitivity of 70% with several false negative CTs because of inability to detect small aldosteronomas (49,157). With better quality, thin-section CT, a sensitivity of 80% to 90% has been achieved (38,67). With the 5-mm-section technique, false negatives are uncommon (12% to 14%) (38,54).

Primary adrenal hyperplasia causing aldosteronism may be micronodular or macronodular. The adrenals may appear normal or diffusely thickened on CT (Fig. 18). One or more discrete nodules ranging from 7 to 16 mm may be seen (121) (Fig. 19). Diagnostic errors may occur because of a unilateral nodule that simulates an adenoma on CT. Conversely, tiny bilateral nodules that are present in 25% of patients with aldosteronomas (30) may result in an erroneous diagnosis of hyperplasia. An accuracy of 80% for CT showing lack of lateralization (either both glands are normal, both are enlarged, or there are bilateral nodules) has been reported (54). Because of these potential difficulties, adrenal venous sampling still can be useful in certain patients. Some have advocated routine adrenal venous sampling if bilateral nodules are seen on CT (35). When properly done, biochemical testing of adrenal vein samples can have a diagnostic accuracy of nearly 100% (13,49); however, technical failures are common in unexperienced hands. Misleading information can result if the data are not obtained and interpreted correctly (54). For example, an inadequate sample from the right adrenal

vein would result in apparent lateralization to the left adrenal in a case of bilateral hyperplasia. Obtaining both aldosterone and cortisol levels in all blood samples, and correlation of venous sampling results with CT will help to avoid such errors.

Although aldosteronomas can be shown with MRI, there is no advantage of MRI over CT (67). Because many aldosteronomas are small, the lesser spatial resolution of MRI is a theoretical disadvantage. Aldosteronomas are not distinguishable from other adenomas by any MRI feature.

Adrenal CT should be performed first to evaluate a patient with biochemical evidence of primary hyperaldosteronism. Certain biochemical features are strongly in-

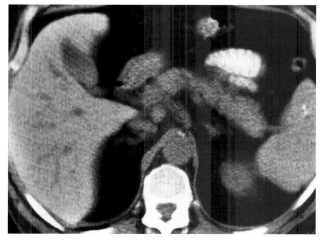

FIG. 18. Conn syndrome due to adrenal hyperplasia. CT shows no focal mass; adrenal venous sampling revealed bilateral elevated aldosterone levels.

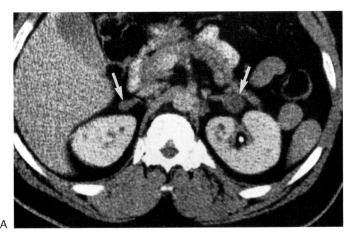
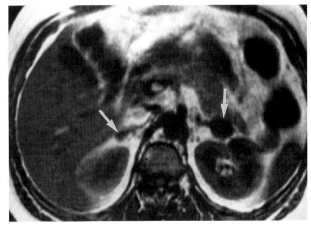

A B

FIG. 19. Conn syndrome due to adrenal hyperplasia. **A:** Bilateral nodular enlargement of the adrenals *(arrows)* is shown by CT. **B:** T1-weighted MRI image also shows bilateral nodularity *(arrows)*. Adrenal venous sampling confirmed bilateral excess aldosterone levels.

dicative of an aldosteronoma (13), and CT should be done to locate the tumor before surgical removal. If the imaging study is inconclusive, adrenal venous sampling should be done and all diagnostic studies correlated prior to surgery.

ADRENAL CARCINOMA

Adrenal carcinoma is a highly malignant neoplasm that arises in the adrenal cortex. It is rare, with an incidence estimated at two cases per million population (65). It can occur at any age, with a median age of about 40 years (45,66,118). Men and women are affected about equally, although there is a slightly greater propensity for women to have functioning neoplasms (66). About 50% of adrenal carcinomas will produce an endocrine disorder. Cushing syndrome is commonest, seen in about 50% of adrenal carcinoma patients, and it accounts for 65% of the functional disorders. Cushing syndrome may be seen alone or in combination with virilization. Virilization alone, feminization, and aldosteronism may be seen, in order of decreasing frequency (10,66,118,143).

Adrenal carcinomas often are very large when first detected. This is especially true of nonfunctioning tumors, which remain clinically silent until very advanced, when they may be discovered because of flank pain, fatigue, palpable mass, or evidence of metastases. Even functioning tumors are usually large when presenting, which may be a result of relatively inefficient production of hormone, so that a very large mass is needed to produce enough functioning hormone to result in a clinical disorder (91). Average size at presentation is 12 cm (range, 3 to 30 cm) (37,45,66). Today, however, with the widespread use of imaging, some of these neoplasms are discovered incidentally (66) and are smaller than previously reported. The histology of adrenocortical carcinoma is variable. It can be difficult to distinguish a well-differentiated carcinoma

from an adenoma, even with a resected specimen. Needle biopsy may be nondiagnostic. Correlation of histology with radiologic features, and sometimes biologic behavior, is needed for diagnosis (27). The overall prognosis is very poor, with 5-year survival of 20% to 25% (10,118). However, prognosis is better (42% to 57%) for localized (stage I) adrenal carcinomas if complete surgical resection can be accomplished (10,66,118). Effective chemotherapy is not available.

Adrenal carcinomas are readily detected by CT. Most often they are seen as large, irregularly shaped, heterogeneous masses in the adrenal region (Figs. 20,21). Both right and left are affected equally, with bilateral disease seen in less than 10% (10). At least some central areas of low attenuation are common (45), because of necrosis. Calcification is found in about 40% (76) (Fig. 21). Hetero-

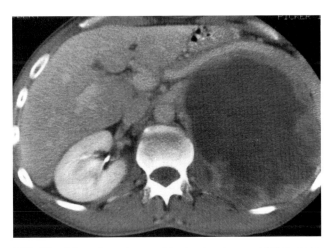

FIG. 20. Adrenal carcinoma. Contrast-enhanced CT reveals a large mass with low-attenuation center and irregular, nodular, enhancing wall which displaced the left kidney inferiorly, the spleen superiorly, and the stomach and pancreas anteriorly.

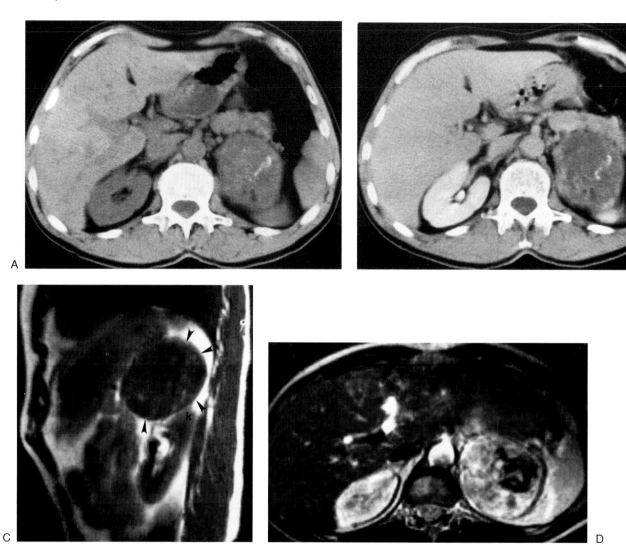

FIG. 21. Adrenal carcinoma. **A:** Precontrast CT shows a heterogeneous 8-cm left adrenal mass containing a small amount of calcification. **B:** The mass shows moderate, heterogeneous enhancement after contrast. **C:** Sagittal T1-weighted image (300/20) shows the mass *(arrowheads)* to be separate from the kidney (k). Note the mass has a few bright foci. **D:** While largely of similar signal intensity to fat, some low-signal areas are present on T2-weighted image (1600/80).

geneous enhancement after intravenous contrast is typical, with strong enhancement of the periphery and little enhancement centrally (45). The tumors may be poorly marginated, or they may show local invasion. Invasion of the inferior vena cava, liver metastases, and retroperitoneal lymph adenopathy may be seen. In general, especially in functioning cases, adrenal carcinomas can be diagnosed by CT, as the above features are clearly different from those of an adenoma or hyperplasia. If an incidental tumor is seen, however, it may be more difficult to discriminate from an adenoma on CT, as both may be less than 5 cm, well circumscribed, and homogeneous (45).

On MRI, adrenal carcinomas are easily seen as large heterogeneous masses in the adrenal bed, with areas isointense or hypointense to liver on T1-weighted images, and isointense or hyperintense to fat on T2-weighted images

(21,124,140) (Figs. 21,22). Areas of hemorrhage may result in variable signal intensity dependent on the age of the hemorrhage. With multiplanar capability and the high tissue contrast of T2-weighted images, MRI can be useful to define the adrenal origin and the extent of disease (Fig. 21). After injection of gadolinium, bright heterogeneous enhancement is seen (84) (Fig. 22). The high sensitivity of MRI for venous involvement and liver disease make it helpful for staging; venous extension is a poor prognostic sign (127), and if metastases are present surgery is not indicated. Although poorly differentiated malignant tissue does not contain lipid, more well-differentiated areas in functioning tumors may show a slight decrease in signal on the opposed phase images, thereby simulating adenoma (131). However, a correct diagnosis can be made confidently when all imaging features are taken into account.

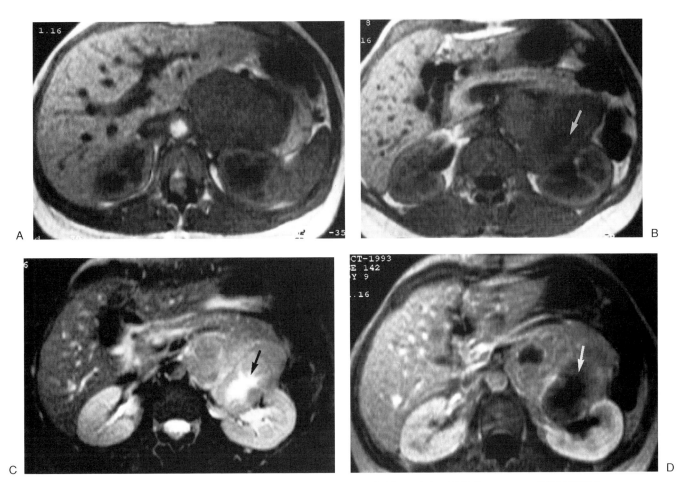

FIG. 22. Cushing syndrome due to adrenal carcinoma. **A:** T1-weighted GRE sequence (150/6/70°7) shows a large (6 ×1 8 ×1 11 cm) lobular left adrenal mass; note the left renal cortex is clearly intact. **B:** At a slightly more caudal level, a low signal area is present *(arrow)*. **C:** On T2-weighted sequence (2800/80) (with fat suppression) most of the mass is moderately hyperintense, with a very hyperintense area *(arrow)* corresponding to the low signal area on T1. **D:** Following intravenous administration of Gd-DTPA (150/6/70°7), there is early heterogeneous enhancement; note the non-enhancing region *(arrow)*, which corresponds to the area that was low signal on T1 and high on T2, representing an area of necrosis.

PHEOCHROMOCYTOMA

A pheochromocytoma is a neoplasm of the adrenal medulla that contains chromaffin cells and causes excess catecholamine production. When such a tumor arises outside the adrenal, it is properly labeled a paraganglioma, because such lesions arise from paraganglia, neural crest cell derivatives that are in close proximity to the sympathetic chain. Most are benign, although about 10% are malignant. Sporadic cases are usually unilateral, affecting the right adrenal slightly more frequently; about 5% are bilateral (95) (Fig. 23). Most patients are hypertensive. Although paroxysmal hypertensive episodes, including symptomatic hypertensive crises, are considered classic, 15% have sustained hypertension without paroxysms (95). Between paroxysmal episodes, some patients are normotensive and others have sustained hypertension (95). The increased catecholamine production is usually

reflected by elevated serum or urinary catecholamine levels, or by urine vanillylmandelic acid (VMA) or metanephrine levels. There are more false negative results with VMA than metanephrines. In most cases, diagnosis of pheochromocytoma can be established with biochemical testing, especially if the plasma catecholamine levels are markedly elevated (over 2,000 pg/ml) (14). However, biochemical tests are expensive, time consuming, and fraught with difficulty, because such factors as episodic catecholamine production, concurrent medication, stress, inadequate urine collection for 24-hour samples, and other factors can contribute to both false positive and false negative results for every known test. Detection and localization are important because surgical resection is curative, and because there is no effective medical therapy. Unrecognized and untreated pheochromocytoma often results in untimely death due to complications of surgery, or due to long-term complications such as myocardial

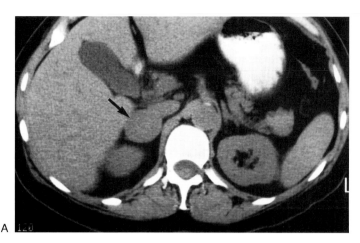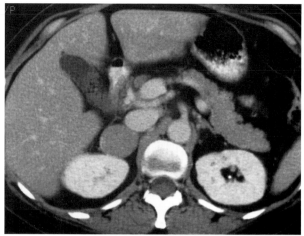

FIG. 23. Pheochromocytoma. **A:** Precontrast CT shows a 3-cm right adrenal mass *(arrow)*; note the left adrenal is normal. **B:** The mass shows mild enhancement after intravenous contrast.

infarction and cerebral vascular disease (145). Thus, imaging can play an important role in evaluation of patients suspected of pheochromocytoma.

Pheochromocytoma is found in less than 1% of the hypertensive population, and in 0.3% of autopsies (145). Clinical signs suggestive of the diagnosis include labile hypertension, including paroxysms of hypertension and tachycardia, headache, palpitation, diaphoresis, pallor, and weight loss (145). There is an increased likelihood of pheochromocytoma in patients with neurofibromatosis, von Hippel-Lindau disease, and multiple endocrine neoplasia (MEN) syndromes (50% in MEN 2 and 90% in MEN 2b). In such syndromes and in children, multiple or bilateral cases are more likely. In MEN 2b, bilateral tumors are so common that bilateral adrenalectomy is recommended, because lesions may recur after unilateral surgery (16,70) (Fig. 24).

Although 90% of pheochromocytomas arise in the ad-

renal, up to 10% are extra-adrenal (Figs. 24–26), with many such lesions (7%) in the infrarenal portion of the retroperitoneum, arising in the organ of Zuckerkandl (60) (Fig. 26). Paragangliomas can be single or multiple, and they may have greater malignant potential (60). Paragangliomas also can be found in the neck, the mediastinum, and the wall of the urinary bladder. The latter patients can present with a distinct clinical picture of headache, diaphoresis, and hypertension related to a distended bladder, or to urination.

Pheochromocytomas are usually over 3 cm at presentation and invariably should be identified by CT (155). If small, the tumors are round and have homogeneous soft-tissue-attenuation values (Fig. 23). Because pheochromocytomas are hypervascular neoplasms, they have a propensity to undergo hemorrhagic necrosis even when benign, accounting for the central low attenuation seen in large neoplasms (Fig. 27). Central necrosis may be so

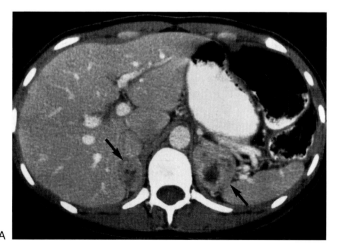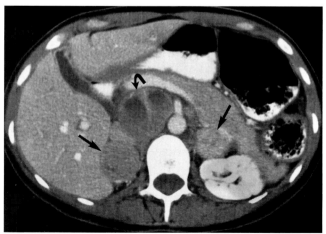

FIG. 24. Multiple pheochromocytomas in MEN2b. **A:** CT shows bilateral heterogeneous adrenal tumors *(arrows)*. **B:** At a more inferior level, additional bilateral adrenal tumors *(arrows)* are seen, as well as an extra-adrenal lesion *(curved arrow)*.

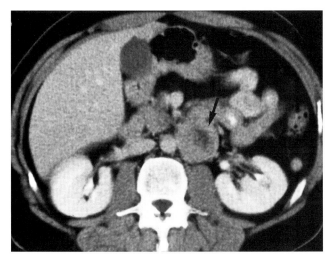

FIG. 25. Paraganglioma. The adrenals (not shown) were normal in this hypertensive man with a 3.3-cm heterogeneous retroperitoneal mass *(arrow).*

extensive as to simulate a cyst (18,40). Calcification is uncommon; when present, it may have an egg-shell pattern (29,56,77). After intravenous administration of iodinated contrast medium, pheochromocytomas exhibit heterogeneous enhancement, a pattern indistinguishable from a malignant adrenal neoplasm. Correlation with biochemical function is required to establish the correct diagnosis.

Because pheochromocytomas are large, they can be detected even with unenhanced CT (121). Some concern has been raised about the use of intravenous contrast in patients with pheochromocytoma. Plasma catecholamine levels can be raised by intravenous injection of iodinated contrast medium, but symptomatic blood pressure eleva-tions do not usually result (122). Only if a patient has known hypertensive episodes and has not had adequate pharmacologic adrenergic blockade is it necessary to avoid contrast. Contrast is especially useful for detection of extra-adrenal lesions. Although paragangliomas can usually be identified on CT (Fig. 25), they have a nonspecific appearance. The CT features of malignant paragangliomas in particular overlap with those of other retroperitoneal malignancies (60). Radionuclide metaiodobenzylguanidine (MIBG) scintigraphy can be useful to document whether a retroperitoneal mass is in fact a paraganglioma (60,120).

Pheochromocytomas have a rather characteristic appearance on MRI (42,51,124). They are readily detected [with a sensitivity of 100% in one report (149)], because they are several centimeters in diameter. When small, they usually are homogeneous and isointense to muscle, hypointense to liver on T1-weighted images, and markedly hyperintense to fat on T2-weighted images (42,149) (Figs. 28,29). As they grow and develop central necrosis, there may be central areas that are hyperintense on both T1- and T2-weighted images (126) (Fig. 27). Exuberant, persistent enhancement after intravenous gadolinium is typical (84,149) (Fig. 29). Because no lipid is found in pheochromocytoma, there is no decrease in signal on opposed phase images. Paragangliomas have similar distinctive imaging characteristics; as a result, MRI is superior to CT for diagnosis of paragangliomas (120), and nearly as sensitive as MIBG (149). Because most such tumors lie in the adrenal or retroperitoneum, coronal MRI can quickly and effectively show the area of abnormality (126) (Fig. 26).

Because the prevalence of pheochromocytoma/paraganglioma is low, no imaging should be done unless there

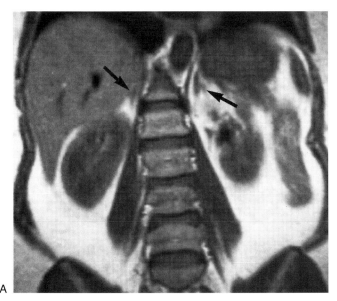

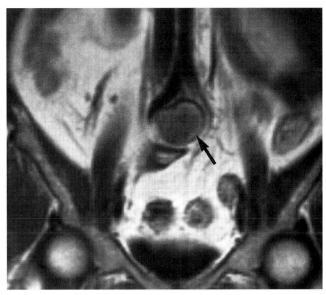

A B

FIG. 26. Organ of Zuckerkandl paraganglioma. **A:** Coronal T1-weighted image (500/20) shows the adrenals *(arrows)* are normal. **B:** A mass is present at the aortic bifurcation *(arrow).*

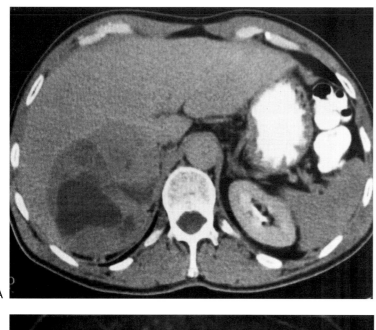

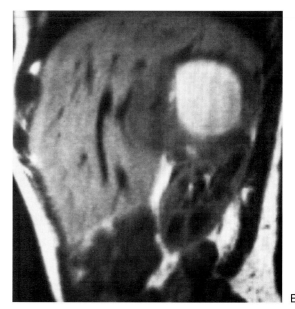

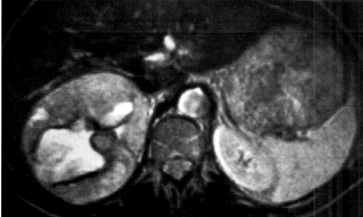

FIG. 27. Pheochromocytoma. **A:** Contrast CT shows a 10-cm right suprarenal mass with marked heterogeneity. **B:** Sagittal T1-weighted image (366/20) show the mass is clearly separate from the kidney, as the renal cortex is intact. Note the areas with signal as intense as fat that correspond to the low-attenuation areas on CT, probably representing hemorrhage. **C:** T2-weighted MRI (1800/80)shows most of the mass is more intense than liver, similar to fat, but the hemorrhagic areas are more intense than fat.

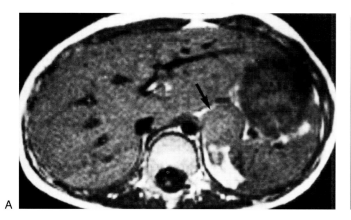

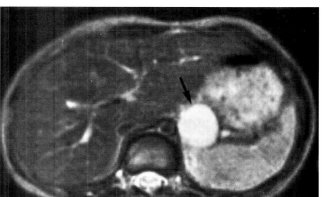

FIG. 28. Pheochromocytoma in a 10-year-old boy with episodic hypertensive crises. **A:** On T1-weighted image (366/26), the 3-cm mass *(arrow)* has signal intensity similar to liver. **B:** On T2-weighted image (2500/80), the mass *(arrow)* is homogeneous and more intense than fat.

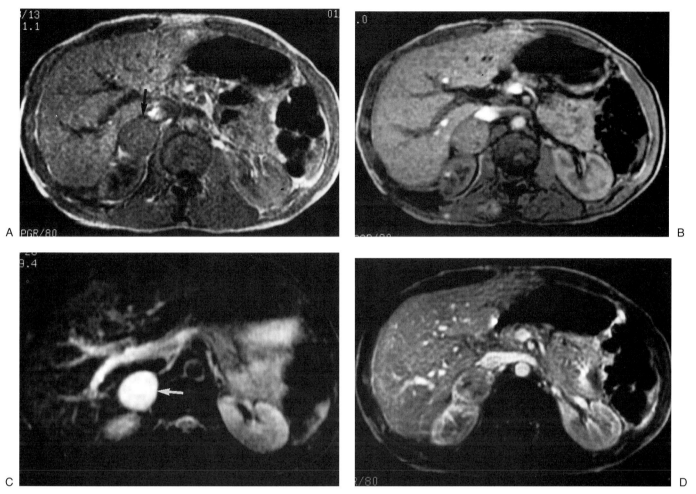

FIG. 29. Pheochromocytoma. **A:** T1-weighted GRE image (150/4.2/80°) during suspended respiration shows a 4-cm right adrenal mass *(arrow)* isointense with liver. **B:** The mass does not lose signal on the opposed phase image (TE 6.3 msec). **C:** On fat-suppressed T2-weighted image (2500/70), the mass *(arrow)* is markedly hyperintense. **D:** Following intravenous Gd-DTPA, the mass shows marked heterogeneous enhancement which persisted for several minutes (150/4.2/80°).

is some clinical or biochemical evidence of its existence. Either CT or MRI can effectively detect or exclude an adrenal pheochromocytoma. If adrenal CT or MRI is negative, no further imaging should be done without strong biochemical findings. If there is strong clinical or biochemical evidence, imaging of the entire retroperitoneum as well as the adrenals should be done; either CT or MRI can be used, although MRI may be preferred because of greater specificity and less concern about contrast effects. Biopsy of a mass suspected to be a pheochromocytoma is not recommended, especially if adequate hypertensive control has not been achieved, because several episodes of severe hemorrhage and even death have resulted following percutaneous biopsy (19,93). MIBG has both high sensitivity and high specificity, and it can detect a paraganglioma in any part of the body (47). However, it is an expensive test that requires up to 72 hours to complete and is not widely available. Furthermore, it does not provide sufficient anatomic detail for surgical planning. It is

most useful in evaluating patients with a strong clinical suspicion and in whom CT or MRI is normal or equivocal, or for follow-up of malignant lesions.

NONHYPERFUNCTIONING NEOPLASMS

Nonhyperfunctioning adrenal neoplasms are clinically silent until they become very large, although they may present with pain if they hemorrhage. Currently, most such masses are found incidentally on studies performed for other reasons. About 30% of all adrenal masses are incidentally detected by CT (2). An adrenal mass is seen in about 4% of all abdominal CT scans, with one third being serendipitous findings; the remainder are either metastases in patients with known malignancies, or they are functioning lesions (2). Most incidental adrenal masses are benign and of no clinical significance, especially in patients with no known malignancy. In two large series, only 6.7% and 9% of serendipitous adrenal masses were subsequently proven malignant (3,48). Although historically size has been considered an important factor, larger tumors having a greater likelihood of malignancy, size is an imperfect criterion. Although malignant neoplasms were all larger than 6.5 cm in one study (3), and although most benign masses are less than 5 cm (2,22), there is considerable overlap. The majority of incidental masses greater than 5 cm are still benign in patients with no history of malignancy (78), and lesions as small as 1 cm may be metastases (81). Thus, it is imperative to use imaging features other than size to make a diagnosis.

NONHYPERFUNCTIONING ADENOMAS

Adrenal adenomas that do not produce clinically significant excess hormones are not infrequent, being found in some 2% to 8% of autopsies (2,62) and in 1% to 2% of abdominal CT scans (2,6,53). They are commonly unilateral, although bilateral adenomas do occur (Fig. 30). Although nonhyperfunctioning adenomas may be 6 cm or larger (81), the majority are 3 cm or less, with only 5% exceeding 5 cm³. The incidence is slightly higher in diabetics (16%) and hypertensives (12%) (81). Because of the fact that they do function, they are "warm nodules" on adrenal scintigrams.

Nonhyperfunctioning adenomas have a CT appearance indistinguishable from other adenomas, except that contralateral atrophy is not present. They are smooth, round or oval, with a well-defined margin. These adenomas are usually homogeneous without a perceptible wall on noncontrast scans. Usually, they have an attenuation value similar to or lower than that of muscle [+50 Hounsfield

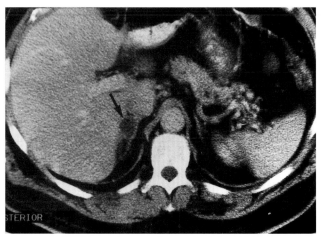

FIG. 31. Adenoma. An 18-mm low-attenuation (−18 HU) right adrenal adenoma *(arrow)* was discovered incidentally in this asymptomatic man. The CT finding of a mass with attenuation this low excludes malignancy.

units (HU)]. However, they may be of water attenuation or lower (−35 HU) if enough lipid is present (53,100) (Fig. 31). If the lesion measures 0 HU or less, its benign nature is assured (87). Calcification may be present (76,98). Nonhyperfunctioning adenomas usually exhibit mild, homogeneous enhancement after intravenous administration of iodinated contrast material (98). Sometimes, a few tiny, brightly enhancing areas are seen, giving a somewhat speckled appearance on early dynamic enhanced scans (8) (Fig. 32). A thin, enhancing rim also may be seen. Using all CT features, including pre- and postcontrast densities, correct diagnosis of nonhyperfunctioning adenoma can be made in most cases (8,87).

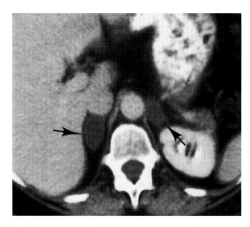

FIG. 30. Biopsy-proved bilateral nonhyperfunctioning adenomas in a patient with bronchogenic carcinoma. Postcontrast CT image demonstrates bilateral adrenal masses *(arrows)*, each measuring 1.5 cm in diameter. Both masses have homogeneous near-water attenuation values. This CT appearance is fairly characteristic of a nonhyperfunctioning adenoma.

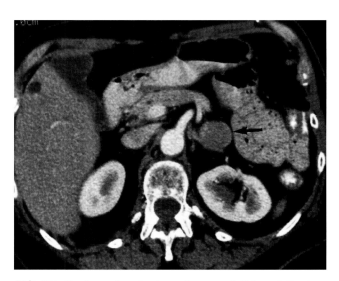

FIG. 32. Nonhyperfunctioning adenoma. A 2.8 cm left adrenal mass *(arrow)* was found incidentally in this 75-year-old woman with no history of malignancy and no endocrine disorder. The lesion is somewhat heterogeneous. Follow-up CT 1 year later showed no change.

Nonhyperfunctioning adenomas also have characteristic MRI features. On MRI, the mass is homogeneous with signal intensity usually less than that of fat but greater than that of muscle on all sequences (21). In most cases, the signal intensity is similar to that of normal liver on both T1- and T2-weighted images (21,24,42,51,124) (Fig. 33). However, signal intensities are affected by many factors and can be variable, such that diagnosis based only on signal intensities may be indeterminate in as much as 21% to 31% (4,24,79,123). After intravenous administration of gadolinium compounds, adenomas show limited enhancement (<100% [signal intensity] SI increase over baseline) with rapid washout (<30% residual enhancement at 10 min) (84,85). Many adenomas contain a significant amount of intracellular lipid, which accounts for the relatively low attenuation value on CT (100). MRI is even more sensitive than CT to the presence of lipid and can be used to document the presence of lipid, thus excluding malignancy (88). This can be achieved by showing a decrease in signal intensity comparing the same gradient echo sequence with TE in or out of phase (97,147) (Fig. 34). However, some adenomas do not contain large amounts of lipid, so lack of signal drop does not prove malignancy. Using all these MRI features, correct diagnosis can be made in most cases.

METASTATIC DISEASE

Metastases to the adrenals are common from a variety of primary malignancies, including thyroid, renal, gastric, colon, pancreatic, and esophageal carcinomas, and melanoma. Lung and breast cancer, however, are the most common sources, with adrenal metastases found on CT in approximately 19% of lung cancer patients (136,150). Because adrenal metastases are so common in lung cancer, and because the adrenals may be the only site of metastasis (113,129), the adrenal glands should be included in the CT examination of all patients presenting with a lung cancer (50,106). Surgery is not indicated if adrenal metastases are present in non-small-cell lung cancer; accurate staging can help determine the prognosis in patients with small cell cancer (150). Not all adrenal masses found in cancer patients, however, are metastases (Fig. 30). Even in patients with lung cancer, about one third of adrenal masses are benign (50,110). Thus, the

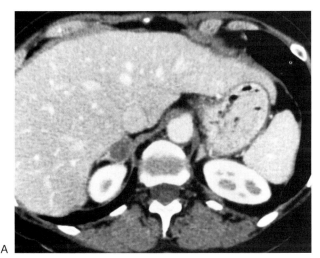

A

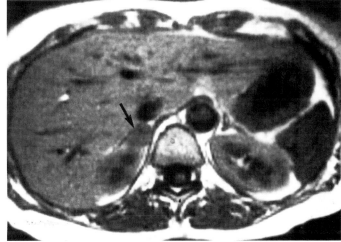

B

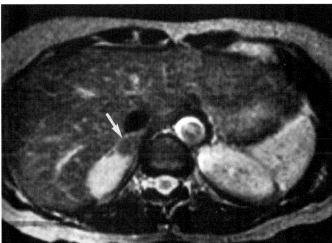

C

FIG. 33. Nonhyperfunctioning adenoma. A: A right adrenal nodule was an incidental finding in this asymptomatic 68-year-old woman. B: On T1-weighted MRI image (300/20), the nodule (arrow) is slightly less intense than the liver. C: The mass (arrow) is isointense with liver on T2-weighted image (2500/80).

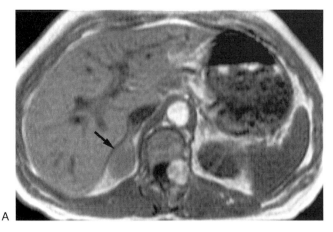

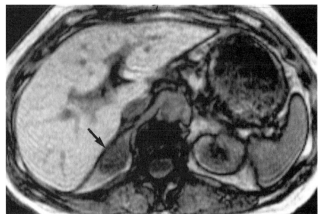

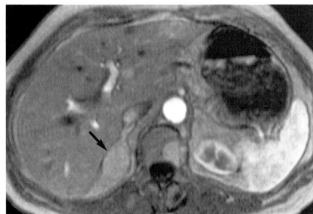

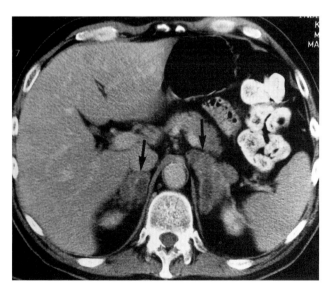

FIG. 34. Nonhyperfunctioning adenoma. **A:** On T1-weighted GRE MRI image (2-D FLASH), a right adrenal mass *(arrow)* isointense with liver is shown. **B:** Opposed-phase T1-weighted GRE image shows the mass *(arrow)* with signal intensity less than the liver. **C:** Following intravenous Gd-DTPA, the mass *(arrow)* shows moderate homogeneous enhancement.

FIG. 35. Adrenal metastases from primary non-small-cell bronchogenic carcinoma. Bilateral adrenal masses *(arrows)* with focal low attenuation areas are noted on this contrast CT.

imaging features must be used to help make the correct diagnosis. If the imaging findings are equivocal, a percutaneous CT-guided biopsy should be performed to establish a histologic diagnosis (Fig. 35). A baseline CT at the time of presentation of patients with lung cancer is a useful aid in follow-up. Detection of a new small adrenal mass on follow-up is clear evidence of metastasis if the baseline showed normal adrenals (Fig. 36).

Adrenal metastases can vary considerably on CT. A normal appearance does not absolutely exclude metastasis, especially with lung cancer (20,112), but most often careful examination will reveal some focal bulge of the adrenal contour. Size can range from less than a centimeter to extremely large; the size, however, overlaps with that of adenomas (81) (Figs. 36–38). Adrenal metastases may be unilateral or bilateral. When small (<5 cm), they commonly are fairly well circumscribed, round or oval, and of soft-tissue density (Fig. 36). They may have smooth or irregular, lobulated contours. They may show local invasion, a sign of malignancy. Calcification is rare (76), and they may hemorrhage (137) (Fig. 39).

Small adrenal metastases are solid tumors and thus usually have homogeneous soft-tissue-attenuation values, similar to or higher than that of muscle on noncontrast scans (Fig. 36). Larger metastases may develop central necrosis and thus are heterogeneous (Figs. 37,38); if hem-

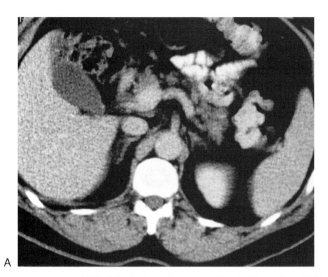
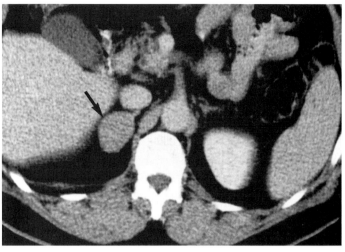

A

B

FIG. 36. Adrenal metastasis. **A:** Baseline CT in this patient presenting with lung cancer shows normal adrenals. **B:** Follow-up 8 months later shows a homogeneous 4-cm mass in the right adrenal *(arrow)*. The appearance is not inconsistent with an adenoma, but because it is new, it is clearly a metastasis.

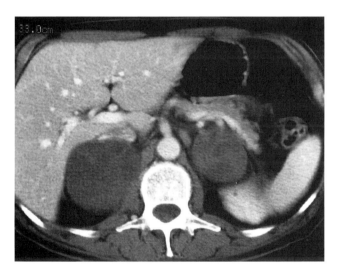

FIG. 37. Adrenal metastases. Large heterogeneous adrenal masses are present bilaterally (right, 8 cm; left, 5 cm) in this man with bronchogenic carcinoma.

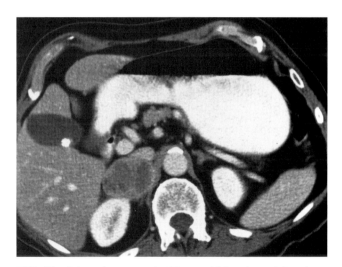

FIG. 38. Adrenal metastasis. The ovoid 3 × 4 cm right adrenal mass in this patient with lung cancer shows an irregular enhancing rim on this CT image done with rapid scanning after bolus intravenous contrast.

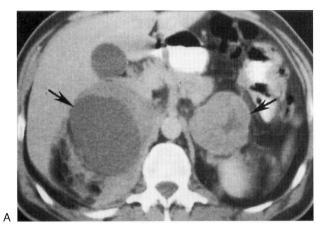

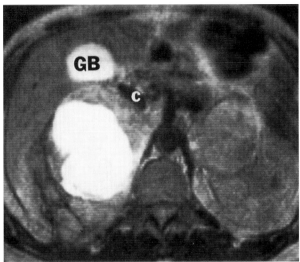

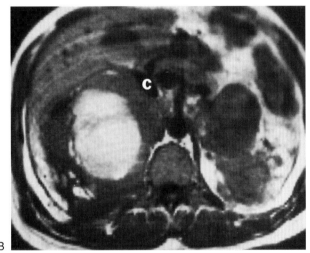

FIG. 39. Hemorrhagic adrenal metastases due to melanoma. **A:** Postcontrast CT image demonstrates bilateral, inhomogeneous adrenal masses *(arrows)*, the right being more irregular than the left. **B:** T1-weighted image (500/35) shows basically the same findings as CT. The extremely high signal intensity seen in the right adrenal mass is due to subacute hemorrhage. **C:** T2-weighted image (2100/90). With the exception of hemorrhage, both adrenal masses have signal intensities similar to that of fat. C, inferior vena cava; GB, gallbladder.

orrhage has occurred, slightly high density areas may be seen on noncontrast scans (Fig. 39). Even if there is central necrosis, however, the density is not lower than that of water, because malignant tumors do not produce lipid (87). Following intravenous administration of iodinated contrast material, there may be homogeneous enhancement, but commonly enhancement is heterogeneous, especially with larger tumors. A thick, nodular enhancing rim also may be seen (8) (Fig. 38).

Adrenal metastases can vary in size and appearance on MRI. On T1-weighted images, metastases usually have signal intensity similar to or lower than that of normal liver tissue, not distinctly different from that of adenomas. They may be heterogeneous (21,42,51,124). On T2-weighted images, they are often heterogeneous, and they are usually hyperintense compared to normal liver, often similar to or of higher intensity than fat, unlike the typical adenoma (21,42,124) (Figs. 40,41). Numerous calculations based on signal intensity ratios, or calculated T2 values, have been investigated, but none have been found to be reliable in practice for distinguishing metastases from adenomas (21,24,51,79,124). Because metastases do not produce lipid, there is no decrease in signal on opposed phase images (92,97,146). This has been shown to be a more consistent finding than T2 values (147). After

intravenous administration of gadolinium compounds, metastases exhibit exuberant and heterogeneous enhancement that persists for several minutes, an enhancement pattern quite different from that of adenomas (85) (Fig. 41). MRI is readily able to demonstrate or exclude local invasion because of the great contrast between neoplastic and normal tissue, especially on fat-suppressed T2-weighted images.

Computed tomography is the most cost-effective method for screening and following patients with malignancies. In most cases, adrenal metastases can be diagnosed or excluded by a well-performed CT. MRI can be valuable in cases in which CT findings are indeterminate and in which treatment may be altered. Percutaneous biopsy under CT guidance can be very effective, with accuracy and negative predictive value of over 90% (61,139,151). However, complications can occur (72,151), and biopsy is not needed if the imaging findings are diagnostic. Follow-up by CT can be diagnostic, because adenomas are very slow growing and will not change in size over a period of a few months, while metastases will show growth.

ADRENAL LYMPHOMA

Adrenal masses occasionally result from involvement by lymphoma, with diffuse non-Hodgkin disease the com-

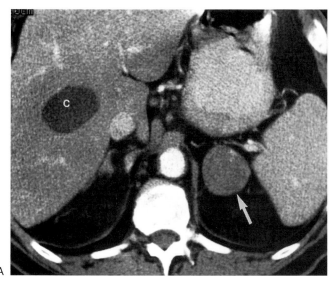

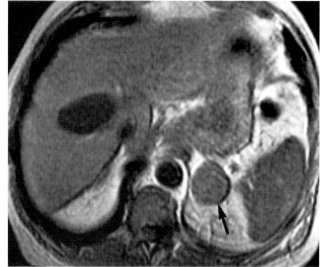

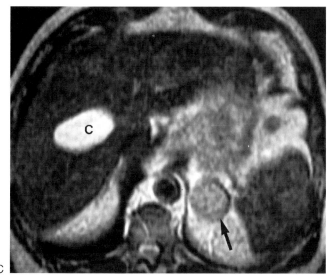

FIG. 40. Adrenal metastasis from a primary esophageal carcinoma. **A:** A 4-cm left adrenal mass *(arrow)* is homogeneous except for a few tiny high-attenuation foci, a pattern that could represent a nonhyperfunctioning adenoma. C, incidental liver cyst. **B:** The mass *(arrow)* is isointense with liver on T1-weighted GRE image (50/5/35°). **C:** On T2-weighted MRI image (2000/80/), the mass *(arrow)* is more intense than liver, but not as intense as the cyst (C).

monest type (52,69,114). This may be found at presentation or at follow-up, with adrenal lymphoma reported in 1% to 4% of patients being followed for lymphoma (52,69,114). Adrenal involvement is most commonly seen in conjunction with an extra-adrenal disease site (43). Primary adrenal lymphoma is rare and is believed to arise from hematopoietic cells in the adrenal (41). Lymphomatous adrenal masses are bilateral in one third of cases; when bilateral, the patient may develop Addison disease (64,96,114) (Fig. 42).

On CT, adrenal lymphomas usually are seen as large soft-tissue masses (40 to 60 HU) replacing the adrenal. They usually alter the shape of the adrenal, but the adrenal may markedly expand while retaining a somewhat adreniform shape. Mild to moderate enhancement is seen after intravenous administration of iodinated contrast (Fig. 42). The lesions may be homogeneous, but they are often heterogeneous with low attenuation areas even before therapy (5,41). Sometimes the growth

pattern can suggest lymphoma, as it is more likely to infiltrate or insinuate around the upper pole of the kidney than displace it, as would be typical of carcinoma (Fig. 43). There may be hemorrhage, and calcification can be found, especially after chemotherapy (41). On MRI, adrenal lymphomas are indistinguishable from other malignancies. They are usually heterogeneous, with low signal on T1-weighted images (less intense than normal liver, but more intense than muscle) and more intense than fat on T2-weighted images (21,51,86) (Fig. 44).

MYELOLIPOMA

Myelolipoma is an uncommon, benign, nonfunctioning neoplasm of the adrenal, found in less than 1% of autopsies (111). It is composed of variable amounts of fat and hematopoietic tissue, including myeloid and erythroid

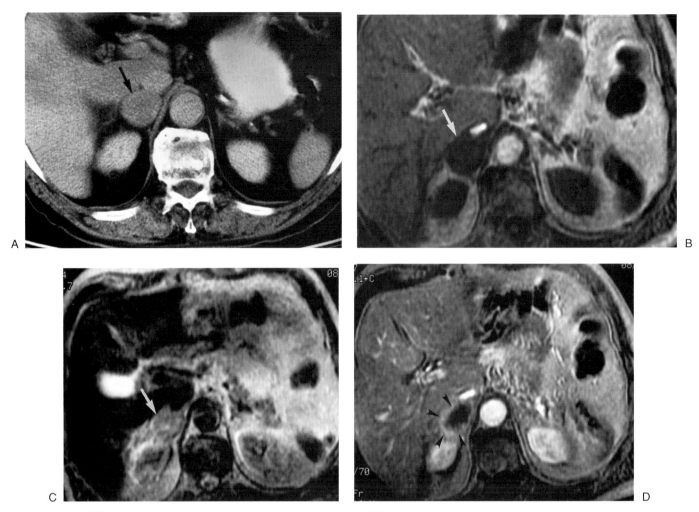

FIG. 41. Adrenal metastasis. **A:** Contrast-enhanced CT shows a fairly homogeneous right adrenal mass *(arrow)* in this patient with a history of bladder cancer; no other abnormality was found in the chest or abdomen. **B:** The mass *(arrow)* has lower signal than liver on T1-weighted GRE image (114/4.2/70°). **C:** The mass *(arrow)* is nearly isointense with fat on T2-weighted spin echo image. **D:** There is heterogeneous enhancement *(arrowheads)* after intravenous Gd-DTPA (114/4.2/70°).

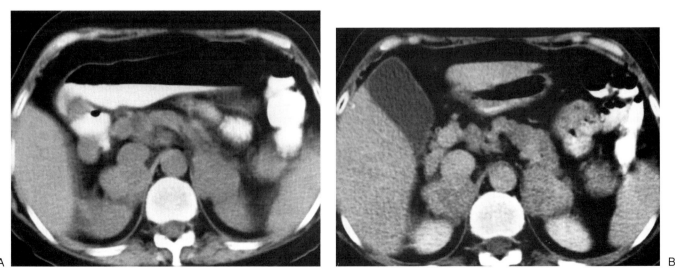

FIG. 42. Adrenal lymphoma. **A:** Bilateral lobular adrenal masses (40 HU) are present on noncontrast CT in this patient presenting with adrenal insufficiency. **B:** Contrast-enhanced scan shows slightly heterogeneous, mild enhancement (88 HU). The patient was Addisonian.

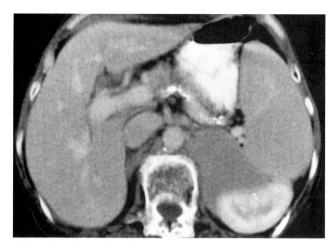

FIG. 43. Adrenal lymphoma. A homogeneous mass arising in the region of the left adrenal insinuates itself around the left kidney without deforming it.

cells and megakaryocytes. The etiology is unclear, but myelolipoma may be a result of metaplasia of cells in the adrenal, possibly myeloid cells misplaced during embryogenesis (28). It affects men and women equally. Although this is a nonfunctioning tumor, in 10% it is associated with endocrine disorders, including Cushing syndrome (7,154), congenital adrenal hyperplasia (109), and Conn syndrome (156). Most myelolipomas (80%) are asymptomatic and are of no clinical significance. Some (10%) become large and cause vague symptoms or pain (44). Large myelolipomas may hemorrhage, which can be the cause of pain. Size ranges from 1 to 15 cm, with a mean of about 4 cm.

On CT, most myelolipomas are well-circumscribed masses, sometimes with a discrete thin apparent capsule (Fig. 45). Occasionally, the mass may appear to extend into the retroperitoneum (152). Nearly all contain some definite fat density (<−20 HU). However, the amount of fat is widely variable, ranging from nearly all fat, to more than

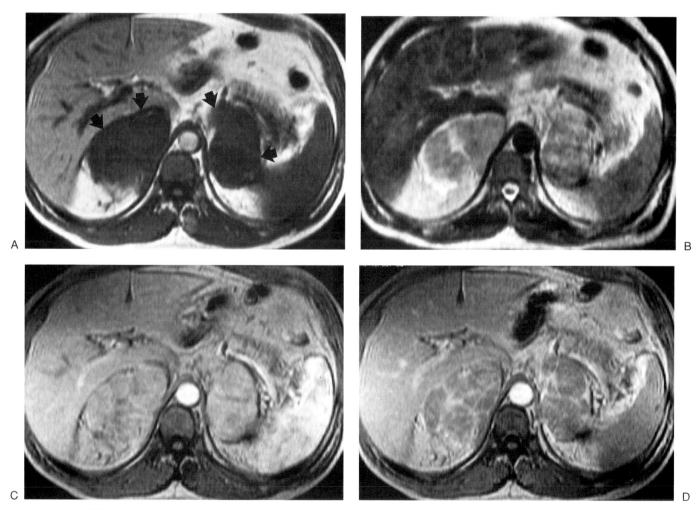

FIG. 44. Primary adrenal lymphoma: MRI appearance. **A:** T1-weighted image (500/35) shows two oblong-shaped adrenal masses (M). **B:** T2-weighted image (2100/90). The masses are slightly inhomogeneous and have a signal intensity similar to that of fat. Based on MRI signal characteristics, adrenal lymphoma cannot be distinguished from metastases. K, kidney; c, inferior vena cava; L, liver; S, spleen. **C:** TI GRE image immediately after gadolinium DTPA injection shows bright heterogeneous enhancement of both masses. **D:** Thirteen minutes after gadolinium DTPA injection, the enhancement is not as bright.

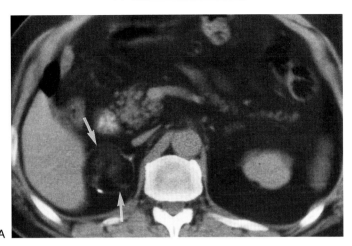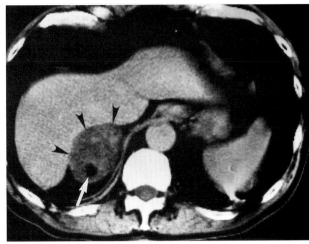

A B

FIG. 45. Myelolipoma. **A:** The right adrenal contains a partly fatty mass *(arrows)* with a capsule; note the calcification. **B:** In another patient, the right adrenal mass is predominantly soft tissue density *(arrowheads)* with only a 1 cm area *(arrow)* that measured −65 HU.

half fat (50%), to only a few tiny foci of fat in a soft-tissue mass (10%) (103,128) (Fig. 45). Occasionally, the mass has an attenuation value between that of fat and water because the fat and myeloid elements are diffusely mixed. Calcification is seen in 30%, often punctate (128) (Fig. 45). With hemorrhage, high density areas can be seen (Fig. 46). Bilateral myelolipomas occur in about 10%.

The presence of fat in an adrenal mass also can be recognized on MRI, because fat is typically bright on both T1- and T2-weighted images (104) (Fig. 47). Decrease in signal with fat suppression or phase cancellation is confirmatory (97) (Fig. 47). However, if the mass is nearly all mature fat, there will not be loss of signal with opposed phase images, because the loss of signal occurs only with

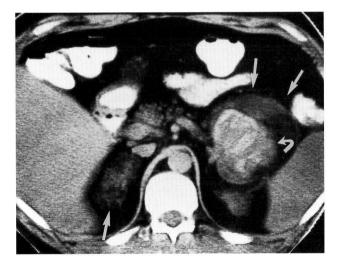

FIG. 46. Bilateral myelolipomas with hemorrhage. CT, done because of acute left flank pain, shows bilateral fat containing adrenal masses *(arrows)*. The left mass contains a high-attenuation area *(curved arrow)*, confirmed to be an acute hemorrhage at surgery.

phase cancellation in areas with an admixture of fat and water protons (146). Overall, myelolipomas are often heterogeneous because the nonfatty areas will have signal intensity similar to that of hematopoietic bone marrow (104). The lesions enhance brightly after intravenous administration of gadolinium (Fig. 47).

The presence of fat in an adrenal mass is the key to the diagnosis of myelolipoma, because virtually no other adrenal lesion contains fat. Teratoma and liposarcoma of the adrenals are extraordinarily rare. An angiomyolipoma of the upper pole of a kidney may be mistaken to be an adrenal myelolipoma. However, this is of no clinical significance, because both these lesions are benign. If necessary, diagnosis can be confirmed by percutaneous needle biopsy (26,55). If the biopsy reveals bone marrow elements and the mass contains fat, the diagnosis is assured, because extramedullary hematopoiesis does not contain fat (80). The presence of megakaryocytes also is an important diagnostic histologic feature (26). A definite diagnosis is important because surgical resection is not indicated unless there has been significant hemorrhage. In nearly all cases, a diagnosis of adrenal myelolipoma can be made confidently based on CT or MRI findings alone.

ADRENAL CYSTS

Adrenal cysts are rare, found in only 1 of 1,400 autopsies (153). They are nonfunctional and usually found incidentally. The commonest type (45%) are endothelial cysts (23), which are predominantly lymphangiomatous cysts, typically small and asymptomatic (74). Thirty-nine percent are pseudocysts, which lack an endothelial lining and are most often a sequela of remote adrenal hemorrhage (46,74,115). These are the type most often detected by

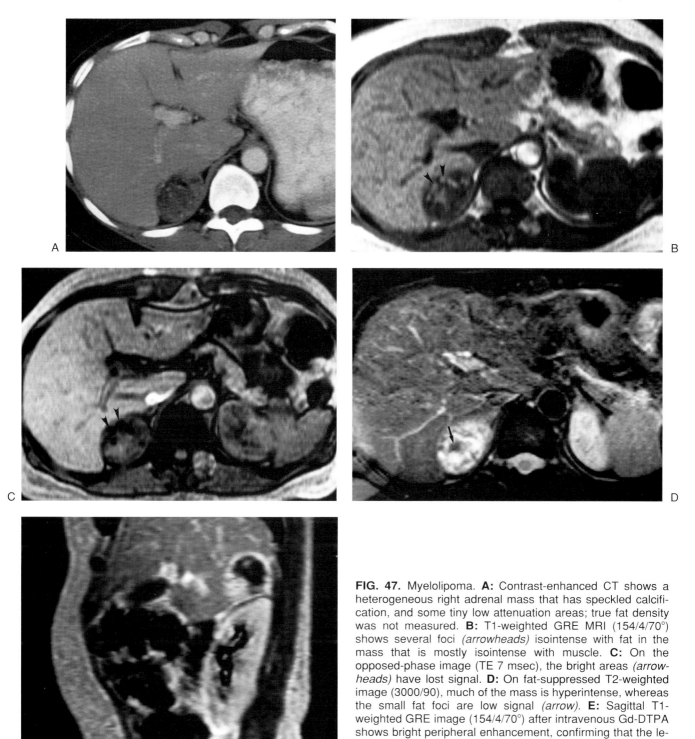

FIG. 47. Myelolipoma. **A:** Contrast-enhanced CT shows a heterogeneous right adrenal mass that has speckled calcification, and some tiny low attenuation areas; true fat density was not measured. **B:** T1-weighted GRE MRI (154/4/70°) shows several foci *(arrowheads)* isointense with fat in the mass that is mostly isointense with muscle. **C:** On the opposed-phase image (TE 7 msec), the bright areas *(arrowheads)* have lost signal. **D:** On fat-suppressed T2-weighted image (3000/90), much of the mass is hyperintense, whereas the small fat foci are low signal *(arrow)*. **E:** Sagittal T1-weighted GRE image (154/4/70°) after intravenous Gd-DTPA shows bright peripheral enhancement, confirming that the lesion does not arise from the kidney.

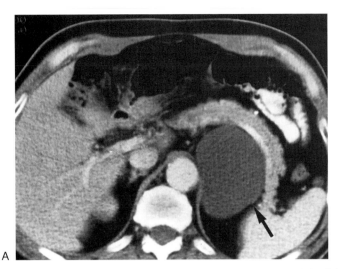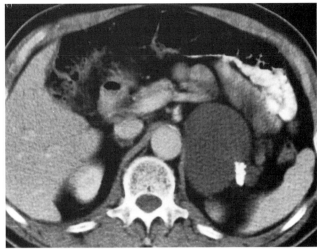

A

B

FIG. 48. Adrenal cyst. **A:** In the region of the left adrenal, a homogeneous water-density mass is seen *(arrow)*. **B:** More inferiorly, there is thick focal calcification in the wall.

CT. These can be quite large and may produce symptoms because of their size. The remaining cystic lesions of the adrenals are parasitic cysts (7%), caused by *Echinococcus,* and true epithelial cysts (9%) (115).

On CT, adrenal cysts are large masses (5 to 20 cm) that are well circumscribed and round. They are suprarenal in location, but it may be difficult on CT to recognize that they arise in the adrenal rather than the kidney or liver. Sonography or MRI may better show their true origin. They usually are of near-water attenuation, but they can have higher or mixed attenuation values resulting from old hemorrhage. The wall may be thick and can show contrast enhancement. Calcification is common (75%) (76), and it is usually curvilinear in shape and often limited to the inferior aspect of the wall (76,148) (Fig. 48). Although MRI may show typical cystic features (homogeneous low intensity on T1-weighted images and extreme hyperintensity on T2-weighted images), signal intensity can vary depending on the age of hemorrhage. There is no central enhancement on either CT or MRI. Adrenal cysts are of no clinical significance, and surgical removal is unnecessary if the diagnosis can be established by imaging. Concern about malignancy is reasonable only in complicated cysts, which may have high attenuation values, a thick enhancing wall, and septations. In such cases, percutaneous needle aspiration may be helpful for both diagnosis and treatment (148).

INFLAMMATORY DISEASE

Inflammatory processes in the adrenals are uncommon. Adrenal abscesses occur rarely; they sometimes represent

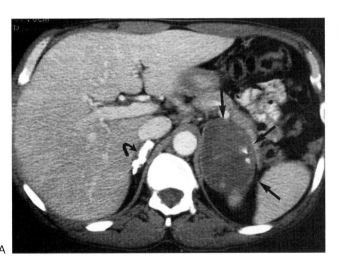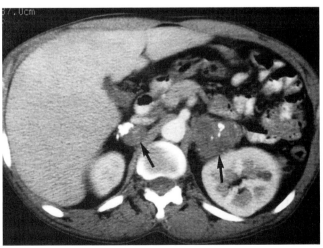

A

B

FIG. 49. Adrenal tuberculosis. **A:** CT reveals a densely calcified right adrenal *(curved arrow)* and a heterogeneous left adrenal mass *(arrows)* in this patient with disseminated tuberculosis. **B:** More inferiorly, both adrenals show heterogeneous, somewhat low-attenuation small masses *(arrows)*. The patient was Addisonian.

adrenal hematomas that became infected (107). More often, adrenal inflammation is due to chronic granulomatous disease, with tuberculosis (TB) and histoplasmosis most common, although North American blastomycosis has been reported to involve the adrenals (58). Granulomatous disease of the adrenals can cause a variety of appearances depending on the stage of disease. In most cases, there is bilateral enlargement of the adrenals (31,59,94,161). Bilateral adrenal enlargement in a patient with a reactive tuberculin skin test, or with chest radiographic changes of TB or histoplasmosis, should suggest the diagnosis, even if pulmonary cultures are nondiagnostic (161).

With active adrenal TB, both glands are usually enlarged to some degree (Fig. 49). The masses are frequently heterogeneous, with heterogeneous enhancement and low-attenuation central areas representing caseous necrosis (159). Calcification is present in nearly half of cases of adrenal TB (144). In some cases, at a late stage of disease, dense calcification with no soft-tissue mass may be seen (31). Active adrenal histoplasmosis most often presents with mild to marked symmetrical enlargement of both adrenals, which retain the normal shape (89,161). There is low attenuation in the center with higher peripheral density, because of caseous necrosis (89,161) (Fig. 50). Calcification is not usually seen in the acute phase, but it may be seen with healing (161).

With both TB and histoplasmosis, there may be associated lymphadenopathy. Both may cause adrenal insufficiency. The diagnosis usually is suggested because of the CT appearance of the glands and the clinical presentation, especially when there is adrenal insufficiency. Percutaneous biopsy can be done to confirm the diagnosis (31,58,161).

The MRI signal intensity of inflammatory adrenal masses is nonspecific. It has signal intensity similar to spleen on T1-weighted images, and similar to or higher than fat on T2-weighted images (4) (Fig. 50). Enhancement patterns have not been described. Calcification is difficult to recognize.

ADRENAL HEMORRHAGE

Adrenal hemorrhage occurs in three distinct settings: neonatal hemorrhage, spontaneous (atraumatic) hemorrhage in the adult, and severe trauma. Neonatal hemorrhage is the most common, resulting partly from the large fetal adrenal that is prone to injury during birth trauma. Because it is primarily the regressing fetal adrenal tissue that is involved, such patients do not develop adrenal insufficiency, and in the adult the only sequela is calcification of the adrenal without an associated mass (76).

Adrenal hemorrhage in the adult is seen usually in the setting of severe illness, such as sepsis, including but not limited to meningococcemia, burns, hypotension, and other life threatening illnesses. In these circumstances, it is likely the stress-related hyperplasia makes the adrenal prone to spontaneous rupture. About one third of cases of adrenal hemorrhage are associated with anticoagulant therapy. Commonly, the bleeding occurs in the first 3 weeks of anticoagulation (108,163). This is probably not caused by excessive anticoagulation but is partly a result of stress-related hyperplasia due to the illness that necessitated the anticoagulation (90).

On CT, adrenal hemorrhage results in unilateral or bilateral adrenal masses that are usually ovoid, about 3 cm in diameter, and of about muscle density or higher with poor enhancement, if any, after intravenous administration of iodinated contrast (Fig. 51). With larger hemorrhages, the masses may be heterogeneous and may have ill defined margins (Fig. 52). The size and attenuation value decrease over time if followed with CT (91,162). Calcification may develop in several weeks to months. If the hemorrhage is bilateral, adrenal insufficiency may occur. It may be important to suggest this possibility so that an ACTH stimulation test can be done to confirm adrenal insufficiency, because the clinical signs may be subtle. As mentioned previously, small metastases rarely cause adrenal insufficiency.

Posttraumatic adrenal hemorrhage is not common, occurring in 2% of patients with severe abdominal injury (17) (Fig. 53). Because of this, 95% of patients also have other injuries, such as hepatic and splenic lacerations (17). Because of lack of specific clinical signs for acute traumatic adrenal hemorrhage, the condition usually is detected as an incidental finding in CT studies performed for evaluation of acute blunt trauma. The right adrenal is more commonly involved (17,135), perhaps because acute elevation of pressure in the inferior vena cava can be directly transmitted to the right adrenal (135), or perhaps because of compression of the adrenal between the liver and spine (160). Bilateral hematomas are uncommon (17), but they must be identified because of the risk of adrenal insufficiency. Again, on CT these lesions appear as ovoid masses, sometimes with higher attenuation values than muscle (50 to 75 HU) due to acute bleeding. There may be ill-defined margins or soft-tissue strands in the surrounding fat, which distinguish them from incidental adenomas (17,160) (Fig. 53)

One distinctive type of surgical trauma may result in an adrenal hematoma. When orthotopic liver transplantation is performed, a segment of the recipient's inferior vena cava must be excised, requiring ligation and division of the right adrenal vein, which can result in infarction and sometimes hemorrhage in the right adrenal region (11,141) (Fig. 54).This may be seen in 2% of patients with such surgery and should be recognized as a surgical complication of no clinical significance as long as the contralateral adrenal is intact (11).

Metastases to the adrenal will hemorrhage, but only rarely. This usually can be distinguished from other adrenal hemorrhages because there is a large heterogeneous

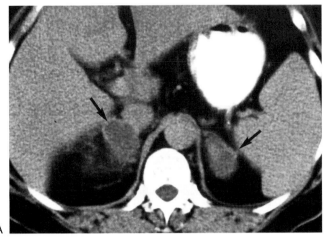

A

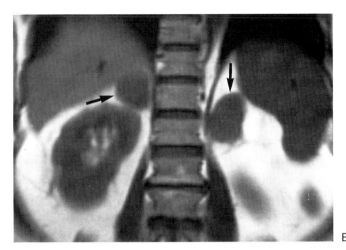

B

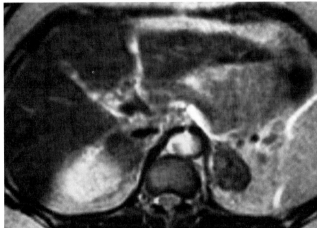

C

FIG. 50. Bilateral adrenal enlargement due to histoplasmosis. **A:** Bilateral heterogeneous adrenal masses with low-attenuation centers and denser rims are seen on CT *(arrows)*. **B:** On T1-weighted coronal MRI image (416/2.0) the masses *(arrows)* are isointense with the spleen. **C:** The masses are of mixed signal on T2 (1600/80), with some central areas isointense with fat, presumably the areas of caseous necrosis.

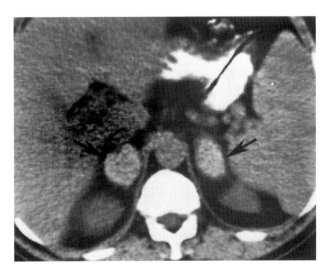

FIG. 51. Acute adrenal hemorrhage. Noncontrast CT image demonstrates bilateral adrenal masses *(arrows)*, each measuring 3.5 cm in diameter. The attenuation value of both masses is uniformly higher than that of paraspinal muscle.

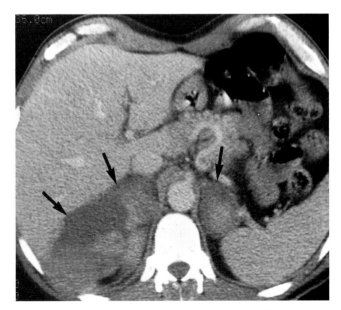

FIG. 52. Spontaneous adrenal hemorrhage. Bilateral heterogeneous adrenal masses *(arrows)* with some high-attenuation areas were found in this patient with severe heart disease who was recently anticoagulated.

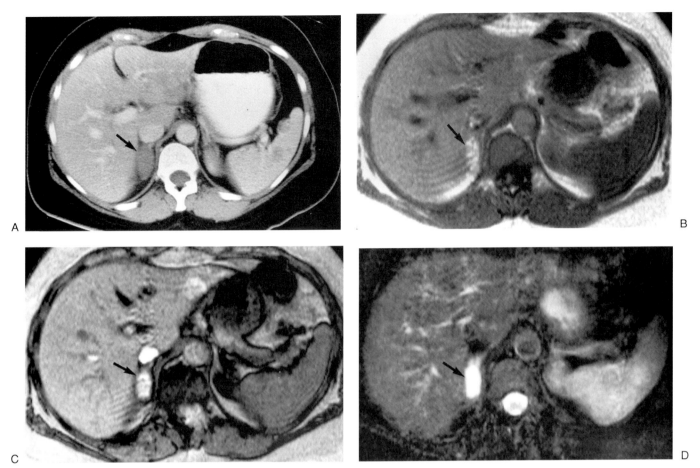

FIG. 53. Traumatic adrenal hematoma. **A:** Contrast-enhanced CT in a patient who was in a motor vehicle accident shows ovoid right adrenal mass *(arrow)* (and incidental splenic hemangioma). **B:** T1-weighted GRE image (2-D FLASH) 3 weeks after the injury shows the mass is more intense than liver. **C:** Persistent hyperintensity on opposed-phase image indicates the hyperintensity is not due to lipid. **D:** The hematoma *(arrow)* is very intense on T2-weighted image with fat suppression.

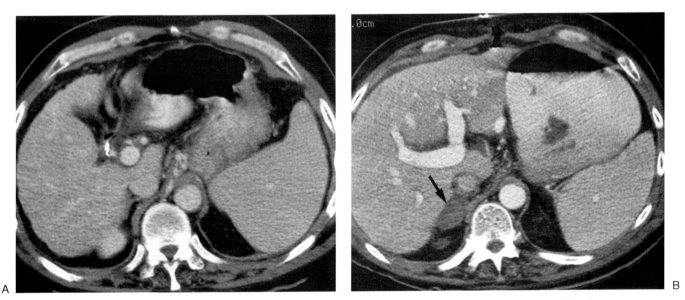

FIG. 54. Iatrogenic adrenal hematoma. **A:** The right adrenal is normal in this preoperative CT. **B:** After liver transplantation, a right adrenal mass *(arrow)* with slightly ill-defined margins has developed.

mass, with more extensive infiltrative retroperitoneal bleeding (137). Because these patients usually have advanced disease, neoplasm elsewhere is also usually evident.

On MRI, adrenal hemorrhage will produce a mass that can have varying signal intensities dependent on the age of the blood. They can be recognized because they usually have a pattern different from that of adenoma or malignancy. A subacute hematoma usually has a high signal intensity on both T1- and T2-weighted images (82) (Fig. 53). In some cases of subacute hematoma, on T1-weighted images the center may be low intensity because of the presence of intracellular deoxyhemoglobin, and the periphery may have high signal because of free methemoglobin; because both substances are high signal on T2, the mass is all high signal on T2. In chronic adrenal hematoma, the center consists of methemoglobin and thus this is of high signal on T1- and T2-weighted images, whereas the periphery contains hemosiderin, which is low signal on both T1- and T2-weighted images. This ring pattern is quite distinctive and suggestive of the diagnosis (68).

ADDISON DISEASE

Adrenal insufficiency may result from a variety of causes including bilateral hemorrhage, inflammatory disease, and idiopathic autoimmune primary Addison disease. Although metastases to the adrenal are common, they rarely lead to Addison disease. When it occurs, the disease is either in advanced stages or is associated with spontaneous hemorrhage (136). Another rare cause is hemochromatosis, which can be recognized on CT, as the adrenals are normal or small in size but have increased attenuation values (31).

CT is indicated in evaluation of patients with Addison disease. In one study, all cases of idiopathic Addison disease could be distinguished from other etiologies (144). Adrenal atrophy that results from autoimmune disease will result in small glands without calcification (31,63,144) (Fig. 55). This must be distinguished from adrenal atrophy due to exogenous steroids, which has a similar appearance, by careful history. Conversely, either adrenal hemorrhage, neoplasms, or inflammatory disease will show either adrenal masses or calcification, as discussed previously (91,94,161) (Figs. 42,49). Small adrenals that are partly or completely calcified suggest old granulomatous disease (particularly TB), whereas very dense calcifications with no soft tissue component suggest remote adrenal hemorrhage.

CT AND OTHER IMAGING TECHNIQUES

Except in a pediatric population, ultrasound is not used as a primary imaging method for adrenal disease, because

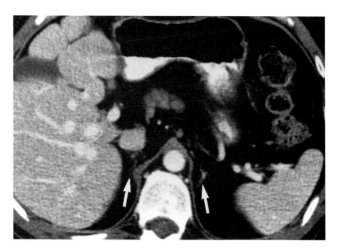

FIG. 55. Idiopathic Addison disease. In this patient presenting with adrenal insufficiency, both adrenals (arrows) are markedly atrophic.

it has both lower sensitivity and specificity than CT or MRI. The adrenals are often difficult to identify on sonography: the left adrenal in particular is frequently obscured by bowel gas. Sonography can be useful in limited circumstances, such as to help determine the exact origin of a large upper abdominal mass, or to determine whether a mass is cystic or solid.

Adrenal angiography and venography have been replaced by CT and MRI. Adrenal venous sampling remains useful in certain cases. In patients with hyperaldosteronism and equivocal CT findings, adrenal venous sampling is helpful in distinguishing aldosteronoma from bilateral hyperplasia. Venous sampling, however, is almost never necessary in evaluation of Cushing syndrome or suspected pheochromocytoma. Adrenal venography and venous sampling nevertheless do have potential for inadequate samples and complications, including hemorrhage and infarction of the adrenal (49).

Despite many years of investigation, adrenal scintigraphy remains little utilized. Compared to CT, it is expensive and requires several days before results are available. There is limited availability of the radiopharmaceuticals, some of which are still investigational. Radioiodine-labeled MIBG does have some usefulness in certain clinical circumstances, although both CT and MRI are highly accurate and more widely available. One advantage of ^{131}I-MIBG is that images of the entire body can be produced in a patient suspected of having primary extra-adrenal or malignant metastatic pheochromocytomas. While MIBG could be used to screen patients suspected of having pheochromocytoma, it is quicker and more cost effective to image the adrenals and retroperitoneum with CT or MRI, because most pheochromocytomas are found there. MIBG can be done in patients with strong clinical and biochemical evidence of a catecholamine-producing neoplasm but negative CT or MRI. Nevertheless, MIBG does not provide enough anatomic detail to allow surgical planning, and some imaging study must be done even if MIBG is positive.

Although MRI is able to demonstrate both normal and abnormal adrenal glands accurately, it remains limited in utility by its longer examination time, greater cost, and more stringent patient requirements, as compared with CT. However, MRI is extremely useful in selected cases. As stated previously, MRI can distinguish between non-hyperfunctioning adenoma and metastasis better than CT. Regarding functional disorders, MRI is probably preferable to CT for evaluation of suspected pheochromocytoma, because it is as accurate for adrenal mass detection (and better for paraganglioma detection), but the findings are more specific. MRI is equivalent to CT in evaluation of Cushing syndrome. However, CT is preferred for evaluation of hyperaldosteronism or adrenal insufficiency. MRI can be very useful to further characterize lesions detected on CT, including more clearly demonstrating the extent of a mass, its exact organ of origin, and detection of vascular or other local extension. MRI can be useful in evaluating an adrenalectomy bed for possible recurrence of a malignancy, because spin echo images show less degradation by clip artifact than CT. Last, pregnant patients suspected of having adrenal disease can be more safely studied with MRI than with CT.

ACKNOWLEDGMENT

We thank David Ling, co-author of this chapter in the previous edition, for his valuable assistance.

REFERENCES

1. Abrams, HI, Siegelman SS, Adams DF. Computed tomography versus ultrasound of the adrenal gland: a prospective study. *Radiology* 1982;143:121–128.
2. Abecassis M, McLoughlin MJ, Langer B, Kudlow JE. Serendipitous adrenal masses: prevalence, significance and management. *Am J Surg* 1985;149:783–788.
3. Aso Y, Homma Y. A survey on incidental adrenal tumors in Japan. *J Urol* 1992;147:1478–1481.
4. Baker ME, Spritzer C, Blinder R, Herfkens J, Leight GS, Dunnick NR. Benign adrenal lesions mimicking malignancy on MR imaging: report of two cases. *Radiology* 1987;163:669–671.
5. Baskal NN, Erdogan G, Kamel AN, Dagci SS, Akyar S, Ekinci C. Localized non-Hodgkin's lymphoma of the adrenal and thyroid glands. *Endocrinol Jpn* 1992;39:269–276.
6. Belldegrun A, Hussain S, Seltzer SE, Loughlin KR, Gittes RF, Richie JP. Incidentally discovered mass of the adrenal gland. *Surg Gynecol Obstet* 1986;163:203–208.
7. Bennett DB, McKenna TJ, Hough AJ, Dean R, Page DL. Adrenal myelolipoma associated with Cushing's disease. *Am J Clin Pathol* 1980;73:443–447.
8. Berland LL, Koslin DB, Kenney PJ, Stanley RJ, Lee JY. Differentiation between small benign and malignant adrenal masses with dynamic incremented CT. *AJR* 1988;151:95–101.
9. Berliner L, Bosniak MA, Megibow A. Adrenal pseudotumors on computed tomography. *J Comput Assist Tomogr* 1982;6:281–285.
10. Bodie B, Novick AC, Pontes JE, et al. The Cleveland Clinic experience with adrenal cortical carcinoma. *J Urol* 1989;141:257–260.
11. Bowen A, Keslar PJ, Newman B, Hashida Y. Adrenal hemorrhage after liver transplantation. *Radiology* 1990;176:85–88.
12. Brady TM, Gross BH, Glazer GM, Williams DM. Adrenal pseudomasses due to varices: angiographic-CT-MRI-pathologic correlations. *AJR* 1985;145:301–304.
13. Bravo EL, Tarazi RC, Dustan HP, et al. The changing clinical spectrum of primary aldosteronism. *Am J Med* 1983;74:641–651.
14. Bravo EL. Adrenal medullary function. In: Moore WT, Eastman RC, eds. *Diagnostic endocrinology*. Philadelphia: BC Becker, 1990;218–226.
15. Brink JA, Heiken JP, Balfe DM, Sagel SS, DiCroce J, Vannier MW. Spiral CT: decreased spatial resolution in vivo due to broadening of section-sensitivity profile. *Radiology* 1992;185:469–474.
16. Brunt LM, Wells SA Jr. The multiple endocrine neoplasia syndromes. *Invest Radiol* 1985;20:916–927.
17. Burks DW, Mirvis SE, Shanmuganathan K. Acute adrenal injury after blunt abdominal trauma: CT findings. *AJR* 1992;158:503–507.
18. Bush WH, Elder JS, Crane RE, Wales LR. Cystic pheochromocytoma. *Urology* 1985;25:332–334.
19. Casola G, Nicolet V, van Sonnenberg E, et al. Unsuspected pheochromocytoma: risk of blood-pressure alterations during percutaneous adrenal biopsy. *Radiology* 1986;159:733–735.
20. Cedermark BJ, Ohlsen H. Computed tomography in the diagnosis of metastases of the adrenal glands. *Surg Gynecol Obstet* 1981;152:13–16.
21. Chang A, Glazer HS, Lee JKT, Ling D, Heiken JP. Adrenal gland: MR imaging. *Radiology* 1987;163:123–128.
22. Chang SY, Lee S, Ma CP, Lee SK. Non-functioning tumors of the adrenal cortex. *Br J Urol* 1989;63:462–464.
23. Cheema P, Cartagena R, Staubitz W. Adrenal cysts: diagnosis and treatment. *J Urol* 1981;120:396.
24. Chezmar JL, Robbins SM, Nelson RC, Steinberg HV, Torres WE, Bernardino ME. Adrenal Masses: characterization with T1-weighted MR imaging. *Radiology* 1988;166:357–359.
25. Davis PL, Hricak H, Bradley WG Jr. Magnetic resonance imaging of the adrenal glands. *Radiol Clin North Am* 1984;22:891–895.
26. DeBlois GG, DeMay RM. Adrenal myelolipoma diagnosis by computed-tomography-guided fine-needle aspiration. *Cancer* 1985;55:848–850.
27. Desai MB, Kapadia SN. Feminizing adrenocortical tumors in male patients: adenoma versus carcinoma. *J Urol* 1988;139:101–103.
28. Dieckmann KP, Hamm B, Pickartz H, Jonas D, Bauer HW. Adrenal myelolipoma: clinical, radiologic and histologic features. *Urology* 1987:29:1–8.
29. Disler DG, Chew FS. Adrenal pheochromocytoma. *AJR* 1992;158:1056.
30. Doppman JL, Gill JR, Miller DL, et al. Distinction between hyperaldosteronism due to bilateral hyperplasia and unilateral aldosteronoma: reliability of CT. *Radiology* 1992;184:677–682.
31. Doppman JL, Gill JR Jr, Nienhuis AW, Earll JM, Long JA Jr. CT findings in Addison's disease. *J Comput Assist Tomogr* 1982;6:757–761.
32. Doppman JL, Miller DL, Dwyer AJ, et al. Macronodular adrenal hyperplasia in Cushing disease. *Radiology* 1988;166:347–352.
33. Doppman JL, Nieman LK. Travis WD, et al. CT and MR imaging of massive macronodular adrenocortical disease: a rare cause of autonomous primary adrenal hypercortisolism. *J Comput Assist Tomogr* 1991;15:773–779.
34. Doppman JL, Travis WD, Nieman L, et al. Cushing syndrome due to primary pigmented nodular adrenocortical disease: findings at CT and MR imaging. *Radiology* 1989;172:415–420.
35. Doppman JL. The dilemma of bilateral adrenocortical nodularity in Conn's and Cushing's syndromes. *Radiol Clin North Am* 1993;31:1039–1050.
36. Dunnick NR, Doppman JL, Gill JR, Strott CA, Keiser HR, Brennan MF. Localization of functional adrenal tumors by computed tomography and venous sampling. *Radiology* 1982;142:429–433.
37. Dunnick NR, Heaston D, Halvorsen R, Moore AV, Korobkin M. *J Comput Assist Tomogr* 1982:6:978–982.
38. Dunnick NR, Leight GS Jr, Roubidoux MA, Leder RA, Paulson E, Kurylo L. CT in the diagnosis of primary aldosteronism: sensitivity in 29 patients. *AJR* 1993;160:321–324.
39. Eghrari M, McLoughlin MJ, Rosen IE, et al. The role of computed tomography in assessment of tumoral pathology of the adrenal glands. *J Comput Assist Tomogr* 1980;4:71–77.

40. Falappa P, Mirk P, Rossi M, Troncone L, Butti A, Colagrande C. Case report. Bilateral pseudocystic pheochromocytoma. *J Comput Assist Tomogr* 1980;4:860–862.

41. Falchook FS, Allard JC. Case report. CT of primary adrenal lymphoma. *J Comput Assist Tomogr* 1991;15:1048–1050.

42. Falke TH, te-Strake L, Shaff MI, et al. MR imaging of the adrenals: correlation with computed tomography. *J Comput Assist Tomogr* 1986;10:242–253.

43. Feldberg MAM, Hendriks MJ, Klinkhamer AC. Massive bilateral non-Hodgkin's lymphomas of the adrenals. *Urol Radiol* 1986;8:85–88.

44. Fink DW, Wurtzebach LR. Symptomatic myelolipoma of the adrenal. *Radiology* 1980;134:451–452.

45. Fishman EK, Deutch BM, Hartman DS, Goldman SM, Zerhouni EA, Siegelman SS. Primary adrenocortical carcinoma: CT evaluation with clinical correlation. *AJR* 1987;148:531–535.

46. Foster DG. Adrenal cysts. *Arch Surg* 1966;92:131–143.

47. Francis IR, Glazer GM, Shapiro B, Sisson JC, Gross BH. Complementary roles of CT and ^{131}I-MIBG scintigraphy in diagnosing pheochromocytoma. *AJR* 1983;141:719–725.

48. Gajraj H, Young AE. Adrenal incidentaloma. *Br J Surg* 1993;80:422–426.

49. Geisinger MA, Zelch MG, Bravo EL, Risius BF, O'Donovan PB, Borkowski GP. Primary hyperaldosteronism: comparison of CT, adrenal venography, and venous sampling. *AJR* 1983;141:299–302.

50. Gillams A, Roberts CM, Shaw P, Spiro SG, Goldstraw P. The value of CT scanning and percutaneous fine needle aspiration of adrenal masses in biopsy-proven lung cancer. *Clin Radiol* 1992;46:18–22.

51. Glazer GM, Woolsey EJ, Borrello J, et al. Adrenal tissue characterization using MR imaging. *Radiology* 1986;158:73–79.

52. Glazer HS, Lee JKT, Balfe DM, Mauro MA, Griffeth R, Sagel SS. Non-Hodgkin lymphoma: computed tomographic demonstration of unusual extranodal involvement. *Radiology* 1983;149:211–217

53. Glazer HS, Weyman PJ, Sagel SS, Levitt RG, McClennan BL. Nonfunctioning adrenal masses: incidental discovery on computed tomography. *AJR* 1982;139:81–85.

54. Gleason PE, Weinberger MH, Pratt JH, et al. Evaluation of diagnostic tests in the differential diagnosis of primary aldosteronism: unilateral adenoma versus bilateral micronodular hyperplasia. *J Urol* 1993;150:1365–1368.

55. Gould JD, Mitty HA, Pertsemlidis D, Szporn AH. Adrenal myelolipoma: diagnosis by fine needle aspiration. *AJR* 148:921–922.

56. Grainger RG, Lloyd GAS, Williams JL. Egg-shell calcification: a sign of pheochromocytoma. *Clin Radiol* 1967;18:282–286.

57. Grant CS, Carpenter P, Van Heerden JA, Hamberger B. Primary aldosteronism. Clinical management. *Arch Surg* 1984;119:585–590.

58. Halvorsen RA Jr, Heaston DK, Johnston WW, Ashton PR, Burton GM. Case report. CT guided thin needle aspiration of adrenal blastomycosis. *J Comput Assist Tomogr* 1982;6:389–391.

59. Hauser H, Gurret JP. Miliary tuberculosis associated with adrenal enlargement: CT appearance. *J Comput Assist Tomogr* 1986;10:254–256.

60. Hayes WS, Davidson AJ, Grimley PM, Hartman DS. Extraadrenal retroperitoneal paraganglioma: clinical, pathologic, and CT findings. *AJR* 1990;155:1247–1250.

61. Heaston DK, Handel DB, Ashton PR, Korobkin M. Narrow gauge needle aspiration of solid adrenal masses. *AJR* 1982;138:1143–1148.

62. Hedeland H, Östberg G, Hökfelt B. On the prevalence of adrenocortical adenomas in an autopsy material in relation to hypertension and diabetes. *Acta Med Scand* 1968;184:211–214.

63. Huebener KH, Treugut H. Adrenal cortex dysfunction: CT findings. *Radiology* 1984;150:195–199.

64. Huminer D, Garty M, Lapidot M, Leiba S, Borohov H, Rosenfeld JB. Lymphoma presenting with adrenal insufficiency. *Am J Med* 1988;84:169–172.

65. Hutler AM, Kayhoe E. Adrenal cortical carcinoma: clinical features in 138 patients. *Am J Med* 1966;41:572.

66. Icard P, Chapuis Y, Andreassian B, Bernard A, Proye C. Adrenocortical carcinoma in surgically treated patients: a retrospective study on 156 cases by the French Association of Endocrine Surgery. *Surgery* 1992;112:972–980.

67. Ikeda DM, Francis IR, Glazer GM, Amendola MA, Gross MD, Aisen AM. The detection of adrenal tumors and hyperplasia in patients with primary aldosteronism: comparison of scintigraphy, CT and MR imaging. *AJR* 1989;153:301–306.

68. Itoh K, Yamashita K, Satoh Y, Sawada H. Case report. MR imaging of bilateral adrenal hemorrhage. *J Comput Assist Tomogr* 1988;12:1054–1056.

69. Jafri SZ, Francis IR, Glazer GM, Bree RL, Amendola MA. CT detection of adrenal lymphoma. *J Comput Assist Tomogr* 1983;7:254–256.

70. Jansson S, Tisell LE, Fjalling M, Lindberg S, Jacobsson L, Zachrisson F. Early diagnosis of and surgical strategy for adrenal medullary disease in MEN II gene carriers. *Surgery* 1988;103:11–18.

71. Kamilaris TC, Chrousos GP. Adrenal diseases. In: Moore WT, Eastman RC, eds. *Diagnostic endocrinology.* Philadelphia: BC Becker, 1990:79–109.

72. Kane NM, Korobkin M, Francis IR, Quint LE, Cascade PN. Percutaneous biopsy of left adrenal masses: prevalence of pancreatitis after anterior approach. *AJR* 157:777–780.

73. Karstaedt N, Sagel SS, Stanley RJ, Melson GL, Levitt RG. Computed tomography of the adrenal gland. *Radiology* 1978;129:723–730.

74. Kearny GP, Mahoney EM, Maher E, Harrison JH. Functioning and nonfunctioning cysts of the adrenal cortex and medulla. *Am J Surg* 1977;134:363–368.

75. Kenney PJ, Robbins GL, Ellis DA, Spirt BA. Adrenal glands in patients with congenital renal anomalies: CT appearance. *Radiology* 1985;155:181–182.

76. Kenney PJ, Stanley RJ. Calcified adrenal masses. *Urologic Radiol* 1987;9:9–15.

77. Kenney PJ. Letters to the editor. Adrenal pheochromocytoma. *AJR* 1993;160:209–210.

78. Khafagi FA, Gross MD, Shapiro B, Glazer GM, Francil I, Thompson NW. Clinical significance of the large adrenal mass. *Br J Surg* 1991;78:828–833.

79. Kier R, McCarthy S. MR characterization of adrenal masses: field strength and pulse sequence considerations. *Radiology* 1989;171:671–674.

80. King BF, Kopecky KK, Baker MK, Clark SA. Extramedullary hematopoiesis in the adrenal glands: CT characteristics. *J Comput Assist Tomogr* 1987;11:342–343.

81. Kobayshi S, Seki T, Nonomura K, Gotoh T, Togashi M, Koyanagi T. Clinical experience of incidentally discovered adrenal tumor with particular reference to cortical function. *J Urol* 1993;150:8–12.

82. Koch KJ, Cory DA. Simultaneous renal vein thrombosis and bilateral adrenal hemorrhage: MR demonstration. *J Comput Assist Tomogr* 1986;10:681–683.

83. Korobkin M, White EA, Kressel HY, Moss AA, Montage JP. Computed tomography in the diagnosis of adrenal disease. *AJR* 1979;132:231–238.

84. Krestin GP, Stenbrich W, Friedman G. Adrenal masses: evaluation with fast gradient-echo MR imaging and Gd-DTPA-enhanced dynamic studies. *Radiology* 1989;171:675–680.

85. Krestin GP, Friedmann G, Fischbach R, Neufang KFR, Allolio B. Evaluation of adrenal masses in oncologic patients: dynamic contrast-enhanced MR vs CT. *J Comput Assist Tomogr* 1991;15:104–110.

86. Lee FT, Thornbury JR, Grist TM, Kelcz. MR imaging of adrenal lymphoma. *Abdom Imaging* 1993;18:95–96.

87. Lee MJ, Hahn PF, Papanicolaou N, et al. Benign and malignant adrenal masses: CT distinction with attenuation coefficients, size, and observer analysis. *Radiology* 1991;179:415–418.

88. Leroy-Willig A, Bittoun J, Luton JP, et al. In vivo MR spectroscopic imaging of the adrenal glands: distinction between adenomas and carcinomas larger than 15 mm based on lipid content. *AJR* 1989;153:771–773.

89. Levine E. CT evaluation of active adrenal histoplasmosis. *Urol Radiol* 1991;13:103–106.

90. Ling D, Korobkin M, Silverman PM, Dunnick NR. CT demonstration of bilateral adrenal hemorrhage. *AJR* 1983;141:307–308.

91. Lipsell MB, Hertz R, Ross GT. Clinical and pathophysiologic aspects of adrenocortical carcinoma. *Am J Med* 1963;35:374–383.

92. Lombardi TJ, Korobkin M, Aisen AM, et al. *Differentiation of adrenal adenomas from nonadenomas using chemical shift and gadolinium enhanced MR imaging.* Presented at the annual meeting of the Society of Uroradiology, Laguna Niguel, CA. January, 1994.

93. McCorkell SJ, Niles NL. Fine-needle aspiration of catecholamine-producing adrenal masses: a possible fatal mistake. *AJR* 1985;145:113–114.

94. McMurray JF Jr, Long D, McClure R, Kotchen TA. Addison's disease with adrenal enlargement on computed tomographic scanning. Report on two cases of tuberculosis and review of the literature. *Am J Med* 1984;77:365–368.

95. Melicow MM. One hundred cases of pheochromocytoma (107 tumors) at the Columbia-Presbyterian Medical Center, 1926–1976: a clinicopathological analysis. *Cancer* 1977;40:1987–2004.

96. Mersey JH, Bowers B, Jezic DV, Padgett CA. Adrenal insufficiency due to invasion by lymphoma: documentation by CT scan. *South Med J* 1986;79:71–73.

97. Mitchell DG, Crovello M, Matteucci T, Petersen RO, Miettinen MM. Benign adrenocortical masses: diagnosis with chemical shift MR imaging. *Radiology* 1992;185:345–351.

98. Mitnick JS, Bosniak MA, Megibow AJ, Naidich DP. Non-functioning adrenal adenomas discovered incidentally on computed tomography. *Radiology* 1983;148:495–499.

99. Mitty HA, Cohen BA, Sprayregen S, Schwartz K. Adrenal pseudotumors on CT due to dilated portosystemic veins. *AJR* 1983;141:727–730.

100. Miyake H, Maeda H, Tashiro M, et al. CT of adrenal tumors: frequency and clinical significance of low-attenuation lesions. *AJR* 1989;152:1005–1007.

101. Montagne JP, Kressel HY, Korobkin M, Moss AA. Computed tomography of the normal adrenal gland. *AJR* 1978;130:963–966.

102. Moon KL, Hricak H, Crooks LE, et al. Nuclear magnetic resonance imaging of the adrenal gland: a preliminary report. *Radiology* 1983;147:155–160.

103. Musante F, Derchi LE, Zappasodi F, et al. Myelolipoma of the adrenal gland: sonographic and CT features. *AJR* 1988;151:961–964.

104. Musante F, Derchi LE, Bazzocchi M, Avataneo T, Grandini G, Mucelli RSP. MR imaging of adrenal myelolipomas. *J Comput Assist Tomogr* 1991;15:111–114.

105. Newhouse JH. MRI of the adrenal gland. *Urol Radiol* 1990;12:1–6.

106. Nielsen ME Jr, Heaston DK, Dunnick NR, Korobkin M. Preoperative CT evaluation of adrenal glands in non-small-cell bronchogenic carcinoma. *AJR* 1982;139:317–320.

107. O'Brien WM, Choyke PL, Copeland J, Klappenbach RS, Lyunch JH. Computed tomography of adrenal abscess. *J Comput Assist Tomogr* 1987;11:550–551.

108. O'Connell TX, Aston SJ. Acute adrenal hemorrhage complicating anticoagulant therapy. *Surg Gynecol Obstet* 1974;139:355–357.

109. Oliva A, Duarte B, Hammadeh R, Ghosh L, Baker RJ. Myelolipoma and endocrine dysfunction. *Surgery* 1988;103:711–715.

110. Oliver TW, Bernardino ME, Miller JI, Mansour K, Greene D, Davis WA. Isolated adrenal masses in non-small-cell bronchogenic carcinoma. *Radiology* 1984;153:217–218.

111. Olsson CA, Krane RJ, Klugo RC, Selikowitz SM. Adrenal myelolipoma. *Surgery* 1973;73:665–670.

112. Pagani JJ. Normal adrenal glands in small cell lung carcinoma: CT-guided biopsy. *AJR* 1983;140:949–951.

113. Pagani JJ. Non-small-cell lung carcinoma adrenal metastases. Computed tomography and percutaneous needle biopsy in their diagnosis. *Cancer* 1984;53:1058–1060.

114. Paling MR, Williamson BRJ. Adrenal involvement in non-Hodgkin lymphoma. *AJR* 1983;141:303–305.

115. Pasciak RM, Cook WA. Case report. Massive retroperitoneal hemorrhage owing to a ruptured adrenal cyst. *J Urol* 1988;130:98–100.

116. Perry RR, Nieman LK, Cutler GB, et al. Primary adrenal causes of Cushing's syndrome: diagnosis and surgical management. *Ann Surg* 1989;210:59–68.

117. Pojunas KW, Daniels DL, Williams AL, Thorsen MK, Haughton VM. Pituitary and adrenal CT of Cushing syndrome. *AJR* 1986;146:1235–1238.

118. Pommier RF, Brennan MF. An eleven-year experience with adrenocortical carcinoma. *Surgery* 1992;112:963–971.

119. Potter EL. *Pathology of the fetus and newborn.* Chicago, Year Book Medical Publishers, 1952.

120. Quint LE, Glazer GM, Francis IR, Shapiro B, Chenevert TL. Pheochromocytoma and paraganglioma: comparison of MR imaging with CT and I-131 MIBG scintigraphy. *Radiology* 1987;165:89–93.

121. Radin DR, Manoogian C, Nadler JL. Diagnosis of primary hyperaldosteronism: importance of correlating CT findings with endocrinologic studies. *AJR* 1992;158:553–557.

122. Raisanen J, Shapiro B, Glazer GM, Desai S, Sisson JC. Plasma catecholamines in pheochromocytoma: effect of urographic contrast media. *AJR* 1984;143:43–46.

123. Reinig JW, Doppman JL, Dwyer AJ, Frank J. MRI of indeterminate adrenal masses. *AJR* 1986;147:493–496.

124. Reinig JW, Doppman JL, Dwyer AJ, Johnson AR, Knop RH. Adrenal masses differentiated by MR. *Radiology* 1986;158:81–84.

125. Remer EM, Weinfeld RM, Glazer GM, et al. Hyperfunctioning and nonhyperfunctioning benign adrenal cortical lesions: characterization and comparison with MR imaging. *Radiology* 1989;171:681–685.

126. Rink IJ, Reinig JW, Dwyer AJ, Doppman JL, Linehan WM, Keiser HR. MR imaging of pheochromocytomas. *J Comput Assist Tomogr* 1985;9:454–458.

127. Ritchey ML, Kinard R, Novicki DE. Adrenal tumors: involvement of the inferior vena cava. *J Urol* 1987;138:1134–1136.

128. Rofsky NM, Bosniak MA, Megibow AJ, Schlossberg P. Adrenal myelolipomas: CT appearance with tiny amounts of fat and punctate calcification. *Urol Radiol* 1989;11:148–152.

129. Sandler MA, Perlberg JL, Madrazo BL, Gitschlag KF, Gross SC. Computed tomographic evaluation of the adrenal gland in the preoperative assessment of bronchogenic carcinoma. *Radiology* 1982;145:733–736.

130. Schaner EG, Dunnick NR, Doppman JL, Strott CA, Gill JR, Javadpour N. Adrenal cortical tumors with low attenuation coefficients: a pitfall in computed tomography diagnosis. *J Comput Assist Tomogr* 1978;2:11–15.

131. Schulund JF, Kenney PJ, Brown ED, Archer SM, Brown JJ, Semelka RC. Adrenal cortical carcinoma: MRI appearance using current tecnique. *JMRI* 1995;5:171–174.

132. Schultz CL, Haaga JR, Fletcher BD, Alfidi RJ, Schultz MA. Magnetic resonance imaging of the adrenal glands: a comparison with computed tomography. *AJR* 1984;143:1235–1240.

133. Schwartz AN, Goiney RC, Graney DO. Gastric diverticulum simulating an adrenal mass: CT appearance and embryogenesis. *AJR* 1986;146:553–554.

134. Schwartz JM, Bosniak MA, Megibow AJ, Hulnick DH. Case report. Right adrenal pseudotumor caused by colon: CT demonstration. *J Comput Assist Tomogr* 1988;12:153–154.

135. Scully RE, Mark EJ, McNeeley BU. Case 28, case records of the Massachusetts General Hospital: weekly clinicopathological exercises. *N Engl J Med* 1984;311:783–790.

136. Seidenwurm DJ, Elmer EB, Kaplan LM, Williams EK, Morris DG, Hoffman AR. Metastases to the adrenal glands and the development of Addison's disease. *Cancer* 1984;54:552–557.

137. Shah HR, Love L, Williamson MR, Buckner BC, Ferris EJ. Hemorrhagic adrenal metastases: CT findings. *J Comput Assist Tomogr* 1989;13:77–81.

138. Silverman PM. Gastric diverticulum mimicking adrenal mass: CT demonstration. *J Comput Assist Tomogr* 1986;10:709–710.

139. Silverman SG, Mueller PR, Pinkney LP, Koenker RM, Seltzer SE. Predictive value of image-guided adrenal biopsy: analysis of results of 101 biopsies. *Radiology* 1993;187:715–718.

140. Smith SM, Patel SK, Turner DA, Matalon TAS. Magnetic resonance imaging of adrenal cortical carcinoma. *Urol Radiol* 1989;11:1–6.

141. Solomon N, Sumkin J. Right adrenal gland hemorrhage as a complication of liver transplantation: CT appearance. *J Comput Assist Tomogr* 1988;12:95–97.

142. Sommers SC. Adrenal glands. In: Anderson WAD, Kissane JM, eds. *Pathology*, vol 2. St. Louis: Mosby, 1977;1658–1679.

143. Stone NN, Janoski A, Muakkassa W, Shpritz L. Mineralocorticoid excess secondary to adrenal cortical carcinoma. *J Urol* 1984;132: 962–965.

144. Sun ZH, Nomura K, Toraya S, et al. Clinical significance of adrenal computed tomography in Addison's disease. *Endocrinol Japon* 1992;39:563–569.

145. St. John Sutton MG, Sheps SG, Lie JT. Prevalence of clinically unsuspected pheochromocytoma: review of a 50-year autopsy series. *Mayo Clin Proc* 1981;56:354–360.

146. Tsushima Y, Ishizaka H, Matsumoto K, Matsumoto M. Differential diagnosis of adrenal masses using out-of-phase flash imaging. A preliminary report. *Acta Radiologica* 1992;33:262–265.

147. Tsushima Y, Ishizaka H, Matsumoto M. Adrenal masses: differentiation with chemical shift, fast low-angle shot MR imaging. *Radiology* 1993;186:705–709.

148. Tung GA, Pfister RC, Papanicolaou N, Yoder IC. Adrenal cysts: imaging and percutaneous aspiration. *Radiology* 1989;173:107–110.

149. van Gils APG, Falke THM, van Erkel AR, et al. MR imaging and MIBG scintigraphy of pheochromocytomas and extraadrenal functioning paragangliomas. *Radiographics* 1991;11:37–57.

150. Vas W, Zylak CJ, Mather D, Figueredo A. The value of abdominal computed tomography in the pre-treatment assessment of small cell carcinoma of the lung. *Radiology* 1981;138:417–418.

151. Vassiliades VG, Bernardino ME. Percutaneous renal and adrenal biopsies. *Cardiovasc Intervent Radiol* 1991;14:50–54.

152. Vick CW, Zeman RK, Mannes E, Cronan JJ, Walse JW. Adrenal myelolipoma: CT and ultrasound findings. *Urol Radiol* 1984;6:7–13.

153. Wahl HR. Adrenal cysts. *Am J Pathol* 1951;27:758.

154. Weiner SN, Bernstein RG, Lowy S, Karp H. Combined adrenal adenoma and myelolipoma. *J Comput Assist Tomogr* 1981;5:440–442.

155. Welch TJ, Sheedy PJ, van Heerden JA, Sheps SG, Hattery RR, Stephens DH. Pheochromocytoma: value of computed tomography. *Radiology* 1983;148:501–503.

156. Whaley D, Becker S, Presbrey T, Shaff M. CT evaluation. *J Comput Assist Tomogr* 1985;9:959–960.

157. White EA, Schambelan M, Rost CR, Biglieri EG, Moss AA, Korobkin M. Use of computed tomography in diagnosing the cause of primary aldosteronism. *N Engl J Med* 1980;303:1503–1508.

158. Wilms G, Baert A, Marchal G, Goddeeris P. Computed tomography of the normal adrenal glands: correlative study with autopsy specimens. *J Comput Assist Tomogr* 1979;3:467–469.

159. Wilms GE, Baert AL, Lint EJ, Pringot JH, Goddeeris PG. Computed tomographic findings in bilateral adrenal tuberculosis. *Radiology* 1983;146:729–730.

160. Wilms G, Marchal G, Baert A, Adisoejoso B, Mangkuwerdojo S. CT and ultrasound features of post-traumatic adrenal hemorrhage. *J Comput Assist Tomogr* 1987;11:112–115.

161. Wilson DA, Muchmore HG, Tisdal RG, Fahmy A, Pitha JV. Histoplasmosis of the adrenal glands studied by CT. *Radiology* 1984; 150:779–783.

162. Wolverson MK, Kannegiesser H. CT of bilateral adrenal hemorrhage with acute adrenal insufficiency in the adult. *AJR* 1984;142: 311–314.

163. Xarli VP, Steele AA, Davis PJ, Buescher ES, Rios CN, Garcia-Bunuel R. Adrenal hemorrhage in the adult. *Medicine* 1978;57: 211–221.

CHAPTER 20

Pelvis

Joseph K. T. Lee, Ann Bagley Willms, and Richard C. Semelka

Computed tomography (CT) is an essential imaging tool for evaluating patients with suspected pelvic disease, because it provides excellent cross-sectional display of bony and soft-tissue pelvic structures regardless of body habitus. In recent years, the clinical utility of magnetic resonance imaging (MRI) in pelvic imaging has been better defined. MRI has several unique features that make it an ideal method for imaging the pelvis. First, its ability to produce images in multiple planes without degradation that results from CT reconstruction is especially helpful with complex pelvic anatomy. Second, MRI has superior contrast sensitivity, causes no known biologic effects, and can distinguish vascular from nonvascular structures without the use of intravenous contrast material. Finally, respiratory motion, which often degrades the quality of upper abdominal and thoracic MR images, is virtually absent in the pelvis.

TECHNIQUES

Computed tomography

A successful CT examination of the pelvis depends on careful patient preparation. Because multiple small bowel loops reside in the pelvis, complete opacification of the alimentary tract is essential lest they be misinterpreted as mass lesions. This is usually achieved by giving the patient 800 to 1,000 ml of dilute oral contrast at least 1 hour before the examination. Although the rectosigmoid and descending colon may be recognized by location and fecal content, their opacification often is desirable. Opacification of these segments may be achieved via the oral route if contrast is administered 6 to 12 hours before the study; a contrast-material enema (200 ml) is routinely given at some institutions to expedite opacification of this region. Although a vaginal tampon may facilitate the identification of the vaginal canal (46), such practice is not necessary.

Because the pelvis is often included as part of the abdominal CT study, and because there is great variability in location and diameter of the pelvic arteries and veins which makes differentiating them from pelvic lymph nodes difficult, intravenous contrast material is now routinely administered for pelvic CT in most institutions. Using a power injector, 150 to 200 ml of 60% iodine solution is intravenously administered, either as a uniphasic (e.g., 2 ml/sec) or as a biphasic (e.g., 2 ml/sec for the initial 50 ml, followed by 1 ml/sec for the remainder) injection. A delay of 3 minutes between the initiation of injection and the performance of scanning is desirable to allow maximal enhancement of pelvic veins, thereby facilitating their differentiation from enlarged pelvic lymph nodes (277) (Fig. 1).

Because of the speed that the entire abdomen and pelvic can be imaged with modern CT scanners, the urinary bladder usually has not yet been opacified by iodinated contrast material excreted from the kidneys at the completion of the initial study. Therefore, an additional set of delayed images through the urinary bladder is routinely obtained at some institutions to allow better assessment of the bladder wall when staging patients with bladder neoplasms or other genitourinary neoplasms.

For routine pelvic studies, contiguous 1-cm transaxial scans will suffice. When staging pelvic neoplasms, contiguous 5-mm scans usually are obtained through the area of interest, with the remainder of the pelvis imaged using 10-mm slice collimation.

Although direct coronal scanning with the patient sitting on a specially designed support device provides a

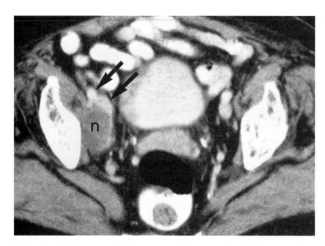

FIG. 1. Enlarged right external iliac nodes (n) secondary to vulvar carcinoma are easily distinguished from vessels *(arrows)* with the use of intravenous contrast.

clear display of the pelvic floor and its adjacent structures (293), it has not gained widespread acceptance because of the additional time required to assemble such a device and because of the ease with which such images can be obtained with MRI. The improved quality of coronal images reconstructed from data through helical acquisition also will make direct coronal CT scanning unnecessary.

Magnetic Resonance Imaging

The pelvis likewise can be successfully examined with MRI. As in the case of CT, an MR oral contrast agent can aid in the differentiation of bowel from other normal or pathologic tissues. Perflurbon (perfluoroctylbromide or PFOB, Imagent, Alliance Pharmaceutical, San Diego, California), which causes darkening of bowel lumen, has been shown to facilitate differentiation between a normal bowel loop and a pelvic mass. The image quality of MR studies also is improved when PFOB is used in conjunction with intramuscular administration of glucagon (28). However, PFOB, one of the few FDA-approved MR oral contrast agents to date, has not achieved widespread clinical acceptance, largely because of its high cost.

A variety of radiofrequency (RF) receiver coils can be used to examine the pelvis. Although a body coil provides the largest field of view and an intraluminal coil yields the best anatomic details, phased-array multicoils combine adequate spatial coverage with improved anatomic resolution (137,240) and have become the receiver of choice for imaging the pelvis.

Both T1- and T2-weighted sequences are required for lesion detection and characterization. T1-weighted imaging can be achieved with either a breath-hold gradient refocused echo (GRE) sequence (FLASH or spoiled GRASS) or a conventional spin-echo (SE) sequence (TR 300 to 1,000 msec, TE as short as possible). Because breathing artifacts are not as problematic in the pelvis as in the abdomen, we generally use T1-weighted spin echo for studies limited to the pelvis because of the higher signal-to-noise ratio of spin echo sequences. We prefer GRE when more extensive imaging requires examination of the abdomen in detail, because it allows multiple sections to be obtained with a single breath-hold, resulting in shorter imaging time and high quality images without respiratory-related artifacts. At 1.5 tesla, with a TR of 130 msec, TE of 4 msec, flip angle of 80°, and one excitation, a total of 14 sections can be obtained in 19 seconds. The relatively short acquisition time required for a GRE sequence allows serial dynamic imaging immediately after intravenous administration of a gadolinium (Gd) compound. T2-weighted imaging (TR > 1,500 msec, TE > 70 msec) can be achieved with a fast spin-echo (FSE) or a turbo spin-echo technique. The advantage of FSE is a substantial reduction in imaging time. The faster imaging time can be used to improve spatial resolution (by increasing imaging matrix elements) and stronger T2-weighting (by increasing TR and obtaining later echoes) within a reasonable data acquisition time. T1- or T2-weighted spin echo technique (or FSE technique) combined with fat saturation results in reduction of ghosting artifact, increased contrast range of nonfatty tissues, and elimination of chemical shift artifact. Fat saturation is especially useful for distinguishing a fat-containing structure from a hemorrhagic lesion (136,266).

Transaxial images are performed in every case, usually with 8- to 10-mm collimation at 10- to 12-mm intervals. The use of a 2-mm interslice gap reduces cross talk between consecutive sections. Thinner slices (e.g., 5 mm) may be obtained through the area of interest for initial staging of patients with known pelvic neoplasms. In most cases, additional views are performed in either the coronal or sagittal plane. Coronal images are useful for evaluating the seminal vesicles and bladder neoplasms that involve the lateral wall. Sagittal views are best for defining the uterine body, cervix, and vaginal canal, and for evaluating the rectum and sacrum. Sagittal images also are necessary in cases in which the bladder neoplasm is located along the anterior or posterior wall.

NORMAL ANATOMY

The pelvis is a complex structure composed of an osseous ring formed by the innominate bones and sacrum, with numerous attached muscles for support and ambulation. Within this musculo-osseous skeleton reside various internal organs and major blood vessels, lymphatics, and nerves. Most of these structures are either midline or bilaterally symmetrical within this skeletal framework. This section will cover the essential CT and MR features of the internal pelvic organs. Information concerning the relationship between the peritoneal and extraperitoneal spaces of the pelvis can be found in Chapter 10.

Computed Tomography

The pelvic muscles (psoas, iliacus, obturator internus, pyriformis, and levator ani) are well delineated on CT scans and are symmetrical in the normal individual (see Figs. 57 and 63 in Chapter 10). Pelvic lymph nodes can be found in close proximity to the pelvic blood vessels. Although lymph nodes smaller than 5 mm cannot be confidently identified as such in the pelvis, lymph nodes that are enlarged, are calcified, or contain fibrolipomatous

changes are readily recognized on CT. Small bowel loops are easily identified if they contain oral contrast material; unopacified bowel loops may simulate a mass lesion. Although the rectum and the ascending, descending, and sigmoid colon can be recognized even if they are not opacified by oral contrast because they are relatively fixed in their location and because they often contain various amounts of air or feces, thereby allowing their distinction from other structures, the wall of these bowel loops can be better assessed if the lumen is distended with contrast material.

The urinary bladder is a homogeneous midline structure whose size and configuration vary greatly depending on the amount of urine it contains. Although urine is of near-water density, the bladder wall has a soft-tissue attenua-

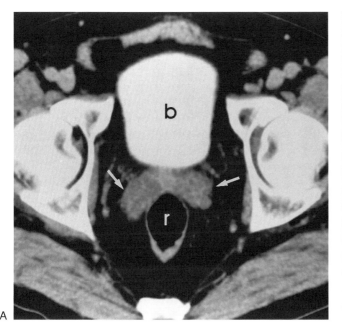

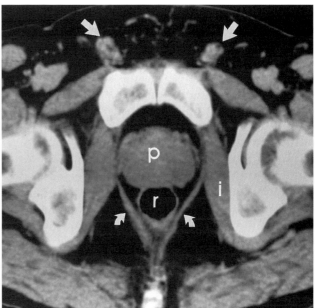

FIG. 2. Normal male pelvis. **A:** The seminal vesicles *(arrows)* lie between the bladder (b) and the rectum (r) and have a "bow-tie" configuration. Fat separates the seminal vesicles from adjacent structures. **B:** Three centimeters caudad, the prostate gland (p) lies posterior to the pubic symphysis. The spermatic cords *(straight arrows)* contain vessels, fat, and the vas deferens. *Curved arrows,* levator ani; r, rectum; i, obturator internus. **C:** Contrast-enhanced CT scan in an older patient with benign prostatic hypertrophy shows greater enhancement of the central gland *(straight arrows)* than of the peripheral zone *(curved arrows).*

tion value. In contrast-enhanced CT scans, opacified urine usually occupies the dependent portion of the bladder, and unopacified urine layers above it. However, this relationship may be reversed in patients with glycosuria or infectious debris in the bladder: here, the unopacified urine has a higher specific gravity than the excreted opacified urine (142,236).

In the male pelvis, the seminal vesicles are seen posterior to the urinary bladder, cephalad to the prostate gland, and anterior to the rectum (Fig. 2). They are oval to tear-shaped structures. A small amount of fat is usually present between the seminal vesicles and the posterior wall of the bladder. This relationship may be distorted by a distended rectum or when the patient is prone (249). The prostate gland is located just posterior to the symphysis pubis and anterior to the

rectum (Fig. 2). It usually has a homogeneous soft-tissue density on non-contrast-enhanced CT scans. However, zonal anatomy can be appreciated in some contrast-enhanced CT studies because the peripheral zone may enhance to a lesser degree than the central gland (182). Zonal anatomy is often more evident in older patients and in patients whose glands are larger in size (182) (Fig. 2). The spermatic cords are seen anterolateral to the symphysis pubis and medial to the femoral vein (Fig. 2). They may appear either as small, oval soft-tissue structures or as thin-walled, ring-like elements, containing several soft-tissue densities representing the vas deferens and the spermatic vessels. The spermatic cord can be traced to the scrotum. The testes and the epididymis are of soft-tissue density; they cannot be separated from each other.

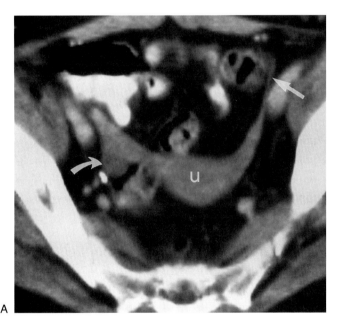

A

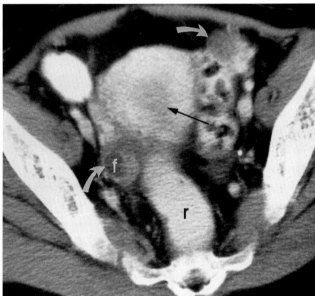

B

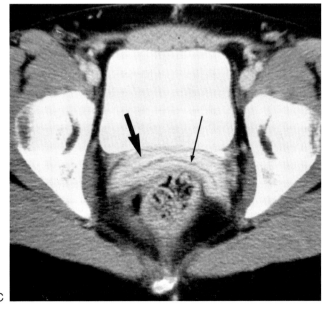

C

FIG. 3. Normal female pelvis. **A:** Contrast-enhanced CT scan in a 27-year-old woman shows an oval uterine fundus (u); note follicle *(curved arrow)* in normal right ovary; round ligament *(straight arrow)* is seen as a thin line of soft-tissue density curving anteriorly from left fundus. **B:** In a different patient, the lower-density endometrial cavity *(straight arrow)* is distinguishable from the myometrium. Both ovaries are well visualized *(curved arrows)*. A follicle (f) is seen in the right ovary. r, rectosigmoid colon. **C:** Contrast-enhanced CT image shows intense enhancement of the vaginal mucosa *(thick arrow)*. The thin line of lower attenuation demarcates the opposed mucosal surfaces *(thin arrow)*.

In the female pelvis, the uterus is seen as an oval or triangular soft-tissue mass located posterior to the urinary bladder (Fig. 3). A central area of lower attenuation, which probably represents secretions within the endometrial cavity, sometimes can be seen on non-contrast-enhanced scans. Although the myometrium cannot be differentiated from the endometrium on contrast-enhanced scans because both exhibit intense enhancement, the endometrial cavity is often better delineated after intravenous contrast administration (78).

Although demarcations between the vagina, cervix, and uterus are not clearly shown by CT scans, they can nevertheless be separated from one another by their configurations. The uterine body usually is triangular in shape, whereas the cervix has a more rounded appearance. At the level of the fornix, the vagina is seen as a flat rectangle. On contrast-enhanced CT studies, the intensely enhancing central portion of the cervix, believed to represent cervical epithelium, can be differentiated from the moderately enhancing peripheral portion made of fibrous stroma. Likewise, the intense central vaginal enhance-

ment, which probably corresponds to vaginal mucosa, can be separated from the poorly enhancing vaginal wall (Fig. 3). The normal adult premenopausal ovaries usually can be seen. Although their position is highly variable, they are most often found slightly posterolateral to the body of the uterus. They may be of uniform soft-tissue density; more commonly, the ovaries contain soft-tissue stroma admixed with small cystic areas representing normal follicles (Fig. 3). The broad ligaments are formed by two layers of peritoneum that drape over the uterus and extend laterally from the uterus to the pelvic side wall. Between the two leaves of the broad ligament is loose extraperitoneal connective tissue, smooth muscle, and fat known as the parametrium, which contains the fallopian tube, round ligament, ovarian ligament, uterine and ovarian blood vessels, nerves, lymphatic vessels, and a portion of the ureter. Although the broad ligament is rarely seen unless ascites is present, its position can be determined by structures that it abuts or contains. The round ligament is frequently seen on CT scans as a thin soft-tissue band that extends laterally from the fundus and gradually tapers in a curved

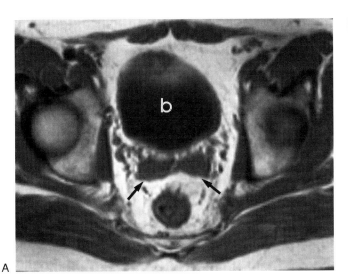

A

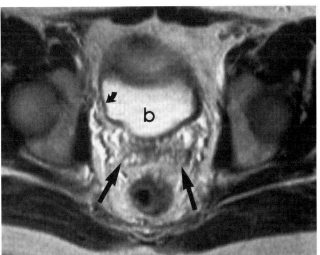

B

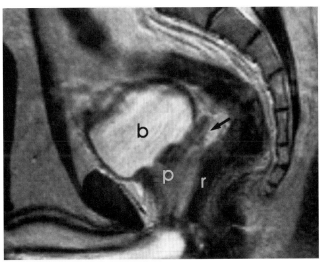

C

FIG. 4. Normal urinary bladder. **A:** Transaxial T1-weighted SE image (600/15) of the bladder (b) and seminal vesicles *(arrows)*. Note that the low-intensity bladder wall cannot be clearly distinguished from urine with this sequence. The seminal vesicles are of medium-to-low signal intensity. Transaxial **(B)** and sagittal **(C)** T2-weighted spin echo images (2500/90). The bladder wall *(curved arrow)* is now easily distinguished from the high-intensity urine. The seminal vesicles *(arrows)* show increased signal intensity due to fluid content; sagittal image not as convincing. b, bladder; p, prostate; r, rectum.

course to enter the internal inguinal ring, terminating in the labia majora (Fig. 3). The cardinal ligament (lateral cervical ligament) forms the base of the broad ligament and is usually seen on CT as a triangular soft-tissue structure extending from the cervix and upper vagina laterally. With high resolution CT, uterosacral ligaments can be seen as arc-like structures extending from the cervix to the sacrum.

Magnetic Resonance Imaging

Normal pelvic anatomy similarly can be depicted with MRI. With the exception of differences in gray scale, the pelvic anatomy as displayed on T1-weighted or proton-density MR images is quite similar to that obtained with CT. The cortical bone has an extremely low signal intensity because of the lack of mobile protons; fat, whether inside or outside the marrow, has a high signal intensity. Pelvic musculature and visceral organs have low to medium signal intensities. Because of the ''time of flight'' phenomenon, pelvic vessels usually are seen as areas of signal void on SE images but as bright foci on GRE images (24). Vessels containing more sluggish blood flow are identified as structures with high signal intensity on a second echo image of a spin-echo technique.

The urinary bladder appears as a homogeneous low signal intensity structure, and the bladder wall possesses minimal signal intensity difference from urine on a T1-weighted image (Fig. 4) (29,72). The signal intensity of urine relative to adjacent perivesical structures increases with prolongation of TR and TE. Therefore, on a T2-weighted image, urine that has a high signal intensity can be easily distinguished from the low-signal-intensity muscular layer of the bladder wall but not the high-signal-intensity mucosa and lamina propria (Fig. 4). With high resolution MRI and in patients with bladder wall hypertrophy, a low-intensity inner muscular layer may be differentiated from an intermediate-signal-intensity outer muscular layer on a T2-weighted image (195). The low-intensity bladder wall may be obscured by the chemical shift artifact that results from the difference in resonance frequency between fat and water protons. The chemical shift artifact occurs at the water–fat interface (bladder–perivesical fat) in the direction of the readout (frequency) gradient which is different for different imaging planes (i.e., with some imagers, the chemical shift artifact would affect lateral walls on transaxial views; it would affect the superior and inferior bladder wall on sagittal sections) (11). The chemical shift artifact can be recognized on a transverse image as a dark band along the lateral wall on one side, and a bright band along the lateral wall on the opposite side. If the pixel bandwidth stays the same, this artifact is more pronounced with increasing field strength. In extreme cases, the chemical shift artifact may lead to apparent thickening of the bladder wall on one side and

absence of the bladder wall on a contralateral side (Fig. 5). As stated previously, chemical shift artifact can be eliminated using a fat-saturation technique. On T1-weighted images obtained immediately after intravenous administration of a Gd compound, the mucosa and lamina propria can be differentiated from the muscle layer of the bladder wall because the former shows earlier and greater enhancement (16).

The prostate gland has a homogeneous low signal intensity, similar to that of skeletal muscle, on T1-weighted images. The neurovascular bundles, which have a low signal and are located posterolateral to the prostate gland at the 5- and 7-o'clock positions, can be identified and separated from the surrounding high-signal periprostatic fat on images obtained with endorectal coils. On post-Gd T1-weighted images, the central/transitional zone of the prostate can be distinguished from the peripheral zone because the latter has a more uniform and less intense enhancement (181). Zonal anatomy of the prostate is best depicted on T2-weighted images. Using a T2-weighted sequence, the central and transitional zones cannot be differentiated from each other but can be distinguished from the peripheral zone because the latter has a higher signal intensity (106,208,261) (Fig. 6). The higher signal intensity of the peripheral zone has been attributed to its more abundant glandular components and its more loosely interwoven muscle bundles. The anterior fibromuscular

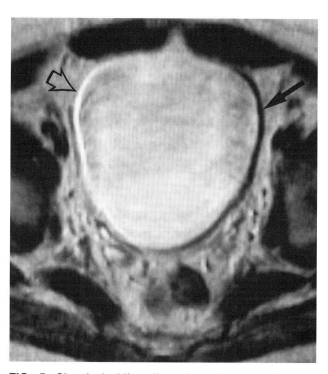

FIG. 5. Chemical shift artifact obscuring normal urinary bladder wall. Transaxial T2-weighted SE image (2500/90) obtained with a 1.5T MR imager shows a thick low-signal-intensity band *(arrow)* replacing the normally thin bladder wall. The opposite bladder wall is replaced by a high-signal-intensity band *(arrow)*.

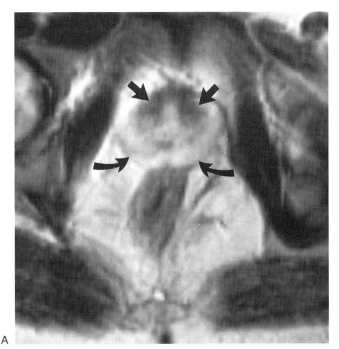

A

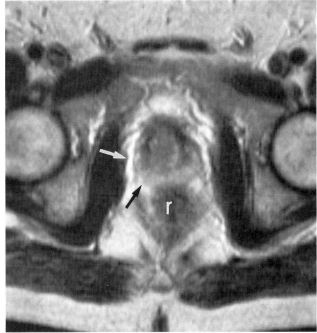

B

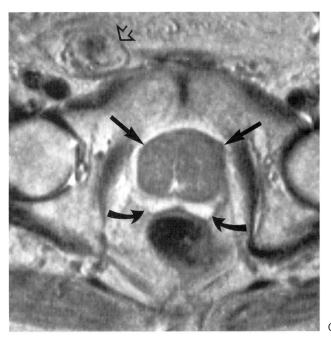

C

FIG. 6. Male pelvis. **A:** Transaxial T2-weighted FSE image (3500/93) through the pubic symphysis in a 34-year-old man shows the high-signal-intensity peripheral zone *(curved arrows)* of the prostate and the lower signal intensity central gland *(straight arrows)*. **B:** Transaxial T2-weighted SE image (2500/90) in another patient with normal prostate again shows the peripheral zone *(black arrow)* to be of higher signal intensity than the central gland (central and transitional zone). The periprostatic venous plexus is seen as a high-signal-intensity rim along the prostatic margins *(white arrow)*. r, rectum. **C:** Transaxial T2-weighted FSE image (3500/93) through the pubic symphysis shows the high-signal-intensity peripheral zone of the prostate *(curved arrows)* is easily distinguished from the hypertrophied transitional zone *(straight arrows)* in this patient with benign prostatic hypertrophy. Note right inguinal hernia *(hollow arrow)*.

band is seen as a low-intensity structure. Although the true (anatomic) capsule of the prostate and the rectoprostatic interface (Denonvilliers' fascia) are infrequently seen on the body coil images, they can be readily identified as low signal intensity bands with endorectal coils (242). The periprostatic venous plexus is seen as a high-signal-intensity rim around the prostate on the second echo of a T2-weighted image (214) (Fig. 6).

The seminal vesicles have a medium-to-low signal intensity on a T1-weighted image (Fig. 7). On T2-weighted images, the fluid within the tubules of the seminal vesicles has a high signal intensity, whereas their walls have a

low signal (Fig. 7). On Gd-enhanced T1-weighted images, the wall of the tubules enhances whereas the fluid remains unenhanced (181) (Fig. 7).

Normal scrotal contents can be seen when imaged with a surface coil (13,229,250). The signal intensity of the testes is similar to that of thigh muscle on T1-weighted images and greater than that of subcutaneous fat on T2-weighted images (Fig. 8). The tunica albuginea has a low signal intensity on both T1- and T2-weighted images; the epididymis has an intensity similar to that of the testis on T1-weighted images but much less than that of the testis on T2-weighted images. The pampiniform plexus can of-

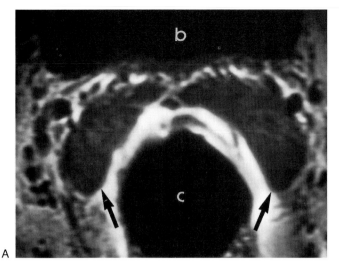

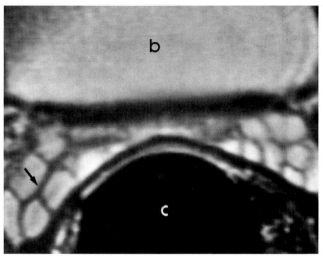

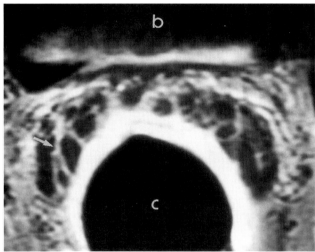

FIG. 7. MR images of normal seminal vesicles obtained with endorectal coil. **A:** T1-weighted SE image (500/25) shows low signal intensity of the teardrop-shaped seminal vesicles *(arrows).* **B:** T2-weighted SE image (2200/80) shows low-signal-intensity tubule walls *(straight arrow)* and high signal intensity of fluid within. **C:** Gadolinium-enhanced T1-weighted SE image (500/25) shows enhancement of tubule walls *(straight arrow)* and nonenhancing tubular fluid. b, bladder; c, endorectal coil. (Courtesy of S. Mirowitz, M.D., St. Louis, Missouri.)

ten be seen as a convoluted structure located cephalad to the epididymal head. The wall of the plexus has a low signal intensity on both T1- and T2-weighted images, whereas the internal structure contains both medium- and high-signal areas, the latter undoubtedly related to slow blood flow. The skin, the dartos muscle, and different scrotal fascia cannot be separated from one another and are imaged as a band of medium-to-low intensity.

Although the uterus has a homogeneous low-to-medium signal intensity on a T1-weighted image, it exhibits three different signal intensities on a T2-weighted image (Fig. 9) (103,148). On a T2-weighted image, the central portion of the uterus (endometrium) has a signal intensity higher than that of subcutaneous fat, whereas the peripheral myometrium has a signal intensity higher than that of striated muscle. Between these two layers is a narrow low intensity band called the junctional zone, which corresponds to the inner myometrium. The junctional zone has a low signal intensity similar to that of striated muscle, because it has a short T1, a short T2, and a low water content (173). Histologic studies have demonstrated that this zone contains an increased number

of myometrial cells with little extracellular matrix compared with the outer myometrium (246).

The MR appearance of the normal uterus is influenced by hormonal changes. In women of reproductive age, the central high-signal-intensity zone is thin immediately after menstruation and achieves its maximal thickness at the midcycle (52,100,175). Likewise, the signal intensity of the myometrium and uterine volume reaches a maximal value during the secretory phase. In women taking oral contraceptive pills, the endometrium is atrophic and the zonal anatomy is indistinct. Such an appearance also is seen in premenarchal and postmenopausal uteri.

Like the uterus, the cervix has a homogeneous low-to-medium signal intensity on T1-weighted images. On T2-weighted images, the central zone in the cervix has a high signal intensity similar to that of the central uterine signal. This corresponds to the secretions in the canal, the cervical mucosa, and the plical palmatae (54,103,148,248). Two distinct signal intensities can be seen in the peripheral cervical zone: an inner low-intensity band and an outer medium-intensity layer (148,319). The inner zone correlates with a region of tightly packed stroma (fibro-

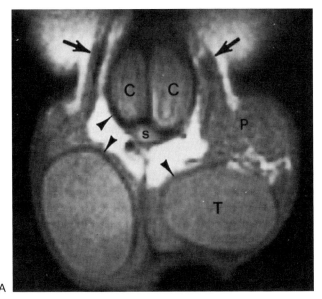

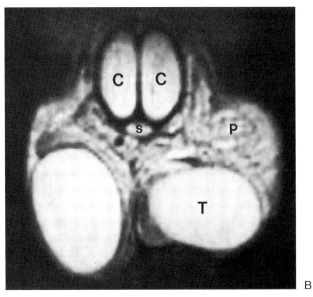

FIG. 8. Normal scrotum. **A:** Coronal T1-weighted SE image (500/15). The testis (T) has a lower signal intensity than subcutaneous fat. *Arrow*, spermatic cord; P, pampiniform plexus; *arrowhead*, tunica covering the testis and penis; C, corpus cavernosum; s, corpus spongiosum. **B:** Coronal T2-weighted SE image (2100/90) obtained at a slightly more posterior level than (A). Note that the signal intensity of the testis is higher than that for fat.

blasts and smooth muscle cells), whereas the outer zone corresponds to a region of more loosely packed stroma (54).

Like the uterus and cervix, the vagina is intermediate in signal intensity on T1-weighted images. The vagina can be distinguished from the surrounding structures on a T2-weighted image. It has a high-signal-intensity center representing the vaginal epithelium and mucus, surrounded by a low-signal-intensity wall (Fig. 10). A prominent venous plexus surrounds the vagina and is of very high signal intensity on T2-weighted images.

The normal reproductive-age ovaries are routinely demonstrated on MRI performed with phased-array mul-

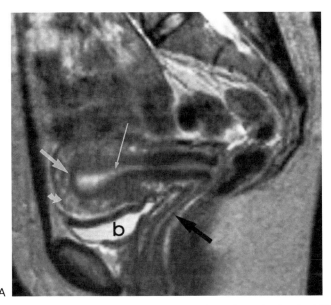

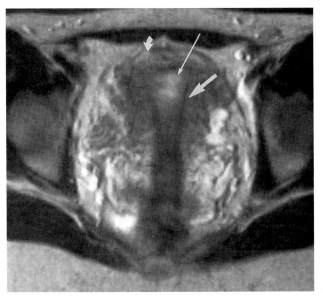

FIG. 9. Normal uterine body and cervix. Sagittal **(A)** and transaxial **(B)** T2-weighted SE images (2500/90) of the female pelvis demonstrate anteverted uterus with high-signal-intensity endometrial layer *(long thin arrow)* contiguous with endocervical layer, low-signal-intensity junctional zone *(straight arrow)* contiguous with inner cervical stroma, and intermediate signal intensity (SI) outer myometrial layer *(curved arrow)* contiguous with outer cervical stroma. *Black arrow*, vagina; b, bladder.

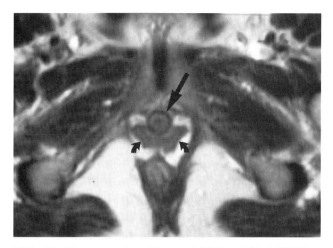

FIG. 10. Normal vagina. Transaxial T2-weighted FSE image (3500/93) shows the H-shaped vagina *(curved arrows)* outlined by high-signal-intensity fat, posterior to the urethra *(straight arrow)* and anterior to the rectum. Note low-signal-intensity outer layer (muscle) and higher-signal-intensity inner layer (mucosa).

ticoils (260). They are isointense relative to uterine myometrium on T1-weighted images; on T2-weighted images, the ovarian stroma is isointense with fat, and follicles are hyperintense (Fig. 11) (59). Frequently, the ovarian cortex appears hypointense to the ovarian medulla on T2-weighted images (202).

The normal female urethra is intermediate in signal intensity on T1-weighted images, but it possesses a characteristic target-like appearance on T2-weighted images, with a middle zone of higher signal intensity sandwiched between a low-signal-intensity center and periphery (see Fig. 10).

Because the parametrium is mainly composed of fat, it has an intermediate-to-high signal intensity on T1-weighted images. However, the parauterine ligaments and vessels have a low signal intensity. The parametrium is intermediate in signal on T2-weighted images, which contrasts well with low signal intensity cervical stroma. Because of slow blood flow, parauterine vessels are imaged as extremely high-signal-intensity structures on second echo images.

The normal zonal anatomy of the uterus and the cervix can be seen on dynamic immediate post-Gd-enhanced T1-weighted images (108,281). Although somewhat variable, myometrial enhancement is usually greater than that of the endometrium; the degree of cervical enhancement is similar to that of the myometrial tissue.

The rectosigmoid colon, which is often surrounded by abundant high signal pelvic fat, has a medium signal intensity on T1- and T2-weighted images. It may be either collapsed or distended with air, which appears as an area of extremely low signal intensity.

STAGING OF PELVIC NEOPLASMS

Urinary Bladder

Most neoplasms of the urinary bladder are of uroepithelial origin, with transitional cell carcinoma much more common than the squamous cell and adenocarcinoma variety. Squamous cell carcinoma most frequently is found in patients with chronic bladder infection and schistosomiasis. Adenocarcinoma typically occurs in patients with cystitis glandularis or urachal abnormality. Urachal carcinoma is an extravesical neoplasm, but it may invade the bladder and be confused with a primary bladder neoplasm (26,197). Although the prognosis depends on the extent of the tumor involvement at presentation, the degree of cellular differentiation affects the rate of bladder wall invasion. The poorly differentiated tumors have a higher tendency to infiltrate the bladder wall than the well-differentiated types (1,85).

Because cystoscopy is very sensitive in detecting small bladder neoplasms and biopsy of these lesions at cystoscopy often can define the depth of tumor extension into the submucosa and muscular layers, these methods remain the primary diagnostic procedures in patients with suspected bladder carcinomas. The role of any imaging method in bladder cancer is, therefore, to determine the presence or absence of invasion into the surrounding perivesical fat, adjacent viscera, and pelvic lymph nodes. Accurate determination of the extent of a bladder tumor is important because it dictates the treatment and prognosis of such a patient (85,132). One of the more commonly used staging systems for bladder carcinomas is listed in

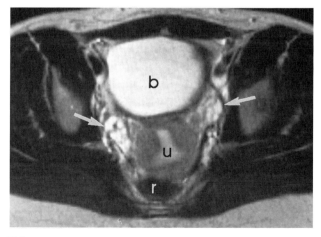

FIG. 11. Normal ovaries in a woman of reproductive age. Transaxial T2-weighted SE image (2500/90) shows high-signal-intensity follicles in both ovaries *(arrows)*. Note retroverted uterus (u) with high-signal-intensity endometrial cavity, low-signal-intensity zone, and medium-signal-intensity outer myometrium. b, bladder; r, rectum.

TABLE 1. *Staging of bladder tumors according to the Marshall system*

O:	Epithelium
A:	Lamina propria
B$_1$:	Superficial muscle
B$_2$:	Deep muscle
C:	Perivesical fat
D$_1$:	Adjacent organs, lymph nodes
D$_2$:	Distant metastases

From ref. 169, with permission.

Table 1. In general, stage A lesions can be treated adequately with fulguration or transurethral resection; low-grade stage B$_1$ lesions may be treated with segmental cystectomy. Radical cystectomy is the procedure of choice for stage B$_2$ or stage C lesions, whereas palliative radiation therapy with an ileal loop is the common management for stage D disease (61).

Computed Tomography

On CT scans, a bladder neoplasm appears as a sessile or pedunculated soft-tissue mass projecting into the bladder lumen (191,196,249) (Fig. 12). It also can present as a focal or diffuse thickening of the bladder wall (Fig. 13). When a neoplasm causes diffuse thickening of the bladder wall, it can be confused with cystitis, although the thickening is usually more uniform in the latter entity (Fig. 14). Similarly, inflammatory pseudosarcoma (pseudotumor) of

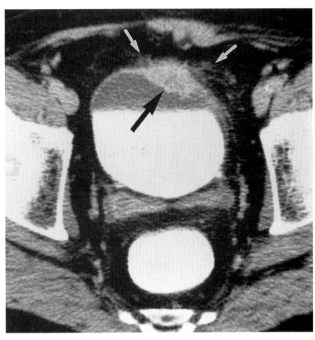

FIG. 13. Bladder carcinoma with extension into perivesical fat. Contrast-enhanced CT scan of the bladder shows an infiltrative mass *(black arrow)* arising in the left anterior bladder wall. Wispy streaks of soft tissue *(white arrows)* infiltrate the perivesical fat.

the bladder may present as a polypoid mass or focal wall thickening and therefore be indistinguishable from a bladder neoplasm on CT scans (92). The density of a bladder neoplasm is similar to that of normal bladder wall on noncontrast scans but is higher than that of normal bladder wall immediately after bolus injection of iodinated con-

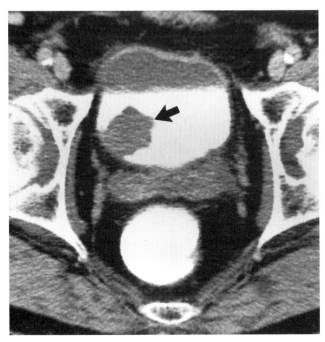

FIG. 12. Bladder carcinoma. Contrast-enhanced CT image shows pedunculated mass *(arrow)* arising from the right posterior bladder wall. The remainder of the bladder wall is uniformly thin.

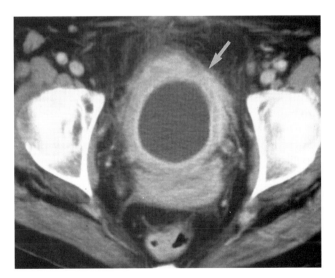

FIG. 14. Torulopsis cystitis. Contrast-enhanced CT scan shows diffuse thickening and heterogeneous enhancement of bladder wall *(arrow)* as well as inflammatory changes in the perivesical fat. (Courtesy of J. Hiken, M.D., Louisville, Kentucky.)

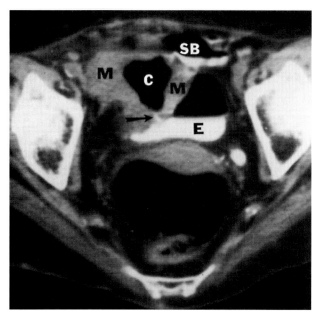

FIG. 15. Bladder carcinoma with bowel invasion. A large right anterior bladder mass (M) has eroded into small bowel (SB) and has cavitated (C). Enteric contrast material (E) has entered the bladder via a neoplastic enterovesical fistula *(arrow)*; intravenous contrast material was not given for this CT examination.

trast material (233). Calcification within the tumor may be seen on rare occasions. In one study (190), calcifications in transitional cell carcinomas were mostly on the surface of the tumor and nodular in appearance, whereas calcifications in mucinous adenocarcinoma tend to be fine, punctate, and scattered throughout the mass.

Extravesical extension of tumor is recognized on CT scans as blurring or obscuration of the perivesical fat planes (see Fig. 13). In more advanced cases, a soft-tissue mass can be seen extending from the bladder into adjacent viscera (Fig. 15) or muscles (e.g., the obturator internus). However, it is often difficult to determine whether actual tumor invasion is present or whether the tumor is merely contiguous with the pelvic wall muscle. When invasion of pelvic bone is present, the diagnosis frequently can be made by CT. Invasion of the seminal vesicles can be predicted when the normal angle between the seminal vesicle and the posterior wall of the bladder is obliterated (249). Caution must be taken not to overuse this sign, as the normal seminal vesicle angle can be distorted by a distended rectum or when the patient is prone (249). Because no distinct fat plane is present between the urinary bladder and the vagina or prostate in normal subjects, a confident CT diagnosis of early invasion into the neighboring structures is difficult. Metastases into the pelvic lymph nodes can be diagnosed only when the involved nodes are enlarged (155,301). Because of the improved scanning technology resulting in better spatial resolution,

nodes greater than 1.0 cm now are considered pathologic (298). Nodes smaller than 1 cm in size usually are considered to be normal unless they are within the expected course of lymphatic spread. In these cases, CT-guided needle aspiration of the suspicious node is often performed, and the aspirate sent for cytologic examination. In the lymphatic spread from bladder cancer, the medial (obturator) and the middle groups of the external iliac nodes are often affected first (Fig. 16), followed by the internal iliac and the common iliac nodes (1). Obturator nodal metastases are best seen on slices obtained 1 to 3 cm superior to the acetabulum.

Computed tomography is capable of differentiating bladder neoplasms with extravesical extension from those confined to the wall, but it is incapable of distinguishing tumors with superficial or deep invasion within the latter group (stages 0, A, B_1 and B_2) from each other (119,139,191,249). The overall accuracy of CT in detecting perivesical and seminal vesicular involvement is in the range of 65% to 85% (119,139,234); the accuracy in detecting lymph node metastases ranges from 70% to 90%, with a false negative rate of 25% to 40% (155,191,301). The major limitation of CT in staging bladder cancer lies in its inability to detect microscopic invasion of the perivesical fat and to recognize normal-sized but neoplastically involved lymph nodes as abnormal. False positive cases usually result from confusion produced by normal contiguous extravesical structures mimicking tumor spread or asymmetrical perivesical fat planes caused by inflammation or fibrosis.

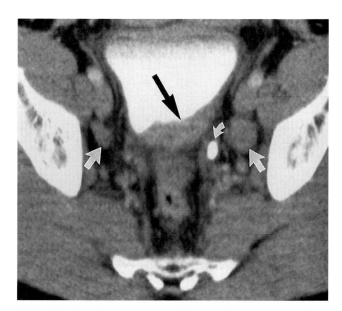

FIG. 16. Bladder carcinoma with nodal metastases. Contrast-enhanced CT scan of the bladder shows a broad-based infiltrative mass *(black arrow)* arising from the left posterior bladder wall with left hydroureter *(curved arrow)* and bilateral external iliac adenopathy *(straight white arrows)*.

Magnetic Resonance Imaging

Tumors of the bladder, whether infiltrative, sessile, or pedunculated, can be detected if they exceed 8 mm (16). The signal intensity of a bladder neoplasm is higher than that of urine but lower than that of fat on both T1-weighted and proton-density images; the signal of a bladder neoplasm is moderately high but slightly lower than that of urine on T2-weighted images. Bladder neoplasms not uncommonly are better seen on SE sequences with a short TE than a long TE (73,154). Because the bladder neoplasm exhibits earlier and greater enhancement than the bladder wall and urine, it can be easily identified on T1-weighted images obtained within the first 2 minutes after intravenous administration of Gd compounds (194,199,275). Gd-enhanced dynamic MR imaging allows detection of smaller bladder lesions than by other MR techniques (273,275) (Figs. 17,18).

Neoplastic infiltration of bladder wall can be differentiated from bladder wall hypertrophy secondary to bladder outlet obstruction because the former has a signal intensity higher than that of normal wall, whereas the latter has a signal intensity similar to that of normal wall (72). However, both mucosal edema and inflammation of the bladder wall have high signal intensity on T2-weighted images, and this overlaps the appearance of bladder neoplasms (73). Furthermore, inflammation of the bladder wall secondary to prior radiation or other causes may be indistinguishable from neoplastic infiltration even on post-Gd images, as both may enhance substantially (99).

Magnetic resonance imaging cannot differentiate stage 0 from stage A tumors (2,30,72,228). However, MRI can detect superficial (stage B_1) and deep muscular invasion (stage B_2). On a T2-weighted or a Gd-enhanced T1-weighted image, superficial muscle invasion is suspected if the inner aspect of the low-intensity bladder wall is irregular, whereas deep muscle invasion is diagnosed if the low-intensity line is disrupted (72,139,228,275). The low-intensity bladder wall is usually preserved in stage 0 and A bladder neoplasms.

Tumor extension into the perivesical fat (stage C) also can be detected and is seen as an area of diminished signal relative to the pelvic fat on a T1-weighted image. It often has a wispy appearance but occasionally may be more confluent. It is best appreciated on T1-weighted images because of sharp contrast between fat and tumor (Fig. 19). Because of the reduced contrast between bladder neoplasm and perivesical fat on T2-weighted or Gd-enhanced T1-weighted images, tumor invasion into perivesical fat is often obscured unless fat saturation is used in conjunction with these sequences (99). Tumor invasion into adjacent organs, such as the seminal vesicles and the rectum, similarly can be detected (Fig. 20). The diagnosis of seminal vesicular involvement can be made by noting not only changes in its size or morphology but also its signal intensity. Normal seminal vesicles have a high sig-

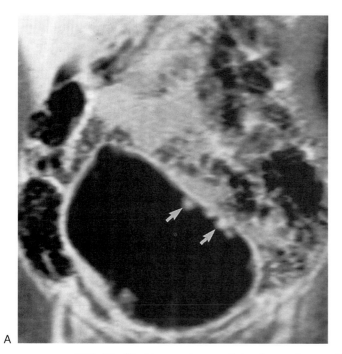
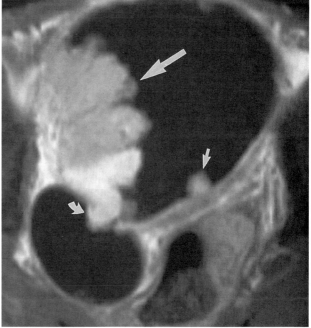

A B

FIG. 17. Bladder carcinoma. Gd-enhanced coronal FLASH (140/4/80°) **(A)** and transaxial T1-weighted fat-saturated (600/15) **(B)** images of the bladder show a large sessile mass *(large arrow)* arising from the right posterolateral wall, and several smaller superficial masses arising from the superior and left posterior bladder wall *(small arrows)*. Note extension of a large mass into bladder diverticulum *(curved arrow)*.

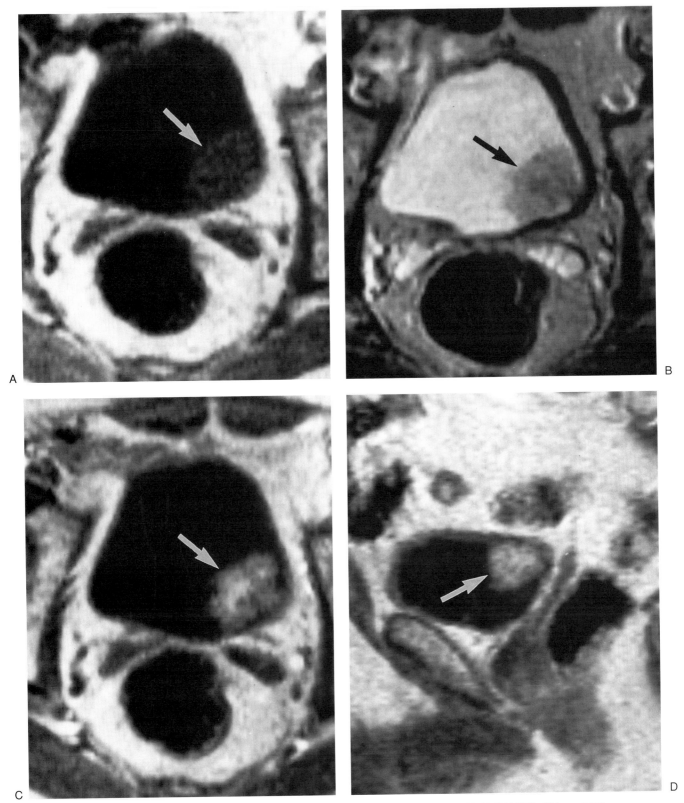

FIG. 18. Bladder carcinoma. Transaxial precontrast T1-weighted FLASH (140/4/80°) **(A)** and T2-weighted SE (2500/90) **(B)** images show a sessile mass *(arrow)* arising from the left posterior bladder wall that is slightly hyperintense to urine and hypointense to fat on T1-weighted image. The mass is hypointense to urine on T2-weighted image. Post-Gd transaxial **(C)** and sagittal **(D)** T1-weighted FLASH images (140/4/80°) show enhancement of the tumor *(arrow)*, making it more visible against unenhanced urine. The underlying bladder wall is preserved.

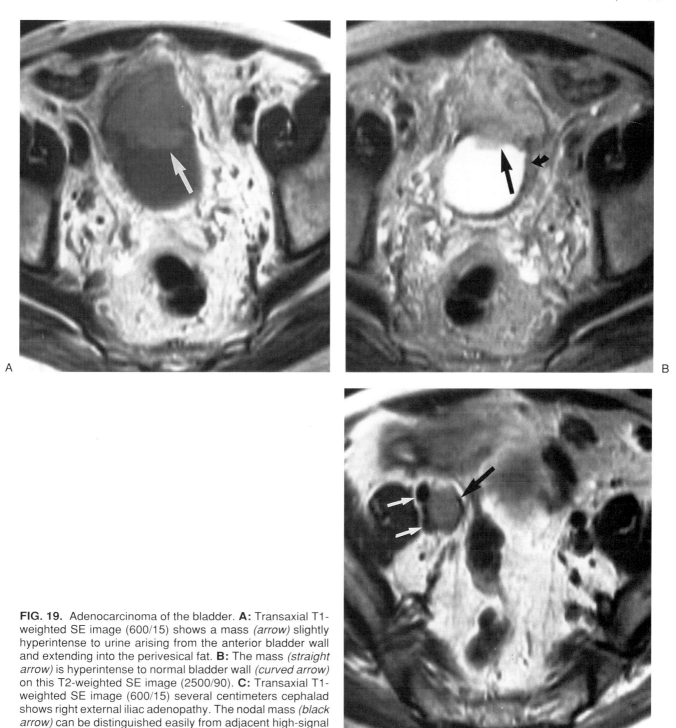

FIG. 19. Adenocarcinoma of the bladder. **A:** Transaxial T1-weighted SE image (600/15) shows a mass *(arrow)* slightly hyperintense to urine arising from the anterior bladder wall and extending into the perivesical fat. **B:** The mass *(straight arrow)* is hyperintense to normal bladder wall *(curved arrow)* on this T2-weighted SE image (2500/90). **C:** Transaxial T1-weighted SE image (600/15) several centimeters cephalad shows right external iliac adenopathy. The nodal mass *(black arrow)* can be distinguished easily from adjacent high-signal fat and flow voids of the iliac vessels *(white arrows).*

nal intensity on T2-weighted images; invasion of the seminal vesicles by carcinomas may lead to a lower signal intensity. Other conditions, such as atrophy, fibrosis, and amyloid deposit may cause a similar decrease in seminal vesicular signal intensity (130). However, these diffuse conditions usually result in bilateral signal intensity loss in the seminal vesicles, compared to cancer, which is usually unilateral or asymmetrical.

Lymph node metastases can be seen if the involved nodes are enlarged. Lymphadenopathy is best appreciated on T1-weighted images. Unfortunately, tissue characterization based on MR signal is not possible. Lymphadenopathy from benign causes cannot be distinguished from malignant disease. Likewise, a normal-sized lymph node replaced with tumor cannot be recognized as abnormal by MRI (58,151). MRI has a reported accuracy of between 58% to 90% in staging bladder neoplasms (2,30,37,73,119,139,228,273,275). The use of specialized

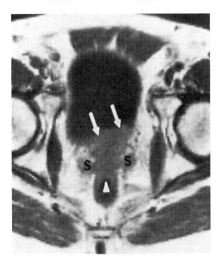

FIG. 20. Bladder carcinoma invading the rectum. Transaxial T1-weighted SE image (500/30) shows invasion of the anterior wall of the rectum *(arrowhead)* by a posterior bladder carcinoma *(arrows)*. s, seminal vesicles.

surface coils results in more accurate staging of bladder compared to imaging in the body coil (15). Although some investigators found Gd-enhanced dynamic MR and oblique imaging to be significantly better than conventional noncontrast MR studies for staging of bladder neoplasms (139,194,275), others reported such improvement to be not statistically significant. MRI is slightly more sensitive than CT in detecting invasion of perivesical fat, the prostate, and the seminal vesicles. It is also superior to CT in distinguishing an enlarged lymph node from a small blood vessel (151). However, like CT, MRI is not able to detect microscopic invasion of the perivesical fat or lymph nodes. Furthermore, asymmetrical perivesical fat planes caused by inflammation may lead to false positive MR interpretations. MRI is more time consuming than CT. Because of the lack of inexpensive and optimal oral contrast agents, small bowel loops may be mistaken for lymphadenopathy on MR images.

Clinical Application

Arteriography, triple-contrast cystography, and lymphangiography have all been used in the past in the preopera-

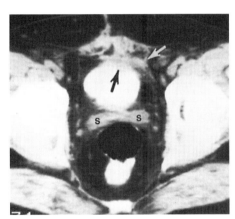

A

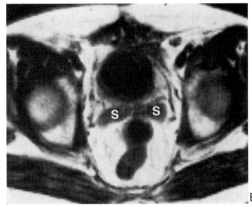

B

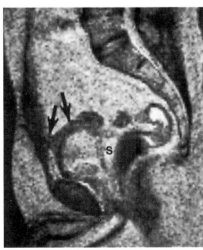

C

FIG. 21. Postoperative scar simulating extravesical tumor invasion: use of MRI. **A:** Contrast-enhanced CT image. A plaque-like tumor *(black arrow)* is noted in the anterior portion of the urinary bladder. A band of soft-tissue density *(white arrow)* is seen between the tumor and abdominal wall, a finding suggestive of extravesical tumor extension. **B:** Transaxial T1-weighted SE image (500/35) shows findings similar to those of CT. **C:** Sagittal T2-weighted SE image (2100/90). The extravesical soft tissue *(arrows)* noted superior and anterior to the bladder has a signal intensity similar to that of the anterior abdominal wall; this finding is compatible with fibrosis rather than tumor extension. Note that the bladder neoplasm is invisible on this image because it has a signal intensity similar to that of urine. s, seminal vesicles. (From ref. 221.)

TABLE 2. *Clinical staging classification for prostatic carcinoma*

A: Occult cancer
B: Cancer nodule confined within prostatic capsule
C: Cancer with extracapsular extension into surrounding structures or confined within capsule with elevation of serum alkaline phosphatase; pelvic nodes may be involved
D: Bone or extrapelvic involvement

From ref. 124, with permission.

tive staging of bladder neoplasms (129,146,299). The first two procedures are invasive and have produced variable results (129,146); lymphangiography evaluates the status of only the pelvic and retroperitoneal lymph nodes, not that of the visceral organs (299). None of these procedures have been routinely applied. Computed tomography provides a noninvasive method of differentiating early from advanced stages of bladder neoplasms and, therefore, helps avoid needless radical surgery in advanced cancers. In spite of its limitations, CT is routinely used in the preoperative evaluation of patients with biopsy-proven bladder neoplasms. Although several recent studies have shown MRI to be more accurate than CT in staging bladder neoplasms, most of the improvements are result from the increased detection of superficial or small bladder neoplasms on dynamic Gd-enhanced MR images (275), information readily obtainable through cystoscopy. The disadvantages of MRI, including higher cost, longer examination time, and more stringent patient requirements, have limited its use. Other than being used to clarify equivocal CT findings or in patients who have contraindications to receive intravenous iodinated contrast agents (Fig. 21), the role of MRI in bladder neoplasms remains to be established.

Prostate

Prostatic carcinoma is an exceedingly common malignancy. More than 95% of malignant prostatic neoplasms are adenocarcinomas, with the rest being transitional or squamous cell carcinoma or sarcomas (41). It is now the most common nonskin malignancy (21) and the second leading cause of death in American men. Prostatic carcinoma is found more frequently in blacks than in whites, and less commonly in the Asian population (326). Screening for the presence of prostatic carcinoma is based on measurement of the prostate-specific antigen (PSA) level (normal, ≤4 ng/dl), performance of digital rectal examination, and biopsy of suspicious lesions (47). Although in the past approximately 65% of newly diagnosed cases were found to have advanced disease, the current routine use of PSA as a screening test has resulted in detection of disease at an earlier stage. The prognosis and treatment depend on the stage of the disease when first seen. A commonly used staging classification for prostatic carcinoma is listed in Table 2 (124). For patients with disease

confined to the capsule and a life expectancy of more than 15 years, radical prostatectomy is the preferred method of treatment. For patients with disease confined to the capsule and a life expectancy of less than 15 years, radiation therapy (external beam or interstitial implant) is preferred (237). For patients with disease outside the capsule without known metastatic disease, radiation therapy is recommended. For patients with widely metastatic disease, hormonal therapy (orchiectomy, diethylstilbestrol, leuprolide acetate) is preferred.

Clinical staging based on bimanual rectal examination, serum acid phosphatase, and radionuclide bone scintigraphy may underestimate the extent of disease in 40% to 50% of cases. The purpose of preoperative diagnostic imaging evaluation is to increase the accuracy of the assigned clinical stage. Detection of more advanced disease (stage C or D) than clinically suspected, eliminates unnecessary surgical procedures.

Computed Tomography

Computed tomography is not used as a screening procedure for the detection of prostatic carcinoma because of its inability to differentiate among normal, hyperplastic, and cancerous glands (219,271,291). Nevertheless, CT does provide useful information as to the extent of the tumor once a histologic diagnosis is established. Computed tomography is capable of differentiating patients with stage A and B disease from those with stage C and D disease (Figs. 22,23). The criteria used to diagnose extracapsular extension from prostatic carcinomas are essentially the same as those used in the staging of bladder carcinomas, namely, lack of symmetry of peripelvic fat

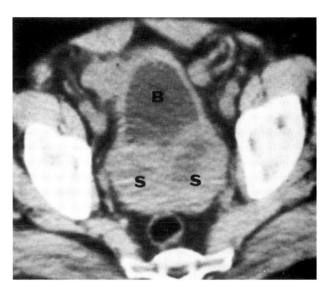

FIG. 22. Prostatic carcinoma, stage C. Unenhanced CT scan shows that the seminal vesicles (S) are markedly enlarged because of direct invasion by an adjacent prostatic carcinoma. B, bladder.

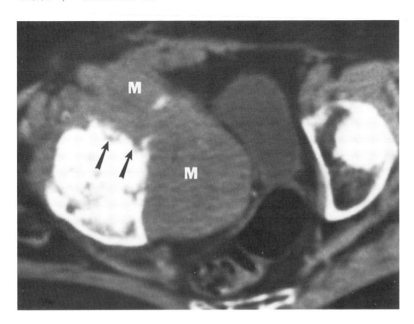

FIG. 23. Prostatic carcinoma, stage D. Unenhanced CT scan demonstrates a large soft-tissue mass (M) involving the right pelvic side-wall and inguinal area due to metastatic prostate cancer. Note the associated sclerosis and cortical destruction *(arrows)* of the acetabulum.

planes and obliteration of the seminal vesicle angles. Metastases to pelvic lymph nodes also can be detected if they cause nodal enlargement. The size criterion (1 cm) used to differentiate a normal from an abnormal pelvic lymph node in prostatic carcinoma is similar to that used in bladder carcinoma. However, in one prospective CT study of 285 patients with prostatic carcinoma, nodes 6 mm or greater in cross-sectional diameter were considered pathologic and biopsied with a fine needle under CT guidance (205). CT-guided aspiration biopsy improved the specificity and accuracy of CT in diagnosing lymph node metastases from 96.7% and 93.7% to 100% and 96.5%, respectively, whereas the sensitivity remained unchanged at 77.8%. CT was falsely negative in only ten patients, who had microscopic metastasis in a solitary lymph node. As with urinary bladder neoplasms, lymphatic drainage of the prostate is mainly into external and internal iliac nodal groups. The overall accuracy of CT in detecting pelvic lymph node metastases from prostatic cancer is in the range of 67% to 93% with sensitivities varying from 0% to 100% (75,89,158,191,211,306). Although the sensitivity in detecting extracapsular extension is low, the specificity is high, with no false positive CT interpretations reported in some series (89). Because of its low sensitivity in detecting extracapsular extension of the prostatic carcinoma (213), especially in early clinical stages, CT should be performed only for cases in which there is a high clinical suspicion of advanced disease (stages C and D). In patients who are scheduled to receive radiation therapy for prostatic carcinoma, CT can also be used to help design radiation ports because of its high accuracy in assessing the size and precise location of the prostate gland (56,211). CT is also valuable in the evaluation of patients with suspected recurrent disease.

Magnetic Resonance Imaging

There have been conflicting reports on the ability of MRI to differentiate prostatic carcinoma from benign hyperplasia. Although studies performed on low-field units (0.04 to 0.15T) have shown that prostatic carcinoma can be differentiated from benign hyperplasia because of its longer T1 and T2 (147,268), the results based on medium-

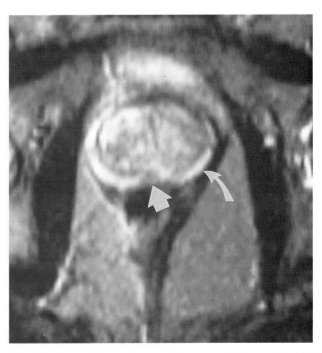

FIG. 24. Prostatic carcinoma. Transaxial T2-weighted SE image (2500/90) of the prostate gland shows a small intermediate-signal-intensity nodule *(straight arrow)* within the high-signal-intensity peripheral zone *(curved arrow)*.

field (0.3 to 0.6T) superconducting imagers have been less encouraging. With the exception of one report (117), most investigators found it difficult to distinguish between these two entities (31,162,209).

Prostatic carcinoma typically appears as a focus of low signal, either poorly or well defined, in the peripheral zone on T2-weighted images (238) (Fig. 24). Rarely, adenocarcinoma, especially the mucinous type, may display a signal intensity similar to or higher than that of normal peripheral zone on T2-weighted images (204). Besides prostatic carcinoma, benign prostatic hyperplasia also may appear as hypointense nodules in the peripheral zone and thus simulate carcinoma (164,221,238). Other benign conditions, such as prostatitis, granulomatous disease, and postbiopsy blood, all may appear as low-signal-intensity lesions (19,237). In fact, the signal intensity observed on T2-weighted images correlates better with the tissue optical density than a specific tissue type (221). Therefore, tissues with more open space (lumen with mucus) have a higher signal intensity on T2-weighted images than tissues with fewer glands and more stroma. In spite of the nonspecific signal characteristics, low-signal abnormalities identified in the posterior half of the outer gland are more likely to be cancers (39,66). Furthermore, cancers

that are larger, more poorly differentiated, or located in the posterior half of the outer gland are easier to detect. Cancers arising in the central gland are isointense to the surrounding glandular tissue and are thus difficult to detect (121). Larger carcinomatous nodules may demonstrate many internal septations that do not form complete rings, the so-called broken septa sign. This pattern has not been reported with benign prostatic hyperplasia (237). Because Gd does not improve the detection of prostatic carcinoma, it is not routinely used (181,220).

Because of the overlapping signal intensities of benign and malignant prostatic nodules, accurate determination of tumor volume has been difficult with images obtained with either body coils (222) or endorectal coils (121, 203,237). In one study performed with an external phased-array coil (multicoils), a more accurate depiction of tumor volume was achieved (262). In spite of the difficulty in precise delineation of intraprostatic tumor volume, MRI is capable of demonstrating gross capsular invasion and extracapsular tumor extension. Capsular invasion often leads to an irregular bulge, with a square or rectangular edge, and less commonly it results in a smooth curvilinear bulge (243). Asymmetry of the neurovascular bundle with retraction of the ipsilateral neurovascular

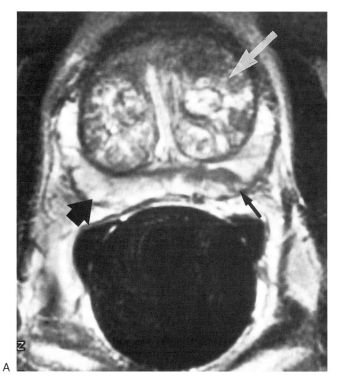 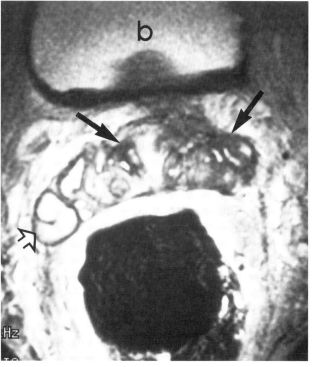

A   B

FIG. 25. Prostatic carcinoma with seminal vesical invasion. **A:** Transaxial T2-weighted SE image (2200/80) of the prostate obtained with an endorectal coil shows enlargement of the central gland, consistent with benign prostatic hypertrophy *(white arrow)*. Within the high-signal peripheral zone *(thick black arrow)*, the tumor appears as a bandlike focus of intermediate signal intensity *(thin black arrow)*. **B:** At a more superior level, tumor is seen infiltrating the left seminal vesicle diffusely with minimal involvement of the right seminal vesicle *(black arrows)*. Note appearance of normal, spared right seminal vesicle seen as tubular structures of high signal intensity with low-signal-intensity walls *(hollow arrow)*. b, bladder. (Courtesy of S. Mirowitz, M.D., St. Louis, Missouri.)

bundle is also associated with capsular invasion (278). Criteria for tumor extension beyond the capsule into the neurovascular bundles include direct posterolateral extension of low-signal-intensity tumor into the neurovascular bundle, and obliteration of the rectoprostatic angle by a focus of low signal intensity. Extracapsular tumor extension likewise can be predicted when there is disruption of either periprostatic fat or periprostatic venous plexus, which appears on the anterior and the lateral aspects of the prostate as a high-signal-intensity rim on a second echo image (20,216). Early involvement of the seminal vesicles is evidenced by thickening of tubal walls; at later stages, intraluminal low-signal-intensity foci can be identified on T2-weighted images (20,241). On Gd-enhanced T1-weighted images, tumors in both the lumen of the seminal tubules and the septae exhibit contrast enhancement leading to the disruption of normal ''honeycomb'' pattern (181). Other signs of seminal vesicular invasion include asymmetrical enlargement of the seminal vesicle and obliteration of the ipsilateral seminal vesicle angle. While recognition of changes in the signal intensity of seminal vesicles is a more sensitive indicator of tumor invasion than changes in their size (Fig. 25), postbiopsy hemorrhage (180,312) (Fig. 26), postradiation or hormonal therapy (42), and, rarely, amyloid deposits or calculi all may cause the signal intensity of the seminal vesicles to be lower than normal on T2-weighted images. Low-signal-intensity nodules of benign prostatic hyperplasia can protrude into the medial aspect of the seminal vesicles and thereby simulate tumor invasion. Awareness of these conditions coupled with appropriate clinical history will reduce false positive interpretations. Furthermore, blood in the seminal vesicles can be differentiated from neoplastic infiltration, because the former may have a high signal intensity on T1-weighted images (Fig. 26).

Extension of prostatic carcinoma into adjacent pelvic organs can be detected by MRI. Because of the Denonvilliers' fascia, tumor often grows around the rectum to occupy the presacral space rather than invading the rectum directly (Fig. 27). As in the case of bladder neoplasm, metastases to lymph nodes can be seen on MRI if the involved nodes are enlarged.

In spite of the exquisite anatomic details displayed by MR images obtained with endorectal coils, some studies have shown that endorectal MRI has a low sensitivity for detecting capsular and extracapsular tumor invasion and an overall staging accuracy similar to that of body coils (203,279). However, pooled data from all published reports show a definite improvement in the overall staging accuracy of MRI for prostatic carcinoma with endorectal coils (237). Based on 399 patients studied with body coils and 212 patients evaluated with endorectal coils, the sensitivity is 65% and specificity 69% for body coils, whereas it is 87% and 81%, respectively, for endorectal coils. Considerable interobserver variability is noted in interpreting images obtained with body coils (239) compared to

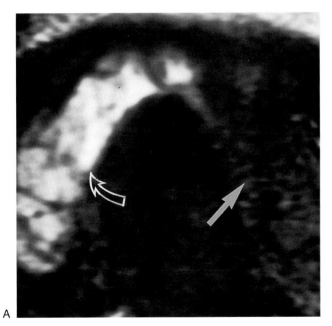
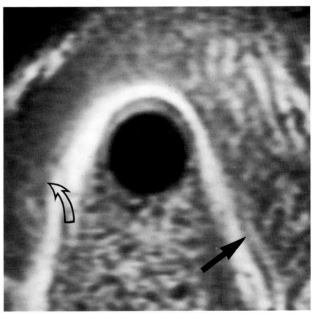

A   B

FIG. 26. Seminal vesicle hemorrhage post biopsy. **A:** Transaxial T2-weighted SE image (3000/80) obtained with endorectal coil shows the left seminal vesicle *(solid arrow)* to be enlarged and diffusely low in signal intensity suggestive of tumor invasion. Note high-signal-intensity appearance of normal right seminal vesicle *(hollow arrow)*. **B:** Transaxial T1-weighted SE image (600/20) shows high signal intensity in the left seminal vesicle *(black arrow)*, consistent with hemorrhage rather than tumor. Normal right seminal vesicle *(open arrow)* is low in signal intensity. (Courtesy of S. Mirowitz, M.D., St. Louis, Missouri.)

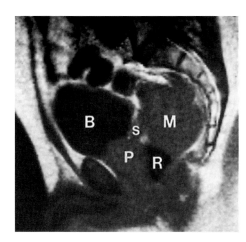

FIG. 27. Prostatic carcinoma, with rectal invasion; sagittal T1-weighted SE image (500/30). A large mass (M) representing contiguous spread of prostatic carcinoma lies posterior to the rectum (R). B, urinary bladder; s, seminal vesicles; P, prostate. (From ref. 151.)

those obtained with endorectal coils (203). Furthermore, more experienced readers perform better than less experienced ones, with the former achieving a much higher receiver operating characteristic (ROC) area (0.79) for the detection of periprostatic invasion compared to the latter (0.49) in one study (279). In any case, understaging (false negative interpretations) usually results from the inability of MRI to detect microscopic or early extracapsular invasion. Overstaging (false posi tive interpretations) is often a result of misinterpreting inflammatory or other benign processes as tumor infiltration.

Clinical Application

Although the overall accuracy of MRI for staging prostatic carcinoma is not high, it is still more sensitive than clinical staging, transrectal ultrasound, and CT (105, 218,230). The increased experience in interpretation of MRI examinations, and the combined use of endorectal and body coil coupled with FSE technique, which allows examination of the prostate with a T2-weighted sequence in more than one plane, will further improve the diagnostic accuracy of MRI. Whereas improvement in MRI technology is unlikely to allow detection of microscopic disease, fortunately, the presence of minimal extracapsular tumor invasion is not believed to represent a contraindication for radical prostatectomy (177). Furthermore, the prognosis of patients with minimal extracapsular tumor invasion after surgery has been found to be similar to that of patients in whom tumor is completely confined within the prostate capsule (177,263). In spite of its limitations, the ability of endorectal coil MRI to reliably depict the presence of gross extraprostatic tumor spread makes it the best imaging tool currently available for local staging of prostatic carcinoma.

Whereas CT can be used to confirm the extent of tumor in patients with clinically suspected advanced disease and to provide information useful for radiotherapy planning (56), CT is not recommended for local staging of prostatic carcinoma because of its inability to depict intraprostatic tumor, as well as its low sensitivity and specificity (67).

Cervix

Carcinoma of the cervix is the fifth most common form of cancer in American women, after breast, colorectum, lung, and endometrium. The incidence rises after the age of 20 years, reaching its maximum for the group between 45 and 55 years of age. The overwhelming majority of carcinomas of the cervix are epidermoid. Most arise at the transformation zone (squamocolumnar junction), where squamous epithelium undergoes replacement through metaplasia. In women under the age of 35, the junction is usually outside the endocervical canal on the ectocervix. In women over the age of 35, the squamocolumnar junction generally lies within the endocervical canal. Carcinomas involving the ectocervix tend to grow in a polypoid, not infiltrative, fashion. Extension is often directly into the vagina. Carcinomas arising from the endocervical canal tend to expand the canal and extend through the cervical wall. Direct lateral spread can invade the parametrium and eventually the pelvic side wall. Lymphatic spread to the iliac lymph nodes is followed by involvement of the para-aortic nodal chains. In general, grading (degree of histologic differentiation) of epidermoid carcinoma is of little prognostic value (1). After the histologic diagnosis of cervical carcinoma is established, assessment of actual extent of the disease will dictate the method of treatment. Whereas treatment options include radical hysterectomy with lymph node sampling or radiation therapy in stages I to IIa (Table 3), radiation therapy is the

TABLE 3. *Staging classification for cervical carcinoma*

Stage 0	Carcinoma *in situ.*
Stage I	Carcinoma strictly confined to the cervix.
Stage Ia	Microinvasive carcinoma.
Stage Ib	All other cases of stage I.
Stage II	The carcinoma extends beyond the cervix.
Stage IIa	No obvious parametrial involvement.
Stage IIb	Obvious parametrial involvement.
Stage III	The carcinoma involves the lower third of the vagina.
Stage IIIa	No extension to the pelvic wall.
Stage IIIb	Extension to the pelvic wall and/or hydronephrosis or nonfunctioning kidney.
Stage IV	The carcinoma has extended beyond the true pelvis or has involved the mucosa of the bladder or rectum.
Stage IVa	Spread to adjacent organs.
Stage IVb	Spread to distant organs.

From ref. 145, with permission.

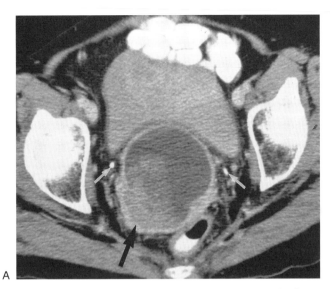 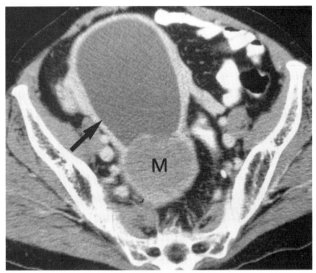

FIG. 28. Cervical carcinoma, stage IIa. **A:** Contrast-enhanced CT shows a bulky low-density cervical mass with cavitation *(large arrow)*. The ureters are not dilated *(small arrows)*. **B:** Four centimeters cephalad, note dilated, fluid-filled endometrial cavity *(arrow)*. M, tumor mass.

treatment of choice in stages IIb to IVb. Clinical staging procedures involve bimanual pelvic examination and conventional radiologic methods, such as excretory urography, barium enema, and lymphangiography. Cystoscopy and proctoscopy are also used in cases where there is a clinical suspicion of direct invasion to the urinary bladder and the rectum.

Computed Tomography

Carcinoma of the cervix may be recognized on noncontrast CT scans as a large cervix with regular or irregular borders. On postcontrast CT scans, the tumor may appear as a soft-tissue mass enlarging the cervix with diminished intravenous contrast enhancement compared to normal

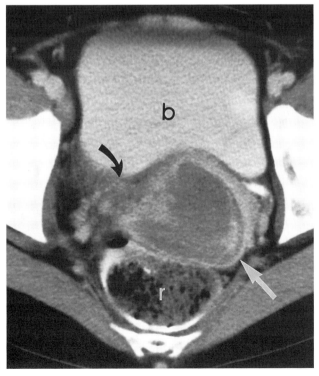 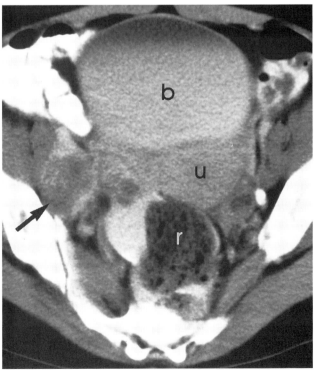

FIG. 29. Cervical carcinoma, stage IIIb. **A:** Contrast-enhanced CT shows large hypodense mass expanding cervix *(straight arrows)*. Note right parametrial extension *(curved arrow)* that caused distal ureteral obstruction and hydronephrosis (seen on other images). b, bladder; r, rectum. **B:** Scan at the level of the uterus (u) shows right external iliac adenopathy *(arrow)*. b, bladder; r, rectosigmoid colon.

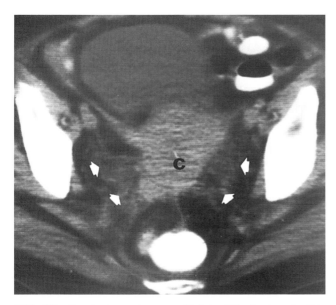

FIG. 30. Cervical carcinoma: pitfall in CT staging. In this case, wispy, soft-tissue infiltration in the parametrial fat *(arrows)* was due to inflammation. The tumor was confined to the cervix (C).

cervical tissue (Fig. 28). Fluid collections in the endometrial cavity and uterine enlargement are frequently seen as a result of tumor obstruction of the endocervical canal. CT is capable of differentiating tumor confined to the cervix from tumor that has invaded the parametrium (138,282,302,313).

Computed tomographic criteria for parametrial tumor invasion are: (a) irregularity or poor definition of the lateral cervix margins, (b) prominent parametrial soft-tissue strands or eccentric soft-tissue mass, and (c) obliteration of the periureteral fat plane (296) (Fig. 29). A parametrial soft-tissue mass and loss of the periureteral fat plane are essential for a definitive CT diagnosis of parametrial tumor extension. Caution must be taken not to overinterpret loss of the cervical border and minimal soft-tissue infiltration of the paracervical fat as parametrial tumor invasion, because parametritis secondary to prior instrumentation may result in similar CT findings (Fig. 30). Furthermore, parauterine vessels, and normal broad, round, cardinal, and uterosacral ligaments, should not be mistaken for lateral tumor extension.

Pelvic side-wall tumor extension (stage IIIb) is characterized by confluent, irregular, linear parametrial soft-tissue strands extending to and/or enlarging the obturator internus and pyriformis muscle (302). When a parametrial mass is within 2 to 3 mm of the pelvic side wall, even though there is small intervening fat plane, the tumor should be staged as IIIb. In these cases, the gynecologist usually cannot interpose his or her examining fingers between the bulky tumor and the pelvic side wall and stages the tumor as IIIb. CT demonstration of hydronephrosis resulting from distal ureteral obstruction with or without

pelvic side-wall extension indicates a stage IIIb tumor (see Fig. 29). Tumor extension into the urinary bladder or rectum (stage IVa) can be suggested if there is focal loss of the perivesical/perirectal fat plane accompanied by asymmetric wall thickening. Additional features include nodular indentation or serrations along the bladder/rectal wall and intraluminal tumor mass (Fig. 31).

Besides local invasion, carcinoma of the cervix metastasizes primarily by the lymphatic system. Although clinical staging classification does not recognize pelvic lymph node metastases, demonstration of such lymph node metastases by CT precludes surgical salvage. While CT is reported to be slightly more accurate than clinical examination in detecting tumor extension into the parametrium and the pelvic side wall in some studies (302,313), it is found to be less accurate in others (144,295). The reported accuracy for CT ranges from 58% to 88% (23,91, 138,144,302,313), whereas the accuracy of clinical staging is generally cited as 60% to 78% (128,144). Both false positive and false negative CT interpretations may occur. False positive CT diagnoses are often a result of misinterpreting normal or inflammatory parametrial soft-tissue strands as tumor invasion; false negative diagnoses are usually a result of CTs inability to detect microscopic or early disease. In addition, CT may not be able to determine whether invasion of a structure is present or whether the tumor is just contiguous, especially in the rectal area.

The overall accuracy for CT in detecting pelvic nodal metastases from cervical carcinoma is in the range of 70% to 80% (84,138,297,302). As with other pelvic malignant neoplasms, false negative cases are mostly a result of microscopic disease or metastases less than 1 cm in size; false

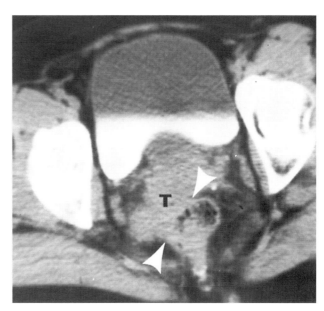

FIG. 31. Cervical carcinoma, stage IV. Contrast-enhanced CT scan shows extension of parametrial tumor almost to the right pelvic side wall. The rectum also is invaded *(arrowheads).*

positive cases are largely a result of misinterpretation of hyperplastic lymph nodes as metastatic disease. Because metastases from cervical carcinoma often replace a portion of a lymph node without enlarging it, the reported false negative rates for CT vary from 20% to 80% (70,170,297). Because lymphangiography is capable of delineating intranodal architecture, and hyperplastic changes usually can be differentiated from metastatic disease, lymphangiography is more accurate than CT in diagnosing lymph node involvement from cervical carcinoma (84).

Magnetic Resonance Imaging

Cervical carcinoma can be accurately depicted by MRI (27,33,148,160,210,232,284,319). On T2-weighted images, cervical carcinoma most often appears as a mass of high signal intensity, distorting or disrupting the normal zonal anatomy of the cervix (Fig. 32).

When the cervical carcinoma is large (greater than 4 cm), additional MR findings may be noted (Fig. 33). These include blurring and widening of the uterine junctional low-intensity band, as well as broadening of the central uterine high-intensity zone. The latter finding is caused by uterine secretions retained within an enlarged uterine cavity—the

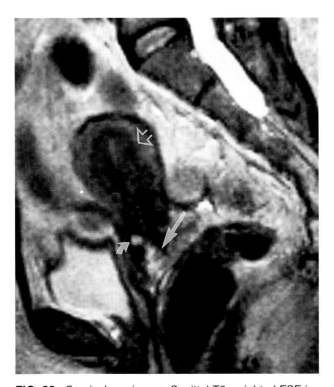

FIG. 32. Cervical carcinoma. Sagittal T2-weighted FSE image (3500/93) shows the tumor as an irregular area of high signal intensity in the posterior lip of the cervix *(white arrow)*. Note round, well-defined focus of high signal intensity in the anterior lip, consistent with a Nabothian cyst *(curved arrow)*. The uterine junctional zone is broadened, consistent with adenomyosis *(open arrow)*.

so-called obstructed uterus (319). When the retained uterine secretions are nonbloody, problems can arise in differentiating uterine secretions in an obstructed uterus from merely thickened endometrium on noncontrast MR images. This difficulty arises because both entities have low signal intensity on T1-weighted images and high signal intensity on T2-weighted images. However, differentiation of the two can be made on postcontrast images because the endometrium enhances, whereas secretions do not. Furthermore, if the retained uterine secretions are bloody, they will have a high signal intensity on both T1- and T2-weighted images. This allows differentiation between sequestered bloody uterine secretions and thickened endometrium on unenhanced images.

Besides being able to image the primary cervical carcinoma, MRI is also able to detect extension of the tumor into the parametria and pelvic side walls. Because fat has an intermediate T2 and cervical carcinoma has a long T2, tumor extension into the parametria is best evaluated on T2-weighted images. Parametrial extension is diagnosed by either an asymmetric appearance of the parametria or by abnormally high signal intensity tumor extending into the parametrial ligaments through a disrupted low-signal-intensity ring of the cervix on T2-weighted images (284). Whereas preservation of the low-signal-intensity ring of the cervical stroma on T2-weighted images reliably indicates that the tumor is confined to the cervix, parametrial extension is difficult to exclude when there is full-thickness stromal invasion as evidenced by total disruption of the low-intensity ring (110). Problems in evaluating parametrial status also may be encountered in patients with a prominent anteverted uterus that makes it difficult to obtain a true cross section of the cervix or in patients with a large exophytic tumor that distends the vaginal fornix (288). Invasion of the vagina appears as segmental disruption of low-intensity vaginal wall on T2-weighted images. Infiltration of adjacent pelvic muscles and the rectum similarly can be detected because the affected structures have abnormally high signal intensity on T2-weighted images. MR findings that suggest vesical invasion include nodularity and irregularity of the bladder wall, masses protruding into the bladder lumen, and high signal intensity of the anterior aspect of the posterior wall of the bladder (141). Metastases to lymph nodes and bone also can be detected by MRI (Fig. 33). As stated previously, the diagnosis of malignant lymphadenopathy by MRI is similar to that of CT and is based on recognition of enlargement of the involved node. It has been shown that the minimum axial diameter is a more accurate size criterion than the maximum axial diameter. In one study (143), MRI had an accuracy of 93%, with 62% sensitivity and 98% specificity, using 1 cm as the cutoff for the minimum axial diameter.

The reported accuracy for MRI in detecting parametrial invasion ranges from 87% to 92% (141,144,255,288); the overall staging accuracy varies from 77% to 83% (141,144,288). Although the endorectal coil images can

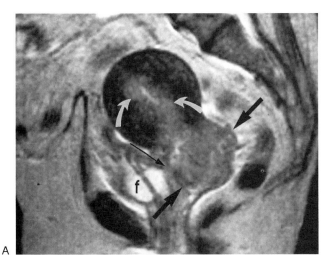
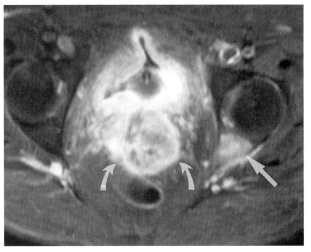

A

B

FIG. 33. Cervical carcinoma. **A:** Sagittal T2-weighted FSE image (3500/93) shows bulky cervical mass *(arrows)* with loss of fat plane between mass and bladder *(thin arrow)*. Involvement of the endometrium is also noted *(curved arrows)*. f, Foley catheter. **B:** Transaxial T1-weighted fat-saturated post-Gd SE image (600/15) shows enhancement of cervical mass *(curved arrows)*. Note high-signal-intensity focus in the posterior left acetabulum *(arrow)*, consistent with osseous metastasis.

provide increased anatomic details and can demonstrate tissue planes between tumor and normal structures that are not seen on the body coil images (178), it is not known whether the increased anatomic resolution will improve the accuracy of MRI for staging cervical carcinoma. Whereas post-Gd T1-weighted SE images are at best equal to, and usually inferior to, unenhanced T2-weighted sequence for evaluating cervical carcinoma (109, 115,257), dynamic MR imaging using GRE sequence after bolus injection of Gd may improve assessment of stromal invasion and tumor size (322). Gadolinium also can be used to improve the display of tumor invasion of the bladder and rectum (108) (Fig. 34).

Besides being used for the initial staging, MRI also can be used to monitor the effect of radiation or chemotherapy (140). An early (2 to 3 months) and significant decrease in the signal intensity and volume of a tumor indicates a favorable response (76). Large primary tumors (>50 cm^3) may show a delayed response. Pathologically low-signal-intensity areas on T2-weighted images correspond to low cellularity, prominent fibrosis, and hemosiderin deposits in the necrotic tissue (76,256). The MR findings of reconstitution of the normal zonal anatomy of the cervix and the presence of homogeneous low-signal-intensity cervical stroma are reliable indicators that the cervix is normal (115). However, high signal intensity on T2-weighted im-

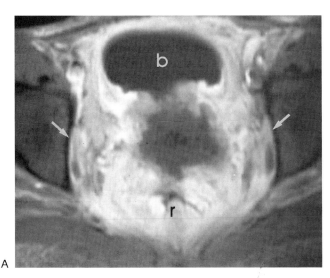
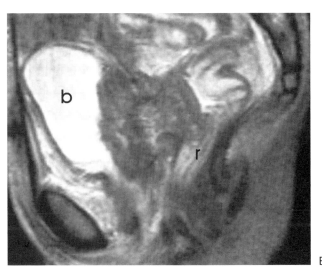

A

B

FIG. 34. Recurrent advanced-stage cervical carcinoma after radiation therapy. Transaxial T1-weighted fat-saturated post-Gd SE (600/15) **(A)** and sagittal T2-weighted fast SE (3500/100) **(B)** images show a bulky pelvic mass with invasion of the bladder (b) and rectum (r). Increased signal of obturator internus muscle *(arrows)* and presacral area are consistent with postradiation changes.

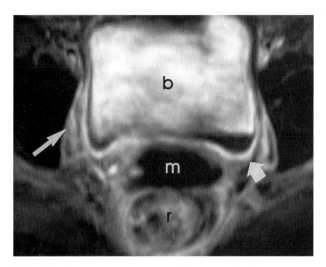

FIG. 35. Cervical carcinoma with postradiation changes. Transaxial T1-weighted fat-saturated Gd-enhanced SE image (600/15) shows intense enhancement of the bladder wall *(short arrow),* obturator internus muscles *(long arrow),* and perirectal tissue. The necrotic cervical mass (m) is of low signal intensity. b, bladder; r, rectum.

ages after treatment may represent either residual tumor or peritumoral edema/inflammatory tissue (76,86,115,256). Posttreatment inflammation/edema is especially prominent within the first 6 months of treatment (64,115) (Fig. 35). Whereas the unenhanced T2-weighted images are the best sequence to demonstrate posttreatment changes, Gd-enhanced T1-weighted images are helpful in evaluating patients with adnexal or pelvic side wall recurrence and patients with treatment complications (e.g., fistula formation) (115).

Clinical Application

Accurate staging of cervical carcinoma is crucial in determining the mode of treatment. Clinical evaluation is often inaccurate, with reported discrepancy of 34% to 39% between clinical and surgical staging (292). In spite of several limitations, CT has been used by some to evaluate all patients having more than microinvasive disease (138) and by others to assess patients with tumors of suspected clinical stage IIb and above (84,88,167,297). CT also has been used to evaluate patients with suspected recurrence (300,302).

Magnetic resonance imaging is superior to CT for delineating the primary tumor and extracervical extension (110,144,288). MRI stage shows better correlation with complete tumor regression, local tumor control, and disease-free survival at 12 months than clinical stage (112). Furthermore, MRI can differentiate between posttreatment tumor, fibrosis, and local recurrent tumor. Because of these advantages, MRI has replaced CT for the initial staging and follow-up evaluation of patients with

cervical carcinoma in several institutions. The use of MRI as the initial examination often obviates other invasive procedures and results in net cost savings (111). CT is reserved for patients in whom there is contraindication to the performance of an MRI examination or in institutions where MRI is less available. Cytoscopy and sigmoidoscopy are performed in patients with hematuria or guaiac-positive stool.

Uterus

Endometrial carcinoma is the most common invasive malignancy of the female genital tract. Approximately 70% of endometrial cancers are adenocarcinoma, 15% are adenoacanthomas, and 15% are adenosquamous carcinomas. Uterine sarcomas are rare: they are either mixed müllerian tumors or leiomyosarcomas. The prognosis of this neoplasm, which usually affects women in the fifth decade, depends on the histology, the grade (degree of cellular differentiation), and the stage (anatomic extent) of the tumor. Whereas well-differentiated adenocarcinomas of the endometrium are often localized on initial presentation, poorly differentiated adenocarcinomas and endometrial sarcomas tend to metastasize widely. In addition, the incidence of distant metastases increases with increasing depth of myometrial invasion. If the myometrium is not invaded, nodal metastases are present in about 3% of patients. If the invasion reaches the outer half of the myometrium, nodal metastases are present in about 40% of cases (22). In the lymphatic spread from neoplasms of the uterine body, the para-aortic and paracaval groups are most frequently involved, followed by external iliac and inguinal nodes (1). Local spread to the cervix, the broad ligament, and adnexal structures, as well as metastases to the omentum and peritoneum, also may occur.

The clinical management of patients with endometrial cancer varies from institution to institution. At our institution, the treatment of stage I (Table 4) disease depends on the degree of cellular differentiation: low-grade tumors are managed by hysterectomy; high-grade tumors receive staging laparotomy after brief intracavitary radiation. In addition to hysterectomy, random sampling of pelvic

TABLE 4. *Staging classification for endometrial carcinoma*

I. Tumor confined to the corpus
A. Uterine cavity less than 8 cm
B. Uterine cavity greater than 8 cm
II. Tumor involving corpus and cervix
III. Involvement of parametria, adnexae, pelvic sidewall, or pelvic nodes
IV. A. Bladder or rectal involvement
B. Metastases outside the true pelvis

From ref. 120, with permission.

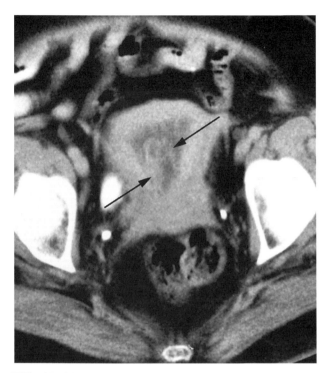

FIG. 36. Mucinous adenocarcinoma of the endometrium and cervix. Contrast-enhanced CT image shows a dilated endometrial cavity secondary to cervical portion of tumor (not shown). Enhancing endometrial tumor mass *(arrows)* is outlined by luminal fluid.

lymph nodes and peritoneal washing are also performed. The subsequent therapy depends on the operatively determined tumor extent. Treatment of stage II disease depends on the extent of cervical involvement: patients with macroscopic tumors undergo a staging laparotomy as described for high-grade stage I patients. In patients with stage III and IV tumors, palliative radiation or surgery is often the only treatment rendered.

Computed Tomography

On noncontrast CT scans, focal or diffuse enlargement of the uterine body can be seen. After contrast administration, endometrial neoplasm appears as a mass that enhances to a lesser degree than normal myometrium but to a greater degree than nonenhancing uterine secretions (Fig. 36) (95,98,245,303). In some cases, the primary tumor may occlude the internal cervical os, resulting in hydrometra, hematometra, or pyometra. When this occurs, CT demonstrates a symmetrically enlarged uterus containing a central low-attenuation mass surrounded by a large amount of fluid (245). Such an appearance may be confused with a cystic ovarian cancer. Occlusion of the internal os also may result from senile contraction, primary or recurrent carcinoma of the cervix, radiation therapy, or postsurgical scarring. The depth of myometrial invasion can be determined from postcontrast scans (Fig.

37) (60,95,98). Endometrial tumor involvement of the cervix by CT is characterized by cervical enlargement and hypodense areas within the fibromuscular stroma of the cervix (14,98). CT findings of parametrial and pelvic side-wall extension from endometrial carcinoma are similar to those seen in cervical carcinoma.

The reported accuracy for CT in staging patients with endometrial cancer ranges from 58% to 88% (14,294, 303). CT often correctly upstages clinical stage I and II tumors by detecting occult metastases to pelvic and para-aortic lymph nodes or the omentum (Fig. 38). Most of the staging errors by CT are caused by its failure to identify microscopic tumor spread to the parametria, lymph nodes, or other pelvic viscera. False positive staging errors are largely the result of misinterpretation of inflammatory changes as neoplastic involvement. Furthermore, false positive interpretations of deep myometrial invasion may occur when large exophytic tumors fill the endometrial cavity and stretch the myometrium to a very thin layer (60,294).

Magnetic Resonance Imaging

Endometrial carcinoma has a variable MRI appearance. On T1-weighted images, most endometrial carcinomas will be isointense to the uterus unless they contain hemorrhagic areas. On T2-weighted images, tumor nodules ranging from a few millimeters to a few centimeters in size can be identified within the uterine cavity on T2-weighted images. They usually have a signal intensity intermediate between that of normal endometrium and

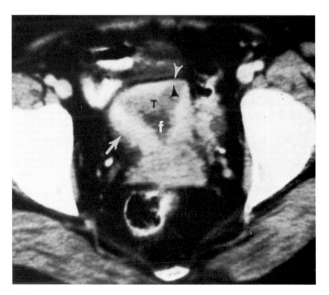

FIG. 37. Endometrial carcinoma, with deep myometrial invasion. Contrast-enhanced CT image demonstrates that the tumor (T) is enhanced to a lesser degree than normal myometrium *(arrow)*, but more than endometrial fluid (f). Marked thinning of the anterior myometrium *(arrowheads)* is due to tumor invasion.

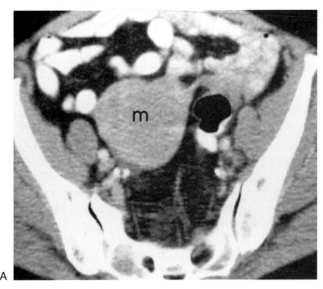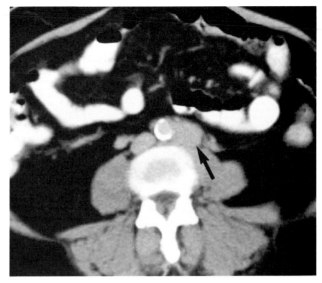

A | B

FIG. 38. Endometrial carcinoma. **A:** Contrast-enhanced CT scan shows the uterine body largely replaced and expanded by a hypodense mass (m). **B:** At a higher level, note left para-aortic adenopathy *(arrow)*.

that of myometrium (Fig. 39) (114,148,294,319). In some patients with endometrial carcinoma, especially those studied with low-field units (0.35T or lower), MRI will only show expansion of the central high-signal-intensity area of the uterus (294,319) without discrete nodules. Although the expanded central high-signal-intensity usually corresponds to the tumor mass/thickened endometrium, it correlates with increased uterine secretion in some cases. As stated previously, differentiation between nonbloody uterine secretions and the underlying endometrium can be achieved only on post-Gd T1-weighted images. Because endometrial carcinoma occurs predominantly in postmenopausal women, and because normal postmenopausal uteri have a very thin central high signal intensity (often less than 5 mm in width), expansion of the central high-intensity zone in this age group should raise the suspicion of uterine pathology.

The appearance of endometrial carcinoma is variable after intravenous administration of Gd (Fig. 39C). Most tumors enhance less than myometrium on both dynamic and delayed postcontrast images (108,321). However, some may show early enhancement compared to the myometrium, and others may appear isointense or hyperintense to the myometrium on delayed images. Contrast-enhanced images improve tumor detection and differentiation between a viable tumor and retained debris in the endometrial cavity.

Although uterine sarcomas often appear as a large mass of inhomogeneous signal intensity, totally obscuring the uterine contour (148,252,319), the MRI findings are nonetheless nonspecific and mimic invasive endometrial carcinoma (252).

Magnetic resonance imaging has proven to be useful

for staging endometrial carcinoma and for assessing the depth of myometrial invasion (114,216,319). On T2-weighted images, preservation of the low-intensity junctional band usually implies the absence of myometrial invasion; focal disruption or total obliteration of this band suggests myometrial involvement (Fig. 39). However, caution must be taken not to overinterpret this finding, because the entire junctional zone may not be visible in some healthy postmenopausal women (52). In patients without visible zonal anatomy, presence of myometrial invasion must be determined on the basis of the appearance of the interface between the endometrium and the myometrium. If the interface is irregular, invasion may be presumed to be present and if the interface is smooth, invasion is presumed to be absent. However, these findings do not have a high predictive value. Furthermore, patients with large intraluminal polypoid tumors can have a significant expansion of the endometrial cavity with thinning of the myometrium over it, thereby simulating deep myometrial invasion (161). In patients with leiomyomata, congenital uterine anomalies, or small uteri, assessment of myometrial invasion by MRI also may be difficult (247). Although MRI can detect tumor extension into the cervix reliably, it is less accurate in detecting metastases to the adnexa, the peritoneum, and the lymph nodes (114). In one study, the accuracy of MRI decreased from 92%, if all stages of endometrial carcinomas were included, to 57% when the data were analyzed separately for only more advanced disease (stages II to IV) (114).

The reported accuracy of MRI for staging endometrial carcinoma ranges from 75% to 88% (108,113,294); the accuracy for determining the depth of myometrial invasion varies from 68% to 82% (50,108,113,161,258,294,

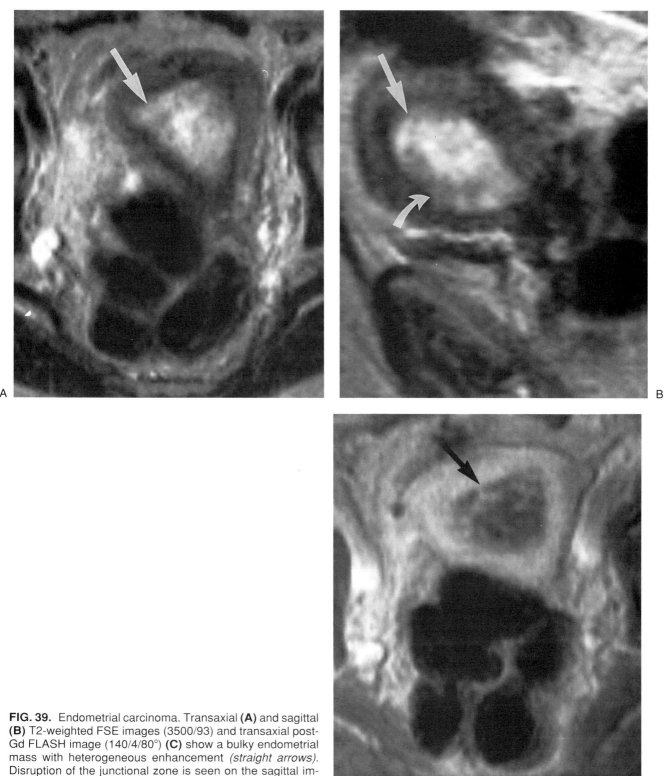

FIG. 39. Endometrial carcinoma. Transaxial **(A)** and sagittal **(B)** T2-weighted FSE images (3500/93) and transaxial post-Gd FLASH image (140/4/80°) **(C)** show a bulky endometrial mass with heterogeneous enhancement *(straight arrows)*. Disruption of the junctional zone is seen on the sagittal image at the inferior aspect of the endometrial cavity *(curved arrow)*, consistent with superficial myometrial invasion.

321). Preliminary data have shown that Gd-enhanced MRI improves both the overall staging (75% to 95%) and the determination of the depth of myometrial invasion (72% to 94%) (113,321).

Clinical Application

Because initial symptoms are postmenopausal bleeding, most patients with endometrial cancer normally seek medical care when the disease is at an early stage. Diagnosis is established by fractional dilatation and curettage. In patients with well-differentiated stage I adenocarcinoma, total hysterectomy is usually performed with staging of the disease carried out at the time of surgery. Besides bimanual pelvic examination, preoperative evaluation is limited to sonographic determination of the depth of the uterine cavity, chest radiographs, and excretory urography. In patients with high-grade endometrial carcinomas (grade III or above) or sarcomas, additional imaging studies should be performed preoperatively to determine the depth of myometrial invasion and clinically unsuspected extrauterine metastases. Demonstration of deep myometrial invasion often necessitates preoperative radiation and intraoperative lymphadenectomy. Documentation of extrauterine metastases will preclude surgery as the curative treatment. Because MRI can more clearly demonstrate the primary neoplasm and more accurately determine the depth of myometrial invasion than CT, it has replaced CT as the imaging procedure of choice in the preoperative evaluation of patients with high-grade endometrial carcinoma and uterine sarcomas in some institutions (108,294). In institutions where MRI is less available and in patients in whom there are contraindications to the performance of MRI examinations, CT remains a valuable imaging tool for detecting clinically unsuspected extrauterine metastases, such as the omentum and lymph nodes. CT also is useful in patients with suspected recurrence and for following the response to chemotherapy or radiation therapy. Although transvaginal sonography had an accuracy similar to MRI in determining the depth of myometrial invasion in one study (50), it has a limited field of view compared to either MRI or CT and is therefore not widely used for staging purposes.

Ovary

Ovarian cancer is the most lethal of all gynecologic malignancies. The peak incidence is in women between 40 and 65 years of age. The prognosis depends on the clinical stage, the degree of cellular differentiation, and the histologic type of ovarian cancer. Because of a paucity of symptoms in early stages, most patients present with advanced disease. Approximately 85% of ovarian cancers are epithelial in origin, with the remaining 15% derived from germ or stroma cells (1). In patients with epithelial ovarian carcinomas, the great majority (90%) are either serous or mucinous cystadenocarcinomas, with the rest being endometrial or solid carcinomas. Stage for stage (Table 5), the prognosis for patients with solid carcinomas is worse than that for either serous or mucinous tumors.

Ovarian carcinomas usually spread by implanting widely on the omental and peritoneal surfaces. Although not pathognomonic, demonstration of an omental "cake" is highly suggestive of an ovarian malignancy (Fig. 40) (159). An omental cake appears as an irregular sheet of nodular soft-tissue densities beneath the anterior abdominal wall on CT, and as masses of medium signal intensities on MRI. Peritoneal tumor implants are recognized as soft-tissue or medium-signal-intensity nodules/plaques along the lateral peritoneal surfaces of the abdomen (123) (Fig. 41). Subdiaphragmatic peritoneal nodules are most easily detected between the abdominal wall and the liver in the presence of ascites (123). Rarely, peritoneal and omental metastases may calcify (Fig. 42) (184). Although intraperitoneal seeding is the almost exclusive metastatic mode in mucinous carcinomas, lymphatic metastases to the para-aortic lymph nodes, and occasionally to the inguinal nodes, do occur in serous and other types of ovarian carcinomas (Fig. 43).

In most centers, neither CT nor MRI plays a primary role in the initial evaluation of ovarian carcinoma. When the diagnosis of an ovarian carcinoma is suspected, based on physical examination or sonographic findings, exploratory laparotomy usually follows. Because the sensitivity of CT and MRI in detecting small intraperitoneal implants (<1 cm) is low, surgical exploration is necessary to document the exact stage of the disease in all cases (3,45,77,127). Surgical debulking of the neoplasm is particularly helpful in patients with stage III or IV ovarian cancer (90). Cytoreductive surgery not only allows for greater drug exposure and penetration, it also may favorably affect tumor cell kinetics allowing for greater cell

TABLE 5. *Staging classification for ovarian carcinoma*

Stage I:	Growth limited to the ovaries
Stage IA:	One ovary; no ascites
Stage IB:	Both ovaries; no ascites
Stage IC:	One or both ovaries; ascites present with malignant cells in the fluid
Stage II:	Growth involving one or both ovaries with pelvic extension
Stage IIA:	Extension and/or metastases to the uterus and/or tubes only
Stage IIB:	Extension to other pelvic tissues
Stage III:	Growth involving one or both ovaries with widespread intraperitoneal metastases (the omentum, the small intestine, and its mesentery), limited to the abdomen
Stage IV:	Growth involving one or both ovaries with distant metastases outside the peritoneal cavity

From ref. 120, with permission.

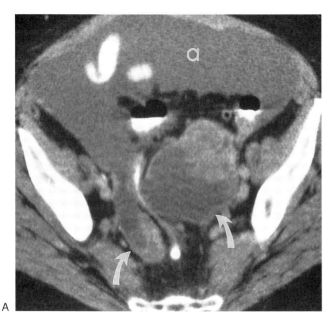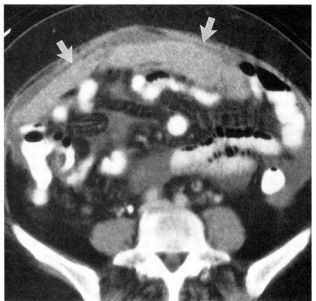

FIG. 40. Ovarian carcinoma. **A:** Contrast-enhanced CT shows bilateral complex solid and cystic masses *(arrows)* in the mid pelvis, associated with ascites (a). **B:** At a more superior level, note omental "cake" of tumor anteriorly *(arrows)*.

kill with chemotherapeutic agents (90). Whereas CT is valuable in following treatment response in patients with ovarian malignancy by demonstrating residual or recurrent tumor (3,176,217,226), it cannot replace second-look laparotomy for accurate assessment of disease status, because of its low accuracy in detecting small peritoneal metastases (25,45,254). Whereas CT performed after intraperitoneal administration of iodinated contrast material (CT-IP) was similar to conventional CT for detecting

small peritoneal metastases in one study (198), CT-IP detected residual tumor in most patients with a prior negative conventional CT exam in another study (79). However, even in the latter study, CT-IP had a sensitivity of only 77%. Preliminary data have shown that MRI performed with Gd-enhanced GRE and fat-suppressed T1-weighted SE sequences may be superior to CT for detecting peritoneal metastases (165,251) (Figs. 44,45).

CLARIFICATION OF KNOWN AND SUSPECTED PELVIC ABNORMALITY

Evaluation of Urinary Bladder Deformity

When the lateral aspect of the urinary bladder is noted to be compressed on an excretory urogram, either unilaterally or on both sides, the differential diagnosis usually includes pelvic lipomatosis, pelvic lymph node enlargement, hypertrophic iliopsoas muscles (43), lymphocele, urinoma, hematoma, or pelvic venous thrombosis. Documentation of a urinoma/hematoma or pelvic lymphadenopathy can be accomplished quickly with sonography (187). Pelvic lipomatosis is often suspected from apparent increased lucency on the plain radiograph. A diagnosis of venous thrombosis and pelvic collateral venous congestion causing bladder deformity has required venography previously. Because of the superior contrast sensitivity of CT and MRI, both are capable of differentiating among fat, water, and soft tissues (Fig. 46). Because mature fat has a characteristic CT and MRI appearance, a definitive diagnosis of pelvic lipomatosis can be made by either method and surgical exploration or percu-

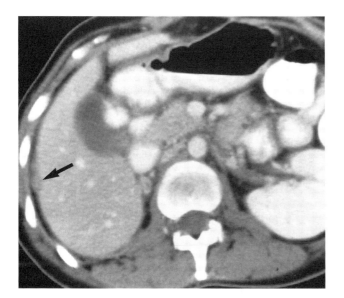

FIG. 41. Peritoneal metastasis from ovarian carcinoma. Contrast-enhanced CT scan through the abdomen shows a small hypodense mass *(arrow)* along the lateral aspect of the right hepatic lobe consistent with peritoneal implantation.

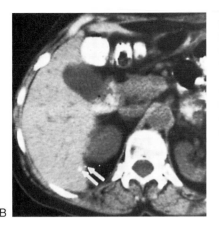 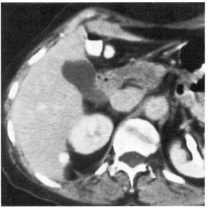

A,B

FIG. 42. Calcified peritoneal metastases due to recurrent ovarian carcinoma. **A:** Noncontrast CT image shows two specks of calcification *(arrows)* near the surface of the liver. **B:** Postcontrast CT study obtained 6 months later demonstrates interval increase in the size of the calcification. Percutaneous biopsy confirmed ovarian metastasis.

taneous biopsy obviated (44,97,272,311). In this entity, coronal and sagittal MR images can clearly demonstrate cephalad displacement of the bladder base, elongation of the bladder neck and posterior urethra, and elevation of the prostate gland (51). Likewise, characteristic medial and superior displacement of the seminal vesicles and increased separation between the prostate gland and the rectum by fatty tissue can be shown. The true nature of venous collaterals can be established on CT scans by administering iodinated contrast medium intravenously. Such a diagnosis also can be made by MRI without the use of intravenous contrast medium. In cases in which the bladder deformity is caused by compression by enlarged pelvic lymph nodes, either CT or MRI can be used to assess the status of the retroperitoneal and mesenteric lymph nodes as well.

Characterization of Presacral Masses

Ultrasonography is not as accurate in detecting presacral masses as in diagnosing gynecologic masses. Sono-

graphic studies are often suboptimal in obese patients because of marked attenuation of the sound beam by abundant subcutaneous fat. Furthermore, ultrasound is incapable of evaluating bony abnormalities, which are often associated with presacral masses. Both CT and MRI are useful in these circumstances in confirming the presence of a pelvic mass when one is suspected either by physical examination or by other radiologic tests (e.g., barium enema). In general, CT is superior to MRI in evaluating the integrity of cortical bone and in demonstrating gas bubbles and calcifications. In contradistinction, MRI is more sensitive than CT in detecting marrow alteration, and it provides a better topographic display of a presacral mass because of its direct multiplanar imaging capability. When a mass is detected, either CT or MRI can characterize many lesions and give an accurate assessment of possible bony involvement. Air, fat, fluid, and soft tissue are easily differentiated. An air-containing mass suggests an abscess cavity (6), whereas a mass with the density of fat is compatible with a benign lipoma. Masses with near-

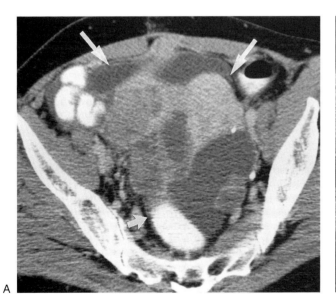 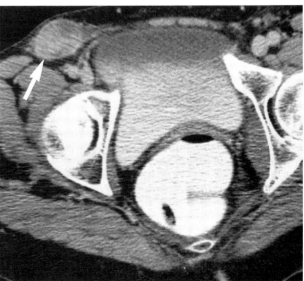

A   B

FIG. 43. Ovarian carcinoma, stage IV. **A:** Contrast-enhanced CT scan shows a bulky complex mass with solid and cystic areas *(large arrows)*. Long interface with colon *(short arrow)* is consistent with invasion. **B:** Right inguinal adenopathy *(arrow)* is noted on this more caudal scan.

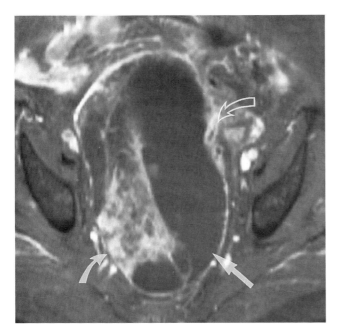

FIG. 44. Advanced ovarian carcinoma. Transaxial T1-weighted fat-saturated post-Gd SE image (600/15) shows large complex mass in the pelvis *(arrows)*. Note excellent characterization of internal architecture of the mass, with cystic portion appearing low in signal intensity *(straight arrow)*, and solid portion enhancing heterogeneously *(curved solid arrow)*. Sigmoid colon *(open arrow)* is closely applied to the tumor and was invaded at surgery.

water density or signal intensity include seroma, urinoma, and cystic teratoma, although a teratoma often contains areas of fatty and calcific elements and usually has a thick wall. When the mass is composed of soft tissue, definitive histologic diagnosis by CT or MRI is not possible. Although both CT and MRI are capable of delineating the size and the shape of the mass as well as its effect on neighboring viscera, differentiation between a benign and a malignant tumor may be difficult unless secondary findings such as lymph node metastases or bony destruction are also present. The attenuation value of an abscess, a hematoma, and a necrotic tumor also may overlap, and distinguishing among these entities often depends on the clinical history and physical findings. Likewise, the signal intensity of an abscess overlaps that of a necrotic tumor.

Evaluation of Gynecologic Abnormalities

Although some studies have shown CT and MRI to be more sensitive than ultrasonography for detecting ovarian masses (36,55), others report endovaginal sonography to be more accurate than MRI performed with a body coil (83% versus 70%) for diagnosing adnexal masses (122). In spite of these disparate results, sonography remains the primary imaging method in the evaluation of patients with suspected gynecologic pathology, largely because of its lower cost, absence of ionizing radiation, and ease in obtaining longitudinal and transverse scans. Ultrasonography can accurately differentiate cystic from solid lesions and uterine from ovarian masses (304). Also, sonography is superior to CT in detecting internal septations within a cystic mass (69). However, CT can be helpful when sonography is suboptimal, either because of abundant intestinal gas or because of marked obesity. Because a successful pelvic sonographic study is dependent on the presence of a distended urinary bladder, CT also can be beneficial in patients with a small irritable bladder and in patients with prior cystectomy. Although MRI is more time consuming and more costly than sonography or CT, it provides superior soft-tissue contrast beyond that obtainable by either of these two modalities. MRI now has become a valuable adjunct to sonography in many nonobstetric cases for which ultrasound does not provide sufficient diagnostic information (244). It is most useful in determining the organ of origin in large pelvic masses (Fig. 47), differentiation between uterine leiomyoma and adenomyosis, characterization of pelvic masses in women of child-bearing age, and assessment of congenital uterine anomalies (207,289,307). The role of MRI is expected to increase further with the use of phased-array coils and FSE sequences.

Leiomyomas

Computed Tomography

Leiomyomas most commonly appear as an enlarged uterus with a deformed contour (40,274). They usually are of homogeneous soft-tissue density similar to that of normal uterus. Necrosis or degeneration may result in a low-attenuation mass, sometimes simulating adnexal abnormality. Calcification, occurring up to 10% of uterine leiomyomas, is a more specific CT sign (Fig. 48). It can be mottled, rimlike, whorled, or streaked (40). Alterations in contour or lobulations are identified more often in the uterine fundus; such changes may be seen in the body or in the lower uterine segment. Leiomyomas also may occur as an intracavitary mass obliterating the uterine cavity, thus simulating an endometrial polyp or carcinoma. A leiomyoma may be distinguished from an endometrial carcinoma because the former tends to exhibit contrast enhancement similar to that of normal myometrium, whereas the latter enhances to a lesser degree and appears as a hypodense mass (98). However, the reliability of this potentially distinctive CT feature is unknown. In our experience, a noncalcified uterine leiomyoma cannot be distinguished from a malignant uterine neoplasm based on the CT attenuation value alone (Fig. 49).

Magnetic Resonance Imaging

Most leiomyomas are round or oval, have clear margins, and do not infiltrate the myometrium. They have

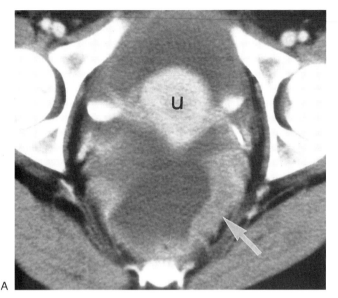 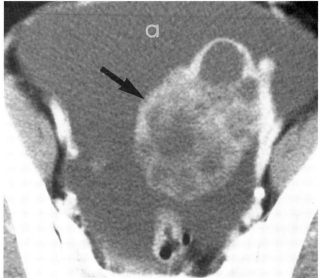

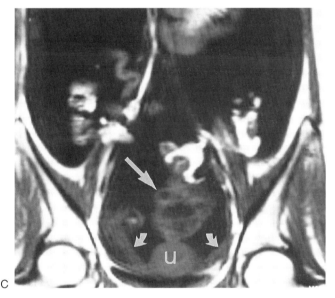

FIG. 45. Ovarian and peritoneal metastases secondary to a primary sinus rhabdomyosarcoma. **A:** Contrast-enhanced CT at the level of the uterus (u) shows pelvic ascites and soft-tissue mass *(arrow)* along the posterolateral pelvic wall. **B:** Scan several centimeters craniad shows complex solid and cystic mass *(arrow)* consistent with ovarian metastasis. a, ascites. **C:** Coronal T1-weighted SE image (600/15) shows complex ovarian mass *(straight arrow)*, pelvic wall implants *(curved arrows)* and massive ascites. u, uterus.

intermediate-to-low signal intensity on T1-weighted images, and low signal intensity on T2-weighted images (116) (Fig. 50). Leiomyomas that are found in pregnant women or have undergone torsion and infarction may have increased signal areas on T1-weighted images (186). A peripheral high-signal rim, corresponding to the dilated lymphatic vessels, dilated veins, or edema, may be seen on T2-weighted images (116,188,327). Leiomyomas that have undergone cystic degeneration or necrosis often have areas of high signal intensity on T2-weighted images (116,307) (Fig. 51). Leiomyomas with relatively increased cellularity may have intermediate-to-high signal intensity on T2-weighted images, and they show increased enhancement after intravenous administration of Gd (148,325). There is yet no reliable MRI feature for detecting malignant degeneration within a benign leiomyoma.

Leiomyomas must be differentiated from other causes of low-signal-intensity myometrial masses such as sustained uterine contractions and adenomyosis. Sustained uterine contractions can be differentiated from leiomyomas by their changing shape and location on successive imaging sequences (283). Adenomyosis, a common condition in which foci of endometrium, usually basalis, are located ectopically within myometrium, usually can be distinguished from a leiomyoma because the former appears as an ill-defined mass whereas the latter is often well defined (Fig. 52) (10,168,289). Focal or diffuse adenomyosis also may appear as thickening of the junctional zone ($\geq$12 mm) (224); tiny foci of high signal, which probably represent islands of endometrium, can be seen within the myometrium on T2-weighted images. T2-weighted SE images are more accurate than Gd-enhanced T1-weighted images for identifying and differentiating between leiomyomas and adenomyosis (107).

As with CT, a majority of leiomyomas are discovered

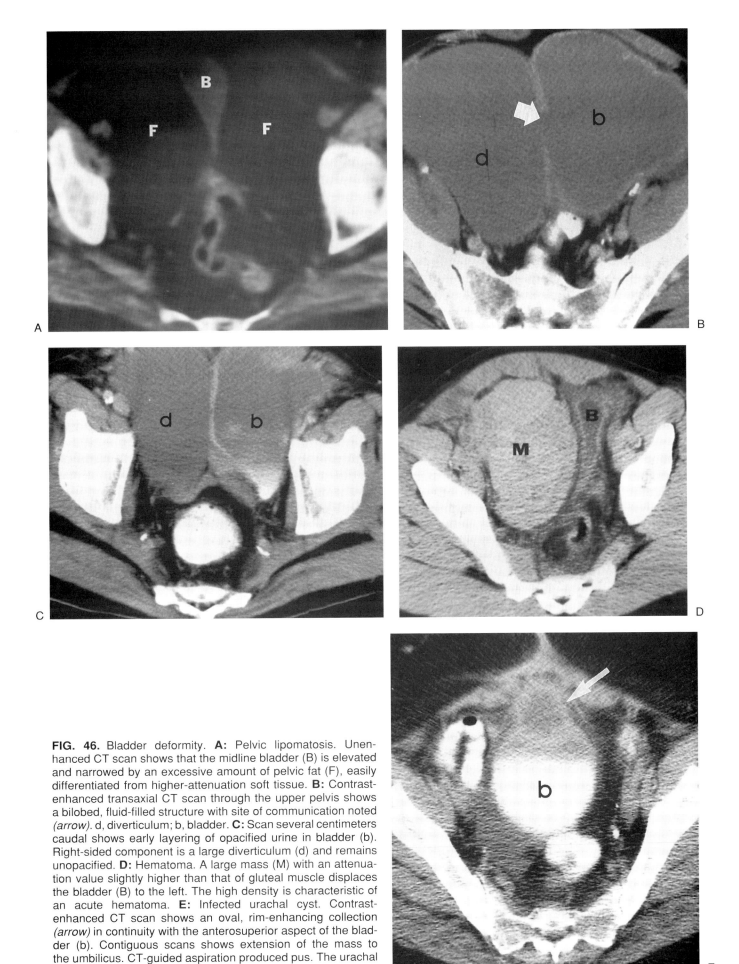

FIG. 46. Bladder deformity. **A:** Pelvic lipomatosis. Unenhanced CT scan shows that the midline bladder (B) is elevated and narrowed by an excessive amount of pelvic fat (F), easily differentiated from higher-attenuation soft tissue. **B:** Contrast-enhanced transaxial CT scan through the upper pelvis shows a bilobed, fluid-filled structure with site of communication noted *(arrow)*. d, diverticulum; b, bladder. **C:** Scan several centimeters caudal shows early layering of opacified urine in bladder (b). Right-sided component is a large diverticulum (d) and remains unopacified. **D:** Hematoma. A large mass (M) with an attenuation value slightly higher than that of gluteal muscle displaces the bladder (B) to the left. The high density is characteristic of an acute hematoma. **E:** Infected urachal cyst. Contrast-enhanced CT scan shows an oval, rim-enhancing collection *(arrow)* in continuity with the anterosuperior aspect of the bladder (b). Contiguous scans shows extension of the mass to the umbilicus. CT-guided aspiration produced pus. The urachal remnant was surgically resected after resolution of the infection.

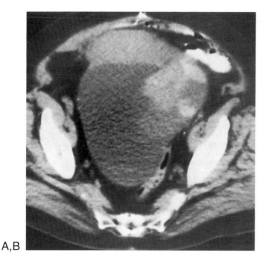 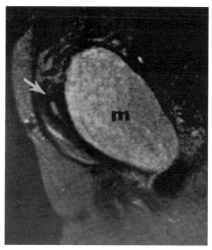 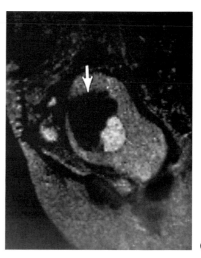

A,B   C

FIG. 47. Ovarian cystadenocarcinoma. **A:** Postcontrast CT image demonstrates a large, complex pelvic mass with both cystic and solid components. The exact location of the uterus is difficult to determine. **B:** Sagittal T2-weighted SE image (1500/90) shows the uterus *(arrows)*, with its characteristic high-intensity endometrium, to be displaced anteriorly by the mass (m). This portion of the mass is filled with fluid. **C:** Sagittal T2-weighted SE image (1500/90) 2 cm lateral to (B) shows solid components *(arrow)* of the mass, convincingly demonstrating that the mass is extrauterine in origin.

incidentally on MRI examinations performed for other indications. Although MRI is the most accurate imaging modality for detecting and localizing leiomyomas, transabdominal or endovaginal sonography is still the preferred screening procedure (62,327). MRI is reserved for cases in which sonographic findings are indeterminate (307). In addition, MRI is performed to obviate laparoscopy and/ or hysterosalpingography for mapping of leiomyomas in women who do not require evaluation of their fallopian tubes before myomectomy (62,206,327).

Magnetic resonance imaging also may be used to document the regression of leiomyomas after treatment by gonadotropin-releasing hormone (GnRH) analogs (329). Because the primary effect of these agents is on undegenerated myoma cells, and because undegenerated leiomyomas enhance more than degenerated ones, intravenous administration of a Gd compound may help select patients who are more likely to respond to GnRH therapy (325).

FIG. 48. Calcified uterine leiomyomata. Contrast-enhanced CT scan through the pelvis shows the uterus to be lobulated, containing several calcified leiomyomata *(arrows)* as well as a pedunculated noncalcified leiomyoma (l) in the right cul-de-sac. b, bladder.

Ovarian Masses

Computed Tomography

Both benign and malignant ovarian tumors have been diagnosed by CT. A benign ovarian cyst appears as a well-circumscribed, round, near-water-density structure with an almost imperceptible wall (Fig. 53). It does not enhance after intravenous administration of water-soluble iodinated contrast medium. The CT appearance of an ovarian cyst is quite similar to cysts in other organs (e.g., renal cysts, hepatic cysts). A follicular cyst cannot be differentiated from a corpus luteum cyst based on CT appearances alone, and both may involute without treatment. In patients with the Stein-Leventhal syndrome, both ovaries are enlarged and contain numerous cysts. The diagnosis usually can be made by CT. On occasion, the

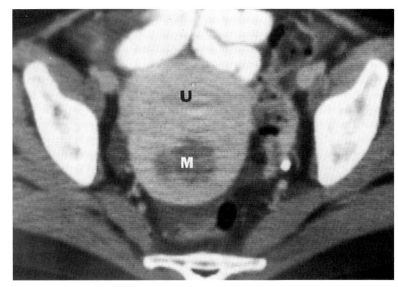

FIG. 49. Uterine leiomyoma. An irregular mass (M) with central low attenuation enlarges the posterior uterine fundus (U) in this contrast-enhanced CT image. By CT criteria, this leiomyoma is indistinguishable from uterine malignancy.

cysts are too small to be discernible by CT and the ovaries may simply appear as two enlarged soft-tissue masses (Fig. 54). Under these circumstances, polycystic ovarian disease cannot be differentiated from other solid ovarian neoplasms.

Dermoid cysts (cystic teratomas) occur in young women and are bilateral in 25% of patients. They are composed of ectodermal, mesodermal, and endodermal elements. They are predominantly cystic tumors with varying amounts of fat. When calcific (or osseous) and fatty elements are present within the tumor, diagnosis by CT is accurate (Fig. 55). In one study of 43 cystic teratomas of the ovary (41 benign, two with malignant transformation), fat was present in 93%, tooth or calcification noted in 56%, and a fat–fluid level in 12% of all cases (35). In one case report, mobile fat balls were noted within a cystic teratoma (192). Whereas most benign cystic teratomas contain some soft-tissue components, the presence of a large (>10 cm), irregular soft-tissue mass within the tumor should raise the suspicion of malignant transformation (35). Although an ovarian lipoleiomyoma also may contain fat, it is predominantly of soft-tissue density (57).

Endometriosis is a disease affecting a substantial proportion of the menstruating population. Symptoms have classically been characterized as the triad of dysmenorrhea, dyspareunia, and infertility. On CT, an endometrioma may have soft-tissue density, near-water density, or a mixture of the two (Fig. 56) (74). In one series, 15% of endometriomas shown on CT had a hyperdense (90 to 140 Hounsfield units), round or crescent-shaped focus located close to the inner border of the cystic lesion (34). The hyperdense area measures between 2 to 15 mm and corresponds to a blood clot pathologically. The CT appearance of diffuse peritoneal endometriosis may simulate peritoneal carcinomatosis (193).

Ovarian cystadenomas often are quite large when they first present. They appear as well-defined, uni- or multilocular, low-density masses. The walls and internal septae are of varying thickness and regularity (Fig. 57) (304). Papillary projections of soft-tissue density may be seen within the tumor. Whereas serous cystadenoma has a CT density approaching that of water, mucinous cystadenoma has a density slightly less than that of soft tissue. Amorphous, coarse calcifications sometimes can be seen in

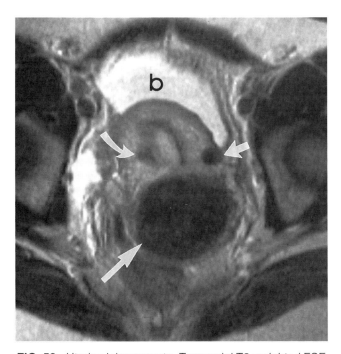

FIG. 50. Uterine leiomyomata. Transaxial T2-weighted FSE image (3500/93) shows three well-defined low-signal-intensity masses arising from the uterus: a large intramural mass posteriorly *(large arrow)*, a smaller subserosal mass to the left *(small arrow)*, and small submucosal mass on the right *(curved arrow)* b, bladder. (Courtesy of S. Ascher, M.D., Washington, DC.)

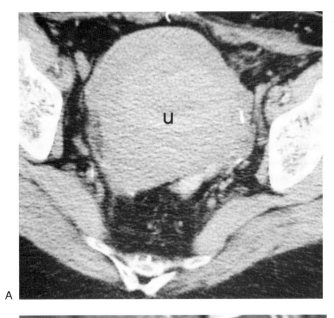

A

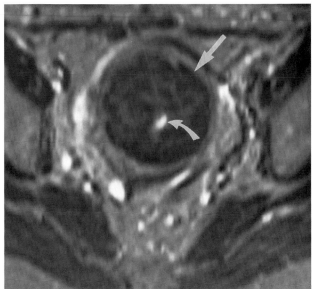

B

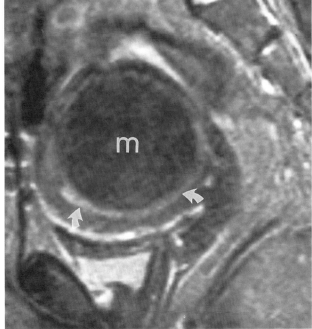

C

FIG. 51. Noncalcified uterine leiomyoma. **A:** CT scan shows enlarged, lobulated uterus (u) of slightly heterogeneous density. **B:** Transaxial T2-weighted SE image (2100/90) at same level as (A) shows large low-signal-intensity mass *(arrow)*, with central focus of high signal intensity *(curved arrow)*, likely related to degeneration. **C:** Sagittal T2-weighted SE image (2100/90) shows low-signal-intensity mass (m) compressing endometrial stripe *(arrows)* inferiorly.

the wall or within the soft-tissue component of a serous cystadenoma. Although the presence of a thick, irregular wall, irregular septa, and enhancing soft-tissue projections or nodules suggests malignancy, malignant ovarian cystadenocarcinomas cannot be reliably distinguished from benign cystadenomas unless metastases are present (36,83). In one study (36), 69% of benign serous cystadenomas and 62% of benign mucinous cystadenomas were correctly characterized based on CT findings.

The CT appearances of primary solid ovarian carcinomas are similar to those of their benign counterparts. Concomitant metastases to the lymph nodes, other organs, and omentum may be detected.

The CT appearance of a tubo-ovarian abscess is similar to that of abscesses occurring in other parts of the body. It appears as a soft-tissue mass with central areas of lower density and a thick irregular wall (Fig. 58). An associated hydrosalpinx, which appears as a tubular fluid-density adnexal mass, sometimes also may be seen (Fig. 59). Other ancillary CT findings include anterior displacement of the mesosalpinx, hydroureter, and increased density of the fat and ligaments anterior to the sacrum (315). If the abscess contains air, a precise diagnosis can be provided (Fig. 60). In the absence of gas bubbles, a tubo-ovarian abscess cannot be differentiated from a necrotic tumor or a hematoma based on the CT findings alone. Pelvic inflammatory disease that does not present as a discrete abscess also has a nonspecific CT appearance. The normal

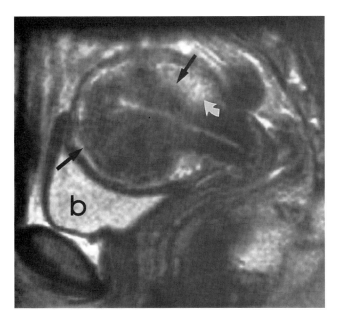

FIG. 52. Adenomyosis. Sagittal T2-weighted image (2100/90) shows marked broadening of the junctional zone *(arrows)*. Note normal myometrial intermediate signal intensity *(curved arrow)*. b, bladder. (Courtesy of S. Ascher, M.D., Washington, DC.)

pelvic structures are poorly defined because of obliteration of fat planes by the inflammatory process.

Magnetic Resonance Imaging

The MRI appearance of an uncomplicated ovarian cyst is similar to that of cyst elsewhere in the body (59,96,185). An ovarian cyst usually has an extremely

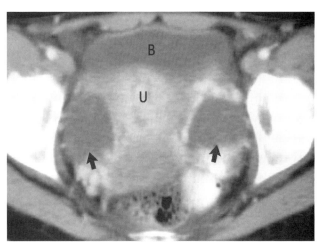

FIG. 54. Polycystic ovaries. Contrast-enhanced CT scan shows symmetrical enlargement of both ovaries *(arrows)*. Note that the attenuation of both ovaries is similar to the urine within the urinary bladder (B) and much lower than the pelvic musculature. U, uterus.

low signal intensity on T1-weighted images and a very high signal intensity on T2-weighted images (Figs. 61,62). Hemorrhage into an ovarian cyst may result in higher signal intensity on T1-weighted images (Fig. 63). In patients with polycystic ovary disease, T2-weighted images often show multiple, small peripheral cysts of high signal intensity surrounding abundant low-intensity central stroma (183).

Dermoid cysts (cystic teratomas) vary in signal intensity depending on their tissue composition (Fig. 64) (33,103,185,286). The majority of cystic teratomas have

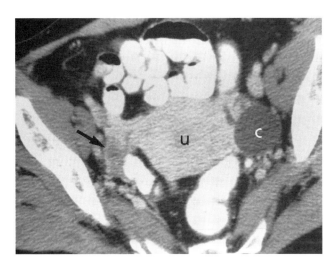

FIG. 53. Benign ovarian cyst. Contrast-enhanced CT scan of the pelvis shows a well-circumscribed, nonenhancing structure of water density (c) arising from the left ovary consistent with benign cyst. Note right ovary *(arrow)* and uterus (u).

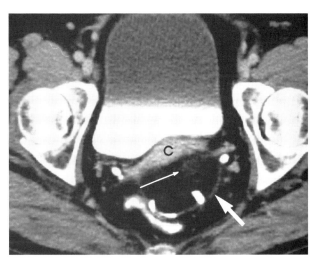

FIG. 55. Ovarian dermoid. Contrast-enhanced CT shows a well-defined mass of mostly fat attenuation in the left recto-uterine fossa *(thick arrow)*. Feathery-appearing soft-tissue density corresponding to hair *(thin arrow)*, and both rim- and tooth-like calcifications are seen within the mass. c, cervix.

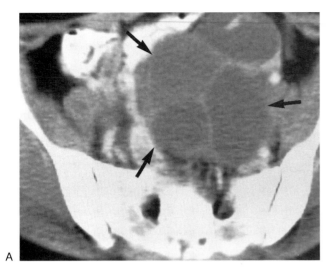 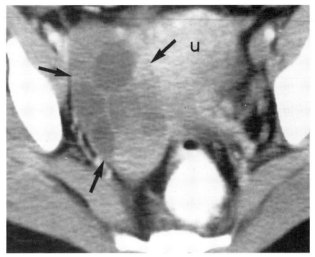

A   B

FIG. 56. A,B: Endometriomas. Contrast-enhanced CT scans through the pelvis of a 32-year-old woman show multiple rounded low- to soft-tissue-density structures in both adnexal regions *(arrows)*. Although the appearance simulates that of ovarian neoplasm, the masses were found to represent endometriomas at surgery. u, uterus.

appeared as masses with high signal intensity as a result of their large fat content. However, calcifications, bone, hair, and fibrous tissue, all of which are frequently found in teratomas, appear as low-intensity foci. A unique chemical shift artifact that is the exact reverse of what can be seen around the urinary bladder may be seen in some cases of cystic teratomas (286). Proton-selective fat-saturation technique or phase-shift GRE (i.e., comparison of in-phase image with the opposed-phase image) is supe-

rior to the conventional SE sequence for demonstrating minute amounts of fat and for differentiating fat from subacute blood, both of which may have similarly high signal intensities on T1 and T2-weighted SE images (136,266,320,324). Additional MRI findings of cystic teratomas include gravity-dependent layering, floating debris or fat, and complex mural protrusions (dermoid plugs) (286).

Endometriomas may appear as a uni- or multilocular cystic mass (33,96,103,200). On T1-weighted images, the signal intensity of an endometrioma may be similar to that of urine (low signal intensity) or fat (high signal intensity) depending on the amount and age of hemorrhage within the lesion

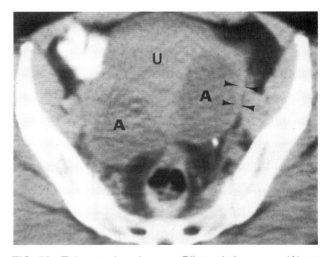

FIG. 57. Ovarian cystadenoma. Non-contrast-enhanced CT scan shows a complex mass representing the cystadenoma (C) posterior to the uterus (U). Two soft-tissue nodules *(arrows)* lie in the wall. The attenuation value of the fluid component is between that of soft tissue and water. b, urinary bladder.

FIG. 58. Tubo-ovarian abscess. Bilateral abscesses (A) are present. Thick, nonuniform walls *(arrowheads)* surround the low-density masses. Correlation of the CT findings with clinical history is necessary to distinguish abscess from other ovarian lesions. U, uterus.

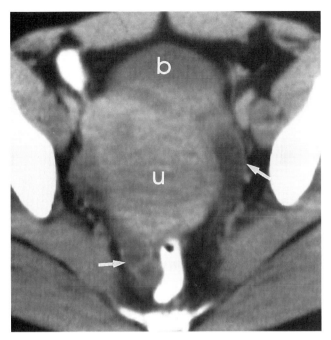

FIG. 59. Hydrosalpinx. Contrast-enhanced CT scan demonstrates dilated, fluid-filled fallopian tubes bilaterally *(arrows)*, adjacent to the uterus (u). b, bladder.

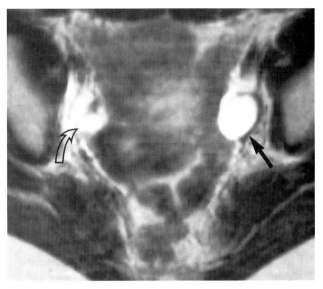

FIG. 61. Ovarian cyst. Transaxial T2-weighted FSE image (3500/93) shows homogeneously high signal intensity, sharply marginated structure arising from the left ovary *(solid arrow)*. Several small follicles are seen within the right ovary *(hollow arrow)*.

(96). A distinct low-intensity capsule has been seen in some cases (200). Although endometriomas share many MRI features with hemorrhagic ovarian cysts, these two entities usually can be distinguished from each other. Multiplicity, distorted shape, and "shading" on T2-weighted images favor the diagnosis of endometriomas, whereas hemorrhagic ovarian cysts are more often solitary and round (287). *Shading*

refers to the shortening of T2 of the cyst contents, producing lower signal intensity than that expected for simple fluid on T2-weighted images within the cyst. This is caused by blood by-products and may produce a gradient of lower signal intensity across the cyst.

Endometriosis also may present as solid fibrotic nodules implanted on the peritoneum, simulating ovarian peritoneal metastases. They have an intermediate signal intensity

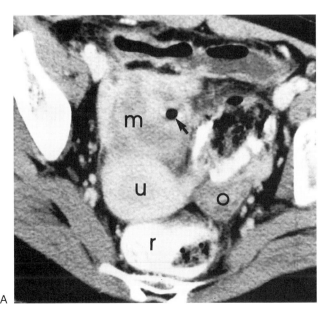

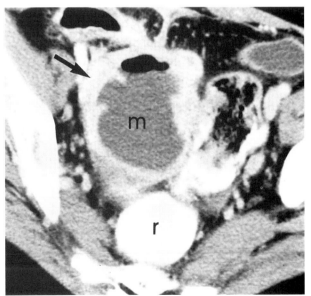

A B

FIG. 60. Tubo-ovarian abscess. A: Contrast-enhanced CT scan at the level of the uterus (u) shows a complex mass (m) in the right adnexal region that contains gas *(arrow)*. o, left ovary. B: Scan 2 cm craniad shows more cystic component of mass (m). Note thick enhancing rim *(arrow)* and gas. r, rectum.

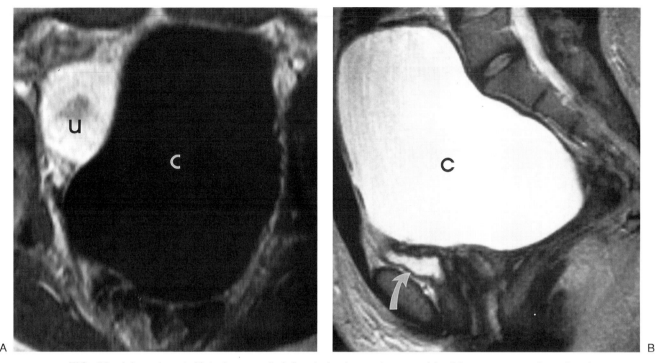

FIG. 62. Adnexal cyst. Note large well defined simple cystic mass (c) of homogeneous low signal intensity on transaxial post-Gd T1-weighted FLASH (140/4/80°) **(A)** and high signal intensity on sagittal T2-weighted FSE images (3500/100) **(B)** arising in the pelvis and extending into the abdomen. *Arrow,* urinary bladder.

mixed with punctate foci of high signal intensity on T1-weighted images, and low signal intensity on T2-weighted images, and they exhibit enhancement after intravenous administration of contrast material (253). Low-signal-intensity fibrotic nodules seen with endometriosis are uncommon for ovarian malignant neoplasms (267). Although MRI is extremely accurate (90% sensitivity, 98% specificity in one series) for the diagnosis of endometriomas, especially if fat-saturated T1-weighted MR images are used (94,270,287), it is as insensitive as CT and ultrasonography for identifying

most peritoneal implants (less than 5 mm) and adhesions (9,328). Therefore, laparoscopy remains the definitive test for diagnosis and evaluation of endometriosis in most patients. MRI is used to detect changes in endometriomas in women with a known diagnosis of endometriosis and to detect response to treatment by GnRH analogs (329).

Ovarian cystadenomas often appear as large pelvic masses (96,185). The signal characteristics of these masses differ depending on the chemical composition of the cyst fluid and the amount of solid components contained within the

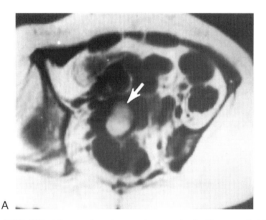
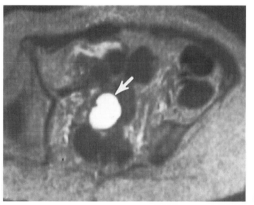

FIG. 63. Hemorrhagic ovarian cyst. **A:** Transaxial T1-weighted SE image (500/17) shows a relatively high-signal-intensity mass *(arrow)* in the right ovary. The pelvis is deformed in this patient with a congenital neuromuscular disorder. **B:** On T2-weighted SE image (2100/90), the mass *(arrow)* has a higher signal intensity than fat.

tumor (Fig. 65). Although the accuracy for distinguishing between benign and malignant ovarian lesions improves with the addition of Gd-enhanced MR images (323), malignant ovarian cystadenocarcinomas cannot be reliably differentiated from benign cystadenomas unless metastases are present (Figs. 65,66).

Congenital Uterine Anomalies

Computed tomography is not routinely performed to evaluate patients with suspected congenital uterine anomalies because it uses ionizing radiation. However, congenital uterine abnormalities may be detected in the course of CT evaluation for other clinical indications, such as pelvic pain or a palpable pelvic mass. Anomalies such as absent uterus with ectopic ovaries, uterine didelphys, bicornuate uterus, and hydrometrocolpos, all have been diagnosed on CT scans (Fig. 67) (71,223).

Both endovaginal ultrasonography and MRI are extremely accurate in the detection and characterization of various uterine anomalies. They allow noninvasive differentiation among septate uterus, uterine didelphys, and bicornuate uterus, thus obviating diagnostic laparoscopy and hysteroscopy (Fig. 68) (38,179,207,285).

The septum in a septate uterus may be composed of fibrous tissue, myometrium, or a combination of both (38,207). The diagnosis of septate uterus is made on the basis of demonstration of a convex outer surface of the uterine fundus, or a minimal (less than 1 cm) concavity (Fig. 69). The diagnosis of bicornuate uterus is made on

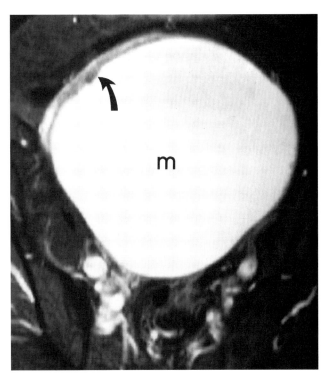

FIG. 65. Ovarian cystadenocarcinoma. T1-weighted fat-saturated post-Gd SE image (600/15) shows large cystic mass (m) of homogeneous high signal intensity consistent with hemorrhage. Nodular thickening of right anterior wall of mass *(arrow)* is consistent with malignant neoplasm.

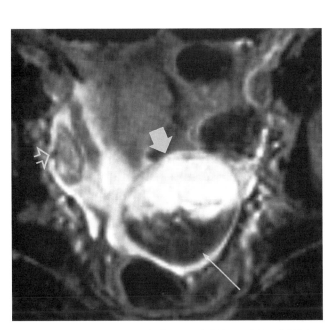

FIG. 64. Ovarian dermoid. Transaxial T2-weighted SE image (2500/90) shows a complex cystic structure in the left pelvis *(thick arrow)*. The lower-signal-intensity material seen posteriorly was hair *(thin arrow)*; the higher-signal-intensity material was proteinaceous fluid. *Open arrow*, right ovary.

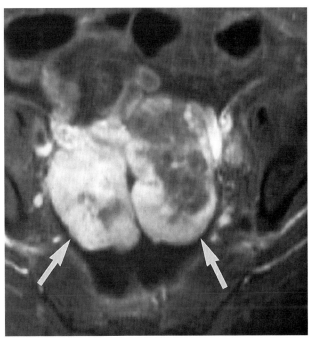

FIG. 66. Metastatic appendiceal carcinoma to ovaries. Transaxial T1-weighted fat-saturated post-Gd SE image (600/15) shows bilateral complex enhancing adnexal masses *(arrows)*.

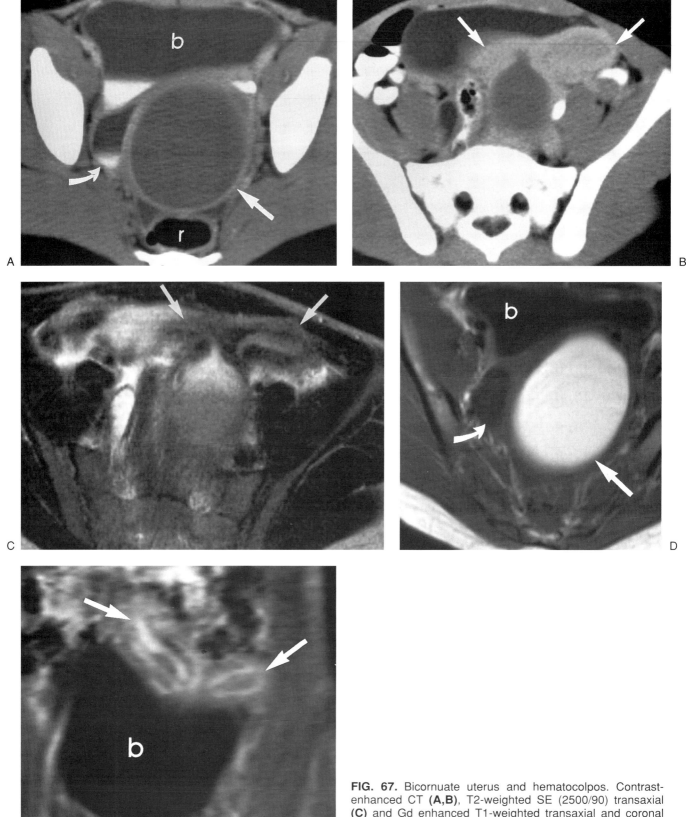

FIG. 67. Bicornuate uterus and hematocolpos. Contrast-enhanced CT **(A,B)**, T2-weighted SE (2500/90) transaxial **(C)** and Gd enhanced T1-weighted transaxial and coronal **(D,E)** FLASH (140/4/80°) images. Large low-density mass *(straight arrow)* between rectum (r) and bladder (b) on CT in (A) is of high signal intensity on corresponding T1-weighted MR image (D), consistent with hematocolpos. Note bladder diverticulum *(curved arrow)*. At a more craniad level, two widely separated uterine horns are seen, consistent with bicornuate uterus *(arrows)* in (B,C). Coronal MR image (E) also shows the divergent uterine horns *(arrows)* superior to the bladder (b).

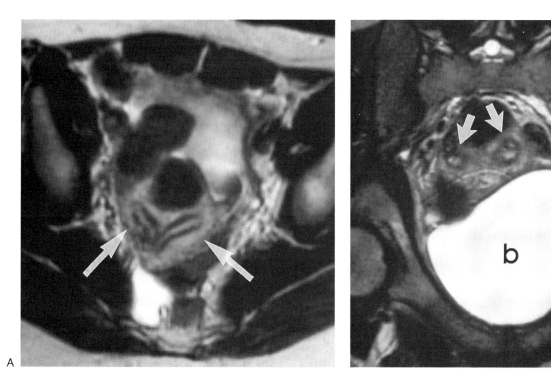

FIG. 68. Duplicated uterus. Transaxial **(A)** and coronal **(B)** T2-weighted FSE images (3500/100) show two separate uterine cavities *(arrows)*. b, bladder. (Courtesy of S. McCarthy, New Haven, Connecticut.)

the basis of a greater than 1-cm concavity, and the tissue separating the cornua is composed entirely of myometrium and therefore has a medium signal intensity on T1-weighted images and a higher signal intensity on T2-weighted images (see Fig. 67).

The choice between MRI and endovaginal sonography as the initial imaging method depends on a number of factors including cost, availability, and local expertise. Because of its higher cost, MRI usually is reserved for cases in which the results of endovaginal sonography

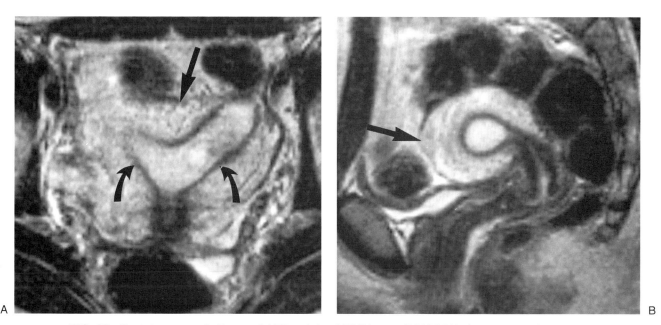

FIG. 69. Septate uterus. **A:** Transaxial T2-weighted FSE image (3500/100) shows two uterine cornua *(curved arrows)* with no indentation of the myometrium separating them *(straight arrow)*, consistent with septate rather than bicornuate uterus. **B:** Sagittal T2-weighted FSE image (3500/100) shows thick myometrium at midline *(arrow)*.

are not conclusive. Because normal zonal anatomy of the uterus is best shown on T2-weighted images, a combination of T2-weighted transaxial and sagittal images is often used to delineate uterine anomalies. Evaluation of fundal contour may be facilitated by the use of off-axis scanning (18).

Localization of Undescended Testes

Gray-scale sonography is the procedure of choice in the evaluation of patients with suspected testicular pathology when the testis lies within the scrotal sac. However, CT or MRI can almost always accurately depict the presence and location of the testis when it is not palpable on physical examination.

The testis develops from the elongated embryonic gonad lying ventral to the mesonephric ridge. It migrates from its intra-abdominal position to the scrotal sac during the latter third of gestation (5). Interruption of this normal migratory process results in ectopic positioning of the testis. Because malignant neoplasms occur 12 to 40 times more commonly in the undescended (intra-abdominal) than in the descended testis, it is widely agreed that orchiopexy be performed in patients younger than 10 years of age and orchiectomy be performed in patients who are seen after puberty (212). Preoperative localization of a nonpalpable testis by radiologic methods often helps in planning the surgical approach and shortens the anesthesia time.

Detection of an undescended testis by CT is based on recognition of a mass that is of soft-tissue density and oval in shape, along the expected course of testicular descent (Figs. 70–73) (149,153,317). However, the pars infravaginalis gubernaculi (the terminal end of the gubernaculum) can be similar in appearance to the undescended testis on CT (231).

Five different CT patterns have been encountered in patients with undescended testis: (a) spermatic cord absent, testis absent; (b) spermatic cord in the inguinal canal, testis absent; (c) spermatic cord in the canal, testis in the canal; (d) spermatic cord in the canal, testis in the abdomen; (e) spermatic cord not seen, testis in the abdomen (149). When the undescended testis is unusually large or contains areas of low attenuation (163), it may be either because of malignant transformation or epididymitis. In general, it is easier to detect an undescended testis in the inguinal canal or in the lower pelvis where structures are usually bilaterally symmetrical. An undescended testis as small as 1 cm has been accurately located in these areas. Detection of such an atrophic testis and differentiation from adjacent structures are more difficult in the upper pelvis and lower abdomen because bowel loops, vascular structures, and lymph nodes are more abundant. Despite these limitations, CT has proven accurate in localization of nonpalpable testes (149).

Other radiologic methods that have been used to local-

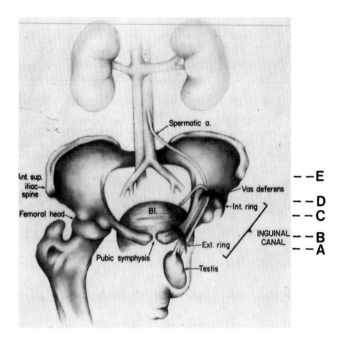

FIG. 70. Schematic drawing showing the relationships among the inguinal canal, the spermatic cord (containing spermatic vessels and vas deferens), and adjacent bony landmarks. The inguinal canal is a superficial structure that runs parallel to the iliac wing. The internal inguinal ring is located halfway between the pubic symphysis and the anterior superior iliac spine (i.e, approximately 5 to 6 cm caudad to the anterior superior iliac spine). The external inguinal ring is just cephalad to the pubic ramus. Letters A–E correspond to planes of imaging in Figure 71. (From ref. 150.)

ize an undescended testis include testicular arteriography, venography, gray-scale ultrasound, and MRI (81,87,133, 166). Testicular arteriography is not only technically difficult but also painful. Although testicular venography is less traumatic than arteriography, it is also associated with a high radiation dose and some morbidity, although the false negative rate is relatively low. Selective catheterization of the right testicular vein is technically difficult; selective venography of either testicular vein can be unsuccessful because of the presence of venous valves. Although ultrasound is useful in localizing an undescended testis within the inguinal canal, it is usually not reliable in the pelvis or abdomen (166). MRI may have a problem similar to that of sonography in detecting intra-abdominal testis, unless an oral contrast agent is used to facilitate the identification of the bowel loops (81,134). On MRI, undescended testes, which are often atrophic, may have a lower signal intensity than the contralateral normal testis (Fig. 74). Because of its availability, ease of performance, and noninvasive nature, CT has remained the procedure of choice in the preoperative localization of a nonpalpable testis. MRI may be preferred in institutions where the equipment is more available and in patients in whom ionizing radiation is a major concern. In cases in which neither CT nor MRI can demonstrate the testis, testicular

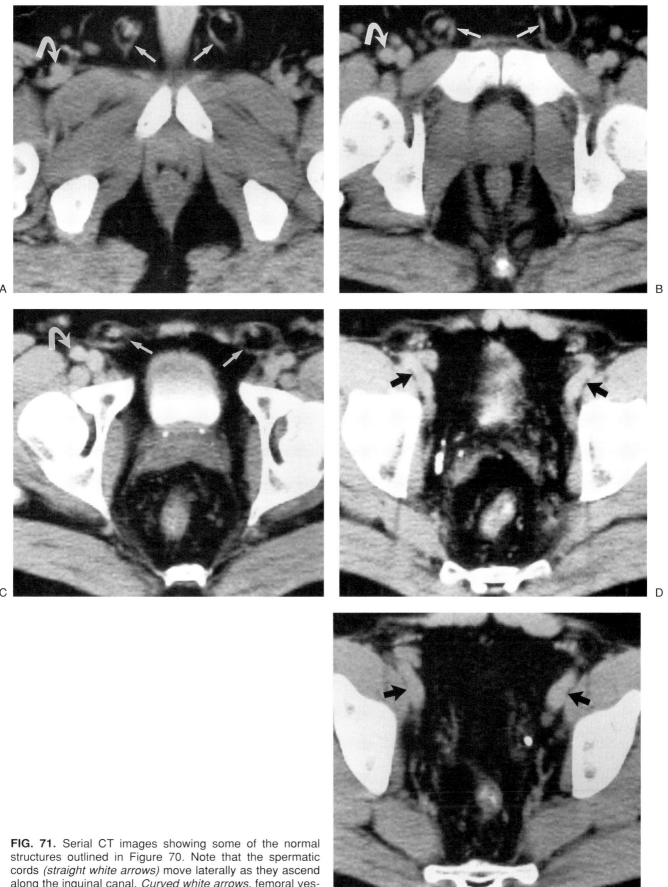

FIG. 71. Serial CT images showing some of the normal structures outlined in Figure 70. Note that the spermatic cords *(straight white arrows)* move laterally as they ascend along the inguinal canal. *Curved white arrows*, femoral vessels; *black arrows*, iliac vessels.

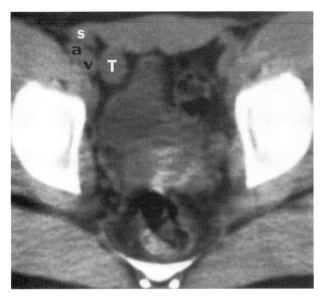

FIG. 72. Intra-abdominal testis. Unenhanced CT scan shows that the slightly atrophic right testis (T) lies medial to the right iliac artery (a) and vein (v). This is a common site for an intra-abdominal testicle. The spermatic cord (s) is anterior to the vessels.

venography or arteriography may still be employed for further evaluation.

Evaluation of Scrotal Pathology

Computed tomography is not used to primarily evaluate scrotal pathology, because testicular lesions are poorly defined on CT scans. However, in some studies obtained for other indications, CT may reveal herniation of fat and bowel loops into the scrotum (Fig. 75) or a hydrocele.

In contradistinction, MRI is capable of differentiating an intratesticular from an extratesticular lesion (Figs. 76–80) (12,80,229,250). Because of the long T2 of normal testis, most intratesticular disease processes appear iso- or hypointense to normal testicular tissue on T2-weighted images. Based on the MRI signal intensity, a cystic lesion can be differentiated from a solid neoplasm, and a simple fluid collection (e.g., spermatocele, hydrocele) can be distinguished from one complicated by infection or hemorrhage. Although MRI features have been described that allow distinction of tubular ectasia of the testis, a benign condition, from a testicular neoplasm, and differentiation of nonseminomatous (heterogeneous signal intensity with a dark fibrous capsule) from seminomatous neoplasms (homogeneous hypointense signal without a capsule) (126,276), the features are usually nonspecific and often do not even permit differentiation of benign from malignant disorders (79,280).

At present, MRI provides information similar to that obtained with sonography in most cases. Therefore, sonography remains the procedure of choice for evaluating scrotal pathology because of its ease of performance and lower cost. However, MRI is helpful in patients with painful scrotal lesions. Whereas sonographic examination requires good contact with the scrotal surface, MRI can be performed with a minimum of patient discomfort. The ability of MRI to clearly delineate the tunica albuginea is also helpful in the evaluation of scrotal trauma, because surgical intervention is often needed in cases in which the tunica is disrupted (12,250).

Assessment of the Postoperative Pelvis

Postcystectomy

The detection of possible surgical complications and local neoplastic recurrences has been difficult by conven-

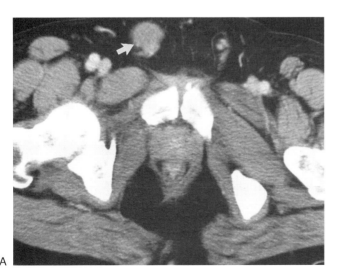
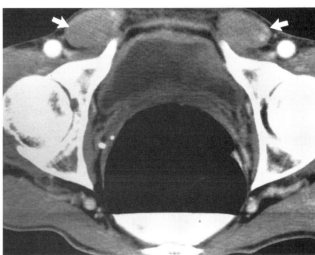

FIG. 73. Intracanalicular testicles. Contrast-enhanced CT scans through the pelvis in two different male patients show an ovoid soft-tissue-density structure in the right inguinal canal **(A)** *(arrow)*, and in both inguinal canals **(B)** *(arrows)*.

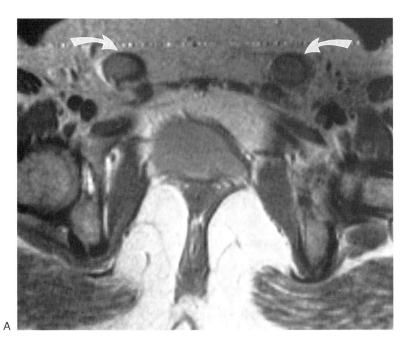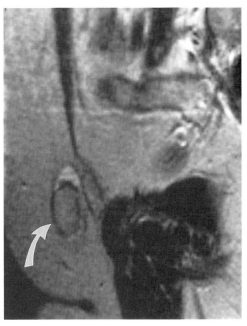

FIG. 74. Bilateral undescended testicles. Transaxial proton-density-weighted (2500/20) **(A)** and sagittal T2-weighted (2500/80) **(B)** SE images show ovoid, intermediate-signal-intensity structures in both inguinal canals *(arrows)*. Extrascrotal testes are lower in signal intensity than intrascrotal testes as a result of ischemic changes.

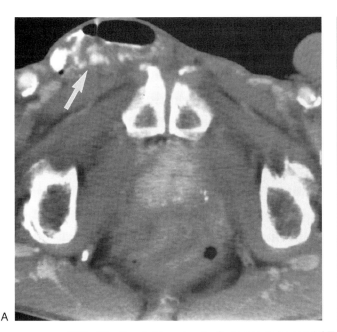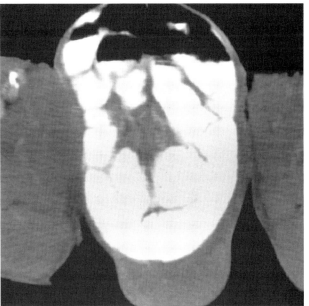

FIG. 75. Scrotal hernia. **A:** Contrast-enhanced CT scan through the symphysis pubis shows several contrast-filled bowel loops in the right inguinal canal *(arrow)*. **B:** Scan several centimeters caudally shows multiple bowel loops within the scrotum.

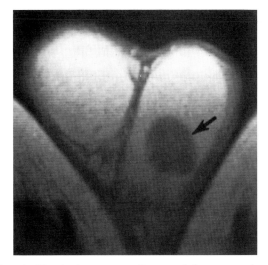

FIG. 76. Testicular cyst. Transaxial proton-density-weighted SE image (1500/35) shows a well-defined, low-intensity mass *(arrow)* in the left testis. The increased signal intensity in the anterior portions of both testes is due to nonuniform response of a single-loop surface coil.

tional radiologic methods in patients with prior cystectomy for bladder cancers. Barium gastrointestinal studies are insensitive for detecting masses not closely related to the bowel; gallium radionuclide imaging is of little help in the immediate postoperative period. Because the ability to detect pelvic pathology by sonography is highly dependent on the presence of a distended urinary bladder, sonography also is of limited use in postcystectomy patients. Furthermore, the presence of surgical wounds, with or without drains, further constrains its usefulness.

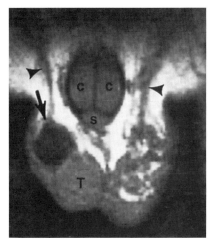

FIG. 77. Simple spermatocele. Coronal T1-weighted SE image (500/35) shows a round, low-intensity mass *(arrow)* superior and lateral to the right testis (T). *Arrowheads,* spermatic cords; c, corpora cavernosum; s, corpus spongiosum.

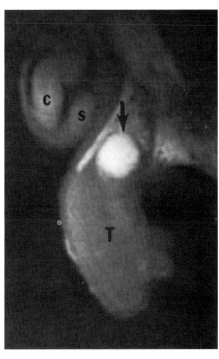

FIG. 78. Hemorrhagic epididymal cyst. Sagittal T1-weighted SE (500/35) image shows a high-intensity lesion *(arrow)* in the region of left epididymal head. T, testis; c, corpora cavernosum; s, corpus spongiosum.

Computed tomography is well suited for evaluation of such patients (152). Normal surrounding anatomy and pathologic alterations can be delineated in patients with prior cystectomy. In male patients after radical cystectomy, the bladder, the prostate, and the seminal vesicles are absent. In female patients, the uterus and both fallopian tubes as well as the urinary bladder are absent. Small bowel loops and, rarely, a loop of sigmoid colon fill in the space previously occupied by these structures (Fig. 81). Although the perivesical fat plane often is disrupted in postcystectomy patients, the muscle groups lining the pelvic side wall, namely the obturator internus in the lower pelvis and the iliopsoas in the upper pelvis, remain symmetrical. Recognition of alterations in the symmetry of the remaining structures enables diagnosis of pathologic conditions at a relatively early stage. Local recurrences, surgical complications (e.g., urinoma, lymphoceles, abscesses), and distant metastases all may be recognized on postoperative CT examinations (Figs. 82,83). Recurrent tumor often appears as a mass of soft-tissue density, separate from bowel, with or without central necrosis. Although unopacified bowel loops and other normal pelvic structures may masquerade as recurrent disease, routine use of oral and intravenous contrast medium has largely eliminated this potential problem. In one study of 27 postcystectomy patients with recurrent transitional cell carcinoma of the bladder, CT demon-

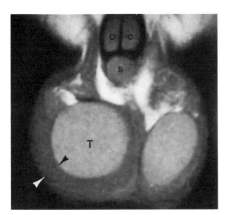

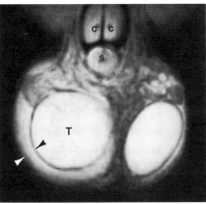

FIG. 79. Simple hydrocele. **A:** Coronal proton-density-weighted SE image (1500/35) shows a crescentic collection with homogeneous signal intensity *(arrowheads)* in the right hemiscrotum. T, testis; c, corpora cavernosum; s, corpus spongiosum. **B:** Coronal T2-weighted SE image (2100/90) shows that the collection *(arrowheads)* has a signal intensity similar to that of the testis, thereby confirming its fluid nature.

needed for such a differentiation. The role of MRI for evaluating patients with prior cystectomy has not been determined.

Post Abdominoperineal Resection:

Abdominoperineal (AP) resection of the rectum and distal sigmoid colon is the standard surgical procedure in treating patients with mid to distal rectal carcinoma. The incidence of tumor recurrence following AP resection is high in patients initially presenting with advanced stage disease. In one study (305), more than half of the patients with Dukes' B and C rectal carcinoma (Table 6) developed recurrent disease within 5 years. Approximately 50% of patients with recurrence manifested only distant metastases; the rest had local recurrence either alone or in conjunction with distant metastases.

Because conventional radiologic methods, including contrast gastrointestinal studies, are insensitive in detecting pelvic recurrence, the ability to detect local recurrence has relied largely on the presence of a palpable mass on physical examination or the development of severe pelvic pain. Knowledge of the size of the recurrent tumor is essential in designing radiation ports so that maximal dose can be given to the tumor with sparing of adjacent normal structures.

Because of its ability to provide detailed cross-sectional images of the pelvic anatomy easily, CT has become the imaging method of choice in following these patients for

strated that the pelvis was the most common site for recurrence (65). Recurrence at cystectomy site or retroperitoneal nodes are usually accompanied by pelvic lymphadenopathy, but the reverse is not as common. An abscess cavity can be confidently diagnosed if an extra-alimentary-tract mass containing gas is shown on CT scans (6). However, in the absence of gas bubbles, an abscess cavity may be confused with a necrotic tumor based on the CT findings alone. Correlation with clinical history and physical examination, or biopsy of the lesion directly at surgery or via a percutaneous needle, is often required. A urinoma is seen as a low-density mass with an imperceptible wall located outside the genitourinary tract. Although the density of a urinoma is close to that of water in most cases, it varies with the specific gravity of the urine (264); enhancement may occur after intravenous contrast medium administration. A urinoma could be confused with a seroma, lymphocele, or even an abscess on CT. Correlation again, with clinical information and sometimes chemical analysis of the aspirated fluid, is

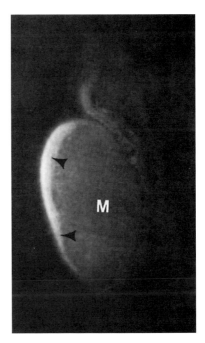

FIG. 80. Testicular seminoma. Sagittal T2-weighted SE image (2100/90) shows a large hypointense mass (M) almost completely replacing the right testis. A crescentic layer of normal parenchyma is seen anteriorly *(arrowheads)*.

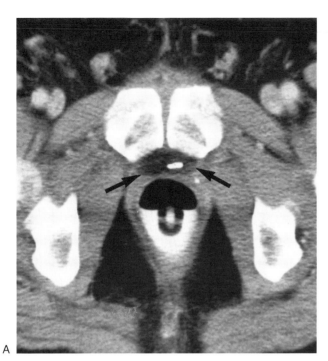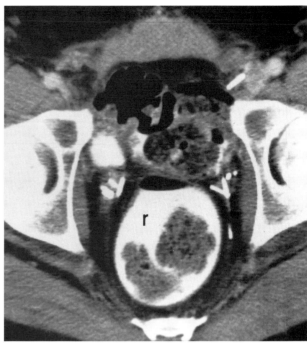

FIG. 81. Normal appearance after radical cystectomy in a male patient. **A:** Contrast-enhanced CT scan at the level of the pubic symphysis shows a surgical clip in the prostatic bed *(arrows)* posterior to the symphysis. **B:** Scan at the level of the acetabuli shows multiple bowel loops occupying the postcystectomy space anterior to the rectum (r).

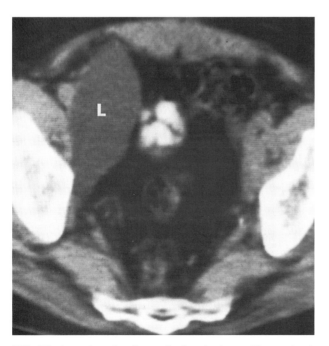

FIG. 82. Lymphocele after radical cystectomy. Noncontrast-enhanced CT scan shows the ellipsoid, well-defined, water-density lymphocele (L) in the extraperitoneal space along the right pelvic side wall. The diagnosis was established by chemical analysis of the aspirated fluid.

possible recurrence. In the immediate postoperative period, amorphous soft tissue densities, felt to represent edema or hemorrhage, can be seen in the surgical bed (Fig. 84). The normal fascial planes and contours of the remaining pelvic organs are often obscured. Although the exact duration of the postoperative changes probably varies from patient to patient, such changes resolve within several months, in most cases. In some instances, postoperative changes may persist and appear as masslike lesions in the presacral area (123,131,227).

Several months after AP resection, the urinary bladder can be seen on CT scan to occupy a presacral (precoccygeal) location. Although the prostate gland remains fixed in its preoperative position, the seminal vesicles in men and the uterus in women move with the bladder and can be seen in a presacral location (Fig. 85) (156). In addition, loops of small bowel also may be seen in the previous rectal fossa if the surgical procedure does not include restoration of the peritoneal floor or if the surgical sutures are disrupted.

On CT scans, recurrent tumor appears as an irregular soft-tissue mass with or without central necrosis. When the recurrence is large or is associated with metastases to other organs such as lymph nodes, bones, and the liver, the diagnosis can be confidently made. When the local recurrent tumor is small, difficulty in the differentiation between recurrent tumor and postoperative fibrosis has been reported (118,131,227). However, our own studies have shown that

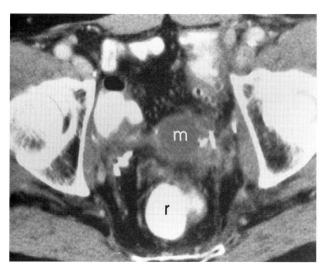

FIG. 83. Recurrent bladder carcinoma after cystectomy. Contrast-enhanced CT scan shows hypodense soft-tissue mass (m) adjacent to surgical clips. r, rectum.

pelvic CT scans in patients without local recurrence usually contained no detectable abnormality, or contained minimal streaky densities located anterior to the sacrococcygeal bone (156). Thus, postoperative changes usually are quite distinct and can be confidently distinguished from a local recurrent tumor, which often appears as a masslike lesion (Fig. 86). Because our patients had uncomplicated postoperative courses, it is conceivable that surgical complications, including prolonged wound infection, may lead to extensive scar formation and, therefore, result in a masslike lesion on CT scans. Because postoperative changes could theoretically simulate recurrent neoplasm, a baseline CT study several months after the AP resection may be beneficial. Changes detected on subsequent CT evaluations will then be more readily identified as recurrent tumor or as evolving postoperative tissue alterations. Percutaneous biopsy of any visible mass lesion in the operative bed is valuable to confirm recurrent neoplasms (32). Alternatively, MRI can be used to differentiate between recurrent neoplasm and postoperative fibrosis. Whereas recurrent neoplasm usually has a medium-to-high signal intensity on T2-weighted images, mature fibrosis (scar) has a very low signal intensity similar to that of skeletal muscle (64,86,150). However, fibrosis as a response to benign or malignant neoplasms (desmoplastic reaction) also has a very low signal intensity on T2-weighted images, simulating postoperative fibrosis (53). Likewise, postsurgical edema, usually present within the first 6 months after the operation, often has a high signal intensity on T2-weighted images and should not be mistaken for recurrent tumor (64,150).

Postirradiated Pelvis

The recognition of changes in the irradiated pelvis is important lest they be mistaken for recurrent neoplasms.

The extent of changes after radiation therapy is dependent on multiple factors including the total dose administered and the volume of tissue irradiated. Concurrent or prior surgery or chemotherapy may further increase the risk of radiation toxicity. Acute radiation leads to endarteritis of small blood vessels and increased endothelial permeability, resulting in the formation of interstitial edema and congestion. Chronic radiation effect is caused by ischemia and fibrosis, resulting in impaired organ function, stricture, or fistula formation (102).

On CT, symmetrical thickening of the perirectal fascia and widening of the presacral space are commonly seen in patients who have received a total radiation dose of 5,400 cGy or more (Fig. 87). Symmetrical thickening of the walls of the urinary bladder and rectum also can be seen in some cases (201). These changes usually become stable 12 weeks after radiotherapy. In rare cases, enterovesical fistula may develop as a complication of pelvic radiotherapy and can be demonstrated on CT studies (157).

Radiation-induced changes have been studied more extensively by MRI (Fig. 88). The severity of these changes is graded based on both the MRI signal intensity and the thickness of the wall of the involved organ. In general, radiation leads to higher signal intensity of the mucosa and submucosa on T2-weighted images before it affects the outer muscular layer of the bladder and rectum (269). Thickening of perirectal fascia and widening of presacral space also can be seen. The irradiated premenopausal uterus not only is smaller in size but also lacks normal zonal differentiation (8). The endometrium undergoes atrophy; the myometrium demonstrates a diffuse decrease in signal intensity on the T2-weighted image. After intravenous administration of contrast media, the irradiated uterus shows diffuse enhancement (115). The irradiated premenopausal uterus has an MR appearance similar to that of the postmenopausal uterus. Likewise, the ovaries become smaller in size and demonstrate a homogeneous, decreased signal intensity on T2-weighted images, reflecting atrophy of the ovarian follicles, increased fibrosis, and vascular sclerosis. In the acute phase, the wall of the vagina exhibits an increased signal intensity on T2-weighted images, whereas the vagina becomes atrophic with a homogeneously low signal intensity in the chronic phase. After irradiation, the obturator internus and iliopsoas muscles both will demonstrate a high signal intensity on T2-weighted images. Radiation will result in myeloid depletion and an increase in fat content, accounting

TABLE 6. *Dukes' classification of colon cancer*

A:	Confined to the bowel wall
B:	Tumor invasion through the muscularis into the serosa or into the mesenteric fat
C:	Tumor distant from the bowel

From ref. 63, with permission.

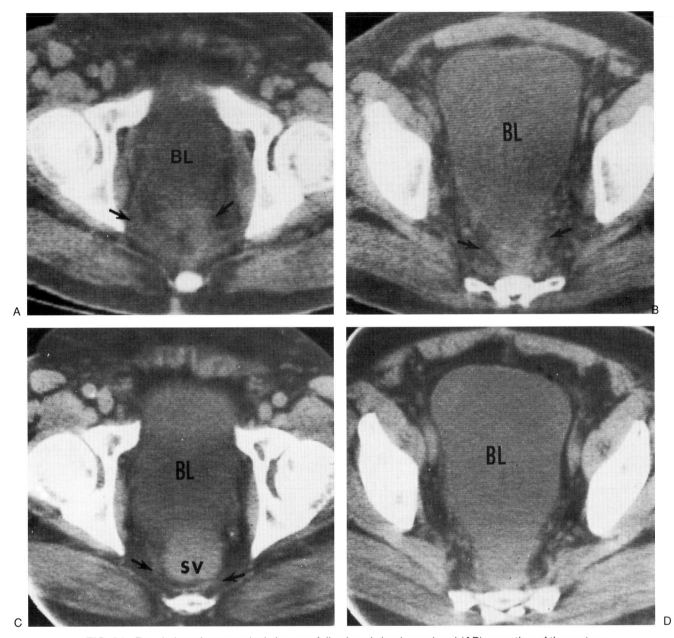

FIG. 84. Resolution of postsurgical changes following abdominoperineal (AP) resection of the rectum. **A,B:** Precontrast CT images obtained 1 month after AP resection show amorphous soft-tissue densities *(arrows)* obliterating normal fascial planes in the operative bed. **C,D:** Follow-up images obtained 8 months after surgery demonstrate much clearer delineation of the seminal vesicles (SV), with only minimal streaky densities *(arrows)* in the postsurgical space in front of the coccyx. BL, urinary bladder. (From ref. 153.)

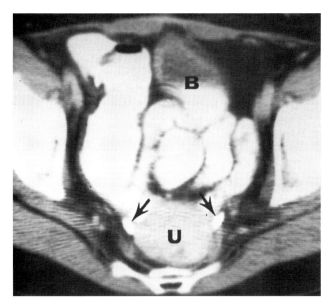

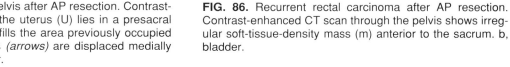

FIG. 85. Normal female pelvis after AP resection. Contrast-enhanced CT shows that the uterus (U) lies in a presacral position, and small bowel fills the area previously occupied by the uterus. The ureters *(arrows)* are displaced medially and posteriorly. B, bladder.

FIG. 86. Recurrent rectal carcinoma after AP resection. Contrast-enhanced CT scan through the pelvis shows irregular soft-tissue-density mass (m) anterior to the sacrum. b, bladder.

for the high signal intensity of irradiated bone marrow on T1-weighted images.

Obstetrical Application

General

Sonography is the procedure of choice in imaging the gravid uterus because of its lack of ionizing radiation,

high accuracy, lower cost, flexibility, and real time capability. Ideally, the gravid uterus should never be examined using CT. However, when the gravid uterus is scanned inadvertently, intrauterine pregnancies can be demonstrated by CT (Fig. 89). On rare occasion, CT is used to confirm an equivocal sonographic finding of fetal anomaly, such as ancephaly or traumatic uterine rupture with extrusion of the fetus (48).

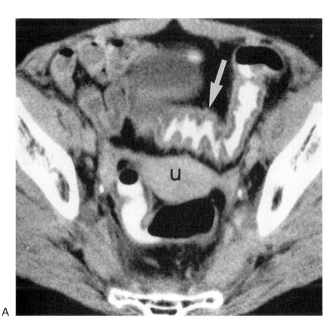

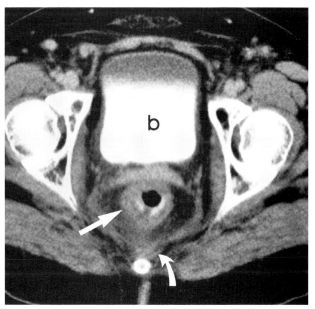

FIG. 87. Changes after radiation therapy in the pelvis, on CT. **A:** Contrast-enhanced CT of the mid pelvis in a patient who underwent radiation therapy for cervical carcinoma shows irregular fold thickening in a small bowel loop *(arrow)*. u, uterus. **B:** At a lower level, note rectal wall thickening *(arrow)* and amorphous soft-tissue density in the presacral space *(curved arrow)*. b, bladder.

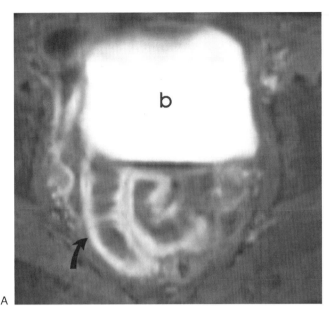

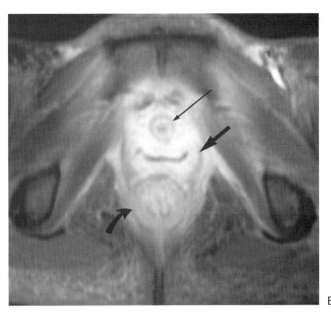

A

B

FIG. 88. Changes after radiation therapy in the pelvis on MR. **A:** Transaxial T1-weighted fat-saturated post-Gd SE image (600/15) shows thickening and intense enhancement of small bowel loops in the pelvis *(arrow)*. b, bladder. **B:** Gd-enhanced transaxial T1-weighted fat-saturated SE image (600/15) in another patient shows intense enhancement of structures in the pelvic floor, including urethra *(thin arrow)*, vagina *(arrow)*, and rectum *(curved arrow)*.

In some institutions, digital CT pelvimetry is performed to assess the feasibility of vaginal breech delivery. This method includes obtaining two digital radiographs (anteroposterior and lateral) and a transaxial CT scan at the level of the ischial spines (68). The ischial spines, through which the transaxial CT scan is obtained, usually can be determined from either the AP or the lateral digital radiograph. When they are not visible on either radiograph, a CT scan should be obtained through the inferior margin of the fovea of the femoral heads followed by

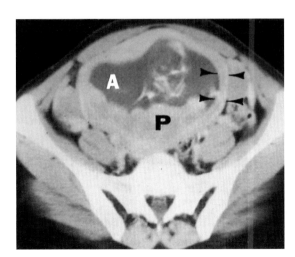

FIG. 89. Intrauterine pregnancy. Contrast-enhanced CT scan shows that the enlarged endometrial cavity contains the fetus, floating in amniotic fluid (A), and the posteriorly placed placenta (P). The myometrium is thin *(arrowheads)*.

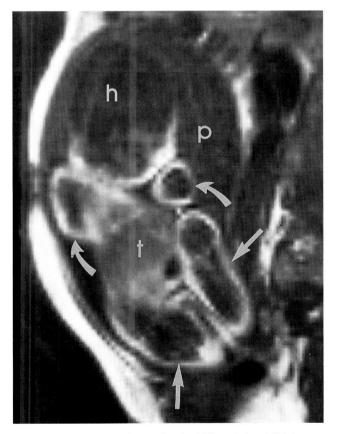

FIG. 90. Intrauterine fetus. Sagittal T1-weighted SE image (600/15) shows the fetus in breech position. Note head (h), trunk (t), upper extremities *(curved arrows)*, lower extremities *(arrows)*, placenta (p).

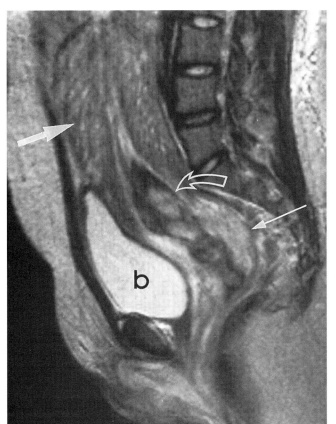

A

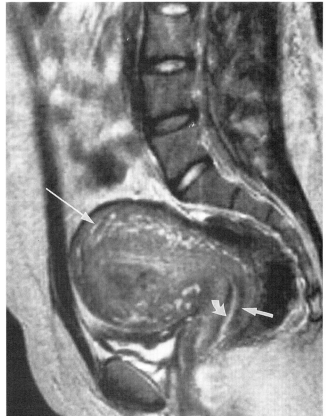

B

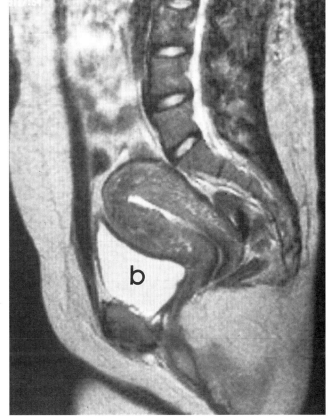

C

FIG. 91. Postpartum uterus. Sagittal T2-weighted FSE images (3500/100) at 1 day (A), 1 week (B), and 2 weeks (C). b, bladder. Field of view is identical in all images to illustrate decrease in uterine size. **A:** The uterine body and cervix are enlarged. The myometrium *(solid white arrow)* is of diffuse heterogeneous signal intensity with no definable junctional zone. Collection *(open arrow)* of mixed high and low signal intensity in lower uterine segment and cervical canal is consistent with blood. The outer cervical stroma *(thin arrow)* is of high signal intensity, consistent with high fluid content. **B:** At 1 week, the uterus has decreased in size. Note persistent enlarged myometrial vessels *(long thin arrow)*. The cervix shows decrease in signal intensity of outer cervical stroma. The inner cervical stroma *(short arrow)* is of low signal intensity and cervical mucosa/secretions are of high signal intensity *(curved arrow)*. **C:** At 2 weeks, there is further decrease in size of uterine body. The junctional zone is still not visible.

another scan 10 mm caudad, if the ischial spines are not included on the initial transaxial scan (7). The three standard measurements obtained are the anteroposterior pelvic inlet, transverse pelvic inlet, and the interspinous distance. Because the x-ray beam diverges across the CT table (transverse direction) and causes geometric distortion, the transverse diameter measured from the anteroposterior digital radiograph is only accurate at gantry isocenter. Error resulting from geometric distortion can be reduced either by placing the patient within the CT gantry so that the transverse measurement points are at the gantry isocenter (68) or by using established correction factors (259,314).

Although there are yet no known hazards associated with MRI, women in their first trimester of pregnancy generally are not imaged because of concern of inducing fetal anomalies. Furthermore, fetal anatomy is less well delineated at this stage of pregnancy as a result of rapid fetal motion (125,309). Fetal anatomy is better demonstrated during the last part of the first trimester and in patients with severe oligohydramnia resulting from restricted fetal motion. The heart and major vessels are seen as areas of signal void; the fluid-filled lungs are seen as high-signal-intensity structures on T2-weighted images. The brain and some of the major abdominal organs also can be seen (172,309,310). Intracranial and extracranial fetal anomalies can likewise be demonstrated by MRI (171,310). One study suggests that assessment of fetal subcutaneous fat by MRI may be a better indicator for detecting intra-uterine growth retardation than sonographic measurement of fetal growth parameters (265). MRI is most useful in the diagnosis of extra-uterine gestation, evaluation of placental position (Fig. 90), and determination of extent or nature of maternal pelvic masses (4,93,135,174,215,308,310).

While ultrasound remains the primary obstetric imaging method, MRI can provide important data about fetal anomalies, growth, and development when sonographic evaluation is limited by oligohydramnios or maternal obesity. It also can be used to confirm fetal abnormalities when sonography is equivocal, and to demonstrate maternal pelvic structures when sonography is unsuccessful because of bowel gas or obesity.

Both CT and MRI have been used to evaluate the postpartum pelvis after vaginal delivery or Caesarean section. Normal changes in the pelvis demonstrable by CT after uncomplicated term vaginal delivery include enlargement of the uterus, intrauterine blood, widening of the pubic symphysis and sacroiliac joints, and gas in the sacroiliac joints (82).

Magnetic resonance images obtained within 30 hours after a normal vaginal delivery show that the myometrium has a heterogeneous, intermediate signal intensity without a demonstrable low-signal-intensity junctional zone (316). Additional findings include a high-signal-intensity outer cervical stroma, prominent myometrial vessels (>5

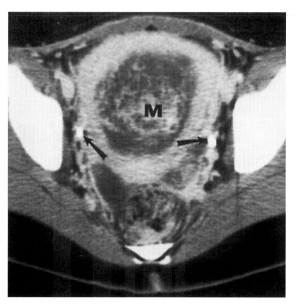

FIG. 92. Gestational trophoblastic disease. Contrast-enhanced CT scan demonstrates a large hydatidiform mole (M) within the uterine cavity. The mole is enhanced inhomogeneously with intravenous contrast material and contains numerous small cystic spaces. The ureters *(arrows)* are dilated because of extrinsic compression. Vascular engorgement accounts for soft-tissue strands in the parametrial fat.

mm), bloody fluid in the endometrial cavity of the lower uterine segment, and occasionally a small amount of free pelvic fluid. Most of these changes resolve completely over the ensuing weeks, with the exception of the junctional zone, which is only incompletely reconstituted by the end of a 6-month period (Fig. 91).

In patients with Caesarean section, the uterine incision site can be identified by CT and MRI in the immediate postpartum period. The incision site appears as uterine discontinuity on CT and manifests as subacute hematoma within the myometrium on MRI (290,318). Hematoma, fluid collections, and air bubbles all may be seen in the endometrial cavity and the parametrium in normal post-Caesarean-section patients.

Gestational Trophoblastic Disease

Gestational trophoblastic disease represents a spectrum of gynecologic pathology from benign hydatiform mole to choriocarcinoma (101). Sonography is effective in the initial diagnosis of molar disease but is not as useful in staging patients with invasive molar disease or choriocarcinoma [sometimes referred to as gestational trophoblastic neoplasia (GTN)] (225). Both CT and MRI have been used to evaluate this group of patients (49,104,189,235).

Although the uterus in patients with GTN is often diffusely enlarged, it may also be normal in size or focally enlarged. Although the size of the uterus does not correlate with the serum level of human chorionic gonadotropin (HCG), patients with an enlarged uterus are more likely to have distant metastases and to require hysterectomy for successful treatment. On CT, the uterus often exhibits inhomogeneous contrast enhancement with multiple areas of lower density (Fig. 92). Myometrial tumor nodules appear as hypodense areas on postcontrast CT scans. The ovaries are often enlarged and contain numerous thecal-lutein cysts. Local invasion as well as distant metastases to the liver and lung can be seen on CT scans. On MRI, the GTNs appear as masses of heterogeneous signal intensities obliterating normal uterine zonal anatomy. Numerous, tortuous, dilated vessels appearing as areas of signal void are often seen within the tumor.

Although MRI features of gestational trophoblastic disease overlap with those seen in incomplete abortion and ectopic pregnancy, MRI is useful in depicting the extent of disease in patients known to have it, information that may alter therapeutic management (17).

REFERENCES

1. Ackerman LV, delRegato JA. *Cancer, diagnosis, treatment and prognosis*, 4th ed. St. Louis: Mosby, 1970.
2. Amendola MA, Glazer GM, Grossman HB, Aisen AM, Francis R. Staging of bladder carcinoma: MRI-CT-surgical correlation. *AJR* 1986;146:1179–1183.
3. Amendola MC, Walsh JW, Amendola BE, Tisnado J, Hall DJ, Goplerud DR. Computed tomography in the evaluation of carcinoma of the ovary. *J Comput Assist Tomogr* 1981;5:179–186.
4. Angtuaco TL, Shah HR, Mattison DR, Quirk JG Jr. MR imaging in high-risk obstetric patients: a valuable complement to US. *Radiographics* 1992;12:91–109.
5. Arey LB. *Developmental anatomy*, 7th ed. Philadelphia: Saunders, 1965;315–341.
6. Aronberg DJ, Stanley RJ, Levitt RG, Sagel SS. Evaluation of abdominal abscess with computed tomography. *J Comput Assist Tomogr* 1978;2:384–387.
7. Aronson D, Kier R. CT pelvimetry: the foveae are not an accurate landmark for the level of the ischial spines. *AJR* 1991;156:527–530.
8. Arrive L, Chang YC, Hricak H, Brescia RJ, Auffermann W, Quivey JM. Radiation-induced uterine changes: MR imaging. *Radiology* 1989;170:55–58.
9. Arrive L, Hricak H, Martin MC. Pelvic endometriosis: MR imaging. *Radiology* 1989;171:687–692.
10. Ascher SM, Arnold LL, Patt RH, Schruefer JJ, Bagley AS, Semelka RC, Zeman RK, Simon JA. Adenomyosis: prospective comparison of MR imaging and transvaginal sonography. *Radiology* 1994;190:803–806.
11. Babcock EE, Brateman L, Weinreb JL, Horner SD, Nunnally RL. Edge artifacts in MR images: chemical shift effect. *J Comput Assist Tomogr* 1985;9:252–257.
12. Baker LL, Hajek PC, Burkhard TK, Dicapua L, Landa HM, Leopold GR, Hesselink JR, Mattrey RF. MR imaging of the scrotum: pathologic conditions. *Radiology* 1987;163:93–98.
13. Baker LL, Hajek PC, Burkhard TK, Dicapua L, Leopold GR, Hesselink JR, Mattrey RF. MR imaging of the scrotum: normal anatomy. *Radiology* 1987;163:89–92.
14. Balfe DM, van Dyke J, Lee JKT, Weyman PJ, McClennan BL. Computed tomography in malignant endometrial neoplasms. *J Comput Assist Tomogr* 1983;7:677–681.
15. Barentsz JO, Lemmens JAM, Ruijs SHJ, Boskamp EB, Hendrikx AJM, Karthaus HFM, Kaanders JHAM, Rosenbusch G. Carcinoma of the urinary bladder: MR imaging with a double surface coil. *AJR* 1988;151:107–112.
16. Barentsz JO, Ruijs SHJ, Strijk SP. The role of MR imaging in carcinoma of the urinary bladder. *AJR* 1993;160:937–947.
17. Barton JW, McCarthy SM, Kohorn EI, Scoutt LM, Lange RC. Pelvic MR imaging findings in gestational trophoblastic disease, incomplete abortion, and ectopic pregnancy: are they specific? *Radiology* 1993;186:163–168.
18. Baumgartner BR, Bernardino ME. MR imaging of the cervix: off-axis scan to improve visualization of zonal anatomy. *AJR* 1989;153:1001–1002.
19. Bezzi M, Kressel HY, Allen KS, Schiebler ML, Altman HG, Wein AJ, Pollack HM. Prostatic carcinoma: staging with MR imaging at 1.5T. *Radiology* 1988;169:339–349.
20. Biondetti PR, Lee JKT, Ling D, Catalona WJ. Clinical stage B prostate carcinoma: staging with MR imaging. *Radiology* 1987;162:325–329.
21. Boring CC, Squires TS, Tong T. Cancer statistics 1992. *Cancer* 1992;42:19–43.
22. Boronow RC, Morrow CP, Creasman WT, et al. Surgical staging in endometrial cancer: clinical-pathological findings of a prospective study. *Obstet Gynecol* 1984;63:825–832.
23. Botsis D, Gregoriou O, Kalovidouris A, Tsarouchis K, Zourlas PA. The value of computed tomography in staging cervical carcinoma. *Int J Gynaecol Obstet* 1988;27(2):213–218.
24. Bradley WG, Waluch V. Blood flow: magnetic resonance imaging. *Radiology* 1985;154:443–450.
25. Brenner DE, Shaff MI, Jones HW, Grosh WW, Greco FA, Burnett LS. Abdominopelvic computed tomography: evaluation in patients undergoing second-look laparotomy for ovarian carcinoma. *Obstet Gynecol* 1985;65:715–719.
26. Brick SH, Friedman AC, Pollack HM, Fishman EK, Radecki PD, Siegelbaum MH, Mitchell DG, Lev-Toaff AS, Carolina DF. Urachal carcinoma: CT findings. *Radiology* 1988;169:377–381.
27. Bries JR, Ellis JH, Kopecky KK, Sutton GP, Klatte EC, Stehman FB, Ehrlich CE. Assessment of primary gynecologic malignancies: comparison of 0.15T resistive MRI with CT. *AJR* 1984;143:1249–1257.
28. Brown JJ, Duncan JP, Heiken JP, Balfe DM, Corr AP, Mirowtiz SA, Eilenberg SS, Lee JKT. Perfluoroctylbromide as a gastrointestinal contrast agent for MR imaging: use with and without glucagon. *Radiology* 1991;181:455–460.
29. Bryan PJ, Butler HE, LiPuma JP, Haaga JR, Yousef SJE, Resnick MI, Cohen AM, Malviya VK, Nelson AD, Clampitt M, Alifid RJ, Cohen J, Morrison SC. NMR scanning of the pelvis: initial experience with a 0.3T system. *AJR* 1983;141:1111–1118.
30. Bryan PJ, Butler HE, LiPuma JP, Resnick MI, Kursh ED. CT and MR imaging in staging bladder neoplasms. *J Comput Assist Tomogr* 1987;11:96–101.
31. Bryan PJ, Butler HE, Nelson AD, LiPuma JP, Kopiwoda SY, Resnick MI, Cohen AM, Haaga JR. Magnetic resonance imaging of the prostate. *AJR* 1986;146:543–548.
32. Butch RJ, Wittenberg J, Mueller PR, Meyer JE, Ferrucci JT, Jr. Presacral masses after abdominoperineal resection for colorectal carcinoma: the need for needle biopsy. *AJR* 1985;144:309–312.
33. Butler H, Bryan PJ, LiPuma JP, Cohen AM, El Yousef S, Andriole JG, Lieberman J. Magnetic resonance imaging of the abnormal female pelvis. *AJR* 1984;143:1259–1266.
34. Buy JN, Ghossain MA, Mark AS, Deligne L, Hugol D, Truc JB, Poitout P, Vadrot D. Focal hyperdense areas in endometriomas: a characteristic finding on CT. *AJR* 1992;159:769–771.
35. Buy JN, Ghossain MA, Moss AA, Bazot M, Doucet M, Hugol D, Truc JB, Poitout P, Ecoiffier J. Cystic teratoma of the ovary: CT detection. *Radiology* 1989;171(3):697–701.
36. Buy JN, Ghossain MA, Sciot C, Bazot M, Guinet C, Prevot S, Hugol D, Laromiguiere M, Truc JB, Poitout P, Vadrot D, Ecoiffier J. Epithelial tumors of the ovary: CT findings and correlation with US. *Radiology* 1991;178:811–818.
37. Buy JN, Moss AA, Guinet C, Ghossain MA, Malbee L, Arrive L, Vadrot D. MR staging of bladder carcinoma: correlation with pathologic findings. *Radiology* 1988;169:695–700.
38. Carrington BM, Hricak H, Nuruddin RN, Secaf E, Laros RK Jr, Hill EC. Mullerian duct anomalies: MR imaging evaluation. *Radiology* 1990;176:715–720.
39. Carter HB, Brem RF, Tempany CM, Yang A, Epstein JI, Walsh

PC, Zerhouni EA. Nonpalpable prostate cancer: detection with MR imaging. *Radiology* 1991;178:523–525.

40. Casillas J, Joseph RC, Guerra JJ. CT appearance of uterine leiomyomas. *Radiographics* 1990;10:999–1007.

41. Catalona WJ, Scott WW. Carcinoma of the prostate: a review. *J Urol* 1978;119:1–8.

42. Chan TW, Kressel HY. Prostate and seminal vesicles after irradiation: MR appearance. *J Magn Reson Imaging* 1991;1:503–511.

43. Chang SF. Pear-shaped bladder caused by large iliopsoas muscles. *Radiology* 1978;128:349–350.

44. Church PA, Kazam E. Computed tomography and ultrasound in diagnosis of pelvic lipomatosis. *Urology* 1979;14:631–633.

45. Clarke-Pearson DL, Bandy LC, Dudzinski M, Heaston D, Creasman WT. Computed tomography in evaluation of patients with ovarian carcinoma in complete clinical remission. Correlation with surgical-pathologic findings. *JAMA* 1986;255:627–630.

46. Cohen WN, Seidelmann FE, Bryan PJ. Use of a tampon to enhance vaginal localization in computed tomography. *AJR* 1977;128:1064–1065.

47. Cupp MR, Oesterling JE. Prostate specific antigen, digital rectal examination, and transrectal ultrasonography: their roles in diagnosing early prostate cancer. *Mayo Clin Proc* 1993;689:297–306.

48. Dash N, Lupetin AR. Uterine rupture secondary to trauma: CT findings. *J Comput Assist Tomogr* 1991;15(2):329–331.

49. Davis WK, McCarthy S, Moss AA, Braga C. Computed tomography of gestational trophoblastic disease. *J Comput Assist Tomogr* 1984;8:1136–1139.

50. DelMaschio A, Vanzulli A, Sironi S, Spagnolo D, Belloni C, Garancini P, Taccagni GL. Estimating the depth of myometrial involvement by endometrial carcinoma: efficacy of transvaginal sonography vs MR imaging. *AJR* 1993;160:533–538.

51. Demas BE, Avallone A, Hricak H. Pelvic lipomatosis: diagnosis and characterization by magnetic resonance imaging. *Urol Radiol* 1988;10(4):198–202.

52. Demas BE, Hricak H, Jaffe RB. Uterine MR imaging: effects of hormonal stimulation. *Radiology* 1986;159:123–126.

53. deLange EE, Fechner RE, Wanebo HJ. Suspected recurrent rectosigmoid carcinoma after abdominoperineal resection: MR imaging and histopathologic findings. *Radiology* 1989;170:323–328.

54. deSouza NM, Hawley IC, Schwieso JE, Gilderdale DJ, Soutter WP. The uterine cervix on in vitro and in vivo MR images: a study of zonal anatomy and vascularity using an enveloping cervical coil. *AJR* 1994;163:607–612.

55. DiSantis DJ, Scatarige JC, Kempt G, Given FT, Hsiu J-G, Cramer MS. A prospective evaluation of transvaginal sonography for detection of ovarian disease. *AJR* 1993;161:91–94.

56. Dobbs HJ, Husband JE. The role of CT in the staging and radiotherapy planning of prostatic tumours. *Br J Radiol* 1985;58:429–436.

57. Dodd GD III, Lancaster KT, Moulton JS. Ovarian lipoleiomyoma: a fat-containing mass in the female pelvis. *AJR* 1989;153:1007–1008.

58. Dooms GC, Hricak H, Moseley ME, Bottles K, Fisher M, Higgins CB. Characterization of lymphadenopathy by magnetic resonance imaging and tissue characterization. *Radiology* 1985;155:691–697.

59. Dooms GC, Hricak H, Tscholakoff D. Adnexal structures: MR imaging. *Radiology* 1986;158:639–646.

60. Dore R, Moro G, D'Andrea F, Fianza AL, Franchi M, Bolis PF. CT evaluation of myometrium invasion in endometrial carcinoma. *J Comput Assist Tomogr* 1987;11:282–289.

61. Droller MJ. Transitional cell cancer: upper tracts and bladder. In: Walsh PC, Gittes RF, Perlmutter AD, Stamey TA, eds. *Campbell's urology*, New York: Saunders, 1986;1343–1440.

62. Dudiak CM, Turner DA, Patel SK, Archie JT, Silver B, Norusis M. Uterine leiomyomas in the infertile patient: preoperative localization with MR imaging versus US and hysterosalpingography. *Radiology* 1988;167:627–630.

63. Dukes CE. The classification of cancer of the rectum. *J Pathol Bacteriol* 1932;35:323–332.

64. Ebner F, Kressel HY, Mintz MC, Carlson JA, Cohen EK, Schiebler M, Gefter W, Axel L. Tumor recurrence versus fibrosis in the female pelvis: differentiation with MR imaging at 1.5T. *Radiology* 1988;166:333–340.

65. Ellis JH, McCullough NB, Francis IR, Grossman HB, Platt JF. Transitional cell carcinoma of the bladder: patterns of recurrence after cystectomy as determined by CT. *AJR* 1991;157:999–1002.

66. Ellis JH, Tempany C, Sarin MS, Gatsonis C, Rifkin MD, McNeil BJ. MR imaging and sonography of early prostatic cancer: pathologic and imaging features that influence identification and diagnosis. *AJR* 1994;162:865–872.

67. Engeler CE, Wasserman NF, Zhang G. Preoperative assessment of prostatic carcinoma by computed tomography: weaknesses and new perspectives. *Urology* 1990;40:346–350.

68. Federle MP, Cohen HA, Rosenwein MF, Brant-Zawadzki MN, Cann CE. Pelvimetry by digital radiography: a low-dose examination. *Radiology* 1982;143:733–735.

69. Federle MP, Filly RA, Moss AA. Cystic hepatic neoplasms: complementary roles of CT and sonography. *AJR* 1981;136:345–348.

70. Feigen M, Crocker EF, Read J, Crandon AJ. The value of lymphoscintigraphy, lymphangiography and computer tomography scanning in the preoperative assessment of lymph nodes involved by pelvic malignant conditions. *Surg Gynecol Obstet* 1987;165:107–110.

71. Fields SE, Katz S, Beyth Y. Computed tomography of unilateral hematometrocolpos. *J Comput Assist Tomogr* 1988;12(3):530–531.

72. Fisher MR, Hricak H, Crooks LE. Urinary bladder MR imaging: Part I. Normal and benign conditions. *Radiology* 1985;157:467–470.

73. Fisher MR, Hricak H, Tanagho EA. Urinary bladder MR imaging: Part II. Neoplasm. *Radiology* 1985;157:471–477.

74. Fishman EK, Scatarige JC, Saksouk FA, Rosenshein NB, Siegelman SS. Computed tomography of endometriosis. *J Comput Assist Tomogr* 1983;7:257–264.

75. Flanigan RC, Mohler JL, King CT, Atwell JR, Umer MA, Loh FK, McRoberts JW. Preoperative lymph node evaluation in prostatic cancer patients who are surgical candidates: the role of lymphangiography and computerized tomographic scanning with directed fine needle aspiration. *J Urol* 1985;134:84–87.

76. Flueckiger F, Ebner F, Poschauki H, Tamussino K, Einspieler R, Renner G. Cervical cancer: serial MR imaging before and after primary radiation therapy—a 2-year follow-up study. *Radiology* 1992;184:89–93.

77. Forstner R, Hricak H, Occhipinti KA, Powell CB, Frankel SD, Stern JL. Ovarian cancer: staging with CT and MR imaging. *Radiology* 1995;197:619–626.

78. Foshager MC, Walsh JW. CT anatomy of the female pelvis: a second look. *Radiographics* 1994;14:51–66.

79. Frasci G, Contino A, Iaffaioli RV, Mastrantonio P, Conforti S, Persico S. Computerized tomography of the abdomen and pelvis with peritoneal administration of soluble contrast (IPC-CT) in detection of residual disease for patients with ovarian cancer. *Gynecol Oncol* 1994;52(2):154–160.

80. Fritzsche PJ. MRI of the scrotum. *Urol Radiol* 1988;10(1):52–57.

81. Fritzsche PJ, Hricak H, Kogan BA, Winkler ML, Tanagho EA. Undescended testis: value of MR imaging. *Radiology* 1987;164:169–173.

82. Garagiola DM, Tarver RD, Gibson L, Rogers RE, Wass JL. Anatomic changes in the pelvis after uncomplicated vaginal delivery: a CT study in 14 women. *AJR* 1989;153:1239–1241.

83. Ghossain MA, Buy JN, Ligneres C, Bazot M, Hassen K, Malbec L, Hugol D, Truc JB, Decroix Y, Poitout P, Vadrot D. Epithelial tumors of the ovary: comparison of MR and CT findings. *Radiology* 1991;181:863–870.

84. Ginaldi S, Wallace S, Jing BS, Bernardino ME. Carcinoma of the cervix: lymphangiography and computed tomography. *AJR* 1981;136:1087–1091.

85. Gittes RF. Tumors of the bladder. In: Harrison JH, Gittes RF, Perlmutter AD, Stamey TA, Walsh PC, eds. *Urology*. Philadelphia: Saunders, 1970;1033–1070.

86. Glazer HS, Lee JKT, Levitt RG, Heiken JP, Ling D, Totty WG, Balfe DM, Emami B, Wasserman TH, Murphy WA. Radiation fibrosis: differentiation from recurrent tumor by MR imaging. *Radiology* 1985;156:721–726.

87. Glickman MG, Weiss RM, Itzchalk Y. Testicular venography for undescended testes. *AJR* 1977;129:71–75.

88. Goldman SM, Fishman EK, Rosenshein NB, Gatewood OMB, Siegelman SS. Excretory urography and computed tomography in the initial evaluation of patients with cervical cancer: are both examinations necessary? *AJR* 1984;143:991–996.

89. Golimbu M, Morales P, Al-Askari S, Shulman Y. CAT scanning in staging of prostatic cancer. *Urology* 1981;18:305–308.

90. Griffiths CT, Parker LM, Fuller AF Jr. Role of cytoreductive surgical treatment in the management of advanced ovarian carcinoma. *Cancer Treat Rep* 1979;63:235–240.

91. Grumbine FC, Rosenshein NB, Zerhouni EA, Siegelman SS. Abdominopelvic computed tomography in the preoperative evaluation of early cervical cancer. *Gynecol Oncol* 1981;12:286–290.

92. Gugliada K, Nardi PM, Borenstein MS, Torno RB. Inflammatory pseudosarcoma (pseudotumor) of the bladder. *Radiology* 1991;179:66–68.

93. Ha HK, Jung JK, Kang SJ, Koong SEN, Kim SJ, Kim JY, Shinn KS. MR imaging in the diagnosis of rare form of ectopic pregnancy. *AJR* 1993;160:1229–1232.

94. Ha HK, Lim YT, Kim HS, Suh TS, Song HH, Kim SJ. Diagnosis of pelvic endometriosis: fat-suppressed T1-weighted vs conventional MR images. *AJR* 1994;163:127–131.

95. Hamlin DJ, Burgener FA, Beechman JB. CT of intramural endometrial carcinoma: contrast enhancement is essential. *AJR* 1981;137:551–554.

96. Hamlin DJ, Fitzsimmons JR, Pettersson H, Riggall RC, Morgan L, Wilkinson EJ. Magnetic resonance imaging of the pelvis: evaluation of ovarian masses at 0.15T. *AJR* 1985;145:585–590.

97. Harris RD, Bendon JA, Robinson CA, Seat SG, Herwig KR. Computed tomographic evaluation of pear-shaped bladder. *Urology* 1979;14:528–530.

98. Hasumi K, Matsuzawa M, Chen HF, Takahashi M, Sakura M. Computed tomography in the evaluation and treatment of endometrial carcinoma. *Cancer* 1982;50:904–908.

99. Hawnaur JM, Johnson RJ, Read G, Isherwood I. Magnetic resonance imaging with gadolinium-DTPA for assessment of bladder carcinoma and its response to treatment. *Clin Radiol* 1993;47:302–310.

100. Haynor DR, Mack LA, Soules MR, Shuman WP, Montana MA, Moss AA. Changing appearance of the normal uterus during the menstrual cycle: MR studies. *Radiology* 1986;161:459–462.

101. Hilgers RD, Lewis JL. Gestational trophoblastic disease. In: Danforth DN, ed. *Obstetrics and gynecology*. Philadelphia: Harper & Row, 1982;393–406.

102. Hricak H. Magnetic resonance imaging evaluation of the irradiated female pelvis. *Semin Roentgenol* 1994;29:70–80.

103. Hricak H, Alpers C, Crooks LE, Sheldon PE. Magnetic resonance imaging of the female pelvis: initial experience. *AJR* 1983;141:1119–1128.

104. Hricak H, Demas BE, Braga CA, Fisher MR, Winkler ML. Gestational trophoblastic neoplasm of the uterus: MR assessment. *Radiology* 1986;161:11–16.

105. Hricak H, Dooms GC, Jeffrey RB, Avallone A, Jacobs D, Benton WK, Narayan P, Tanagho EA. Prostatic carcinoma: staging by clinical assessment, CT, and MR imaging. *Radiology* 1987;162:331–336.

106. Hricak H, Dooms GC, McNeal JE, Mark AS, Marotti M, Avallone A, Pelzer M, Proctor EC, Tanagho EA. MR imaging of the prostate gland: normal anatomy. *AJR* 1987;148:51–58.

107. Hricak H, Finck S, Honda S, Goranson H. MR imaging in the evaluation of benign uterine masses: value of gadopentetate dimeglumine-enhanced T1-weighted images. *AJR* 1992;158:1043–1050.

108. Hricak H, Hamm B, Semelka RC, Cann CE, Nauert T, Secaf E, Stern JL, Wolf KJ. Carcinoma of the uterus: use of gadopentetate dimeglumine in MR imaging. *Radiology* 1991;181:95–106.

109. Hricak H, Kim B. Contrast-enhanced MR imaging of the female pelvis. *J Magn Reson Imaging* 1993;3:297–306.

110. Hricak H, Lacey CG, Sandles LG, Chang YCF, Winkler ML, Stern JL. Invasive cervical carcinoma: comparison of MR imaging and surgical findings. *Radiology* 1988;166:623–631.

111. Hricak H, Powell CB, Yu KK, Washington E, Subak LL, Stern JL, Cisternas MG, Arenson RL. Invasive cervical carcinoma: role of MR imaging in pretreatment work-up—cost minimization and diagnostic efficacy analysis. *Radiology* 1996;198:403–409.

112. Hricak H, Quivey JM, Campos Z, Gildenborin V, Hindmarsh T, Bis KG, Stern JL, Phillips TL. Carcinoma of the cervix: predictive value of clinical and magnetic resonance (MR) imaging assessment of prognostic factors. *Int J Radiat Oncol Biol Phys* 1993;27:791–801.

113. Hricak H, Rubinstein LV, Gherman GM, Karstaedt N. MR imaging evaluation of endometrial carcinoma: results of an NCI cooperative study. *Radiology* 1991;179:829–832.

114. Hricak H, Stern JL, Fisher MR, Shapeero LG, Winkler ML, Lacey CG. Endometrial carcinoma staging by MR imaging. *Radiology* 1987;162:297–305.

115. Hricak H, Swift PS, Campos Z, Quivey JM, Gildengorin V, Goranson H. Irradiation of the cervix uteri: value of unenhanced and contrast-enhanced MR imaging. *Radiology* 1993;189:381–388.

116. Hricak H, Tscholakoff D, Heinrichs L, Fisher MR, Dooms GC, Reinhold C, Jaffe JB. Uterine leiomyomas: correlation of MR, histopathologic findings and symptoms. *Radiology* 1986;158:385–391.

117. Hricak H, Williams RD, Spring DB, Moon KL Jr, Hedgcock MW, Watson RA, Crooks LE. Anatomy and pathology of the male pelvis by magnetic resonance imaging. *AJR* 1983;141:1101–1111.

118. Husband JE, Hodson NJ, Parsons CA. The use of computed tomography in recurrent rectal tumors. *Radiology* 1980;134:677–682.

119. Husband JE, Olliff JFC, Williams MP, Heron CW, Cherryman GR. Bladder cancer: staging with CT and MR imaging. *Radiology* 1989;173:435–440.

120. International Federation of Gynecology and Obstetrics: Classification and staging of malignant tumors in the female pelvis. *J Int Fed Gynecol Obstet* 1965;3:204.

121. Jager GJ, Ruijter ETG, van de Kaa CA, de la Rosette JJMCH, Oosterhof GOH, Thornbury JR, Barentsz JO. Local staging of prostate cancer with endorectal MR imaging: correlation with histopathology. *AJR* 1996;166:845–852.

122. Jain KA, Friedman DL, Pettinger TW, Alagappan R, Jeffrey RB Jr, Sommer FG. Adnexal masses: comparison of specificity of endovaginal US and pelvic MR imaging. *Radiology* 1993;186:697–704.

123. Jeffrey RB Jr. CT demonstration of peritoneal implants. *AJR* 1980;135:323–326.

124. Jewett JH. The present status of radical prostatectomy for stages A and B prostatic cancer. *Urol Clin North Am* 1975;2:105–124.

125. Johnson IR, Symonds EM, Worthington BS, Pipkin FB, Hawkes RC, Gyngell M. Imaging of pregnant human uterus with nuclear magnetic resonance. *Am J Obstet Gynecol* 1984;148:1136–1139.

126. Johnson JO, Mattrey RF, Phillipson J. Differentiation of seminomatous from nonseminomatous testicular tumors with MR imaging. *AJR* 1990;154(3):539–543.

127. Johnson RJ, Blackledge G, Eddleston B, Crowther D. Abdominopelvic computed tomography in the management of ovarian carcinoma. *Radiology* 1983;146:447–452.

128. Kademian MT, Bosch A. Staging laparotomy and survival in carcinoma of the uterine cervix. *Acta Radiol* 1977;16:314–324.

129. Kafkas M. Study and diagnosis of bladder tumors by triple contrast cystography. *J Urol* 1973;109:32–34.

130. Kaji Y, Sugimura K, Nagaoka S, Ishida T. Amyloid deposition in seminal vesicles mimicking tumor invasion from bladder cancer: MR findings. *J Comput Assist Tomogr* 1992;16(6):989–991.

131. Kelvin FM, Korobkin M, Heaston DK, Grant JP, Akwari O. The pelvis after surgery for rectal carcinoma: serial CT observations with emphasis on nonneoplastic features. *AJR* 1983;141:959–964.

132. Kenny GM, Hardner GJ, Moore RM, Murphy GP. Current results from treatment of stages C and D bladder tumors at Roswell Park Memorial Institute. *J Urol* 1972;107:56–59.

133. Khademi M, Seebode JJ, Falla A. Selective spermatic arteriography for localization of impalpable undescended testis. *Radiology* 1980;136:627–634.

134. Kier R, McCarthy S, Rosenfield AT, Rosenfield NS, Rapoport S, Weiss RM. Nonpalpable testes in young boys: evaluation with MR imaging. *Radiology* 1988;169(2):429–433.

135. Kier R, McCarthy SM, Scoutt LM, Viscarello RR, Schwartz PE. Pelvic masses in pregnancy: MR imaging. *Radiology* 1990;176(3):709–713.

136. Kier R, Smith RC, McCarthy SM. Value of lipid- and water-suppression MR images in distinguishing between blood and lipid within ovarian masses. *AJR* 1992;158:321–325.

137. Kier R, Wain S, Troiano R. Fast spin-echo MR images of the pelvis obtained with a phased-array coil: value in localizing and staging prostatic carcinoma. *AJR* 1993;161(3):601–606.

138. Kilcheski TS, Arger PH, Mulhern CB Jr, Coleman BG, Kressel HY, Mikuta JI. Role of computed tomography in the presurgical evaluation of carcinoma of the cervix. *J Comput Assist Tomogr* 1981;5:378–383.

139. Kim B, Semelka SC, Ascher SM, Chalpin DB, Carroll PR, Hricak H. Bladder tumor staging: comparison of contrast-enhanced CT, T1- and T2-weighted MR imaging, dynamic gadolinium-enhanced imaging, and late gadolinium-enhanced imaging. *Radiology* 1994; 193:239–245.

140. Kim KH, Lee BH, Do YS, Chin SY, Park SY, Kim BG, Jang JJ. Stage IIb cervical carcinoma: MR evaluation of effect of intraarterial chemotherapy. *Radiology* 1994;192:61–65.

141. Kim SH, Han MC. Invasion of the urinary bladder by uterine cervical carcinoma: evaluation with MR imaging. *AJR* 1997;168: 393–397.

142. Kim SH, Han MC. Reversed contrast-urine levels in urinary bladder: CT findings. *Urol Radiol* 1992;13(4):249–252.

143. Kim SH, Kim SC, Choi BI, Han MC. Uterine cervical carcinoma: evaluation of pelvic lymph node metastasis with MR imaging. *Radiology* 1994;190:807–811.

144. Kim SY, Choi BI, Lee HP, Kang SB, Choi YM, Han MC, Kim CW. Uterine cervical carcinoma: comparison of CT and MR findings. *Radiology* 1990;175:45–51.

145. Kottmeier HL. *Annual report on the results of treatment in carcinoma of the uterus, vagina, and ovary,* vol 16. Stockholm: International Federation of Gynecology and Obstetrics, 1976.

146. Lang EK. The use of arteriography in the demonstration of staging of bladder tumors. *Radiology* 1963;80:62–68.

147. Larkin BT, Berquist TH, Utz DC. Evaluation of the prostate by magnetic resonance imaging. *Magn Reson Imaging* 1986;4:53–58.

148. Lee JKT, Gersell DJ, Balfe DM, Worthington JL, Picus D, Gapp G. The uterus: in vitro MR—anatomic correlation of normal and abnormal specimens. *Radiology* 1985;157:175–179.

149. Lee JKT, Glazer HG. CT in the localization of the nonpalpable testis. *Urol Clin North Am* 1982;9:397–404.

150. Lee JKT, Glazer HS. Controversy in the MR imaging appearance of fibrosis. *Radiology* 1990;177:21–22.

151. Lee JKT, Heiken JP, Ling D, Glazer HS, Balfe DM, Levitt RG, Dixon WT, Murphy WA Jr. Magnetic resonance imaging of abdominal and pelvic lymphadenopathy. *Radiology* 1984;153:181–188.

152. Lee JKT, McClennan BL, Stanley RJ, Levitt RG, Sagel SS. Use of CT in evaluation of postcystectomy patients. *AJR* 1981;136: 483–487.

153. Lee JKT, McClennan BL, Stanley RJ, Sagel SS. Utility of computed tomography in the localization of the undescended testis. *Radiology* 1980;135:121–125.

154. Lee JKT, Rholl KS. MRI of the bladder and prostate. *AJR* 1986; 147:732–736.

155. Lee JKT, Stanley RJ, Sagel SS, McClennan BL. Accuracy of CT in detecting intraabdominal and pelvic lymph node metastases from pelvic cancers. *AJR* 1978;131:675–679.

156. Lee JKT, Stanley RJ, Sagel SS, Levitt RG, McClennan BL. CT appearance of the pelvis after abdomino-perineal resection for rectal carcinoma. *Radiology* 1981;141:737–741.

157. Levenback C, Gershenson DM, McGehee R, Eifel PJ, Morris M, Burke TW. Enterovesical fistula following radiotherapy for gynecologic cancer. *Gynecol Oncol* 1994;52(3):296–300.

158. Levine MS, Arger PH, Coleman BG, Mulhern CB, Pollack HM, Wein AJ. Detecting lymphatic metastases from prostatic carcinoma: superiority of CT. *AJR* 1981;137:207–211.

159. Levitt RG, Sagel SS, Stanley RJ. Detection of neoplastic involvement of the mesentery and omentum by computed tomography. *AJR* 1978;131:835–838.

160. Lien HH, Blomlie V, Kjorstad K, Abeler V, Kaalhus O. Clinical stage I carcinoma of the cervix: value of MR imaging in determining degree of invasiveness. *AJR* 1991;156:1191–1194.

161. Lien HH, Blomlie V, Trope C, Kaern J, Abeler VM. Cancer of the endometrium: value of MR imaging in determining depth of invasion into the myometrium. *AJR* 1991;157:1221–1223.

162. Ling D, Lee JKT, Heiken JP, Balfe DM, Glazer HS, McClennan BL. Prostatic carcinoma and benign prostatic hyperplasia: inability of MR imaging to distinguish between the two diseases. *Radiology* 1986;158:103–107.

163. Lorigan JG, Shirkhoda A, Dexeus FH. CT and MR imaging of malignant germ cell tumor of the undescended testis. *Urol Radiol* 1989;11(2):113–117.

164. Lovett K, Rifkin MD, McCue PA, Choi H. MR imaging characteristics of noncancerous lesions of the prostate. *J Magn Reson Imaging* 1992;2:35–39.

165. Low RN, Carter WD, Saleh F, Sigeti JS. Ovarian cancer: comparison of findings with perfluorocarbon-enhanced MR imaging, In-111-CYT-103 immunoscintigraphy, and CT. *Radiology* 1995;195: 391–400.

166. Madrazo BL, Klugo RC, Parks JA, DiLoreto R. Ultrasonographic demonstration of undescended testis. *Radiology* 1979;133:181–183.

167. Marincek B, Devaud MC, Triller J, Fuchs WA. Value of computed tomography and lymphography in staging carcinoma of the uterine cervix. *Eur J Radiol* 1984;4:118–121.

168. Mark AS, Hricak H, Heinrichs LW, Hendrickson MR, Winkler ML, Bachica JA, Stickler JE. Adenomyosis and leiomyoma: differential diagnosis with MR imaging. *Radiology* 1987;163:52–529.

169. Marshall VF. The relation of the preoperative estimate to the pathologic demonstration of the extent of vesical neoplasm. *J Urol* 1952;68:714–723.

170. Matsukuma K, Tsukamoto N, Matsuyama T, Ono M, Nakano H. Preoperative CT study of lymph nodes in cervical cancer—its correlation with clinical findings. *Gynecol Oncol* 1989;33(2):168–171.

171. McCarthy SM, Filly RA, Stark DD, Callen PW, Golbus MS, Hricak H. Magnetic resonance imaging of fetal anomalies in utero: early experience. *AJR* 1985;145:677–682.

172. McCarthy SM, Filly RA, Stark DD, Hricak H, Brant-Zawadski MN, Callen PW, Higgins CB. Obstetrical magnetic resonance imaging: fetal anatomy. *Radiology* 1985;154:427–432.

173. McCarthy SM, Scott G, Majumdar S, Shapiro B, Thompson S, Lange R, Gore J. Uterine junctional zone: MR study of water content and relaxation properties. *Radiology* 1989;171:241–243.

174. McCarthy SM, Stark DD, Filly RA, Callen PW, Hricak H, Higgins CB. Obstetrical magnetic resonance imaging: maternal anatomy. *Radiology* 1985;154:421–425.

175. McCarthy SM, Tauber C, Gore J. Female pelvic anatomy: MR assessment of variations during the menstrual cycle and with use of oral contraceptives. *Radiology* 1986;160:119–123.

176. Megibow AJ, Bosniak MA, Ho AG, Beller U, Hulnick DH, Beckman EM. Accuracy of CT in detection of persistent or recurrent ovarian carcinoma: correlation with second-look laparotomy. *Radiology* 1988;166:341–345.

177. Middleton RG, Smith JA Jr, Melzer RB, Hamilton PE. Patient survival and local recurrence rate following radical prostatectomy for prostate carcinoma. *J Urol* 1986;136:422–424.

178. Milestone BN, Schnall MD, Lenkinski RE, Kressel HY. Cervical carcinoma: MR imaging with an endorectal surface coil. *Radiology* 1991;180:91–95.

179. Mintz MC, Thickman DI, Gussman D, Kressel HY. MR evaluation of uterine anomalies. *AJR* 1987;148:287–290.

180. Mirowitz SA. Seminal vesicles: biopsy-related hemorrhage simulating tumor invasion at endorectal MR imaging. *Radiology* 1992; 185(2):373–376.

181. Mirowitz SA, Brown JJ, Heiken JP. Evaluation of the prostate and prostatic carcinoma with gadolinium-enhanced endorectal coil MR imaging. *Radiology* 1993;186:153–157.

182. Mirowitz SA, Hammerman AM. CT depiction of prostatic zonal anatomy. *J Comput Assist Tomogr* 1992;16(3):439–441.

183. Mitchell DG, Gefter WB, Spritzer CE, Blasco L, Nulson J, Livolsi V, Axel L, Arger PH, Kressel HY. Polycystic ovaries: MR imaging. *Radiology* 1986;160:425–429.

184. Mitchell DG, Hill MC, Hill S, Zaloudek C. Serous carcinoma of the ovary: CT identification of metastatic calcified implants. *Radiology* 1986;158:649–652.

185. Mitchell DG, Minta MC, Spritzer CE, Gussman D, Arger PH, Coleman BG, Axel L, Kressel HY. Adnexal masses: MR imaging

observations at 1.5T, with US and CT correlation. *Radiology* 1987; 162:319–324.

186. Mitchell DG, Outwater EK. Benign gynecologic disease: applications of magnetic resonance imaging. *Top Magn Reson Imaging* 1995;70(1):26–43.

187. Mittelstaedt CA, Gosink BB, Leopold GR. Gray scale patterns of pelvic disease in the male. *Radiology* 1977;123:727–732.

188. Mittl RL Jr, Yeh IT, Kressel HY. High-signal-intensity rim surrounding uterine leiomyomas on MR images: pathologic correlation. *Radiology* 1991;180:81–83.

189. Miyasaka Y, Hachiya J, Furuya Y, Seki T, Watanabe H. CT evaluation of invasive trophoblastic disease. *J Comput Assist Tomogr* 1985;9:459–462.

190. Moon WK, Kim SH, Cho JM, Han MC. Calcified bladder tumors: CT features. *Acta Radiol* 1992;33:440–443.

191. Morgan CL, Calkins RF, Cavalcanti EJ. Computed tomography in the evaluation, staging and therapy of carcinoma of the bladder and prostate. *Radiology* 1981;140:751–761.

192. Muramatsu Y, Moriyama N, Takayasu K, Nawano S, Yamada T. CT and MR imaging of cystic ovarian teratoma with intracystic fat balls. *J Comput Assist Tomogr* 1991;15(3):528–529.

193. Nardi PM, Ruchman RB. CT appearance of diffuse peritoneal endometriosis. *J Comput Assist Tomogr* 1989;13(6):1075–1077.

194. Narumi Y, Kadota T, Inoue E, Kuriyama K, Fujita M, Hosomi N, Sawai Y, Kuroda M, Kotake T, Koruda C. Bladder tumors: staging with gadolinium-enhanced oblique MR imaging. *Radiology* 1993; 187:145–150.

195. Narumi Y, Kadota T, Inoue E, Kuriyama K, Horinouchi T, Kasai K, Maeda H, Kuroda M, Kotake T, Ishiguro S, Kuroda C. Bladder wall morphology: in vitro MR imaging—histopathologic correlation. *Radiology* 1993;187:151–155.

196. Narumi Y, Sato T, Hori S, Kuriyama K, Fukita M, Kadowaki K, Inoue E, Maeshima S, Fujino Y, Saiki S, Kuroda M, Kotake T. Squamous cell carcinoma of the uroepithelium: CT evaluation. *Radiology* 1989;173:853–856.

197. Narumi Y, Sato T, Kuriyama K, Fujita M, Saiki S, Kuroda M, Miki T, Kotake T. Vesical dome tumors: significance of extravesical extension on CT. *Radiology* 1988;169:383–385.

198. Nelson RC, Chezmar JL, Hoel MJ, Buck DR, Sugarbaker PH. Peritoneal carcinomatosis: preoperative CT with intraperitoneal contrast material. *Radiology* 1992;182:133–138.

199. Neuerberg JM, Bohndorf K, Sohn M, Teufl F, Guenther RW, Daus HJ. Urinary bladder neoplasms: evaluation with contrast-enhanced MR imaging. *Radiology* 1989;172:739–743.

200. Nishimura K, Togashi K, Itoh K, Fujisawa I, Noma S, Kawamura Y, Nakano Y, Itoh H, Torizuka K, Ozasa H. Endometrial cysts of the ovary: MR imaging. *Radiology* 1987;162:315–318.

201. Ohtomo K, Shuman WP, Griffin BR, Steward GR, Laramore GE, Moss AA. CT manifestation in the pararectal area following fast neutron radiotherapy. *Radiat Med* 1987;5(6):198–201.

202. Outwater EK, Mitchell DG. Normal ovaries and functional cysts: MR appearance. *Radiology* 1996;198:397–402.

203. Outwater EK, Petersen RO, Siegelman ES, Gomella LG, Chernesky CE, Mitchell DG. Prostate carcinoma: assessment of diagnostic criteria for capsular penetration on endorectal coil MR images. *Radiology* 1994;193:333–339.

204. Outwater E, Schiebler ML, Tomaszewski JE, Schnall MD, Kressel HY. Mucinous carcinomas involving the prostate: atypical findings at MR imaging. *J Magn Reson Imaging* 1992;2(5):297–600.

205. Oyen RH, Van Poppel JP, Ameye FE, Van de Voorde WA, Baert AL, Baert LV. Lymph node staging of localized prostatic carcinoma with CT and CT-guided fine-needle aspiration biopsy: prospective study of 285 patients. *Radiology* 1994;190:315–322.

206. Panageas E, Kier R, McCauley TR, McCarthy S. Submucosal uterine leiomyomas: diagnosis of prolapse into the cervix and vagina based on MR imaging. *AJR* 1992;159:555–558.

207. Pellerito JS, McCarthy SM, Doyle MB, Glickman MG, DeCherney AH. Diagnosis of uterine anomalies: relative accuracy of MR imaging, endovaginal sonography, and hysterosalpingography. *Radiology* 1992;183:795–800.

208. Phillips ME, Kressel HY, Spritzer CE, Arger PH, Wein AJ, Axel L, Gefter WB, Pollack HM. Normal prostate and adjacent structures: MR imaging at 1.5T. *Radiology* 1987;164:381–385.

209. Phillips ME, Kressel HY, Spritzer CE, Arger PH, Wein AJ, Ma-

rinelli D, Axel L, Gefter WB, Pollack HM. Prostatic disorders: MR imaging at 1.5T. *Radiology* 1987;164:386–392.

210. Picus D, Lee JKT. Magnetic resonance imaging of the female pelvis. *Urol Radiol* 1986;8:166–174.

211. Pilepich MV, Perez CA, Prasad S. Computed tomography in definitive radiotherapy of prostatic carcinoma. *Int J Radiat Oncol Biol Phys* 1980;6:923–926.

212. Pinch L, Aceta T, Meyer-Hahlbung HFL. Cryptorchidism. A pediatric review. *Urol Clin North Am* 1974;1:573–592.

213. Platt JF, Bree RL, Schwab RE. The accuracy of CT in the staging of carcinoma of the prostate. *AJR* 1987;149(2):315–318.

214. Poon PY, Bronskill MJ, Poon CS, McCallum RW, Bruce AW, Henkelman RM. Identification of the periprostatic venous plexus by MR imaging. *J Comput Assist Tomogr* 1991;15(2):265–268.

215. Powell MC, Buckley J, Price H, Worthington BS, Symonds EM. Magnetic resonance imaging and placenta previa. *Am J Obstet Gynecol* 1986;154:565–569.

216. Powell MC, Womack C, Buckley J, Worthington BS, Symonds EM. Pre-operative magnetic resonance imaging of Stage I endometrial adenocarcinoma. *Br J Obstet Gynecol* 1986;93:353–360.

217. Prayer L, Kainz C, Kramer J, Stiglbauer R, Schurawitzki H, Baldt M, Schima W, Poelzleitner D, Reinthaller A, Koelbl H, Imhof H. CT and MR accuracy in the detection of tumor recurrence in patients treated for ovarian cancer. *J Comput Assist Tomogr* 1993; 17(4):626–632.

218. Presti JC Jr, Hricak H, Narayan PA, Shinohara K, White S, Carroll PR. Local staging of prostatic carcinoma: comparison of transrectal sonography and endorectal MR imaging. *AJR* 1996;166:103–108.

219. Price JM, Davidson AJ. Computed tomography in the evaluation of the suspected carcinomatous prostate. *Urol Radiol* 1979;1:38–42.

220. Quinn SF, Franzini DA, Demlow TA, Rosencrantz DR, Kim J, Hanna RM, Szumowski J. MR imaging of prostate cancer with an endorectal surface coil technique: correlation with whole-mount specimens. *Radiology* 1994;190:323–327.

221. Quint LE, Van Erp JS, Bland PH, Del Buono EA, Mandell SH, Grossman HB, Gikas PW. Prostate cancer: correlation of MR images with tissue optical density at pathologic examination. *Radiology* 1991;179:837–842.

222. Quint LE, Van Erp JS, Bland PH, Mandell SH, DelBuono EA, Grossman HB, Glazer GM, Gikas PW. Carcinoma of the prostate: MR images obtained with body coils do not accurately reflect tumor volume. *AJR* 1991;156:511–516.

223. Reed DH, Dixon AK, Braude PR. Ectopic ovaries associated with absent uterus and pelvic kidney: CT findings. *J Comput Assist Tomogr* 1990;14(1):157–158.

224. Reinhold C, McCarthy S, Bret PM, Mehio Am, Atri M, Zakarian R, Glaude Y, Liang L, Seymour RJ. Diffuse adenomyosis: comparison of endovaginal US and MR imaging with histopathologic correlation. *Radiology* 1996;199:151–158.

225. Requard C, Mettler F. The use of ultrasound in the evaluation of trophoblastic disease and its response to therapy. *Radiology* 1980; 135:419–422.

226. Reuter KL, Griffin T, Hunter RE. Comparison of abdominopelvic computed tomography results and findings at second-look laparotomy in ovarian carcinoma patients. *Cancer* 1989;63(6):1123–1128.

227. Reznek RH, White FE, Young JWR, Fry IK. The appearances on computed tomography after abdomino-perineal resection for carcinoma of the rectum: a comparison between the normal appearances and those of recurrence. *Br J Radiol* 1983;56:237–240.

228. Rholl KS, Lee JKT, Heiken JP, Ling D, Glazer HS. Primary bladder carcinoma: evaluation with MR imaging. *Radiology* 1987;163:117–121.

229. Rholl KS, Lee JKT, Ling D, Heiken JP, Glazer HS. MR imaging of the scrotum with a high-resolution surface coil. *Radiology* 1987; 163:99–103.

230. Rifkin MD, Zerhouni EA, Gatsonis CA, et al. Comparison of magnetic resonance imaging and ultrasonography in staging early prostate cancer: results of a multi-institutional cooperative trial. *N Engl J Med* 1990;323:621–626.

231. Rosenfield AT, Blair DN, McCarthy S, Glickman MG, Rosenfield NS, Weiss R. Society of Uroradiology Award paper. The pars

infravaginalis gubernaculi: importance in the identification of the undescended testis. *AJR* 1989;153(4):775–778.

232. Rubens D, Thornbury JR, Angel C, Stoler MH, Weiss SL, Lerner RM, Beecham J. Stage IB cervical carcinoma: comparison of clinical, MR, and pathologic staging. *AJR* 1988;150:135–138.

233. Sager EM, Fossa SD, Kaalhus O, Talle K. Contrast-enhanced computed tomography in carcinoma of the urinary bladder: the use of different injection methods. *Acta Radiol* 1987;28(1):67–70.

234. Sager EM, Talle K, Fossa S, Ous S, Stenwig AE. The role of CT in demonstrating perivesical tumor growth in the preoperative staging of carcinoma of the urinary bladder. *Radiology* 1983;146:443–446.

235. Sanders C, Rubin E. Malignant gestational trophoblastic disease: CT findings. *AJR* 1987;148:165–168.

236. Savit RM, Udis DS. ''Upside-Down'' contrast—Urine level in glycosuria: CT features. *J Comput Assist Tomogr* 1987;11(5):911–912.

237. Schiebler ML, Schnall MD, Pollack HM, Lenkinski RE, Tomaszewski JE, Wein AJ, Whittington R, Rauschning W, Kressel HY. Current role of MR imaging in the staging of adenocarcinoma of the prostate. *Radiology* 1993;189:339–352.

238. Schiebler ML, Tomaszewski JE, Bezzi M, Pollack HM, Kressel HY, Cohen EK, Altman HG, Gefter WB, Wein AJ, Axel L. Prostatic carcinoma and benign prostatic hyperplasia: correlation of high-resolution MR and histopathologic findings. *Radiology* 1989;172:131–137.

239. Schiebler ML, Yankaskas BC, Tempany C, Spitzer CE, Rifkin MD, Pollack HM, Holtz P, Zerhouni EA. MR imaging in adenocarcinoma of the prostate: interobserver variation and efficacy for determining stage C disease. *AJR* 1992;158:559–562.

240. Schnall MD, Connick T, Hayes CE, Lenkinski RE, Kressel HY. MR imaging of the pelvis with an endorectal-external multicoil array. *Magn Reson Imaging* 1992;2(2):229–232.

241. Schnall MD, Imai Y, Tomaszewski J, Pollack HM, Lenkinski RE, Kressel HY. Prostate cancer: local staging with endorectal surface coil MR imaging. *Radiology* 1991;178(3):797–802.

242. Schnall MD, Lenkinski RL, Pollack HM, Imai Y, Hressel HY. Prostate: MR imaging with an endorectal surface coil. *Radiology* 1989;172:570.

243. Schnall MD, Tomaszewski J, Pollack HM, Wein AJ, Kressel HY. The bulging prostate gland: a sign of capsular involvement *(abstr)*. *J Magn Reson Imaging* 1991;1:279.

244. Schwartz LB, Panageas E, Lange R, Rizzo J, Comite F, McCarthy SM. Female pelvis: impact of MR imaging on treatment decisions and net cost analysis. *Radiology* 1994;192:55.

245. Scott WW Jr, Rosenshein NB, Siegelman SS, Sanders RC. The obstructed uterus. *Radiology* 1981;141:767–770.

246. Scoutt LM, Flynn SD, Luthringer DJ, McCauley TR, McCarthy SM. Junctional zone of the uterus: correlation of MR imaging and histologic examination of hysterectomy specimens. *Radiology* 1991;179:403–407.

247. Scoutt LM, McCarthy SM, Flynn SD, Lange RC, Long F, Smith RC, Chambers SK, Kohorn E, Schwartz P, Chambers JT. Clinical stage 1 endometrial carcinoma: pitfalls in preoperative assessment with MR imaging. *Radiology* 1995;194:567–572.

248. Scoutt LM, McCauley TR, Flynn SD, Luthringer DJ, McCarthy SM. Zonal anatomy of the cervix: correlation of MR imaging and histologic examination of hysterectomy specimens. *Radiology* 1993;186:159–162.

249. Seidelmann FE, Cohen WN, Bryan PJ, Temes SP, Kraus D, Schoenrock G. Accuracy of CT staging of bladder neoplasms using the gas-filled method: report of 21 patients with surgical confirmation. *AJR* 1978;130:735–739.

250. Seidenwurm D, Smathers RL, Lo RK, Carrol CL, Basset J, Hoffman AR. Testes and scrotum: MR imaging at 1.5T. *Radiology* 1987;164:393–398.

251. Semelka RC, Lawrence PH, Shoenut JP, Heywood M, Kroeker MA, Lotocki R. Primary ovarian cancer: prospective comparison of contrast-enhanced CT and pre- and postcontrast, fat-suppressed MR imaging, with histologic correlation. *J Magn Reson Imaging* 1993;3:99–106.

252. Shapeero LG, Hricak H. Mixed mullerian sarcoma of the uterus: MR imaging findings. *AJR* 1989;153:317–319.

253. Siegelman ES, Outwater E, Wang T, Mitchell DG. Solid pelvic masses caused by endometriosis: MR imaging features. *AJR* 1994;163:357–361.

254. Silverman PM, Osborne M, Dunnick NR, Bandy LC. CT prior to second-look operation in ovarian cancer. *AJR* 1988;150:829–832.

255. Sironi S, Belloni C, Taccagni GL, DelMaschio A. Carcinoma of the cervix: value of MR imaging in detecting parametrial involvement. *AJR* 1991;156:753–756.

256. Sironi S, Belloni C, Taccagni G, DelMaschio A. Invasive cervical carcinoma: MR imaging after preoperative chemotherapy. *Radiology* 1991;180:719–722.

257. Sironi S, De Cobelli F, Scarfone G, Columbo E, Bolis G, Ferrari A, DelMaschio A. Carcinoma of the cervix: value of plain and gadolinium-enhanced MR imaging in assessing degree of invasiveness. *Radiology* 1993;188:797–801.

258. Sironi S, Taccagni G, Garancini P, Belloni C, DelMaschio A. Myometrial invasion by endometrial carcinoma: assessment by MR imaging. *AJR* 1992;158:565–569.

259. Smith RC, McCarthy S. Improving the accuracy of digital CT pelvimetry. *J Comput Assist Tomogr* 1991;15(5):787–789.

260. Smith RC, Reinhold C, McCauley TR, Lange RC, Constable RT, Kier R, McCarthy S. Multicoil high-resolution fast spin-echo MR imaging of the female pelvis. *Radiology* 1992;184:671–675.

261. Sommer FG, McNeal JE, Carrol CL. MR depiction of zonal anatomy of the prostate at 1.5T. *J Comput Assist Tomogr* 1986;10:983–989.

262. Sommer FG, Nghiem HV, Herfkens R, McNeal J, Low RN. Determining the volume of prostatic carcinoma: value of MR imaging with an external array coil. *AJR* 1993;161:81–86.

263. Stamey TA, McNeal JE. Adenocarcinoma of the prostate. In: Walsh PC, Retik AB, Stamey TA, Vaughan ED Jr, eds. *Campbell's urology*, 6th ed. Philadelphia: Saunders, 1992;1180.

264. Stanley RJ. Fluid characterization with computed tomography. In: Moss AA, Goldberg HI, eds. *Computed tomography, ultrasound and x-ray: an integrated approach*. San Francisco: University of California, Department of Radiology, 1980;65–66.

265. Stark DD, McCarthy SM, Filly RA, Callen PW, Hricak H, Parer JT. Intrauterine growth retardation: evaluation by magnetic resonance. *Radiology* 1985;155:425–427.

266. Stevens SK, Hricak H, Campos Z. Teratomas versus cystic hemorrhagic adnexal lesions: differentiation with proton-selective fat-saturation MR imaging. *Radiology* 1993;186:481–488.

267. Stevens SK, Hricak H, Stern LL. Ovarian lesions: detection and characterization with gadolinium-enhanced MR imaging at 1.5 T. *Radiology* 1991;181:481–488.

268. Steyn JH, Smith FW. Nuclear magnetic resonance imaging of the prostate. *Br J Urol* 1982;54:726–728.

269. Sugimura K, Carrington BM, Quivey JM, Hricak H. Postirradiation changes in the pelvis: assessment with MR imaging. *Radiology* 1990;175:805–813.

270. Sugimura K, Okizuka H, Imaoka I, Kaji Y, Takahashi K, Kitao M, Ishida T. Pelvic endometriosis: detection and diagnosis with chemical shift MR imaging. *Radiology* 1993;188(2):435–438.

271. Sukov RJ, Scardino PT, Sample WF, Winter J, Confer DJ. Computed tomography and transabdominal ultrasound in the evaluation of the prostate. *J Comput Assist Tomogr* 1977;1:281–289.

272. Susmano DE, Dolin EH. Computed tomography in diagnosis of pelvic lipomatosis. *Urology* 1979;13:215–220.

273. Tachibana M, Baba S, Deguchi N, et al. Efficacy of gadolinium diethylenetrimine-pentaacetic acid-enhanced magnetic resonance imaging for differentiation between superficial and muscle-invasive tumor of the bladder: a comparative study with computerized tomography and transurethral ultrasonography. *J Urol* 1991;145:1169–1173.

274. Tada S, Tsukioka M, Ishii C, Tanaka H, Mizunuma K. Computed tomographic features of uterine myoma. *J Comput Assist Tomogr* 1981;5:866–869.

275. Tanimoto A, Yuasa Y, Imai Y, Izutsu M, Hiramatsu K, Tachibana M, Tazaki H. Bladder tumor staging: comparison of conventional and gadolinium-enhanced dynamic MR imaging and CT. *Radiology* 1992;185:741–747.

276. Tartar VM, Trambert MA, Balsara ZN, Mattrey RF. Tubular ectasia of the testicle: sonographic and MR imaging appearance. *AJR* 1993;160(3):539–542.

277. Teefey SA, Baron RL, Schulte SJ, Shuman WP. Differentiating

pelvic veins and enlarged lymph nodes: optimal CT techniques. *Radiology* 1990;175:683–685.

278. Tempany CM, Rahmouni AD, Epstein JI, Walsh PC, Zerhouni EA. Invasion of the neurovascular bundle by prostate cancer: evaluation with MR imaging. *Radiology* 1991;181:107–112.

279. Tempany CM, Zhou X, Zerhouni EA, Rifkin MD, Quint LE, Piccoli CW, Ellis JH, McNeil BJ. Staging of prostate cancer: results of radiology diagnostic oncology group project comparison of three MR imaging techniques. *Radiology* 1994;192:47–54.

280. Thurnher S, Hricak H, Carroll PR, Pobiel RS, Filly RA. Imaging of the testis: comparison between MR imaging and US. *Radiology* 1988;167(3):631–636.

281. Thurnher SA. MR imaging of pelvic masses in women: contrast-enhanced vs. unenhanced images. *AJR* 1992;159:1243–1250.

282. Tisnado J, Amendola MA, Walsh JW, Jordan RL, Turner MA, Krempa J. Computed tomography of the perineum. *AJR* 1981;136:475–481.

283. Togashi K, Kawakami S, Kimura I, Asato R, Okumura R, Fukuoka M, Mori T, Konishi J. Uterine contractions: possible diagnostic pitfall at MR imaging. *J Magn Reson Imaging* 1993;3(6):889–893.

284. Togashi K, Nishimura K, Itoh K, Fujisawa I, Asato R, Nakano Y, Itoh H, Torizuka K, Ozasa H, Mori T. Uterine cervical cancer: assessment with high field MR imaging. *Radiology* 1986;160:431–435.

285. Togashi K, Nishimura K, Itoh K, Fujisawa I, Nakano Y, Torizuka K, Ozasa H, Ohshima M. Vaginal agenesis: classification by MR imaging. *Radiology* 1987;162:675–677.

286. Togashi K, Nishimura K, Itoh K, Fujisawa I, Sago T, Minami S, Nakano Y, Itoh H, Torizuka K, Ozasa H. Ovarian cystic teratomas: MR imaging. *Radiology* 1987;162:669–673.

287. Togashi K, Nishimura K, Kimura I, Tsuda Y, Yamashita K, Shibata T, Nakano Y, Konishi J, Konishi I, Mori T. Endometrial cysts: diagnosis with MR imaging. *Radiology* 1991;180:73–78.

288. Togashi K, Nishimura K, Sagoh T, Minami S, Noma S, Fujisawa I, Nakano Y, Konishi J, Ozasa H, Konishi I, Mori T. Carcinoma of the cervix: staging with MR imaging. *Radiology* 1989;171:245–251.

289. Togashi K, Ozasa H, Konishi I, Itoh H, Nishimura K, Fujisawa I, Noma S, Sagoh T, Minami S, Yamashita K, Nakano Y, Konishi J, Mori T. Enlarged uterus: differentiation between adenomyosis and leiomyoma with MR imaging. *Radiology* 1989;171:531–534.

290. Twickler DM, Setiawan AT, Harrell RS, Brown CEL. CT appearance of the pelvis after cesarean section. *AJR* 1991;156:523–526.

291. Van Engelshoven JMA, Kreel L. Computed tomography of the prostate. *J Comput Assist Tomogr* 1979;3:45–51.

292. Van Nagel JR Jr, Roddick JW Jr, Lowin DM. The staging of cervical cancer: inevitable discrepancies between clinical staging and pathologic findings. *Am J Obstet Gynecol* 1971;110:973–978.

293. VanWaes PFGM, Zonneveld FW. Direct coronal body computed tomography. *J Comput Assist Tomogr* 1982;6:58–66.

294. Varpula MJ, Klemi PJ. Staging of uterine endometrial carcinoma with ultra-low field (0.02 T) MRI: a comparative study with CT. *J Comput Assist Tomogr* 1993;17(4):641–647.

295. Vercamer R, Janssens J, Usewils R, Ide P, Baert A, Lauwerijns J, Bonte J. Computed tomography and lymphography in the presurgical staging of early carcinoma of the uterine cervix. *Cancer* 1987;60:1745–1750.

296. Vick CW, Walsh JW, Wheelock JB, Brewer WH. CT of the normal and abnormal parametria in cervical cancer. *AJR* 1984;143:597.

297. Villasanta U, Whitley NO, Haney PJ, Brenner D. Computed tomography in invasive carcinoma of the cervix: an appraisal. *Obstet Gynecol* 1983;62:218–224.

298. Vinnicombe SJ, Norman AR, Nicolson V, Husband JE. Normal pelvic lymph nodes: evaluation with CT after bipedal lymphangiography. *Radiology* 1995;194:349–355.

299. Wajsman Z, Baumgartner G, Murphy GP, Merrin C. Evaluation of lymphangiography for clinical staging of bladder tumors. *J Urol* 1975;114:714–724.

300. Walsh JW, Amendola MA, Hall DJ, Tisnado J, Goplerud DR. Recurrent carcinoma of the cervix: CT diagnosis. *AJR* 1981;136:117–122.

301. Walsh JW, Amendola MA, Konerding KF, Tisnado J, Hazra TA. Computed tomographic detection of pelvic and inguinal lymph node metastases from primary and recurrent pelvic malignant disease. *Radiology* 1980;137:157–166.

302. Walsh JW, Goplerud DR. Prospective comparison between clinical and CT staging in primary cervical carcinoma. *AJR* 1981;137:997.

303. Walsh JW, Goplerud DR. Computed tomography of primary, persistent, and recurrent endometrial malignancy. *AJR* 1982;139:1149.

304. Walsh JW, Rosenfield AT, Jaffe CC, Schwartz PE, Simeone J, Dembner AG, Taylor KJW. Prospective comparison of ultrasound and computed tomography in the evaluation of gynecologic pelvic masses. *AJR* 1978;131:955–960.

305. Walz BJ, Lindstrom ER, Butcher HR, Baglan RJ. Natural history of patients after abdominal-perineal resection: implications for radiation therapy. *Cancer* 1977;39:2437–2442.

306. Weinerman PM, Arger PH, Coleman BG, Pollack HM, Banner MP, Wein AJ. Pelvic adenopathy from bladder and prostate carcinoma: detection by rapid-sequence computed tomography. *AJR* 1983;140:95–99.

307. Weinreb JC, Barkoff NC, Megibow A, Demopoulos R. The value of MR imaging in distinguishing leiomyomas from other solid pelvic masses when sonography is indeterminate. *AJR* 1990;154(2):295–299.

308. Weinreb JC, Brown CE, Lowe TW, Cohen JM, Erdman WA. Pelvic masses in pregnant patients: MR and US imaging. *Radiology* 1986;159:717–724.

309. Weinreb JC, Lowe T, Cohen JM, Kutler M. Human fetal anatomy: MR imaging. *Radiology* 1985;157:715–720.

310. Weinreb JC, Lowe TW, Santos-Ramos R, Cunningham FG, Parkey R. Magnetic resonance imaging in obstetric diagnosis. *Radiology* 1985;154:157–161.

311. Werboff LH, Korobkin M, Klein RS. Pelvic lipomatosis: diagnosis using computed tomography. *Urology* 1979;122:257–259.

312. White S, Hricak H, Forstner R, Kurhanewicz J, Vigneron DB, Zaloudek CJ, Weiss JM, Narayan P, Carroll PR. Prostate cancer: effect of postbiopsy hemorrhage on interpretation of MR images. *Radiology* 1995;195:385–390.

313. Whitley NO, Brenner DE, Francis A, Villasanta U, Aisner J, Wiernik PH, Whitley J. Computed tomographic evaluation of carcinoma of the cervix. *Radiology* 1982;142:439–446.

314. Wiesen EJ, Crass JR, Bellon EM, Ashmead GG, Cohen AM. Improvement in CT pelvimetry. *Radiology* 1991;178:259–262.

315. Wilbur AC, Aizenstein RI, Napp TE. CT findings in tuboovarian abscess. *AJR* 1992;158:575–579.

316. Willms AB, Brown ED, Kettritz UI, Kuller JA, Semelka RC. Anatomic changes in the pelvis after uncomplicated vaginal delivery: evaluation with serial MR imaging. *Radiology* 1995;195:91–94.

317. Wolverson MK, Jagannadharao B, Sundaram M, Riaz A, Nalesnik WJ, Houttiun E. CT in localization of impalpable cryptochid testes. *AJR* 1980;134:725–729.

318. Woo GM, Twickler DM, Stettler RW, Erdman WA, Brown CE. The pelvis after cesarean section and vaginal delivery: normal MR findings. *AJR* 1993;161(6):1249–1252.

319. Worthington JL, Balfe DM, Lee JKT, Gersell DJ, Heiken JP, Ling D, Glazer HS, Jacobs AJ, Kao MS, McClennan BL. Uterine neoplasms: MR imaging. *Radiology* 1986;159:725–730.

320. Yamashita Y, Hatanaka Y, Torashima M, Takahashi M, Miyazaki K, Okamura H. Mature cystic teratomas of the ovary without fat in the cystic cavity: MR features in 12 cases. *AJR* 1994;163:613–616.

321. Yamashita Y, Harada M, Sawada T, Takahashi M, Miyazaki K, Okamura H. Normal uterus and FIGO stage I endometrial carcinoma: dynamic gadolinium-enhanced MR imaging. *Radiology* 1993;186:495–501.

322. Yamashita Y, Takashi M, Sawada T, Miyazaki K, Okamura H. Carcinoma of the cervix: dynamic MR imaging. *Radiology* 1992;182:643–648.

323. Yamashita Y, Torashima M, Hatanaka Y, Harada M, Higashida Y, Takahashi M, Mizutani H, Tashiro H, Iwamasa J, Miyazaki K, Okamura H. Adnexal masses: accuracy of characterization with transvaginal US and precontrast and postcontrast MR imaging. *Radiology* 1995;194:557–565.

324. Yamashita Y, Torashima M, Hatanaka Y, Harada M, Sakamoto Y, Takahashi M, Miyazaki K, Okamura H. Value of phase-shift

gradient-echo MR imaging in the differentiation of pelvic lesions with high signal intensity at T1-weighted imaging. *Radiology* 1994;191:759–764.

325. Yamashita Y, Torashima M, Takahashi M, Tanaka N, Katabuchi H, Miyazaki K, Ito M, Ikamura H. Hyperintense uterine leiomyoma at T2-weighted MR imaging: differentiation with dynamic enhanced MR imaging and clinical implications. *Radiology* 1993; 189:721–725.

326. Yatani R, Chigusa I, Akazaki K, Stemmerman GN, Welsh RA, Correa P. Geographic pathology of latent prostatic carcinoma. *Int J Cancer* 1982;29:611–616.

327. Zawin M, McCarthy S, Scoutt L. High-field MRI and US evaluation of the pelvis in women with leiomyomas. *Magn Reson Imaging* 1990;8:371–376.

328. Zawin M, McCarthy S, Scoutt L, Comite F. Endometriosis: appearance and detection at MR imaging. *Radiology* 1989;171: 693–696.

329. Zawin M, McCarthy S, Scoutt L, Lange R, Lavy G, Vulte J, Comite F. Monitoring therapy with a gonadotropin-releasing hormone analog: utility of MR imaging. *Radiology* 1990;175:503–506.

CHAPTER 21

Computed Tomography of Thoracoabdominal Trauma

Paul L. Molina, David M. Warshauer, and Joseph K. T. Lee

Trauma is the fifth leading cause of death in the United States. In 1991, 89,347 deaths were attributed to trauma, and it was the leading cause of death in persons under the age of 35 (371). Potential life years lost due to trauma exceed those due to heart disease and cancer (334). Trauma also results in approximately 100,000 permanent disabilities annually (129), and the cost of trauma in this country is estimated at $84 billion per year (334).

Blunt trauma, also called wide impact trauma, accounts for the majority of injuries and is most commonly the result of motor vehicle accidents. Other common causes include home and work-related accidents such as crush injuries, blast injuries, and falls from a height. Multisystem trauma is a characteristic of motor vehicle accidents, with the extremities involved most frequently (90%), followed by injury to the head (70%), chest (50%), abdomen (30%), and pelvis (25%) (334).

In recent years, improved triage using telecommunication and expedited transport to designated trauma centers has enhanced survival of major trauma victims (11). Trauma centers effectively reduce morbidity and mortality of the accident patient, and the nationwide development of the Emergency Medical Service System, which identifies trauma centers by a process of categorization, regionalization, and verification, has markedly improved the care of trauma patients (216). Another significant advancement in modern trauma care has been the intensive use of computed tomography (CT) for immediate patient evaluation. CT accurately depicts craniocerebral, facial, spinal, abdominal, and pelvic injuries and in these areas has largely replaced other diagnostic imaging modalities (216). CT facilitates rapid, efficient evaluation of the ma-

jor trauma victim and now plays an essential role in trauma center operations.

BLUNT THORACIC TRAUMA

Blunt chest trauma is much more common than penetrating chest trauma and is responsible for almost 90% of the chest injuries that occur in civilian populations (131). Chest injury, alone or in combination with other injuries, accounts for nearly half of all traumatic deaths. The overall death rate is 2% to 12% for isolated chest injuries. For patients with chest injuries associated with polytrauma, the mortality rate rises to 35% (129). Most patients with blunt chest trauma have associated extrathoracic injuries. In a representative large series of 515 cases of blunt chest trauma, 431 patients (84%) had extrathoracic injuries, and nearly half of these patients had involvement of two or more extrathoracic sites (314). The most common associated injuries were head trauma, extremity fractures, and intraabdominal injuries. These extrathoracic injuries in conjunction with thoracic trauma can lead to additional impairment of respiratory function. Head injuries, for example, can result in aspiration or neurogenic pulmonary edema. Skeletal trauma combined with hypovolemic shock can produce the fat embolism syndrome. Abdominal injuries resulting in hemorrhagic shock (i.e., hepatic or splenic lacerations) may also compound the effects of blunt chest trauma (335).

Blunt chest injury results from the transfer of kinetic energy to the chest wall and thoracic contents through a number of synergistic mechanisms, including (a) direct impact, (b) sudden inertial deceleration, (c) spallation, and (d) implosion. Direct impact, as occurs with forceful, direct blows to the chest, causes a sudden release of local kinetic energy that may fracture bony structures and contuse, crush, and shear underlying soft tissues. If the chest wall is compressed substantially by the force of the impact, the resultant increase in intrathoracic pressure may also lead to rupture of alveoli and supporting structures. Sudden inertial deceleration at the time of impact is a major injury factor in high-speed motor vehicle accidents. Inertial deceleration imparts differential moments of rotation to chest tissues and causes mobile or elastic structures to rotate about points of fixation. The resulting torsional deformation and shearing stresses at internal thoracic interfaces (i.e., interface between the relatively mobile alveolar tissues and the more fixed bronchovascular interstitium) can cause microscopic tears or gross lacerations. Spallation occurs when a broad kinetic shock wave from sudden compression is partially reflected at gas–fluid interfaces, such as at the alveolocapillary surface. The resulting release of energy causes local disruption of tissue near the point of shock wave impact. Spallation injury is typically manifest in the anterior lung during sudden compression of the anterior chest wall in steering wheel injuries. Implosion is the low-pressure decompressive wave that follows the high-pressure compressive shock wave of spallation, causing disruption of lung tissue through rebound overexpansion of gas bubbles within alveoli. In most cases, blunt thoracic injury is the result of a combination of these major energy transfer mechanisms (114,129).

Indications

Although CT is the examination of choice in trauma of the head and abdomen, its precise role in the evaluation of blunt chest trauma continues to evolve. This is largely due to the remarkable amount of information provided by chest radiography, which remains the principal diagnostic screening examination in patients with blunt thoracic trauma. Many traumatic abnormalities of the thorax (e.g., tension pneumothorax, hemothorax, pulmonary contusion) can be diagnosed or suggested with reasonable confidence by conventional radiographic methods. In stable posttraumatic patients, thoracic CT can be performed in order to confirm and/or more precisely define the full extent of thoracic injury, which is often underestimated by chest radiography (173,211,217,240,286,324,350). CT can be particularly beneficial in patients with equivocal radiographic findings or technically inadequate radiographic examinations. CT may also be used to diagnose radiographically inapparent or clinically unsuspected injuries such as parenchymal lacerations or occult pneumothoraces. In selected patients with possible aortic injury, CT can assist in screening for aortography. In the later postinjury stage, additional indications for use of CT include demonstration of sites of thoracic infection (237), differentiation of pleural from parenchymal abnormalities (125), and guidance of therapeutic interventions such as empyema drainage (29) or revision of malpositioned and occluded thoracostomy tubes (237). In general, MRI is not used routinely to assess acute chest or abdominal trauma.

Technique

Posttraumatic thoracic CT examinations generally should be performed at 8- to 10-mm intervals with 8- to 10-mm collimation through the entire thorax following the bolus administration of intravenous contrast material. In select cases, depending on the nature of the injury, clinical setting, and chest film findings, contiguous 5-mm sections may be obtained through an appropriate region of interest (e.g., from above the aortic arch down through the carina in patients with suspected mediastinal injury). In patients already undergoing head CT or abdominal CT, some investigators add a ''limited'' chest CT examination regardless of clinical or chest film findings. For such ''limited'' studies, a total of five to ten additional slices are obtained to survey several axial levels: the aortic knob region for mediastinal hemorrhage and sternoclavicular dislocation; the base of the heart for pericardial effusion and retrosternal hematoma possibly indicating myocardial injury; and the diaphragmatic dome and costovertebral sulcus for evaluation of occult pneumothorax and diaphragmatic tears (344).

Whenever performing trauma CT, the patient should be closely monitored throughout the examination by trained medical personnel, and emergency resuscitative equipment must be immediately available in the CT scanning room. If possible, the patient's arms should be positioned above the head rather than along the sides in order to reduce streak artifacts. Artifacts can also be minimized by removing as many nonessential tubes and other foreign objects from the scanning field as possible prior to imaging.

Specific Trauma Sites

Chest Wall

The chest wall is commonly injured in blunt thoracic trauma. For the majority of chest wall injuries, a combination of physical examination and radiographs is sufficient to define their nature and extent. Chest wall contusion, with or without rib fracture, can produce a reticular pattern of increased density in the usually homogeneous subcutaneous fat. Soft tissue hematomas can obliterate fat–tissue planes between muscles and produce a focal mass-like bulge (193) (Fig. 1). Both contusions and hema-

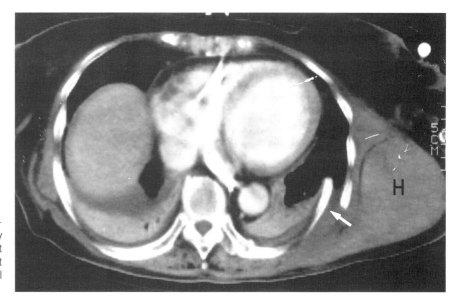

FIG. 1. Chest wall hematoma secondary to lacerated thoracodorsal artery following blunt trauma. Note large left chest wall hematoma (H) and adjacent displaced rib fracture (*arrow*). Bilateral lower lobe atelectasis is also present.

tomas of the chest wall are readily demonstrated by CT but are generally of little clinical significance.

Subcutaneous or intramuscular chest wall emphysema is also readily demonstrated by CT because of the significant contrast difference between air and soft tissue. Subcutaneous emphysema appears on CT as bands of air within the subcutaneous fat and along or between the chest wall muscles (Fig. 2). Following blunt chest trauma, the finding of subcutaneous emphysema can indicate the presence of underlying pneumothorax or pneumomediastinum, particularly if skin lacerations or open soft tissue wounds are absent. Detection of mottled subcutaneous air and/or soft tissue swelling days to weeks following trauma should suggest the possibility of an abscess, the extent of which can be easily delineated with CT (125).

Rib fractures occur in over 50% of patients with significant chest trauma and most commonly affect the fourth through ninth ribs (334). Although rib fractures are a common sequelae of blunt chest trauma, major internal thoracic injury can occur in the absence of rib fractures or other evident injury to the chest wall, particularly in younger individuals with compliant chest walls. There is a much greater incidence of rib fractures in older adults, whose ribs are relatively inelastic, compared with the incidence of rib fractures in children, whose ribs are generally more pliable and resilient (131). Rib fractures in and of themselves are usually of little clinical significance and are not accurate predictors of serious injury. However, they do reflect the magnitude of force imparted and can provide clues as to the type and location of underlying

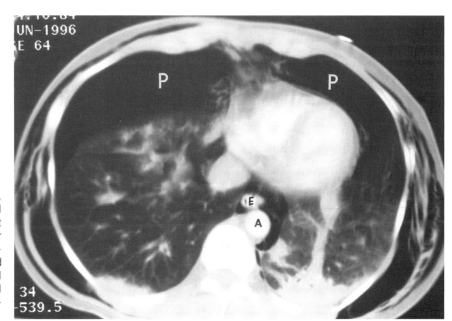

FIG. 2. Subcutaneous emphysema, pneumomediastinum, and bilateral pneumothoraces following blunt chest trauma. CT image through the lower chest demonstrates extensive subcutaneous emphysema in the anterior and lateral chest wall. There are bilateral pneumothoraces (P) and mediastinal air outlines the esophagus (E) and descending aorta (A).

injuries (129). Fractures of the first three ribs indicate significant energy transfer because these ribs are protected by the shoulder girdles and by heavy surrounding musculature. Their association with aortic or tracheobronchial injury is not as constant as previously believed, however, and they are not, as isolated findings, reliable predictors of aortic rupture. Several studies have shown that aortography should be performed only if associated radiologic signs of mediastinal hemorrhage accompany the first rib fractures (102,191,378). Extrapleural hematomas may accompany fractures of the upper ribs or trauma to the subclavian vessels over the apex of the lung. Such extrapleural hematomas or "pleural caps" can mimic a large hemothorax on supine chest radiographs. CT readily distinguishes between an extrapleural collection of blood over the apex of the lung and a hemothorax. Fractures of the lower ribs, particularly the tenth through twelfth ribs, should increase suspicion of hepatic, splenic, or renal injury, as well as associated intraperitoneal and retroperitoneal hemorrhage. Confirmation of such injuries should then be sought by appropriate diagnostic investigations such as CT (193).

Fractures of three or more sequential ribs or costal cartilages in multiple places can lead to an unstable, isolated segment of chest wall that exhibits paradoxical respiratory motion, the so-called "flail chest." The flail segment of chest wall is sucked in with inspiration and blown out with expiration, moving in a direction opposite to the usual and leading to impaired pulmonary ventilation. The diagnosis of flail chest is made clinically and it represents a very severe form of chest wall injury. Because significant force is needed to produce a flail segment, multiple associated injuries are frequently encountered, many of which can be documented by CT if necessary (e.g., lung contusion, lung laceration, sternal fracture) (334). Rarely, a segment of lung may herniate through a defect in the chest wall created by the flail segment and this too can be easily detected by CT (239).

Additional fractures of the bony thorax discovered by CT, including scapular (Fig. 3), sternal, or thoracic spine fractures, may be of considerable value in clarifying radiographic findings, elucidating the mechanism of injury,

and initiating investigation for important associated injuries. Thoracic spine fractures most often involve the lower thoracic spine (T9 through T11 vertebrae) and are of particular clinical significance because the thoracic spinal cord is unusually susceptible to injury. In comparison to the cervical or lumbar spinal cord, the thoracic spinal cord occupies a greater percentage of the total cross-sectional area of its surrounding spinal canal and it is easily injured by displaced fragments of bone or disk material. The blood supply to the midthoracic spinal cord is also very tenuous and when disrupted can result in devastating neurologic deficits. CT can accurately determine the presence, extent, and stability of thoracic spine fractures. Vertebral body fractures are readily demonstrated on CT, as are the relationships of fracture fragments and displaced disk material to the spinal cord (131).

Sternal fractures, occurring in 8% to 10% of patients after severe blunt trauma, are more easily diagnosed on CT than on supine chest radiographs. CT is also superior for detection of retrosternal hematoma, which may result from laceration of the internal mammary vessels by sternal fracture fragments. Sternal fractures should elicit concern about associated myocardial injury such as myocardial contusion, which can lead to significant arrhythmias and hemodynamic instability (334).

Posterior dislocation of the clavicle at the sternoclavicular joint is another injury best visualized by CT. Although less common than anterior dislocations, posterior dislocations of the sternoclavicular joint are more difficult to diagnose clinically and can result in compression or laceration of the trachea, esophagus, and great vessels (198,336). Prompt reduction of such dislocations can decrease the likelihood of visceral injury (112).

Pleural Space

Pneumothorax

Pneumothorax, with or without an associated rib fracture, is a common complication of blunt chest trauma, occurring in up to 40% of blunt trauma victims (75).

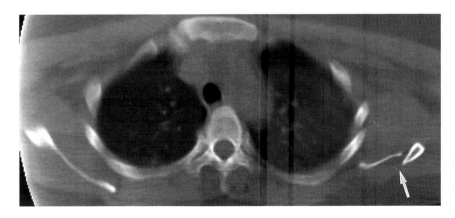

FIG. 3. Scapular fracture. CT image through the upper chest reveals a scapular fracture (*arrow*) not appreciated on the chest radiograph. Left upper lobe parenchymal contusion is also evident.

Pneumothoraces secondary to trauma are often bilateral and associated with hemothorax (129). When a rib fracture is present with a pneumothorax (70% of cases), laceration of the visceral pleura by rib fragments is usually the cause. When no fracture is present (30% of cases), the mechanism is likely that of parenchymal lung injury, including laceration, with subsequent interstitial emphysema. Pneumomediastinum and subcutaneous emphysema may also develop (193,334). Additional causes of posttraumatic pneumothorax include alveolar compression in crushing injuries, tracheobronchial or esophageal tears, and barotrauma.

The supine chest radiograph can detect most pneumothoraces large enough to require immediate thoracostomy. However, it has been reported that as many as 30% of pneumothoraces in critically ill patients are not detected on supine radiographs and that half of these progress to tension pneumothoraces (346). In the supine position, small amounts of pleural air tend to collect in the anteromedial and subpulmonic pleural spaces and may be difficult to detect on supine chest radiographs. The use of lateral decubitus radiography of the uppermost lung with a horizontal beam, as well as chest CT, has been recommended to improve detection of pneumothoraces.

Computed tomography is an exquisitely sensitive method for detecting a pneumothorax in the supine position. Occult pneumothorax, defined as pneumothorax evident by CT but not by clinical examination or chest radiography, has been reported in 2% to 12% of patients undergoing abdominal CT scanning for blunt trauma (281,362,374) (Fig. 4). A much higher percentage of occult pneumothorax (44%) has been reported in a select group of patients with severe head trauma undergoing limited chest CT examination in addition to cranial CT scanning (347).

Although CT is capable of demonstrating pneumothoraces that are not evident on clinical examination or plain radiographs, the clinical significance of, and definitive indications for, CT detection of occult pneumothorax are not entirely clear. As a general rule, a careful search for pneumothoraces in major trauma patients with seemingly normal supine chest radiographs is appropriate. In patients already undergoing abdominal CT scanning for blunt trauma, images of the upper abdomen (lower thorax) should be viewed at lung windows (level −500 to −600 H, width 1000 H) in addition to the usual soft tissue windows in order to enhance detection of small pneumothoraces (362).

Recognition of even a small, occult pneumothorax is sometimes critical, particularly in patients requiring mechanical ventilation or general anesthesia for emergent surgery. Barotrauma from mechanical ventilation and induction of anesthesia may produce enlargement of a pneumothorax resulting in significant respiratory or cardiovascular compromise (78,155). Animal studies have shown that inspiration of 75% nitrous oxide will double a 300-ml pneumothorax in 10 min and triple it in 45 min (78). In order to prevent progression to a tension pneumothorax, prophylactic tube thoracostomy is generally recommended for occult pneumothoraces in trauma patients needing to undergo mechanical ventilation or general anesthesia (27,347). Patients with a small, occult pneumothorax who are hemodynamically stable and not ventilated may be followed with close clinical observation and serial

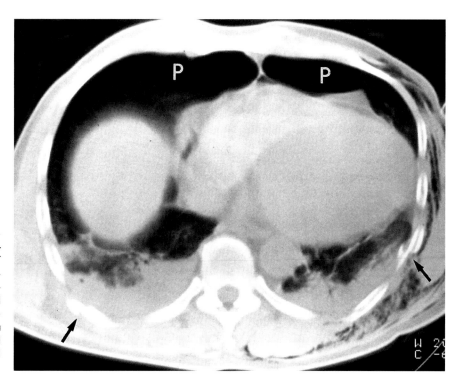

FIG. 4. Bilateral occult pneumothoraces in a patient with splenic rupture following blunt abdominal trauma. CT image at the level of the right hemidiaphragm reveals bilateral pneumothoraces (P) and left chest wall subcutaneous emphysema. The pneumothoraces were not identified on an AP supine chest radiograph. Bilateral rib fractures (*arrows*) and bilateral lower lobe atelectasis are also evident.

chest radiography to detect an increase in size of the pneumothorax. Tube thoracostomy may then be performed when appropriate (27,49,107, 374).

In patients treated with a chest tube for pneumothorax, CT may be helpful in assessing the adequacy of chest tube placement and pneumothorax drainage. A large percentage of thoracostomy tubes placed for acute chest trauma lie within a pleural fissure, but they may still function as effectively as those located elsewhere in the pleural space (62). At times, unsuspected extrapleural location of a chest tube and/or significant residual pneumothorax is detected on CT. In such situations, CT can be used to guide chest tube repositioning or additional chest tube insertion.

CT may also be of value in characterizing a number of potentially confusing posttraumatic air collections noted on chest radiography. Medial pneumothorax, for example, can be distinguished from pneumomediastinum, paramediastinal pneumatocele, or air within the pulmonary ligament on CT. A narrow air collection with a fluid level occurring after blunt trauma suggests medial pneumothorax, whereas a broad or spherical gas collection without a fluid level suggests posterior pneumomediastinum, particularly when occurring in association with respiratory distress and mechanical ventilation (121). Underlying pneumothorax in patients with extensive subcutaneous emphysema can also be reliably identified with CT.

Pleural Effusion/Hemothorax

Posttraumatic pleural effusions may be composed of transudate, exudate, blood, or chyle, or some mixture of these fluids. Transudative effusions can occur with acute pulmonary atelectasis or with vigorous resuscitation and overhydration of the patient (300). Exudative effusions are often due to infection of the pleural space. Chylous pleural fluid may follow a crush or penetrating injury to the thorax or neck with resultant damage to the thoracic duct. The overwhelming majority of pleural effusions developing after trauma represent hemothorax.

Hemothorax occurs in 50% of patients with blunt thoracic trauma and is often bilateral. It can be caused by many different injuries such as lung contusion, lung laceration, intercostal vessel laceration, and mediastinal or diaphragmatic tears (129). When hemothorax is due to bleeding from the lung (e.g., lung contusion) it is usually mild and self-limited. The low perfusion pressures and rich thromboplastin content of the lung favors hemostasis, as does the tamponade effect of associated collapsed lung (24). A large, rapidly expanding hemothorax is more likely due to injury to higher pressure arterial sources in the chest wall, diaphragm, or mediastinum. Laceration of systemic vessels such as the intercostal arteries, internal mammary arteries, aorta, and great vessels can lead to massive hemothorax and resultant shock.

Computed tomography and sonography are more sensitive than radiographs to the presence of pleural fluid collections. In a study evaluating the frequency and significance of thoracic injuries detected on abdominal CT scans of multiple trauma patients, hemothorax was recognized by CT alone in 23 (88%) of 26 patients (281). Although most pleural fluid collections apparent only at CT are small and may not require emergent drainage, possible increases in their size need to be assessed, and they may require sampling to determine their cause. The CT density of the fluid collection sometimes can suggest its origin. Acute hemothorax, for example, can measure 70 to 80 Hounsefield units (HU), compared to 10 to 20 HU for most transudates (350). Because of the tendency for hemothorax to produce pleural fibrosis, chest tube drainage is often indicated.

Occasionally, even large pleural effusions, particularly if symmetric and bilateral, may not be apparent on supine chest radiographs. The same is true of fluid collections located at the bases or trapped behind stiff, noncompliant lung (such as develops with posttraumatic adult respiratory distress syndrome). Both CT and sonography can readily identify such collections as well as guide their aspiration and/or drainage (337).

In patients treated with catheter or thoracostomy tube drainage, CT may be particularly beneficial in assessing the adequacy of pleural drainage. Persistent loculated collections and/or malpositioned chest tubes can be reliably detected with CT (Fig. 5). When appropriate, CT can be used to guide chest tube repositioning or additional chest tube insertion (237,333). CT is also of value in detection and drainage of associated complications such as empyema (Fig. 6) or lung abscess. CT can better delineate complex pleuroparenchymal opacities, distinguishing pleural fluid from other components causing radiographic density such as atelectasis, consolidation, or contusion (239).

Lung Parenchyma

Pulmonary Contusion

Pulmonary contusion is the most common injury resulting from blunt chest trauma (372), occurring in 30% to 75% of patients sustaining blunt trauma to the chest (177). Contusion results in exudation of blood and/or edema fluid into the airspaces and interstitium of the lung. Although often mild and localized, pulmonary contusion may be widespread and associated with respiratory failure. Massive contusion can lead to the development of adult respiratory distress syndrome (ARDS). The mortality rate from pulmonary contusion ranges from 14% to 40%, depending on the severity and extent of lung damage and other injuries (129,177).

Radiologically, pulmonary contusion generally results

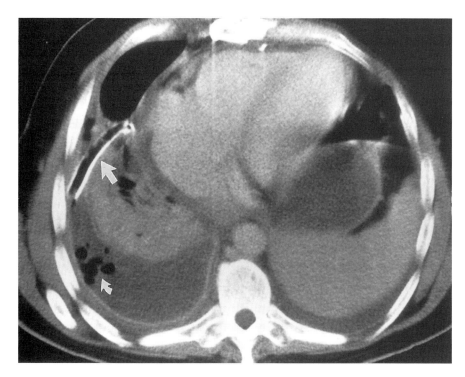

FIG. 5. Malpositioned chest tube. CT image through the lower chest demonstrates that the right chest tube (*straight arrow*) is well anterior to the right pleural fluid collection. Locules of air (*curved arrow*) within the pleural fluid collection were introduced at the time of chest tube placement.

in nonsegmental airspace consolidation, which may vary from patchy, faint, ill-defined areas of increased parenchymal density to extensive homogeneous opacification in one or both lungs. Contusions are frequently peripheral in distribution and tend to occur near the site of blunt impact and adjacent to solid structures such as the ribs, spine, heart, or liver (278). Contusions may also be seen in areas remote from the injured site due to the contrecoup effect (372). Usually, contusions appear within 4 to 6 hours after injury and clear within 3 to 8 days. The abrupt onset and relatively rapid clearing of areas of parenchymal opacification are characteristic of pulmonary contu-

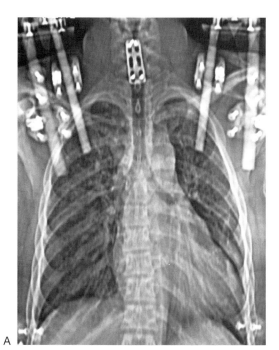

A

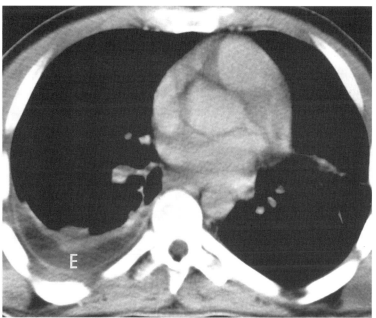

B

FIG. 6. Occult empyema in a febrile patient following blunt trauma. **A:** Scout view from the CT examination is unremarkable except for hardware related to a halo fixation device that overlies the upper chest. **B:** CT image though the lower chest reveals an occult empyema (E).

sion. Contusion may increase in size and become more visible for up to 48 hours after injury. Progressive increase in parenchymal opacification after 48 hours, or delayed resolution beyond 6 to 10 days, suggests either the wrong initial diagnosis or superimposition of another pathologic process such as pneumonia, atelectasis, aspiration, or ARDS (193,239,335,339). Intraalveolar blood and edema fluid within contused lung, coupled with impaired clearance of secretions and regional diminished lung compliance, provides a nidus for the development of infection and sepsis. In addition, because of disruption of alveolar/capillary membranes, contused lung is more susceptible to pulmonary edema (142). Administration of large amounts of intravenous fluids may accentuate the degree of edema and result in worsening radiographic opacification (129,142).

The overall severity and extent of contusion are often underestimated at initial clinical and radiographic examination (21). Rib fractures or other external signs of chest wall injury may be absent, even when extensive life-threatening contusion has occurred. Animal studies suggest that contusion involving up to one third of the lung may go undetected with plain radiography (80).

Computed tomography is much more sensitive than chest radiography in determining the presence and extent of pulmonary contusion (297, 359,361). On CT, contusion appears as an ill-defined area of hazy ground-glass density or consolidation, usually with a peripheral, nonsegmental distribution (Fig. 7). As with chest radiography, the CT appearance of contusion initially may be indistinguishable from other causes of consolidation such as aspiration, edema, and pneumonia. CT demonstration of localized, patchy infiltrates neighboring a rib fracture or chest wall hematoma suggests contusion, whereas infiltrates predominantly located in the superior segments of both lower lobes and other dependent segments suggests aspiration (344).

Although CT is capable of demonstrating earlier, as well as more extensive, pulmonary contusion than chest radiography, several investigators have questioned the clinical significance of this improved detection (274,328). In some studies, only those contusions diagnosed by chest radiography proved clinically significant (328), and it has been stated that the detection of pulmonary contusion on CT should not dictate a change in clinical management in the absence of hypoxemia or other respiratory disturbances (274). Nevertheless, other investigators have shown that CT quantitation of pulmonary contusion may be useful in the management of patients with blunt chest injury. In a review of 69 patients with severe blunt chest trauma examined by CT within 24 hours of admission, it was found that when there was CT evidence of pulmonary contusion involving >28% of the total lung volume, ventilatory support was invariably required (360).

Pulmonary Laceration, Pneumatocele, and Hematoma

Pulmonary laceration is a tear in the lung parenchyma that develops through any of the four major mechanisms of blunt injury described earlier (i.e., direct impact, inertial deceleration, spallation, implosion) or from any penetrating injury, such as from sharp, depressed rib fragments. The initial linear or stellate tear of a laceration tends to form an ovoid or elliptical postlaceration space due to elastic recoil of the adjacent intact lung (243). Concomitant tears of bronchi and blood vessels may fill the postlaceration space with air (pneumatocele), blood (hematoma), or both (hematopneumatocele) (129). Pathologically, lacerations are lined by compressed alveoli and connective tissue remnants, and may be uni- or multilocular, generally varying from 2 to 14 cm in diameter (236,243).

Radiographically, pulmonary lacerations appear as circumscribed areas containing air, fluid, or both. They are often obscured initially by surrounding pulmonary contusion and may become more apparent as the contusion resolves. If the laceration becomes filled with blood and a pulmonary hematoma forms, it can present as a focal mass on chest radiography, mimicking a primary lung cancer.

Computed tomography is considerably more sensitive than chest radiography in detecting pulmonary laceration. In a series of 85 consecutive chest trauma victims, CT detected 99 lacerations compared to only 5 detected by radiography (359). Because of the frequent CT identification of pulmonary laceration following blunt trauma, it has been suggested that pulmonary laceration is the basic mechanism of injury in pulmonary contusion, pulmonary hematoma, and traumatic pulmonary cyst, as well as the cause of most cavities in areas of pulmonary contusion (359) (Fig. 8).

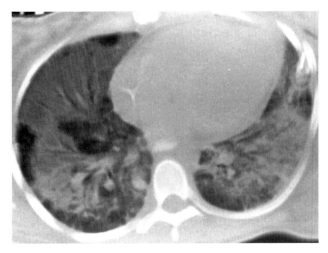

FIG. 7. Pulmonary contusion. CT image through the lower chest of a young woman struck by an automobile demonstrates bilateral, nonsegmental areas of parenchymal consolidation and ground-glass density.

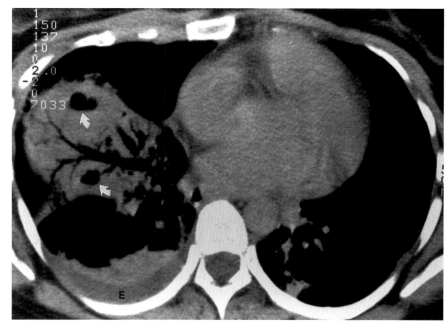

FIG. 8. Pulmonary laceration and contusion. CT image through the lower chest in a young woman involved in a motor vehicle accident demonstrates several air-filled cavities (*arrows*) representing pulmonary lacerations within an area of pulmonary contusion. The lacerations were obscured by the surrounding contusion on plain chest radiographs. A small right pleural effusion (E) is also present.

Pulmonary lacerations can be divided into four types on the basis of CT criteria and mechanism of injury. Type 1 lacerations, the most common type seen on CT, result from sudden compression of a pliable chest wall, causing rupture of air-containing lung. They usually appear on CT as intraparenchymal cavities with or without an air–fluid level (Fig. 9). On occasion, they may appear as air-filled linear structures extending through the visceral pleura resulting in a pneumothorax. Type 2 lacerations are relatively uncommon and present as air-containing cavities or intraparenchymal air–fluid levels within the basilar paravertebral lung (Fig. 10). They result from sudden compression of the more pliable lower chest wall, which causes the lower lobe to shift suddenly across the spine, producing a shearing-type injury. Type 3 lacerations appear as small peripheral cavities or linear lucencies neighboring a fractured rib that has punctured the underlying lung. These lacerations are usually associated with a pneumothorax. Type 4 lacerations are rare and occur at sites of pleuroparenchymal adhesion, which cause the lung to tear when the overlying chest wall is violently moved inward or is fractured. These lacerations can be diagnosed only surgically or at autopsy (359).

Most pulmonary lacerations resolve completely in a period of several weeks to months after injury, with air-filled lacerations (pneumatoceles) resolving more quickly than blood-filled lacerations (hematomas) (42). In mechanically ventilated patients, postlaceration spaces/pneumatoceles can progressively enlarge and communicate with the pleural space, resulting in pneumothorax. Rarely, they can become infected. CT has been shown to be superior to chest radiography in identifying and following the evolution of these lesions and in establishing the presence of complications such as infection or hemorrhage (19,168,312) (Fig. 11).

Aorta and Great Vessels

Laceration of the thoracic aorta and brachiocephalic arteries is a significant cause of morbidity and mortality secondary to blunt chest trauma. The majority of these injuries result from high-speed motor vehicle accidents. Most of the remainder are due to falls from heights and crush or blast injuries. Of all autopsied auto accident victims, about 16% have aortic laceration (128). Laceration is thought to result from shearing stress on the aorta produced by differential deceleration (whiplash) of the aortic root, aortic arch, and descending aorta at the time of impact. Sudden increases in intraaortic pressure produced by chest or abdominal wall compression may also contribute to aortic injury (204). A more recent hypothesis suggests that compression of the aorta between the sternum and the thoracic spine results in an "osseous pinch" of the aorta that causes laceration (47,48,58). Whatever the mechanism of injury, the result is that one or more layers of the aortic wall are torn, usually in a transverse fashion. Though the tear may be short (few millimeters) and superficial (limited to the intima), most are circumferential and transmural, constituting a complete transection. When only part of the aortic circumference is involved, the tear tends to be posterior (269).

In clinical series, over 90% of aortic tears occur at the aortic isthmus (i.e., the distal aortic arch at the insertion of the ligamentum arteriosum just after the origin of the left subclavian artery), which is the site of maximum

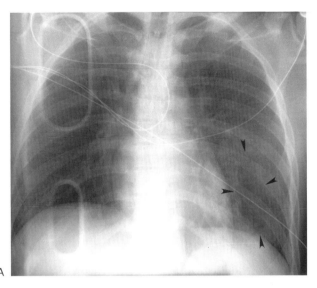

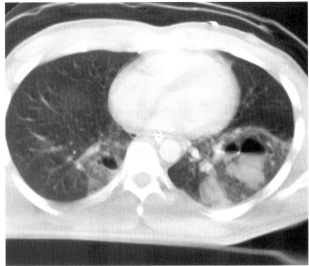

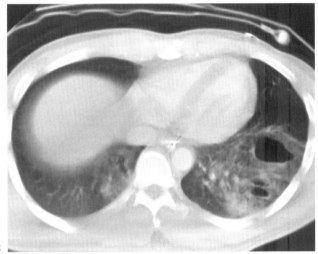

FIG. 9. Pulmonary lacerations following blunt chest trauma. **A:** Supine chest radiograph demonstrates subtle, focal air lucency (*arrowheads*) at the left lung base. **B, C:** CT images reveal multiple, bilateral lower lobe intraparenchymal cavities containing air–fluid levels. Surrounding parenchymal contusion is also evident.

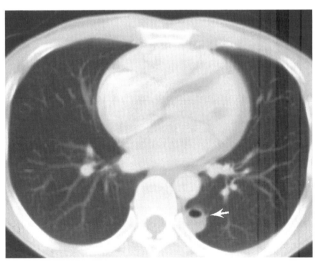

FIG. 10. Pulmonary laceration following fall from a height. CT image demonstrates intraparenchymal air–fluid level (*arrow*) within the basilar paravertebral lung.

aortic wall shear stress. Approximately 5% of tears involve the ascending aorta, usually just above the aortic valve (64,175,203,292). In autopsy series, the incidence of ascending aortic tears is higher (20% to 25%), reflecting the fact that tears of the ascending aorta are almost always immediately fatal (269,340). Death is usually due to associated cardiac injuries. Severe cardiac injuries such as myocardial contusion, aortic valve rupture, coronary artery laceration, and hemopericardium with cardiac tamponade are present in 75% of patients with ascending aortic laceration, compared to only 25% of patients with aortic isthmus laceration (269). Most victims of combined ascending aortic laceration and cardiac injury have been pedestrians, ejected passengers, or sufferers of falls, including airplane crashes and elevator accidents (128, 269,340). Injuries to the descending aorta from blunt trauma are rare. When laceration of the descending aorta does occur, it is usually at the level of the aortic hiatus where the distal descending aorta exits the thorax through the diaphragm (335). Multiple aortic tears occur in 6% to 19% of cases (128,269), and associated injury or avul-

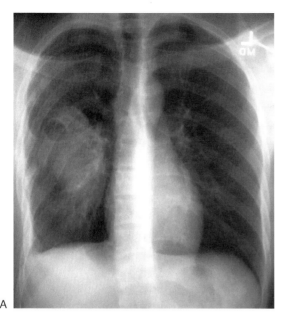 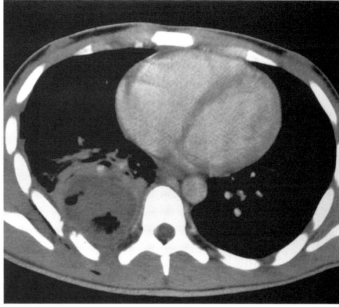

A   B

FIG. 11. Infected hematoma. **A:** Chest radiograph in febrile patient 3 weeks after rollover motor vehicle accident demonstrates multiple right rib fractures and a large, rounded opacity containing multiple locules of air in the right midlung field. **B:** CT image shows large intraparenchymal mass containing fluid and air compatible with an infected hematoma or lung abscess. A small amount of subcutaneous air is present in the right posterior chest wall.

sion of the brachiocephalic arteries has been reported in 4% of cases (101). Brachiocephalic injuries are often multiple, occurring much more commonly in association with other aortic or brachiocephalic lacerations than as single-artery insults (101).

Eighty to ninety percent of all patients with aortic laceration die at the scene of the accident or before they can be transported to a hospital and treated (269). For the remaining 10% to 20% who arrive at a hospital alive, expedient diagnosis and immediate surgical repair generally are essential to prevent exsanguinating hemorrhage at the site of the aortic tear. The importance of rapid diagnosis and treatment in this group of patients is underscored by the fact that survival rates ranging from 68% to 80% have been reported if timely surgical repair can be performed (44,53,175,179,298). It is estimated that without treatment <5% of patients survive. These are usually patients with only partial aortic transection in whom the pulsating hematoma is contained by the adventitia or the periaortic tissues (269).

Clinical findings in patients with traumatic aortic laceration are frequently absent, and the possibility of aortic injury is often initially raised solely on the basis of a history of trauma involving significant deceleration (i.e., high-speed motor vehicle accident). More than 50% of patients with aortic laceration may have no visible external signs of chest trauma. Furthermore, it may be impossible to elicit symptoms in a substantial number of these patients because of altered mental status due to concomitant head trauma (183). The most common complaint in

the immediate postinjury period is retrosternal or interscapular pain, thought to be due to mediastinal dissection of blood. Less frequently encountered signs and symptoms include dyspnea, dysphagia, upper extremity hypertension, lower extremity hypotension, and a harsh systolic murmur over the precordium or interscapular area (due to turbulent flow across the area of transection). Unfortunately, none of these clinical findings are sufficiently sensitive or specific to be considered diagnostic of aortic injury (175).

The diagnosis of aortic injury is usually suggested by findings on chest radiography and then confirmed by thoracic aortography. Radiographic findings suggestive of acute aortic trauma primarily reflect the presence of mediastinal hematoma and may include (a) widening of the superior mediastinum; (b) fullness, deformity, or obscuration of the aortic contour, particularly in the region of the aortic arch, isthmus, or aortopulmonary window; (c) deviation of the trachea or nasogastric tube in the esophagus to the right; (d) caudal displacement of the left main stem bronchus; (e) widening of the right paratracheal stripe; (f) widening of the paravertebral stripes; and (g) extrapleural extension of hemorrhage over the lung apex (apical cap) (228,318,343,379). Of these numerous findings, widening of the mediastinum with loss of the aortic contour is the most sensitive predictor of aortic injury, and the most frequent indication for aortography (10,133,183,304). Isolated fractures of the first and/or second ribs, once thought to indicate severe mediastinal trauma, do not correlate with aortic rupture and are not by themselves an indication for aortography in the absence of radiographic or CT evidence of mediastinal hematoma (102,191,378).

Although the chest radiograph has a high sensitivity for mediastinal hematoma, it is frequently falsely positive due to a variety of factors, including shallow inspiration, supine anteroposterior positioning, vascular ectasia, pulmonary disease adjacent to the mediastinum, and mediastinal fat. It is important to note that even when mediastinal hemorrhage is correctly diagnosed it is most commonly caused by disruption of small arteries and veins in the mediastinum rather than by aortic injury (6,263). Mediastinal hematoma may also result from nonaortic hemorrhage associated with other mediastinal injuries, such as tracheobronchial tears, or fractures of the lower cervical and upper thoracic spine (69). A completely normal chest radiograph is of greater diagnostic significance than an abnormal chest radiograph because it has a 98% negative predictive value for traumatic aortic or brachiocephalic artery rupture (212,229,377).

Aortography remains the definitive method of establishing the diagnosis of traumatic aortic laceration and of defining its anatomic extent. It is used liberally in trauma patients because the consequences of missing an aortic rupture are grave, the clinical findings are frequently absent, and the radiographic findings are nonspecific. Only 10% to 20% of patients with clinical and radiographic findings suggestive of aortic trauma have angiographic confirmation of an aortic tear (133,229,341). Angiographically, lacerations appear as sharply defined linear lucencies, produced by the infolded, torn edges of the intima.

Associated irregularity of the aortic wall and/or a false aneurysm may also be seen. Conventional aortography has been reported to have a 100% sensitivity and 99% specificity for the diagnosis of traumatic aortic injury, with a positive predictive value of 97% and a negative predictive value of 100% (341). Similar success rates have been achieved using intraarterial digital subtraction aortography, which in comparison to conventional aortography can reduce both the amount of time and the amount of intravascular contrast material needed to obtain a diagnostically accurate study (235).

The role of CT in the evaluation of patients with suspected injury of the aorta remains controversial. Some advocate the use of CT as an adjunct to chest radiography in determining the need for aortography (2,208,234, 249,277,282). Others have questioned the accuracy of CT findings and the validity of CT usage in this regard (224,368). It is generally agreed that patients who are clinically unstable or who have definite clinical or radiographic evidence of mediastinal injury require emergency aortography or direct surgical intervention. CT generally is performed only on hemodynamically stable patients with a low to moderate clinical suspicion of aortic tear, and in whom chest radiographic findings are equivocal (249). In such patients, CT can accurately exclude the presence of mediastinal hemorrhage or provide alternative explanations for equivocal radiographic findings, thus eliminating the need for aortography. Apparent mediastinal widening on chest radiographs, for example, may be shown on CT to represent excessive mediastinal fat (Fig. 12), paravertebral pleural effusion, atelectatic/contused

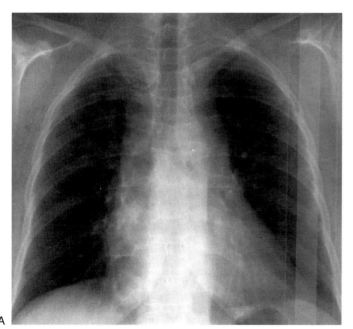
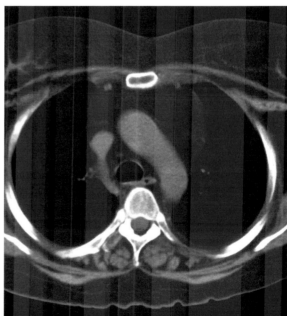

FIG. 12. Mediastinal lipomatosis. **A:** Chest radiograph demonstrates mediastinal widening in a 40-year-old woman following a motor vehicle accident. **B:** CT image at the level of the aortic arch demonstrates abundant mediastinal fat accounting for the mediastinal widening.

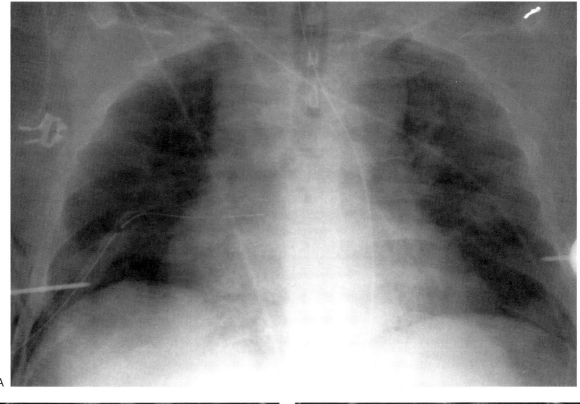

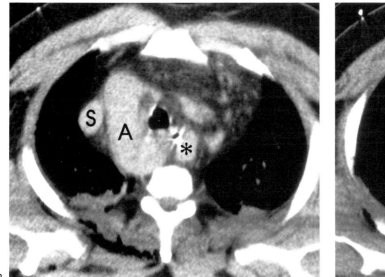

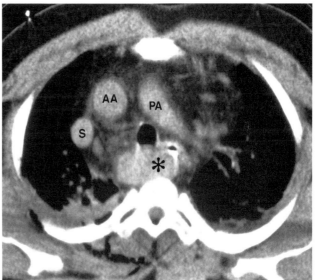

FIG. 13. Right aortic arch and aberrant left subclavian artery. **A:** Chest radiograph demonstrates mediastinal widening and right chest wall subcutaneous emphysema in a 37-year-old man following a fall from 30 feet. Endotracheal tube, nasogastric tube, and right chest tube are in place. **B, C:** CT images demonstrate anterior mediastinal fat and a right aortic arch (A) with aberrant left subclavian artery (*asterisk*) accounting for the mediastinal widening. The right aortic arch displaces the superior vena cava (S) laterally. The aberrant left subclavian artery originates from the posterior portion of the right aortic arch and courses posterior to the air-filled trachea and esophagus. High-attenuation streak artifact emanates from the nasogastric tube in the esophagus. Subcutaneous air is noted in the right posterior and lateral chest wall; (AA) ascending aorta; (PA) pulmonary artery.

lung adjacent to the mediastinum, vascular ectasia, or congenital vascular anomalies such as right aortic arch (Fig. 13), persistent left superior vena cava, or hemiazygous continuation of the inferior vena cava (293,330, 345,348). Chest CT has also been used as an ancillary screening modality for aortography in clinically stable patients requiring CT examination for another indication (e.g., evaluation of intracranial or abdominal trauma). In patients already undergoing abdominal CT examination, the limited additional CT sections required for the detection of mediastinal hematoma adds less than 10 min to the study and may eliminate the need for aortography (249,277). In a recent meta-analysis study evaluating the

cost effectiveness of using CT for triage of patients to aortography, the addition of dynamic chest CT in patients requiring CT for evaluation of other injuries following blunt trauma was found to be both medically effective and cost reducing (82,154).

Most studies to date suggest that an unequivocally normal chest CT reliably excludes aortic injury, with an overall false negative CT rate of approximately 1% (2,98, 100,208,224,234,249,277,282,369). False negative CT studies have been attributed to contained intimal and/or medial tears unassociated with mediastinal hemorrhage, or to technically suboptimal examinations degraded by motion artifact or inadequate contrast material administra-

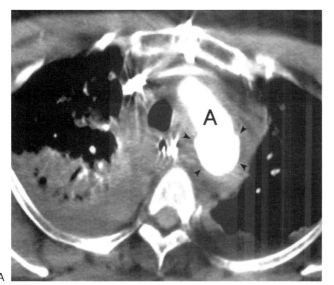

A

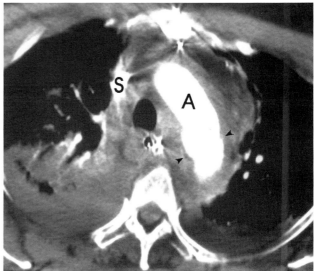

B

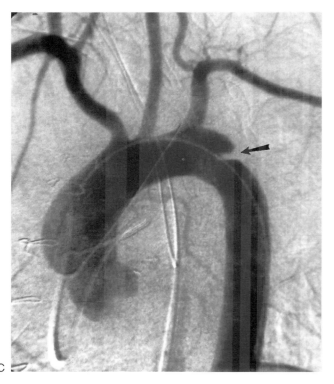

C

FIG. 14. Aortic laceration in 56-year-old woman involved in a motor vehicle accident. **A, B:** Contiguous 8-mm CT sections through the aortic arch (A) and proximal descending thoracic aorta demonstrate periaortic mediastinal hemorrhage and focal increase in caliber of the aortic lumen with marked irregularity of the aortic margins (*arrowheads*). Right lung contusion and small left pleural effusion are also evident. There is streak artifact from the nasogastric tube in the esophagus and from multiple median sternotomy suture wires; (S) superior vena cava. **C:** Angiography confirms the presence of aortic laceration (*arrow*) just distal to the origin of the left subclavian artery.

tion (249). By excluding mediastinal hemorrhage or providing alternative explanations for mediastinal widening, CT has been reported to reduce the need for aortography in selected trauma patients by 50% to 73% (156,208,234,249,277,282). A more recent study, however, reported that the "absolute exclusion" of mediastinal hemorrhage by CT was often difficult and resulted in only a 25% reduction in the use of aortography (100).

CT can demonstrate both direct and indirect (i.e., mediastinal hemorrhage) evidence of aortic injury. The presence of mediastinal hemorrhage on CT is an indication for aortography, even in the absence of direct signs of aortic injury (234,282). The mediastinal hemorrhage may be focal or diffuse and appears on CT as homogeneous areas of fluid within the mediastinum or as streaky tissue density fluid infiltrating the mediastinal fat (100,249,277) (Fig. 14). Difficulties in interpretation may arise due to confusion of mediastinal hemorrhage with thymic tissue in the anterior mediastinum, partial volume averaging of the pulmonary artery in the aortopulmonary window, periaortic atelectasis in the left lower lobe, or motion artifact producing haziness in the mediastinum (276,282,368). In-

terpretive errors may be minimized by obtaining 5-mm contrast-enhanced dynamic (249) or helical CT sections through the mediastinum. The majority of patients with CT evidence of mediastinal hemorrhage will not have angiographic evidence of an aortic tear (100,249,277, 282). As mentioned previously, mediastinal hemorrhage is merely a marker of significant mediastinal trauma and is not specific for aortic injury. Most commonly, the bleeding is from disruption of mediastinal veins and/or small arteries rather than from aortic rupture (6).

Direct CT findings of aortic injury include a false aneurysm and the presence of a linear lucency within the opacified aortic lumen caused by the torn edge of the aortic wall (Fig. 15). The false aneurysm may be focal or circumferential, and can be identified on CT as a saccular outpouching or increase in caliber of the aortic lumen compared to the more proximal normal aorta (139, 141,213) (Figs. 14 and 15). Direct assessment of aortic injury can be improved with the use of helical CT. In a recent large series using helical scanning exclusively to screen 1518 patients with blunt chest trauma, helical CT with overlapping reconstruction was found to be 100%

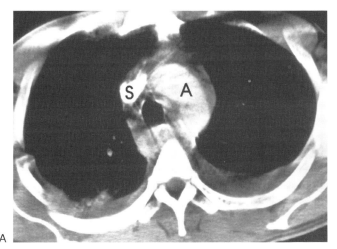
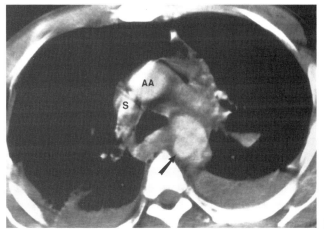
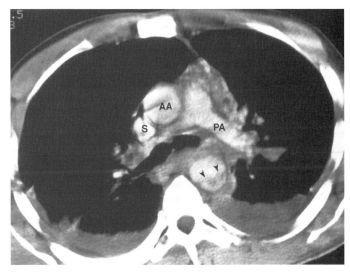

FIG. 15. Aortic laceration in young man involved in rollover MVA. **A–C:** CT images from the aortic arch (A) through the left pulmonary artery (PA) demonstrate a focal aortic pseudoaneurysm (*arrow*) with adjacent periaortic hemorrhage. Irregular linear lucency (*arrowheads*) within the opacified aortic lumen in C represents the torn edge of the aortic wall. There is considerable streak artifact in the ascending aorta (AA) and proximal aortic arch from high-density contrast material in the superior vena cava (S). Bilateral pleural effusions are also present.

sensitive and 81.7% specific in detecting aortic injury (109).

Although a small number of patients with mediastinal hemorrhage and direct CT evidence of aortic injury have undergone surgery without aortography, preoperative confirmatory aortography is usually performed (141,156). Less specific CT findings, such as marginal irregularity of the aortic wall or a periaortic hematoma, also generally warrant aortography (Fig. 16). It remains to be seen as to whether the use of newer CT techniques such as helical CT angiography or electron beam CT angiography can further improve the direct assessment of aortic injury, and possibly even replace transcatheter aortography (108, 276,299,353). Magnetic resonance imaging has not assumed a major role in the evaluation of acute traumatic aortic injury, primarily because it is relatively difficult to monitor trauma patients undergoing MR examination. Transesophageal echocardiography and intravascular ultrasound may be useful in selected cases of aortic trauma, but experience to date has been limited to a few case reports (30,308,367).

If the aorta is only partially transected following blunt trauma and the patient survives without recognition and treatment, a localized false (pseudo-) aneurysm may subsequently develop over a period of months to years. These lesions, which continue to communicate with the aortic lumen through the tear and tend to expand with time, are most commonly found immediately distal to the origin of the left subclavian artery, in the region of the aortic isthmus. They have been estimated to occur in 2% to 5% of patients with aortic injury and may be detected incidentally on plain chest radiography or because of symptoms related to their expansion (14,99,269). Contrary to the assessment of acute traumatic injury of the aorta, either CT or MRI usually is adequate for diagnostic confirmation of a chronic traumatic pseudoaneurysm suspected on plain chest radiography, and aortography is rarely required. On CT or MRI, a chronic traumatic pseudoaneurysm appears as saccular or fusiform dilatation of the aortic isthmus (Fig. 17). Peripheral calcification of the wall of the pseudoaneurysm may be seen on CT (41) (Fig. 18). Sagittal MR images have been reported to be helpful in defining the exact relationship of the pseudoaneurysm to the left subclavian artery and in determining the size of its communication to the aortic lumen (246). Because of the persistent risk of rupture of these posttraumatic aneurysms and their low operative mortality, elective surgical excision is generally recommended (14, 99,143).

Heart and Pericardium

Blunt chest trauma can result in a spectrum of cardiac injuries ranging in severity from inconsequential, asymptomatic lesions that are detectable only by serial electrocardiograms to rapidly fatal cardiac rupture. Acute heart injuries include contusion, transmural myocardial necrosis, and laceration or rupture of the pericardium, myocardium, septa, papillary muscles, cardiac valves, and coronary arteries (76,177,268). Although the exact incidence of cardiac injury from blunt chest trauma is unknown, autopsy series have demonstrated that >10% of highway fatalities have evidence of cardiac damage, and that in approximately 5%, the cardiac injury is lethal (261,327). In clinical series, estimates of cardiac injury as high as 76% have been reported among selected groups of severely injured patients (317).

Myocardial contusion represents the most common manifestation of cardiac trauma and has been reported to occur in 8% to 76% of patients following severe chest injury (147). It results in myocardial edema, hemorrhage, and necrosis, and an increase in the MB fraction of the enzyme creatine phosphokinase (CPK). Electrocardiogram (ECG) changes are similar to those of myocardial ischemia and infarction. Delayed onset of right ventricular contractions, localized wall motion abnormalities, and depressed ejection fraction on ECG-gated radionuclide blood pool scans has also been observed (192,289). The right ventricle is the most frequently injured because it makes up the majority of the exposed anterior surface of the heart directly behind the sternum. Clinically, myocardial contusion usually is well tolerated. However, the resultant myocardial damage can lead to functional cardiac abnormalities such as diminished cardiac output or acute cardiac arrhythmias in up to 20% of patients (150).

Cardiac dysfunction resulting from blunt trauma is frequently missed or detected late because the cardiac injury

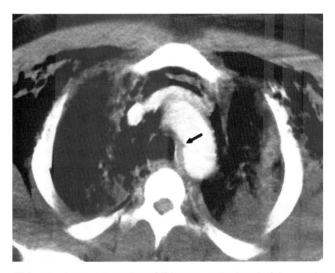

FIG. 16. Aortic laceration. CT image at the level of the aortic arch demonstrates marginal irregularity of the aortic wall (*arrow*) with adjacent periaortic hemorrhage. Subsequent angiography confirmed the presence of aortic laceration. Extensive pneumomediastinum and subcutaneous emphysema were from concomitant laceration of the proximal left main stem bronchus.

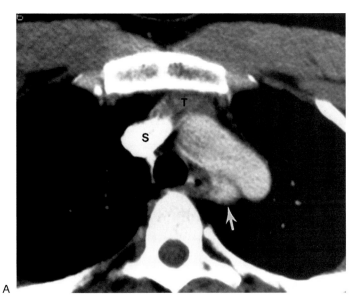

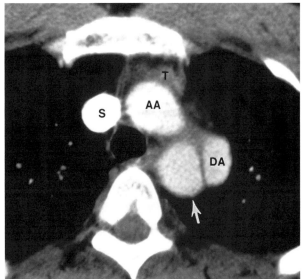

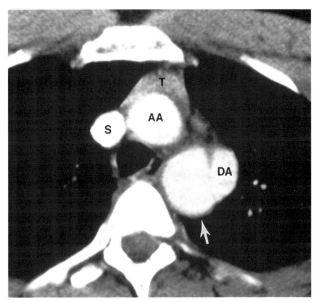

FIG. 17. Posttraumatic aortic pseudoaneurysm in a 21-year-old man approximately 2 years following MVA and repair of a ruptured left hemidiaphragm. **A–C:** CT images demonstrate a pseudoaneurysm (*arrow*) projecting medially from the proximal descending aorta (DA). The distal aortic arch and descending aorta are displaced superiorly and laterally by the pseudoaneurysm. The patient underwent successful surgical repair with placement of an aortic tube graft; (AA) ascending aorta; (S) superior vena cava; (T) thymus.

(e.g., contusion) is often masked by other more obvious multisystem injury and because routine tests such as ECGs and CPK isoenzyme determinations are nonspecific following severe trauma (21,289). Chest radiography and CT play only a minor role in the evaluation of myocardial injury. Radiographic findings may include evidence of congestive failure such as cardiac enlargement and pulmonary edema. The presence of anterior rib fractures and sternal fractures should increase clinical suspicion of myocardial injury, although there is no clear relationship between the extent of chest wall injury and the degree of underlying cardiac damage (239). Ventricular aneurysms may develop as a sequela of cardiac injury such as contusion or infarction, and can be detected on CT or conventional chest radiographs by a change in cardiac contour and by the presence of calcification within the wall of the aneurysm (125).

Acute hemopericardium can occur following injury to the heart or pericardium. CT is very sensitive for detecting pericardial space fluid and may indicate the presence of pericardial hemorrhage by the high CT attenuation (i.e., near soft tissue density) of the fluid (338) (Fig. 19). Small hemorrhagic pericardial effusions of no functional significance are sometimes seen as incidental findings on posttraumatic CT examinations. Rapid accumulation of blood in the pericardial space can lead to cardiac tamponade and severe hemodynamic compromise. The diagnosis of acute tamponade is usually established by the presence of clinical signs such as tachycardia, elevated central venous pressure, distended neck veins, muffled cardiac sounds, and diminished cardiac output. Emergency bedside sonographic evaluation of the heart can document the presence of pericardial effusion prior to prompt pericardiocentesis or pericardiotomy. CT findings of acute

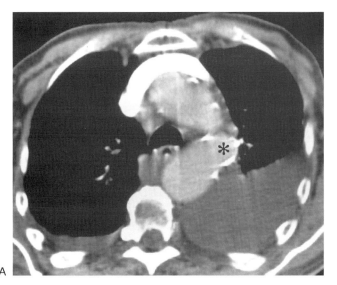
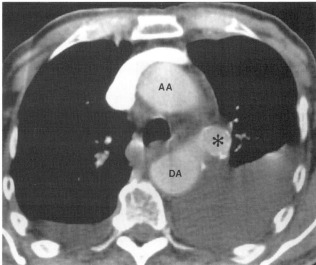

FIG. 18. Posttraumatic aortic pseudoaneurysm in a patient with a remote history of MVA requiring hospitalization. **A, B:** CT images demonstrate focal aortic pseudoaneurysm with peripheral calcification (*asterisk*). There are bilateral pleural effusions, left greater than right; (AA) ascending aorta; (DA) descending aorta.

tamponade following blunt trauma include hemorrhagic pericardial fluid, distended central veins (e.g., vena cavae, hepatic veins, renal veins), and periportal lymphedema in the liver (123).

Pneumopericardium is an uncommon manifestation of blunt chest trauma and is thought to result from dissection of air along perivascular and/or peribronchial sheaths into the pericardium. Air from ruptured alveoli, for example, can track along the adventitia of the pulmonary veins and enter the pericardial space (206,210). Moderately small amounts of pericardial air are generally of little clinical significance and may be detected incidentally on CT (Fig.

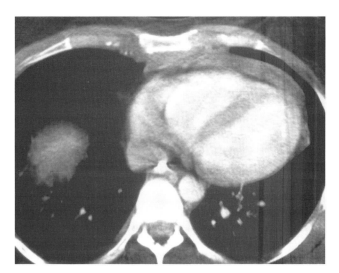

FIG. 19. Acute traumatic hemopericardium. CT image demonstrates high-attenuation anterior pericardial effusion consistent with pericardial hemorrhage.

20). Rarely, larger amounts of air can compress the heart and lead to the development of tension pneumopericardium. Radiographically this is manifest by a sudden, substantial decrease in size of the cardiac silhouette in the presence of pneumopericardium and clinical signs of cardiac tamponade (232). Prolonged positive airway pressure in combination with pulmonary contusion, pneumothorax, or tracheobronchial tear may increase the development of this complication.

Pericardial rupture is a rare sequela (<0.5%) of severe blunt chest trauma (106). Rupture may involve the diaphragmatic pericardium and/or the pleuropericardium, most commonly on the left. The diagnosis is usually made intraoperatively or at autopsy. Antemortem diagnosis may be suggested by chest radiographic or CT findings of herniation of air-containing abdominal viscera into the pericardium accompanying diaphragmatic rupture (239). Additional CT findings that have been reported in patients with traumatic pericardial rupture include pneumopericardium, posterolateral rotation of the cardiac apex, and extrusion of the heart through the pericardial tear (174).

Trachea and Bronchi

Tracheobronchial tear is an uncommon but serious complication of blunt chest trauma with an estimated overall mortality of 30% (176). Most tears involve the distal trachea (15%) or proximal main stem bronchi (80%) (372), with >80% of all tears occurring within 2.5 cm of the carina (176). The clinical and radiographic findings vary, depending on the site and extent of the tear. Complete tears of the right main stem and distal left main

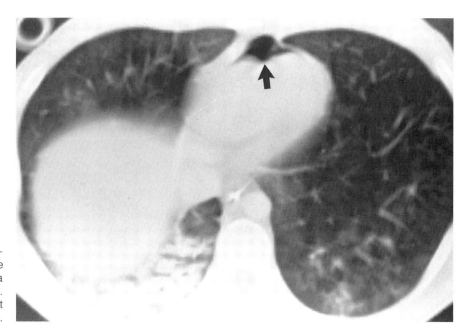

FIG. 20. Posttraumatic pneumopericardium. CT image at the level of the right hemidiaphragm demonstrates a small amount of pericardial air (*arrow*). Parenchymal contusion is evident at both lung bases, right greater than left.

stem bronchi generally manifest as pneumothorax. The pneumothorax tends to be large and unrelieved by chest tube drainage. Tears of the trachea and proximal left main stem bronchus usually result in pneumomediastinum. The pneumomediastinum is often severe, persistent, and progressive, with widespread dissection of air into the neck and subcutaneous tissues. Incomplete tracheobronchial tears with intact peritracheal and peribronchial adventitia may not be associated with pneumothorax, pneumomediastinum, or other radiographic findings. This is because the integrity of the airway is initially maintained, preventing passage of air into the mediastinum or pleura. Such partial tears may remain occult until subsequent high-pressure mechanical ventilation causes mediastinal emphysema or delayed massive pneumothorax (129).

Although the findings of tracheobronchial tear are sometimes subtle and overshadowed by other injuries, the diagnosis is usually suggested by the presence of dyspnea, persistent pneumothorax or air leak following chest tube drainage, and massive or rapidly increasing mediastinal or subcutaneous emphysema (148). Abnormalities in position and configuration of an endotracheal tube, including overdistention of the balloon cuff or extraluminal position of the tip, may be seen in patients with tracheal rupture (288,357). In complete bronchial tear with associated pneumothorax, the collapsed lung may fall away from the hilum toward the most dependent portion of the hemithorax, giving rise to the so-called falling lung sign (184,258) (Fig. 21). This is the reverse of the usual finding in uncomplicated pneumothorax, where the lung is tethered by the hilum and collapses toward it. The disrupted bronchus may be deformed (i.e., sharply angulated) and/or obstructed. Both the presence of the falling lung sign and endotracheal tube abnormalities such as an overdistended

balloon cuff are considered reliable though uncommon indicators of airway injury (357).

Computed tomography can diagnose tracheal tears in patients with indwelling endotracheal tubes by demonstrating extraluminal tip position or by showing an overdistended balloon protruding through the tracheal tear into the mediastinum (344). The actual rent in the tracheal wall may be seen even in the absence of endotracheal tube abnormality (264). Associated mediastinal and subcutaneous emphysema are also well depicted on CT. Bronchial rupture has been recognized on CT by abrupt tapering of the injured bronchus, coupled with shift of the mediastinum toward the compromised lung and retraction of the trachea in the opposite direction (364). Although CT is capable of demonstrating tracheobronchial injury, the standard chest radiograph and appropriate clinical findings are usually enough to suggest urgent bronchoscopy, which generally is required for definitive diagnosis prior to surgery (125). In a few select cases of tracheal rupture, diagnostic findings on CT examination have led to immediate surgical repair without bronchoscopy (344).

Esophagus

Injury to the esophagus from blunt chest trauma is extremely uncommon. When it does occur, it is usually secondary to severe chest and/or abdominal compression and is frequently associated with other thoracic injuries such as aortic rupture and cardiac contusion (358). Proposed mechanisms of esophageal injury in blunt trauma include sudden elevation in esophageal hydrostatic pressure, crushing of the esophagus between the spine and

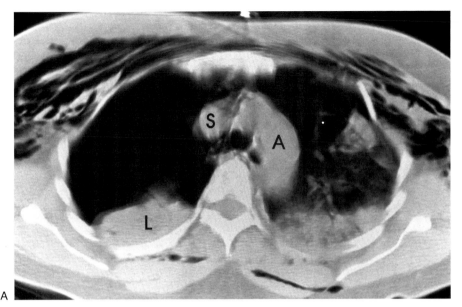

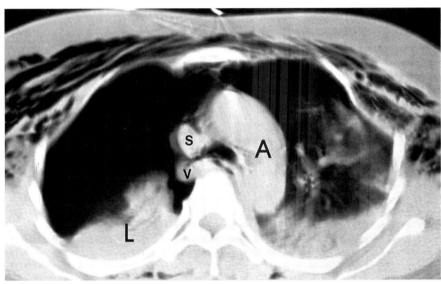

FIG. 21. Traumatic rupture of the right main stem bronchus. **A, B:** CT images at the level of the aortic arch (A) demonstrate bilateral pneumothoraces, pneumomediastinum, and extensive subcutaneous emphysema. The collapsed right lung (L) has fallen away from the hilum toward the most dependent portion of the hemithorax. Patchy areas of parenchymal contusion are noted in the left lung; (S) superior vena cava; (V) azygous vein arch. (Case courtesy of Paul Barry, M.D., Greensboro, North Carolina)

trachea, tearing due to hyperextension (particularly at the level of the diaphragmatic hiatus), and direct penetration by cervical spine fracture fragments (236). Other causes of esophageal injury in the acute trauma setting include inadvertent esophageal intubation or traumatic nasogastric tube placement. The vast majority of traumatic esophageal perforations are caused by iatrogenic interventions such as endoscopy, tube placement, or esophageal dilatation (125).

Radiologic manifestations of esophageal rupture include pneumomediastinum, cervical emphysema, pneumothorax, pleural effusion, and an abnormal mediastinal contour resulting from hemorrhage or leakage of gastroesophageal contents into the mediastinum. Early recognition and prompt medical and surgical intervention is critical, as esophageal rupture may rapidly progress to fulminant mediastinitis and septic shock (380). If there is associated rupture of the mediastinal pleura, acute empy-

ema may also develop (130). Occasionally, a tracheoesophageal fistula develops either from the initial trauma or as a sequela of the acute mediastinitis. In such cases, the fistula may protect against mediastinal abscess formation by providing a route of drainage for esophageal contents (380). Contrast esophagography is >90% sensitive in the diagnosis of esophageal rupture, and is the procedure of choice for establishing its presence and extent (20). Esophagoscopy has similar diagnostic sensitivity and may provide complementary diagnostic information in select cases (236).

Computed tomographic scanning has been reported to be useful in suggesting the diagnosis of esophageal perforation in patients with atypical or confusing clinical signs and symptoms (8,365). CT findings indicative of esophageal perforation include esophageal thickening, periesophageal fluid, extraluminal air, and pleural effusion (Fig. 22). Identification of extraesophageal air is the most

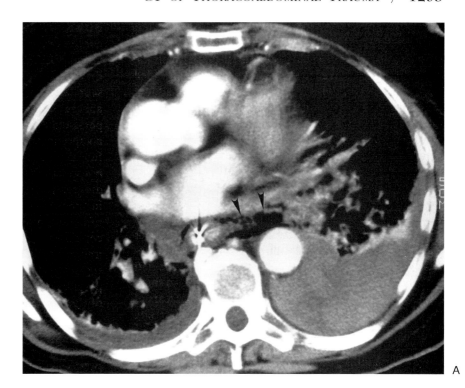

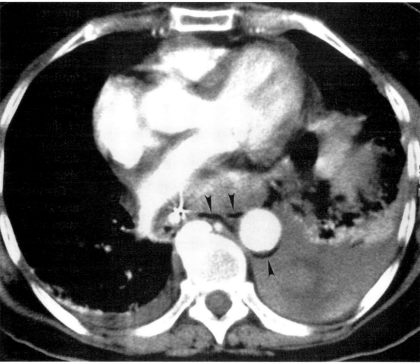

FIG. 22. Esophageal rupture. **A, B:** CT images demonstrate a thick-walled distal esophagus and periesophageal mediastinal air (*arrowheads*) tracking into the left pleural space. The left pleural effusion is heterogeneous and high in attenuation (40 to 50 HU), consistent with leakage of gastroesophageal contents. Small, low-attenuation (10 HU) right pleural effusion is also present. There is considerable streak artifact from a nasogastric tube in the distal esophagus.

useful finding and is demonstrated on CT with greater sensitivity than on plain chest radiographs (365). In some cases, leakage of oral contrast material from the disrupted esophagus into the mediastinum or pleural space may be seen (239). CT is also useful for defining extraluminal manifestations of esophageal rupture such as mediastinitis, mediastinal abscess, and empyema (365). Such information often has important implications for medical and/or surgical management.

Diaphragm

Diaphragmatic rupture occurs in approximately 5% of patients who have experienced major blunt trauma (222), and 65% to 85% of diaphragmatic ruptures are on the left side (169,222,248,287,366). Left-sided injury predominates because of the protective effect of the liver on the right hemidiaphragm and/or underdiagnosis of right-sided injuries (81,144). Proposed mechanisms of injury in blunt diaphragmatic rupture include shearing of a stretched membrane, avulsion of the diaphragm from its points of attachment, and abrupt increase in transdiaphragmatic pressure following severe compression of the upper abdomen and lower thorax (169). Injury can also result from direct laceration of the diaphragm by fractures of the lower thoracic ribs. The diaphragm most frequently ruptures in the area of the central tendon or at its transition to the muscular portion of the diaphragm. The posterior and posterolateral diaphragmatic segments are most commonly involved (300,335). With laceration of the left hemidiaphragm, the omentum, stomach, spleen, and small and large bowel can herniate into the thorax. With tears of the right hemidiaphragm, the liver is usually the offending organ.

Diaphragmatic rupture is often unrecognized at the time of trauma because of lack of early herniation of abdominal organs into the thorax and because the diaphragmatic injury is often obscured or overshadowed by other associated injuries. Diaphragmatic rupture rarely occurs in isolation, and a high percentage of patients sustain serious concomitant intraabdominal (59%) or intrathoracic (45%) injuries (248). In the absence of characteristic clinical signs and radiologic findings at the time of injury, the correct initial diagnosis may be made in <50% of cases. The diagnosis is most readily made when the injury is recent and the tear is large and left-sided with herniation of hollow abdominal organs. If the trauma is remote or unknown and the tear is right-sided with herniation of solid organs such as the liver, the diagnosis is less likely to be made (9). Not uncommonly, recognition of diaphragmatic tears may be delayed for hours to years, allowing time for progressive herniation of abdominal contents into the thorax. Such tears may only be discovered when the patient presents with complications of post-traumatic herniation such as intestinal obstruction, visceral strangulation, and respiratory impairment (56,61, 127,138). Delayed presentation of diaphragmatic rupture with visceral herniation and strangulation is associated with higher morbidity and mortality (30%) than when the diagnosis is made and managed acutely (56,335).

The diagnosis of diaphragmatic rupture is usually suggested on the basis of abnormalities on chest radiography or is made incidentally at the time of an exploratory laparotomy (131). Diagnostic or strongly suggestive radiographic findings include the presence of air-filled viscera (i.e., stomach, bowel) or the tip of a nasogastric tube above the diaphragm. The nasogastric tube may be seen to extend inferiorly below the normal gastroesophageal junction and then form an upward curve into herniated gastric fundus within the left hemithorax (272). Other abnormalities suggestive but not diagnostic of diaphragmatic injury are more commonly seen and include an indistinct or elevated hemidiaphragm, an irregular or lumpy diaphragm contour, a persistent basilar opacity that resembles atelectasis or a supradiaphragmatic mass, an unexplained pleural effusion, and fractures of the lower ribs (4,113,225). The nonspecificity of these findings results in the chest radiograph being inconclusive for diaphragmatic injury in most cases. Diaphragmatic rupture with herniation of abdominal contents can be mimicked or masked by concurrent pulmonary abnormalities such as multiple traumatic lung cysts, lower lobe contusion and/or atelectasis, pleural effusion, loculated hemopneumothorax, phrenic nerve paresis, and total or partial eventration of the hemidiaphragm (113,239).

Computed tomography has been used to diagnose diaphragmatic rupture in patients with equivocal chest radiographs. A recent study reported that CT is highly specific (87%) in diagnosing diaphragmatic rupture and that it detects approximately two thirds of acute diaphragmatic ruptures after blunt trauma (251). On transverse CT images, the diaphragm appears as a thin, curvilinear structure of soft tissue density outlined centrally by subdiaphragmatic fat and peripherally by lung. The posterolateral portions of the diaphragm are usually best demonstrated and tears at those sites are readily detected. Tears involving the dome of the diaphragm or portions of the diaphragm in contact with structures of similar density such as the liver, spleen, and stomach are more difficult to detect, unless there is associated herniation of abdominal contents (140).

Computed tomographic findings of diaphragmatic rupture include abrupt discontinuity of the diaphragm, herniation of abdominal viscera or fat into the thorax, and focal constriction of the stomach or bowel at the site of herniation (67,134,140,381) (Fig. 23). A large gap between the torn ends of the diaphragm may be seen, giving rise to the "absent diaphragm sign" (252). A diagnosis of herniation is indicated by the presence of abdominal viscera and/or fat posterior-lateral (i.e., peripheral) to the diaphragm and thus within the thoracic cavity. On occasion, CT can demonstrate diaphragmatic disruption before visceral herniation, leading to early surgical intervention and averting the potentially life-threatening complications of an undiagnosed herniation (146). In patients with suboptimal diaphragmatic visualization or equivocal findings of diaphragmatic rupture, use of thin-section CT (e.g., 3 to 5 mm) may help improve diagnostic accuracy (146,381) (Fig. 24). Accuracy may be further improved by the performance of coronal and sagittal reformations using helical CT (28,157) (Fig. 24). In a small number of patients, direct coronal and sagittal MRI has also been

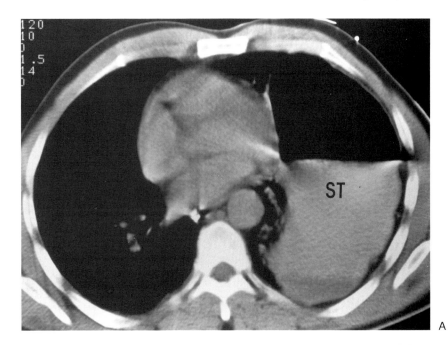

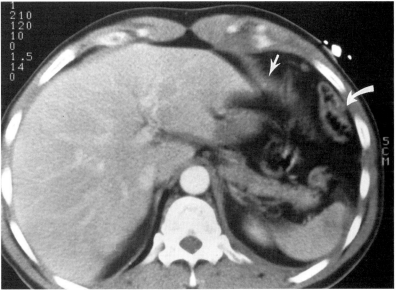

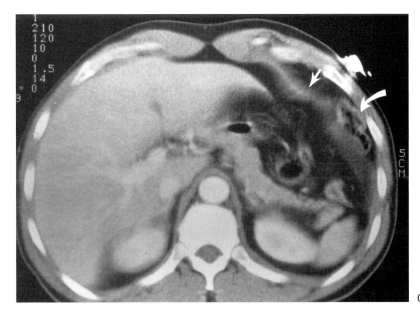

FIG. 23. Diaphragmatic rupture. **A:** CT image at the level of the heart demonstrates an air–contrast level within stomach (ST) which is herniated into the thorax. **B, C:** CT images more caudally demonstrate thickened, disrupted left hemidiaphragm (*straight arrow*) with herniated intraabdominal fat and descending colon (*curved arrow*) located lateral to the diaphragm.

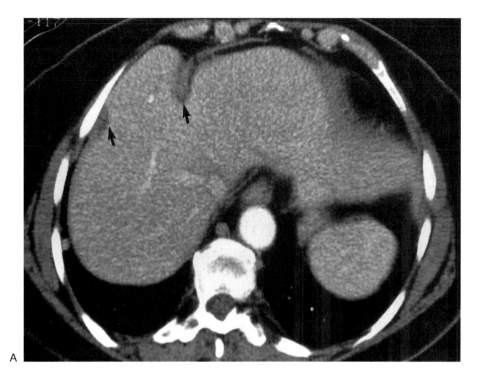

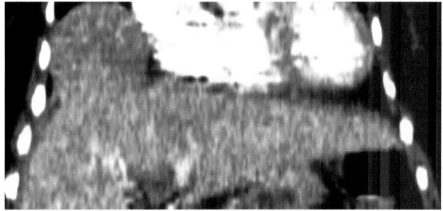

FIG. 24. Diaphragmatic rupture. **A:** A 5-mm helical CT section demonstrates herniation of a portion of the right lobe of the liver through the diaphragmatic defect (*arrows*). Small, incidental pulmonary nodule is noted in the right posterolateral lung base. **B:** Coronal reformation demonstrates herniated liver in the right lower chest.

performed to demonstrate traumatic diaphragmatic rupture (23,233).

BLUNT ABDOMINAL TRAUMA

Trauma to the abdomen accounts for approximately 10% of the traumatic deaths that occur annually in the United States (152). Most civilian abdominal injuries are caused by blunt trauma secondary to high-speed motor vehicle accidents, although penetrating injuries are common in urban settings. Mortality rates are generally higher in patients sustaining blunt trauma than in those with penetrating wounds (313). Solid abdominal organs are most frequently injured from blunt trauma, as the sudden application of pressure to the abdomen is more likely to rupture a solid organ than a hollow viscus. Rapid acceleration-deceleration of abdominal viscera at the time

of impact generates shearing forces that result in transection or laceration of the underlying parenchyma and vessels, most commonly at points of relative fixation or attachment (e.g., along the ligamentum teres of the liver) (152). Prompt recognition and management of bleeding from intraabdominal organs is essential to minimize morbidity and mortality.

Computed tomography has become an integral part of the clinical evaluation and management of patients with blunt abdominal trauma. It has been shown to be highly sensitive, specific, and accurate in detecting the presence and extent of injury to the abdomen in acutely traumatized patients (3,94,95,271,370). CT also often provides important additional information regarding associated extraabdominal injuries (e.g., pulmonary contusion, pneumothorax, fractures of the thoracolumbar spine and pelvis) (216). The use of CT in the evaluation of patients with blunt abdominal trauma, along with a general trend toward more conservative management of abdominal injuries, has decreased the need for exploratory surgery and reduced the frequency of nontherapeutic laparotomies (94,95,216,370). The overall trend toward nonoperative management of abdominal trauma is due in part to the ability of CT not only to define injury but to exclude significant injury, thereby avoiding unnecessary surgery (95,216,373).

Indications

Computed tomography is indicated in hemodynamically stable patients with signs, symptoms, or history of severe abdominal trauma requiring further diagnostic assessment (94). Particularly suitable candidates for CT scanning include alert patients with localizing symptoms or signs, or patients with laboratory findings suggesting intraabdominal injury (e.g., decreasing hematocrit, leukocytosis, elevated serum amylase). CT is also performed in patients in whom clinical abdominal examination is either equivocal or unreliable, often due to altered mental status from concomitant head injury, drug abuse, or ethanol intoxication (94,271).

Computed tomography generally is not performed in hemodynamically unstable patients or in patients with overt, life-threatening neurologic, thoracic, or abdominal injury (90,111). Patients who manifest such injuries or who are unstable usually require immediate surgery.

The use of CT in the evaluation of blunt abdominal trauma has replaced the use of other abdominal imaging methods, including radionuclide scanning, angiography, and sonography. CT has also replaced diagnostic peritoneal lavage (DPL) for the initial evaluation of suspected abdominal injury in hemodynamically stable patients (370, 373). CT has several significant advantages in comparison to DPL. First, it can more precisely define the location and extent of organ injury. Second, CT can assess both intraperitoneal and retroperitoneal injury, and third, CT is noninvasive. In addition, CT often is able to provide valuable information regarding associated extraabdominal injury (i.e., skeletal fractures, pulmonary contusion, pneumothorax) (111,122). DPL is now essentially performed only in patients who are too unstable to have abdominal CT evaluation or who are undergoing emergent extraabdominal surgery (370). In the latter group, DPL may be performed either immediately before or during surgery to help determine the need for laparotomy (111,373). Limited four-quadrant abdominal ultrasound looking for intraperitoneal fluid has recently been proposed as a screening test in blunt abdominal trauma patients. Unfortunately, it suffers from many of the same drawbacks as DPL. Although it is noninvasive, it lacks the capability for assessment of the retroperitoneum, and with it injury to the pancreas, duodenum, and kidneys. It also is of limited value in defining the location and extent of intraperitoneal

injury. Thus, patients with significant abdominal trauma are best evaluated by rapid, efficient CT examination.

Technique

Close attention to proper patient preparation and scanning technique is critical to accurate abdominal CT examination in patients with blunt abdominal trauma. To opacify the bowel so that it is not mistaken for localized hematoma or fluid collection, dilute (1% to 2%), water-soluble contrast material is administered orally or via a nasogastric tube prior to CT scanning. Bowel leaks related to bowel perforation also can then be identified. Use of dilute (1% to 2%), water-soluble contrast material minimizes streak artifacts produced by more concentrated solutions and eliminates the risk of barium spillage into the peritoneal cavity. If a nasogastric tube is present, it should first be used to decompress the stomach of gas and fluid contents prior to installation of the water-soluble contrast material. This helps minimize streak artifact produced by the gastric air–fluid level. The nasogastric tube should then be withdrawn into the distal esophagus prior to scanning to avoid artifact from the radiopaque markers used in most tubes (89).

All extraneous objects such as ECG leads, intravenous lines, and other monitoring or support apparatus should be repositioned out of the scanning field whenever possible because the streak artifacts they produce degrade image quality and may simulate or obscure traumatic lesions (89). The patient's arms should be placed over the chest or above the head. If this cannot be done, then the arms should be positioned next to the trunk because allowing an air gap to remain between the arm and the body causes worse artifact than securing the limb against the abdomen (111). If the arms must remain over the abdomen, a larger scanning field of view may be utilized to decrease artifact (91).

Posttraumatic abdominal CT examinations should be performed utilizing intravenous contrast material, unless contraindicated by known major contrast allergy or severe renal insufficiency. Intravenous infusion of contrast material maximizes the difference between contrast-enhancing parenchyma and nonenhancing hematomas and lacerations (89) (Fig. 25). It also aids in detection of extravasation of contrast-opacified urine (89) and in visualization of sites of active arterial hemorrhage (159,307). Some have suggested performing non-contrast-enhanced CT in addition to contrast-enhanced CT in order to visualize hematomas that may become isodense after intravenous contrast administration (171). In one study addressing the value of non-contrast-enhanced CT in blunt abdominal trauma, such hematomas were generally found to be small and inconsequential (171). As contrast-enhanced scanning alone accurately depicts the vast majority of clinically significant injuries, most authors do not perform a preliminary noncontrast examination (226,373).

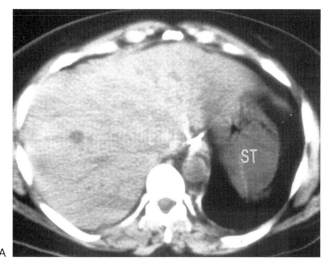 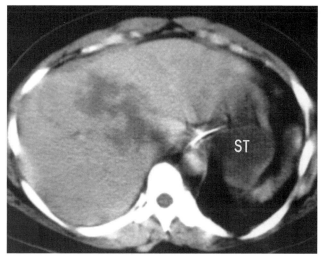

A

B

FIG. 25. Liver laceration prior to (**A**) and during the administration of intravenous contrast material (**B**). Bolus intravenous administration of contrast material markedly improves the conspicuity of liver lacerations by increasing the difference in attenuation between normal contrast-enhancing parenchyma and nonenhancing lacerations. Streak artifact is noted from the nasogastric tube coursing into the stomach (ST).

Intravenous contrast material is preferably administered with a power injector via a large-bore peripheral venous line or central venous catheter. A total of approximately 150 ml of contrast material can be given intravenously as an initial bolus of 50 to 75 ml at a rate of 2 to 3 ml/sec, followed by rapid infusion of the remaining contrast material at 1 ml/sec. Alternatively, the contrast material may be administered as a single sustained bolus at a rate of 2 to 4 ml/sec. Dynamic or helical scanning at the rate of six or more scans per minute should be initiated 60 to 70 sec after the start of contrast infusion. With helical scanning, motion artifacts are minimized, as data acquisition can be rapidly completed in less than 1 min of scanning time. Contiguous 1-cm CT sections are obtained from the dome of the diaphragm to the pubic symphysis. The entire pelvis is scanned in order to assess the presence and extent of hemoperitoneum (90). More narrowly collimated, contiguous images may be obtained through the pelvis if there is particular concern about bladder injury or pelvic fractures.

Patients are closely monitored throughout the examination, and adequate equipment and personnel for emergency resuscitation should be readily available. Ideally, the CT scanning area should be located as near as possible to the trauma room to allow rapid transport to and from the scanner. The CT images are all printed at standard soft tissue windows (level 40 HU, width 350 HU). Lung windows (level −500 to −600 HU, width 1500 to 2000 HU) are printed of all sections that include lung to evaluate the lower chest/upper abdomen for pneumothorax, parenchymal lung injury, or free peritoneal air indicating hollow viscus injury. When pelvic or spine fractures are suspected, images should be printed at bone windows (level 400 HU, width 1500 HU) as well. It is also useful

to adjust window and level settings of the images directly on the console video monitor to enhance detection of subtle but potentially significant findings (373). At the conclusion of the study, oral contrast material can be withdrawn from the stomach via nasogastric suction so as to minimize the risk of aspiration, particularly in obtunded patients or in those patients likely to undergo surgery (91).

Hemoperitoneum

Hemoperitoneum is a common result of blunt abdominal trauma, and its identification on CT should prompt a thorough search for injury to visceral organs. At times, small quantities of hemoperitoneum may be the only sign of subtle or occult visceral injury, particularly those involving the bowel or mesentery (230,373). CT is highly sensitive and specific for diagnosing hemoperitoneum (97), which initially tends to collect near the source of bleeding and then spills over into more dependent portions of the peritoneal cavity. Morison's pouch, the most dependent peritoneal recess in the upper abdomen, is the most common site of blood collection seen on CT in upper abdominal trauma (89) (Fig. 26). Blood in Morison's pouch (also known as the hepatorenal fossa or posterior subhepatic space) was seen in 97% of cases of hepatic and splenic lacerations in one large series (97). Other common sites of blood accumulation include the perihepatic (right subphrenic) and perisplenic (left subphrenic) spaces, the paracolic gutters (peritoneal recesses lateral to the ascending and descending colon), and the pelvis, particularly adjacent to the urinary bladder. Blood from any intraabdominal source typically flows

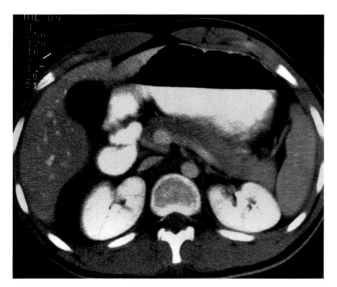

FIG. 26. Hemoperitoneum. Blood is present in Morison's pouch (*asterisk*), the most dependent peritoneal recess in the upper abdomen. Note that the acute hemoperitoneum appears relatively low in attenuation compared with the attenuation of enhanced liver and renal parenchyma.

down along the root of the mesentery and the right paracolic gutter into the pelvis (223). With extensive hemorrhage, large collections of blood may fill the pelvis, even when relatively little blood is seen in the paracolic gutters or other upper abdominal sites (97) (Fig. 27); this is because the pelvis is the most dependent portion of the peritoneal cavity and contains up to one third of its volume. It is important, therefore, that the entire pelvis be scanned in patients following blunt abdominal trauma in order to accurately assess the presence and extent of hemoperitoneum (89).

The CT appearance of blood in the peritoneal cavity is variable and depends on the location, age, and physical state (clotted versus lysed) of extravasated blood. Immediately after hemorrhage, intraperitoneal blood has the same attenuation as circulating blood, but within hours its attenuation increases as hemoglobin is concentrated during clot formation (16,254,256). Clotted blood usually measures between 50 and 75 HU attenuation, whereas lysed blood flowing freely within the peritoneal cavity has attenuation values generally ranging from 30 to 45 HU. Densely clotted blood may have attenuation values of greater than 100 HU (91). Clots within the peritoneal cavity tend to lyse rapidly due to repetitive respiratory motion and adjacent bowel peristalsis, whereas clots within solid viscera such as the liver remain intact for longer periods (97). In most cases, the attenuation value of blood begins to decrease within several days as clot lysis takes place (16). The attenuation value continues to decrease steadily with time and often approaches that of water (0 to 20 HU) after 2 to 3 weeks (181).

Acute hemoperitoneum may be low attenuation (<30 HU) in patients with severe anemia or in patients who have undergone peritoneal lavage prior to CT scanning (230). Other factors that may cause low attenuation values for posttraumatic fluid collections include CT scanner miscalibration, volume averaging of peritoneal fat adjacent to fluid, and a delay between trauma and CT scanning of 24 to 48 hr or more. The problem of volume averaging can be minimized by placing the region of interest (ROI) cursor in the center of each fluid collection measured and by making certain that fluid appears on CT images above and below the area measured whenever possible. Beam-hardening artifacts also may artificially lower attenuation values, particularly of pelvic fluid collections located between the dense bones of the lower pelvis (195). In a recent study of 42 consecutive patients with hepatic or splenic lacerations and intraperitoneal fluid after blunt abdominal trauma, low attenuation measurements (<20 HU) for acute hemoperitoneum represented a common finding that was not attributable to technical factors or underlying anemia (195). The authors suggested that low-attenuation acute hemoperitoneum may be explained by hemoperitoneum-induced peritonitis resulting in sufficient peritoneal transudation to dilute acute hemoperitoneum to attenuation values similar to those of simple fluid. It is also important to note that acute hemoperitoneum often appears relatively low in attenuation compared with the attenuation of enhanced liver or spleen (70 to 80 HU) following bolus administration of intravenous contrast material (111) (see Fig. 26).

Recent intraperitoneal hemorrhage can exhibit a variety of morphologic features. The fluid collection may be homogeneously hyperdense or it may be inhomogeneous, with linear or nodular areas of high attenuation intermixed with

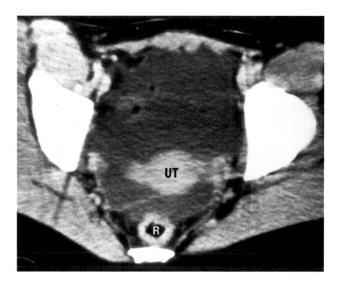

FIG. 27. Hemoperitoneum secondary to hepatic laceration. CT image through the lower pelvis demonstrates a large amount of blood pooling in the pelvis. If CT sections through the pelvis had not been obtained, the extent of hemoperitoneum would have been seriously underestimated; (UT) uterus; (R) rectum.

lower attenuation fluid. The inhomogeneity may result from irregular clot resorption or intermittent bleeding leading to repeated episodes of clot formation and retraction (375). Occasionally, fresh blood within a hematoma or confined within a peritoneal space may demonstrate a hematocrit effect, with layering of serous fluid on dependent, sedimented erythrocytes and clot (97) (Fig. 28). More frequently, a localized collection of highattenuation clotted blood, referred to as the sentinel clot, is seen in close proximity to a site of visceral injury (260) (Fig. 29). The sentinel clot is a sensitive sign of visceral injury, and it may be the only sign indicating the source of peritoneal hemorrhage in a significant percentage of cases. When present, it should prompt careful examination of the adjacent viscera for subtle or occult injury. In some patients, especially those with small capsular lacerations, the localized perivisceral hematoma may be more evident than the underlying intraparenchymal hematoma or laceration (97). As such, the sentinel clot sign has been noted to be particularly useful in the diagnosis of subtle bowel, mesenteric, and splenic injuries (111,260,373).

It must be remembered that the presence of hemoperitoneum on CT does not necessarily indicate that active hemorrhage is present. Rather, the quantity of hemoperitoneum on a single CT study merely reflects the amount of blood lost since the time of injury (230). Serial CT evaluation of hemoperitoneum may be useful in documenting resolution or in detecting new hemorrhage (104). Hemoperitoneum should resolve significantly in most cases by 1 week after injury. Persistence of hemoperitoneum without change for 3 to 7 days after injury suggests continued intraperitoneal bleeding, even though the pa-

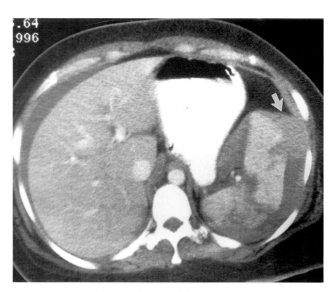

FIG. 29. Splenic lacerations with hemoperitoneum and sentinel clot. Contrast-enhanced CT image demonstrates multiple splenic lacerations and high-attenuation clotted blood, or so-called sentinel clot (*arrow*), along the anterolateral margin of the spleen. Lower attenuation lysed blood is also present in the perisplenic and perihepatic spaces.

tient may remain hemodynamically stable (104). Occasionally, active arterial hemorrhage can be identified on dynamic contrast-enhanced CT as focal or diffuse high-attenuation areas of extravasated contrast-enhanced blood (159,307) (Fig. 30). The areas of extravasation range in

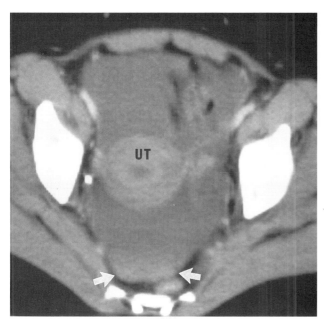

FIG. 28. Hemoperitoneum with hematocrit effect. CT scan through the lower pelvis demonstrates a large amount of blood filling the pelvis. Note hematocrit effect with blood elements layering dependently (*arrows*); (UT) uterus.

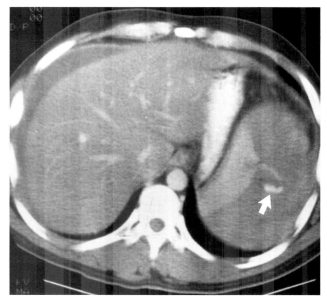

FIG. 30. Active arterial hemorrhage. Dynamic contrast-enhanced CT scan demonstrates a high-attenuation focus of extravasated contrast-enhanced blood (*arrow*) originating from the spleen. The area of active hemorrhage is surrounded by a large perisplenic hematoma which is lower in attenuation than the extravasated contrast material. Perihepatic blood is also evident.

attenuation from 80 to 370 HU (higher attenuation than free or clotted blood), and typically are isodense or hyperdense to the abdominal aorta and adjacent major arteries. Most commonly, the areas of extravasation are surrounded by a large hematoma that is lower in attenuation than the extravasated contrast material. In patients with significant blood loss resulting in hypovolemia, several CT signs may be seen. These include a small, constricted aorta (311), a flattened or collapsed inferior vena cava (160), and abnormally intense contrast enhancement of the bowel wall and kidneys (323).

Specific Trauma Sites

Spleen

The spleen is the most commonly injured abdominal organ (26,285, 355). Injury can occur as a result of blunt or penetrating abdominal trauma. Iatrogenic splenic injury has been reported as a result of intraoperative manipula-

tion, as well as following colonoscopy, thoracentesis, or renal biopsy (126,197,279).

Computed tomography is the modality of choice for evaluation of splenic injury. Its sensitivity and specificity are both high in the setting of blunt abdominal trauma (96,355). Administration of intravenous contrast material is needed for adequate evaluation of splenic trauma, as areas of hematoma and laceration are frequently isodense to splenic parenchyma on non-contrast-enhanced CT (Fig. 31). Occasionally, hematoma may be seen only on a non-contrast scan, although in such cases the injury is usually small (171). Following rapid intravenous injection of contrast material, the spleen may initially exhibit a heterogeneous pattern of parenchymal opacification, reflecting variable blood flow patterns within different compartments of the spleen (116) (Fig. 32). Care must be taken not to misinterpret this early postinjection heterogeneity as representing splenic injury. In questionable cases, repeat scans should be obtained following equilibration of the contrast material. In normal cases, the splenic paren-

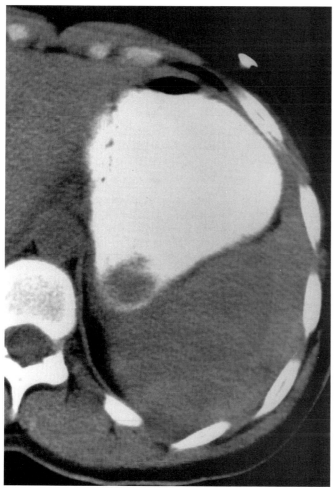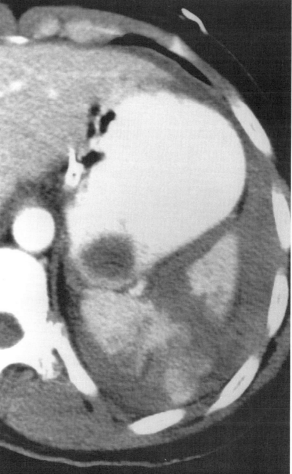

FIG. 31. Shattered spleen prior to (**A**) and during the administration of intravenous contrast material (**B**). The use of intravenous contrast material markedly improves the visualization of splenic injuries. Perisplenic hematoma is also evident.

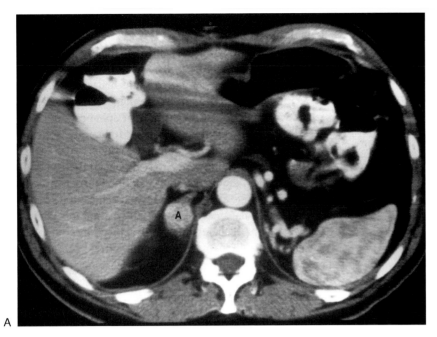

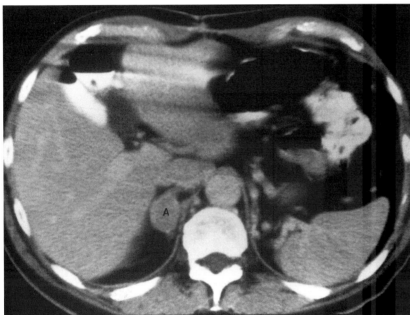

FIG. 32. Heterogeneous early splenic enhancement. **A:** Early-phase dynamic contrast-enhanced CT image demonstrates heterogeneous enhancement of the splenic parenchyma that could be mistaken for splenic injury. Note the absence of perisplenic hematoma. Right adrenal adenoma (A) is incidentally noted. **B:** Delayed scan during equilibrium phase demonstrates homogeneous splenic parenchyma without evidence of splenic injury.

chyma will achieve a uniform, homogeneous appearance with no surrounding hemorrhage.

Injury to the spleen can take the form of laceration, intrasplenic hematoma, subcapsular hematoma, or infarction. In severe cases, the spleen may be shattered into multiple small fragments (Fig. 33). Splenic laceration typically appears as an irregular linear area of hypodensity on contrast-enhanced CT (Fig. 34). Intrasplenic hematoma appears as a broader area of hypodense, nonperfused splenic parenchyma (Fig. 35). Although hypodense relative to the splenic parenchyma on contrast-enhanced CT, an intrasplenic hematoma may appear hyperdense on a noncontrast examination. Subcapsular hematomas appear

as crescentic collections of fluid that flatten or indent the underlying splenic parenchyma (Fig. 36). Splenic infarcts may occur following injury to the splenic vasculature and appear as wedge-shaped areas of nonperfusion that extend to the splenic capsule.

Streak artifact from nasogastric tubes or electrocardiographic leads may mimic splenic laceration and ideally these objects should be repositioned or removed prior to scanning. Beam-hardening artifact from ribs and streak artifact from an air–contrast interface in the stomach may also simulate splenic injury. Such artifacts generally are better defined and more regular in appearance than true lacerations, and often extend beyond the margin of the

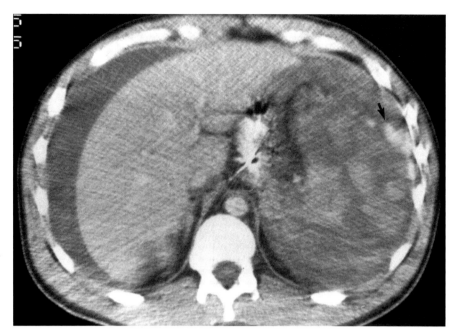

FIG. 33. Shattered spleen. The spleen is shattered into multiple small fragments. There is a large amount of hemoperitoneum, and considerable streak artifact arises from the nasogastric tube within the stomach. Small focus of high-attenuation extravasated contrast material representing active hemorrhage (*arrow*) is also evident.

spleen. Splenic clefts can mimic laceration but typically are more smoothly contoured in appearance (Fig. 37). The absence of associated perisplenic blood is also helpful in distinguishing clefts from true lacerations. Enhancing atelectatic lung, as well as a prominent left lobe of the liver draping around the spleen, may on occasion simulate splenic injury and perisplenic hematoma (43) (see Fig. 35). An overdistended stomach compressing the medial border of the spleen has been reported to obscure superficial lacerations and in such cases gastric decompression has been suggested (115). A decrease in overall splenic

enhancement to less than that of the liver has been noted in traumatized hypotensive patients and should not be interpreted as representing splenic vascular injury. This decrease in splenic enhancement is thought to result from adrenergic effects on splenic blood flow (18,124).

Hemoperitoneum almost always accompanies significant splenic injury (96). In cases where there is significant intraabdominal fluid, the presence of local perisplenic clot, the so-called sentinel clot, suggests splenic injury as the site of bleeding (260) (Figs. 29, 35, 38, and 39). Such clot usually appears denser (greater than 60 HU versus

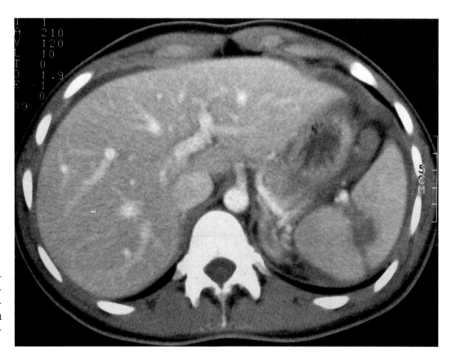

FIG. 34. Splenic laceration. Contrast-enhanced CT scan demonstrates irregular, low-attenuation splenic laceration extending to the splenic hilum. There is a small amount of perisplenic and perihepatic blood.

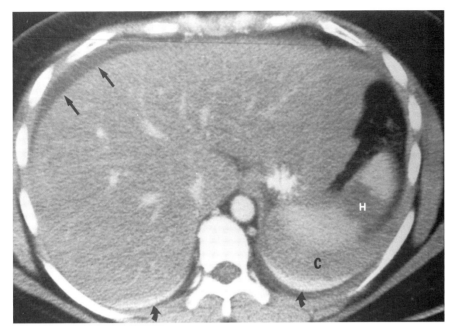

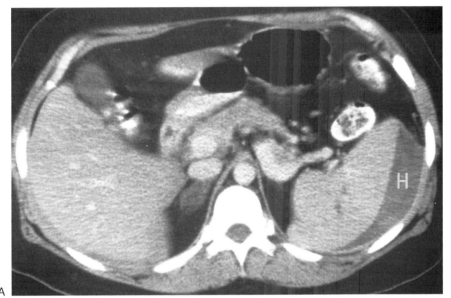

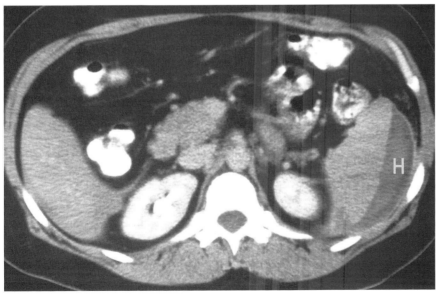

FIG. 35. Splenic hematoma and hemoperitoneum. Contrast-enhanced CT scan demonstrates a broad area of hypodense, nonperfused splenic parenchyma representing intrasplenic hematoma (H). High-attenuation perisplenic clotted blood (C) and lower attenuation perihepatic lysed blood (*straight arrows*) are also present. Markedly enhancing atelectatic lung (*curved arrows*) at both lung bases mimics active hemorrhage.

FIG. 36. Subcapsular splenic hematoma. CT images through the mid- (**A**) and lower spleen (**B**) demonstrate several small low-attenuation splenic lacerations and a lenticular-shaped subcapsular hematoma (H) that flattens the underlying splenic parenchyma. A small amount of perihepatic blood is also present.

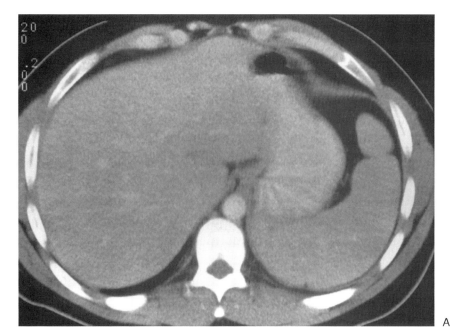

A

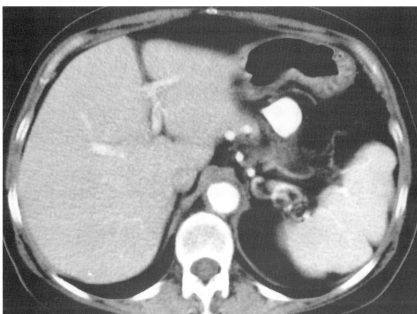

B

FIG. 37. Congenital splenic clefts. **A:** CT image demonstrates a sharply marginated cleft in the anterior tip of the spleen. The smooth, rounded contour of the cleft as it meets the margin of the spleen, as well as the absence of perisplenic hematoma, is helpful in distinguishing a congenital cleft from a parenchymal laceration. **B:** Another patient with multiple splenic clefts along the lateral margin of the spleen.

35–45 HU for hemoperitoneum) and more heterogeneous than the remainder of the intraabdominal blood (96). In one report of 65 cases of splenic injury, a sentinel clot was the only sign present in 6 (9%) patients. These cases were usually those with either a small peripheral laceration or a small parenchymal hematoma around a more central tear (260). Sometimes the perisplenic hematoma has a multilayered or onion-skin appearance (Fig. 39). Blood may also dissect via the peritoneal attachments of the spleen and appear as fluid within the left anterior pararenal space or left lateroconal fascia (342).

Active bleeding may be identified on contrast-enhanced

CT as areas of bright vascular enhancement (Figs. 30, 33, and 40). Pseudoaneurysm formation can occur following trauma and appears as a focal well-circumscribed area of vascular enhancement within the splenic parenchyma that is larger than the normal vessels (Fig. 41). Surrounding hematoma is frequently noted (110,145).

The increased incidence of overwhelming infection in patients following splenectomy has placed emphasis on nonoperative management in hemodynamically stable patients (201). Grading of the severity of splenic injury by CT has been proposed in the hope of separating patients who can be safely managed nonoperatively from those

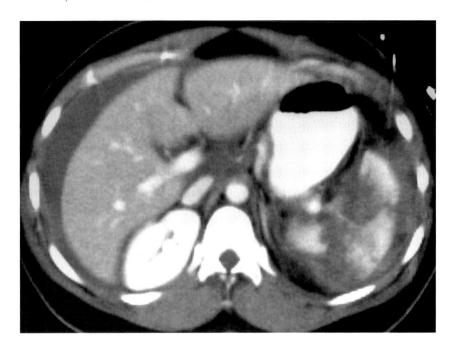

FIG. 38. Ruptured spleen with hemoperitoneum and perisplenic sentinel clot. CT scan through the upper abdomen demonstrates a ruptured spleen and surrounding high-attenuation sentinel clot. Note lower attenuation lysed blood around the liver. The patient was explored and a bleeding vessel was ligated in the splenic hilum. Splenectomy was not required.

who would benefit from immediate surgery (e.g., those with an increased risk of delayed splenic rupture). The desirability of such a predictive grading system is increased by the fact that early surgical intervention more often results in splenic salvage than does delayed operation (280,296,356). Several CT grading systems have been described and evaluated (35,241,245,280). Each assesses the integrity of the splenic capsule, the size of hematoma, the length and number of lacerations, involve-

ment of segmental or hilar vessels, and extent of parenchymal devascularization. The presence and extent of intraabdominal fluid and associated intraabdominal injuries is also included in several classification schemes (Tables 1 and 2). Initial reports suggested that such classification systems would be valuable in predicting which patients were likely to fail nonoperative management (45, 280,296). Later studies have shown that although the incidence of operation may go up with severity of injury,

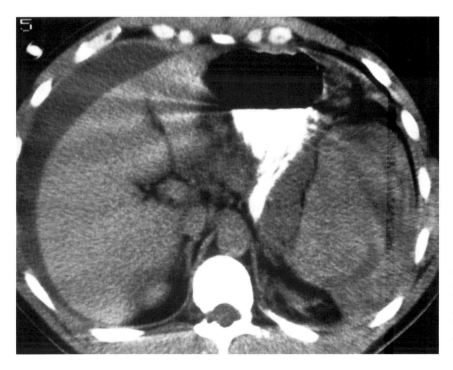

FIG. 39. Splenic laceration with hemoperitoneum and perisplenic sentinel clot. Contrast-enhanced CT scan through the upper abdomen demonstrates low-attenuation splenic laceration and lamellated-appearing perisplenic hematoma. Lower attenuation lysed blood is seen around the liver, and there is considerable streak artifact from the air−contrast interface in the stomach. Beam-hardening artifact is also noted arising from the ribs, particularly on the right.

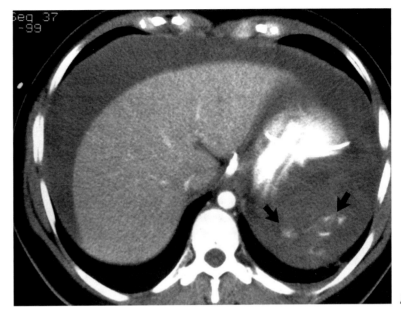

A

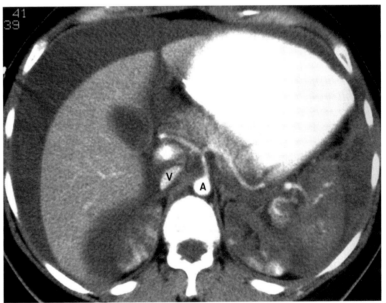

B

FIG. 40. Partial transection of the splenic hilum with active bleeding and massive hemoperitoneum. **A:** CT scan through the upper third of the liver demonstrates large amount of hemoperitoneum, virtually absent perfusion of the splenic parenchyma, and active bleeding (*arrows*) from disrupted hilar vessels. **B:** CT scan at the level of the splenic hilum demonstrates hypoperfused and contused kidneys. Note also the diminutive aorta (A) and collapsed inferior vena cava (V) secondary to hypovolemia. **C:** CT scan through the lower margin of the spleen (S) shows some preservation of splenic enhancement consistent with partial hilar transection.

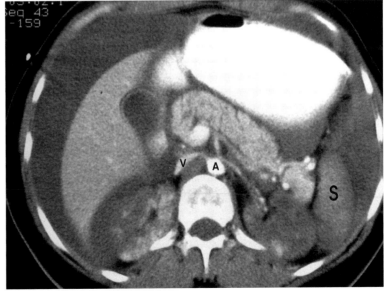

C

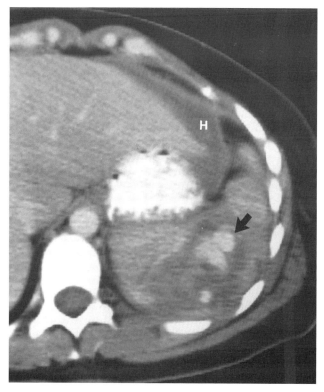

FIG. 41. Splenic hematoma with pseudoaneurysm formation (*arrow*). Note hemoperitoneum (H) adjacent to the left lobe of the liver. The patient was observed closely and transfused but did not require surgery.

there are a significant number of patients with severe splenic injury grades who can be successfully managed nonoperatively as well as a number of patients with low-grade injuries who will fail nonoperative management (13,26,180,241,291,356). The presence of active hemorrhage or a pseudoaneurysm has been associated with an increased failure rate of attempted nonsurgical management (110,301). Even in patients with this negative prognostic factor, however, nonoperative management was successful in approximately 40% (110,301). In general, children have a lower incidence of failed nonoperative management (22,45,209,280,356). The reason for this is unclear but may relate to differences in functional smooth muscle content, elasticity, and thickness of the splenic capsule (209,250). In adults, age greater than 55 to 65 years has also been found to have a negative impact on the success of nonoperative management (79,120,329).

Delayed splenic rupture has been reported in a few patients in whom the initial CT scan was interpreted as normal (85,267,356). This may be secondary to splenic fracture in which there is little initial hemorrhage or in which poor-contrast opacification of the spleen renders hematoma isodense with splenic parenchyma (50,267,356).

An average increase in splenic volume of approximately 25% has been noted following blunt abdominal trauma. This apparent splenic enlargement on CT does not correlate with deteriorating splenic status but rather has been postulated to result from a return to normal splenic size following physiologic contraction in response to the initial injury (124).

Splenic injuries may take several months to fully resolve on follow-up CT examinations (70,275). Severely traumatized spleens took up to 11 months for healing in one study in a pediatric population (15). Typically, intraperitoneal blood and perisplenic hematoma resolve in 1 to 3 weeks. Intrasplenic hematomas gradually decrease in density and become more sharply defined as the clots mature. They may go on to complete resolution leaving only a slightly deformed splenic margin, or they may form a posttraumatic splenic pseudocyst (70,84). Infection may complicate hematoma resolution and produce a splenic abscess. Splenic lacerations usually resolve in a few weeks to a few months depending on their depth and severity. Splenic infarcts generally resolve over several months. Although it has been suggested by some authors that routine follow-up CT may be valuable in demonstrating healing and hence allow earlier return to normal

TABLE 1. *Buntain classification of splenic injury*

Class I	Localized capsular disruption or subcapsular hematoma, without significant parenchymal injury.
Class II	Capsular and parenchymal disruptions that do not extend into the hilum or involve major vessels. Intraparenchymal hematoma may or may not coexist.
Class III	Deep fractures extending into the hilum and involving major blood vessels.
Class IV	Completely shattered or fragmented spleen, or separated from its normal blood supply at the pedicle.
A)	Without other intraabdominal injury
B)	With other associated intraabdominal injury
	B1—solid viscus
	B2—hollow viscus
C)	With associated extraabdominal injury

Adapted from Buntain et al. (35).

TABLE 2. *Mirvis classification of splenic injury*

Grade 1	Capsular avulsion, superficial laceration(s) or subcapsular hematoma <1 cm.
Grade 2	Parenchymal laceration(s) 1-3 cm deep, central/subcapsular hematoma(s) <3 cm.
Grade 3	Laceration(s) >3 cm deep, central/subcapsular hematom(s) >3 cm.
Grade 4	Fragmentation of 3 or more sections, devascularized (nonenhanced) spleen.

From Mirvis et al. (241).

physical activity (93), others report that follow-up CT does not affect clinical management (189,275).

Liver

The liver is the second most commonly injured abdominal organ in patients with blunt abdominal trauma and represents the most common abdominal injury leading to death (25,89). Overall mortality of patients with liver injury ranges from 7% to 26% (247,349). Mortality generally is lower in patients with isolated liver trauma (3% to 4%) and tends to increase with increasing number and severity of associated extrahepatic injuries (>70% mortality with five or more associated injuries) (5,66,354). As with splenic trauma, associated injury to other abdominal organs is a common occurrence (136). Concomitant injuries to the head, chest, and extremities also are frequently present (91).

The right hepatic lobe is most frequently injured, particularly the posterior segment (104,332). This is because the right lobe constitutes most of the volume of the liver and because the posterior segment of the right lobe is readily accessible to blunt impact from the ribs and spine (244,332). Relative fixation of the liver by the coronary ligaments may also contribute to the predilection for right lobe injury (332). Left hepatic lobe injuries are much less common than injuries to the right lobe and tend to occur with a forceful, direct blow to the epigastrium. Left lobe injuries have a much higher association with injuries to the pancreas, duodenum, and transverse colon (162,332).

Computed tomography has proven to be highly sensitive, specific, and accurate in defining and characterizing hepatic injury (104,122, 244). The CT findings of hepatic injury are similar to those seen in the spleen and include laceration or fracture through the hepatic parenchyma, intraparenchymal hematoma, and subcapsular hematoma. Hepatic lacerations appear as irregular linear, branching, or rounded areas of low attenuation within the normally enhancing liver parenchyma (244,351) (Fig. 42). High-attenuation foci of freshly clotted blood may be seen in the areas of laceration. Lacerations commonly parallel the hepatic or portal venous vasculature (104) and often extend to the periphery of the liver. Parallel, linear lacerations on the surface of the liver or radiating out from the hilar region may assume a configuration that has been termed the bear claw pattern due to its radiating, parallel, and jagged appearance (162,230) (Fig. 43). On occasion, hepatic lacerations may demonstrate a branching pattern that superficially simulates the appearance of dilated bile ducts (90,244) (Fig. 44). This resemblance is usually lim-

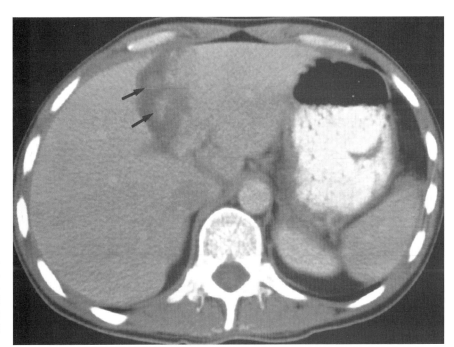

FIG. 42. Hepatic laceration. Note irregular, low-attenuation laceration extending through the left lobe and caudate. High-attenuation foci of clotted blood (*arrows*) are seen within the areas of laceration. Small amount of hemoperitoneum is also present.

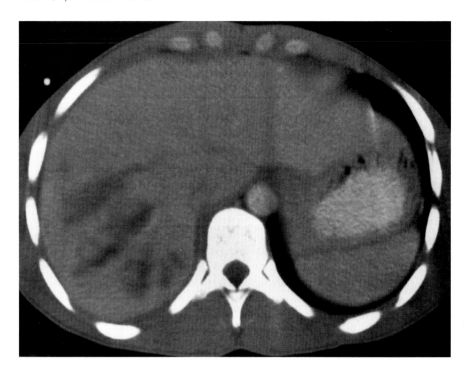

FIG. 43. Bear claw type laceration of the right hepatic lobe. Note roughly parallel, radiating, low-attenuation lacerations in the right lobe of the liver.

ited to a single CT section, and in most cases careful analysis of contiguous sections allows correct diagnosis. Deep lacerations, or lacerations extending between two visceral surfaces, may result in fragmentation of the liver, producing isolated nonperfused fragments. Lacerations extending into the perihilar region of the liver have an increased incidence of bile duct injury and associated complications such as biloma and hemobilia (162,332). Lacerations near the confluence of the hepatic veins or the intrahepatic inferior vena cava (IVC) should suggest the potential for hepatic vein or IVC laceration. Such injuries are of particular concern because they can result in rapid exsanguination, particularly when the liver is mobilized at the time of surgical inspection (17,162). Proper preoperative preparation is essential to prevent a surgical catastrophe (17,162).

Intrahepatic hematomas appear as poorly marginated, confluent areas of low attenuation within the hepatic parenchyma (Fig. 45). They tend to be rounded or oval in configuration, and often display a central high-attenuation area of clotted blood surrounded by a larger low-attenuation region of lysed clot and contused liver parenchyma (162).

Subcapsular hematomas occasionally result from blunt trauma but more frequently are the result of iatrogenic injuries such as percutaneous liver biopsy. Subcapsular hematomas usually appear on CT as peripheral, well-marginated, lenticular or crescent-shaped fluid collections that characteristically flatten or indent the underlying liver parenchyma. Most subcapsular hematomas occur along the parietal surface of the liver, particularly along the

anterolateral aspect of the right hepatic lobe (285). The attenuation of the collection depends on the age of the hematoma, generally being of higher attenuation early when clotted blood is present and then decreasing in attenuation over time as clot lysis takes place.

On occasion, gas may be seen in areas of hepatic laceration or hematoma within 2 to 3 days following blunt abdominal trauma (1,266) (Fig. 46). Although the presence of hepatic gas often indicates the presence of infection (136), such gas may also be a manifestation of severe blunt trauma without infection (1,266). It has been postulated that the gas arises from hepatic ischemia and necrosis (227). In the appropriate clinical setting, such gas-containing injuries usually can be treated conservatively without the need for surgical or percutaneous intervention (266).

Periportal low attenuation surrounding portal venous branches (periportal tracking) is frequently seen on CT scans of patients with hepatic trauma (190,207,270, 306,316,325) (Fig. 47). In patients with hepatic injury, the periportal low attenuation has been attributed to dissection of blood along the course of the portal veins (207). In the absence of direct CT evidence of hepatic disruption, however, the finding of diffuse periportal low attenuation after blunt trauma should not be taken as de facto evidence of hepatic injury (306). In most trauma patients, periportal tracking most likely represents distension of periportal lymphatics and lymphedema associated with elevated central venous pressure produced by rapid expansion of intravascular volume during vigorous intravenous fluid resuscitation (54,306). Other trauma-related pathologic

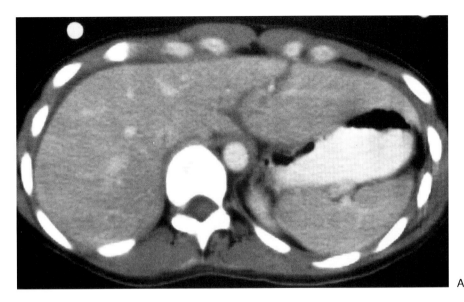

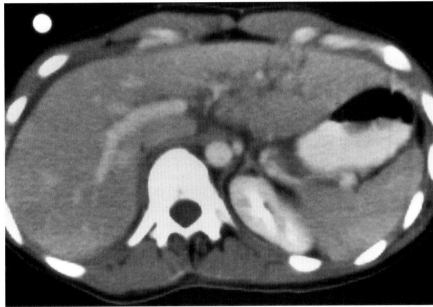

FIG. 44. Left hepatic lobe lacerations mimicking biliary ductal dilatation. **A:** Note left hepatic lobe lacerations along the plane of the ligamentum teres. Small amount of perihepatic blood is also evident. **B:** On a CT scan several centimeters caudal to A, the branching, reticular appearance of the left lobe lacerations superficially simulates the appearance of dilated bile ducts.

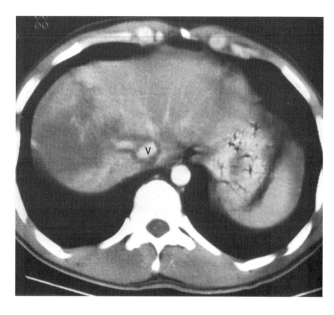

FIG. 45. Intrahepatic hematoma. Contrast-enhanced CT scan demonstrates a poorly marginated, confluent area of low attenuation within the dome of the liver consistent with an intraparenchymal hematoma. Dissection of blood along the right hepatic vein and around the inferior vena cava (V) is also noted.

changes leading to elevated central venous pressure such as tension pneumothorax, pericardial tamponade, or hematoma obstructing hepatic venous outflow also may result in diffuse periportal low attenuation (182,306).

Lacerations or hematomas of the hepatic parenchyma can be simulated by beam-hardening artifact from adjacent ribs or streak artifacts from air–contrast interfaces. Rib artifacts can usually be identified by their typical location deep to the rib and by their tendency to fade and become more diffuse as they proceed into the liver (111). Artifacts from air–contrast interfaces in stomach and bowel generally are more regular and linear in appearance than true lacerations. Lacerations also can be simulated by congenital clefts or fissures (Fig. 48). A laceration or hematoma can be missed in cases of fatty liver in which the low-attenuation fatty-infiltrated parenchyma, even when enhanced, remains isodense with the areas of low-attenuation injury (Fig. 49). Associated hemoperitoneum should remain evident, however, and may be the only readily identifiable sign suggesting hepatic injury. In such cases, it may be helpful to view images of the liver at narrow window widths (100–200 HU) in order to enhance

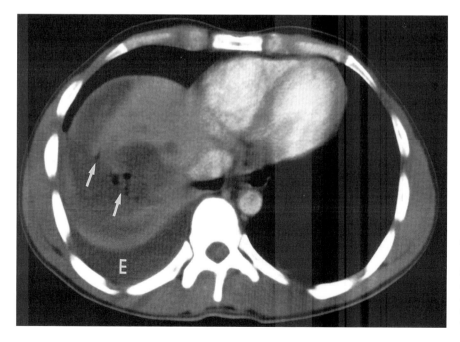

FIG. 46. Intrahepatic hematoma with sterile necrosis. Contrast-enhanced CT scan 3 days following blunt abdominal trauma demonstrates intraparenchymal hematoma containing several small bubbles of gas (*arrows*), presumably secondary to necrosis within the area of injury. The patient had no evidence of infection and recovered uneventfully; (E) pleural effusion.

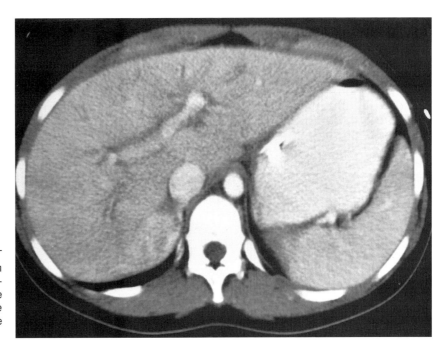

FIG. 47. Periportal low attenuation. CT image at the level of the portal bifurcation demonstrates diffuse periportal low attenuation surrounding the portal triads. Subtle laceration in the posterior segment of the right lobe of the liver was noted on more caudal images.

detection of subtle parenchymal findings, such as alteration of the course of intrahepatic vessels and/or ducts within the areas of parenchymal injury (244,285).

Although a significant percentage of patients (22% to 61%) with hepatic injury have obvious signs of shock or peritonitis at the time of admission and require immediate surgery without preliminary imaging studies (194,354), there are also a large number of patients with significant hepatic trauma who are hemodynamically stable that may be best managed nonoperatively. Previous surgical series have noted that up to 70% of hepatic injuries had stopped bleeding at the time of laparotomy and could have been managed conservatively (63,259,303). This observation, coupled with the use of abdominal CT scanning in the initial assessment and subsequent follow-up of hepatic injuries, has led to an increasing trend toward nonsurgical management of hepatic trauma in hemodynamically stable patients (60,87,88,104,220).

Conservative management of stable patients with minor, isolated hepatic trauma and limited or no hemoperitoneum has been in place for some time now. More recently, several studies have shown that even extensive hepatic parenchymal injuries (CT severity grades 3 and 4) with significant hemoperitoneum on CT scans also can be successfully managed nonoperatively (12,60,242). Keys to successful nonoperative management include constant hemodynamic monitoring, serial clinical and laboratory assessment, blood replacement as necessary, and ready availability of nursing, surgical, and imaging facilities in the event of hemodynamic deterioration (104,220,242).

Management decisions in the setting of hepatic injury should be based primarily on the clinical status of the patient rather than on CT findings (12,26,59). Although injury grading with CT may reflect the degree of hepatic parenchymal damage, it does not reliably indicate patients in whom complications may develop or in whom surgery will be necessary (12). Furthermore, as nearly all hemodynamically stable patients with hepatic trauma have an excellent prognosis with nonoperative management, CT grading of blunt hepatic injuries is of limited discriminatory value in predicting the outcome of conservative treatment (158). Nonetheless, CT is useful in monitoring the healing of hepatic injuries, confirming the resorption of hemoperitoneum, and detecting complications such as hepatic infarction, enlarging hematoma, biloma, or abscess formation (12,33,104,351).

Hemoperitoneum normally is resorbed from the peritoneal cavity and in most cases is either significantly reduced or absent by 1 week after injury (104). Persistence of hemoperitoneum or increase in the volume of intraperitoneal fluid on repeat CT scans 3 to 7 days after injury suggests either ongoing intraperitoneal bleeding or bile leakage (104). Delayed hemorrhage, or progression of initially stable parenchymal injuries, appears to be much less common with hepatic trauma than with splenic injury (158,242,259).

Subcapsular liver hematomas usually resolve in 6 to 8 weeks (295). Intraparenchymal hematomas heal much more slowly, often requiring 6 months to several years to resolve completely, as bile in the hematoma prolongs clot resorption and adversely affects parenchymal healing (295). Lacerations appear to heal more rapidly, with evidence of significant healing generally noted on serial CT examinations over a 2- to 3-week period (104) (Fig. 50).

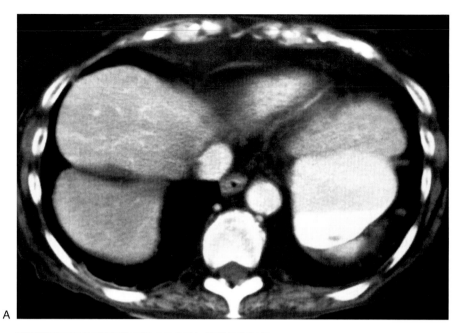

A

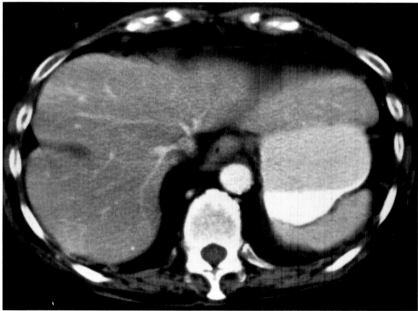

B

FIG. 48. Congenital hepatic cleft. **A:** CT scan through the dome of the liver demonstrates a deep cleft in the hepatic parenchyma. **B:** On a CT image 1 cm caudal to A, the peripheral cleft mimics a parenchymal laceration. Note the absence of perihepatic blood.

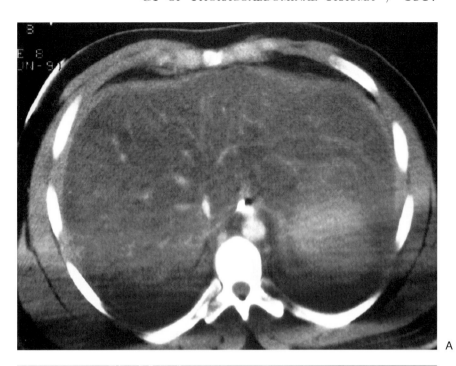

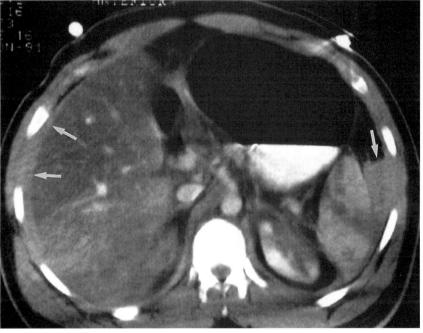

FIG. 49. Hepatic lacerations obscured by fatty liver. Diffuse fatty infiltration of the liver hides multiple long-segment lacerations (up to 15 cm) noted at surgery in both lobes of the liver. Patient exsanguinated during emergency surgery. **A:** CT scan through the upper third of the liver demonstrates diffuse low-attenuation of the liver parenchyma from fatty infiltration but no definite lacerations. High-attenuation fluid representing acute hemoperitoneum surrounds the liver. There is considerable streak artifact over the posterior portion of the scan. **B:** CT scan through the lower third of the liver demonstrates vague areas of increased attenuation in the right hepatic lobe presumably secondary to hepatic contusion and/or hemorrhage. Perihepatic and perisplenic blood (*arrows*) is present, and there is evidence of splenic laceration and left renal contusion.

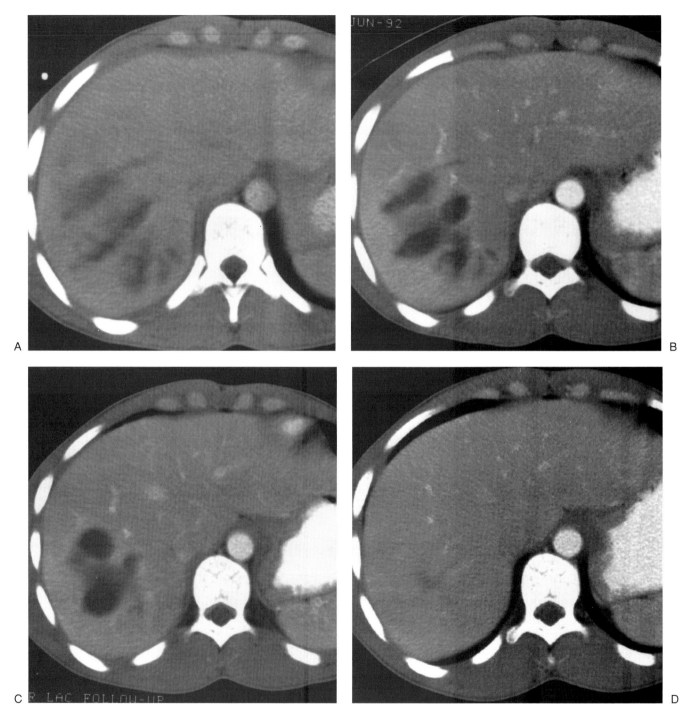

FIG. 50. Healing hepatic lacerations on serial CT examinations. **A:** Initial scan obtained in the same patient as illustrated in Fig. 43 demonstrates bear claw type of laceration in the right lobe of the liver. **B:** Scan 4 days later shows decrease in CT attenuation value and slight increase in size of the hepatic lacerations, probably due to osmotic absorption of fluid. **C:** On a scan 3 weeks later, the lacerations have assumed a more rounded configuration, and the margins of the lacerations are better defined. **D:** Follow-up scan 3 months after the initial injury demonstrates virtually complete resolution of the liver lacerations.

Hepatic lacerations and hematomas typically demonstrate a decrease in CT attenuation value, as well as a slight increase in size on initial follow-up CT studies (i.e., 7 days post injury), probably due to osmotic absorption of fluid (104,230). Irregular margins of lacerations and hematomas become better defined with healing and tend to assume a rounded or ovoid configuration with resolution (104,230). Such lesions may progressively decrease in size or they may persist as well-defined hepatic cysts or bilomas (295).

Pancreas

Pancreatic injuries from blunt trauma are relatively uncommon, accounting for only 3% to 12% of all abdominal injuries (7,74,105, 164). The mechanism of injury to the pancreas in blunt trauma is thought to be compression of the pancreas between the vertebral column and the anterior abdominal wall, often due to a direct steering wheel injury (in adults) or bicycle handlebar injury (in children) to the midepigastrium (74,165). Pancreatic injuries are frequently associated with injuries to other intraabdominal organs, and they result in a mortality rate of approximately 20% (74,165). Most deaths within the first 48 hr are due to hemorrhage from extrapancreatic injuries (105, 165). Delays in diagnosis can lead to increased late (>48 hr post injury) morbidity and mortality related to the pancreatic injuries alone (199).

The diagnosis of blunt pancreatic injury can be extremely difficult because the clinical, laboratory, and radiographic findings are highly variable and nonspecific (7). Clinical manifestations of pancreatic injury such as abdominal pain and leukocytosis frequently are mild, absent, or masked by associated injuries (57,253). Serum amylase levels may be elevated, but this is not invariably the case, as initial serum amylase determinations have been reported to be normal in up to 40% of patients with pancreatic injury (165). Even with total disruption of the pancreatic ductal system, amylase levels may not be elevated until 24 to 48 hr post injury. In addition, the degree of serum amylase elevation does not correlate with the degree of pancreatic injury (105). Because pancreatic injuries may be clinically occult or unrecognized, they often are discovered at the time of laparotomy for other known intraabdominal injuries (46,163, 262).

Pancreatic injuries can range from minor parenchymal contusions and hematomas to major lacerations or fractures with associated pancreatic duct disruption. Computed tomography has been reported to diagnose pancreatic injury in 67% to 85% of cases (161,322). On contrast-enhanced CT, contusions generally appear as focal low-attenuation areas within the normally enhancing pancreatic parenchyma (Fig. 51). Lacerations or fractures appear as linear, irregular regions of low attenuation, often oriented perpendicular to the long axis of the pancreas (Fig. 52). Fractures most commonly occur in the pancreatic neck or body where the pancreas overlies the spine, although a few fractures have been reported in the pancreatic head or tail (71). Additional suggestive but nonspecific signs of pancreatic injury include infiltration of the peripancreatic fat and mesentery, thickening of the left

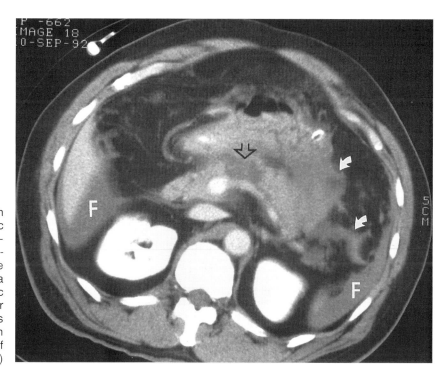

FIG. 51. Pancreatic contusion. CT scan at the level of the superior mesenteric vein–splenic vein confluence demonstrates a sharply demarcated region of diminished enhancement in the body of the pancreas (*open arrow*) consistent with a pancreatic contusion. Note peripancreatic infiltration of the mesentery and anterior pararenal space (*curved arrows*). There is fluid (F) in the hepatorenal fossa and in the left paracolic gutter. (Case courtesy of Dr. Holly Burge, Raleigh, North Carolina.)

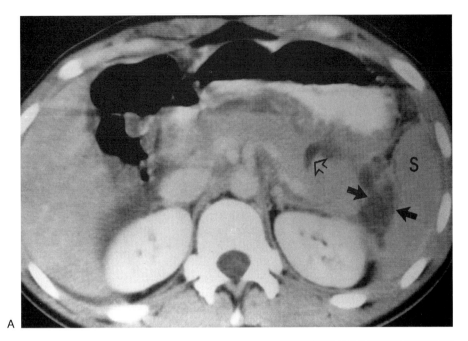

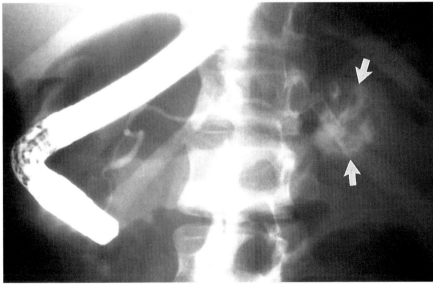

FIG. 52. Pancreatic laceration with disruption of the pancreatic duct. **A:** CT scan demonstrates laceration through the tail of the pancreas (*open arrow*). Fluid is seen about the tail of the pancreas (*solid arrows*) adjacent to the spleen (S). **B:** Endoscopic retrograde cholangiopancreatography (ERCP) demonstrates disruption of the main pancreatic duct in the tail of the pancreas with extravasation of contrast material (*arrows*).

anterior renal fascia (161), tracking of fluid between the splenic vein and pancreas (186), and fluid in the anterior pararenal space or lesser sac (320).

Pancreatic laceration or fracture may be difficult to identify acutely (<12 hr post injury) with CT due to obscuration of the fracture plane by hemorrhage and/or close apposition of the lacerated parenchymal fragments (161). As the time from injury progresses, edema, inflammation, and autodigestion by exuded pancreatic enzymes often make the CT findings of pancreatic injury more apparent. Thus, if suspicion of pancreatic injury persists despite initially normal CT findings, repeat CT scans in 12 to 24 hr may be warranted (71,219).

False positive diagnosis of pancreatic laceration or fracture may result from streak artifacts, physiologic thinning of the pancreatic neck (Fig. 53), or misinterpretation of unopacified proximal jejunal loops as the pancreatic body, separated from the pancreatic head and neck region by a fat plane around the mesenteric vessels (91) (Fig. 54). In questionable cases, repeat delayed scans with additional oral contrast material usually demonstrates changes in shape and opacification of the bowel loops, allowing correct diagnosis.

CT cannot directly assess the integrity of the pancreatic duct, which is the principal determinant in the management of pancreatic injuries (51). A recent study assessing CT grading of blunt pancreatic injuries suggested that ductal disruption was likely to be present if CT scans demonstrated a deep laceration or transection of the pancreas (376). In general, however, definitive determination

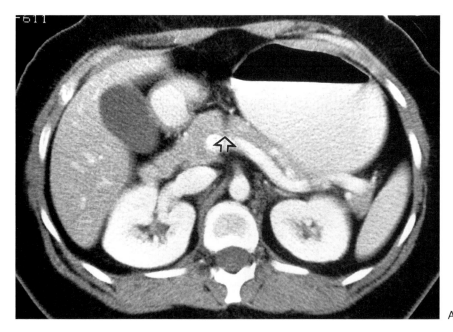

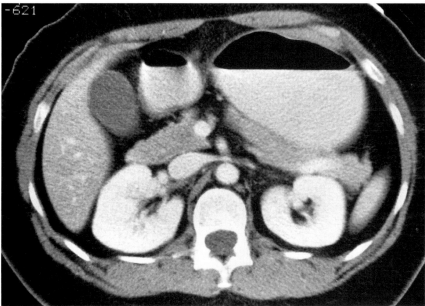

FIG. 53. Pseudofracture of the pancreas due to physiologic thinning of the pancreatic neck. **A:** CT scan at the level of the superior mesenteric vein–splenic vein confluence demonstrates apparent fracture of the pancreatic neck (*open arrow*). **B:** CT scan 1 cm caudal to A shows fat in the region of the neck consistent with physiologic thinning. Note also the absence of peripancreatic fluid.

of pancreatic duct integrity requires either endoscopic retrograde cholangiopancreatography (ERCP) (see Fig. 52) or intraoperative evaluation (40,89).

Bowel and Mesentery

Injuries to the bowel and mesentery are reported to occur in 3% to 5% of patients sustaining blunt abdominal trauma (32,309). They are most often associated with motor vehicle accidents, and their prevalence has increased with the use of lap-type seat-belt restraints, particularly in children (65,305,326). Mechanisms of injury include direct compression of the bowel between the vertebral column and the anterior abdominal wall, sudden marked increase in intralu-minal pressure, and shearing-type injury near sites of mesenteric fixation such as the ligament of Treitz and the ileocecal junction (55,68). Bowel injuries can range from focal mural contusions or hematomas to complete transections. They most commonly involve the duodenum, usually the second and third portions. Colonic injuries following blunt abdominal trauma are less common than either duodenal or other small bowel injuries (151).

Prompt diagnosis of intestinal or mesenteric injury is often difficult because signs and symptoms may be delayed and physical examination is neither sensitive nor specific (36,72). Early clinical findings are frequently subtle, and the classic triad of tenderness, rigidity, and absent bowel sounds only occurs in about 30% of patients (36). Clear-cut peritoneal signs and symptoms can take hours

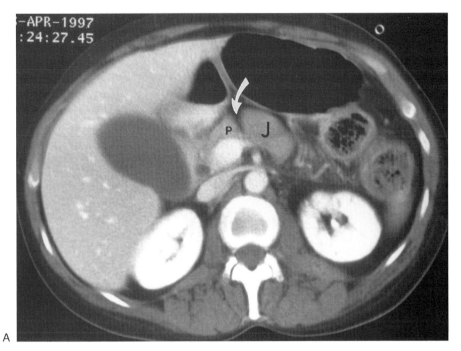

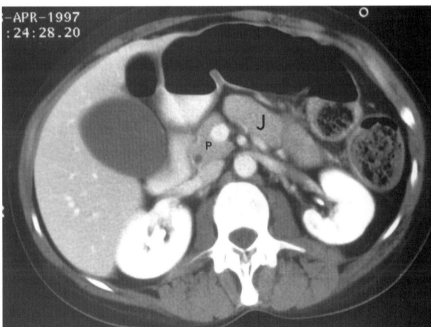

FIG. 54. Pancreatic pseudofracture secondary to unopacified small bowel loops. CT images through the pancreatic head (**A**) and uncinate process (**B**) demonstrate a pseudofracture (*curved arrow*) due to close apposition of unopacified proximal jejunal loops (J) simulating the pancreatic body separated from the normal head and neck region by fat around the mesenteric vessels; (P) pancreatic parenchyma.

or days to develop in stable patients with intestinal injury because of minimal blood loss, contained retroperitoneal involvement in some duodenal and colonic injuries, and the nonirritative composition (i.e., neutral pH) and low bacterial counts of small bowel chyme (72, 309). If undiagnosed, bowel perforation can lead to fatal peritonitis. A delay of more than 24 hr in diagnosis and surgical repair of bowel perforation results in a significant increase in morbidity and mortality (117,202,284).

Computed tomography has been shown to be useful for detecting bowel and mesenteric injuries caused by blunt trauma, but careful inspection and meticulous scanning technique are required to detect often subtle findings (231,255,309). Although many earlier studies found poor sensitivity of CT for detection of bowel injuries (39,51, 170,214,221,310), more recent studies have reported higher sensitivity of CT for diagnosing bowel and mesenteric injuries and for distinguishing those injuries that are likely to require surgical intervention (34,73,77, 231, 283,309).

CT signs of bowel and mesenteric injury include extraluminal air, extravasation of oral contrast material, free intraabdominal fluid, thickened and/or discontinuous bowel wall, high-attenuation clot (sentinel clot) adjacent to the involved bowel, and streaky soft tissue infiltration of the mesenteric fat (73,231,255,260,283) (Fig. 55). Free air in either the peritoneal cavity or the retroperitoneum is a relatively specific sign of bowel perforation but is seen in only 50% of cases (117,283) (Figs. 56 and 57). The volume of air may be quite small and subtle. To optimize detection of extraluminal air and to facilitate its differentiation from intraluminal air or from fat, images should be viewed at

wide window settings (i.e., lung windows) (55,309). Pneumoperitoneum is most commonly seen in the subdiaphragmatic area, along the anterior peritoneal surfaces of the liver and spleen (Fig. 56). Extraluminal air also may be present within the leaves of the mesentery (Figs. 55 and 58) or in the retroperitoneum, particularly in the anterior pararenal space (255,373) (Fig. 57). Occasionally, intraperitoneal or retroperitoneal gas results from extraperitoneal dissection of air from traumatic injuries of the thorax (pneumothorax, pneumomediastinum) or bladder (bladder rupture) and is not related to bowel trauma (34,51). Extravasation of oral contrast material from the bowel lumen is considered diagnostic

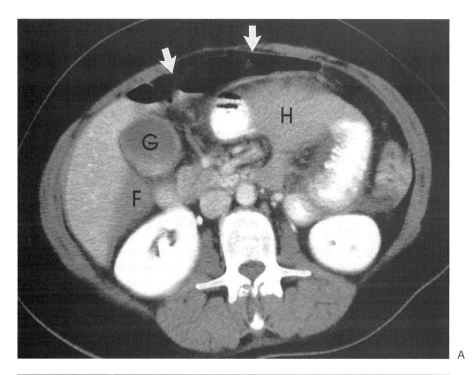

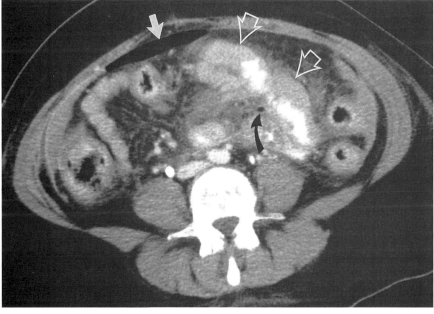

FIG. 55. Jejunal perforation and mesenteric hematoma. **A:** CT scan at the level of the gallbladder (G) demonstrates free intraperitoneal air anteriorly (arrows) and mesenteric/jejunal hematoma (H). Free fluid (F) is present in the hepatorenal fossa. **B:** CT scan several centimeters caudal to A demonstrates jejunal wall thickening (*open arrows*), infiltration of the adjacent mesenteric fat, and a single dot of extraluminal mesenteric air (*curved black arrow*). Free air is again noted anteriorly (*solid white arrow*).

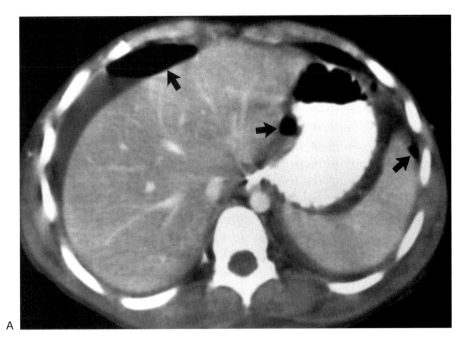

A

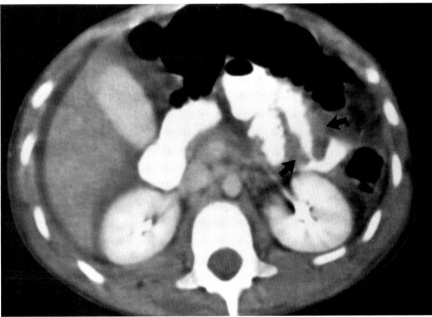

B

FIG. 56. Jejunal hematoma and perforation. **A:** CT scan at the level of the gastroesophageal junction demonstrates free intraperitoneal air (*arrows*) and fluid along the anterior peritoneal surfaces of the liver and spleen and in the lesser sac. **B:** CT scan several centimeters caudal to A demonstrates jejunal wall thickening (*arrows*). Perihepatic peritoneal fluid is again noted.

of bowel perforation but is seen in only a minority of cases (55,283) (Fig. 59).

Intraabdominal fluid is a very common but nonspecific CT finding of bowel or mesenteric injury (231,283). The fluid may be of low attenuation, representing extravasated small bowel contents, or of intermediate to high attenuation from acute hemorrhage. Free intraperitoneal fluid in the absence of an apparent solid visceral source of hemorrhage should heighten suspicion of a bowel or mesenteric injury (231,283). Occasionally, small quantities of intraperitoneal fluid, particularly when localized in the small bowel mesentery or between loops of bowel, may be the only CT sign of bowel perforation. Moderate or large amounts of fluid are less common as the sole CT abnormality but have a higher likelihood of being associated with bowel or mesenteric injury (196). Other suggestive but nonspecific abnormalities such as focal bowel wall thickening or strandy soft tissue infiltration of the mesenteric fat can improve diagnostic accuracy when combined with other CT scan findings (34,73). In one recent study, the CT finding of mesenteric bleeding and bowel wall thickening associated with mesenteric hematoma or infiltration indicated a high likelihood of a mesentery-bowel injury requiring surgical intervention (77).

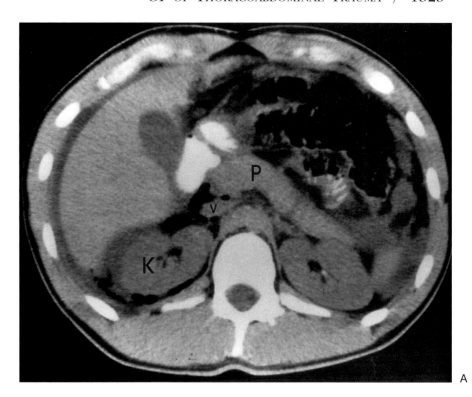

A

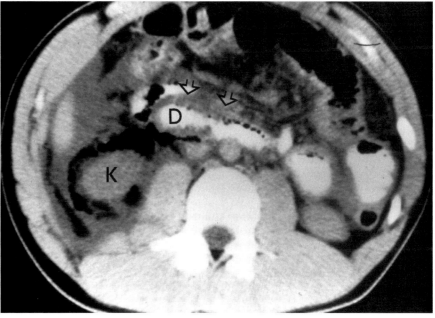

B

FIG. 57. Duodenal hematoma and perforation. **A:** CT scan at the level of the pancreas (P) demonstrates air dissecting in the retroperitoneum around the inferior vena cava (V) and right kidney (K). Peritoneal fluid is also noted around the liver and in the left paracolic gutter. **B:** CT scan several cm caudal to A demonstrates duodenal wall thickening (*open arrows*) and dissection of extraluminal retroperitoneal air around the lower pole of the right kidney (K); (D) duodenum.

Intramural hemorrhage is detected in most patients with bowel injury as circumferential or eccentric thickening of the bowel wall on CT, often with associated luminal narrowing (153,185) (Fig 60). Intense enhancement of the bowel wall has also been reported as a sign of bowel injury (137, 321). When combined with bowel thickening and free peritoneal fluid, intense bowel wall enhancement suggests bowel perforation and peritonitis (137). It should be noted, however, that increased contrast enhancement of the bowel wall is not a specific sign of bowel rupture,

as it can also be seen in children with the hypoperfusion complex (323) and in adults with prolonged hypoperfusion resulting in so-called shock bowel (238).

Kidney

Trauma to the kidney can occur either as an isolated event, or more frequently as concomitant injury in patients with acute abdominal trauma. Worldwide, blunt trauma is

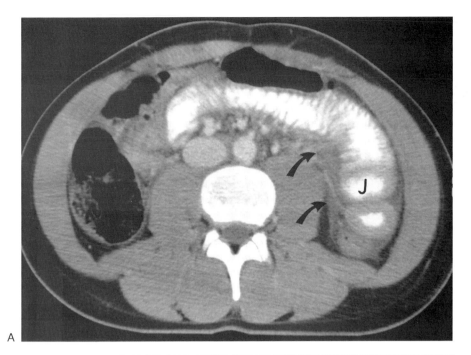

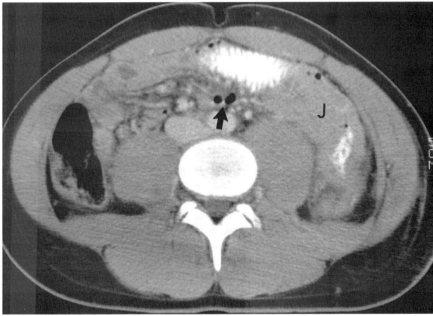

FIG. 58. Jejunal perforation. CT images through the lower abdomen (**A and B**) demonstrate thick-walled jejunum (J), soft tissue infiltration of the adjacent mesenteric fat (*curved arrows*), and extraluminal mesenteric air (*straight arrow*).

responsible for 80% of renal injuries, but the number attributable to penetrating wounds increases dramatically in urban settings with a high rate of violent crime (135). Most closed renal injuries are due to motor vehicle accidents, with contact sports, falls, fights, and assaults accounting for the remainder. With blunt trauma, the kidney may be injured by a direct blow, lacerated by the lower ribs, or torn by rapid acceleration-deceleration (273).

Penetrating injuries are usually secondary to gunshot or stab wounds. Interventional procedures, such as percutaneous nephrostomy and renal biopsy, constitute another group of penetrating injuries. A diseased or anomalous kidney is more susceptible to injury than a healthy one (Fig. 61). Minor or trivial trauma may lead to disruption of a hydronephrotic renal pelvis, fracture of a fragile, infected kidney, or laceration of a poorly protected ectopic or horseshoe kidney. Preexisting renal disease should be suspected whenever the inciting trauma seems disproportionately trivial to the patient's clinical findings (31,103). Underlying renal disease is more common in children with renal injury than in adults (167).

Renal injuries can be divided into four broad categories

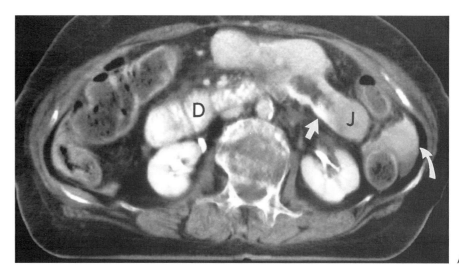

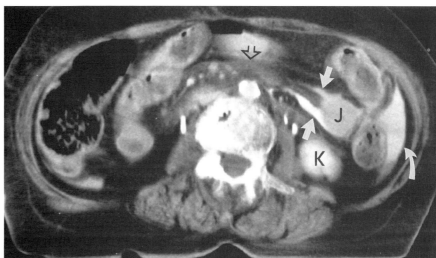

FIG. 59. Small bowel laceration at the ligament of Treitz with extravasation of oral contrast material. CT images at the level of the transverse duodenum (**A**) and lower pole of the left kidney (**B**) demonstrate extravasated oral contrast material along the small bowel mesentery (*straight arrows*) and in the left paracolic gutter (*curved arrow*). Ill-defined hemorrhage is noted at the root of the mesentery (*open arrow*); (D) opacified transverse duodenum; (J) unopacified jejunum; (K) lower pole of left kidney.

based upon a combination of clinical and imaging findings (92). Category I lesions include contusions and small corticomedullary lacerations that do not communicate with the collecting system. They account for 75% to 85% of all renal injuries. Category II lesions consist of lacerations that communicate with the renal collecting system and account for about 10% of cases. Lesions in category III consist of shattered kidneys and injuries to the renal vascular pedicle. They comprise about 5% of the total. Category IV is established for the relatively uncommon entity of ureteropelvic junction (UPJ) avulsion and laceration of the renal pelvis.

Most surgeons agree that category I injuries are best managed nonoperatively, whereas category III and IV injuries require prompt surgery (132). Controversy exists as to the proper management of category II lesions, with opinions ranging from extreme conservatism to aggressive intervention (37,83,382).

Unlike closed renal injuries which generally are managed more conservatively, penetrating renal trauma usu-

ally is an indication for surgery. Gunshot wounds invariably require surgical exploration and debridement because of the prevalence of associated injuries, contamination by foreign material (e.g., clothing) and extensive tissue necrosis produced by their blast effects (132). Stab wounds of the kidney, on the other hand, once an incontrovertible indication for surgery, are now being managed by watchful expectancy in selected cases because of the precise information provided by noninvasive imaging methods (132).

In the absence of associated injuries, clinical findings of the patient with renal injury are dictated by the type and severity of renal trauma. Renal injury must be presumed in every patient with abdominal trauma who has gross or microscopic hematuria. In one report of 38 children after blunt abdominal trauma, the amount of hematuria correlated better than hypotension with the severity of renal injury (331). However, hematuria may be absent in 10% to 28% of patients with renal trauma, especially those with injuries to the renal pedicles (215). Because

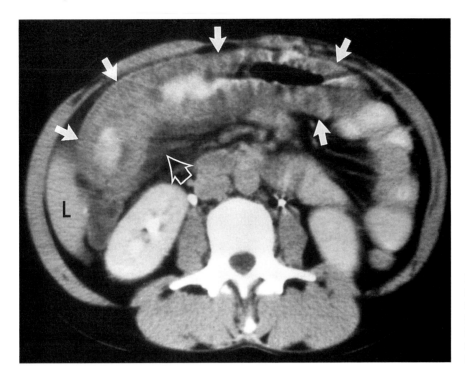

FIG. 60. Jejunal hematoma. CT scan at the inferior margin of the liver (L) demonstrates marked circumferential wall thickening of a loop of jejunum (*solid arrows*). Some infiltration of the adjacent mesentery is also identified (*open arrow*).

rapid deceleration is a common cause of renal pedicle injury, it is prudent to subject all patients with deceleration injuries (e.g., head-on motor vehicle collision, fall from a height) to renal imaging, regardless of the presence or absence of hematuria.

The role of the radiologist in assessing patients with suspected renal trauma is to accurately define the nature and extent of renal damage so that the maximum amount of functioning renal parenchyma can be preserved with the fewest complications. The choice of imaging studies

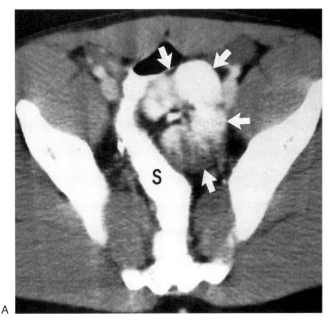
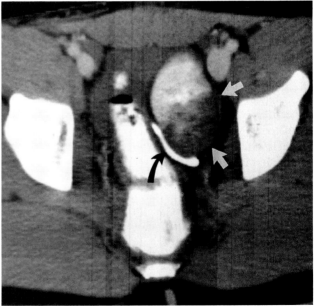

FIG. 61. Devascularization injury of a pelvic kidney. **A:** Pelvic kidney (*straight arrows*) is identified just to the left of the sigmoid colon (S). Ill-defined region of low attenuation along the posterior margin of the kidney represents the superior aspect of an area of devascularization involving the lower pole. **B:** CT image 2 cm caudal to A demonstrates a well-demarcated area of hypoperfusion involving the posterior half of the lower pole of the pelvic kidney (*straight arrows*); (*curved arrow*) ureter from pelvic kidney.

depends on the condition of the patient, the availability of imaging resources and personnel, and the surgeon's approach to management of renal trauma.

Computed tomography is the most informative radiologic study in renal trauma. A complete CT examination of the abdomen and pelvis can be completed with ease and speed (5 to 10 min) using state-of-the-art CT scanners. The use of CT is no longer limited to the evaluation of patients with severe renal trauma, suspected multiorgan trauma, or penetrating trauma. In fact, many have used CT as the initial imaging study in all patients with abdominal and renal trauma (178,370,382). Excretory urography still is used in some institutions for economical reasons to evaluate stable, asymptomatic patients with a history of minor, localized renal trauma (188). A normal urogram obviates further imaging evaluation in this clinical setting. CT is performed only in patients with persistent hematuria or a falling hematocrit. CT also is performed if the prior urogram suggests major injury or is inconclusive.

Ultrasonography and radionuclide scintigraphy have not received wide acceptance as the initial imaging study in renal trauma. However, radionuclide imaging can be used to assess residual renal function after conservative treatment of renal injury (382). Arteriography is reserved for preoperative road mapping and for therapeutic interventions such as embolization of bleeding vessels and arteriovenous fistulas. In spite of its ability to demonstrate vascular patency and parenchymal abnormalities (contusions and lacerations), magnetic resonance imaging (MRI) offers few advantages over well-performed contrast-enhanced CT and is not used in acute situations.

Computed tomography is capable of demonstrating virtually the entire spectrum of renal injury and effectively reveals preexisting renal abnormalities. The mildest form of renal injury is a contusion (Fig. 62). Renal contusion appears on unenhanced scans as diffuse or focal swelling containing scattered foci of high-density fresh blood intermixed with normally homogeneous soft-tissue-attenuation renal parenchyma. The involved area often exhibits delayed and decreased enhancement after intravenous administration of iodinated contrast medium (273). A striated nephrogram, presumably resulting from stasis of urine in blood-filled tubules, also has been encountered (290).

Parenchymal lacerations likewise can be recognized on CT. They appear as unenhanced areas disrupting the normally enhancing renal parenchyma on dynamic contrast-enhanced scans (Fig. 63). Both contusions and small parenchymal lacerations are often accompanied by a small subcapsular or perirenal hemorrhage. Whereas subcapsular hematomas generally appear as lenticular collections that flatten the underlying renal contour, perirenal hematomas infiltrate or displace perirenal fat and may extend to the renal (Gerota's) fascia.

Category II injuries are easily detected on enhanced CT as parenchymal defects extending from the renal surface into the medulla where they may enter the collecting system and/or transect the kidney (Fig. 64). Typically, such renal fractures parallel intervascular tissue planes, often without tearing major arteries or veins (302). The parenchymal margins often enhance inhomogeneously, producing a mottled appearance (302).

Category II injuries are almost always accompanied by perirenal hemorrhage. Extravasation of opacified urine, into either renal parenchyma or the perirenal space, frequently occurs (Fig. 65). An admixture of urine and blood also may be seen in the leaves of renal fascia as well as the anterior pararenal space (315).

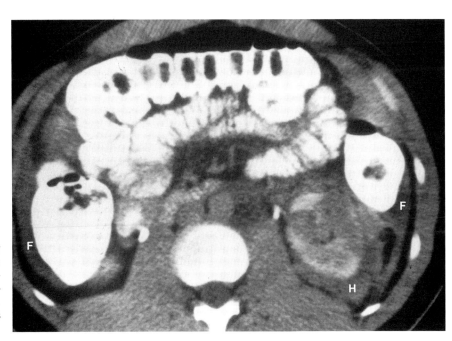

FIG. 62. Renal contusion. Note patchy areas of decreased enhancement in the lower pole of the left kidney representing renal contusion. Small perinephric hematoma (H) is also present. Fluid in the paracolic gutters (F) was related to concomitant splenic injury.

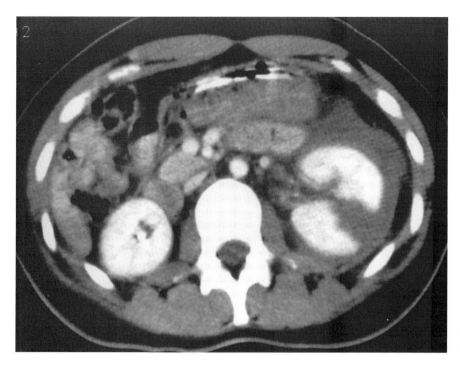

FIG. 63. Renal laceration with perirenal hematoma. Contrast-enhanced CT scan demonstrates large left renal laceration with associated perirenal hematoma confined by the renal (Gerota's) fascia.

Catastrophic renal injuries (category III) include shattered kidney and renal vascular pedicle injury. A shattered or pulverized kidney is recognized on CT as multiple fracture planes separating enhancing or nonenhancing renal fragments (Fig. 66). In contradistinction to the fractures in category II lesions, fractures associated with a shattered kidney generally shear across segmental renal blood vessels. A large perirenal hematoma is invariably present with a shattered kidney.

In renal pedicle injury, the occluded or avulsed main renal artery can be depicted on contrast-enhanced helical CT (257). In such an injury, a normal-sized, nonenhancing kidney is identified (Fig. 67). A rim of cortical tissue may be perfused by subcapsular collateral vessels (118,205), although this finding may not be noted acutely. Other associated findings include hematoma surrounding the renal hilus, abrupt cutoff of the contrast-filled renal artery, small perinephric hematoma, and retrograde filling of the renal vein (38). Disruption of a branch vessel results in a segmental infarct that appears as a wedge- or hemispheric-shaped zone of underperfused renal parenchyma subtending the distribution of the occluded vessel.

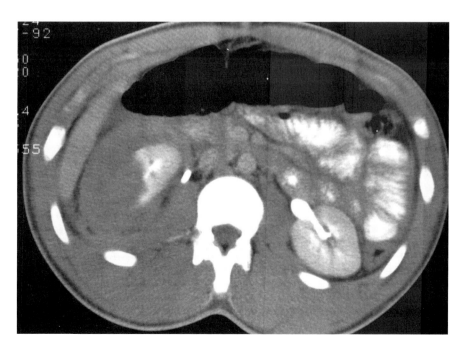

FIG. 64. Renal fracture. Contrast-enhanced CT scan demonstrates fractured right lower renal pole with large perirenal hematoma.

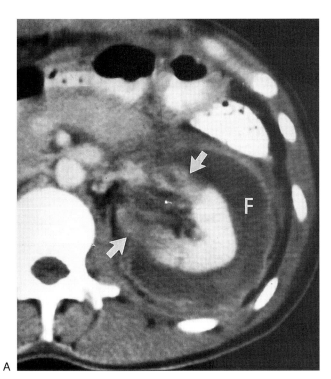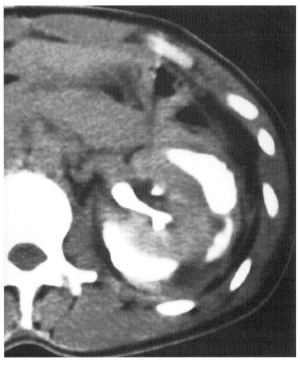

A   B

FIG. 65. Renal contusion with laceration of the collecting system. **A:** Ill-defined areas of decreased parenchymal enhancement consistent with contusion (*arrows*) are seen surrounding the renal pelvis medially. Low-attenuation fluid (F) expands the perirenal space. **B:** Delayed CT image demonstrates extravasation of contrast-opacified urine into the perirenal space consistent with laceration of the collecting system.

A wedge-shaped infarct is typically oriented with its base directed toward the renal capsule and its apex toward the renal hilus (118).

Renal vein injury occurs in 20% of patients with solitary pedicle injury (86). Acute renal vein occlusion may produce an enlarged rather than a normal-sized kidney, and associated cortical rim enhancement is usually thicker than with arterial obstruction (119). Demonstration of thrombus within a dilated renal vein on CT confirms the diagnosis.

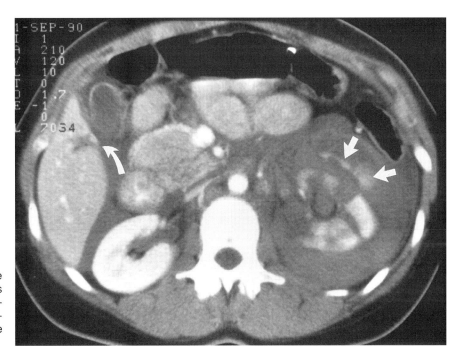

FIG. 66. Shattered kidney with large perirenal hematoma. Active bleeding is noted in the left perirenal space anteriorly (*straight arrows*). Small liver laceration (*curved arrow*) and blood in the hepatorenal fossa are also evident.

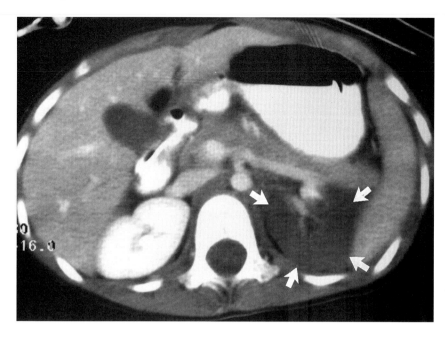

FIG. 67. Renal pedicle injury with devascularization of the left kidney. CT scan at the level of the left renal hilum demonstrates absent perfusion of the left kidney (*arrows*).

CT findings of massive accumulation of extravasated urine in the medial rather than dorsolateral aspect of the perirenal space, absence of renal parenchymal injury, and lack of ureteral opacification should suggest the diagnosis of ureteropelvic junction disruption (category IV injury) (172). Retrograde ureteropyelography should be performed to confirm the diagnosis prior to surgical correction.

Ureter

Iatrogenic trauma secondary to surgical procedures is the leading cause of ureteral injury (187). Penetrating and blunt trauma account for a relatively small number of ureteral injuries. When present, they commonly are associated with renal parenchymal, arterial, and venous injuries (352). Most reported cases are hyperextension inju-

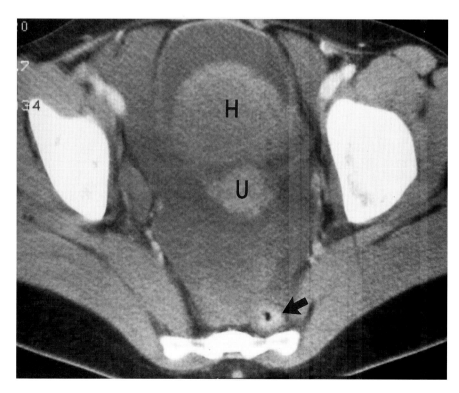

FIG. 68. Bladder hematoma. There is a large mural hematoma (H) involving the bladder base. A large amount of blood is also seen filling the pelvis. Note the hematocrit effect with denser blood elements layering posteriorly adjacent to the rectum (*arrow*). The patient had multiple liver lacerations on CT scans of the abdomen; (U) Uterus.

ries sustained by children in motor vehicle collisions. As described in the previous section, CT findings of isolated ureteral disruption in adults include nonvisualization of the ureter distal to the point of disruption, intact renal parenchyma, and confinement of extravasated urine to the medial perirenal space (172). In children, however, the urine extravasation also expands into leaves of the renal fascia, anterior pararenal space, and the psoas compartment (315).

Bladder

Bladder injuries may occur as a result of blunt, penetrating, or iatrogenic trauma. The susceptibility of the bladder to injury varies with the degree of distension; a distended urinary bladder is much more prone to injury than a nearly empty one. Most patients with bladder rupture complain of suprapubic pain or tenderness; however, the discomfort associated with a fractured bony pelvis often obscures the pain associated with the urinary tract injury. Gross hematuria almost invariably accompanies bladder injury. In one reported series (265), 95% of patients with bladder rupture had gross hematuria, whereas the remainder had microscopic hematuria.

The type of urine extravasation (intraperitoneal versus extraperitoneal) is dependent on the location of the bladder tear and its relationship to the peritoneal reflections (294). With an anterosuperior perforation, extravasation may be either intraperitoneal, into the prevesical space (space of Retzius), or both. With a posterosuperior tear, fluid can spread intraperitoneally, retroperitoneally, or both. Extravasation may also extend inferiorly into the perineum, the scrotum, and the thigh if the urogenital diaphragm is disrupted.

Intraperitoneal rupture usually results from a direct blow (often a kick) to a distended bladder and requires surgical repair. Extraperitoneal rupture often results from a shearing injury at the base of the bladder and is best treated with suprapubic cystostomy (52).

Retrograde cystography has been the preferred radiologic procedure for evaluating patients with suspected bladder injury (294). Earlier reports have shown that bladder rupture may be missed on CT studies if the urinary bladder is not adequately distended (218). More recent studies have demonstrated that a properly performed CT is as sensitive for detecting bladder injuries as conventional cystography (149,166,200). To minimize false negative CT diagnosis of bladder rupture, scans of the pelvis should be obtained with the urinary bladder fully distended either by retrograde or antegrade means (149,166,200). Both delayed scans and repeat scanning of the pelvis after bladder drainage have been used to help detect subtle bladder injury (149,166,319). Because many patients with possible bladder injuries also are suspected of having other organ injuries, and because CT is the procedure of choice for evaluating patients with blunt abdominal and pelvic trauma, the diagnosis of bladder rupture often is made on CT. Retrograde cystography is reserved for cases in which there is persistent suspicion of bladder injury in spite of a negative CT study or in cases where the CT examination is suboptimal or equivocal.

Angiography plays no role in the primary assessment of bladder injury but may be of considerable value in the diagnosis and management of arterial bleeding associated with pelvic fractures. Radionuclide scintigraphy can detect small amounts of extravasation with great sensitivity, but because of its inferior spatial resolution compared to conventional radiography and CT it is rarely used in assessing cases of bladder trauma. Although ultrasonogra-

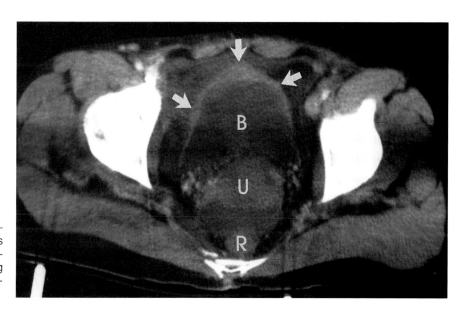

FIG. 69. Intraperitoneal bladder rupture. CT scan through the lower pelvis demonstrates extravasated contrast-opacified urine (*arrows*) surrounding the bladder (B). Fluid is also noted between the uterus (U) and rectum (R).

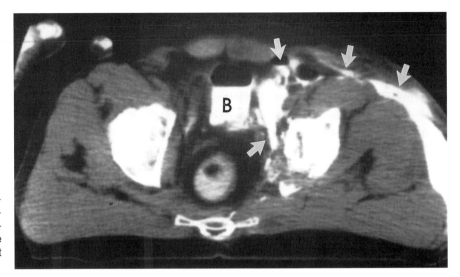

FIG. 70. Extraperitoneal bladder rupture. CT scan at the level of the acetabula demonstrates extravasation of contrast-opacified urine (*arrows*) into the extraperitoneal soft tissues on the left side of the bladder (B).

phy also may demonstrate lacerations of the urinary bladder (363), it is not widely used in the United States for this purpose.

On CT, different types of bladder injuries can be identified and differentiated from one another. Bladder contusion or hematoma appears as focal or diffuse wall thickening without extravasation of contrast medium (Fig. 68). With intraperitoneal rupture of the bladder, extravasated urine, and contrast medium can be found surrounding the bladder or bowel and pooling in the paracolic gutters (294) (Fig. 69). Extraperitoneal rupture results in extravasation of contrast medium and urine into the perivesical fat, anterior thigh, scrotum, penis, and abdominal wall (Fig. 70). Contrast medium also can extend cephalad to the perirenal and pararenal spaces (294).

REFERENCES

1. Abramson SJ, Berdon WE, Kaufman RA, Ruzal-Shapiro C. Hepatic parenchymal and subcapsular gas after hepatic laceration caused by blunt abdominal trauma. *AJR* 1989;153:1031–1032.
2. Agee CK, Metzler MH, Churchill RJ, Mitchell FL. Computed tomographic evaluation to exclude traumatic aortic disruption. *J Trauma* 1992;33:876–881.
3. Ang JGP, Hanslits ML, Clark RA, Hawkins HH. Computed tomography of abdominal and pelvic trauma. *J Emerg Med* 1985; 3:311–325.
4. Aronchick JM, Epstein DM, Gefter WE, Miller WT. Chronic traumatic diaphragmatic hernia: the significance of pleural effusion. *Radiology* 1988;168:675–678.
5. Athey GN, Rahman SU. Hepatic hematoma following blunt injury: nonoperative management. *Injury* 1982;13:302–306.
6. Ayella RJ, Hankins JR, Turney SZ, Cowley RA. Ruptured thoracic aorta due to blunt trauma. *J Trauma* 1977;17:199–205.
7. Bach RD, Frey CF. Diagnosis and treatment of pancreatic trauma. *Am J Surg* 1971;121:20–29.
8. Backer CL, LoCicero J, Hartz RS, Donaldson JS, Shields T. Computed tomography in patients with esophageal perforation. *Chest* 1990;98:1078–1080.
9. Ball T, McCrory R, Smith JO, Clements JL. Traumatic diaphragmatic hernia: errors in diagnosis. *AJR* 1982;138:633–637.
10. Barcia TC, Livoni JP. Indications for angiography in blunt thoracic trauma. *Radiology* 1983;147:15–19.
11. Baxt WG, Moody P. The impact of a rotorcraft aeromedical emergency care service on trauma mortality. *JAMA* 1983;249:3047–3051.
12. Becker CD, Gal I, Baer HU, Vock P. Blunt hepatic trauma in adults: correlation of CT injury grading with outcome. *Radiology* 1996; 201:215–220.
13. Becker CD, Spring P, Glattli A, Schweizer W. Blunt splenic trauma in adults: can CT findings be used to determine the need for surgery? *AJR* 1994;162:343–347.
14. Bennett DE, Cherry JK. The natural history of traumatic aneurysms of the aorta. *Surgery* 1967;61:516–523.
15. Benya EC, Bulas DI, Eichelberger MR, Sivit CJ. Splenic injury from blunt abdominal trauma in children: follow-up evaluation with CT. *Radiology* 1995;195:685–688.
16. Bergstrom M, Ericson K, Levander B, Svendsen P, Larsson S. Variation with time of the attenuation values of intracranial hematomas. *J Comput Assist Tomogr* 1977;1:57–63.
17. Berland LL. CT of blunt abdominal trauma. In: Fishman EK, Federle MP, eds. *Body CT categorical course syllabus.* New Orleans, LA: American Roentgen Ray Society, 1994;207–214.
18. Berland LL, VanDyke JA. Decreased splenic enhancement on CT in traumatized hypotensive patients. *Radiology* 1985;156:469–471.
19. Black WC, Gouse JC, Williamson BRJ, Newman BM. Computed tomography of traumatic lung cyst: case report. *J Comput Tomogr* 1986;10:33–35.
20. Bladergroen MR, Lowe JE, Postlethwait RW. Diagnosis and recommended management of esophageal perforation and rupture. *Ann Thorac Surg* 1986;42:235–239.
21. Blair E, Topuzlu C, Davis JH. Delayed or missed diagnosis in blunt chest trauma. *J Trauma* 1971;11:129–145.
22. Bond SJ, Eichelberger MR, Gotschall CS, Sivit CJ, Randolph JG. Nonoperative management of blunt hepatic and splenic injury in children. *Ann Surg* 1996;223:286–289.
23. Boulanger BR, Mirvis SE, Rodriguez A. Magnetic resonance imaging in traumatic diaphragmatic rupture: case reports. *J Trauma* 1992;32:89–93.
24. Boyd AD. Pneumothorax and hemothorax. In: Hood RM, Boyd AD, Culliford AT, eds. *Thoracic trauma.* Philadelphia: WB Saunders, 1989;133–148.
25. Bresler MJ. Computed tomography of the abdomen. *Ann Emerg Med* 1986;15:280–285.
26. Brick SH, Taylor GA, Potter BM, Eichelberger MR. Hepatic and splenic injury in children: role of CT in the decision for laparotomy. *Radiology* 1987;165:643–646.
27. Bridges KG, Welch G, Silver M, Schinco MA, Esposito B. CT detection of occult pneumothorax in multiple trauma patients. *J Emerg Med* 1993;11:179–186.
28. Brink JA, Heiken JP, Semenkovich J, Teefey SA, McClennan BL,

Sagel SS. Abnormalities of the diaphragm and adjacent structures: findings on multiplanar spiral CT scans. *AJR* 1994;163:307–310.

29. Brooks AP, Olson LK. Computed tomography of the chest in the trauma patient. *Clin Radiol* 1989;40:127–132.

30. Brooks SW, Cmolik BL, Young JC, Townsend RN, Diamond DL. Transesophageal echocardiographic examination of a patient with traumatic aortic transection from blunt chest trauma: a case report. *J Trauma* 1991;31:841–845.

31. Brower P, Paul J, Brosman SA. Urinary tract abnormalities presenting as a result of blunt abdominal trauma. *J Trauma* 1978;18:719.

32. Brown RA, Bass DH, Rode H, Millar AJW, Cywes S. Gastrointestinal tract perforation in children due to blunt abdominal trauma. *Br J Surg* 1992;79:522–524.

33. Bulas DI, Eichelberger MR, Sivit CJ, Wright CJ, Gotschall CS. Hepatic injury from blunt trauma in children: follow-up evaluation with CT. *AJR* 1993;160:347–351.

34. Bulas DI, Taylor GA, Eichelberger MR. The value of CT in detecting bowel perforation in children after blunt abdominal trauma. *AJR* 1989;153:561–564.

35. Buntain WL, Gould HR, Maull KI. Predictability of splenic salvage by computed tomography. *J Trauma* 1988;28:24–34.

36. Burney RE, Mueller GL, Coon GL, Thomas EJ, Mackenzie JR. Diagnosis of isolated small bowel injury. *Ann Emerg Med* 1983;12:71–74.

37. Cass AS. Discussion. In: Guerriero WG, ed. *Problems in Urology,* vol 2. Philadelphia: JB Lippincott, 1988;184.

38. Cates JD, Foley WD, Lawson TL. Retrograde opacification of renal vein: a CT sign of renal artery avulsion. *Urol Radiol* 1986;8:92–94.

39. Ceraldi CM, Waxman K. Computerized tomography as an indicator of isolated mesenteric injury: a comparison with peritoneal lavage. *Am Surgeon* 1990;56:806–810.

40. Chapman WC, Morris JA. Diagnosis and management of blunt pancreatic injury. *J Tenn Med Assoc* 1989;82:84–85.

41. Chew FS, Panicek DM, Heitzman ER. Late discovery of a post-traumatic right aortic arch aneurysm. *AJR* 1985;145:1001–1002.

42. Chiles C, Putman CE. Acute thoracic trauma. In: Goodman LR, Putman CE, eds. *Critical care imaging,* 3rd ed. Philadelphia: WB Saunders, 1992;199–212.

43. Cholankeril JV, Zamora BO, Ketyer S. Left lobe of the liver draping around the spleen: a pitfall in computed tomography diagnosis of perisplenic hematoma. *J Comput Assist Tomogr* 1984;8:261–267.

44. Clark DE, Zeiger MA, Wallace KL, Packard AB, Nowicki ER. Blunt aortic trauma: signs of high risk. *J Trauma* 1990;30:701–705.

45. Cogbill TH, Moore EE, Jurkovich GJ, Morris JA, Mucha P, Shackford SR. Nonoperative management of blunt splenic trauma: a multicenter experience. *J Trauma* 1989;29:1312–1317.

46. Cogbill TH, Moore EE, Morris JA, et al. Distal pancreatectomy for trauma: a multicenter experience. *J Trauma* 1991;31:1600–1606.

47. Cohen AM, Crass JR. Traumatic aortic injuries: current concepts. *Semin Ultrasound CT MR* 1993;14:71–84.

48. Cohen AM, Crass JR, Thomas HA, Fisher RG, Jacobs DG. CT evidence for the ''osseous pinch'' mechanism of traumatic aortic injury. *AJR* 1992;159:271–274.

49. Collins JC, Levine G, Waxman K. Occult traumatic pneumothorax: immediate tube thoracostomy versus expectant management. *Am Surgeon* 1992;58:743–746.

50. Conrad MR. Splenic trauma: false-negative CT diagnosis in cases of delayed rupture (letter). *AJR* 1988;151:200–201.

51. Cook DE, Walsh JW, Vick CW, Brewer WH. Upper abdominal trauma: pitfalls in CT diagnosis. *Radiology* 1986;159:65–69.

52. Corriere JN, Sandler CM. Mechanisms of injury, patterns of extravasation and management of extraperitoneal bladder rupture due to blunt trauma. *J Urol* 1987;139:43–44.

53. Cowley RA, Turney SZ, Hankins JR, Rodriguez A, Attar S, Shankar BS. Rupture of thoracic aorta caused by blunt trauma. A fifteen-year experience. *J Thorac Cardiovasc Surg* 1990;100:652–661.

54. Cox JF, Friedman AC, Radecki PD, Lev-Toaff AS, Caroline DF. Periportal lymphedema in trauma patients. *AJR* 1990;154:1124–1125.

55. Cox TD, Kuhn JP. CT scan of bowel trauma in the pediatric patient. *Radiol Clin North Am* 1996;34:807–818.

56. Cozacov C, Krausz L, Freund U. Emergencies in delayed diaphragmatic herniation due to blunt trauma. *Injury* 1984;15:370–371.

57. Craig MH, Talton DS, Hauser CJ, Poole GV. Pancreatic injuries from blunt trauma. *Am Surgeon* 1995;61:125–128.

58. Crass JR, Cohen AM, Motta AO, Tomashefski JR, Wiesen EJ. A proposed new mechansim of traumatic aortic rupture: the osseous pinch. *Radiology* 1990;176:645–649.

59. Croce MA, Fabian TC, Kudsk KA, et al. AAST organ injury scale: correlation of CT-graded liver injuries and operative findings. *J Trauma* 1991;31:806–812.

60. Croce MA, Fabian TC, Menke PG, et al. Nonoperative management of blunt hepatic trauma is the treatment of choice for hemodynamically stable patients: results of a prospective trial. *Ann Surg* 1995;221:744–755.

61. Cruz CJ, Minagi H. Large-bowel obstruction resulting from traumatic diaphragmatic hernia: imaging findings in four cases. *AJR* 1994;162:843–845.

62. Curtin JJ, Goodman LR, Quebbeman EJ, Haasler GB. Thoracostomy tubes after acute chest injury: relationship between location in a pleural fissure and function. *AJR* 1994;163:1339–1342.

63. Cywes S, Rode H, Millar AJW. Blunt liver trauma in children: nonoperative management. *J Pediatr Surg* 1985;20:14–18.

64. Daniels DL, Maddison FE. Ascending aortic injury: an angiographic diagnosis. *AJR* 1981;136:812–813.

65. Dauterive AH, Flancbaum L, Cox EF. Blunt intestinal trauma: a modern day review. *Ann Surg* 1985;201:198–203.

66. Defore WW, Mattox KL, Jordan GL, et al. Management of 1,590 consecutive cases of liver trauma. *Arch Surg* 1976;111:493–496.

67. Demos TC, Solomon C, Posniak HV, Flisak MJ. Computed tomography in traumatic defects of the diaphragm. *Clin Imag* 1989;13:62–67.

68. Denis R, Allard M, Atlas H, Farkouh E. Changing trends with abdominal injury in seatbelt wearers. *J Trauma* 1983;23:1007–1008.

69. Dennis LN, Rogers LF. Superior mediastinal widening from spine fractures mimicking aortic rupture on chest radiographs. *AJR* 1989;152:27–30.

70. Do HM, Cronan JJ. CT appearance of splenic injuries managed nonoperatively. *AJR* 1991;157:757–760.

71. Dodds WJ, Taylor AJ, Erickson SJ, Lawson TL. Traumatic fracture of the pancreas: CT characteristics. *J Comput Assist Tomogr* 1990;14:375–378.

72. Donohue J, Crass R, Trunkey D. Management of duodenal and small intestinal injury. *World J Surg* 1985;9:904–913.

73. Donohue JH, Federle MP, Griffiths BG, Trunkey DD. Computed tomography in the diagnosis of blunt intestinal and mesenteric injuries. *J Trauma* 1987;27:11–17.

74. Donovan AJ, Turrill F, Berne CJ. Injuries of the pancreas from blunt trauma. *Surg Clin North Am* 1972;52:649–665.

75. Dougall AM, Paul ME, Finley RJ, Holliday RL, Coles JC, Duff JH. Chest trauma: current morbidity and mortality. *J Trauma* 1977;17:547–553.

76. Dow RW. Myocardial rupture caused by trauma. *Surgery* 1982;91:246–247.

77. Dowe MF, Shanmuganathan K, Mirvis SE, Steiner RC, Cooper C. CT findings of mesenteric injury after blunt abdominal trauma: implications for surgical intervention. *AJR* 1997;168:425–428.

78. Eger EI, Saidman LJ. Hazards of nitrous oxide anesthesia in bowel obstruction and pneumothorax. *Anesthesiology* 1965;26:61–66.

79. Elmore JR, Clark DE, Isler RJ, Horner WR. Selective nonoperative management of blunt splenic trauma in adults. *Arch Surg* 1989;124:581–586.

80. Erickson DR, Shinozaki T, Beekman E, Davis JH. Relationship of arterial blood gases and pulmonary radiographs to the degree of pulmonary damage in experimental pulmonary contusion. *J Trauma* 1971;11:689–696.

81. Estrera AS, Landay MJ, McClelland RN. Blunt traumatic rupture of the right hemidiaphragm: experience in 12 patients. *Ann Thorac Surg* 1985;39:525–530.

82. Evens RG. Radiology decision making: the importance of cost-effectiveness analysis (commentary). *AJR* 1995;165:37.

83. Evins SC, Thomason WB, Rosenblaum R. Non-operative management of severe renal lacerations. *J Urol* 1980;123:247–249.

84. Faer MJ, Lynch RD, Lichtenstein JE, Madewell JE, Feigin DS. Traumatic splenic cyst. *Radiology* 1980;134:371–376.

85. Fagelman D, Hertz MA, Ross AS. Delayed development of splenic subcapsular hematoma: CT evaluation. *J Comput Assist Tomogr* 1985;9:815–816.

86. Fanney DR, Casillas J, Murphy BJ. CT in the diagnosis of renal trauma. *RadioGraphics* 1990;10:29–40.

87. Farnell MB, Spencer MP, Thompson E, Williams HJ, Mucha P, Ilstrup DM. Nonoperative management of blunt hepatic trauma in adults. *Surgery* 1988;104:748–755.

88. Federico JA, Horner WR, Clark DE, Isler RJ. Blunt hepatic trauma: nonoperative management in adults. *Arch Surg* 1990;125:905–909.

89. Federle MP. Computed tomography of blunt abdominal trauma. *Radiol Clin North Am* 1983;21:461–475.

90. Federle MP. CT of upper abdominal trauma. *Semin Roentgenol* 1984;19:269–280.

91. Federle MP. CT of abdominal trauma. In: Federle MP, Brant-Zawadzki M, eds. *Computed tomography in the evaluation of trauma*, 2nd ed. Baltimore: Williams and Wilkins, 1986;191–273.

92. Federle MP. Evaluation of renal trauma. In: Pollack HM, ed. *Clinical urography*, vol 2. Philadelphia: WB Saunders, 1990;1472–1494.

93. Federle MP. Splenic trauma: is follow-up CT of value? *Radiology* 1995;194:23–24.

94. Federle MP, Crass RA, Jeffrey RB, Trunkey DD. Computed tomography in blunt abdominal trauma. *Arch Surg* 1982;117:645–650.

95. Federle MP, Goldberg HI, Kaiser JA, Moss AA, Jeffrey RB, Mall JC. Evaluation of abdominal trauma by computed tomography. *Radiology* 1981;138:637–644.

96. Federle MP, Griffiths B, Minagi H, Jeffrey RB. Splenic trauma: evaluation with CT. *Radiology* 1987;162:69–71.

97. Federle MP, Jeffrey RB. Hemoperitoneum studied by computed tomography. *Radiology* 1983;148:187–192.

98. Fenner MN, Fisher KS, Sergel NL, Porter DB, Metzmaker CO. Evaluation of possible traumatic thoracic aortic injury using aortography and CT. *Am Surg* 1990;56:497–499.

99. Finkelmeier BA, Mentzer RMJ, Kaiser DL, Tegtmeyer CJ, Nolan SP. Chronic traumatic thoracic aneurysm. Influence of operative treatment on natural history: an analysis of reported cases, 1950–1980. *J Thorac Cardiovasc Surg* 1982;84:257–266.

100. Fisher RG, Chasen MH, Lamki N. Diagnosis of injuries of the aorta and brachiocephalic arteries caused by blunt chest trauma: CT vs aortography. *AJR* 1994;162:1047–1052.

101. Fisher RG, Hadlock F, Ben-Menachem Y. Laceration of the thoracic aorta and brachiocephalic arteries by blunt trauma. Report of 54 cases and review of the literature. *Radiol Clin North Am* 1981;19:91–110.

102. Fisher RG, Ward RE, Ben-Menachem Y, Mattox KL, Flynn TC. Arteriography and the fractured first rib: too much for too little? *AJR* 1982;138:1059–1062.

103. Fitzgerald JB, Crawford ES, deBakey ME. Surgical considerations of nonpenetrating abdominal injuries. *Am J Surg* 1960;100:22.

104. Foley WD, Cates JD, Kellman GM, et al. Treatment of blunt hepatic injuries: role of CT. *Radiology* 1987;164:635–638.

105. Frey CF. Trauma to the pancreas and duodenum. In: Blaisdell FW, Trunkey DD, eds. *Abdominal trauma*. New York: Thieme-Stratton, 1982;87–122.

106. Fulda G, Rodriguez A, Turney SZ, Cowley RA. Blunt traumatic pericardial rupture. A ten-year experience 1979 to 1989. *J Cardiovasc Surg* 1990;31:525–530.

107. Garramone RR, Jacobs LM. An objective method to measure and manage occult pneumothorax. *Surg Gynecol Obstet* 1991;173:257–261.

108. Gavant ML, Flick P, Menke P, Gold RE. CT aortography of thoracic aortic rupture. *AJR* 1996;166:955–961.

109. Gavant ML, Menke PG, Fabian T, Flick PA, Graney MJ, Gold RE. Blunt traumatic aortic rupture: detection with helical CT of the chest. *Radiology* 1995;197:125–133.

110. Gavant ML, Schurr M, Flick PA, Croce MA, Fabian TC, Gold RE. Predicting clinical outcome of nonsurgical management of blunt splenic injury: using CT to reveal abnormalities of splenic vasculature. *AJR* 1997;168:207–212.

111. Gay SB, Sistrom CL. Computed tomographic evaluation of blunt abdominal trauma. *Radiol Clin North Am* 1992;30:367–388.

112. Gazak S, Davidson SJ. Posterior sternoclavicular dislocations: two case reports. *J Trauma* 1984;24:80–82.

113. Gelman R, Mirvis SE, Gens D. Diaphragmatic rupture due to blunt trauma: sensitivity of plain chest radiographs. *AJR* 1991;156:51–57.

114. Gerblich AA, Kleinerman J. Blunt chest trauma and the lung. *Am Rev Respir Dis* 1977;115:369–370.

115. Ginaldi S. Post-traumatic splenic hematoma hidden by an overdistended stomach: use of nasogastric tube to avoid pitfalls. *Comput Radiol* 1987;11:203–205.

116. Glazer GM, Axel L, Goldberg HI, Moss AA. Dynamic CT of the normal spleen. *AJR* 1981;137:343–346.

117. Glazer GM, Buy JN, Moss AA, Goldberg HI, Federle MP. CT detection of duodenal perforation. *AJR* 1981;137:333–336.

118. Glazer GM, Francis IR, Brady TM, Teng SS. Computed tomography of renal infarction: clinical and experimental observations. *AJR* 1983;140:721–727.

119. Glazer GM, Francis IR, Gross BH, Amendola MA. Computed tomography of renal vein thrombosis. *J Comput Assist Tomogr* 1984;8:288–293.

120. Godley CD, Warren RL, Sheridan RL, McCabe CJ. Nonoperative management of blunt splenic injury in adults: age over 55 years as a powerful indicator for failure. *J Am College Surg* 1996;183:133–139.

121. Godwin JD, Merten DF, Baker ME. Paramediastinal pneumatocele: alternative explanations to gas in the pulmonary ligament. *AJR* 1985;145:525–530.

122. Goldstein AS, Sclafani SJA, Kupferstein NH, et al. The diagnostic superiority of computerized tomography. *J Trauma* 1985;25:938–946.

123. Goldstein L, Mirvis SE, Kostrubiak IS, Turney SZ. CT diagnosis of acute pericardial tamponade after blunt chest trauma. *AJR* 1989;152:739–741.

124. Goodman LR, Aprahamian C. Changes in splenic size after abdominal trauma. *Radiology* 1990;176:629–632.

125. Goodman PC. CT of chest trauma. In: Federle MP, Brant-Zawadzki M, eds. *Computed tomography in the evaluation of trauma*, 2nd ed. Baltimore: Williams and Wilkins, 1986;168–190.

126. Gores PF, Simso LA. Splenic injury during colonoscopy. *Arch Surg* 1989;124:1342.

127. Graivier L, Freeark RJ. Traumatic diaphragmatic hernia. *Arch Surg* 1963;86:363–373.

128. Greendyke RM. Traumatic rupture of aorta. Special reference to automobile accidents. *JAMA* 1966;195:119–122.

129. Greene R. Blunt thoracic trauma. *Syllabus: a categorical course in diagnostic radiology—chest radiology*. Radiological Society of North America. Oak Brook, IL: RSNA Publications 1992;297–309.

130. Grimes OF. Nonpenetrating injuries to the chest wall and esophagus. *Surg Clin North Am* 1972;52:597–609.

131. Groskin SA. Selected topics in chest trauma. *Radiology* 1992;183:605–617.

132. Guerriero WG. Genitourinary trauma. In: Guerriero WG, ed. *Problems in urology*, vol 2. Philadelphia: JB Lippincott, 1988;186–187.

133. Gundry SR, Williams S, Burney RE, MacKenzie JR, Cho KJ. Indications for aortography. Radiography after blunt chest trauma: a reassesment of the radiographic findings associated with traumatic rupture of the aorta. *Invest Radiol* 1983;18:230–237.

134. Gurney J, Harrison NL, Anderson JC. Omental fat simulating pleural fluid in traumatic diaphragmatic hernia: CT characteristics. *J Comput Assist Tomogr* 1985;9:1112–1114.

135. Hai MA, Pontes JE, Pierce JM. Surgical management of major renal trauma: a review of 102 cases treated by conservative surgery. *J Urol* 1977;118:7–9.

136. Haney PJ, Whitley NO, Brotman S, Cunat JS, Whitley J. Liver injury and complications in the postoperative trauma patient: CT evaluation. *AJR* 1982;139:271–275.

137. Hara H, Babyn PS, Bourgeois D. Significance of bowel wall enhancement on CT following blunt abdominal trauma in childhood. *J Comput Assist Tomogr* 1992;16:94–98.

138. Hegarty MM, Bryer JV, Angorn IB, Baker LW. Delayed presentation of traumatic diaphragmatic hernia. *Ann Surg* 1978;188:229–233.

139. Heiberg E, Wolverson MK. CT of traumatic injuries of the aorta. *Semin Ultrasound Comput Tomogr Magn Reson Imag* 1985;6:172–180.

140. Heiberg E, Wolverson MK, Hurd RN, Jagannadharao B, Sundaram M. CT recognition of traumatic rupture of the diaphragm. *AJR* 1980;135:369–372.

141. Heiberg E, Wolverson MK, Sundaram M, Shields JB. CT in aortic trauma. *AJR* 1983;140:1119–1124.

142. Henry DA. Thoracic trauma: radiologic triage of the chest radiograph. Syllabus, Categorical Course on Chest Radiology. *Am Roentgen Ray Soc* 1986;13–22.

143. Heystraten FM, Rosenbusch G, Kingma LM, Lacquet LK. Chronic posttraumatic aneurysm of the thoracic aorta: surgically correctable occult threat. *AJR* 1986;146:303–308.

144. Hill LD. Injuries of the diaphragm following blunt trauma. *Surg Clin North Am* 1972;52:611–624.

145. Hiraide A, Yamamoto H, Yahata K, Yoshioka T, Sugimoto T. Delayed rupture of the spleen caused by an intrasplenic pseudoaneurysm following blunt trauma: case report. *J Trauma* 1994;36:743–744.

146. Holland DG, Quint LE. Traumatic rupture of the diaphragm without visceral herniation: CT diagnosis. *AJR* 1991;157:17–18.

147. Holness R, Waxman K. Diagnosis of traumatic cardiac contusion utilizing single photon-emission computed tomography. *Crit Care Med* 1990;18:1–3.

148. Hood RM, Sloan HE. Injuries of the trachea and major bronchi. *J Thorac Cardiovasc Surg* 1959;38:458–480.

149. Horstman WG, McClennan BL, Heiken JP. Comparison of computed tomography and conventional cystography for detection of traumatic bladdder rupture. *Urol Radiol* 1991;12:188–193.

150. Hossack KF, Moreno CA, Vanway CW, Burdick DC. Frequency of cardiac contusion in nonpenetrating chest injury. *Am J Cardiol* 1988;61:391–394.

151. Howell HS, Bartizal JF, Freeark RJ. Blunt trauma involving the colon and rectum. *J Trauma* 1976;16:624–632.

152. Hoyt DB, Potenza BM. Trauma. In: Greenfield LJ, Mulholland MW, Oldham KT, Zelenock GB, Lillemoe KD, eds. *Surgery: scientific principles and practice,* 2nd ed. New York: Lippincott-Raven, 1997;267–422.

153. Hughes JJ, Brogdon BG. Computed tomography of duodenal hematoma. *J Comput Tomogr* 1986;10:231–236.

154. Hunink MGM, Bos JJ. Triage of patients to angiography for detection of aortic rupture after blunt chest trauma: cost-effectiveness analysis of using CT. *AJR* 1995;165:27–36.

155. Hunter AR. Problems of anesthesia in artificial pneumothorax. *Proc R Soc Med* 1955;48:765–768.

156. Ishikawa T, Nakajima Y, Kaji T. The role of CT in traumatic rupture of the thoracic aorta and its proximal branches. *Semin Roentgenol* 1989;24:38–46.

157. Israel RS, Mayberry JC, Primack SL. Diaphragmatic rupture: use of helical CT scanning with multiplanar reformations. *AJR* 1996;167:1201–1203.

158. Jeffrey RB. CT diagnosis of blunt hepatic and splenic injuries: a look to the future. *Radiology* 1989;171:17–18.

159. Jeffrey RB, Cardoza JD, Olcott EW. Detection of active intraabdominal arterial hemorrhage: value of dynamic contrast-enhanced CT. *AJR* 1991;156:725–729.

160. Jeffrey RB, Federle MP. The collapsed inferior vena cava: CT evidence of hypovolemia. *AJR* 1988;150:431–432.

161. Jeffrey RB, Federle MP, Crass RA. Computed tomography of pancreatic trauma. *Radiology* 1983;147:491–494.

162. Jeffrey RB, Olcott EW. Imaging of blunt hepatic trauma. *Radiol Clin North Am* 1991;29:1299–1310.

163. Jones RC. Management of pancreatic trauma. *Am J Surg* 1985;150:698–704.

164. Jones RC, Shires GT. Pancreatic trauma. *Arch Surg* 1971;102:424–430.

165. Jurkovich GJ. Injuries to the duodenum and pancreas. In: Feliciano DV, Moore EE, Mattox KL, eds. *Trauma,* 3rd ed. Stamford, CT: Appleton and Lange, 1996;573–594.

166. Kane NM, Francis IR, Ellis JH. The value of CT in the detection of bladder and posterior urethral injuries. *AJR* 1989;153:1243–1246.

167. Kass EJ. Renal injury in children. In: Cass AS, ed. *Genitourinary trauma.* Boston: Blackwell Scientific, 1988;58.

168. Kato R, Horinouchi H, Maenaka Y. Traumatic pulmonary pseudocyst. Report of twelve cases. *J Thorac Cardiovasc Surg* 1989;97:309–312.

169. Kearney PA, Rouhana SW, Burney RE. Blunt rupture of the diaphragm: mechanism, diagnosis, and treatment. *Ann Emerg Med* 1989;18:1326–1330.

170. Kearney PA, Vahey T, Burney RE, Glazer G. Computed tomography and diagnostic peritoneal lavage in blunt abdominal trauma. *Arch Surg* 1989;124:344–347.

171. Kelly J, Raptopoulos V, Davidoff A, Waite R, Norton P. The value of non-contrast-enhanced CT in blunt abdominal trauma. *AJR* 1989;152:41–46.

172. Kenney PJ, Panicek DM, Witanowski LS. Computed tomography of ureteral disruption. *J Comput Assist Tomogr* 1987;11:480–484.

173. Kerns SR, Gay SB. CT of blunt chest trauma. *AJR* 1990;154:55–60.

174. Kirsch JD, Escarous A. CT diagnosis of traumatic pericardium rupture. *JCAT* 1989;13:523–524.

175. Kirsh MM, Behrendt DM, Orringer MB, et al. The treatment of acute traumatic rupture of the aorta. A 10-year experience. *Ann Surg* 1976;184:308–316.

176. Kirsh MM, Orringer MB, Behrendt DM, Sloan H. Management of tracheobronchial disruption secondary to nonpenetrating trauma. *Ann Thorac Surg* 1976;22:93–101.

177. Kirsh MM, Sloan H. Blunt chest trauma. General principles of management. Boston: Little, Brown, 1977.

178. Kisa E, Schenk WG. Indications for emergency intravenous pyelography (IVP) in blunt abdominal trauma: a reappraisal. *J Trauma* 1986;26:1086.

179. Kodali S, Jamieson WRE, Leia-Stephens M, Miyagishima RT, Janusz MT, Tyers GFO. Traumatic rupture of the thoracic aorta. A 20-year review: 1969–1989. *Circulation* 1991;84:40–46.

180. Kohn JS, Clark DE, Isler RJ, Pope CF. Is computed tomographic grading of splenic injury useful in the nonsurgical management of blunt trauma? *J Trauma* 1994;36:385–390.

181. Korobkin M, Moss AA, Callen PW, DeMartini WJ, Kaiser JA. Computed tomography of subcapsular splenic hematoma: clinical and experimental studies. *Radiology* 1978;129:441–445.

182. Koslin DB, Stanley RJ, Berland LL, Shin MS, Dalton SC. Hepatic perivascular lymphedema: CT appearance. *AJR* 1988;150:111–113.

183. Kram HB, Appel PL, Wohlmuth DA, Shoemaker WC. Diagnosis of traumatic thoracic aortic rupture: A 10-year retrospective analysis. *Ann Thorac Surg* 1989;47:282–286.

184. Kumpe DA, Oh KS, Wyman SM. A characteristic pulmonary finding in unilateral complete bronchial transection. *AJR* 1970;110:704–706.

185. Kunin JR, Korobkin M, Ellis JH, Francis IR, Kane NM, Siegel SE. Duodenal injuries caused by blunt abdominal trauma: value of CT in differentiating perforation from hematoma. *AJR* 1993;160:1221–1223.

186. Lane MJ, Mindelzun RE, Sandhu JS, McCormick VD, Jeffrey RB. CT diagnosis of blunt pancreatic trauma: importance of detecting fluid between the pancreas and the splenic vein. *AJR* 1994;163:833–835.

187. Lang EK. Ureteral injuries. In: Pollack HM, ed. *Clinical urography,* vol 2. Philadelphia: WB Saunders, 1990;1495–1504.

188. Lang EK, Sullivan J, Frentz G. Renal trauma: radiological studies. Comparison of urography, computed tomography, angiography and radionuclide studies. *Radiology* 1985;154:1–6.

189. Lawson DE, Jacobson JA, Spizarny DL, Pranikoff T. Splenic trauma: value of follow-up CT. *Radiology* 1995;194:97–100.

190. Lawson TL, Thorsen MK, Erickson SJ, Perret RS, Quiroz FA, Foley WD. Periportal halo: a CT sign of liver disease. *Abdom Imag* 1993;18:42–46.

191. Lazrove S, Harley DP, Grinnell VS, White RA, Nelson RJ. Should

all patients with first rib fracture undergo arteriography? *J Thorac Cardiovasc Surg* 1982;83:532–537.

192. Lee VW, Allard JC, Berger P, et al. Right ventricular tardokinesis in cardiac contusion: a new observation on phase images. *Radiology* 1988;167:737–741.

193. Leitman BS, Birnbaum BA, Naidich DP. Radiologic evaluation of thoracic trauma. In: Hood RM, Boyd AD, Culliford AT, eds. Thoracic trauma. Philadelphia: WB Saunders, 1989;67–100.

194. Levin A, Gover P, Nance FC. Surgical restraint in the management of hepatic injury: a review of charity hospital experience. *J Trauma* 1978;16:399–404.

195. Levine CD, Patel UJ, Silverman PM, Wachsberg RH. Low attenuation of acute traumatic hemoperitoneum on CT scans. *AJR* 1996; 166:1089–1093.

196. Levine CD, Patel UJ, Wachsberg RH, Simmons MZ, Baker SR, Cho KC. CT in patients with blunt abdominal trauma: clinical significance of intraperitoneal fluid detected on a scan with otherwise normal findings. *AJR* 1995;164:1381–1385.

197. Levine E, Wetzel LH. Splenic trauma during colonoscopy. *AJR* 1987;149:939–940.

198. Levinsohn EM, Bunnell WP, Yuan HA. Computed tomography in the diagnosis of dislocations of the sternoclavicular joint. *Clin Orthop* 1979;140:12–16.

199. Linos DA, King RM, Mucha P, Farnell MB. Blunt pancreatic trauma. *Minn Med* 1983;66:153–160.

200. Lis LE, Cohen AJ. CT cystography in the evaluation of bladder trauma. *J Comput Assist Tomogr* 1990;14:386–389.

201. Lucas CE. Splenic trauma: choice of management. *Ann Surg* 1991; 213:98–112.

202. Lucas CE, Ledgerwood AM. Factors influencing outcome after blunt duodenal injury. *J Trauma* 1975;15:839–846.

203. Lundell CJ, Quinn MF, Finck EJ. Traumatic laceration of the ascending aorta: angiographic assessment. *AJR* 1985;145:715–719.

204. Lundevall J. The mechanism of traumatic rupture of the aorta. *Acta Pathol Microbiol Scand* 1964;62:34–46.

205. Lupetin AR, Mainwaring BL, Daffner RH. CT diagnosis of renal artery injury caused by blunt abdominal trauma. *AJR* 1989;153: 1065–1068.

206. Macklin CC. Transport of air along sheaths of pulmonic blood vessels from alveoli to mediastinum. *Arch Intern Med* 1939;64: 913–926.

207. Macrander SJ, Lawson TL, Foley WD, Dodds WJ, Erickson SJ, Quiroz FA. Periportal tracking in hepatic trauma: CT features. *J Comput Assist Tomogr* 1989;13:952–957.

208. Madayag MA, Kirshenbaum KJ, Nadimpalli SR, Fantus RJ, Cavallino RP, Crystal GJ. Thoracic aortic trauma: role of dynamic CT. *Radiology* 1991;179:853–855.

209. Malangoni MA, Cue JI, Fallat ME, Willing SJ, Richardson JD. Evaluation of splenic injury by computed tomography and its impact on treatment. *Ann Surg* 1990;211:592–599.

210. Mansfield PB, Graham CB, Beckwith JB, Hall DG, Sauvage LR. Pneumopericardium and pneumomediastinum in infants and children. *J Pediatr Surg* 1973;8:691–699.

211. Manson D, Babyn PS, Palder S, Bergman K. CT of blunt chest trauma in children. *Pediatr Radiol* 1993;23:1–5.

212. Marnocha KE, Maglinte DDT. Plain-film criteria for excluding aortic rupture in blunt chest trauma. *AJR* 1985;144:19–21.

213. Marotta R, Franchetto AA. The CT appearance of aortic transection. *AJR* 1996;166:647–651.

214. Marx JA, Moore EE, Jorden RC, Eule J. Limitations of computed tomography in the evaluation of acute abdominal trauma: a prospective comparison with diagnostic peritoneal lavage. *J Trauma* 1985;25:933–937.

215. McAninch JW. *Urogenital trauma*. New York: Thieme-Stratton, 1985.

216. McCort JJ. Caring for the major trauma victim: the role for radiology. *Radiology* 1987;163:1–9.

217. McGonigal MD, Schwab CW, Kauder DR, Miller WT, Grumbach K. Supplemental emergent chest computed tomography in the management of blunt torso trauma. *J Trauma* 1990;30:1431–1435.

218. Mee SL, McAninch JW, Federle MP. Computerized tomography in bladder rupture: diagnostic limitations. *J Urol* 1987;137:207–209.

219. Meredith JW, Trunkey DD. CT scanning in acute abdominal injuries. *Surg Clin North Am* 1988;68:255–268.

220. Meyer AA, Crass RA, Lim RC, Jeffrey RB, Federle MP, Trunkey DD. Selective nonoperative management of blunt liver injury using computed tomography. *Arch Surg* 1985;120:550–554.

221. Meyer DM, Thal ER, Weigelt JA, Redman HC. Evaluation of computed tomography and diagnostic peritoneal lavage in blunt abdominal trauma. *J Trauma* 1989;29:1168–1172.

222. Meyers BF, McCabe CJ. Traumatic diaphragmatic hernia. Occult marker of serious injury. *Ann Surg* 1993;218:783–790.

223. Meyers MA. Intraperitoneal spread of infections. In: Meyers MA, ed. *Dynamic radiology of the abdomen: normal and pathologic anatomy*, 4th ed. New York: Springer-Verlag, 1994;55–113.

224. Miller FB, Richardson JD, Thomas HA, Cryer HM, Willing SJ. Role of CT in diagnosis of major arterial injury after blunt thoracic trauma. *Surgery* 1989;106:596–603.

225. Minagi H, Brody WR, Laing FC. The variable roentgen appearance of traumatic diaphragmatic hernia. *J Can Assoc Radiol* 1977;28: 124–128.

226. Mindell HJ. On the value of non-contrast-enhanced CT in blunt abdominal trauma. *AJR* 1989;152:651–652.

227. Mindelzun RE. Abnormal gas collections. In: McCort JJ, ed. *Abdominal radiology*. Baltimore: Williams and Wilkins, 1981;204–206.

228. Mirvis SE, Bidwell JK, Buddemeyer EU, Diaconis JN, Pais SO, Whitley JE. Imaging diagnosis of traumatic aortic rupture. A review and experience at a major trauma center. *Invest Radiol* 1987; 22:187–196.

229. Mirvis SE, Bidwell JK, Buddemeyer EU, et al. Value of chest radiography in excluding traumatic aortic rupture. *Radiology* 1987; 163:487–493.

230. Mirvis SE, Dunham CM. Abdominal/Pelvic trauma. In: Mirvis SE, Young JWR, eds. *Imaging in trauma and critical care*. Baltimore: Williams and Wilkins, 1992;148–242.

231. Mirvis SE, Gens DR, Shanmuganathan K. Rupture of the bowel after blunt abdominal trauma: diagnosis with CT. *AJR* 1992;159: 1217–1221.

232. Mirvis SE, Indeck M, Schorr RM, Diaconis JN. Posttraumatic tension pneumopericardium: the "small heart" sign. *Radiology* 1986;158:663–669.

233. Mirvis SE, Keramati B, Buckman R, Rodriguez A. MR imaging of traumatic diaphragmatic rupture. *J Comput Assist Tomogr* 1988; 12:147–149.

234. Mirvis SE, Kostrubiak I, Whitley NO, Goldstein LD, Rodriguez A. Role of CT in excluding major arterial injury after blunt thoracic trauma. *AJR* 1987;149:601–605.

235. Mirvis SE, Pais SO, Gens DR. Thoracic aortic rupture: advantages of intraarterial digital subtraction angiography. *AJR* 1986;146: 987–991.

236. Mirvis SE, Rodriguez A. Diagnostic imaging of thoracic trauma. In: Mirvis SE, Young JWR, eds. *Imaging in trauma and critical care*. Baltimore: Williams and Wilkins, 1992;93–147.

237. Mirvis SE, Rodriguez A, Whitley NO, Tarr RJ. CT evaluation of thoracic infections after major trauma. *AJR* 1985;144:1183–1187.

238. Mirvis SE, Shanmuganathan K, Erb R. Diffuse small-bowel ischemia in hypotensive adults after blunt trauma (shock bowel): CT findings and clinical significance. *AJR* 1994;163:1375–1379.

239. Mirvis SE, Templeton P. Imaging in acute thoracic trauma. *Semin Roentgenol* 1992;27:184–210.

240. Mirvis SE, Tobin KD, Kostrubiak I, Belzberg H. Thoracic CT in detecting occult disease in critically ill patients. *AJR* 1987;148: 685–689.

241. Mirvis SE, Whitley NO, Gens DR. Blunt splenic trauma in adults: CT-based classification and correlation with prognosis and treatment. *Radiology* 1989;171:33–39.

242. Mirvis SE, Whitley NO, Vainwright JR, Gens DR. Blunt hepatic trauma in adults: CT-based classification and correlation with prognosis and treatment. *Radiology* 1989;171:27–32.

243. Moolten SE. Mechanical production of cavities in isolated lungs. *Arch Pathol* 1935;19:825–832.

244. Moon KL, Federle MP. Computed tomography in hepatic trauma. *AJR* 1983;141:309–314.

245. Moore EE, Shackford SR, Pachter HL, et al. Organ injury scaling: spleen, liver and kidney. *J Trauma* 1989;29:1664–1666.

246. Moore EH, Webb WR, Verrier ED, et al. MRI of chronic posttraumatic false aneurysms of the thoracic aorta. *AJR* 1984;143:1195–1196.

247. Moore FA, Moore EE, Seagraves AS. Nonresectional management of major hepatic trauma. *Am J Surg* 1985;150:725–729.

248. Morgan AS, Flancbaum L, Esposito T, Cox EF. Blunt injury to the diaphragm: an analysis of 44 patients. *J Trauma* 1986;26:565–568.

249. Morgan PW, Goodman LR, Aprahamian C, Foley WD, Lipchik EO. Evaluation of traumatic aortic injury: does dynamic contrast-enhanced CT play a role? *Radiology* 1992;182:661–666.

250. Morgenstern L, Uyeda RY. Nonoperative management of injuries of the spleen in adults. *Surg Gynecol Obstet* 1983;157:513–518.

251. Murray JG, Caoili E, Gruden JF, Evans SJ, Halvorsen RA, Mackersie RC. Acute rupture of the diaphragm due to blunt trauma: diagnostic sensitivity and specificity of CT. *AJR* 1996;166:1035–1039.

252. Naidich DP, Zerhouni EA, Siegelman SS. *Computed tomography and magnetic resonance of the thorax,* 2nd ed. New York: Raven Press, 1991;473–502.

253. Nelson MG, Jones DR, Vasilakis A, Timberlake GA. Computed tomographic diagnosis of acute blunt pancreatic transection. *W V Med J* 1994;90:274–278.

254. New PF, Aronow S. Attenuation measurements of whole blood and blood fractions in computed tomography. *Radiology* 1976;121:635–640.

255. Nghiem HV, Jeffrey RB, Mindelzun RE. CT of blunt trauma to the bowel and mesentery. *AJR* 1993;160:53–58.

256. Norman D, Price D, Boyd D, Fishman R, Newton TH. Aspects of computed tomography of the blood and cerebrospinal fluid. *Radiology* 1977;123:335–338.

257. Nunez D, Becerra JL, Fuentes D, Pagson S. Traumatic occlusion of the renal artery: helical CT diagnosis. *AJR* 1996;167:777–780.

258. Oh KS, Fleischner FG, Wyman SM. Characteristic pulmonary finding in traumatic complete transection of a main-stem bronchus. *Radiology* 1969;92:371–372.

259. Oldham KT, Guice KS, Ryckman F, Kaufman RA, Martin LW, Noseworthy J. Blunt liver injury in childhood: evolution of therapy and current perspective. *Surgery* 1986;100:542–549.

260. Orwig D, Federle MP. Localized clotted blood as evidence of visceral trauma on CT: the sentinel clot sign. *AJR* 1989;153:747–749.

261. Osborn GR, Meld MB. Findings in 262 fatal accidents. *Lancet* 1943;245:277–284.

262. Pachter HL, Hofstetter SR, Liang HG, Hoballah J. Traumatic injuries to the pancreas: the role of distal pancreatectomy with splenic preservation. *J Trauma* 1989;29:1352–1355.

263. Pais SO. Assessment of vascular trauma. In: Mirvis SE, Young JWR, eds. Imaging in trauma and critical care. Baltimore: Williams and Wilkins, 1992;485–515.

264. Palder SB, Shandling B, Manson D. Rupture of the thoracic trachea following blunt trauma: diagnosis by CAT scan. *J Pediatr Surg* 1991;26:1320–1322.

265. Palmer JK, Benson GS, Corriere JN. Diagnosis and initial management of urological injuries associated with 200 consecutive pelvic fractures. *J Urol* 1983;130:712–714.

266. Panicek DM, Paquet DJ, Clark KG, Urrutia EJ, Brinsko RE. Hepatic parenchymal gas after blunt trauma. *Radiology* 1986;159:343–344.

267. Pappas D, Mirvis SE, Crepps JT. Splenic trauma: false-negative CT diagnosis in cases of delayed rupture. *AJR* 1987;149:727–728.

268. Parmley LF, Manion WC, Mattingly TW. Nonpenetrating traumatic injury of the heart. *Circulation* 1958;18:371–396.

269. Parmley LF, Mattingly TW, Manion WC, Jahnke EJ. Nonpenetrating traumatic injury of the aorta. *Circulation* 1958;17:1086–1101.

270. Patrick LE, Ball TI, Atkinson GO, Winn KJ. Pediatric blunt abdominal trauma: periportal tracking at CT. *Radiology* 1992;183:689–691.

271. Peitzman AB, Makaroun MS, Slasky BS, Ritter P. Prsopective study of computed tomography in initial management of blunt abdominal trauma. *J Trauma* 1986;26:585–592.

272. Perlman SJ, Rogers LF, Mintzer RA, Mueller CF. Abnormal course of nasogastric tube in traumatic rupture of left hemidiaphragm. *AJR* 1984;142:85–88.

273. Pollack HM, Wein AJ. Imaging of renal trauma. *Radiology* 1989;172:297–308.

274. Poole GV, Morgan DB, Cranston PE, Muakkassa FF, Griswold JA. Computed tomography in the management of blunt thoracic trauma. *J Trauma* 1993;35:296–302.

275. Pranikoff T, Hirschl RB, Schlesinger AE, Polley TZ, Coran AG. Resolution of splenic injury after nonoperative management. *J Pediatr Surg* 1994;29:1366–1369.

276. Raptopoulos V. Chest CT for aortic injury: maybe not for everyone (commentary). *AJR* 1994;162:1053–1055.

277. Raptopoulos V, Sheiman RG, Phillips DA, Davidoff A, Silva WE. Traumatic aortic tear: screening with chest CT. *Radiology* 1992;182:667–673.

278. Ratliff JL, Fletcher JR, Kopriva CJ, Atkins C, Aussem JW. Pulmonary contusion. A continuing mangement problem. *J Thorac Cardiovasc Surg* 1971;62:638–644.

279. Rauch RF, Korobkin M, Silverman PM, Moore AV. CT detection of iatrogenic percutaneous splenic injury. *J Comput Assist Tomogr* 1983;7:1018–1021.

280. Resciniti A, Fink MP, Raptopoulos V, Davidoff A, Silva WE. Nonoperative treatment of adult splenic trauma: development of a computed tomographic scoring system that detects appropriate candidates for expectant management. *J Trauma* 1988;28:828–831.

281. Rhea JT, Novelline RA, Lawrason J, Sacknoff R, Oser A. The frequency and significance of thoracic injuries detected on abdominal CT scans of multiple trauma patients. *J Trauma* 1989;29:502–505.

282. Richardson P, Mirvis SE, Scorpio R, Dunham CM. Value of CT in determining the need for angiography when findings of mediastinal hemorrhage on chest radiographs are equivocal. *AJR* 1991;156:273–279.

283. Rizzo MJ, Federle MP, Griffiths BG. Bowel and mesenteric injury following blunt abdominal trauma: evaluation with CT. *Radiology* 1989;173:143–148.

284. Robbs JV, Moore SW, Pillary SP. Blunt abdominal trauma with jejunal injury: a review. *J Trauma* 1980;20:308–311.

285. Roberts JL, Dalen K, Bosanko CM, Jafir SZ. CT in abdominal and pelvic trauma. *RadioGraphics* 1993;13:735–752.

286. Roddy LH, Unger KM, Miller WC. Thoracic computed tomography in the critically ill patient. *Crit Care Med* 1981;9:515–518.

287. Rodriguez-Morales G, Rodriguez A, Shatney CH. Acute rupture of the diaphragm in blunt trauma: analysis of 60 patients. *J Trauma* 1986;26:438–444.

288. Rollins RJ, Tocino I. Early radiographic signs of tracheal rupture. *AJR* 1987;148:695–698.

289. Rosenbaum RC, Johnston GS. Posttraumatic cardiac dysfunction: assessment with radionuclide ventriculography. *Radiology* 1986;160:91–94.

290. Rubin BE, Schliftman R. The striated nephrogram in renal contusion. *Urol Radiol* 1979;1:119–121.

291. Ruess L, Sivit CJ, Eichelberger MR, Taylor GA, Bond SJ. Blunt hepatic and splenic trauma in children: correlation of a CT injury severity scale with clinical outcome. *Pediatr Radiol* 1995;25:321–325.

292. Sanborn JC, Hietzman ER, Markarian B. Traumatic rupture of the thoracic aorta. Roentgen—pathological correlations. *Radiology* 1970;95:293–298.

293. Sanchez FW, Greer CF, Thomason DM, Vujic I. Hemiazygous continuation of a left inferior vena cava: misleading radiographic findings in chest trauma. *Cardiovasc Intervent Radiol* 1985;8:140–142.

294. Sandler CM, Hall JT, Rodriguez MB, Corriere JN. Bladder injury in blunt pelvic trauma. *Radiology* 1986;158:633–638.

295. Savolaine ER, Grecos GP, Howard J, White P. Evolution of CT findings in hepatic hematoma. *J Comput Assist Tomogr* 1985;9:1090–1096.

296. Scatamacchia SA, Raptopoulos V, Fink MP, Silva WE. Splenic trauma in adults: impact of CT grading on management. *Radiology* 1989;171:725–729.

297. Schild HH, Strunk H, Weber W, et al. Pulmonary contusion: CT vs plain radiograms. *J Comput Assist Tomogr* 1989;13:417–420.

298. Schmidt CA, Wood MN, Razzouk AJ, Killeen JD, Gan KA. Primary repair of traumatic aortic rupture: a preferred approach. *J Trauma* 1992;32:588–592.

299. Schnyder P, Chapuis L, Mayor B, et al. Helical CT angiography for traumatic aortic rupture: correlation with aortography and surgery in five cases. *J Thorac Imag* 1996;11:39–45.

300. Schnyder P, Gamsu G, Essinger A, Duvoisin B. Trauma. In: Moss AA, Gamsu G, Genant HK, eds. *Computed tomography of the body with magnetic resonance imaging,* 2nd ed. Philadelphia: WB Saunders, 1992;311–323.

301. Schurr MJ, Fabian TC, Gavant M, et al. Management of blunt splenic trauma: computed tomographic contrast blush predicts failure of nonoperative management. *J Trauma* 1995;39:507–513.

302. Sclafani SJA, Becker JA. Radiological diagnosis of renal trauma. *Urol Radiol* 1985;7:192–200.

303. Sclafani SJA, Shaftan GW, McAuley J, et al. Interventional radiology in the management of hepatic trauma. *J Trauma* 1984;24:256–262.

304. Sefczek DM, Sefczek RJ, Deeb ZL. Radiographic signs of acute traumatic rupture of the thoracic aorta. *AJR* 1983;141:1259–1262.

305. Shalaby-Rana E, Eichelberger M, Kerzner B, Kapur S. Intestinal stricture due to lap-belt injury. *AJR* 1992;158:63–64.

306. Shanmuganathan K, Mirvis SE, Amoroso M. Periportal low density on CT in patients with blunt trauma: association with elevated venous pressure. *AJR* 1993;160:279–283.

307. Shanmuganathan K, Mirvis SE, Sover ER. Value of contrast-enhanced CT in detecting active hemorrhage in patients with blunt abdominal or pelvic trauma. *AJR* 1993;161:65–69.

308. Shapiro MJ, Yanofsky SD, Trapp J, et al. Cardiovascular evaluation in blunt thoracic trauma using transesophageal echocardiography (TEE). *J Trauma* 1991;31:835–840.

309. Sherck J, Shatney C, Sensaki K, Selivanov V. The accuracy of computed tomography in the diagnosis of blunt small-bowel perforation. *Am J Surg* 1994;168:670–675.

310. Sherck JP, Oakes DD. Intestinal injuries missed by computed tomography. *J Trauma* 1990;30:1–7.

311. Shin MS, Berland LL, Ho K-J. Small aorta: CT detection and clinical significance. *J Comput Assist Tomogr* 1990;14:102–103.

312. Shin MS, Ho K-J. Computed tomography evaluation of posttraumatic pulmonary pseudocysts. *Clin Imag* 1993;17:189–192.

313. Shires GT, Thal ER, Jones RC, et al. Trauma. In: Schwartz SI, ed. *Principles of surgery,* 5th ed. New York: McGraw-Hill, 1989;217–284.

314. Shorr RM, Crittenden M, Indeck M, Hartunian SL, Rodriguez A. Blunt thoracic trauma. Analysis of 515 patients. *Ann Surg* 1987;206:200–205.

315. Siegel MJ, Balfe DM. Blunt renal and ureteral trauma in childhood: CT patterns of fluid collections. *AJR* 1989;152:1043–1047.

316. Siegel MJ, Herman TE. Periportal low attenuation at CT in childhood. *Radiology* 1992;183:685–688.

317. Sigler LH. Traumatic injuries of the heart. Incidence of its occurrence in 42 cases of severe accidental bodily injury. *Am Heart J* 1945;30:459–478.

318. Simeone JF, Minagi HM, Putman CE. Traumatic disruption of the thoracic aorta: significance of the left apical extrapleural cap. *Radiology* 1975;117:265–268.

319. Sivit CJ, Cutting JP, Eichelberger MR. CT diagnosis and localization of rupture of the bladder in children with blunt abdominal trauma: significance of contrast material extravasation in the pelvis. *AJR* 1995;164:1243–1246.

320. Sivit CJ, Eichelberger MR. CT diagnosis of pancreatic injury in children: significance of fluid separating the splenic vein and the pancreas. *AJR* 1995;165:921–924.

321. Sivit CJ, Eichelberger MR, Taylor GA. CT in children with rupture of the bowel caused by blunt trauma: diagnostic efficacy and comparison with hypoperfusion complex. *AJR* 1994;163:1195–1198.

322. Sivit CJ, Eichelberger MR, Taylor GA, Bulas DI, Gotschall CS, Kushner DC. Blunt pancreatic trauma in children: CT diagnosis. *AJR* 1992;158:1097–1100.

323. Sivit CJ, Taylor GA, Bulas DI, et al. Posttraumatic shock in children: CT findings associated with hemodynamic instability. *Radiology* 1992;182:723–726.

324. Sivit CJ, Taylor GA, Eichelberger MR. Chest injury in children with blunt abdominal trauma: evaluation with CT. *Radiology* 1989;171:815–818.

325. Sivit CJ, Taylor GA, Eichelberger MR, Bulas DI, Gotschall CS, Kushner DC. Significance of periportal low-attenuation zones following blunt trauma in children. *Pediatr Radiol* 1993;23:388–390.

326. Sivit CJ, Taylor GA, Newman KD, et al. Safety-belt injuries in children with lap-belt ecchymosis: CT findings in 61 patients. *AJR* 1991;157:111–114.

327. Slatis P. Injuries in fatal traffic accidents. *Acta Chir Scand* (Suppl) 1962;297:9–39.

328. Smejkal R, O'Malley KF, David E, Cernaianu AC, Ross SE. Routine initial computed tomography of the chest in blunt torso trauma. *Chest* 1991;100:667–669.

329. Smith JS, Wengrovitz MA, Delong BS. Prospective validation of criteria, including age, for safe, nonsurgical management of the ruptured spleen. *J Trauma* 1992;33:363–369.

330. Spouge AR, Burrows PE, Armstrong D, Daneman A. Traumatic aortic rupture in the pediatric population. Role of plain film, CT and angiography in the diagnosis. *Pediatr Radiol* 1991;21:324–328.

331. Stalker HP, Kaufman RA, Stedje K. The significance of hematuria in children after blunt abdominal trauma. *AJR* 1990;154:569–571.

332. Stalker HP, Kaufman RA, Towbin R. Patterns of liver injury in childhood: CT analysis. *AJR* 1986;147:1199–1205.

333. Stark DD, Federle MP, Goodman PC. CT and radiographic assessment of tube thoracostomy. *AJR* 1983;141:253–258.

334. Stark P. Radiology of thoracic trauma. *Invest Radiol* 1990;25:1265–1275.

335. Stark P. *Radiology of thoracic trauma.* Boston: Andover, 1993.

336. Stark P, Jaramillo D. CT of the sternum. *AJR* 1986;147:72–77.

337. Stavas J, van Sonnenberg E, Casola G, Wittich GR. Percutaneous drainage of infected and noninfected thoracic fluid collections. *J Thorac Imag* 1987;2:80–87.

338. Stern EJ, Frank MS. Acute traumatic hemopericardium. *AJR* 1994;162:1305–1306.

339. Stevens E, Templeton AW. Traumatic nonpenetrating lung contusion. *Radiology* 1965;85:247–252.

340. Strassmann G. Taumatic rupture of the aorta. *Am Heart J* 1947;33:508–515.

341. Sturm JT, Hankins DG, Young G. Thoracic aortography following blunt chest trauma. *Am J Emerg Med* 1990;8:92–96.

342. Sutton CS, Haaga JR. CT evaluation of limited splenic trauma. *J Comput Assist Tomogr* 1987;11:167–169.

343. Tisando J, Tsai FY, Als A, Roach JF. A new radiographic sign of acute traumatic rupture of the thoracic aorta: displacement of the nasogastric tube to the right. *Radiology* 1977;125:603–608.

344. Tocino I, Miller MH. Computed tomography in blunt chest trauma. *J Thorac Imag* 1987;2:45–59.

345. Tocino IM, Miller MH. Mediastinal trauma and other acute mediastinal conditions. *J Thorac Imag* 1987;2:79–100.

346. Tocino IM, Miller MH, Fairfax WR. Distribution of pneumothorax in the supine and semirecumbent critically ill adult. *AJR* 1985;144:901–905.

347. Tocino IM, Miller MH, Frederick PR, Bahr AL, Thomas F. CT detection of occult pneumothorax in head trauma. *AJR* 1984;143:987–990.

348. Tomiak MM, Rosenblum JD, Messersmith RN, Zarins CK. Use of CT for diagnosis of traumatic rupture of the thoracic aorta. *Ann Vasc Surg* 1993;7:130–139.

349. Toombs BD, Sandler CM. Acute abdominal trauma. In: Toombs BD, Sandler CM, eds. *Computed tomography in trauma.* Philadelphia: WB Saunders, 1987;27–64.

350. Toombs BD, Sandler CM, Lester RG. Computed tomography of chest trauma. *Radiology* 1981;140:733–738.

351. Toombs BD, Sandler CM, Rauschkolb EN, Strax R, Harle TS. Assessment of hepatic injuries with computed tomography. *J Comput Assist Tomogr* 1982;6:72–75.

352. Townsend M, DeFalco AJ. Absence of ureteral opacification below ureteral disruption: a sentinel CT finding. *AJR* 1995;164:253–254.

353. Trerotola SO. Can helical CT replace aortography in thoracic trauma? *Radiology* 1995;197:13–15.

354. Trunkey DD, Shires GT, McClelland R. Management of liver trauma in 811 consecutive patients. *Ann Surg* 1974;179:722–728.

355. Udekwu PO, Gurkin B, Oller DW. The use of computed tomography in blunt abdominal injuries. *Am Surg* 1996;62:56–59.

356. Umlas S-L, Cronan JJ. Splenic trauma: can CT grading systems enable prediction of successful nonsurgical treatment? *Radiology* 1991;178:481–487.

357. Unger JM, Schuchmann GG, Grossman JE, Pellett JR. Tears of the trachea and main bronchi caused by blunt trauma: radiologic findings. *AJR* 1989;153:1175–1180.

358. Van Moore A, Ravin CE, Putman CE. Radiologic evaluation of acute chest trauma. *CRC Crit Rev Diagn Imag* 1983;19:89–110.

359. Wagner RB, Crawford WO, Schimpf PP. Classification of parenchymal injuries of the lung. *Radiology* 1988;167:77–82.

360. Wagner RB, Crawford WO, Schimpf PP, Jamieson PM, Rao KCVG. Quantitation and pattern of parenchymal lung injury in blunt chest trauma. Diganostic and therapeutic implications. *J Comput Assist Tomogr* 1988;12:270–281.

361. Wagner RB, Jamieson PM. Pulmonary contusion. Evaluation and classification by computed tomography. *Surg Clin North Am* 1989;69:31–40.

362. Wall SD, Federle MP, Jeffrey RB, Brett CM. CT diagnosis of unsuspected pneumothorax after blunt abdominal trauma. *AJR* 1983;141:919–921.

363. Wan YL, Asich H, Lee TY, Tsai CC. Wall defect as a sign of urinary bladder rupture in sonography. *J Ultrasound Med* 1988;7:511.

364. Weir IH, Muller NL, Connell DG. CT diagnosis of bronchial rupture. *J Comput Assist Tomogr* 1988;12:1035–1036.

365. White CS, Templeton PA, Attar S. Esophageal perforation: CT findings. *AJR* 1993;160:767–770.

366. Wiencek RG, Wilson RF, Steiger Z. Acute injuries of the diaphragm. An analysis of 165 cases. *J Thorac Cardiovasc Surg* 1986;92:989–993.

367. Williams DM, Simon HJ, Marx MV, Starkey TD. Acute traumatic aortic rupture: intravascular US findings. *Radiology* 1992;182:247–249.

368. Wills JS, Lally JF. Use of CT for evaluation of possible traumatic aortic injury (letter). *AJR* 1991;157:1123–1124.

369. Wilson D, Voystock JF, Sariego J, Kerstein MD. Role of computed tomography scan in evaluating the widened mediastinum. *Am Surgeon* 1994;60:421–423.

370. Wing VW, Federle MP, Morris JA, Jeffrey RB, Bluth R. The clinical impact of CT for blunt abdominal trauma. *AJR* 1985;145:1191–1194.

371. Wingo PA, Tong T, Bolden S. Cancer statistics, 1995. *CA Cancer J Clin* 1995;45:8–30.

372. Wiot JF. The radiologic manifestations of blunt chest trauma. *JAMA* 1975;231:500–503.

373. Wolfman NT, Bechtold RE, Scharling ES, Meredith JW. Blunt upper abdominal trauma: evaluation by CT. *AJR* 1992;158:493–501.

374. Wolfman NT, Gilpin JW, Bechtold RE, Meredith JW, Ditesheim JA. Occult pneumothorax in patients with abdominal trauma: CT studies. *J Comput Assist Tomogr* 1993;17:56–59.

375. Wolverson MK, Crepps LF, Sundaram M, Heiberg E, Vas WG, Shields JB. Hyperdensity of recent hemorrhage at body computed tomography: incidence and morphologic variation. *Radiology* 1983;148:779–784.

376. Wong Y-C, Wang L-J, Lin B-C, Chen C-J, Lim K-E, Chen R-J. CT grading of blunt pancreatic injuries: prediction of ductal disruption and surgical correlation. *J Comput Assist Tomogr* 1997;21:246–250.

377. Woodring JH. The normal mediastinum in blunt traumatic rupture of the thoracic aorta and brachiocephalic arteries. *J Emerg Med* 1990;8:467–476.

378. Woodring JH, Fried AM, Hatfield DR, Stevens RK, Todd EP. Fractures of first and second ribs: predictive value for arterial and bronchial injury. *AJR* 1982;138:211–215.

379. Woodring JH, Pulmano CM, Stevens RK. The right paratracheal stripe in blunt chest trauma. *Radiology* 1982;143:605–608.

380. Worman LW, Hurley JD, Pemberton AH, Narodick BG. Rupture of the esophagus from external blunt trauma. *Arch Surg* 1962;85:173–178.

381. Worthy SA, Kang EY, Hartman TE, Kwong JS, Mayo JR, Muller NL. Diaphragmatic rupture: CT findings in 11 patients. *Radiology* 1995;194:885–888.

382. Yale-Loehr AJ, Kramer SS, Quinlan DM, LaFrance ND, Mitchell SE, Gearhart JP. CT of severe renal trauma in children: evaluation and course of healing with conservative therapy. *AJR* 1989;152:109–113.

CHAPTER 22

Musculoskeletal CT

William G. Totty, Kevin W. McEnery, Jordan B. Renner, Douglas D. Robertson, Paul S. Hsieh, and Stephen F. Hatem

The application of computed tomography (CT) initially, and of magnetic resonance imaging (MRI) a decade later, to the study of musculoskeleal disease has revolutionized our understanding of disease processes and improved our recognition, description, and staging of many musculoskeletal abnormalities. Each of these complex imaging modalities has particular advantages and disadvantages that can be exploited to best define normal musculoskeletal anatomy and disease conditions. They are best seen as complementary methods that must be wisely used to provide maximum information about the patient quickly, efficiently and at the lowest possible cost and lowest radiation dose. More than ever before, the proper choice and application of imaging technology requires sophisticated knowledge of the specific capabilities of each imaging technique, knowledge of normal human anatomy, knowledge of changes produced by pathology, and knowledge of how each imaging technique can be optimized to demonstrate the expected changes produced by various pathologic conditions.

In this period of multiple imaging methods it is the job of the musculoskeletal radiologist to judiciously choose or recommend to the referring physician the best method for evaluating specific suspected traumatic or nontraumatic pathologic processes. The overall method must define whether or not an abnormality exists, localize its site of origin, define its characteristics so as to suggest or support a suspected diagnosis, estimate the seriousness or aggressiveness of the process, define its local extent and relationship to adjacent vital structures, and, finally, provide any specific anatomic data that may be required by the physician or surgeon to assess prognosis and aid in treatment planning.

Most musculoskeletal abnormalities are initially evaluated using conventional radiographs. Radiographs remain the most important imaging method in the study of many musculoskeletal conditions, especially trauma and bone tumors. Radiographs are generally sensitive for such bone abnormalities and provide the highest specificity available from any imaging method. Although almost always obtained, radiographs frequently do not supply significant information about soft tissue musculoskeletal abnormalities. When skeletal lesions are suspected and radiographs are nonconfirmatory, additional imaging is required. Bone scintigraphy is commonly the second imaging method used for suspected bone abnormalities. It may define bone abnormalities that are not recognizable on radiographs, better establish a known lesion's extent, or identify additional lesions in adjacent or remote areas of the skeleton. Bone scintigraphy is not generally useful in associated soft tissue musculoskeletal abnormalities. It is in the case where radiographs and bone scintigraphy do not supply or are not expected to supply all of the needed information that CT and MRI become most useful.

CT has many advantages as a musculoskeletal imaging technique, including its cross-sectional display of anatomy which easily defines the spatial relationships between organs and allows easy comparison between sides. Compared with radiographs, there is increased contrast sensitivity allowing better definition of nonbone anatomy. Recent advances in spiral CT have optimized the ability to manipulate and reformat imaging data to provide multiplanar visualization of the anatomy. MRI shares many of the advantages of CT and adds many more of its own. Like CT, it provides sectional display of the anatomy, but unlike CT, it has the ability to directly image in any plane. MRI provides superior soft tissue contrast with spatial resolution essentially equal to that of CT.

1343

Because of its increased soft tissue contrast, MRI demonstrates better soft tissue anatomic detail and allows the identification of many more anatomic structures. This is particularly useful in the depiction of muscles, tendons, ligaments, cartilage, and meniscal structures. Similarly, MRI is exquisitely sensitive to changes in bone marrow. Among its disadvantages, MRI is less sensitive than CT in the depiction of soft tissue gas and small amounts of soft tissue calcium. It is somewhat more difficult to recognize subtle changes in bone cortex using MRI, although improved sequences and resolution have made this disadvantage less clinically significant.

Because of its greater soft tissue contrast and the inherent improved visualization of soft tissue anatomy it provides, MRI has largely eclipsed CT in the study of many musculoskeletal abnormalities. The body of information relating to musculoskeletal MRI has thus grown to greatly exceed that relating to musculoskeletal CT. It is not possible to even begin to review the myriad body of data relating to MRI in the musculoskeletal system in a single book chapter. Thus, in this chapter we will concentrate on the current uses of CT in the musculoskeletal system, with references to MRI when needed, to best define CT's role in clinical practice. We will emphasize where CT is best used and where it can be used with success even though MRI might be somewhat better. We will compare the advantages of CT with those of MRI where either may be used. Emphasis will be placed on the developing role of CT for trauma evaluation, prosthesis modeling, and reconstructive surgery planning.

TECHNIQUE

With the availability of MRI, much of musculoskeletal CT has evolved into a problem solving rather than screening modality with scan protocols tailored to address specific clinical questions. The patient's clinical history, current physical status, and prior radiographic studies all serve to focus examinations. Optimal musculoskeletal scanning involves precise positioning and selection of imaging parameters that maximize spatial resolution, minimize field of view (FOV), and utilize thin section collimation and edge-enhancing image- processing algorithms. Image filming with wide window and level is commonly used.

Helical CT offers the musculoskeletal imager the capability to obtain an optimized examination for in-plane images and multiplanar reconstruction while minimizing actual scan time (223,348). The elimination of interslice motion artifacts on multiplanar and three-dimensional (3-D) reconstructions from helical CT offers the potential for improved images and more widespread clinical use.

Review of the plain radiographs is essential to indicate the appropriate scan plane. The primary CT acquisition plane should be perpendicular to the area of greatest interest. With the availability of fast CT scanning and focused scan protocols (discussed below), it may be practical to scan an extremity in two complementary anatomic positions without appreciably increasing scan time. For instance, in the wrist, axial and coronal images are often complementary in the assessment of intercarpal pathology (26).

Patient positioning is guided by a simple tenet: position the area of anatomic interest in an advantageous position while maintaining the patient's comfort. One must consider the desired position in the context of the movement limitations of the patient, whether secondary to cast immobilization or pain. An optimal position is meaningless if a patient cannot keep the extremity motionless. In the proximal articulations (shoulder, hip, knee), for practical purposes, positioning is limited to the axial plane with multiplanar reconstructions providing sagittal or coronal images (Table 1). The wrist can be put into multiple scanning positions (338). The ankle/calcaneus can be easily imaged directly in either the axial or coronal plane. The use of specialized holders and other positioning devices can assist in patient positioning but is not mandatory. Often the blankets or sheets routinely available in the scanner suite can provide the appropriate immobilization bolster.

Spatial resolution is optimized through a combination of thin section collimation and small FOV. With the availability of efficient conventional and helical CT scanners, 2-mm and 3-mm section collimation has become the routine. On some systems 1-mm collimation can substitute for 2-mm imaging. In our opinion, the FOV should generally be limited to the extremity of interest. Whenever possible, the contralateral extremity should be symmetrically positioned to allow comparison images if needed, but imaging of the contralateral side is not often necessary. In selected cases, it is advantageous to store raw image data so that comparison images of the contralateral extremity can be retrospectively reconstructed from the original scan data if needed. This can provide useful information in severe trauma, where inclusion of the contralateral extremity provides an anatomic reference for the normal appearance.

An exception to minimizing FOV exists in acetabular fracture assessment where it may be advantageous to maintain a larger FOV. The inclusion of the sacrum and contralateral acetabulum could demonstrate associated pathology which may not have been originally suspected. Most modern CT scanners provide an elegant solution for the selection of appropriate FOV, especially in the traumatized patient. During postprocessing, two sets of images can be created from the raw data set, one optimized for multiplanar reconstructions of limited FOV and maximal image overlap (e.g., the specific acetabulum) and a second with a larger FOV including the entire body part (e.g., entire pelvis). This postprocessing technique may also be useful for obtaining ''comparison'' images

TABLE 1. *Musculoskeletal exam positioning*

	Acquisition plane	Reconstruction planes
Shoulder	Axial	Coronal
Elbow	Axial—arm flexed	Coronal
	Axial—arm extended	Sagittal
Radius/wrist	Axial	Axial
	Coronal	Coronal
	Sagittal	Sagittal
Scaphoid	Coronal	*not recommended*
	Sagittal—long axis	
Pelvis, hip	Axial	Coronal
		Sagittal
Knee-tibial plateau	Axial	Coronal
	Coronal	Sagittal
ankle, calcaneous	Axial	Coronal
	Coronal	Sagittal
Metatarsals	Axial (gantry tilt)	Coronal
	Coronal	Sagittal

of the contralateral extremity after the patient has left the CT scanner. Unlike conventional comparison radiographs, this does not increase the radiation dose for the patient as the images are produced though additional image processing of the original dataset.

Exact assessment of the computed scout radiogram (topogram) is crucial. A precise limit on scan coverage minimizes scan time, maintains patient throughout, and preserves patient comfort while providing high-quality diagnostic scans. The first step of topogram assessment is the determination that the extremity has been properly positioned. Next, the topogram serves to limit the scan extent to the area of clinical concern. This reduces the number of sections required to completely image a joint or limb.

In helical CT, the required tissue volume necessary to ensure adequate coverage must be prospectively determined. The radiograph can provide an estimate of the tissue volume and the topogram precisely establishes the volume requirement. Tissue volume imaged during a helical CT acquisition is calculated by multiplying table increment (mm/sec) by the time of scanning (Table 2). For instance, a 32- sec scan at 2 mm/sec will image a 6.4-cm tissue volume. The table increment must be sufficient

TABLE 2. *Helical (spiral) CT: volume coverage (mm)*

Table speed (mm/sec)	Scan time			
	20 sec	30 sec	40 sec	60 sec
2	40	60	80	120
3	60	90	120	180
4	80	120	160	240
5	100	150	200	300

Note: There is a direct relationship between table speed and volume coverage. Required coverage can be estimated from plain radiographs. It is recommend that table increment be limited to provide coverage of only the exact area of interest. This allows minimized table increment and high-quality multiplanar reconstructions.

to completely image the area of concern within the constraint of scan time limits mandated by tube heating restrictions.

In helical CT it is advantageous to minimize the table increment. Initial reports of helical CT scanning noted thickening of slice sensitivity profiles producing decreased spatial resolution of multiplanar reconstructions; however, with thin slice collimation and improved image reconstruction algorithms this is no longer a problem (222). As a general rule, articulations can be imaged with a table increment of 2 mm/sec or less. However, for the hip/acetabulum, increasing the table speed (collimation) to 3 mm/sec is routinely required to obtain adequate volume coverage. It is possible to increase the table speed to greater than collimation (pitch >1) to obtain greater volume coverage, but there is usually no need to employ this option for routine musculoskeletal imaging. In most situations where an increased volume of tissue coverage is required, consecutive helical scans are a better option.

An available option with most modern helical scanners is the ability to image an articulation with a combination of thin and slightly thicker collimation. For example, in the evaluation of a complex pelvis fracture, thin collimation (2 to 3 mm) could be utilized through the acetabulum and thicker (5 mm) collimation through the iliac wings. This would provide an optimized examination both for precise evaluation of the acetabulum and for an overview of the entire pelvis as visualized with multiplanar or 3-D reconstructions.

The choice of whether to perform a helical or conventional CT depends on the specific indication for the study requested. For examinations in which precise anatomic detail is required, such as in the determination of fracture union, a nonhelical CT exam in the appropriate anatomic plane is preferred as it produces relatively decreased image noise secondary to greater available milliamperage.

In the acutely traumatized patient, helical CT allows decreased examination time and the capability for high-quality multiplanar reconstructions (92,260). Helical scanning provides for overlapping image sections without increased radiation dose. With conventional CT, the section collimation, table increment, and FOV are specified at the start of scanning. When saving image data, the FOV and image reconstruction algorithm can be modified during postprocessing. With helical CT, the section collimation, table increment, and therefore the volume of tissue imaged are determined prior to scan initiation. Like conventional CT, FOV and image reconstruction algorithm are determined at the conclusion of the examination. However, helical CT allows one to create images at any position within the scan volume.

As mentioned above, tube heating limits restrict the available milliamperage of helical CT compared to conventional CT. During scan monitoring, if image quality of helical CT images proves non-diagnostic, the exam protocol can be changed to standard CT with increased available milliamperage. With larger patients, the increased milliamperage provided with a 2-sec conventional CT scan may be mandatory to limit image degradation secondary to image noise.

When it is anticipated that multiplanar reconstructions will aid in the diagnosis, then helical CT is advised. The highest quality multiplanar reconstructions are derived from thin collimation images and overlapping image sections (222,244,246). A 50% overlap effectively doubles the number of scan images. With conventional CT this also doubles the examination time and radiation exposure. Increased scan time also increases the chance that patient motion will degrade multiplanar reconstructions. For helical CT, the request to overlap section increment is a postprocessing option that does not increase scan time or radiation dose.

Most modern CT scanners come equipped with software to accomplish multiplanar and 3-D reconstructions. The use of multiplanar and 3-D reconstructions in the assessment of complex trauma has been widely investigated (25, 89, 92, 159, 204, 206, 208, 217, 243, 245, 317,347,354,365,378). Several studies have noted that CT with reconstructions positively affects patient outcomes by providing information that alters the plan for surgical treatment both in adults (88,171,203,204,212,364) and in pediatric populations (204). Although multiplanar or 3-D reconstructions may not assist the radiologist in identifying the extent of a fracture, their greatest utility may be in helping the orthopedic surgeon in the overall visualization of a complex fracture that may be difficult for him to comprehend on the multiple axial images. In addition, as trauma patients are not always able to position themselves in the perfect position for true axial images, we often find it useful to create reconstructions in standard anatomic planes. Nonstandard anatomic planes can then supplement the acquired images, especially when the radiologist finds them helpful in explaining the complex pathology.

There are two methods used to create 3-D reconstructions: surface and volumetric renderings. With the surface shading technique, the computer presents the image data referencing distance from the observer to a given surface point as a color value, usually a gray scale. Through manipulation of a "light source," specific surface features are accentuated. Volume rendering techniques require complex image manipulation in assigning different optical transparencies or colors to distinct tissue densities. The examination dataset is manipulated by highlighting specific tissue densities. For trauma assessment, CT attenuation values corresponding to bone density are highlighted and soft tissue densities are rendered transparent.

There are inherent strengths and weaknesses associated with each of these 3-D reconstruction techniques. Surface rendering presents a detailed view of the bone contours. Fractures manifest as contour discontinuities that are accentuated through light source manipulation. The surface rendering method is sensitive for the detection of fractures which disrupt the cortical surface. However, surface rendering has difficulty detecting fractures that are nondisplaced or not perpendicular to the scan plane (197).

Although volume rendering techniques excel in their more realistic representation of anatomic structures, there are instances where the superimposition of structures and the relatively smooth rendering of bone surface make this technique less than optimal for fracture detection (357). For fracture imaging, it has been demonstrated that the surface rendering technique is the preferred 3-D technique for fracture characterization (364).

Metal artifact is a commonly encountered problem in musculoskeletal scanning, especially related to stainless steel internal fixation devices or joint prostheses. Several software methods have been developed to reduce this streak artifact (91,288). Increasing the kilovoltage and using processing algorithms with less edge enhancement can help reduce this artifact. Some manufacturers have developed specific solutions to minimize metal artifacts. In wrist imaging, it is possible to limit artifacts associated with internal screw fixation by carefully aligning the screw parallel to the scan plane (338). Newer titanium internal fixation devices have the advantage of reducing artifacts on both CT and MRI (74).

While MRI has supplanted CT for the routine assessment of soft tissue and bone neoplasm, in patients with specific contraindications to MRI scanning, CT remains an important imaging modality. In such cases, intravenous contrast can assist with tumor definition and is an important adjunct. Fast CT scanning technique can provide information regarding tumor vascularity at maximal contrast intensity. Intra-articular contrast serves to better delineate cartilage integrity especially of the glenoid labrum and assists in the identification of loose bodies.

ANATOMY

Shoulder and Upper Extremity

The upper extremity is supported and kept free from the thoracic cage by the structures of the pectoral, or shoulder, girdle. The osseous shoulder girdle consists of paired dorsal scapulae and ventral clavicles (Fig. 1). The sole articulation with the axial skeleton occurs anteriorly at the sternoclavicular joints; the trapezius muscles suspend the distal clavicles and scapulae.

The scapula is a triangular flat bone with medial, lateral,

and superior margins, sharp inferior and superior angles, and concave costal and dorsal surfaces (Fig. 2). The lateral angle forms the articular process for the humerus. This consists of the shallow, anterolaterally directed glenoid fossa, which is supported by the short, broad scapular neck. From the upper neck, the coracoid projects forward and superiorly. At its base medially is the scapular notch. The dorsal surface is divided into upper and lower parts by the spine. Laterally, the spine expands to form the acromion, which overhangs the glenohumeral joint and articulates with the distal clavicle.

The clavicle is S-shaped with broadened medial and

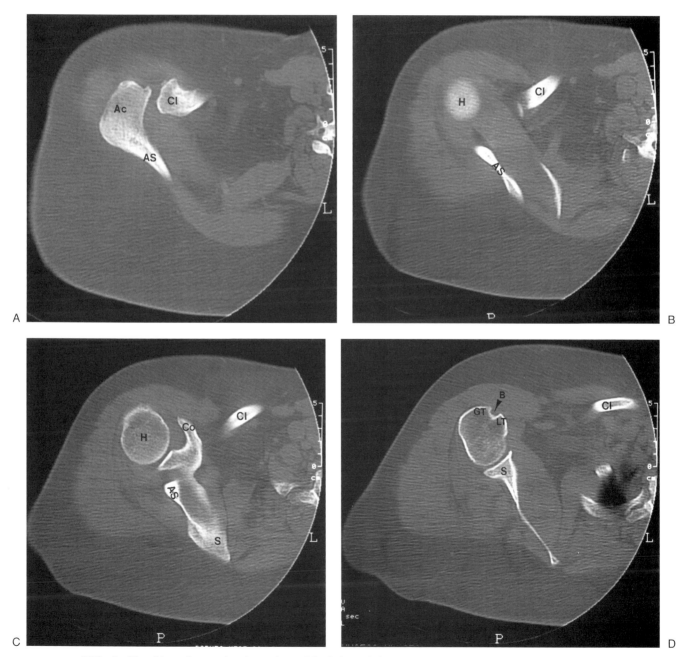

FIG. 1. Shoulder—bone. Ac, Acromium; AS, Spine of the scapula; B, Bicipital groove; Cl, Clavicle; Co, Coracoid process; GT, Greater tuberosity; H, Humerus; LT, Lesser tuberosity; S, Scapula.

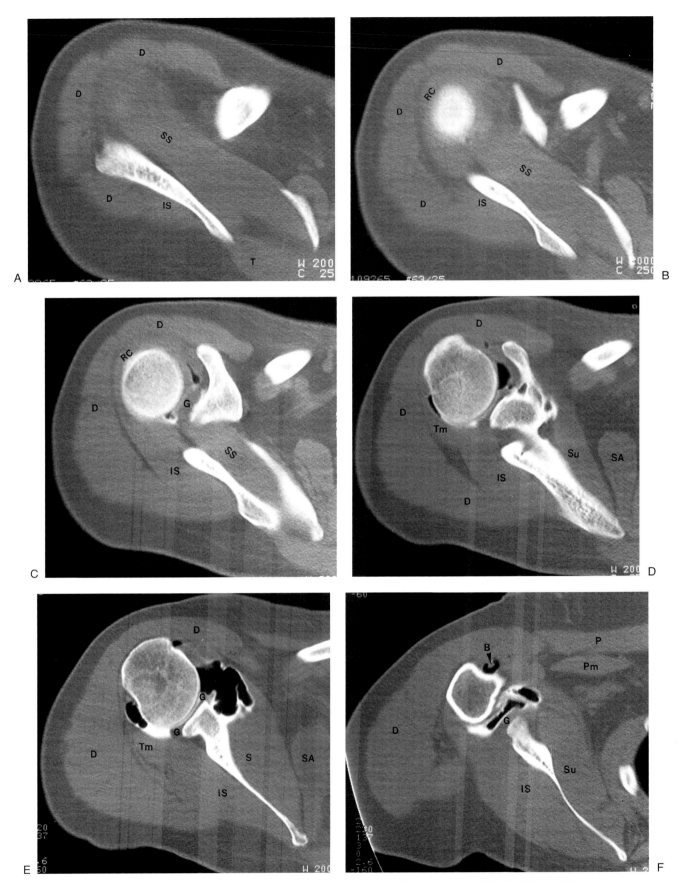

FIG. 2. Shoulder—soft tissue. B, Biceps tendon, long head; D, Deltoid muscle; G, Glenoid labrum; IS, Infraspinatus muscle; P, Pectoralis major muscle; Pm, Pectorialis minor muscle; PL, Posterior glenoid labrum; RC, Rotator cuff; SA, Serratus anterior; SS, Supraspinatus muscle; Su, Subscapularis muscle; T, Trapezius muscle; Tm, Teres minor muscle.

lateral ends. The medial end, or clavicular head, articulates with the sternum and first costal cartilage at the diarthrodial sternoclavicular joint. Attachment to the first rib is via the costoclavicular ligaments. A secondary ossification center is seen medially in the late teenage years, with fusion by the mid-20s. The distal, or acromial, end of the clavicle articulates with the acromion at the synovial acromioclavicular joint. The coracoid attaches to both the acromion and clavicle by the coracoacromial and coracoclavicular ligaments.

On axial images, the humeral head is seen as a spherical osseous structure that is seated in the glenoid fossa. Beneath the level of the coracoid, the bicipital groove, containing the long head of the biceps tendon, is seen anteriorly, flanked by the lateral greater tuberosity and medial lesser tuberosity. Posterolaterally, the margin may appear somewhat flattened. The trabecular pattern of the head can appear quite heterogeneous, particularly in osteopenic patients; this should not be mistaken for a lytic lesion.

The glenohumeral joint is formed by the articulation of the round humeral head and the concave glenoid labrum. On CT arthrography, the fibrocartilaginous labrum is seen as a triangular structure, though its apex may be slightly rounded (Fig. 2). The labrum is firmly attached peripherally; the looser attachment centrally may allow a small amount of air or contrast to collect there, especially superiorly and anteriorly, in the sublabral foramen. The glenohumeral ligaments are variably visualized.

The rotator cuff consists of the supraspinatus superiorly, inserting on the greater tuberosity; the infraspinatus posteriorly, inserting on the greater tuberosity more caudally and posteriorly; the teres minor, inserting most distally on the greater tuberosity; and the subscapularis crosses anterolaterally to insert on the lesser tuberosity

(Fig. 2). The long head of the biceps tendon inserts on the superior glenoid and contributes to the superior labral complex before exiting the joint at the bicipital groove. The deltoid is seen superficial to the rotator cuff musculature. Discrimination of muscle anatomy is largely dependent on the amount of adjacent adipose tissue.

Other than the axillary neurovascular bundle, the scapular notch is the most important neurovascular site evaluated on axial images. Containing fat and transmitting the suprascapular artery and nerve, it is seen posteriorly at the junction of the glenoid and scapular neck. Mass lesions in this area can lead to an entrapment syndrome that can mimic rotator cuff pathology.

The lateral aspect of the midarm is protuberant at the insertion of the deltoid muscle on the deltoid tuberosity. Cortical thickening and irregularity, as well as eccentric lobulation of the marrow space, may be seen. Medial and lateral intermuscular septae divide the arm into ventral flexor and dorsal extensor compartments. The short (medial) and long (lateral) heads of the biceps brachii, coracobrachialis, and brachialis muscles form the flexor compartment; it also transmits the brachial vessels, and the musculocutaneous; median, and ulnar nerves. The extensor compartment contains the triceps, the profunda brachii artery, and the radial nerve (Fig. 3).

The distal humerus flattens and flares at the elbow into medial and lateral epicondyles, the curved articular surfaces of the trochlea and capitellum, and the hollowed concavities of the coronoid and olecranon fossae (Fig. 4). A groove for the ulnar nerve is present dorsally at the level of the medial epicondyle.

The proximal ulna forms the deep concavity of the trochlear notch for its hinge articulation with the trochlea. Anteriorly, the beak-like coronoid process of the ulna

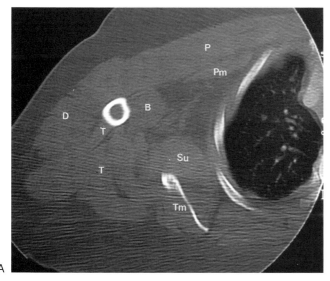

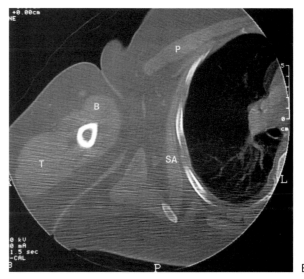

A   B

FIG. 3. Upper arm. B, Biceps brachii muscle; D, Deltoid muscle; P, Pectoralis major muscle; Pm, Pectoralis minor muscle; SA, Serratus anterior muscle; Su, Subscapularis muscle; T, Triceps brachii muscle; Tm, Teres minor.

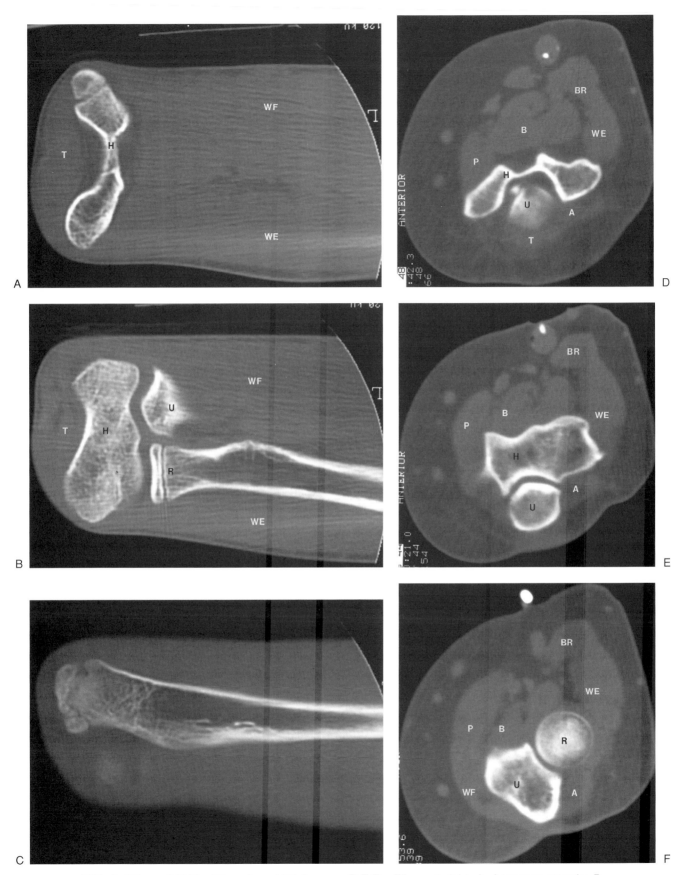

FIG. 4. Elbow. **A,B,C**—Elbow flexed 90 degrees; **D,E,F**—Elbow straight. A, Anconeus muscle; B, Brachialis muscle; BR, Brachioradialis muscle; H, Humerus; P, Pronator teres muscle; R, Radius; U, Ulna; WF, Wrist flexors; WR, Wrist extensors; T, Triceps muscle.

provides coverage. Posteriorly, the olecranon process of the ulna is seen within the olecranon fossa as a roughly triangular structure on axial images. Distally, it broadens symmetrically up to the level of the proximal radioulnar joint, where a prominent concavity, the radial notch, is seen laterally. The smooth, round radial head lies congruently within the notch and is largely uncovered. Its capitellar articular surface is slightly concave. The radial neck is the mild constriction between the radial head and the posteromedial prominence, the radial tuberosity, site of attachment for the biceps.

The medial epicondyle serves as the common flexor origin; the lateral epicondyle, the common extensor origin. Medially, the pronator teres attaches just proximal to the epicondyle. Just proximal to the lateral epicondyle, the extensor carpi radialis muscle originates anteriorly and the anconeus posteriorly. Radial and ulnar collateral ligaments also attach to the lateral and medial epicondyles, respectively, en route to their distal attachments at the annular ligament and coronoid process.

The important neurovascular structures of the arm all pass through the cubital fossa, with the exception of the ulnar nerve, which curves behind the medial epicondyle in the ulnar groove. These include the lateral and medial cutaneous nerves, the median nerve, brachial artery, and radial nerve.

The radius and ulna roughly parallel each other with the wrist supinated in anatomic position, which is also the typical positioning used for CT (Fig. 5). They are connected by a tough interosseous membrane. Each bone is flattened near the attachment of the interosseous membrane, resulting in triangular cross-sections with apices directed to each other centrally.

The interosseous membrane, radius, and ulna divide the forearm into volar and medial flexor and dorsal and lateral extensor compartments. The flexors are further divided into superficial (the pronator teres, flexor carpi radialis, palmaris longus, flexor digitorum longus, and flexor carpi ulnaris from lateral to medial) and deep (flexor pollicis longus, flexor digitorum profundus, and the distal, transversely oriented pronator quadratus) groups. The extensor compartment also is composed of superficial (brachioradialis, extensor carpi radialis longus, extensor carpi radialis brevis, extensor digitorum, extensor digiti minimi, and extensor carpi ulnaris) and deep (supinator, abductor pollicis longus, extensor pollicis longus, extensor pollicis brevis, and extensor indicis) groups.

The principal neurovascular structures of the forearm course between the superficial and deep layers of both compartments. In the ventral compartment, these include the ulnar artery and nerve medially, the median nerve and artery centrally, and the radial artery and superficial branch of the radial nerve laterally. On the extensor side, the posterior interosseous artery and nerve (the deep branch of the radial nerve) are seen.

The wrist and hand are complex structures anatomically, with numerous small, curved bones and their articulations. Standard axial imaging is usually superseded by coronal or, occasionally, sagittal imaging techniques (Figs. 6 and 7). Most patients can be positioned to obtain direct coronal or sagittal images; for others, reconstructions can be performed. Two planes are almost always necessary for optimal evaluation.

The wrist begins at the distal radioulnar joint, best depicted on axial sections. At this level, the radius has broadened in all directions, but more so transversely. Me-

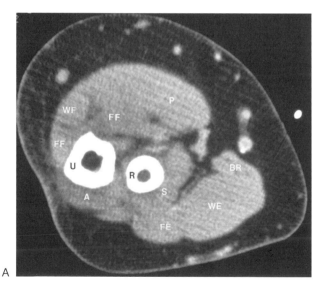
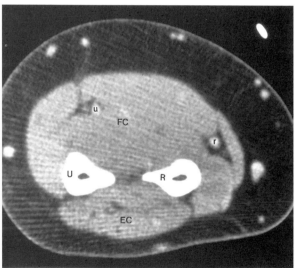

A

B

FIG. 5. Forearm: **A**—proximal, **B**—mid. A, Anconeus muscle; BR, Brachioradialis muscle; EC, Extensor compartment; FC, Flexor compartment; FE, Finger extensor muscles; FF, Finger flexor muscles; P, Pronator teres muscle; R, Radius; r, Radial artery; U, Ulna; u, Ulnar artery; WF, Wrist flexors; WE, Wrist extensors.

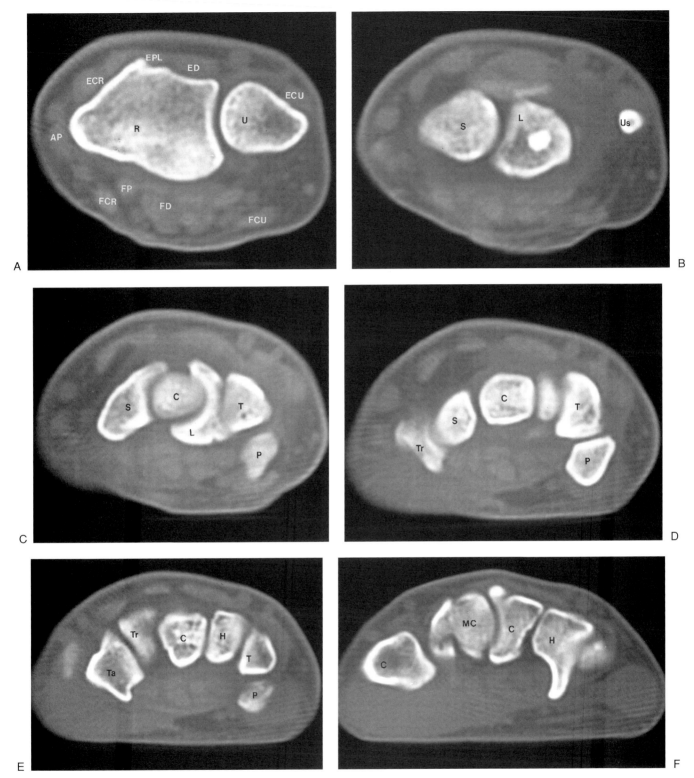

FIG. 6. Wrist: **A–F**—Axial 2 mm sections, **G,H**—Reconstructions from axial images. AP, Adductor pollicis longus / extensor pollicis brevis; C, Capitate; ECU, Extensor carpi ulnaris; ED, Digital extensors; EPL, Extensor pollicis longus; ECR, Extensor carpi radialis longus and brevis; FD, Flexor digitorum superficialis and profundus; FCR, Flexor carpii radialis; FCU, Flexor carpi ulnaris; FP, Flexor pollicis longus; H, Hamate; L, Lunate; MC, Metacarpal; P, Pisiform; R, Radius; S, Scaphoid; T, Triquetrum; Ta, Trapezoid; Tr, Trapezium; U, Ulna; Us, Ulnar styloid.

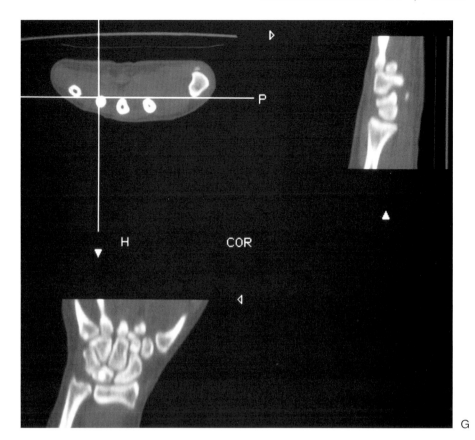

G

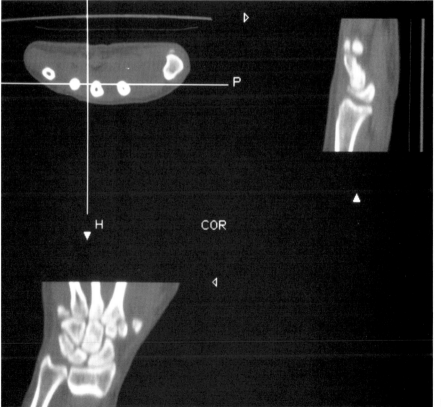

FIG. 6. *Continued.*

H

dially there is a shallow concavity, the ulnar notch, which articulates with the convex distal ulna. Congruence should be maintained throughout the ranges of pronation and supination. The dorsal tubercle of Lister is readily identified and separates the tendons of the extensor pollicis longus medially and the extensor carpi radialis brevis laterally. The radius terminates in the radial styloid process laterally and similarly the ulna ends medially with the ulnar styloid.

The radius extends most distally laterally and dorsally at the radial styloid and dorsal rim. These account for the normal ulnar inclination and volar tilt of the radiocarpal joint. The ulna is separated from the joint by an articular disc, the triangular fibrocartilage. The proximal articular surface is formed by this medial disc, and two fossae in the distal radius: the lunate fossa centrally, often separated from the lateral scaphoid fossa by a small ridge. The distal articular surface consists of the triquetrum, lunate, and proximal pole of the scaphoid, which are interconnected by intrinsic wrist ligaments. Extrinsic wrist ligaments between the radius and ulna carpus additionally support the wrist. These ligamentous structures are not visualized on CT.

The midcarpal joint lies between the scaphoid, lunate, and triquetrum proximally and the trapezium, trapezoid, capitate, and hamate distally. Other intercarpal articulations allow less mobility and do not have separate capsules. The palmar aspects of the carpal bones help define the limits of the carpal tunnel. Ulnarly, the pisiform and hook of the hamate define the osseous limits. Radially, it is the distal pole of the scaphoid and the tubercle of the trapezium. The carpometacarpal, metacarpophalangeal, and interphalangeal joints are best evaluated with coronal and sagittal images due to their predominantly transverse lie.

Lower Extremity

The osseous pelvis consists of a sacrum (located in the posterior midline) as well as two hemipelvic bones (one on each side), each of which are formed from the ilium, the ischium, and the pubis (Fig. 8). Anteriorly, the two pubic bones meet at the pubic symphysis. Posteriorly, the hemipelvic bones articulate with the sacrum at the sacroiliac joints bilaterally. Hence, the osseous pelvis forms a rigid ring, which moves as a single unit. The ilium, the ischium, the pubis, and the sacrum have complex curved shapes and are oriented at oblique angles, which makes them sometimes difficult to evaluate with conventional radiography. However, CT can overcome

these difficulties and display the various structures in exquisite anatomic detail.

The sacroiliac joints consist of a synovial portion (antero-inferior one third) and a fibrous or ligamentous portion (posterior-superior two thirds). The synovial portion is normally 2.5 to 4.0 mm wide, with a smoothly uniform cartilage space surrounded by thin, parallel, uniformly wide bone cortices. The fibrous portion is narrower ventrally (adjacent to the synovial portion) and widens dorsally, in an inverted V shape on transaxial sections. Both the synovial and fibrous portions of the joint should be bilaterally symmetric. Hence, it is possible to evaluate for unilateral widening of a sacroiliac joint by comparing it with the opposite side.

The acetabulum is formed superiorly by the ilium, postero-inferiorly by the ischium and anteroinferiorly by the pubis. In pediatric patients, the triradiate cartilage can also be seen separating these three bones. In an adult, cross-sectional images also reveal a focal concavity within the acetabulum, the acetabular fossa. The adjacent femoral head appears as a spherical osseous structure, residing centrally within the acetabulum. A patient who is in a supine and relaxed position will tend to rotate his or her leg externally, resulting in slight widening of the anterior joint space when compared to the posterior space. This is a normal appearance.

Transaxial images of the femoral head typically show a characteristic star-shaped condensation of trabecular bone in the central medullary cavity. This region of sclerotic bone can be traced inferiorly until it runs into the medial cortex of the femoral neck, forming the calcar. The fovea capitis can also be visualized as a small central depression in the medial surface of the femoral head. This is the insertion site for the femoral ligament. More inferiorly, one can also visualize the greater and lesser trochanters as protuberances from the femur, on the lateral and medial aspects, respectively.

The hip flexors reside anteriorly (Fig. 9). The iliacus and psoas muscles reside anterior to the iliac wing, in the iliac fossa. They combine to form the iliopsoas muscle inferiorly. The rectus femoris is also a major hip flexor. The sartorius acts as a minor hip flexor in addition to its primary function as a knee flexor. More inferiorly, these hip flexors can all be identified anterior to the hip joint and femoral head.

The various thigh abductors reside laterally. These include the tensor fascia lata, as well as the gluteus medius and gluteus minimus. The tensor fascia lata inserts into the iliotibial band, not into an osseous structure. The thigh adductors reside medially. These include the adductor

FIG. 7. Wrist: Direct Coronal and Sagittal. C, Capitate; H, Hamate; L, Lunate; MC, Metacarpal; P, Pisiform; R, Radius; S, Scaphoid; T, Triquetrum; Ta, Trapezoid; Tr, Trapezium; U, Ulna.

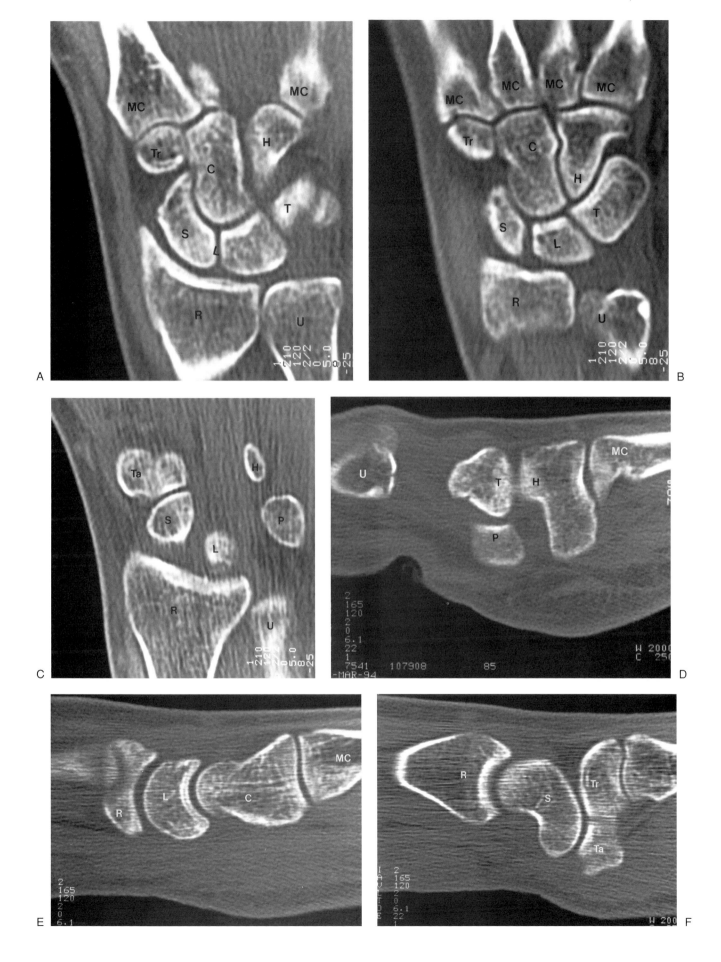

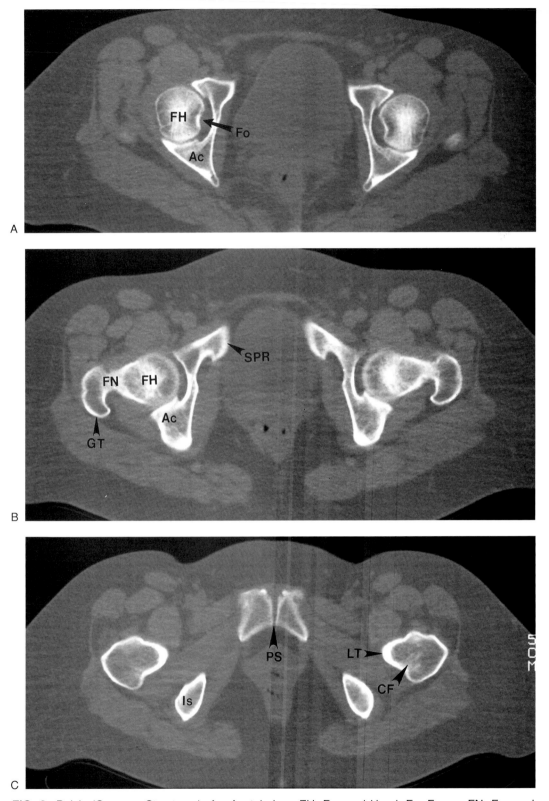

FIG. 8. Pelvis (Osseous Structures). Ac, Acetabulum; FH, Femoral Head; Fo, Fovea; FN, Femoral Neck; GT, Greater Trochanter; LT, Lesser Trochanter; CF, Calcar Femoris; SPR, Superior Pubic Ramus; PS, Pubic Symphysis; Is, Ischium.

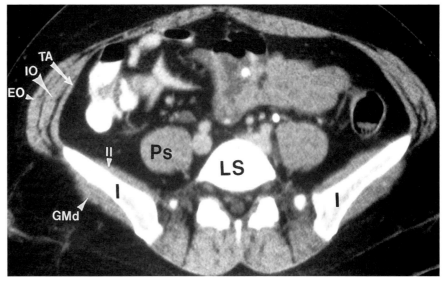

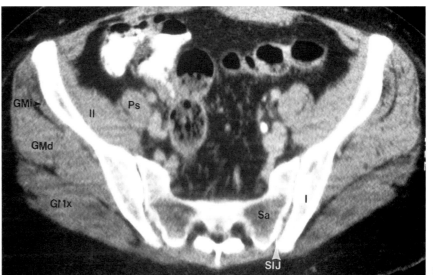

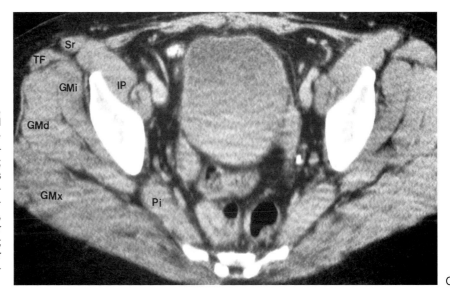

FIG. 9. Pelvis (Soft Tissues). EO, External Oblique; IO, Internal Oblique; TA, Transversus abdominis; II, Iliacus; Ps, Psoas; IP, Iliopsoas; GMx, Gluteus Maximus; GMd, Gluteus Medius; GMi, Gluteus Minimus; Pi, Pyriformis; Sr, Sartorius; RF, Rectus Femoris; TF, Tensor Fascia Lata; Pe, Pectineus; OI, Obturator Internus; OE, Obturator Externus; SG, Superior Gemellus; IG, Inferior Gemellus; LS, Lumbar Spine; I, Ilium; Sa, Sacrum; SIJ, Sacroiliac Joint.

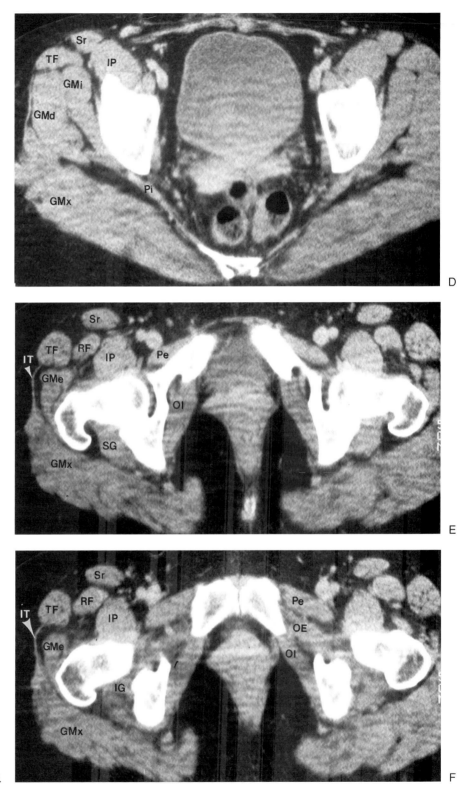

FIG. 9. Continued.

FIG. 10. Thigh. Sr, Sartorius; RF, Rectus Femoris; TF, Tensor Fascia Lata; QF, Quadrator Femoris; Pe, Pectineus; IP, Iliopsoas; GMx, Gluteus Maximus; VL, Vastus Lateralis; VI, Vastus Intermedius; VM, Vastus Medialis; AL, Adductor Longus; AB, Adductor Brevis; AM, Adductor Magnus; Sm, Semimembranosus; St, Semitendinosus; Gr, Gracilis; BF, Biceps Femoris; F, Femur; IsT, Ischial Tuberosity.

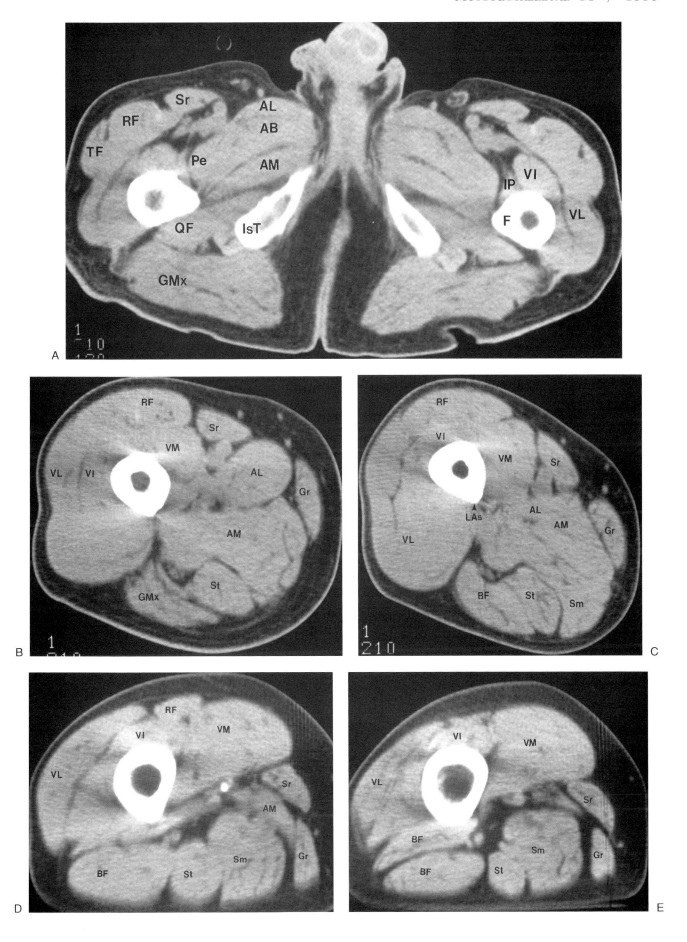

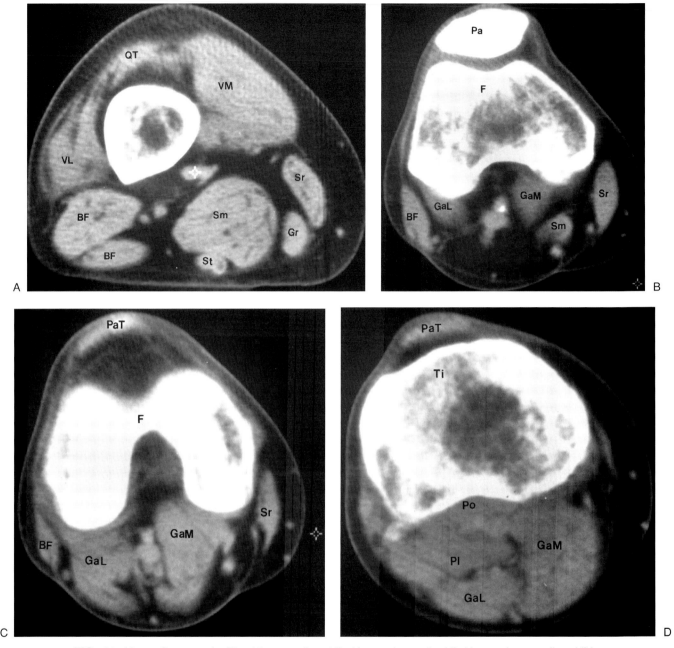

FIG. 11. Knee. Same as in Fig. 10, as well as VL, Vastus Lateralis; VI, Vastus Intermedius; VM, Vastus Medialis; Sr, Sartorius; Sm, Semimembranosus; St, Semitendinosus; Gr, Gracilis; BF, Biceps Femoris; QT, Quadriceps Tendon; GaL, Gastrocnemius (lateral head); GaM, Gastrocnemius (medial head); PaT, Patellar Tendon; Po, Popliteus; Pl, Plantaris; F, Femur; Pa, Patella; Ti, Tibia.

longus, adductor brevis, and adductor magnus. The pectineus muscle is located anterior to the adductor muscles and posteromedial to the femoral artery and nerve.

Posteromedially, there are several deep lateral hip rotators. These include the piriformis, the obturator internus and externus, the superior and inferior gemelli, and the quadratus femoris. The obturator internus and the piriformis arise from inside the pelvis proper. The hip extensors can be visualized posteriorly. These include the gluteus maximus and, more inferiorly, the semimembranosus, the semitendinosus, and the biceps femoris.

Two major neurovascular bundles can be easily identified within the pelvis. The femoral artery, vein, and nerve run in the plane between the adductors (medial group) and the flexors (anterior group). The sciatic nerve, the largest peripheral nerve in the body, exits the pelvis through the greater sciatic foramen below the piriformis muscle, passes lateral to the ischial tuberosity, and takes an inferior course anterior to the gluteus maximus muscle and posterior to the other deep lateral hip rotators.

Located on the posterior aspect of the femoral shaft, the linea aspera is a pointed protuberance of bone cortex

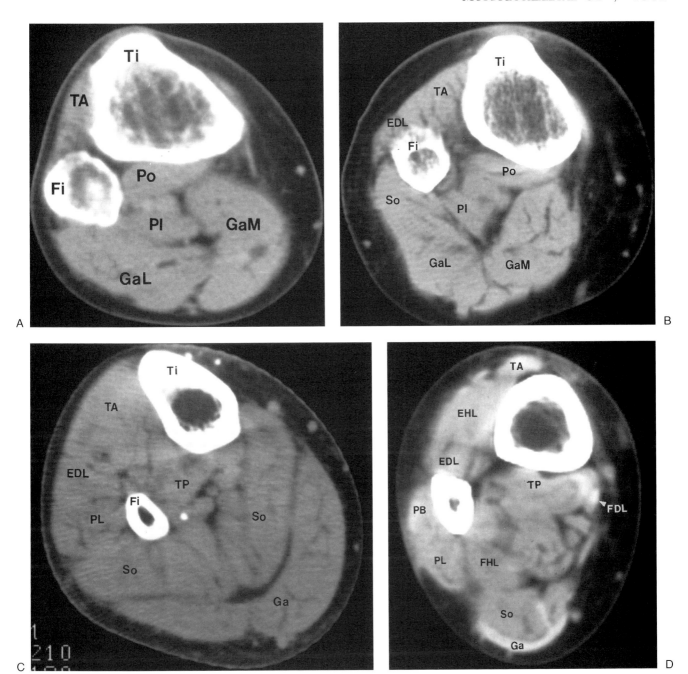

FIG. 12. Calf. GaL, Gastrocnemius (lateral head); GaM, Gastrocnemius (medial head); Ga, Gastrocnemius; Po, Popliteus; Pl, Plantaris; So, Soleus; TA, Tibialis Anterior; EDL, Extensor Digitorum Longus; EHL, Extensor Hallucis Longus; PL, Peroneus Longus; PB, Peroneus Brevis; TP, Tibialis Posterior; FDL, Flexor Digitorum Longus; FHL, Flexor Hallucis Longus; AcT, Achilles Tendon; Ti, Tibia; Fi, Fibula.

extending through most of the length of the shaft (Fig. 10). This is the insertion site of the adductor muscle group and the origin of the vastus lateralis and vastus medialis muscles. The anterior compartment of the thigh contains the knee extensors, including the sartorius as well as the quadriceps femoris (which is composed in turn of the rectus femoris, the vastus lateralis, vastus intermedius, and vastus medialis muscles). The vastus medialis and intermedius are tightly apposed to the anterolateral femoral cortex.

The medial compartment contains the adductor brevis, longus, and magnus muscles, as well as the gracilis. The adductor magnus muscle contains the adductor hiatus. The femoral artery and vein pass through this hiatus as they course inferiorly from the anterior thigh to the posterior. The posterior compartment contains the hamstring muscles, including the semimembranosus, the semitendinosus, and the biceps femoris. These muscles flex the knee joint. In the superior portion of the thigh, the femoral artery, vein, and nerve run between the anterior compart-

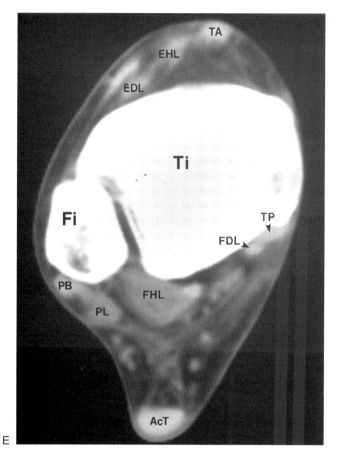

E

FIG. 12. *Continued.*

the gastrocnemius are located more directly posterior to the knee joint. The biceps femoris muscle and tendon reside posterolateral to the knee joint.

At the level of the proximal tibia, two additional muscles are present, deep to the gastrocnemius, and immediately posterior to the tibia. They are the popliteus and plantaris muscles. Slightly more inferiorly, the soleus originates from both the posterior fibula and posterior tibia.

The cruciate ligaments and menisci are typically not well visualized in CT, although they are exquisitely demonstrated with MRI. The popliteal artery and veins reside posteriorly, between the two heads of the gastrocnemius. The tibial nerve runs adjacent to and posterior to the popliteal vessels whereas the common peroneal nerve is located immediately medial to the biceps femoris muscle. More inferiorly, the common peroneal nerve runs lateral and adjacent to the proximal fibula, in a superficial location.

The tibia and fibula are connected by an interosseous membrane (Fig. 12). In addition, several fascial layers attach to the tibia and fibula, separating the calf into three distinct anatomic compartments—anterior, lateral, and posterior. The posterior compartment in turn is separated into superficial and deep subcompartments by another layer of fascia. The anterior compartment contains the following muscles (from medial to lateral): the tibialis anterior, the extensor hallucis longus, the extensor digitorum longus, and (more inferiorly) the peroneus tertius. These muscles all dorsiflex the foot. The lateral compartment contains the peroneus longus and peroneus brevis muscles. These muscles evert the foot.

The superficial posterior compartment contains the gastrocnemius, soleus, and plantaris muscles. These muscles plantar flex the foot. The deep posterior compartment contains the tibialis posterior, the flexor halluces longus, the flexor digitorum longus, and (superiorly) the popliteus muscles.

The anterior tibial artery, vein, and nerve run immediately anterior to the interosseous membrane in the anterior compartment. The posterior tibial artery, vein, and nerve reside between the superficial and deep posterior compartments, anterior to the soleus. The peroneal artery runs between the tibialis posterior and flexor hallucis longus muscles.

The ankle is a hinge joint consisting of the distal tibia, distal fibula, and the talus (Figs. 13 and 14). The tibia and fibula form a slot into which the talar dome fits. The normal ankle permits motion in only one plane, plantarflexion and dorsiflexion. The talus also articulates with the calcaneus inferiorly. There are three separate facets to the subtalar joint, anterior, middle, and posterior. The sustentaculum tali is a shelf of bone along the medial aspect of the calcaneus that articulates with the head of the talus to form the middle subtalar joint. Lateral to this, there is a space between the talus and calcaneus known as the sinus tarsi.

ment and the medial compartment. The sciatic nerve runs between the adductor magnus (in the medial compartment) and the posterior compartment.

Distally, the shaft of the femur flares to form the medial and lateral femoral condyles, separated by the intracondylar notch (Fig. 11). On the anterior surface of the distal femur, the fossa between the condyles is known as the trochlear groove. The patella glides within the trochlear groove and, on transaxial images, its shape parallels the shape of the groove. The patella is the largest sesamoid bone in the body. The tendons for the four quadriceps muscles insert on the superior pole of the patella. A second patellar tendon (or patellar ligament) originates from the inferior pole of the patella and inserts on the tibial tuberosity, at the anterior proximal tibia. The superior surface of the proximal tibia is composed of medial and lateral tibial plateaus that articulate with the medial and lateral femoral condyles, respectively.

Anteriorly, the quadriceps tendons insert on the superior pole of the patella, as described above, although a portion of the vastus medialis can be seen to the level of the mid-patella. Posteromedially, the sartorius, gracilis, and semitendinosus tendons merge to form the pes anserinus, which inserts on the proximal medial tibia. The semimembranosus and the medial and lateral heads of

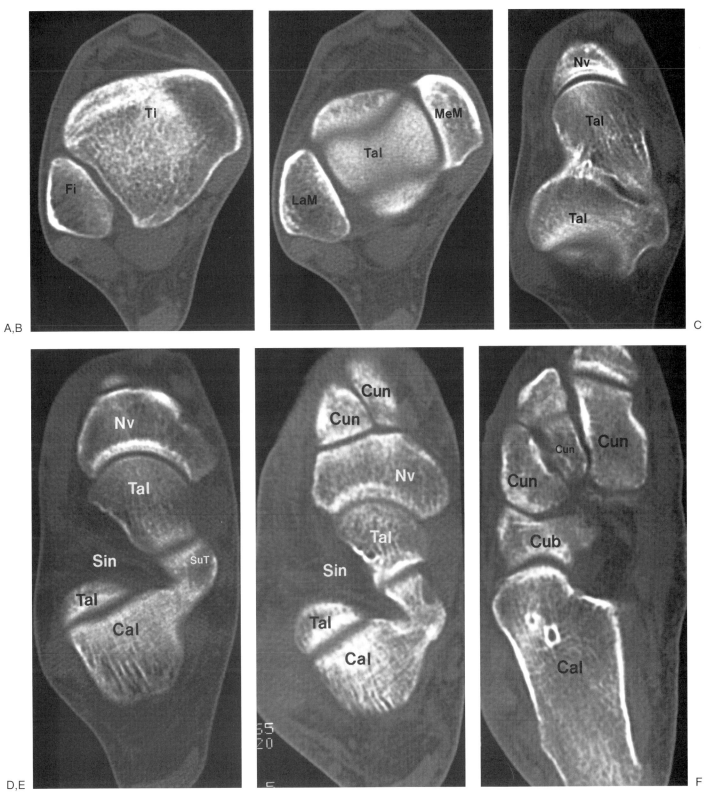

FIG. 13. Ankle: Axial images. Ti, Tibia; Fi, Fibula; LaM, Lateral Malleolus; MeM, Medial Malleolus; Tal, Talus; Nv, Navicular; Cal, Calcaneus; SuT, Sustentaculi Tali; Sin, Sinus Tarsi; Cun, Cuneiform; Cub, Cuboid; Mt, Metatarsal bone.

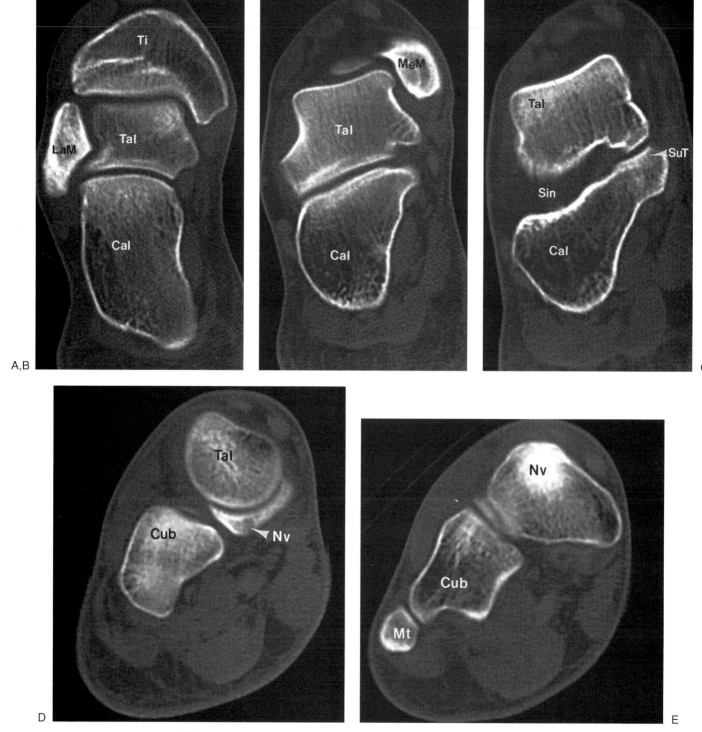

FIG. 14. Ankle: Coronal images. Abbreviations same as in Fig. 13.

The sinus tarsi is roughly cone-shaped, i.e., narrower medially and broader laterally. The midfoot and forefoot bones are also well appreciated on CT.

At the level of the ankle, four groups of tendons cross the joint. These groups correspond to the compartments described within the calf musculature. The anterior group consists of (from medial to lateral) the tibialis anterior, the extensor hallucis longus, and the extensor digitorum longus. The medial tendon group consists of (from anterior to posterior) the tibialis posterior, the flexor digitorum longus, and the flexor halluces longus. The lateral tendon group consists of (from anterior to posterior) the peroneus brevis and peroneus longus. The posterior tendon group consists of the Achilles tendon, formed by a condensation

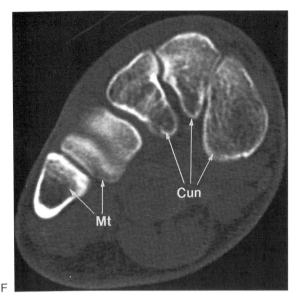
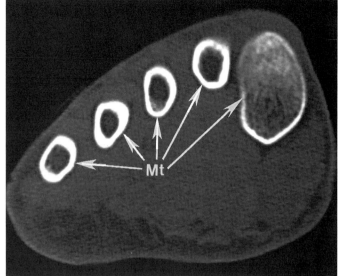

F   G

FIG. 14. *Continued.*

of the tendons for the soleus and gastrocnemius muscles. The plantaris tendon can sometimes be visualized medial to the Achilles tendon. The medial collateral ligament (deltoid ligament), the lateral collateral ligaments, and the sinus tarsi ligaments are generally not well visualized with CT, but can be identified with MRI.

There are three neurovascular bundles at this level. The dorsalis pedis artery is the continuation of the anterior tibial artery, and it runs deep to the extensor hallucis longus. The posterior tibial vessels and nerve run between the flexor digitorum longus and the flexor hallucis longus. The peroneal artery can sometimes be visualized posterior to the inferior tibiofibular articulation.

TRAUMA

The specific indication for CT evaluation of a traumatized articulation is the precise assessment of known fracture extent, the determination of fragment location, and the identification of interarticular fragments. MRI has largely supplanted CT for evaluation of traumatized extremities in the presence of normal plain radiographs. MRI can detect occult fractures (manifest as bone marrow edema) and identify associated ligament injuries better than CT. However, in the acutely traumatized patient, CT remains the examination of choice for the delineation of osseous injury demonstrated on plain radiography. In the presence of a known fracture, CT can precisely determine the relative position of major bone fragments. With addition of multiplanar and 3-D reconstructions, CT can provide the clinician with important information regarding correct fracture classification and appropriate treatment options. In the presence of massive osseous injury, it becomes difficult to distinguish osseous from soft tissue

injury with MRI and therefore one may have difficulty detecting clinically significant fracture fragments. In chronic trauma assessment, CT has advantages over MRI in its depiction of fracture union/healing.

The role of CT in the evaluation of acetabular trauma is well established (3,27,110,118,184,266,302,304,315, 332,351,361) (Fig. 15). Acetabular fractures are classified using the system of Judet and Letournel (191). It is generally possible to group patients in a specific subcategory of this classification scheme by thorough assessment of plain radiographs. CT evaluation can provide precise information regarding relative alignment of fracture components and identification of interarticular fracture fragments. The presence of interarticular fragments can alter the surgical approach and certainly mandates that the specific fragment be identified and either reduced in its displacement or removed from the joint. These fragments may be occult on radiographs and may not be apparent to the surgeon in the operating room.

The axial plane is the standard anatomic plane for visualizing acetabular fractures (Fig. 15A). In the past, 5-mm collimation was considered standard protocol. With the availability of fast CT scanners, we have migrated to acetabulum imaging protocols that employ 3-mm collimation. With spiral CT scanning, the acetabulum can be imaged in <1 min with images reconstructed when the patient is removed from the scanner. While many trauma patients undergo pelvic imaging, one should be cautioned about using standard pelvic trauma acquisitions as an adequate evaluation of acetabular trauma. Most pelvic trauma protocols utilize noncontiguous scanning protocols (5-mm collimation × 8-mm increment). A noncontiguous protocol could allow clinically significant bone fragments of 3 mm or less to go undetected. Given the noncontigu-

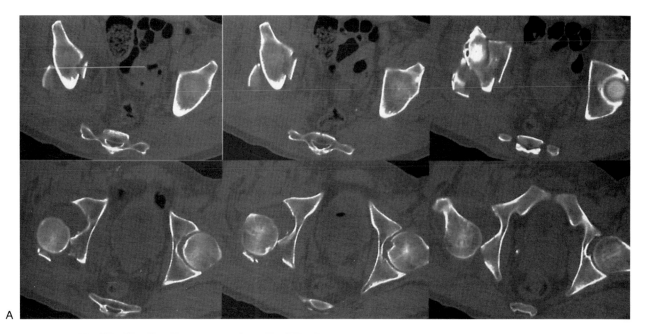

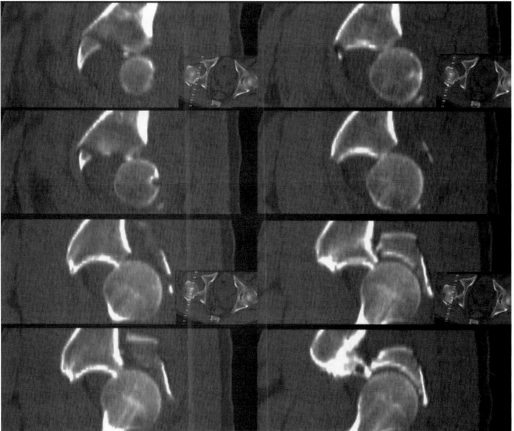

FIG. 15. Posterior hip dislocation/posterior column fracture. **A:** Axial images demonstrate posterior displacement of right hip associated with a fracture of the posterior wall of the acetabulum. A fracture fragment is present within the joint adjacent to the fovea. This fragment could not be seen on radiographs but was identified and removed at surgery. **B:** Sagittal reconstructions again demonstrate the posterior displacement and fractures of both the anterior and posterior acetabular rim.

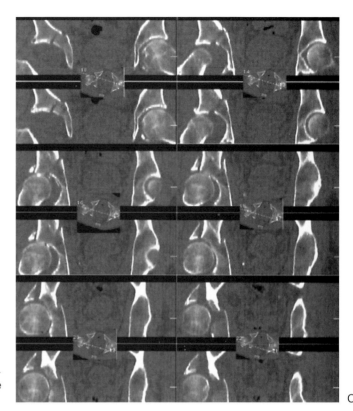

FIG. 15. (*Continued.*) **C:** Coronal reconstructions demonstrate lateral fragment displacement and secondary fracture through the superomedial wall of the acetabulum.

C

ous scanning, resultant multiplanar reconstructions would be of limited clinical value. A separate scan to evaluate acetabular trauma can occur following the pelvic trauma acquisition, assuming that life-threatening injuries were not detected and the patient's clinical condition remains stable.

The usefulness of multiplanar and 3-D reconstructions in acetabular trauma has been extensively studied. Reconstructions allow the visualization of the acetabular wall as well as hip articulation (Fig. 15B, C). Some centers routinely include imaging of the entire pelvis including iliac crests. Although this can be advantageous in the visualization of fractures with 3-D technique, specific evaluation of the acetabulum should not be compromised when planning to image the entire pelvis. We suggest in these instances that lower resolution acquisition be obtained through the iliac crests and high-quality scanning through the acetabular articulation.

In the presence of a dislocated hip, it is better to reduce the hip prior to scanning. Relocation can potentially restore vascular supply to the femoral head and thereby decrease the chance of avascular necrosis. In addition, closed reduction of a dislocated hip can cause a realignment of the acetabular fragments. A possible cause of failure to reduce a dislocation is the presence of bone fragments in the joint. The surgeon needs to have a road map of fragments as they exist after the closed reduction. Some authors have noted the presence of an acetabular "bubble" associated with reduced hip fracture (83). This

information can be useful but in the context of a reduced dislocation without associated fracture it is mostly of academic interest.

Computed tomography is not routinely indicated for the scanning of femoral neck fractures. Intertrocanteric fracture management can be determined by plain radiographs. For occult fracture of the hip, MRI has been shown to be a more sensitive modality than radiography (31,259,279). MRI is also the modality of choice for avascular necrosis whether from trauma or other etiology (15,95,122).

Computed tomographic scanning has a major role in the evaluation and treatment of tibial plateau fractures (68,264) (Figs. 16 and 17). It can also precisely characterize fracture extent in both the tibiofemoral and patellofemoral joints. The advantage of CT over standard tomography is that it can be quickly acquired and allows an examination to be obtained without removal of protective casts or repositioning the extremity. In the traumatized patient, the axial plane is normally imaged. This provides exact information regarding plateau comminution and distraction of fracture fragments. Reconstruction in the sagittal and coronal planes provides additional information regarding fracture extent and characterization of plateau depression.

The goal of orthopedic management is to restore an anatomic configuration to the tibial plateau to provide an optimal long-term outcome. It is a generally accepted principle that displacement of plateau fragments of 5 mm

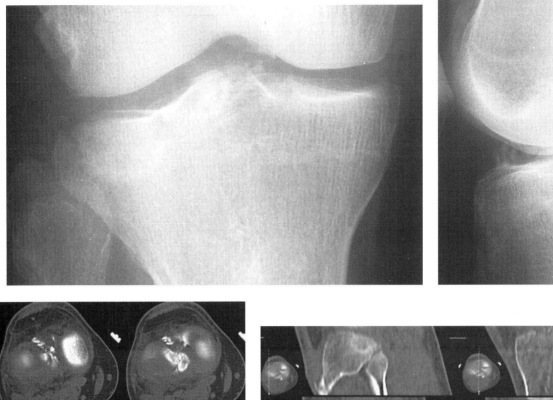

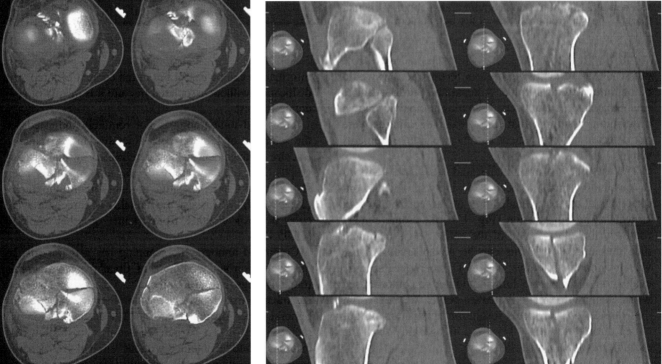

FIG. 16. Tibial plateau fracture. **A, B:** AP and lateral radiographs of the proximal tibia demonstrate a comminuted fracture of the proximal tibia and tibial plateau with numerous bone fragments in the intercondylar notch. **C:** Axial CT reveals extensive comminution of the tibial plateau. **D, E:** Sagittal and coronal reconstructions demonstrate fractures of the medial and lateral plateau. The posterior medial plateau fragment is 3 mm displaced. This patient was treated with realignment of the medial plateau and internal fixation.

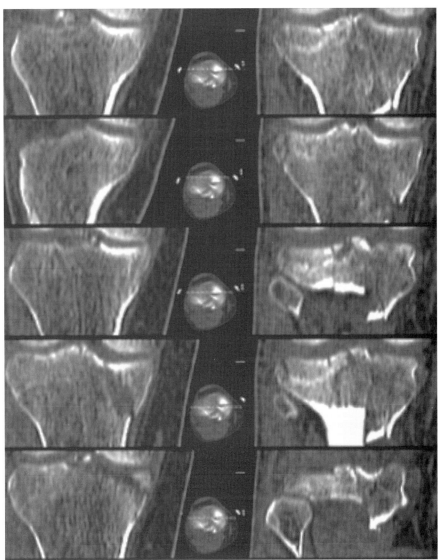

FIG. 16. *Continued.*   E

or greater warrants open reduction (30,232). However, a growing body of orthopedic literature suggests that a depression of 3 mm warrants operative reduction (232) and still other authors argue that any incongruity of the articular surface, especially if subjacent to the menisci, should be operatively reduced (355).

Sagittal and coronal images are required for determination of plateau depression (Fig. 17). These can be derived from a specifically acquired axial image set. We have demonstrated that a spiral CT examination acquired at 2-mm collimation, with images reconstructed at 1-mm intervals, is able to precisely quantify the degree of plateau depression. The 30-sec acquisition of the spiral CT examination provides for efficient management of the traumatized patient. Thicker collimation rapidly decreases the reliability of reconstructed images.

The availability of MRI provides an alternative method to image tibial plateau injuries. Authors have demonstrated that MRI is able to evaluate bone trauma as well as associated soft tissue and ligament injury (14,143, 175,316). The multiplanar capabilities of MRI provide for direct planar images without the need for reconstructions. However, in one series of MRI examinations where there was severe comminution of the tibial plateau, MRI was unable to allow distinction of traumatized plateau from adjacent soft tissue hemorrhage (175).

The selection of CT or MRI to evaluate knee trauma is problematic. There is no argument that MRI better depicts soft tissue injury. In the clinical assessment of the exact degree of plateau comminution, both CT and MRI can provide accurate information. The finding that MRI's usefulness may be limited in cases of severe trauma is of concern because there are no firm criteria as to what degree of trauma excludes the use of MRI.

Although CT cannot determine the extent of soft tissue injury, it can provide criteria for operative versus nonoperative management, namely, the depression of the tibial plateau. In the acute trauma situation, it may be unreason-

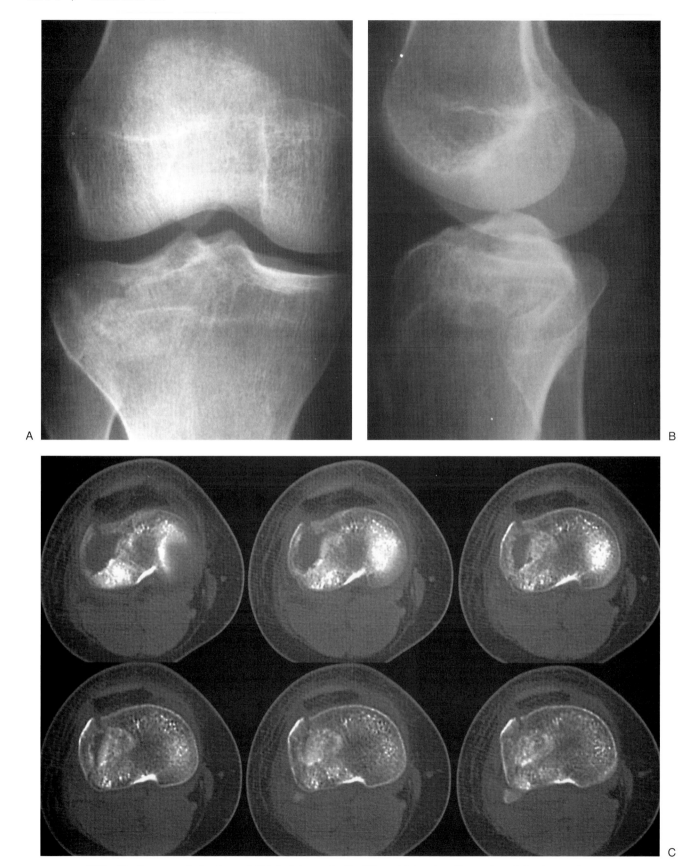

FIG. 17. Dye punch fracture of tibial plateau. **A, B:** AP and lateral radiographs of the knee show a depressed fracture of the lateral tibial plateau. **C:** Axial CT scans through the proximal tibia show a circular defect in the lateral plateau.

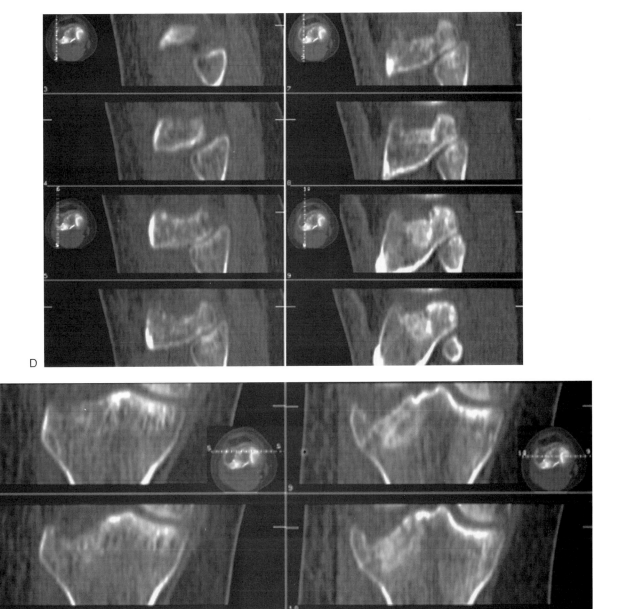

FIG. 17. (*Continued.*) **D, E:** Sagittal and coronal reconstructions directly visualize the 6-mm obliquely depressed fragment. This fracture was treated by elevation of the fragment and bone grafting to support the elevated fragment.

able to expect a patient to remain motionless during the MRI acquisition and the speed of helical CT gives it the advantage. Usually patients can be easily immobilized for the 30 sec needed for a helical CT examination. Once a decision to operate has been made, direct visualization during open reduction of the tibial plateau fracture deter-mines the presence of associated meniscal or ligament injury. MRI is most often used when there is a history of high-velocity knee trauma but minimal plain film find-ings. The fast T1 and T2 sequences increasingly available on modern MRI scanners may soon displace CT in the imaging of the tibial plateau.

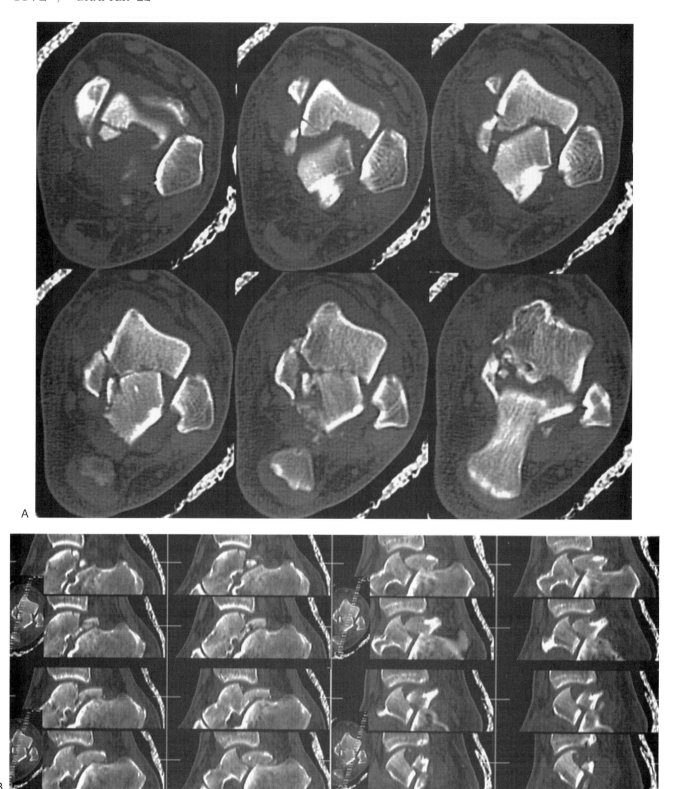

FIG. 18. Talus fracture. **A:** Sequential axial images reveal a communited fracture of the talus with rotation of the posterior fragment. **B,C:** *Continue.*

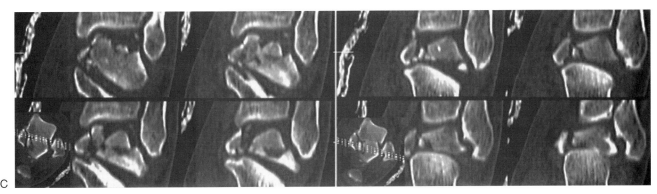

C

FIG. 18. (*Continued.*) **B, C:** Sagittal and coronal reconstructions help to further define that the posterior fragment is inferiorly displaced with discontinuity of the posterior subtalar joint. This discontinuity was difficult to demonstrate on the axial images but clearly shown on the reconstructed images. Fragmentation of the medial talus is seen on both axial and coronal images.

CT evaluation of the tibia is not limited to assessment of the tibial plateau. It has been demonstrated that CT is valuable in the assessment of comminuted fractures of the tibial shaft where there may be rotational deformity and foreshortening of the tibia that must be reduced (377). A problem that can present itself, especially in spiral type fractures of the tibial shaft, is the determination of precise reduction of any rotational deformity following open reduction by pinning or with external fixation. Rather than imaging the fracture, images are taken through the tibial plateau and the lower tibia of both extremities. The relative angulation of the injured tibial shaft can be compared with the normal side, providing the opportunity to adjust fixation before callus formation (33). CT has been shown to assist in the determination of tibial shaft healing through the demonstration of callus formation and subsequent osseous matrix development (316).

Imaging of the foot and ankle focuses on complex talus (Fig. 18), calcaneus (Fig. 19) and midfoot trauma. The value of CT for calcaneus assessment has been well documented (8,115,121,125,139,177,190,202,227,293,307, 325,347). Coronal images are the most valuable for imaging the talus, calcaneus, and subtalar joints. During scan acquisition, the supine patient's knees are bent and the soles of the feet placed flat on the table. The feet are symmetrically positioned because the FOV required to visualize the talocalcaneal joint will be wide enough to visualize both ankles. The coronal plane is particularly advantageous for the visualization of the anterior and posterior subtalar joints and the sustentaculum tali.

Most, if not all complex calcaneous trauma affects the sustentalum tali to some extent. Several calcaneus fracture classification systems have been proposed and are in use (54,73,306); many of these rely on the extent of sustentaculum involvement to determine major stage groupings. As in other joints, determining the exact extent of fracture is crucial for the orthopedic surgeon (Fig. 19). While determining the presence of interarticular fragments is not as essential, knowledge of the fracture extent and relative

displacement(usually impaction) of fragments can guide the surgical approach. It has been noted that one can predict the surgical outcome based on the initial CT evaluation (160). Three-dimensional reconstruction can also contribute to the evaluation of calcaneus fractures (8,347,364).

Whereas the optimal patient position for the hindfoot and subtalar joints is with the feet flat on the table, for the acutely traumatized patient this may be impossible. As a substitute, we find that high resolution spiral CT in the axial plane, 2 mm or less collimation and multiplanar reconstruction in the coronal and sagittal planes are advantageous. The sagittal reconstructions are unique because they are otherwise difficult to routinely obtain without awkward positioning. The diagnostic information of the coronal reconstructions equals that of the direct coronal acquisition with the added benefit of reconstructions in the sagittal plane. As with the hip and knee, a comfortable and still patient imaged in any degree of ankle flexion or leg rotation provides quality image data that can be can be reconstructed in any plane required.

CT can also effectively image complex ankle trauma (76,189,207,218,225,328). As with other articulations, CT is effective in the exact determination of fracture extent. It can assist in treatment planning of complex injuries (207). Specific evaluation of talus fractures (11,75,94, 141,218) can be accomplished with CT (Fig. 18). In the distal tibia, pylon (210), triplane (173,328), and Tillaux fractures (189) can be effectively imaged. CT may even have a role in the relatively common trimalleolar fracture as it has been demonstrated that the size of the posterior tibia fragment is poorly estimated with plain radiography (84).

In imaging of midfoot trauma, we have found the axial plane parallel to the metatarsals to be the most advantageous for precise imaging. Reconstructions perpendicular to this orientation are also of value and again can be easily obtained. The benefit of CT evaluation is in the determination of the exact extent of the fracture. This can

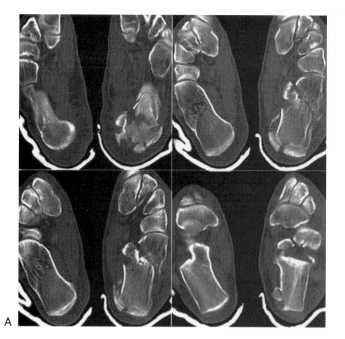

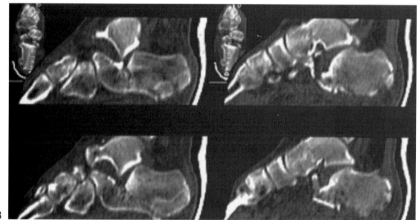

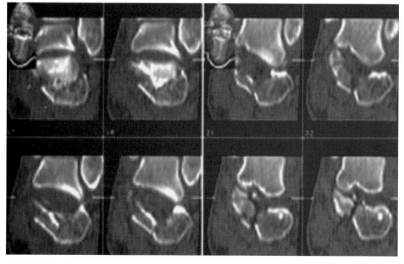

FIG. 19. Comminuted calcaneal fracture. **A:** Axial examination demonstrates a comminuted calcaneus fracture extending from the midportion to posterior aspect of the calcaneus. **B:** Sagittal reconstructions help define the extent of the fracture and demonstrate the degree of incongruity at the calcaneal aspect of the posterior subtalar joint. **C:** Coronal reconstructions demonstrate the extension of the fracture into the sustentaculum tali.

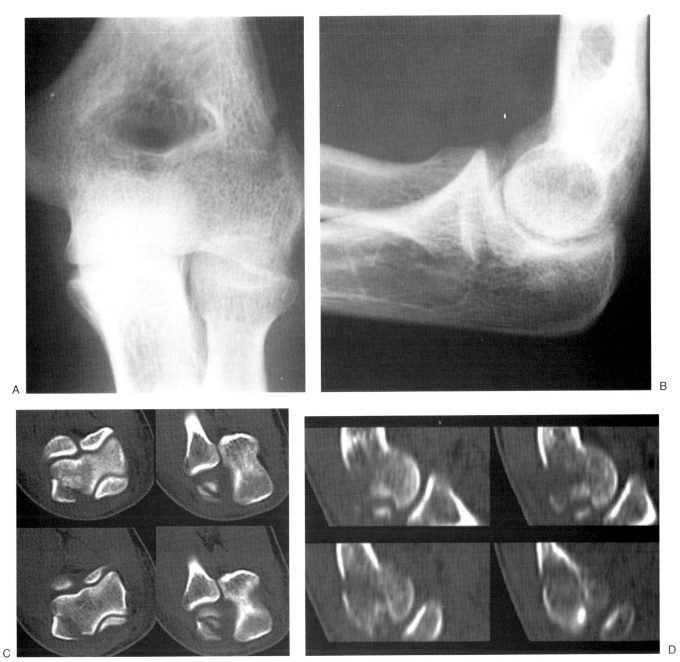

FIG. 20. Capitellum fracture. **A, B:** AP and lateral radiographs shows minimally displaced fracture of the capitellum and associated joint effusion (*arrow*). **C:** Axial CT through elbow shows the capitellar fracture extending upward through the lateral epicondyle. **D:** Sagittal reconstructions demonstrate the coronal plane extension of the fracture through the capitellum and several fragments along the posteroinferior margin of the capitellum.

help the surgeon to determine the best surgical approach and, more important, which bones are stable and can accommodate the internal fixation of adjacent comminuted fractures.

In imaging of shoulder trauma, CT serves as an adjunct to radiography. CT with multiplanar reconstruction can prove useful in determining the exact extent of injuries and orientation of humeral and glenoid fragments post fracture (179). As in the hip, shoulder CT can identify

interarticular fracture fragments. Open reduction of glenoid fractures is practiced with good clinical outcomes described (170,247). CT can provide exact depiction of fracture fragments and their relative position which can guide appropriate operative reduction. Similar use is noted in fractures of the proximal humerus (165). While not routinely needed, CT can identify glenoid rim fractures following shoulder dislocations. This is especially helpful when there is a lipohemarthrosis on postreduction

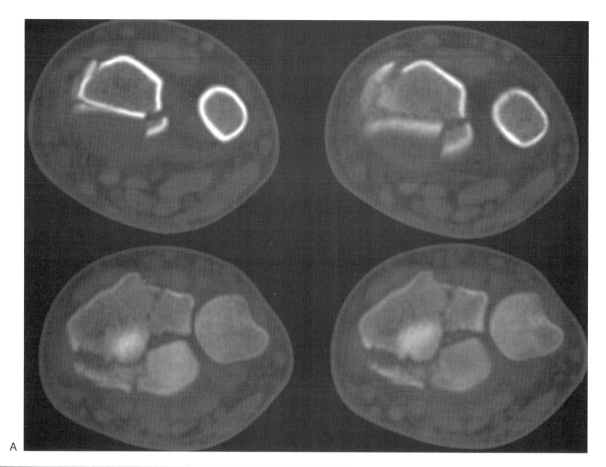

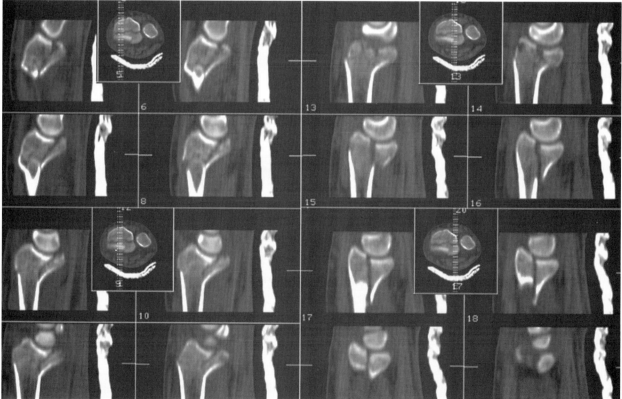

FIG. 21. Distal radial fracture. **A:** Axial images display an intra-articular fracture with extension into the distal radio-ulnar joint and the volar lip. **B, C:** Sagittal and coronal reconstructions precisely demonstrate the incongruity of the distal radial surface as well as the fracture line undermining the radial styloid (*arrow*). The volar lip fragment (*arrowhead*) was difficult to see on radiographs. Based on the CT findings, therapy was changed from closed reduction with casting to open reduction and internal fixation.

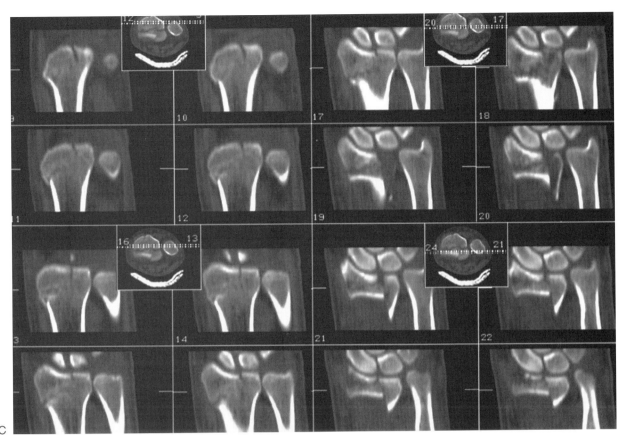

FIG. 21. *Continued.*

radiographs but no fracture is demonstrated. A CT arthrogram can be useful in evaluating the integrity of the joint capsule following shoulder dislocation especially in patients who experience recurrent dislocations.

CT imaging of the elbow (Fig. 20) and wrist (Figs. 21 and 22) plays a role in imaging both acute and chronic trauma, including definition of fracture fragment position and alignment and the identification of posttraumatic complications, such as malunion, nonunion, or avascular necrosis. Optimized wrist CT depends upon understanding the clinical question poised by the clinician and reviewing the patient's radiographs prior to scanning to select an appropriate position for imaging. In general, a "tailored approach" is employed in which the wrist is imaged in two complementary scan planes (338). With efficient positioning, the length of examination can be effectively limited. This is done by positioning the wrist, based on the findings on the radiograph, and then visualizing the area of interest with the topogram. Precise delineation of the area to be scanned can reduce the scanning time required while optimizing diagnostic information. Imaging in the axial, coronal, and sagittal planes is easily accomplished (13,182,338).

In the acutely traumatized patient, the plain radiograph guides the need for scanning. The key information the CT can provide is the precise extent of fracture within the distal radius or carpus. CT scanning can change the management of patients from closed reduction to open reduction based on the visualization of unexpected articular surface displacements or interarticular fracture fragments not appreciated on plain radiographs.

Computed tomography can also assist in the visualization of occult bone injury in the patient with unexplained pain following trauma, although there may be debate over whether MRI examination is more appropriate in this situation. MRI may be more helpful because it can potentially demonstrate occult marrow injury that will not be visualized by CT imaging.

In the assessment of complex distal radial trauma, the goal of the CT is to determine exact extent of the fracture (see Fig. 21). In most instances the articular surface will be well visualized by the surgeon; however, the exact extent of the interarticular fracture line and the degree of impaction of fragments into the distal radius is often difficult to assess. Internal fixation of a fracture to a bone strut that itself has a more proximal fracture is not advantageous. Knowledge of which fragments are, in fact, solid to the proximal radius can assist in the outcome of sur-

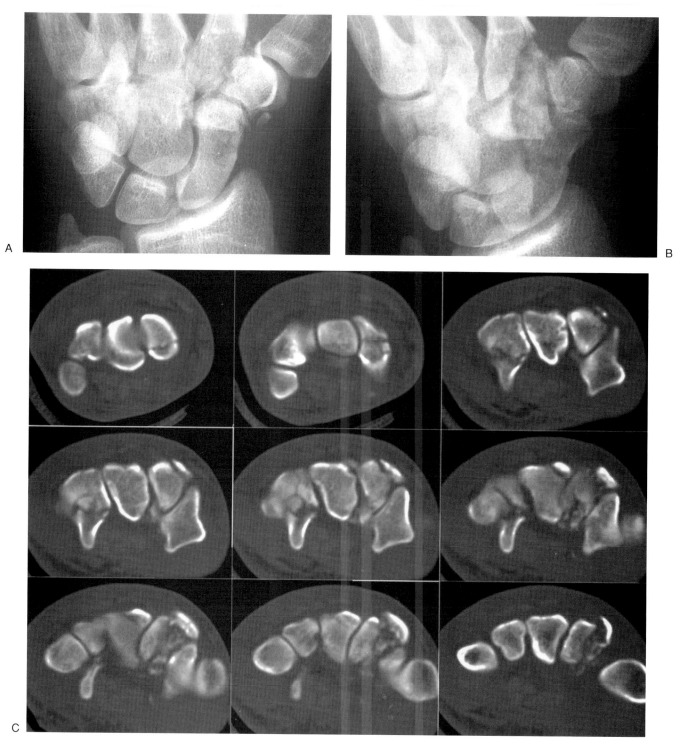

FIG. 22. Complex carpal fracture. **A, B:** AP and oblique radiographs reveal fractures of the scaphoid, trapezoid, hamate and second metacarpal base. **C:** Axial CT scans show the extensive comminution of the trapezoid and hamate.

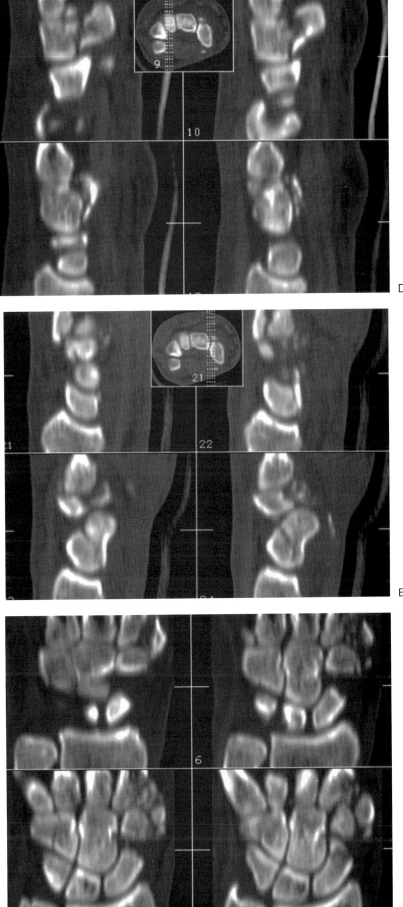

FIG. 22. (*Continued.*) **D–F:** SD agittal and coronal reconstructions further characterize the stellate nature of the hamate and second metacarpal base fractures and show the oblique path of the fracture through the scaphoid. No scaphoid angulation is present.

gery. Identification of impacted "pylon" fragments of the articular surface requires surgical elevation and fixation of the fragments in many cases.

Imaging of the wrist is not limited to the distal radius but can also be useful in assessment of the carpus. Again, plain radiographs are mandatory to guide the selection of the appropriate imaging plane. Although most patients with carpal trauma are imaged with their hand already protected by a plaster cast, this tends to be a short arm cast that will allow positioning in the direct axial, coronal, or sagittal plane. The axial plane provides important information regarding the involvement of individual carpal bones. Sagittal and coronal plane imaging is often important to understand the exact position of fracture lines or fracture fragments. For this reason, when spiral CT is available it can be advantageous to image in the axial plane and then obtain high quality coronal and sagittal images. Fractures of the hamate and triquetrum are well demonstrated on the axial plane with the sagittal plane being complementary. Whatever direct imaging sequence is selected, at least one of the planes should include the entire carpus as there may be unappreciated associated fractures away from the area of clinical interest.

CT has a role in imaging the patient with a scaphoid fracture. Acute scaphoid imaging can demonstrate the amount of displacement or angulation between fracture fragments. A scaphoid waist fracture has a tendency to collapse on itself in an angulated manner. This may be detected on plain radiographs and when seen mandates open reduction with the placement of a bone graft. When there is a clinical question of the degree of displacement or angulation, then CT evaluation of the scaphoid is warranted. For this indication, we suggest a two-plane examination, both acquired using standard 2-mm scans. One plane should be axial and the second plane an oblique sagittal plane parallel to the long axis of the scaphoid. These planes provide the information regarding the extent of the scaphoid fracture and the exact amount of displacement and/or angulation.

Operative reduction of scaphoid fractures requires placement of a triangular wedge graft between the proximal and distal pole fragments, and, often, a Herbert screw or other internal fixator placed through the long axis of the scaphoid to maintain a compressed position of the scaphoid fragments relative to the interposed bone graft. One is often asked to assess healing or degree of fusion in these cases. If there is no evidence of fusion, surgeons are reluctant to remove the cast. Postoperative scaphoid assessment can be effectively accomplished with CT in the presence of the internal fixation. However, one must obtain the long axis scaphoid view with the Herbert screw exactly parallel to the scan plane. Increment images of ×1 mm are acquired and allow the visualization of the fracture healing with the metal artifact minimized. The ideal appearance is the graft in apposition to the adjacent scaphoid and a uniform, homogeneous ossification be-

tween the graft and native scaphoid fragments. This indicates healing and revascularization of the proximal pole. If the ossification of the proximal pole is decreased, this is a good sign. Persistent increased density of the proximal pole suggests decreased vascular supply; however, the designation of necrosis should be reserved for those patients in whom there is collapse of the proximal pole. Cases of delayed revascularization of an otherwise intact scaphoid pole are well known. When there is a gap between the graft and the native scaphoid or a sclerotic proximal pole with collapse, this portends a poor outcome.

PROSTHESIS EVALUATION, MODELING, AND SURGICAL PLANNING

Computed tomography and magnetic resonance imaging have revolutionized the pre- and postoperative evaluations of orthopedic prostheses. Original or reconstructed serial tomographic images from these modalities provide a method for examining joint articulations and the relevant skeleton. However, many would state that CT and MRI's most powerful feature is that they provide for the creation of 3-D depictions of the musculoskeletal system. CT provides accurate representation of the 3-D cortical and cancellous bone geometry and the material properties (density) of these structures, whereas MRI provides detail about cartilaginous surfaces, ligamentous and tendinous attachments and directions, and muscle geometry. The importance of these 3-D renditions is that they provide complete and objective images of the skeleton, from which functional information may be computed. Bone strength, bone stress, and joint range of motion are just a few of the functional mechanical parameters that can be generated from these tomographic studies and provided to the surgeon.

CT Metal Artifact

CT is an important tool in the imaging of bone around prostheses. However, when imaging is performed through prostheses the metal artifact may limit CT's usefulness for examining the bone. Star-burst metal artifacts are produced primarily from missing projection data and also partial volume effects, scatter, and aliasing (167,288,326). When the material of the prosthesis has a high attenuation coefficient or a large cross-section, then the portion of x-ray beam that passes through it is nearly completely absorbed. This produces incomplete data in the respective portions of the projection data. Image reconstructions using these projections produces the star-burst artifacts (Fig. 23).

Metal artifacts may be reduced by at least four tech-

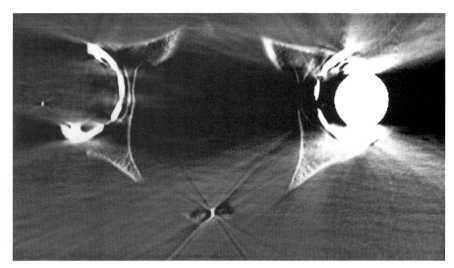

FIG. 23. Axial CT image through a pelvis with bilateral metal-backed acetabular prostheses. The left prosthesis also has a prosthetic femoral head in it. The right acetabular socket is empty. Note the socket screw holes—discontinuities in the bilateral metal arcs.

niques: (a) decreasing the attenuation of the x-ray beam, (b) "averaging out" the artifact in image reformations, (c) artificially generating values for missing projection data, and (d) novel reconstruction mathematics that are less sensitive to incomplete data (241,277,286,289,299, 371,380). While not a metal artifact reduction technique, extended CT scale is a method to improve images of the metal prostheses themselves (174).

Decreasing the attenuation of the x-ray beam may be accomplished by increasing the effective energy of the beam, increasing the photon flux (greater milliamperage, thicker slices) and scanning objects made from less attenuating materials and with smaller cross-sections. Al-

though simple and effective, these approaches are limited by patient dose, the requirement of a low effective energy for optimal bone mineral detection (236), prosthetic materials not being selected based on attenuation coefficients, and the fact that prosthesis size is determined by the patient. In short, patients are imaged with whatever hardware they have. The value in recognizing artifact reduction techniques is that there are prostheses that can be imaged with little or no artifact. Scanning a metal prosthesis does not always mean a terrible artifact-ridden image.

Laboratory studies utilizing cylindrical bone phantoms and cadaveric proximal femurs have demonstrated that by (a) increasing the effective energy of the x-ray beam

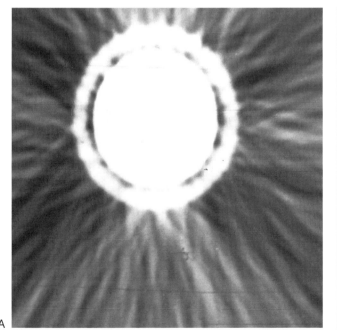

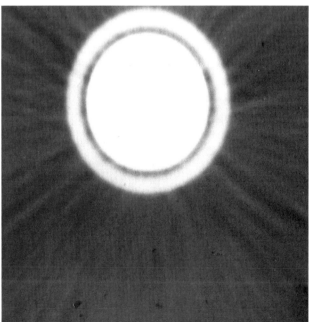

A

B

FIG. 24. CT scans through 42-mm cobalt-chrome alloy (**A**) and titanium 6/4 alloy (**B**) rods. Note the 3-mm acrylic mantle around each rod and the significantly reduced artifact around the titanium rod. The outer ring is cortical bone equivalent.

from 96 to 125 kVp and (b) imaging the titanium 6/4 alloy prostheses as opposed to the cobalt-chrome alloy prostheses, the amount of metal artifact can be decreased (288) (Fig. 24). Rods of titanium 6/4 alloy, cobalt-chrome alloy, and stainless steel alloy were placed in the cylindrical bone phantoms either as a press-fit ("noncemented") or in a 3-mm-thick acrylic sleeve ("cemented"). The dimensional accuracy of the inner and outer bone diameters was tested. At 125 kVp the dimensional errors in the inner (canal) and outer diameter (titanium rods 6 to 42 mm present) averaged 0%. For the cobalt-chrome rods, the errors averaged 5% (range 3% to 8%) for the inner diameters and 0% for the outer diameters. The dimensional errors are largest for the small-diameter cobalt-chrome alloy rods. This is not due to x-ray beam attenuation but to measuring errors having a larger percentage effect on small diameters.

When CT scanning techniques have been optimized and there is still significant artifact, the artifact may be reduced by "averaging it out." Integration of axial CT images, with artifacts within them, into other planes (reformations) will weight the true signal of the image over the "randomly" distributed artifact signal. This technique is easy to perform using either reformation software on the scanner itself or third-party image-processing software packages (Fig. 25).

CT imaging is useful prior to revision surgery of failed total hip replacements (283). CT permitted a 3-D examination of femoral and acetabular bone stock and the relation of the prostheses to internal pelvic structures. Even with substantial metal artifact, axial CT together with reformations was able to answer all pertinent clinical

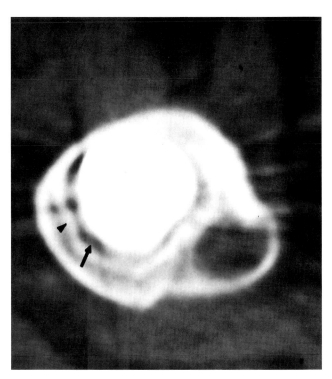

FIG. 26. CT scan through a cemented titanium 6/4 alloy prosthesis. Note the radiolucent line around the prosthesis cement mantle (*arrow*) and the sclerotic, reactive bone (neocortex) formed around the radiolucent line (*arrowhead*). This is a clinically and radiographically loose prosthesis.

questions in the 12 patients. Coronal and sagittal reformation converted six inadequate studies (axial CT images) to six adequate studies (reformations). Only two axial CT studies were judged excellent versus seven for the reformations (Figs. 26 and 27).

It is the missing projection data in the process of image reconstruction that creates the severe image artifacts. If the projections with missing projection are identified and the missing data artificially created (e.g., linear interpolation), then new reconstructions utilizing the complete datasets can be performed (140,167,327). While this method has been around for a while, there is no commercially available software to perform this technique. Figures 28 and 29 demonstrate linear interpolation of the missing CT projection data, as implemented on a Siemens DR-H scanner.

New reconstruction methods are available that are less sensitive to incomplete projection data (Fig. 30). Theoretically, iterative deblurring reconstruction has the potential to create optimal images for a set of incomplete projection data (289,371). An *iterative* reconstruction begins by guessing about the appearance of the image. Subsequent iterations project current guesses along the x-ray paths creating estimated projection profiles. Every physically measured projection profile is then divided point by point by its estimated counterpart. The ratio profiles are then backprojected onto the FOV. The backprojected image is

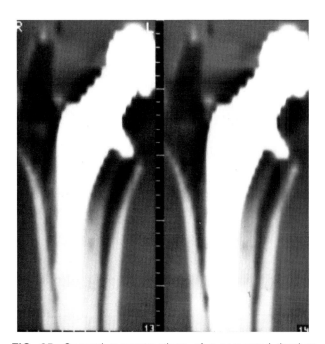

FIG. 25. Coronal reconstructions of a cemented titanium 6/4 alloy prosthesis.

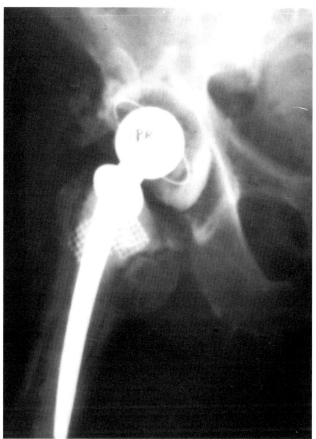

FIG. 27. A: Anteroposterior radiograph of a patient with a loose total hip replacement. **B:** Axial, coronal, and sagittal CT image displayed at soft tissue windows, demonstrating the femoral vessels (*arrows*) immediately adjacent to the protruded acetabular prosthesis. (Reproduced with permission from Robertson DD, Magid D. Poss R, Fishman EK, Brooker AF, Sledge CB. Enhanced computed tomographic techniques for the evalation of total hip arthroplasty. *J Arthroplasty* 1989;4:271–276.)

A

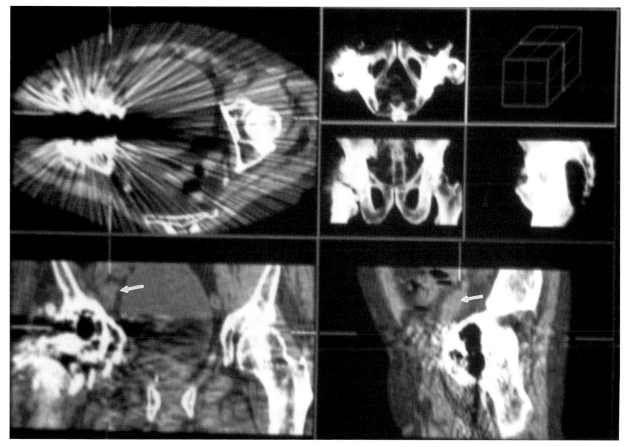

B

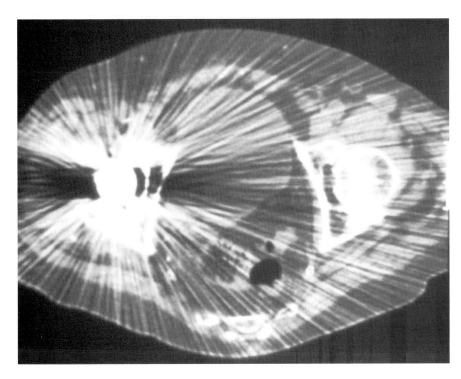

FIG. 28. CT scan through a patient prior to revision joint replacement surgery. (Reproduced with permission from Robertson DD, Magid D. Poss R, Fishman EK, Brooker AF, Sledge CB. Enhanced computed tomographic techniques for the evalation of total hip arthroplasty. *J Arthroplasty* 1989;4: 271–276.)

multiplied point by point by the current guess to produce the next guess. This technique has been implemented and tested using a CT simulator. Comparisons between filtered backprojection, filtered backprojection following linear interpolation of missing projection data, and itera-

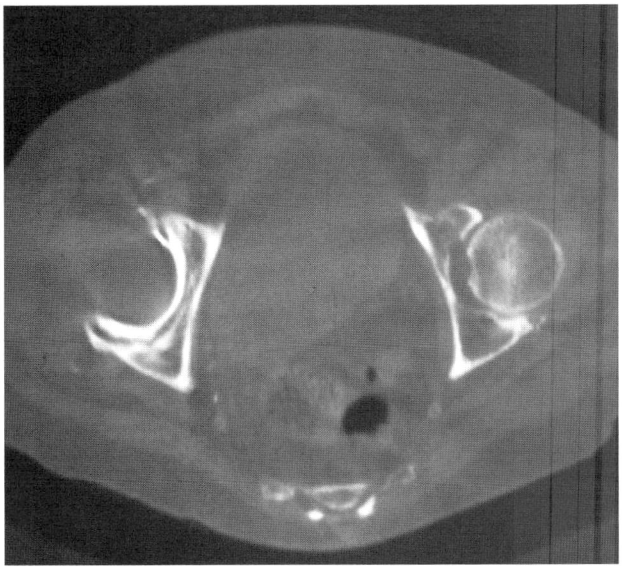

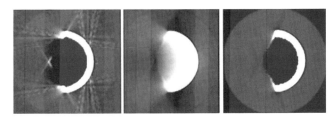

FIG. 29. Identical image slice (as in Fig. 28) after the missing projection has been created by linear interpolation and the new projection data reconstructed. (Reproduced with permission from Robertson DD, Magid D. Poss R, Fishman EK, Brooker AF, Sledge CB. Enhanced computed tomographic techniques for the evalation of total hip arthroplasty. *J Arthroplasty* 1989;4:271–276.)

tive deblurring demonstrated nearly artifact-free images using iterative deblurring (289).

Frequently it is difficult to separate bone cement from the metal prosthesis and to distinguish the actual cross-sectional geometry of the prosthesis, even with appropriate image windowing. Note that the bone cement and prosthesis appear as a central dense object in Fig. 4. The visualization of prosthesis may be improved by extending the range of the CT number scale (174) (Fig. 31). Typically, CT numbers are stored as 12-bit integers and range in value from -1000 Houndsfield units (HU) as a minimum (air) to 3095 HU as a maximum. Any material with an attenuation coefficient corresponding to a Houndsfield unit of 3096 or greater is assigned to 3095. All orthopedic

FIG. 30. Comparison of three reconstruction techniques-filtered backprojection (*left*), filtered back projection following linear interpolation of missing projection data (*center*), and iterative deblurring (*right*). A simulated metal-backed acetabular prosthesis has been used. Note the reduced artifact following iterative deblurring reconstruction. (Reproduced from Robertson DD, Yuan J, Wang G, Vannier MW. Total hip prosthesis metal-artifact suppression using iterative deblurring reconstruction. *Comput Assist Tomogr* 1997;21: 293–298.)

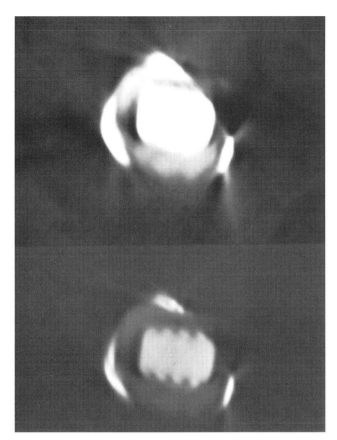

FIG. 31. Identical CT images of an implanted femoral prosthesis without (*above*) and with (*below*) extended CT scale. Note the clarity of the prosthesis with extended scale CT. (Reproduced courtesy of E. Klotz, Siemens, Erlangen, Germany.)

metals have attenuation coefficients that are larger than what can accurately be represented with the standard CT scale. Scalar extension of the CT numbers (up to and beyond 40,000 HU) enables the accurate delineation of the prosthesis, permits automatic contouring of the prosthesis, and allows use of the prosthesis as a relocatable reference system.

Good imaging studies through metal prostheses may be achieved under the proper situations (Fig. 32). Titanium alloy prostheses, especially small to medium-sized ones, produce minimal artifact. Cobalt-chrome alloy prostheses produce significantly more artifact, but even with these prostheses cortical geometry is usually evident. It is important to optimize the CT technique—increase the photon flux by increasing the milliamperage and not using thin slices. For hip prostheses, longer scan times and multiple rotations that produce 480 or more mAs should be used. A slice thickness of 4 mm will improve photon flux and capture anatomic geometric change in large joints.

When the artifact is bad, remember that image reformation is easy, available, and that it will most often provide the imaging detail needed to answer the clinical question. If a joint is being examined, coronal and sagittal reforma-

tions provide a more clinically relevant view while reducing the metal artifact. If axial images are preferred, then new axial images may be interpolated between the scanned slices.

While the artificial generation of missing projections or novel reconstruction mathematics is appealing, there are no commercially available implementations and these techniques represent work in progress. The extended CT scale does improve visualization of the prosthesis and the relationship of the prosthesis to the bone, but by itself it is not an artifact reduction method. Metal artifact may at times be a significant problem, but it is not as significant a problem as is widely believed. CT can provide new and potentially clinically important information regarding the state of the bone around metal prostheses.

Three-dimensional models created from serial CT or MR images and simulations using these models are valuable tools for designing and evaluating joint reconstructions. Clinically, 3-D models are used for surgical planning of osteotomies (238,285,301,376) and prosthetic joint replacements. As an experimental tool the models are used to objectively describe skeletal shape and variability (181,284,276,281,287,367), modify or verify prosthesis design (241,258,277,286,287,299,368,369,380), and perform computational mechanical evaluations of the reconstructed joint (16,39,56,82,98,99,156,157,258,271). The clinical importance of 3-D modeling will continue to grow as the ease of creating the models and performing the simulations improve.

Three-dimensional bone modeling has truly added another dimension to the surgical planning of osteotomies about the hip. In contrast to conventional radiography, 3-D models allow visualization and quantitation of the whole lesion and deformity (238,285,301,376). They also allow the effect of the lesion on the function of the hip to be assessed visually and by computational mechanical analyses. With improved definition of the lesion and its effect, improved selection of the best surgical alternative may be made.

In addition to greatly improving the definition of the pathology, 3-D bone modeling may be used to perform surgical simulations (238,285,301,376). Osteotomies may be simulated by cutting across the outer and inner cortical surfaces using a computer pointing devise, such as a mouse. Osteotomized sections may then be discarded, translated, or rotated. Hardware or grafting materials may be simulated and added. The resultant geometry is then calculated, the new 3-D structure reconstructed and displayed, and visual examination performed for adequacy and ease. The models may also be submitted to kinematic or dynamic computational analyses to predict the effect of the proposed osteotomy. Thus, these 3-D models not only improve the definition of hip lesions and their functional effects, but have the potential of improving surgical selection and planning.

Improved fit appears to be critical to the clinical success

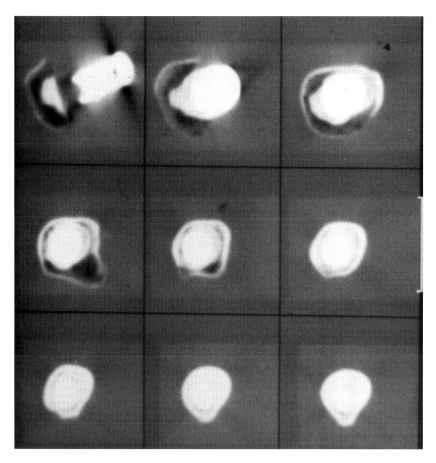

FIG. 32. Multiple axial images through a noncemented titanium alloy proximal femoral prosthesis. Images start at the head and extend distally to the region of the calcar femorale. (Reproduced with permission from Robertson DD, Magid D. Poss R, Fishman EK, Brooker AF, Sledge CB. Enhanced computed tomographic techniques for the evalation of total hip arthroplasty. *J Arthroplasty* 1989;4:271–276.)

of noncemented total joints. Experimental and clinical evidence demonstrates that for noncemented femoral hip prostheses, maximal prosthesis-cortical bone contact, especially proximally, produces more normal strain values, reduces micromotion and sinkage, and improves clinical results (258). In response, off-the-shelf systems have added more sizes, increased modularity of the system, and improved instrumentation. However, a properly designed custom prosthesis will produce an optimal fit for a given individual. Traditionally, custom prostheses have been designed based on anatomic data obtained from two orthogonal planar radiographs. It is only recently that some companies have incorporated cross-sectional data extracted from axial CT images (277). Typically, CT data is used only to extract dimensional measurements or aid in the final approval of a custom design.

An optimal custom design may be produced by using a 3-D model of the bone to determine the shape of a prosthesis, not just to check whether or not a prosthesis fits. The design of an optimal-contact prosthesis requires extraction of the accurate 3-D geometry of the bone canal and incorporation of this geometry with design features that produce an optimal strain environment (258,286). Recreation of the exact canal geometry may be obtained using CT. However, beam hardening, partial volumes, and scatter may introduce errors in single energy x-ray

CT generated images (108,162–164,282,384). Careful selection of scanning techniques, dual-energy scanning, or postprocessing corrective procedures may be used to reduce these errors (9,162,168,282). However, the easiest method is to include a bone sizing reference phantom in the scan field (284) (Fig. 33). Software is then used to extract the various cylindrical cross-sections of the phantom and to correct any dimensional errors. These corrections are then applied to the extracted femoral contours. This method also corrects dimensional errors created by image convolvers and the use of digital image filters.

Following scanning, inner and outer bone contours are extracted from the axial CT slices using software that includes a combination of digital filtering, boundary detection based on a changing CT number threshold, and dimensional error correction. A computer-aided design (CAD) solid model is constructed from the bone contour data (Fig. 34). Model modification simulates the surgical preparation of the bone (Fig. 35).

The actual design of the optimal-contact prosthesis begins by defining the prosthesis as having the same surface geometry as the modified bone canal. However, the design does not end here. Although this would be a maximal-contact prosthesis, it may be an uninsertable prosthesis. This is true in the proximal femur where the complex curvature of the proximal canal would prohibit insertion

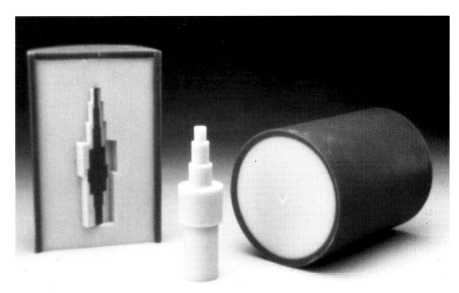

FIG. 33. CT bone sizing reference. Sizing errors are calculated based on the known dimensions of the phantom.

of an exact canal-shaped prosthesis. An exact canal-shaped prosthesis also would not create an optimal bone strain environment if made from the alloys available today. Therefore some prosthesis material must be removed, but it must be removed in an advantageous manner. Optimal-contact design modifies the canal-shaped prosthesis by trying to maintain contact in regions of load transfer and regions important to prosthesis fixation, while removing material in order to make the prosthesis insertable.

Once designed the 3-D prosthesis model is refined and

assessed. Nonpriority regions of the prosthesis are adapted to be easily machined. Prosthesis–bone contact is quantitated and a maximum stress analysis of the final prosthesis performed. If acceptable, the prosthesis surface is translated to computerized, numerically controlled (CNC) machine tool paths and the prosthesis is manufactured. If unacceptable, further redefining of unimportant regions is performed or another design produced correcting the previous problems. For primary arthroplasties, this

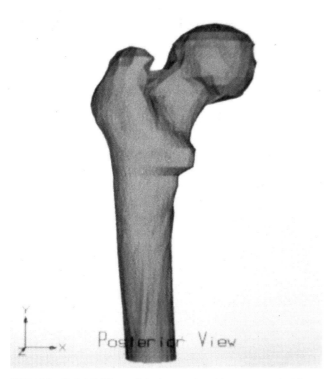

FIG. 34. Solid CAD model of a proximal femur, created from axial CT data.

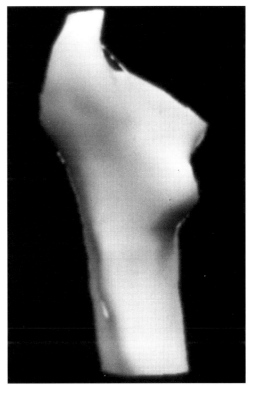

FIG. 35. Solid model after a femoral neck osteotomy has been performed.

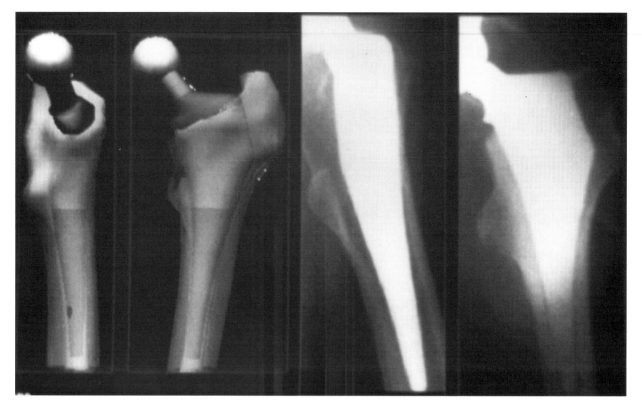

FIG. 36. Radiographs of an actual optimal contact proximal femoral prosthesis (*right*). Note that the prosthesis is visible through the translucent cortex. CAD display of the design (*left*). (Reproduced courtesy of Symbios, SA.)

process is most frequently used to design custom proximal femoral prosthesis and is less frequently used to design custom shoulder, elbow, knee, and ankle prostheses (Fig. 36).

Three-dimensional modeling also assists in the design

of off-the-shelf prostheses. An "average" 3-D femoral geometry may be produced for subpopulations of femurs with common anatomy and pathology. The "average" femur is produced by extracting individual bone contours, scaling them, and averaging the corresponding levels of

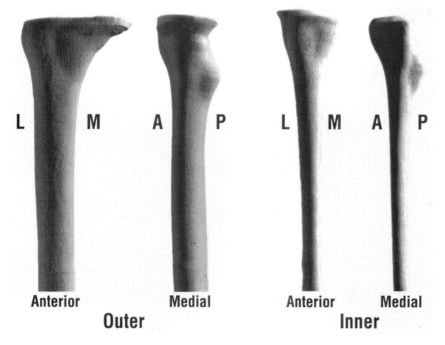

FIG. 37. Average CDH femur model: anterior medial, lateral, and posterior view. Outer = periosteal boundary. Inner = canal boundary. (Reproduced wit permission from Robertson DD, Essinger J, Imura S. Femoral deformity in adults with developmental hip dysplasia. *Clin Orthop* 1996;327:196–206.)

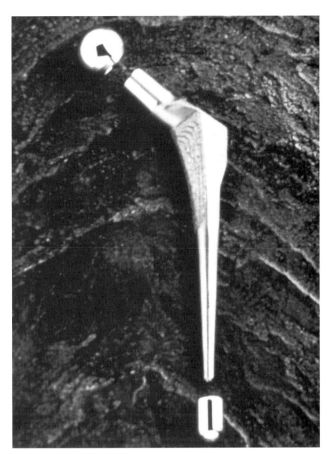

FIG. 38. Actual CDH proximal femoral prosthesis. (Reproduced with permission from Robertson DD, Essinger J, Imura S. Femoral deformity in adults with developmental hip dysplasia. *Clin Orthop* 1996;327:196−206.)

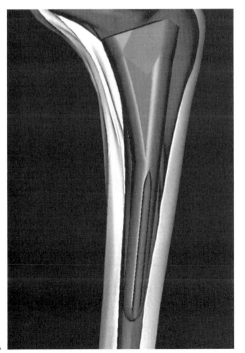

A

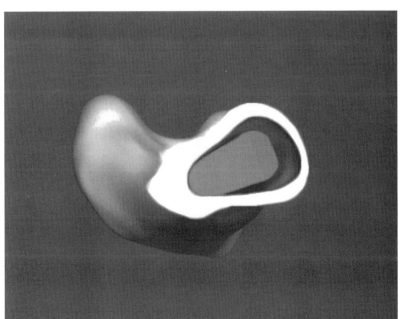

B

FIG. 39. Cutaway view of a CAD model of a proximal femoral prosthesis inserted into an individual femur. **A:** Front view. **B:** Top view.

the individual femurs. The average femur may then be submitted to the optimal contact design process with the expectation that the resultant stem design, when produced in various sizes, would minimize the average stem-bone mismatch for that clinical subpopulation. Three-dimensional average femoral geometries have been produced from CT scans of individuals with congenital dislocation of the hip (281) and individuals in the fifth to eighth decade (258). Both applications have lead to commercially available hip stem systems (Figs. 37 and 38).

CT based 3-D CAD models have also been used to verify and test prosthesis design. Whereas the original design is based on average femur shape data, the final design can be tested within each of the individual femurs that made up the average. The 3-D femur database, created from CT, permits insertion of prostheses into the femurs and nondestructive prosthesis–bone contact analyses (Fig. 39). Material properties of the cortical bone, cancellous bone, and prosthesis materials may be assigned to the 3-D models. The model is then submitted to finite element analysis (FEA) software. This computational stress analysis analyses the mechanical environment of prostheses and bone following joint replacement (16, 39,56,157, 258,271).

Although hip and knee prostheses have only a few percent revision rate at 10 years, the absolute number of revision cases is climbing. Bone loss, both cortical and medullary, and limited revision prosthesis systems make optimal or even successful prosthesis–bone contact and mechanical stability difficult. Knowledge of the extent of bone loss and the structure of the remaining bone allows selection of a prosthesis that contacts cortical bone and is capable of supporting the prosthesis and its loads. Will the remaining bone stock structurally support a prosthesis? Will an off-the-shelf prosthesis work? Is a custom prosthesis or an allograft needed? These are questions a surgeon would like answered preoperatively.

Computed tomography provides a method of obtaining the 3-D bony geometry from which reconstruction plans may be made. Even with its limitations from metal artifact, CT provides a much improved structural description as compared to the crude representations provided by orthogonal radiographs. The models made from CT may be computer models or physically constructed models, created using the techniques described previously. The analysis may be visual, tactile, or quantitative through the use of simple structural analysis methods or finite element analysis methods (Figs. 40 and 41).

CT- and MRI-based 3-D visualization, modeling, and simulation are valuable tools that can provide important functional information to the referring surgeon. Unusual bone geometries from trauma, long- standing dislocation, or prosthesis failure can be objectively and accurately described preoperatively. Mechanical descriptions can be computed from the imaging-based models. All this raises the pre-operative plan to a more sophisticated and accu-

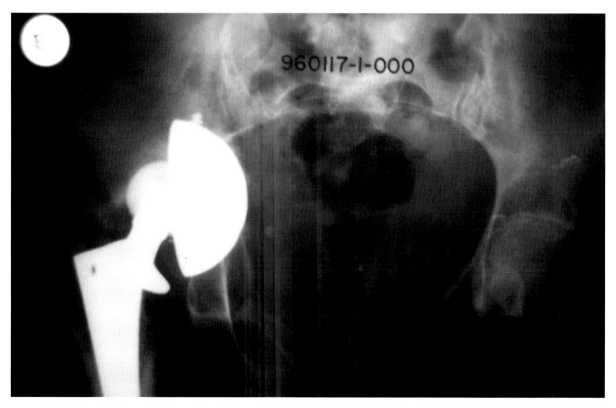

FIG. 40. Radiograph of a patient with a failed total hip replacement and a severe acetabular defect.

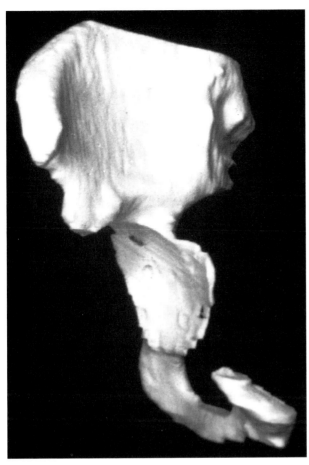

FIG. 41. CNC machined model of the hemipelvis illustrated in Fig. 40. Note the severe bone loss, especially in the anterior column.

rate level. Historically, improved operative planning has resulted in improved patient outcomes. Improved operative planning can also reduce costs if only the prosthesis, instrumentation, and materials that are used are all that are present at surgery. Large inventories of ''just-in-case'' items can be eliminated. The clinical importance of providing these services will continue to grow as improvements are made in imaging adjacent to prostheses, and modeling and simulation software becomes easier to use and more accessible.

JOINTS

Pathologic conditions affecting musculoskeletal articulations can be of many causes. Trauma often alters the structure and function of a joint. Infectious and neoplastic lesions may involve one or more joints as well as adjacent nonarticular osseous structures. Other processes, however, are more confined to musculoskeletal articulations. Such conditions include a wide variety of congenital and developmental disorders that alter the morphology of the articular ends of bones. Other diseases primarily affect articular cartilage, synovium, and capsular structures and include inflammatory, degenerative, traumatic, and metabolic arthropathies and enthesopathies. Collagen vascular disorders such as systemic lupus erythematosus and scleroderma may also have articular manifestations. By altering the morphology of affected bones or by disturbing articular cartilage or osseous metabolism, storage diseases and metabolic disorders may also affect musculoskeletal joints. Other idiopathic processes may affect joints primarily and include synovial osteochondromatosis and pigmented villonodular synovitis. Hematologic disorders such as hemophilia and other blood dyscrasias often produce characteristic articular manifestations. Finally, various surgical procedures, including arthroplasty and arthrodesis, may be performed on joints. The results, both intended and undesirable, may produce distinctive radiologic findings.

Although imaging of articular diseases generally begins with conventional radiographs, further imaging is often required. Such imaging may include arthrography, tomography, ultrasound, nuclear medicine, CT, and MRI. Any joint may be studied with arthrography, and in experienced hands, arthrography is quickly performed, safe, and well tolerated by most patients. Information concerning the integrity of the capsular and internal articular structures may be obtained. Pluridirectional tomography or polytomography may be helpful as an adjunct to arthrography, particularly in the elbow and ankle. Polytomography may also be used in assessing the status of fusion of articular surfaces following attempted arthrodesis, especially in the spine (58). Ultrasound has proven quite helpful in evaluating ligamentous abnormalities such as patellar tendon and Achilles tendon (166,242). Ultrasound is also used as a primary tool to evaluate the rotator cuff in some centers. Dysplastic hip conditions (248) and periarticular fluid conditions may also be evaluated with ultrasound. Nuclear medicine has limited applicability in articular imaging but may be used to assess inflammatory or infectious conditions and to evaluate arthroplasties for possible infection or loosening. With its superior display of intraarticular structures and capsular anatomy, MRI is often the procedure of choice for joint imaging, although accurate delineation of articular structures may require the intraarticular administration of gadolinium. Intraosseous conditions are better displayed by MRI than by the previously mentioned modalities, and MRI depicts extraarticular soft tissue anatomy very well. Conversely, CT displays bone detail better than any modality except conventional radiographs. MRI, for example, cannot match CT's depiction of the extent of cortical or trabecular bone destruction. In cases in which the display of bone detail is important, CT is often preferable over MRI. CT, particularly when enhanced by the intraarticular administration of iodinated contrast and/or air, can be used to evaluate suspected internal derangement of a joint. Arthrographic CT is often improved when supplemented with multipla-

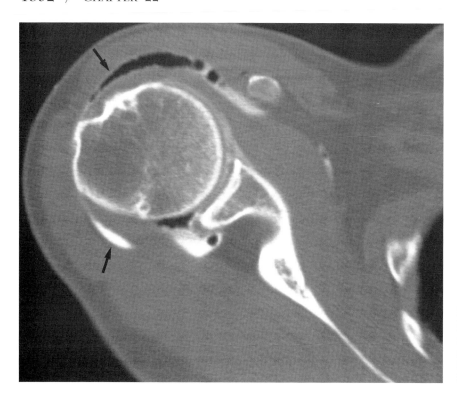

FIG. 42. Axial CT of the shoulder following double-contrast arthrography demonstrates contrast and air in the subacromial-subdeltoid bursa (*arrows*) indicating a full-thickness tear of the rotator cuff.

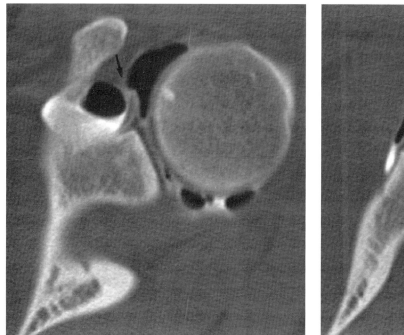

A

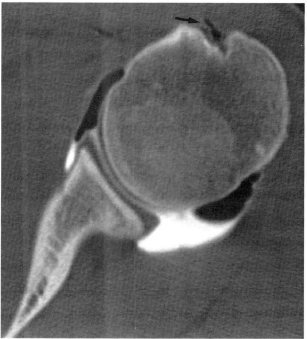

B

FIG. 43. Arthrographic CT of the normal shoulder. **A:** An axial image at the level of the base of the coracoid process reveals the glenoid labrum and articular cartilage of the glenoid and humeral head outlined by contrast and air. The normal superior glenohumeral ligament is seen medially (*arrow*). **B:** An image caudal to A shows the normal smooth appearance of the labrum anteriorly and posteriorly. Air in seen in the bicipital tendon sheath laterally, a normal finding (*arrow*).

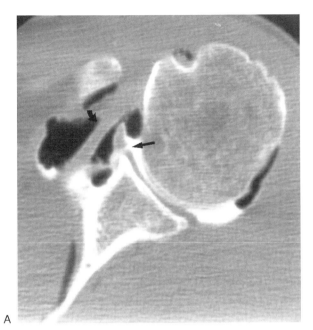

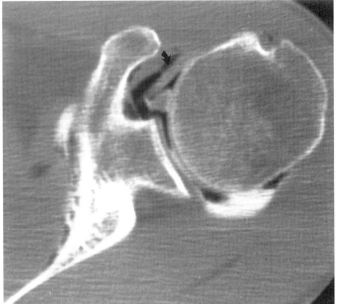

A

B

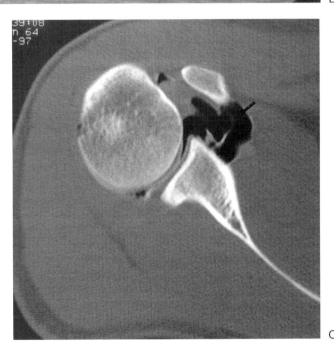

C

FIG. 44. Arthrographic CT demonstrating a tear of the anterior glenoid labrum. **A:** With internal rotation of the glenohumeral joint, contrast is seen traversing the base of the torn anterior labrum (*arrow*) although the fragment of the anterior labrum is approximated with the remainder of the glenoid. **B:** With external rotation the labral fragment is distracted from the remainder of the glenoid. Note the normal subscapularis tendon in both images (*curved arrow*). **C:** In another patient the torn labral fragment is displaced medially. In this case note the ballooned anterior capsule and the middle glenohumeral ligament (*arrow*).

nar reconstruction. However, because of its ability to scan in any plane and its fewer patient positioning restrictions, MRI is often preferred over CT when evaluating internal joint structures.

Other refinements of CT may be applied to articular imaging. Three-dimensional and multiplanar reconstruction, in addition to their accepted applicability in the trauma setting (40,90,354,381) and the spine (107, 278,297), can be very helpful in assessing congenital and developmental conditions (2,12). Helical CT (244) and ultrafast cine-CT (330) permit rapid scanning of most joints in a few seconds, avoiding motion artifacts. Such rapid scanning may also permit scanning a joint in various rotations and positions.

Shoulder

The shoulder girdle is composed of the glenohumeral (GH), acromioclavicular, and sternoclavicular articulations. The shoulder is stabilized by a complex labrocapsular mechanism and by the muscles of the rotator cuff. While shoulder signs and symptoms may be referable to any of these joints, attention is most often directed to the GH joint and its associated soft tissue structures.

Rotator cuff pathology can be assessed with conventional radiographs, conventional arthrography, MRI, ultrasound, and CT (339). Conventional films may show elevation of the humeral head and may strongly suggest the presence of a rotator cuff tear. Ultrasound, as noted

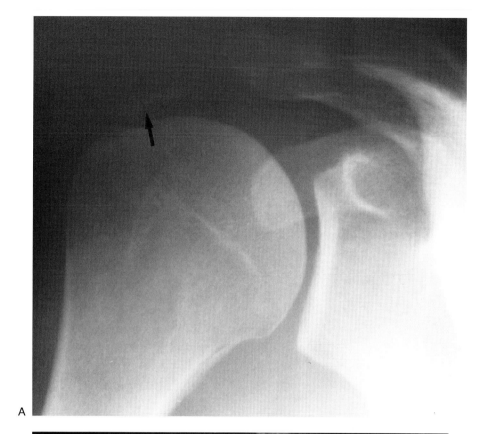

A

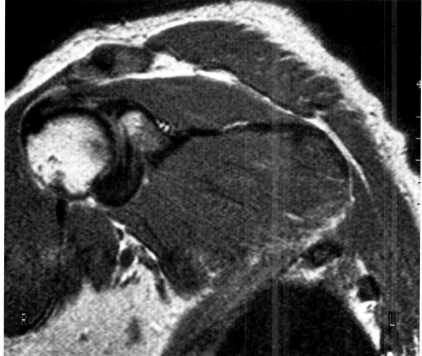

B

FIG. 45. Hydroxyapatite deposition disease in the supraspinatus tendon (calcific tendinitis). **A:** The conventional radiograph demonstrates a typical amorphous deposit in the supraspinatus tendon (*arrow*). **B:** An oblique sagittal MR image shows only decreased signal intensity in the region of the deposit identified on the radiograph.

above, may demonstrate cuff tears. Whereas arthrographic CT (18) (Fig. 42) and MRI (262,268) can demonstrate a rotator cuff tear, confirmation of the presence of a full-thickness rotator cuff tear can be made simply with a traditional arthrogram, avoiding the expense of either MRI or CT (339). CT is able to identify osseous abnormalities contributing to shoulder pain, clinical impingement syndrome, and other rotator cuff symptoms, such as inferior acromial osteophytosis and acromioclavicular overgrowth (67) as well as intraarticular loose bodies (109). The curvature of the acromion may be an important contributor to the development of clinical impingement syndrome. It is best evaluated with properly positioned radiographs or with MRI performed in the oblique sagittal plane (81,253).

Abnormalities of the supporting soft tissues about the shoulder may contribute to shoulder dysfunction. Such lesions include capsular, ligamentous, and labral conditions. Either CT or MRI may be used to demonstrate the normal capsular and labral structures of the shoulder (55) (Fig. 43). Defects in the anterior and posterior labra as well as capsular abnormalities may be seen by MRI (114), but their visualization is improved by the intraarticular administration of gadolinium (46). Similarly, CT following the intraarticular administration of iodinated contrast and air is ideal for demonstrating the status of the normal and abnormal glenoid labrum and the articular capsule (65,265) (Fig. 44). Unlike MRI, however, CT is effectively limited to axial scanning in the shoulder. Some conditions such as the SLAP lesion (superior labral ante-

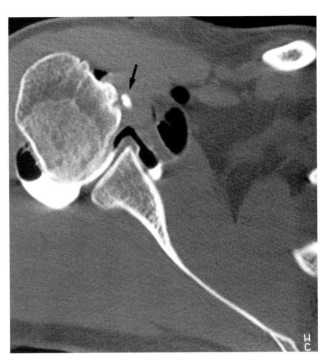

FIG. 47. A CT arthrogram demonstrates a calcification in the subscapularis tendon adjacent to its lesser tuberosity attachment (*arrow*).

rior posterior instability) (231) may be more easily detected by imaging in the oblique sagittal or oblique coronal planes, and in such cases MRI is preferred. MRI in the oblique sagittal plane may afford better visualization of the face of the glenoid and its labrocapsular mechanism than that provided by axial CT. When depiction of calcification and bone detail is particularly important, however, CT may outperform MRI (Fig. 45). Posttraumatic calcification of the posterior labrum, the Bennett lesion, is easily demonstrated with CT (Fig. 46). Calcifications in the rotator cuff, as seen in hydroxyapatite deposition disease or calcium pyrophosphate dihydrate deposition disease, are better shown with CT than with MRI (Fig. 47).

The sternoclavicular (SC) joint is often notoriously difficult to evaluate with conventional radiography. Specialized projections for demonstration of the SC joint have been described but may be difficult to obtain. CT, however, is ideally suited for evaluation of the SC joint (63,67,120) and can display conditions affecting the SC articulation such as sternocostoclavicular hyperostosis (Fig. 48) and septic arthritis of the sternocostoclavicular joint.

Elbow and Wrist

Arthrography of the elbow supplemented with CT can document the presence of intraarticular osteocartilaginous bodies (Fig. 49) and may identify their source (252,334).

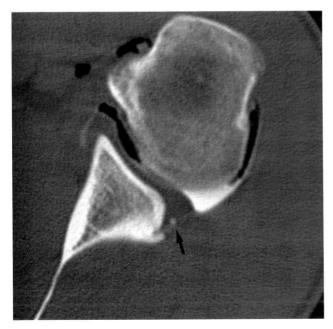

FIG. 46. An axial CT arthrogram of the shoulder reveals contrast and air outlining the posterior labrum. An irregular osteophyte arises from the posterior labrum and the labrum itself contains a small calcification (the Bennett lesion) (*arrow*).

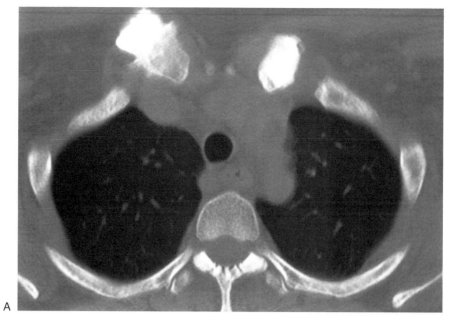

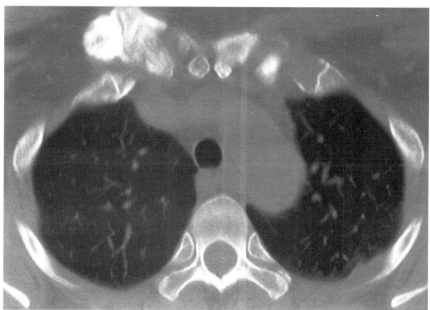

FIG. 48. Sternocostoclavicular hyperostosis. **A:** An axial image of the sternoclavicular articulations exhibits marked sclerosis and overgrowth about the sternocostoclavicular joints bilaterally but more marked on the right. **B:** An image caudal to A again reveals hyperostosis affecting both sternocostoclavicular joints although the right joint is again more severely affected.

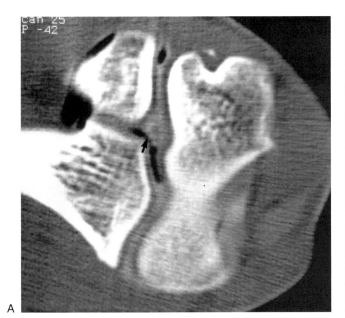

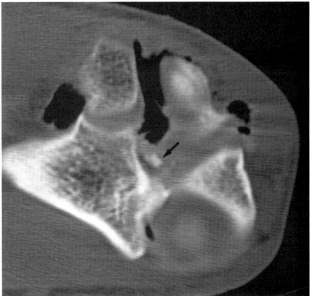

A   B

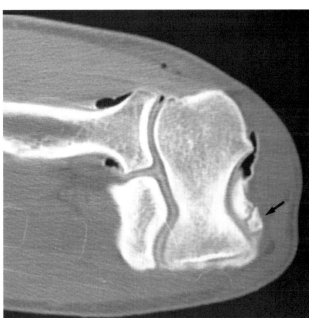

C

FIG. 49. Osteocartilaginous loose bodies identified by elbow CT arthrography. **A:** A cartilaginous intraarticular loose body (*arrow*) is identified between the medial aspect of the radial head and the distal humerus. **B:** Arthrographic CT demonstrates a calcified loose body (*arrow*) adjacent to the olecranon in another patient. **C:** In another patient, a calcified fragment posterior to the distal humerus (*arrow*) was found to be extrasynovial at surgery.

Synovial masses (Fig. 50) can also be shown with arthrographic CT. Other conditions, such as synovial osteochondromatosis, osteochondrosis of the capitellum (Fig. 51), and synovitis (Fig. 52), may be evaluated with arthrographic CT. Abnormalities of the elbow joint capsule, including conditions such as tendinitis and tears of the flexor or extensor attachments to the humerus, are better demonstrated with MRI than with CT. Arthrographic CT shows capsular pathology at the elbow only as contrast extravasation from the joint or as calcifications developing about the traumatized capsule. With MRI, however, such defects may be demonstrated before a complete tear of the structure develops. As in the shoulder, arthrographic MRI may be particularly beneficial in the assessment of elbow capsular lesions (321). CT can easily document the presence of calcified

loose bodies and calcific debris within the cubital tunnel in the setting of ulnar neuropathy.

At the wrist, abnormalities of the distal radioulnar (DRU) joint are difficult to evaluate with conventional films but are easily demonstrated with CT (373). The wrists may be scanned simultaneously in neutral, pronation, and supination, allowing assessment of instability in the symptomatic DRU joint and comparison with the asymptomatic wrist. In this setting, the wrists should be scanned in the degree of pronation or supination that reproduces the patient's complaints. Assessment of DRU stability is best performed by evaluating the relative positioning of the radial sigmoid notch and the center of rotation of the distal ulna in various degrees of wrist rotation (373) (Fig. 53).

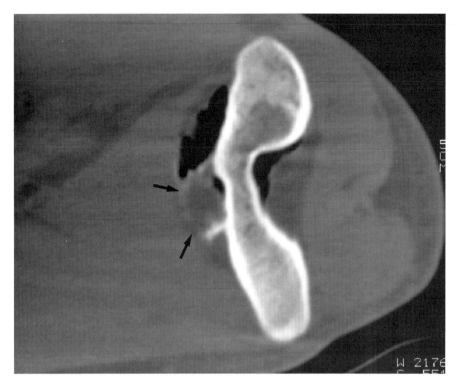

FIG. 50. Elbow CT arthrogram demonstrates a synovial lipoma (*arrows*) anterior to the humerus.

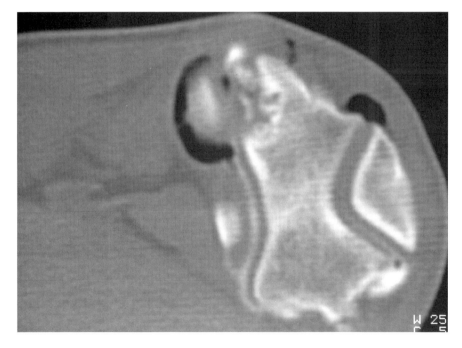

FIG. 51. Arthrographic CT of the elbow shows fragmentation of the capitellum with irregularity and thinning of the overlying articular cartilage representing osteochondrosis (Panner disease).

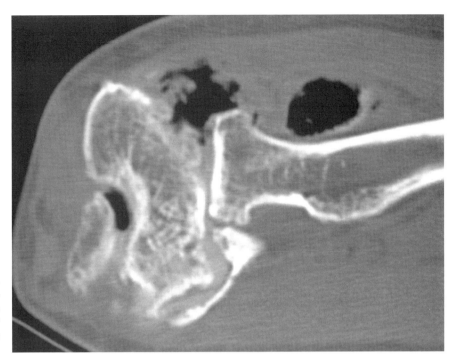

FIG. 52. Elbow CT arthrogram in a patient with rheumatoid arthritis demonstrates marked synovitis, diffuse articular cartilage thinning, and erosions of the radial head and adjacent surfaces of the olecranon and humeral condyles.

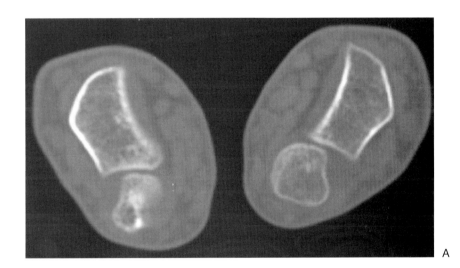

A

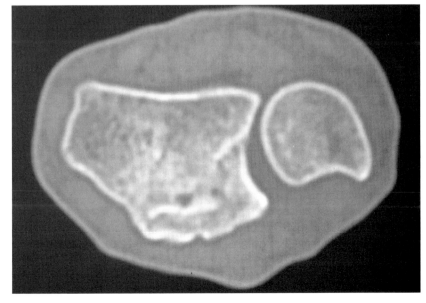

B

FIG. 53. Axial CT of the distal radioulnar joint. **A:** An axial image with the wrists partially supinated demonstrates normal rotational relationships at the DRU joints bilaterally. **B:** In another patient, an axial image of the left wrist with the wrist fully supinated demonstrates widening of the dorsal aspect of the DRU although the center of rotation of the DRU joint remains normal (75).

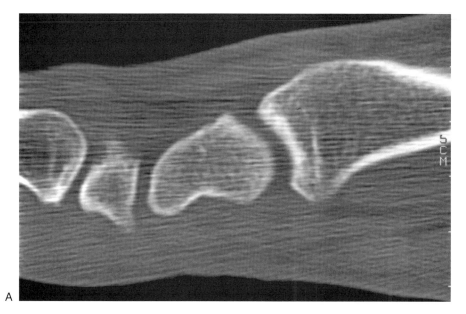

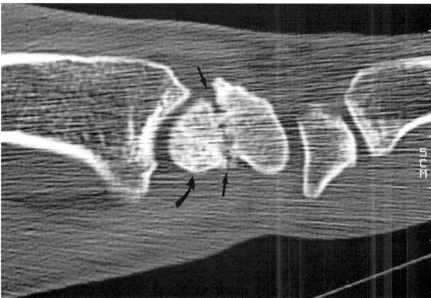

FIG. 54. CT of the scaphoid. **A:** The normal scaphoid demonstrates an intrascaphoid angle of approximately 150°. **B:** Following a fracture of the scaphoid waist (*arrows*) the intrascaphoid angle measures approximately 120°. Osteonecrosis of the proximal pole is manifested by sclerosis (*curved arrow*).

Other symptomatic carpal conditions such as osteonecrosis of the scaphoid and the so-called "humpback" scaphoid are also suitable for evaluation with CT (41). In the evaluation of carpal conditions, the plane of the CT study is crucial (17,26,338). Thin section CT images (1.0 or 1.5 mm) oriented parallel to the long axis of the scaphoid (308) (Fig. 54) are very helpful in the evaluation of the humpback scaphoid (Fig. 55), relative increased volar angulation of the distal pole with respect to the proximal pole. Other conditions, such as the relative alignment of the proximal and distal carpal rows, may be achieved with sagittal or coronal scanning. If the assessment of erosions associated with arthropathies is to be evaluated with CT, coronal or axial images may suffice.

Symptomatic ligamentous conditions such as tears of the scapholunate or lunatotriquetral ligaments or tears of the triangular fibrocartilage complex are better suited for evaluation by arthrography or MRI than by CT (352). Although the diagnosis of carpal tunnel syndrome is often a clinical one, the condition may be imaged by either MRI or CT. The carpal tunnel contents, including the median nerve, may be visualized directly with MRI (Fig. 56), and abnormalities of the median nerve itself can be identified. CT can demonstrate mass lesions within the carpal tunnel.

Imaging of abnormalities of the digits, such as defects in the flexor or extensor mechanisms, usually requires a detailed display of soft tissue anatomy, often in the sagittal or coronal planes parallel to the long axis of the digit. In this case, MRI is superior to CT.

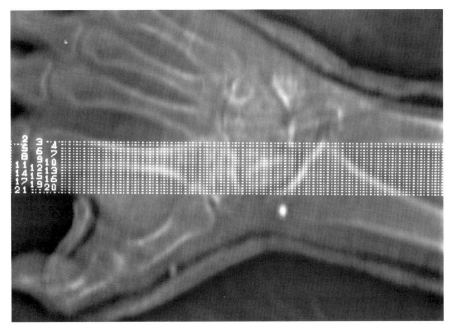

FIG. 55. Scout view of the wrist prior to CT examination of the scaphoid. The patient is prone on the CT table with the shoulder abducted, the elbow flexed, and the hand pronated on the CT table over the patient's head. The plane of the section is parallel to the long axis of the scaphoid.

Hip

As in other sites, CT can be helpful in the hip in evaluating conditions such as inflammatory arthritis (Fig. 57) and other articular conditions such as synovial osteochondromatosis and pigmented villonodular synovitis (PVNS). Calcifications and osseous erosions associated with these conditions are easily demonstrated with CT. Hemosiderin deposition, typical of PVNS, can be identified with CT (294) but is more easily detected with MRI. In synovial osteochondromatosis, intraarticular loose bodies are well demonstrated with CT, particularly when intraarticular

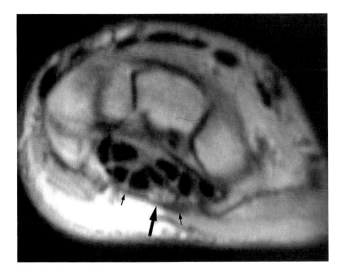

FIG. 56. An axial MR image of the wrist at the level of the carpal tunnel displays the flexor tendons as structures of low signal intensity adjacent to the normal median nerve (*arrow*), deep to the transverse carpal ligament (*small arrows*).

contrast is administered (Fig. 58). MRI also shows osteocartilaginous loose bodies well, especially in the presence of an effusion (Fig. 59). Other localized processes such as iliopsoas bursitis may produce symptoms about the hip or groin and can also be evaluated with CT (254,310).

MRI has replaced CT in the evaluation of other disorders previously studied with CT. Avascular necrosis, for example, can be assessed with CT (69,205). In this case, CT shows the replacement of the normal stellate trabecular architecture of the femoral head by the sclerotic, disordered trabeculae of the necrotic femoral head (69) (Fig. 60). Prior to the advent of MRI, CT was very helpful in this regard. MRI, however, allows direct scanning of the femoral head in the coronal and sagittal planes as well as the axial plane and easily reveals areas of osteonecrosis (Fig. 61). By comparing the MR signal intensity from the area of necrotic bone to surrounding tissues, the avascular process may be characterized with MRI. Unlike CT, MRI can, for example, demonstrate granulation tissue and woven bone formation as an area of increased signal intensity on the inner aspect of the infarction on T2-weighted MR images. MRI can also document the return of marrow fat signal in the reconstituted area of infarction as an indicator of progressive healing. Coronal and sagittal MR images demonstrate subchondral collapse better than does axial CT, but anteroposterior and lateral conventional radiographs are superior to both CT and MRI in this regard.

Congenital and developmental disorders can be analyzed with CT. Combined with 3-D and multiplanar reconstruction, CT demonstrates the deformities associated with developmental hip dysplasia (2,12,136,137) (Fig. 62). Acetabular angles, orientation, and depth are all easily assessed in this manner. CT may also be used to assess

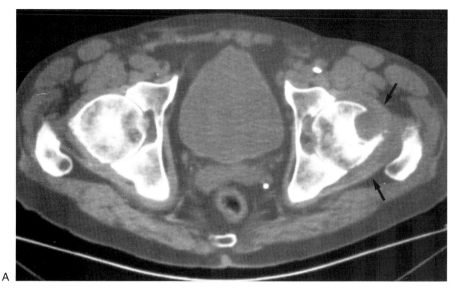

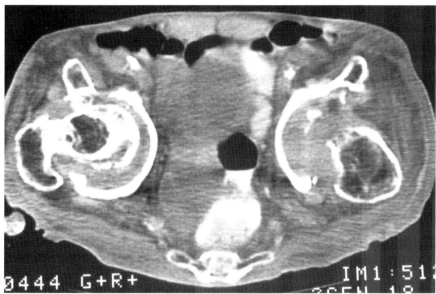

FIG. 57. CT of the hips in rheumatoid arthritis. **A:** A transverse image of the hips shows diffuse narrowing of both hip joints, distension of the left hip joint (*arrows*) and a large erosion of the left femoral neck. **B:** In another patient CT demonstrates bilateral effusions with marked acetabulae protrusio bilaterally.

the adequacy of reduction of congenital dislocation of the hips, even when cast material obscures the hips on conventional radiographs (Fig. 63). Proximal femoral torsion can also be evaluated with CT, and the degree of femoral anteversion with respect to the bicondylar plane of the distal femur can be determined (375) (Fig. 64). In the evaluation of hip arthroplasties, both femoral and acetabular version should be assessed with dedicated conventional radiographic studies (102).

Knee

As in the hip, CT is useful for the assessment of developmental anomalies in the knee. The patellofemoral joint can be studied in various degrees of knee flexion in order to evaluate the patellofemoral joint and patellar tracking (219) (Fig. 65). Tibial torsion can also be analyzed with

CT (137,183). Other developmental conditions such as dysplasia epiphysealis hemimelia (Trevor disease) and the various spondylometaepiphyseal dysplasias can also be evaluated with CT. In such cases, the relationship of the osteochondromatous outgrowth to the remainder of the epiphysis or the conformation of the distorted articular surface is readily displayed by CT.

However, MRI is far superior to CT for the evaluation of internal derangement of the knee. A complete discussion of MRI of the knee is beyond the scope of this chapter, but the menisci, cruciate ligaments, extensor mechanism, and capsular structures are all easily and accurately visualized with MRI. Among the advantages of MRI over CT in this setting are MRI's better soft tissue contrast, its ability to display intraosseous pathology, and its multiplanar capacity. The advantage of multiplanar imaging is particularly important, for example, in coronal imaging of the collateral ligaments, sagittal imaging of

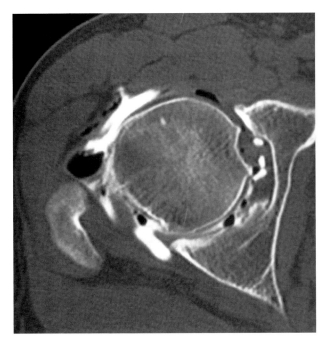

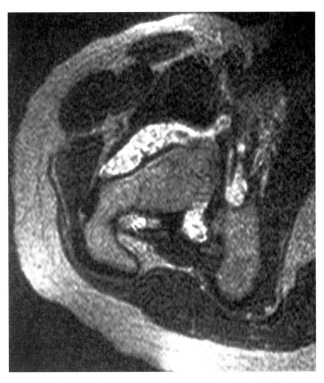

FIG. 58. Synovial osteochondromatosis. An axial image of the hip following double contrast CT arthrography reveals multiple intraarticular fragments best seen adjacent to the femoral head fovea. At arthrotomy, multiple cartilaginous and osseous fragments were evacuated from the joint.

FIG. 59. Synovial osteochondromatosis. An axial MR image of the right hip shows a large effusion containing multiple fragments. At synovectomy, multiple cartilaginous fragment were removed.

the patellar tendon and menisci, and oblique sagittal imaging of the anterior cruciate ligament. Cystic structures such as meniscal cysts and their relationship to meniscal injuries are easily studied with MRI. As noted above, other cystic structures about the knee, such as popliteal cysts and vascular aneurysms, can be evaluated with ultrasound, and the use of ultrasound may be more cost-effective in this setting.

Unlike MRI, unenhanced CT cannot readily differentiate between articular cartilage and the menisci and ligaments. When intraarticular contrast is employed, however, CT's display of intraarticular anatomy is improved. Prior to the widespread availability of MRI, for example, arthrographic CT of the knee was used to identify menis-

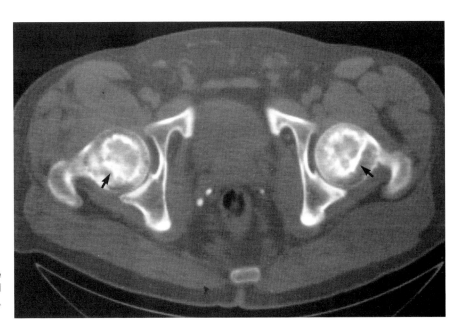

FIG. 60. A transverse CT image of the hips demonstrates bilateral femoral head infarctions indicated by irregular, sclerotic margins (*arrows*).

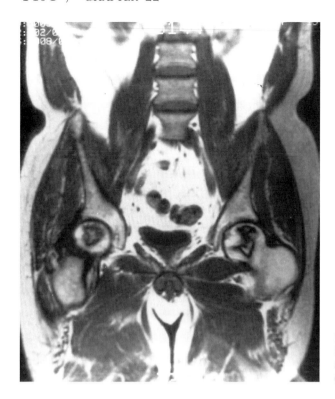

FIG. 61. A coronal MR image of the patient in Fig. 19 reveals irregular areas of low signal intensity in the femoral heads bilaterally replacing the normal fatty marrow, typical in appearance of osteonecrosis.

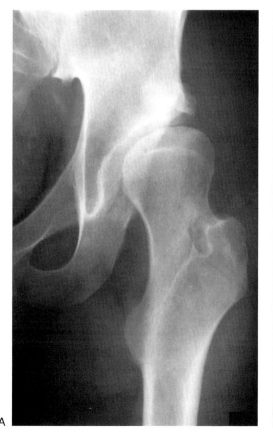 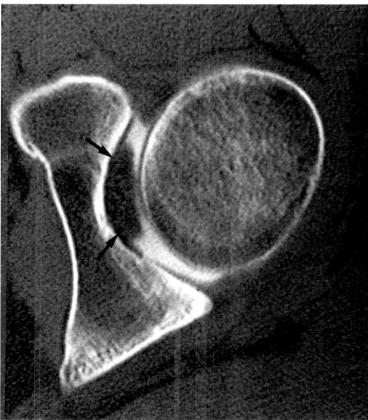

A

B

FIG. 62. Developmental dysplasia of the hip. **A:** An anteroposterior radiograph of the left hip demonstrates a shallow acetabulum and coxa valga. **B:** CT arthrography of the left hip reveals a pulvinar (*arrows*) outlined by contrast.

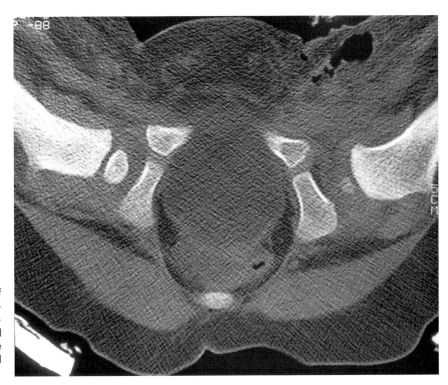

FIG. 63. Developmental dysplasia of the hips. Immediately following open reduction and casting, the right hip is concentrically reduced. The left femoral head is posteriorly subluxed. Note the asymmetric ossification of the femoral heads.

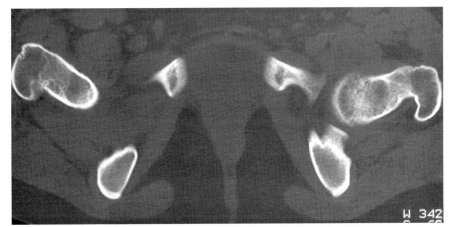

FIG. 64. Femoral neck retroversion. Other images (not shown) established the bicondylar plane of the distal femora. The proximal femora are retroverted bilaterally, especially on the right, with respect to the bicondylar plane.

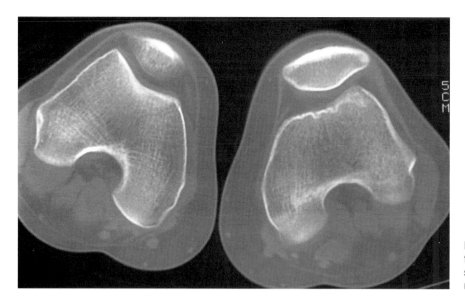

FIG. 65. Axial CT image of the distal femora show a shallow distal femoral sulcus on the left with lateral displacement of the left patella.

cal tears (101,251). Chondromalacia patellae (97,142) and articular cartilage defects and their associated intraarticular loose fragments may be identified by CT in this manner (312) (Fig. 66). Similarly, arthrographic knee CT has been utilized to identify synovial plicae (35,142).

Foot and Ankle

The complex anatomy of the foot and ankle are well demonstrated with cross-sectional imaging studies such

as CT (335,336). MRI is ideal for demonstrating osteonecrosis of the talar dome. CT combined with arthrography can demonstrate osteonecrosis, overlying cartilaginous defects (Fig. 67), intraarticular free fragments, and osteochondritis dessicans (387). In both CT and MRI evaluations of the tibiotalar and subtalar joints, coronal scans are usually most helpful. Posttraumatic degenerative arthrosis affecting the hindfoot and ankle can also be imaged with CT (Figs. 68 and 69). Impingement by articular osteophytes on the contrast-filled peroneal tendon

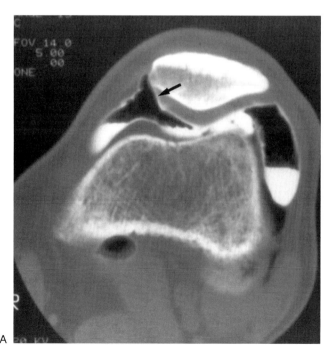
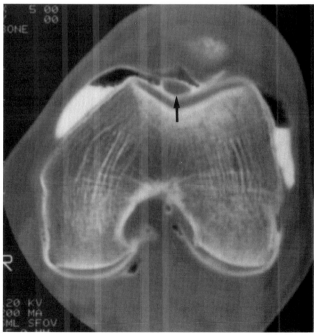

A   B

FIG. 66. CT arthrography of the knee following previous lateral patellar dislocation. **A:** A transverse image through the mid patella shows an oblique defect across the medial patellar cartilage (*arrow*) and thinning and irregularity of the lateral femoral articular cartilage anteriorly. **B:** An image caudal to A demonstrates a triangular intraarticular cartilage fragment (*arrow*).

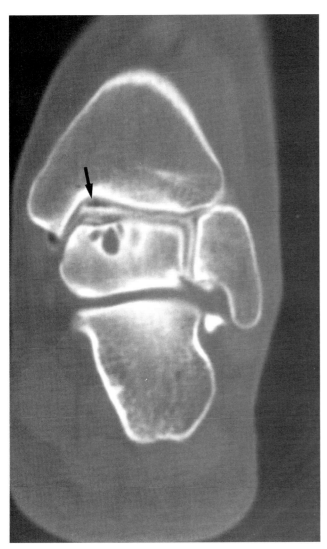

FIG. 67. A coronal CT arthrogram of the tibiotalar joint shows a subchondral defect in the medial talar dome, a small collection of contrast within the overlying articular cartilage and incongruency of the tibiotalar joint with injected air pooling medially (*arrow*).

ous on CT. Fibrous coalitions may be subtle, but careful assessment of adjoining articular surfaces and, if necessary, comparison with the opposite side will usually identify the abnormal articulation. More than one joint may be affected with a coalition, and scanning in two planes is required for complete evaluation of the hindfoot. MRI has been used to assess coalitions but may offer no particular advantage over CT in this regard.

MRI is excellent for the evaluation of abnormal ligaments and tendons about the ankle and hindfoot and is superior to CT in the demonstration of soft tissue and osseous changes of infection. Other inflammatory processes, such as inflammatory enthesopathies, can be seen with MRI but are not well seen with CT. In the setting of neuropathic osteoarthropathy, excluding superimposed infection may be difficult with any imaging modality. In this case, MRI is useful in identifying intraosseous fluid as well as any associated soft tissue abnormalities. CT is excellent for delineating the extent and distribution of bone destruction. In either case, however, complete exclusion of infection may require biopsy or aspiration of suspicious areas.

As in the upper extremity, abnormalities affecting the

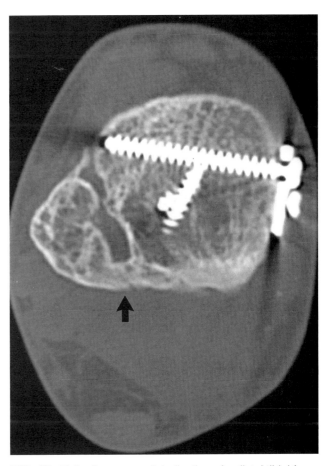

FIG. 68. Following screw-plate fixation of a distal tibial fracture, a solid synostosis (*arrow*) developed posteriorly. On other images (not shown), the synostosis bridged the tibiotalar and subtalar joints.

sheath is readily seen in coronal imaging following peroneal tenography. Similarly, CT may be helpful following tenography of the medial ankle tendons, particularly the posterior tibial tendon.

Coalitions about the hindfoot are a commonly encountered source of hindfoot rigidity and pain. CT is ideal for imaging these conditions (66,218,309), and, as with imaging the subtalar joint, the coronal plane is especially useful. The most common coalition, the calcaneonavicular coalition, may be demonstrated with coronal and axial (parallel to the plantar surface of the foot) images (Fig. 70). Talocalcaneal coalitions involving the sustentaculum tali are best seen on coronal scans (Fig. 71), whereas coalitions of the talonavicular and calcaneocuboid joints are best evaluated with axial scans. Coalitions may be fibrous or osseous (Fig. 70); osseous coalitions are obvi-

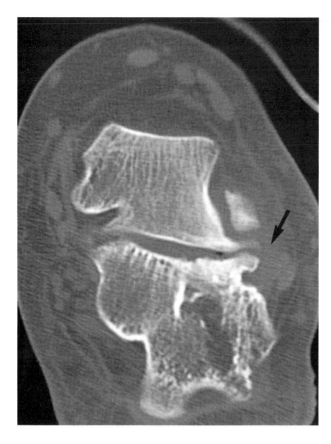

FIG. 69. A coronal CT image of the hindfoot following a fracture of the calcaneus shows union of the fracture. Severe degenerative arthrosis has developed about the lateral aspect of the subtalar joint with osteophyte formation directed laterally toward the peroneal tendons (*arrow*).

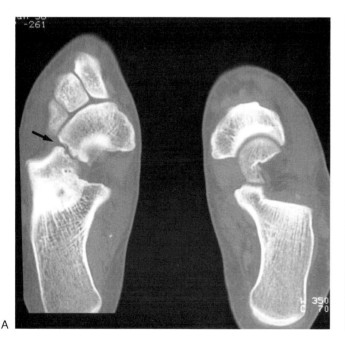
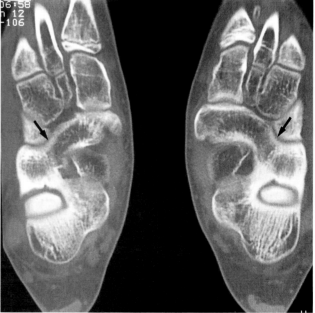

A   B

FIG. 70. Calcaneonavicular coalition. **A:** An axial CT image of the feet (parallel to the plantar surface of the feet) demonstrates a fibrous coalition of the right calcaneonavicular joint (*arrow*). **B:** In another patient, an axial CT image shows bilateral osseous calcaneonavicular coalitions (*arrows*).

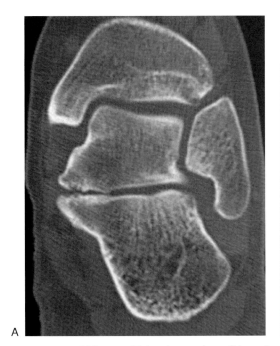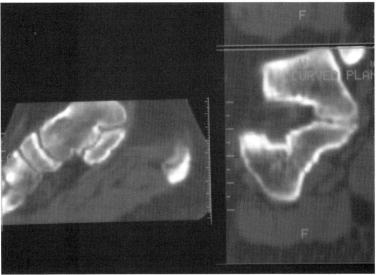

A   B

FIG. 71. Talocalcaneal coalition. **A:** A coronal CT image of the hindfoot shows articular surface irregularity affecting the medial talocalcaneal facet indicating a fibrous coalition. **B:** Sagittal (*left*) and coronal (*right*) multiplanar reconstructions of an axial hindfoot CT in another patient demonstrate a similar fibrous talocalcaneal coalition.

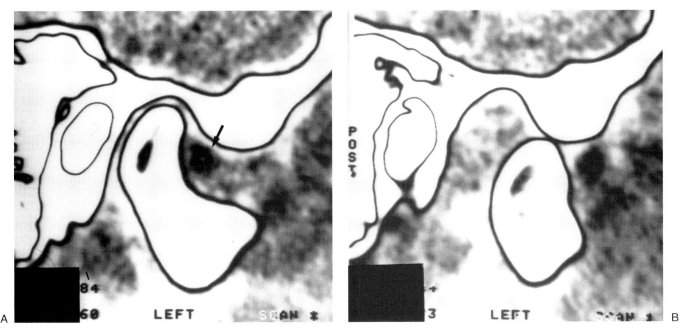

A   B

FIG. 72. CT of the temporomandibular joint. **A:** A direct sagittal CT image with highlight mode windowing shows anterior displacement of the TMJ meniscus (*arrow*). **B:** At the end of mandibular translation the meniscus remains anteriorly displaced.

longitudinal aspect of the rays in the feet include disorders of the flexor and extensor mechanisms. As in the hand, such conditions are better evaluated with MRI than with CT.

Temporomandibular Joint

Imaging the temporomandibular joint (TMJ) for possible internal derangement can be accomplished with conventional films, arthrography, CT, or MRI (131,350). Conventional radiographs with tomography may demonstrate abnormal positioning of the mandibular condyle with respect to the glenoid fossa of the temporal bone. Osseous erosions and osteophytosis associated with inflammatory and degenerative conditions affecting the TMJ can also be demonstrated with radiographs and tomography. Arthrography can demonstrate perforations of the meniscus and can provide dynamic information about the function and motion of the meniscus during mandibular translation (350). With arthrography, the position of the meniscus is inferred by the impression it makes on the contrast-filled lower TMJ articular space. In experienced hands, arthrography is easily and rapidly performed and is well tolerated. Arthrography is, however, invasive and may be rather uncomfortable for the patient.

Computed tomography, particularly using "highlight" or "blink" mode imaging can demonstrate the position of the meniscus directly (47,132,349) (Fig. 72). Direct scanning in the sagittal plane depicts the anteroposterior relationship of the meniscus to the mandibular condyle (216,313). Direct coronal imaging evaluates displacement of the meniscus medially or laterally. The joint can be imaged with the mouth open and closed, providing static information concerning the reduction of the displaced meniscus at the end of the mandibular translation. Osseous anatomy, including erosion and degenerative disease, is better seen with CT than with conventional arthrography. Like CT, MRI visualizes the meniscus directly in the sagittal and coronal planes and shows the relationship of the meniscus and the underlying mandibular condyle (280,349). Unlike CT, MRI can differentiate between the body of the meniscus and its associated ligamentous attachments. Unlike CT, MRI can display fluid collections

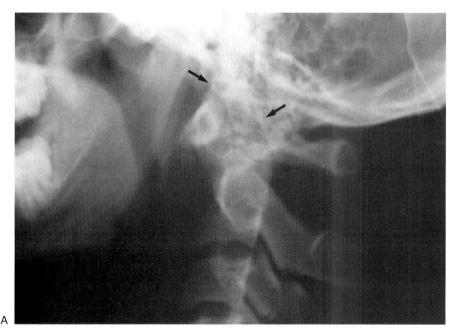

A

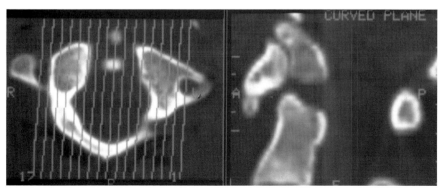

B

FIG. 73. Os odontoideum. **A:** A lateral radiograph shows a typical os odontoideum (*arrows*). Sclerosis and enlargement of the anterior ring of C1 indicate long-term instability at the craniocervical junction related to the os odontoideum. **B:** An oblique sagittal reconstruction (*right*) along the indicated plane (*left*) shows the ununited os odontoideum and the reactive hyperostosis in the C1 ring.

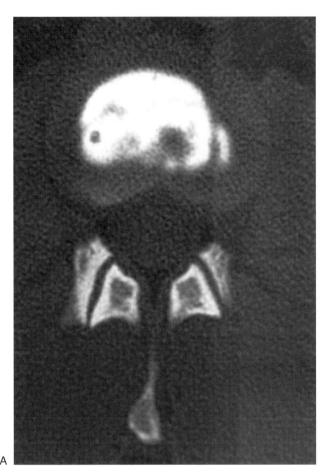 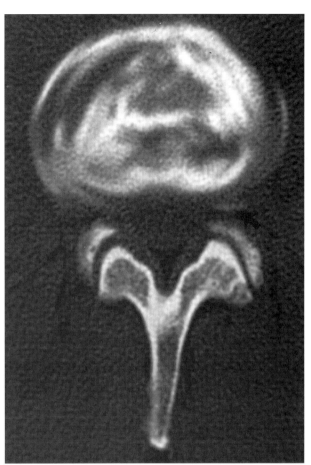

A B

FIG. 74. Postdiscography CT in the lumbar spine. **A:** In the normal disc, contrast is confined to the nucleus pulposus. **B:** In the degenerated disc, contrast spreads throughout the degenerated disc and may enter the epidural space (*arrow*).

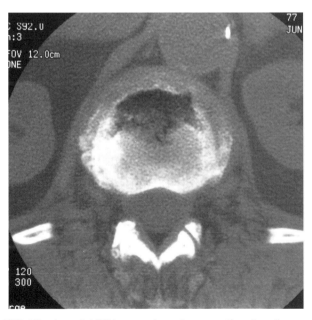

FIG. 75. An axial CT image show degenerative disc disease as well as facet joint hyperostosis and narrowing.

associated with inflammatory conditions affecting the TMJ such as rheumatoid arthritis. Neither CT nor MRI, however, demonstrates perforation of the meniscus, and neither provides the dynamic information afforded by fluoroscopy during arthrography.

Articulations in the Spine

The joints in the spine may be effectively imaged with CT. Abnormalities of the craniocervical junction, the uncovertebral joints in the cervical spine, facet joints in the cervical, thoracic, and lumbar spine, and costovertebral joints in the thoracic spine may be demonstrated. Inflammatory conditions such as rheumatoid arthritis, psoriatic arthritis, ankylosing spondylitis, and multicentric reticulohistiocytosis may affect the craniocervical junction. Erosions associated with these processes can be assessed with CT (44,272). Such disorders may also affect the facet, uncovertebral, and costovertebral articulations and in these sites may also be suited for imaging with CT.

Developmental anomalies may also be encountered in the spine. An os odontoideum, for example, may result

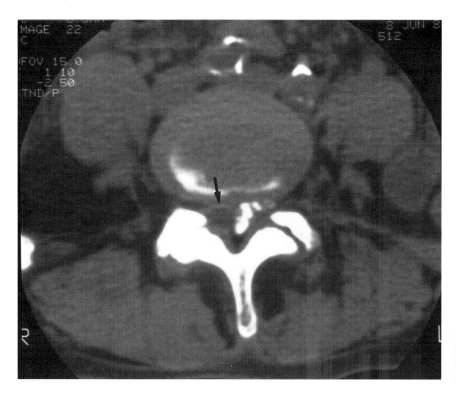

FIG. 76. A CT image of the lumbar spine shows a synovial cyst (*arrow*) adjacent to a lumbar facet joint displacing the contrast-filled thecal sac.

in chronic instability of the atlantoaxial articulation. The abnormality may be demonstrated with conventional radiographs but is effectively imaged with CT, particularly when multiplanar reconstructions are obtained (Fig. 73).

Abnormalities of the discs and discovertebral junctions can be assessed with conventional radiographs, CT, and MRI. Conventional radiographs are limited in this regard and demonstrate only osseous changes secondary to the disc disease, including disc narrowing, discogenic sclerosis, and osteophytosis, but not the position of the disc itself. Computed tomography, occasionally performed after myelography, can demonstrate abnormalities of the

disc contours as well as facet joint disorders. Laterally herniated discs may, however, be difficult to document with CT. Lateral recess stenosis and related overgrowth of the facet joints and ligamentum flavum are well seen with axial CT. Calcifications associated with arachnoiditis ossificans are also easily shown by axial CT scanning.

In many cases, MRI is most helpful and demonstrates the intraosseous compartment, discs, nerve roots, and intracanalicular structures better than the other modalities (229). Abnormalities of MRI signals arising in discs, however, are very common and may not correlate with the patient's pain syndrome. Discography may be requested

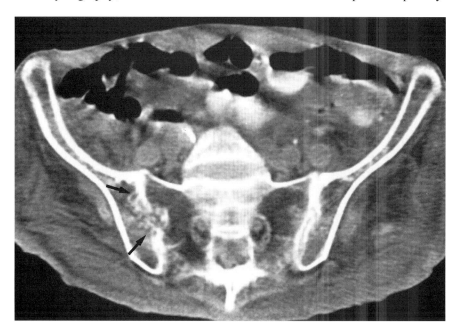

FIG. 77. A CT scan of the sacroiliac joints demonstrates bilateral sacroiliac joint erosion, particularly evident on the right (*arrows*).

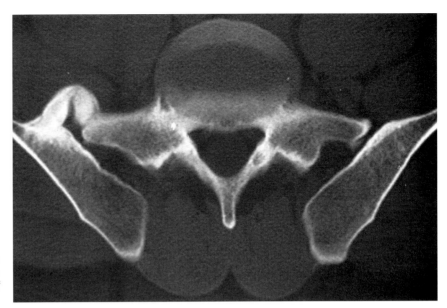

FIG. 78. An axial image of the sacroiliac (SI) joints shows an exuberant osteophyte arising from the anterior aspect of the right SI joint.

to help isolate the source of the patient's pain and to identify symptomatic disc abnormalities. Although the reproduction of the patient's pain syndrome is of primary importance during discography, CT may be used to assess the morphology of the intervertebral discs. Contrast is confined to the nucleus pulposus in the normal disc (Fig. 74). In the abnormal disc, contrast extension posteriorly may be seen in the setting of a herniated nucleus pulposus, and contrast may extravasate from a fissured, degenerated disc (Fig. 74).

Imaging of the abnormally curved spine is usually best accomplished with conventional radiographs and MRI. Conventional radiographs can demonstrate the angular deformities associated with abnormal curvatures in the sagittal and coronal planes and can reveal structural abnormalities contributing to abnormal curvatures such as vertebral dysplasias and neural arch defects. Such vertebral body defects may also be seen with CT. In general, however, MRI provides more information about vertebral body anatomy and intracanalicular pathology than that displayed by CT.

Isolated vertebral body anomalies may be evaluated with CT. Facet joint tropism as well as degenerative osteophytosis and sclerosis of the facet joints are well seen with CT (Fig. 75). When the facet joints are suspected as a source of back pain, facet joint injection may be employed to confirm the clinical impression. CT guidance in this case may be preferred to fluoroscopic guidance. During facet joint arthrography, synovial cysts may be encountered. Such cysts may be a result of inflammatory or degenerative conditions, but their extent may be evaluated with CT (Fig. 76). Other spinal conditions, such as spondylolysis, may also be assessed with CT. As with facet joints, injection of such defects under CT guidance may help confirm their significance in the patient's presentation.

Sacroiliac Joints

The sacroiliac (SI) joints are commonly involved in various arthropathies. The seronegative spondyloarthropathies, in particular, characteristically involve the SI joints, but other disorders such as gout and calcium pyrophosphate dihydrate deposition disease may affect the SI joints. In general, SI involvement in rheumatologic disorders can be adequately evaluated with properly exposed, properly positioned, conventional radiographs, requiring neither CT nor MRI. Occasionally, however, conventional films may not demonstrate the SI joints satisfactorily. In this case, CT has been used to show subtle areas of bone erosion along the margins or subchondral surfaces of the SI joints (43,178,366) (Fig. 77). Degenerative conditions may also affect the SI joints. Sacroiliac joint osteophytes, for example, usually involve the cephalad and caudad portions of the SI joints and appear as sclerotic foci overlying the joints. When the nature of such sclerotic foci is unclear from radiographs, CT can confirm the presence of osteophytes (Fig. 78).

Developmental anomalies of the sacrum and SI joints such as transitional lumbosacral segments or accessory SI joints also occur commonly. Occasionally these may produce low back pain. When needed clinically, they may be evaluated with CT, and the osseous deformity associated with them can be readily displayed. As with facet disorders and spondylolytic defects, such defects may be injected percutaneously under CT guidance to assess their contribution to the patient's pain syndrome.

SKELETAL NEOPLASIA

Bone Tumors

Conventional radiography remains the first technique used for evaluation of skeletal tumors. In most cases,

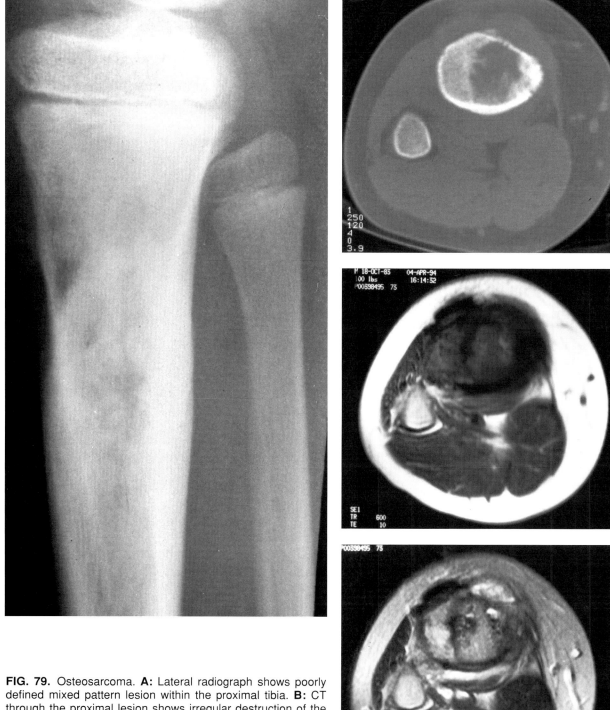

FIG. 79. Osteosarcoma. **A:** Lateral radiograph shows poorly defined mixed pattern lesion within the proximal tibia. **B:** CT through the proximal lesion shows irregular destruction of the normal trabecular pattern by a lytic process. The cortex is breached anteriorly. **C, D:** Axial T1- and T2-weighted MRIs show replacement of marrow fat with a low T1- and heterogeneous high T2-weighted tumor. Soft tissue extension is noted anteriorly where the CT showed interruption of the cortex. The cortex is diffusely increased in signal and thickened indicating involvement with the tumor process.

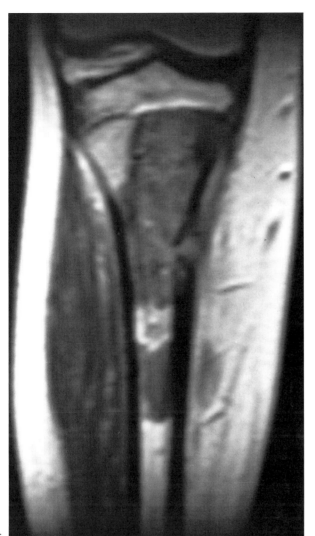
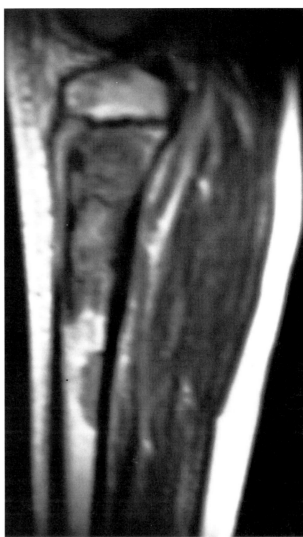

E   F

FIG. 79. (*Continued.*) **E, F:** Coronal and sagittal T1-weighted MRI's show extension of the tumor to the proximal epiphysis of the tibia but not through it and extension down the tibial shaft.

radiographs provide features resulting in the best differential diagnosis and the most probable histopathologic prediction. Occasionally radiographs will yield information clearly indicating that amputation is necessary. In these few cases, no further evaluation is needed. However, current therapeutic approaches emphasize combination chemotherapy and surgery to eradicate tumors and preserve functional anatomy whenever possible (112,213,300,320). Thus, for most tumors, exact determination of the tumor extent is required (80,221,331,333). In such cases, CT and MRI can define the tumor extent and either confirm resectability or clearly show that amputation is necessary (51,100,105,220,211,235, 239, 250,341).

For benign neoplasms, the information on conventional radiography usually is sufficient for both diagnosis and treatment. For malignant osseous neoplasms, staging the extent of the condition requires sectional imaging

(5,61,194). Both CT and MRI can fairly accurately show the location of the primary tumor within the bone, quantify the intramedullary component of the tumor, and define its extraosseous extent (240,385) (Figs. 79–82, 92). CT is more sensitive to subtle cortical erosion and better for identification of small amounts of soft tissue calcification than MRI. The ability of MRI to yield direct coronal and sagittal images and to display higher contrast between the tumor and surrounding normal tissues is a major advantage (19,28,32,274,385) (Figs. 79 and 80). Whereas CT is the preferred method for evaluation of trabecular and cortical integrity and characterization of tumor mineralization (Fig. 81), MRI provides better tissue contrast, which allows easier definition of tumor margins. MRI using marrow-sensitive sequences [short tau inversion recovery (STIR) and fat-saturated T2-weighted] is most often used for estimation of longitudinal intramedullary tumor spread. Exquisite sensitivity to marrow replacement

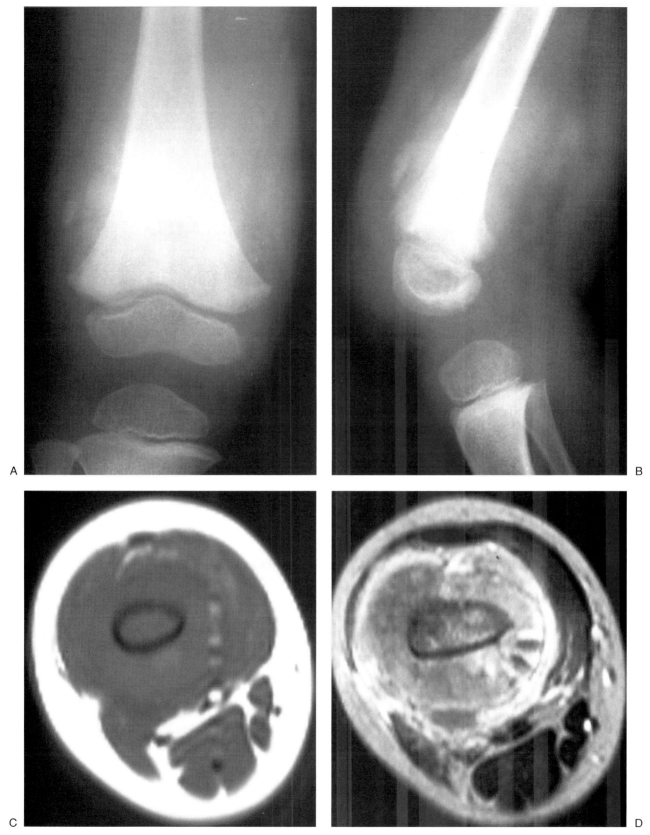

FIG. 80. Osteosarcoma. **A, B:** Radiographs show a classic medullary osteosarcoma with sclerotic density within the marrow and within the large soft tissue mass surrounding the metaphysis. **C, D:** Axial T1- and T2-weighted MRIs show the cloaking soft tissue surrounding the metaphysis. The normally black cortex is thickened and increased in signal. Low signal within the surrounding soft tissue corresponds to the calcification seen on radiographs.

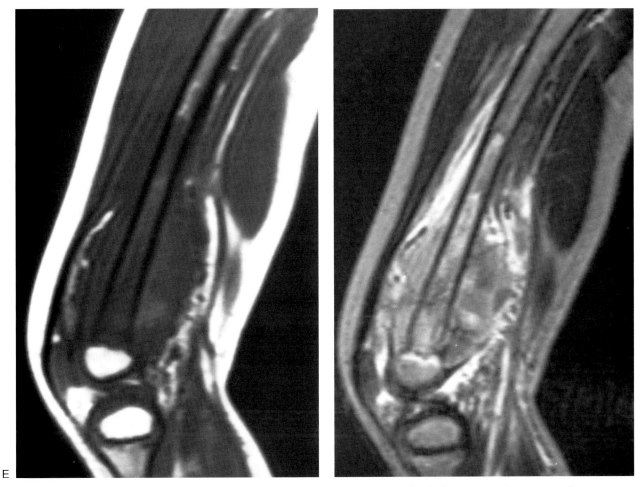

E   F

FIG. 80. (*Continued.*) **E, F:** Direct sagittal and coronal MR images clearly demonstrate the surrounding soft tissue mass and the intramedullary extent of the tumor.

allows detailed evaluation of tumor marrow extension. Using coronal or sagittal imaging, examiners can directly measure the craniocaudal tumor extent in marrow and identify ''skip'' lesions within the marrow cavity that do not erode the endosteal surface (Fig. 82).

Both techniques may be used to identify compartmental anatomy, quantify the number of muscle layers involved by the tumor, and show 3-D spatial relationships in areas of complex skeletal and soft tissue anatomy. Both CT and MRI provide excellent estimates of radial spread of bone tumors into the surrounding soft tissues, but MRI generally shows a more conspicuous interface between tumor and normal tissue (385,386) (see Fig. 79). Likewise, both provide an estimate of major-vessel involvement by tumor, but MRI does so without the need for injection of a contrast agent and with better contrast conspicuity (192). Both accurately show tumor relationships to vital neural and vascular structures, as well as to adjacent articular surfaces— information that is especially important to the surgeon planning conservative, limb-sparing surgery. With both techniques, allowances must be made for the local effects of edema and postbiopsy

hemorrhage, either of which may mimic tumor spread (117). However, these tissue changes have not significantly decreased the accuracy of either imaging method in preoperative tumor staging.

Angiography is reserved for those rare occasions when a preoperative vascular map is required or when intravenous chemotherapeutic agents are to be delivered to a limited area in high doses. Radionuclide scintigraphy provides information regarding multiplicity of the primary tumor and distant metastases.

Sectional imaging is also essential for evaluation of a tumor following therapy (127). If the tumor was not resected, the comparison should be with the study obtained just prior to institution of therapy and any subsequent studies. If the tumor was resected, the comparison should be with a study obtained soon after resection, as well as with any other subsequent examinations. It is advisable to use the same sectional method—CT or MRI—for monitoring therapeutic response, rather than alternating between the methods. This provides better continuity and an improved opportunity to detect an important anatomic change.

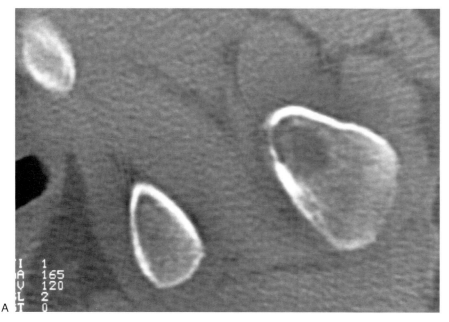

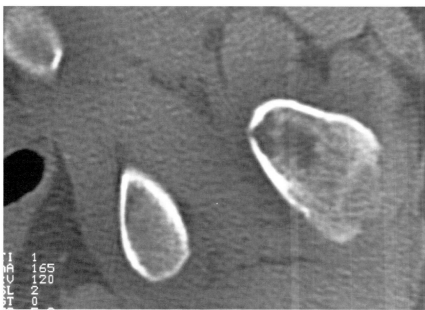

FIG. 81. Eosinophilic granuloma. **A, B:** Sequential CT show erosion of the medial femoral cortex adjacent to a lytic, destructive lesion in the proximal left femoral metaphysis. The lesion is well defined but no sclerotic reaction is seen surrounding the area of destruction.

Benign Skeletal Neoplasms

Benign skeletal tumors usually are identified and easily characterized by conventional radiography. This information is generally sufficient for both probable diagnosis and appropriate treatment decisions. Sectional imaging, usually by CT, may be helpful when radiographs fail to provide sufficient information about a tumor's characteristics to indicate whether or not a biopsy is necessary. Furthermore, sectional imaging may influence management by increasing diagnostic confidence or by better defining spatial relationships (e.g., in the pelvis, to help plan any contemplated operation).

Among benign bone neoplasms, cartilaginous lesions are the most common tumors for which sectional imaging is helpful (146). They occur in most age groups, and at times their radiologic appearances may not allow the radiologist to differentiate benign from malignant lesions. CT can show their mineralization pattern in cross-section, an important advantage compared with radiography (Fig. 83). Benign cartilaginous lesions have matrix calcification that is relatively evenly distributed, without sizable areas of uncalcified soft tissue matrix. Occasionally the nature of calcification in a long-bone lesion may be difficult to classify on radiographs, and the differential diagnosis is between a chondrous lesion and a bone infarct. In these cases, bone infarcts can be recognized on CT by their peripherally marginated calcification, instead of the cen-

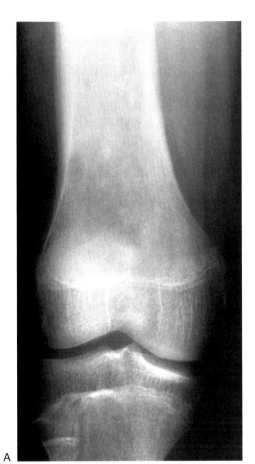

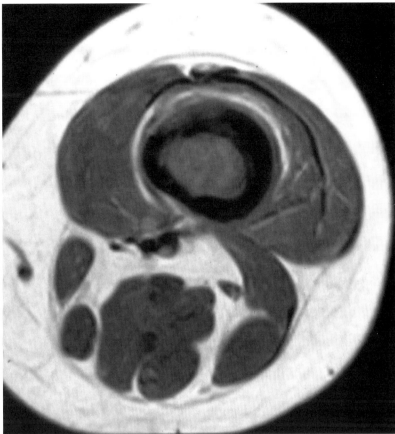

A

B

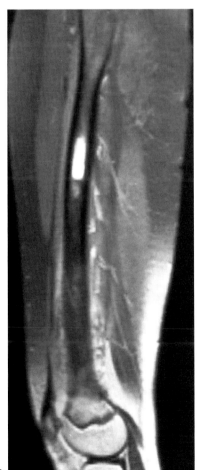

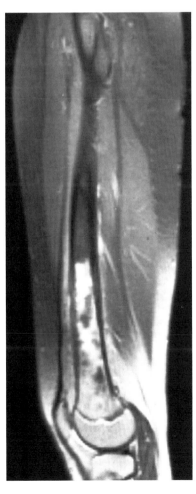

C,D

FIG. 82. Osteosarcoma. **A:** Anteroposterior radiograph shows subtle sclerosis within the metadiaphysis; its proximal extent is not imaged. Thin, layered periostitis is visible along the lateral cortex. **B:** Axial T1-weighted MRI shows thickening and increased signal within the cortex. The normal fatty marrow has been replaced with soft tissue of lower signal than fat (compare marrow with subcutaneous fat). A thin layer of fat surrounds the bone, separating it from the overlying muscle. **C, D:** Sagittal fat saturated T1-weighted images through the long axis of the femur show the proximal extent of the medullary process. Separated from the main lesion is a second focus of increased signal, a "skip" lesion within the marrow (*arrow*).

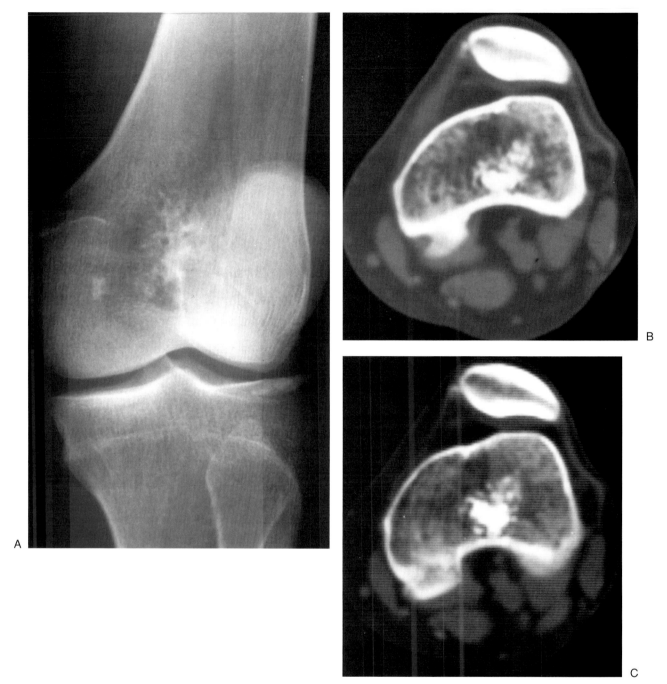

FIG. 83. Enchondroma. **A:** Anteroposterior radiograph shows a coarsely calcified, poorly marginated mass within the metaepiphysis of the left femur. **B, C:** CT through the lesion demonstrates that the calcification is evenly distributed within the center of the lesion. No significant soft tissue component is identifiable beyond the area of calcification.

tral, irregular calcification seen with chondrous tumors (Fig. 84). In addition to showing any medullary calcifications, CT can be used to evaluate the endosteal surface in cross-section; benign lesions generally show no erosion of the endosteal surface.

MRI often cannot detect small calcifications associated with a cartilaginous tumor, but it does show replacement of normal high- signal-intensity marrow with neoplastic

tissue of low signal intensity on T1-weighted images and higher signal intensity than marrow on T2-weighted images. Subtle endosteal surface erosions are more difficult to detect in cross-section by MRI; however, because MRI yields direct coronal and sagittal images, it may better define the longitudinal extent of intramedullary lesions than radiography, scintigraphy, or CT.

Benign osteocartilaginous exostoses that have become

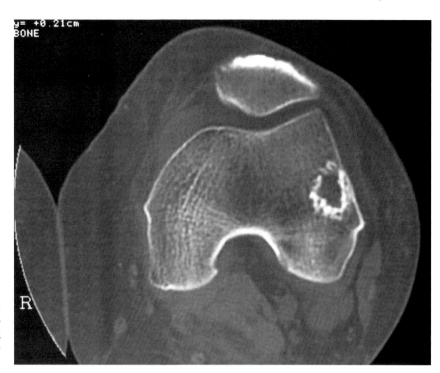

FIG. 84. Bone infarct. CT scan through the distal femur shows a lesion in the lateral femoral condyle. The lesion has a sclerotic rim and a fat density center, characteristic of a mature bone infarct.

symptomatic because of trauma or overlying inflammation may be difficult to distinguish from those in which a chondrosarcoma has developed. CT or MRI of exostoses characteristically shows a bone mass with a sharply defined periphery, an organized central matrix, a medullary cavity and cortex continuous with that of the bone from which it arose, and a thin cartilaginous cap (Fig. 85). When it is otherwise difficult to characterize, localize, and differentiate more sessile osteocartilaginous exostoses (such as those found in the spine or pelvis) from

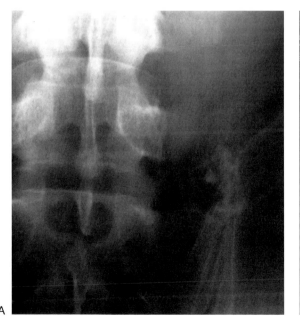

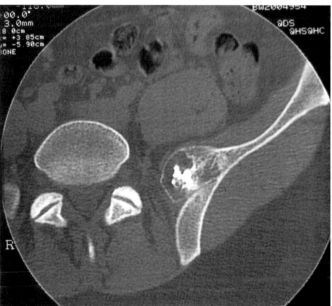

A

B

FIG. 85. Osteocartilagenous exostosis. **A:** Anteroposterior radiograph of the left hemipelvis shows a rounded exostotic lesion extending off the ilium posteriorly. **B:** CT through the largest part of the lesion shows no soft tissue cap. The cortex is smooth and continuous with the cortex of the ilium. The medullary cavity of the lesion flows from the medullary cavity of the ilium.

chondrosarcomas, cross-sectional imaging may be useful (172). The spatial and vascular relationships of pedunculated exostoses are easily demonstrated. Similarly, sectional imaging clearly demonstrates the cortical nature of juxtacortical (periosteal) chondromas.

CT or MRI can be of value for evaluation of many of the less common benign bone lesions in much the same way as for the chondrous lesions. Bone cysts often can be identified on the basis of a thin osseous rim, a near-water-density/intensity central component, and lack of contrast enhancement (Fig. 86). Aneurysmal bone cysts may show fluid–fluid levels and/or multiple compartments on either CT or MRI examination (21,145,155) (Figs. 87 and 88). Cortical margins may be so thinned as to not be appreciable radiographically, but the extent of the cyst may still be identified in sectional images. The thinned cortices are more easily demonstrated with CT than with MRI. Similar features, including high-attenuation components indicative of blood, may be seen in hemophilic pseudotumors (113,133). For each of these fluid- or blood-containing tumors, MRI typically shows bright signal intensity on T2-weighted sections.

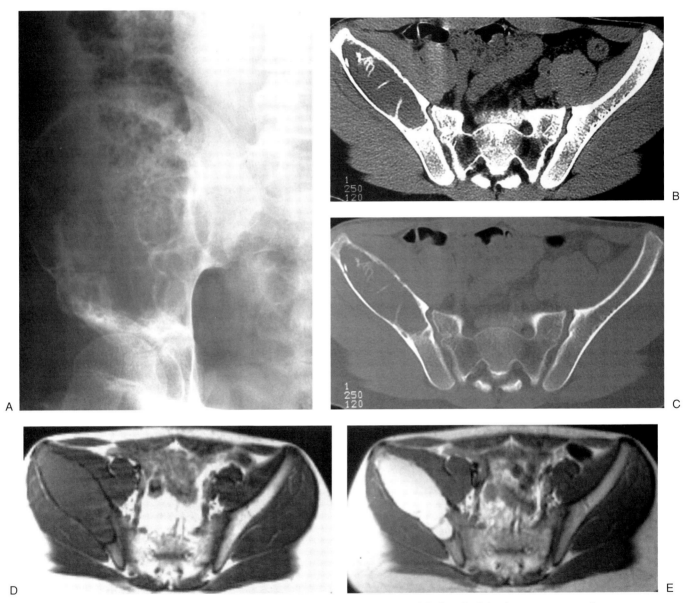

FIG. 86. Simple bone cyst. **A:** Anteroposterior radiograph of the right hemipelvis shows an expansile, lytic lesion of the right iliac wing. Its margins are difficult to define on the radiograph. **B, C:** soft tissue and bone window images through the center of the lesion show it to be sharply defined, with a density slightly higher than that of water but less than that of muscle. Thin bone septae are visible traversing the lesion. **D, E;** T1- and T2-weighted axial MRIs through the lesion again show it to be sharply defined with signal characteristics of a fluid-filled cyst, low to intermediate on T1-weighted images and very high and homogeneous on T2-weighted images.

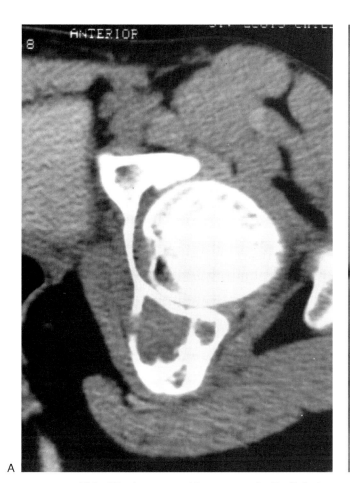
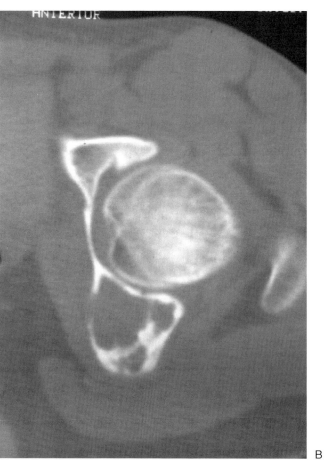

A

B

FIG. 87. Aneurysmal bone cyst. **A, B:** Soft tissue and bone window CT images through the center of an expansile, lytic lesion of the upper ischium. The lesion is sharply marginated and of soft tissue density. The cortex is interrupted along the medial aspect of the lesion.

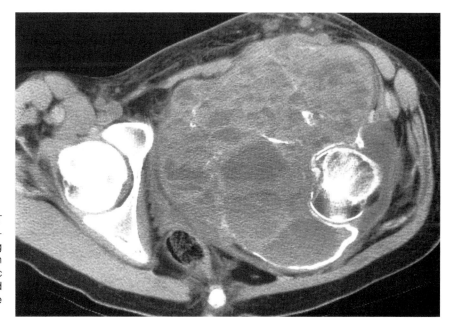

FIG. 88. Aneurysmal bone cyst. CT through the pelvis shows a massive lesion expanding the left ilium, involving the iliac wing, the periacetabular region and both the inferior and superior pubic rami. Its multilocular nature is visible and multiple fluid-debris levels are visible (*arrowheads*).

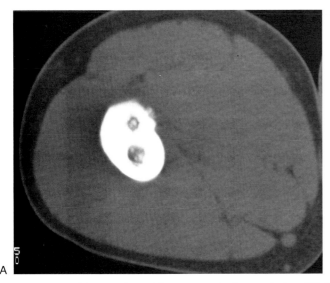 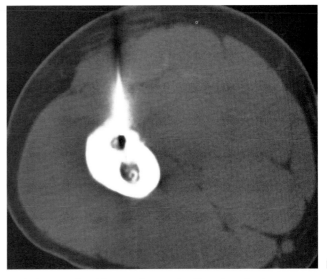

A   B

FIG. 89. Osteoid osteoma. **A:** Bone window CT through the proximal femur shows significant cortical thickening anteriorly. Within the thickened cortex is a sharply defined lucency and within the lucency, a tiny dense focus, the nidus of the osteoid osteoma. **B:** Bone window CT from a localization procedure. Artifact from the localized needle extends to the anterior surface of the lucent lesion.

CT often is of particular value for evaluation of osteoid osteoma and osteoblastoma (6,24,123,372). In these lesions, proper identification of the nidus and/or the lesion extent is critical to complete surgical removal and avoidance of recurrence (Fig. 89). An osteoid osteoma presents as a lucent focus within surrounding sclerosis (86). In some cases, a dense calcified center may be seen. The vascular nature of these lesions results in characteristic enhancement of the nidus following intravenous administration of contrast material (195). Because the nidus often is <1 cm in diameter, it may be obscured by surrounding trabecular bone or reactive sclerosis and thus not be identified by conventional radiographic methods. Thin, contiguous sections may be required in order to detect the nidus by CT (4). MRI also can demonstrate the tumor nidus (106).

Although imaging is not normally needed to characterize benign fibrous lesions, a variety of fibrous lesions can be seen and recognized by CT. Fibrous dysplasia characteristically has sharply defined uninterrupted sclerotic margins on CT images (Fig. 90). A matrix of uniform density may be present; or thick, coarse dense bands may be seen. MRI of fibrous dysplasia shows uniform or heterogeneous low signal marrow replacement on T1-weighted images and a mixed pattern with regions of high signal on T2-weighted sections. Ossifying fibromas are seen as diffusely calcified cortical lesions on CT examination, a characteristic not seen in other benign lesions that

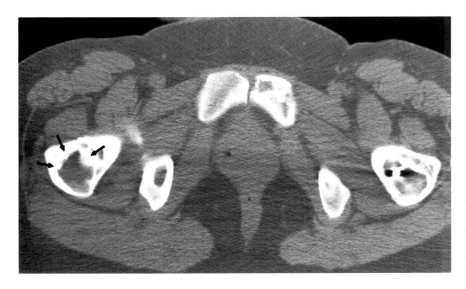

FIG. 90. Fibrous dysplasia. CT scan through the proximal femur show a sharply defined, soft tissue density lesion in the intertrochanteric region. It has a dense sclerotic rim (*arrows*). Radiographs showed a coarse sclerotic rim characteristic of fibrous dysplasia.

involve the cortex. Fibrous cortical defects present as sharply defined, intracortical lucencies with a sclerotic rim (Fig. 91A). Benign fibroosseous lesions may be seen along the posterior distal femur and present as cortically based soft tissue masses with no overlying calcified periostium. A sclerotic margin separates the soft tissue from the medullary cavity (Fig. 91B, C).

CT is important in the evaluation of histologically benign but clinically aggressive lesions such as chondroblastoma and giant cell tumor. It identifies subtle areas of cortical destruction, periosteal reaction, calcification, and soft tissue extent not visible on plain radiographs, thereby helping to characterize either tumor. Chondroblastomas are sharply defined lucent lesions in most cases (29,

146,263). About one third contain calcifications indicating their cartilage nature. CT may disclose certain complications, such as secondary aneurysmal bone cyst formation not identifiable on radiographs. CT of giant cell tumors correlates well with the histologic features (62,150,193,234,356). CT is less effective for detection or exclusion of articular invasion than is arthrotomography or MRI. It helps to combine CT with intraarticular contrast (iodinated or air).

Skeletal angiomatous lesions are common and may have a recognizable appearance on both CT and MRI. Osseous hemangiomas of the spine contain coarse trabeculation visible by CT or MRI. They may contain fat and enhance with contrast. In long bones, hemangiomas are

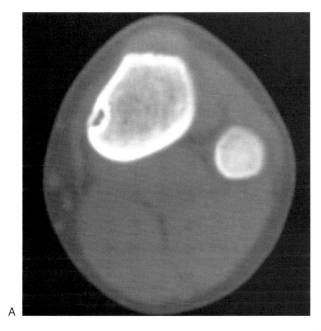

A

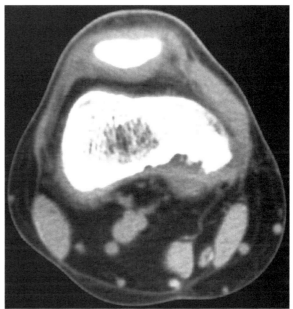

B

FIG. 91. Benign fibrous lesions. **A:** Fibrous cortical defect in the proximal tibia presents as a sharply defined lesion centered within the cortex. It has a sclerotic margin and soft tissue density center. The appearance is most characteristic on radiographs. **B, C:** Bone and soft tissue window CTs through a broad-based soft tissue mass along the posterior distal femur. The mass lies within the expected confines of the cortex but does not have a calcified roof. It is separated from the medullary cavity by an irregular, sclerotic margin. This lesion was biopsied and identified as a benign fibroosseous lesions.

C

lytic and produce a variety of patterns with bubbly, honeycomb, or linear lucent patterns visible (237).

Only limited descriptions of rare lesions such as desmoplastic fibroma (346), osseous hydatid disease (echinococcosis) (34,37), parosteal lipoma (226), and intraosseous lipoma (188,270) have been reported. Except for intraosseous lipoma, CT and MRI provide no histologically specific information about these lesions but may be valuable in better characterizing the process.

Malignant Skeletal Neoplasms

As with benign osseous neoplasms, malignant neoplasms of bone are almost always first identified and initially characterized by conventional radiography (48). In some cases, the radiographs show such extensive bone and soft tissue involvement that therapy can be chosen without further radiologic study. However, in most cases, precise definition of the longitudinal intraosseous and radial soft tissue extent of the lesion is needed to plan adequate resection, while sparing the maximum amount of tissue and retaining as much function as possible (53).

Osteosarcoma

Appropriate therapy for osteosarcoma depends on the extent of the tumor, and it is in the determination of tumor extent that CT and MRI are of most value (64,151, 324,337) (Figs. 79–82). Osteosarcoma has a spectrum of sectional imaging characteristics that parallel its various descriptive clinical and pathologic subtypes. Lytic, sclerotic, and mixed lytic-sclerotic central (medullary) osteosarcomas are most common. Some osteosarcomas have considerable sclerosis because of production of new bone over large areas. Other osteosarcomas produce little bone, presenting as primarily lytic lesions (59). Both cortical destruction and new bone production are easily demonstrated by CT.

Neoplasm replaces the normal, low-attenuation marrow fat in the medullary canal with tumor cells of higher attenuation, allowing direct evaluation of intramedullary tumor extent by CT. Osteosarcoma typically permeates the cortex and extends into the surrounding muscles and fascial planes (see Fig. 79). The radial tumor extent is easily determined by CT when fat planes are prominent but may be unclear when the patient is slender. Occasionally, osteosarcoma margins may be blurred by surrounding reactive edema, although generally this is not of clinical significance. More important problems are the edema and hemorrhage that follow biopsy; these alterations sometimes cannot be distinguished from tumor and may lead to an overestimate of tumor extent. Intravenous contrast enhancement can aid the determination of tumor spread, as it may make tumor margins more easily distinguishable and may facilitate demonstration of vascular

relationships if the tumor is adjacent to the neurovascular bundle (318).

The possible presence of skip metastases is of vital importance in the staging of osteosarcoma; when using CT to identify or exclude such lesions in patients considered candidates for limb sparing surgery, contiguous 1-cm imaging through the entire bone is recommended (318).

MRI is an effective sectional imaging method for staging osteosarcoma (342,386). The sensitivity of T1-weighted, STIR, and fat- saturated images to marrow fat replacement provides a stark outline of the tumor against marrow fat (see Figs. 79, 80, 82). Coronal or sagittal images along the long axis of the involved bone allow precise measurement of longitudinal extent, as well as identification of skip metastases in the marrow.

MRI takes advantage of intermuscular fat planes but, unlike CT, MRI is not fully dependent on them to distinguish between tumor and adjacent normal tissue. Osteosarcoma usually appears on a T2-weighted image as a high-signal mass that is clearly different from muscle (32,36,385,386). Lesions with a large amount of new bone will be of lower signal intensity on T2 images because of the absence of signal from the bone (28). MRI is better than CT for delineating the marrow and soft tissue extent of bone tumors in about one third of cases and equal to CT in the other two thirds (36) (see Fig. 82).

Parosteal osteosarcoma (273,359) is the second important subtype of osteosarcoma. Local resection, with tumor-free margins, is the accepted treatment because parosteal osteosarcoma has a less aggressive clinical course (42). Imaging with CT or MRI provides the same advantages for parosteal osteosarcoma as for medullary (central) osteosarcoma, including more precise definition of tumor spread along the cortex and into the medullary cavity (152,198,249). Radial growth into soft tissues and relationships to the neurovascular bundle are accurately depicted.

Periosteal (116,273,360) and intracortical osteosarcomas are rare. Accurate definition of tumor extent is critical to surgical planning, as local recurrence is common if tumor-free margins are not achieved. CT is accurate for identification of these tumor types and mapping of their extent.

Beyond the initial evaluation of osteosarcomas, CT and MRI have important roles in assessing a tumor's response to therapy and in detecting local and distant metastases. Base line imaging studies of the surgical site after resection are necessary and provide a standard against which follow-up examinations can be compared (49). A response to chemotherapy is evidenced by a decrease in tumor size, tumor necrosis, increased mineralization, and the formation of a calcified rim (305,363). Development of a new soft tissue mass indicates recurrent tumor in most cases. Neither CT nor MRI is effective for demonstration of microscopic foci of residual or recurrent tumor.

Chondrosarcoma

Malignant chondrous tumors are clearly depicted by both CT and MRI (124,147,153,172,295). Malignant exostotic chondrosarcoma may show thickening of the cartilage cap, with development of a soft tissue mass that invades surrounding normal tissues. Irregular calcifications located within the cartilage cap, as shown by CT, suggest malignant transformation. Thin (<2.0 cm) cartilage caps may be more difficult to distinguish from overlying normal soft tissue on CT (153). Other characteristics suggesting a malignant tumor include destruction of adjacent bone and the presence of large unmineralized areas within a partially calcified mass (295).

CT is the better sectional method for evaluation of the calcified or ossified portions of chondrous tumors and has been effective in distinguishing between benign cartilage tumors and chondrosarcomas (172). The increased sensitivity of MRI to soft tissue differences may help distinguish between abnormal cartilage and normal tissue.

Central chondrosarcoma, a neoplasm located within the medullary cavity in long bones, sometimes contains irregular chondrous calcifications that are readily detected by CT but may be missed with MRI. The malignant nature of the lesion is suggested by destruction of the surrounding cortical bone (''pushing'' margins), areas of necrosis in the tumor, and the presence of large noncalcified areas in the lesion (147) (Fig. 92).

The primary value of sectional imaging in evaluation of chondrosarcoma is the definition of tumor extent. CT provides an accurate depiction of tumor extent (124,147). MRI may better define both the intramedullary extent and soft tissue extent of central chondrosarcoma in the same way that it does with osteosarcoma. However, as with osteosarcoma, MRI will not identify small soft tissue calcifications.

Other Sarcomas of Bone

CT also has been used to evaluate the less common primary malignant bone tumors, including chordoma (139,144,296), fibrosarcoma (345), malignant fibrous histiocytoma (72,345), and liposarcoma. In each case, the emphasis is on the ability of sectional studies to define tumor extent. MRI provides a better determination of marrow and soft tissue extent, but a poorer evaluation of tumor calcification and bone mineral integrity, than does CT (138,144,296).

Sarcomas may develop in previously radiated bone. In such cases, CT can clearly demonstrate new bone destruction and the development of a soft tissue mass, strongly suggesting malignant change (200).

Small Cell Neoplasms

CT and MRI have been shown to be of great value for recognition of abnormalities and for therapy planning. Several studies evaluating Ewing sarcoma have emphasized the ability to use CT and MRI to detect tumors in sites of complex anatomy, evaluate the radial extent of the tumor, plan radiation ports and surgery, and evaluate therapeutic responses (36,104,362).

In the evaluation of adult leukemia and lymphoma, CT images display patterns of bone abnormality that parallel those seen on conventional radiographs. These patterns include skeletal permeation, destruction, and sclerosis. Soft tissue may be normal, displaced, or invaded by large or small masses. CT and MRI are particularly helpful in detecting, confirming, and defining the extent of abnormality, especially in areas of complex anatomy such as the chest wall. Such information may be essential in planning CT guided biopsy. Both CT and MRI are useful in identifying recurrent disease.

Similar information may be provided in the evaluation of myeloma and solitary plasmacytoma (129,319). CT may also demonstrate lesions (initial or recurrent) when both radiography and bone scintigraphy findings are normal.

Metastases

Most metastases to the skeleton are detected and confirmed by radiography or bone scintigraphy (119) (Fig. 93). Unsuspected bone metastases sometimes are recognized on CT images obtained for evaluation of another clinical problem. In some cases, metastases can be detected only by assessment of medullary marrow density (128).

CT patterns of metastases are similar to those seen with radiography (Fig. 93). However, in addition to confirmation of a lytic or sclerotic lesion, the radial extent of the metastasis is more easily appreciated. This may be important in planning radiation ports or biopsy sites. Occasionally, CT may be the only imaging procedure to detect and localize a metastasis convincingly, especially in areas of complex anatomy such as the spine (119). CT is particularly useful for detection and characterization of metastases that are suspected because of scintigraphic abnormalities but not confirmed by standard radiography (119).

The high sensitivity of MRI for detection of marrow replacement makes it especially valuable for identifying tumor deposits in marrow (57). Detection of metastases by MRI in the presence of normal findings on bone scintigraphy is valuable, especially when focal bone pain suggests metastases or in the presence of multiple myeloma.

Skeletal Pseudotumors

Hemophiliac patients develop intraosseous hemorrhages that may expand bone (113,133). As with a true neoplasm, CT can display the radial extent of such a

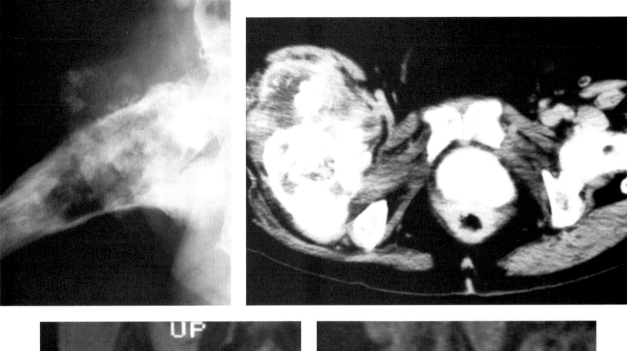

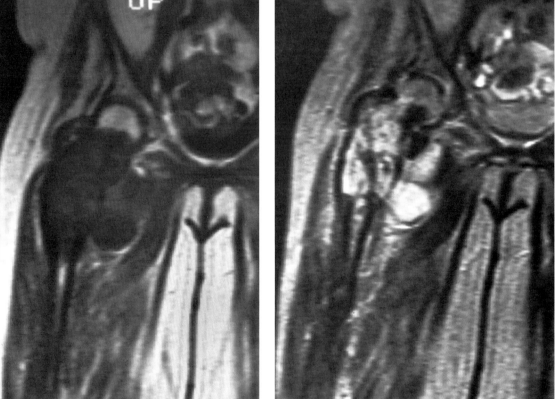

FIG. 92. Chondrosarcoma. **A:** Frog-leg lateral radiograph shows expansion of the proximal right femoral diaphysis and metaphysis associated with a large adjacent soft tissue mass. Coarse calcifications are present within the bone lesion and within the soft tissue mass. The calcifications are irregularly distributed throughout the mass. **B:** CT through the proximal femur shows the central, expansile lesion of the femur and the large anterior soft tissue mass with irregular calcifications visible in both the bone and soft tissue components. **C, D:** Coronal T1- and T2-weighted MRIs clearly demonstrate both the intramedullary and soft tissue extent of the lesion.

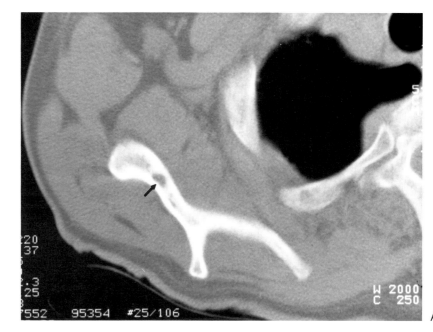

A

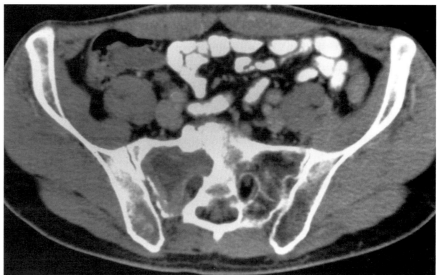

B

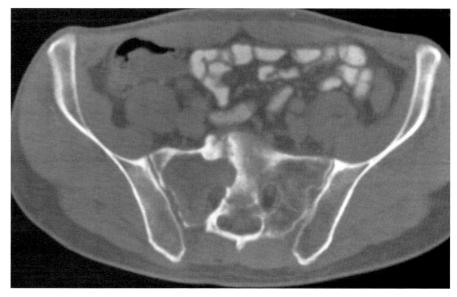

C

FIG. 93. Metastases. **A:** Lung cancer metastasis. Focal lytic lesion in the right scapula (*arrow*) identified by bone scintigraphy but not visible by radiography. **B, C:** Hemangiopericytoma metastasis. Soft tissue and bone window images through the sacrum demonstrate a well defined lytic lesion in the right sacral ala. The lesion is of mixed density.

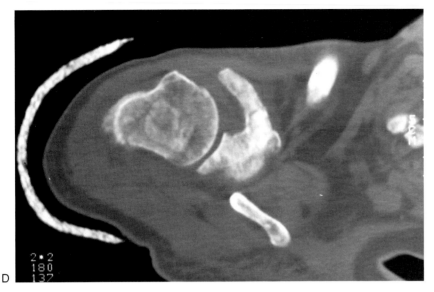

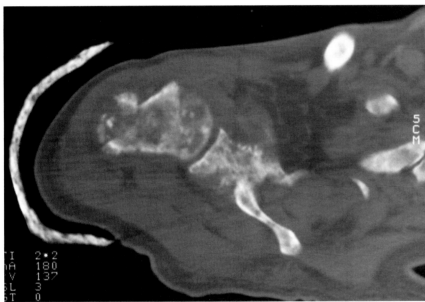

FIG. 93. (*Continued.*) **D, E:** Prostate cancer metastasis. Diffuse mixed pattern (lytic and blastic) metastatic disease throughout the proximal humerus, scapula, and clavicle.

lesion and define its spatial relationships with other important structures. Such information can be important in their management, particularly if surgery becomes necessary. CT also can be used to differentiate between osseous dysplasia associated with neurofibromatosis and bone changes due to benign or malignant neural tumors.

SOFT TISSUE TUMORS

The evaluation of soft tissue masses has been revolutionized, initially by the development of CT (126, 298,348) and subsequently by MRI (51,240,353). The soft tissue contrast resolution and sectional presentation of compartmental anatomy provided by CT and MRI make possible routine identification, characterization, and staging of soft tissue masses.

CT is an effective method for the study of soft tissue masses of many causes (Fig. 94–101). It usually permits distinction between one muscle and another, provides a cross-sectional image of limb compartments, is sensitive to anatomic distortion, localizes neurovascular bundles, and defines both the radial distribution of a mass and its local relationships. In select circumstances, these capabilities are improved by intravascular or intraarticular contrast enhancement (52,256).

CT has several disadvantages (22,61,79,103). In lean parts of the anatomy, there is insufficient fat to permit distinction between normal and pathologic anatomy, and a mass might not be detected because of isodensity with respect to surrounding muscle (Fig. 94). There is also a risk that the size or extent of a mass might be overestimated because of adjacent edema or hemorrhage. Over range artifacts caused by bone or metal in the imaging

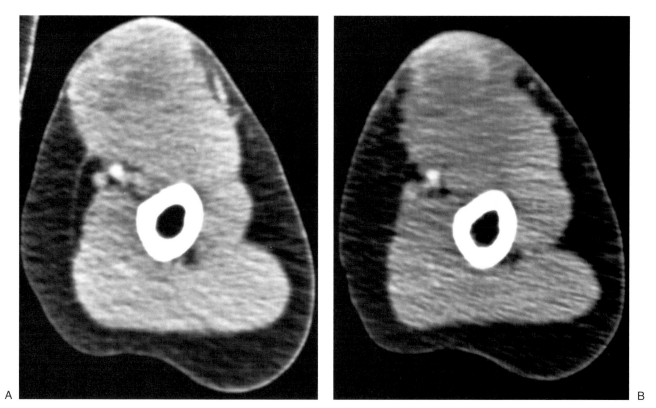

FIG. 94. Undifferentiated sarcoma. **A, B:** Contrast-enhanced CT scans through the upper arm show enlargement and distortion of the biceps muscle and loss of the normal subcutaneous fat plane anteriorly. The mass is heterogeneous and of slightly lower density than muscle.

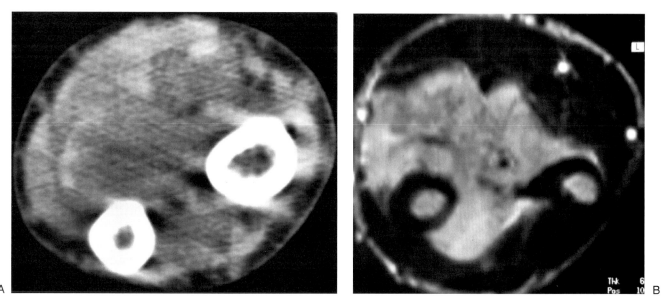

FIG. 95. Rhabdomyosarcoma. **A:** Contrast enhanced CT of the midforearm shows enlargement of the ventral (flexor) compartment due to a large, deeply located soft tissue mass. The mass is heterogenous in density but slightly lower than muscle. The interface between the mass and any normal muscle is difficult to define. **B:** Axial T2-weighted MRI at the same level as the CT again shows the large, deeply located mass. The MRI presents a clearly defined separation between the tumor and the overlying muscle. The tumor passes through the interosseous membrane to enter the extensor compartment, something that is difficult to recognize on the CT.

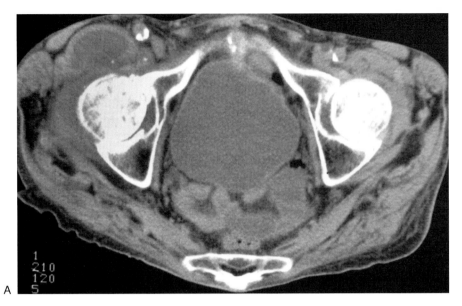

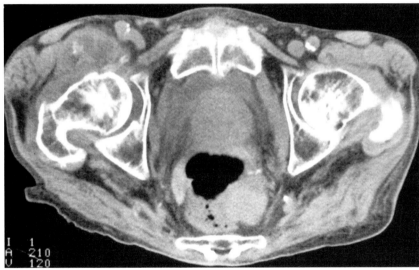

FIG. 96. Distended iliopsoas bursa. A, B: CT scans through the groin demonstrate a large soft tissue mass in the anterior thigh/groin region corresponding to the palpable mass. The mass is smooth with a well defined periphery. Centrally, it is more radiolucent, with a density only slightly higher than urine. It has a relatively thick wall and contains an irregular calcified joint body (B). An associated hip joint effusion is noted.

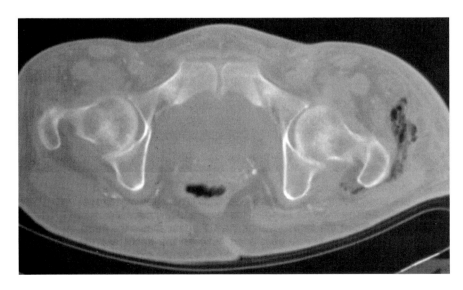

FIG. 97. Hip/buttock abscess. CT scan through the hip region in a patient presenting with a painful left hip mass shows an irregular mass containing a large amount of gas. In the absence of any recent surgery, this indicates an active infectious process producing an abscess.

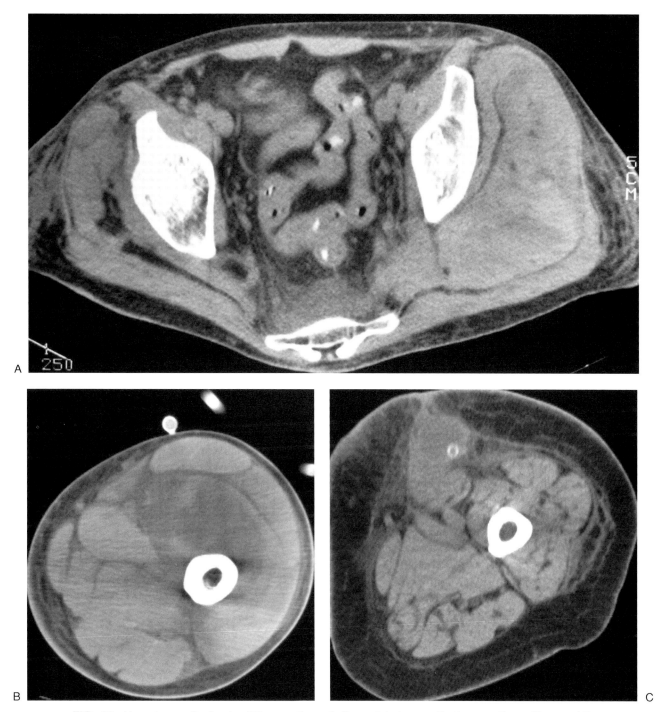

FIG. 98. Hematoma. **A:** Acute. CT scan through the pelvis in a patient presenting with a rapidly expanding left buttock mass. The CT demonstrates a large, hyperdense mass infiltrating between the gluteal muscles. The patient was on anticoagulants. **B:** Subacute. CT scan through the upper thigh shows a heterogeneous soft tissue mass with areas of high and intermediate density involving the vastus medialis and intermedius muscles. Several days prior to the scan the patient experienced a sudden, incapacitating episode of thigh pain while running, indicating an acute muscle tear and hemorrhage. **C:** Chronic. CT scan through the proximal thigh in a patient who has a femoropopliteal bypass graft shows a mass surrounding the graft. The homogeneous mass is of low attenuation and has been present since the immediate postoperative period. It was drained and was sterile, indicating that it is likely a seroma following postoperative bleeding.

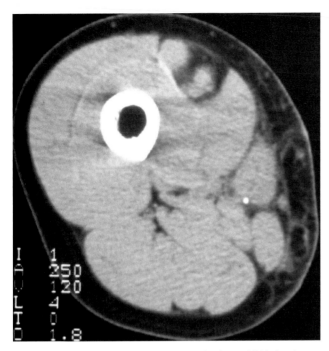

FIG. 99. Lipoma. CT image through the midthigh shows irregular fatty infiltration of the rectus femoris muscle. Biopsy showed an intramuscular lipoma without malignant tissue.

plane may obscure details of the margin or matrix of masses.

MRI is now generally considered the most effective method for detection, localization, and characterization of soft tissue masses (96,111,343). Because of its high contrast sensitivity, MRI will demonstrate the boundaries of tumors with respect to fat, muscle, and bone (Figs. 96 and 101). With the appropriate combination of imaging planes, distinction between the mass and adjacent structures usually can be achieved without difficulty.

MRI has certain disadvantages, the most important of which is insensitivity to small calcifications and collections of gas (353). These features often are diagnostically important but must be detected by conventional radiography or CT (Figs. 96 and 97). MR images are also degraded by metals in the section but to a lesser degree than CT and newer fast spin-echo sequences often decrease artifact sufficiently to allow good images in the presence of large fixation devices or prostheses. As with CT, there is a risk that the size or extent of a mass might be overestimated because of adjacent edema. However, appropriate selection of pulse sequences and selective use of intravenous contrast should resolve most questions.

Comparative studies of CT and MRI show that MRI provides equal or greater information than CT regarding lesion identification, characterization, and determination of extent (353,374). The greater inherent soft tissue contrast resolution of MRI provides clearer definition of tumor margins than does CT. Much has been said about the lack of histologic specificity available with both CT

and MRI. In contrast to the evaluation of bone tumors where most lesion specificity comes from the radiographic data, no such specificity is available for soft tissue tumors. In spite of the actual lack of histologic specificity, remarkable accuracy in defining specific lesion type can be accomplished by clearly defining the epicenter of the lesion and its growth characteristics. Imaging findings that suggest an aggressive growth pattern include marginal irregularity (20,255,353), heterogeneity of internal architecture (214,353), surrounding edema (214), and invasion or encasement of adjacent structures, particularly vessels and nerves, whereas the contrast characteristics of soft tissue masses depend on their compositions. For CT, density depends on the relative proportions of fat, water, and mineral. The MR signal intensity is a more complex phenomenon dependent on the balance of inherent tissue properties of hydrogen density and relaxation factors, blood flow, and pulse-sequence selection (240).

Cysts

Cystic masses usually are associated with a joint and arise from a synovial extension (186,187,261,323,340). These are sharply marginated, homogeneous masses with CT attenuation values or MR signal intensities similar to those for water. If hemorrhagic, their CT attenuation values or their T1-weighted signal intensities may increase. The largest synovial cysts tend to be found about the hip (Fig. 96). Cysts show no enhancement after intravenous administration of contrast material, although this may make their margins more conspicuous because of enhancement of the surrounding tissues. Both CT and MRI are effective methods for demonstration of the nature and origin of cysts. Neither is always effective for distinguishing between a pyogenic cystic collection and a sterile collection; cyst aspiration and fluid culture are necessary.

Abscesses

Soft tissue abscesses infrequently present as masses. When they do, they generally are poorly defined, infiltrating lesions that distort normal muscle anatomy and fascial planes. Although abscesses may occur anywhere in the body, they are most commonly encountered in the paraspinal and pelvic muscles (Fig. 97).

The CT or MRI appearance of an abscess is nonspecific and may be confused with that of hemorrhage or neoplasm unless soft tissue gas is present. In the absence of percutaneous or open surgical intervention, the presence of soft tissue gas is indicative of an inflammatory process. CT is effective for definition of the extent of the abscess, guidance of percutaneous drainage procedures, and documentation of response to therapy. CT is generally preferred when intervention is contemplated. Otherwise, ex-

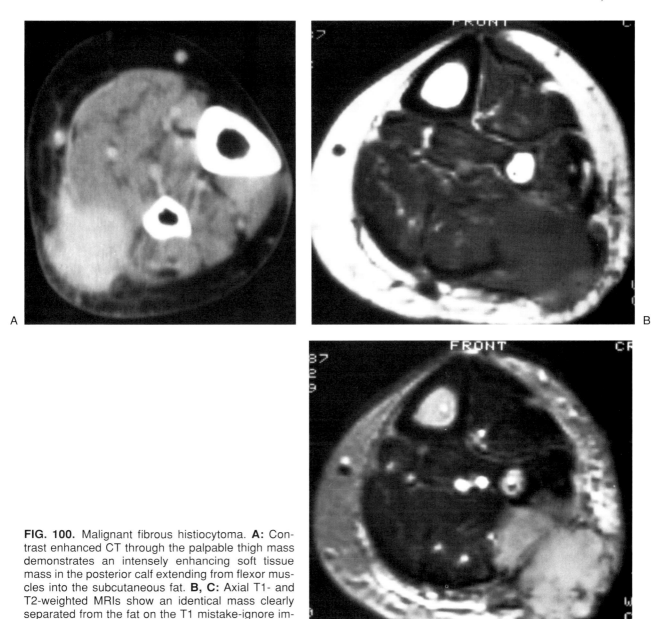

FIG. 100. Malignant fibrous histiocytoma. **A:** Contrast enhanced CT through the palpable thigh mass demonstrates an intensely enhancing soft tissue mass in the posterior calf extending from flexor muscles into the subcutaneous fat. **B, C:** Axial T1- and T2-weighted MRIs show an identical mass clearly separated from the fat on the T1 mistake-ignore images and from normal muscle on T2-weighted images.

cept for the detection of gas, MRI is as effective as CT for demonstration of the abscess (370).

Hematoma

Hemorrhages into soft tissue may have various causes, presentations, localizations, and appearances (Fig. 98). Hemorrhage may occur spontaneously, following trauma, with bleeding diatheses, while a patient is receiving anticoagulants, with inflammatory diseases, into a tumor, and following surgery or percutaneous translumbar aortography. Because of the various causes and possible presentations, a physician may not always consider the diagnosis.

If hemorrhage is suspected, confirmation and precise localization are difficult using radiographic imaging methods.

CT or MRI nearly always shows the location and extent of soft tissue hemorrhage, especially in anatomic regions that are difficult to examine physically. Intramuscular hemorrhage will cause an enlargement of the muscle that is easily recognized when the left and right sides are compared for symmetry (70). Whereas an acute hematoma is characteristically hyperdense (Fig. 98A), a subacute (Fig. 98B) or chronic (Fig. 98C) hematoma may not be readily differentiated from an abscess or a neoplasm on the basis of CT findings alone. Any of these may cause enlargement of a muscle with an isodense or low-density

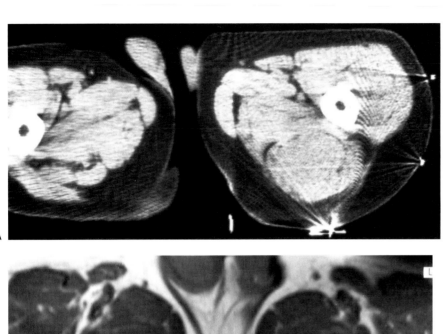

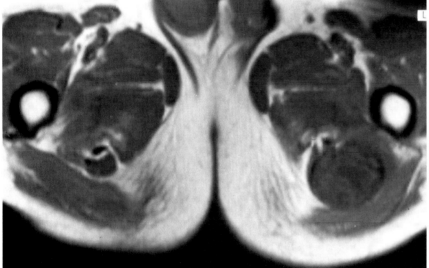

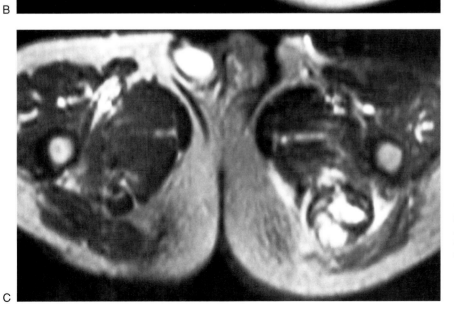

FIG. 101. Malignant nerve sheath tumor. **A:** CT through the palpable mass demonstrates a rounded, poorly marginated mass in the hamstring muscles. **B, C:** T1- and T2-weighted MRIs through the same level as the CT again show the mass. It is relatively homogeneous and low in signal on T1- and very heterogeneous on the T2-weighted image.

mass. With appropriate clinical history, a diagnosis of hemorrhage may be suggested; in selected cases, CT can be used to guide a percutaneous needle aspiration for confirmation.

In addition to localization of soft tissue hemorrhage, CT can characterize and display the various stages in the natural history of hematoma maturation. Initially, the hematoma may be of homogeneous density (Fig. 98A), and then, as liquefaction begins, it may develop a patchy or heterogeneous appearance (Fig. 98B). When completely liquefied, the hematoma will have developed a pseudocapsule and homogeneous density lower than that of muscle (Fig. 98C). If the injury includes muscle necrosis, early mineralization may be detected by CT, indicating ossification of the hematoma or development of myositis ossificans (10). MRI will not identify the soft tissue mineralization on which the specific diagnosis of myositis ossificans depends; it will only show a mass.

The signal characteristics of soft tissue hemorrhage on MRI change as the blood in the mass ages (303,344,358). Acute hemorrhage has a signal intensity close to that of muscle on T1-weighted images and a high signal intensity on T2-weighted images. After about 2 days there is progressive shortening of the T1 relaxation value of the hematoma, and the signal intensity becomes much greater than that of muscle on T1-weighted images. This phenomenon is attributed to sequential changes that occur as the hemoglobin molecules are oxidized to methemoglobin. Within several days, and thereafter for many months, residual hematomas will have very strong signal intensities on both pulse sequences, permitting identification of blood.

Soft Tissue Neoplasms

Benign and aggressive soft tissue tumors can be evaluated by CT or MRI (61). The classic benign mass usually has a well-defined periphery or capsule and a homogeneous matrix. A typical aggressive mass has an ill-defined periphery and a heterogeneous or patchy matrix. On CT examination, tumors usually have an average attenuation value slightly lower than that for normal muscle. In general, on MRI examination, nonfatty tumors are of equal or lower signal intensity than skeletal muscle on T1-weighted sequences and of higher signal intensity than skeletal muscle on T2-weighted images. When compared with fat, most lesions are lower in signal intensity than fat on T1-weighted images and equal to or greater than fat on T2-weighted images. With MRI, lesions tend to be more heterogeneous on T2-weighted images than on T1-weighted images. Unfortunately, in most cases neither CT nor MRI can provide a specific histologic diagnosis. Both benign and malignant lesions may present morphologically as either well-defined or infiltrating masses. Relatively nonaggressive processes include cysts, lipomas,

myositis ossificans, and both benign and malignant neoplasms. Aggressive characteristics may be seen in acute hematomas, abscesses, some benign tumors, and many malignant neoplasms (154).

Soft tissue masses historically were evaluated by a combination of conventional radiography, angiography, radionuclide bone scintigraphy, ultrasonography (38, 185), and sectional imaging (22,134,383). CT and MRI are far superior to conventional radiography for exclusion, confirmation, and characterization of soft tissue masses. Both methods are superior to angiography and have essentially replaced it for lesion localization, definition of margins, determination of vascularity and vascular relationships, and aid in diagnosis (77). Angiography is reserved for those instances when sectional imaging fails to define vascular invasion adequately or when a preoperative vascular map is required. Sectional imaging is also superior to bone scintigraphy for determination of the anatomic relationship of a soft tissue mass to a bone (79). However, bone scintigraphy is more effective for demonstration of a physiologic response of the bone to the adjacent mass (79,148). Radionuclide bone scintigraphy remains the best method to survey the skeleton for metastases. In most instances, CT and MRI are preferred to ultrasonography as the primary imaging tests for extremity masses.

We now employ sectional imaging for preoperative characterization and staging of all soft tissue neoplasia and prefer MRI as the initial or only method in most instances (255). The goal for therapy is complete excision of the tumor, with limb salvage (215) and preservation of function (53,80). Tumors that spare adjacent bone and major vessels and that are limited to a single soft tissue compartment usually can be resected. When the entire tumor, its reactive rim, and a cuff of normal tissue are removed en bloc, local recurrences are few. If the tumor violates a second compartment, enters a joint, or invades major neurovascular structures, amputation may be required. We rely on sectional imaging to provide the necessary anatomic details. Whereas CT is more effective for analysis of soft tissue calcification and bone mineral integrity, MRI is preferred for detailed evaluation of soft tissue and bone marrow.

Sectional imaging also is valuable for evaluation of regional soft tissue anatomy following therapy. Both CT and MRI are effective for demonstration of tumor regression or recurrence. Neither will show microscopic residual or recurrent tumor (149).

Benign Neoplasms

Lipomas are common benign soft tissue tumors (Fig. 99). Most are subcutaneous and need no imaging evaluation. When deep or large or in an unusual location, both CT and MRI can identify and localize the tumors as areas of fatty tissue distorting the surrounding tissues. Lipomas are composed almost exclusively of fatty tissue (-40 to -100 HU), although they may contain recognizable small, thin, soft tissue septae or vessels. In addition, they are well defined and homogeneous (158). When areas of soft tissue density or intensity are present in the lesion, or when the lesion invades surrounding tissue, the possibility of a sarcoma must be considered and a biopsy performed. Larger, more infiltrating lipomatous lesions such as macrodystrophia lipomatosa and infiltrating angiolipomas are rare, but when present, CT or MRI can be used to map their extent and demonstrate where normal muscle is invaded or replaced.

CT and MRI are effective for demonstration of hemangiomas and angiovenous dysplasias of the musculoskeletal system (50,169,196). These are best shown by MRI because the slowly flowing blood in the lesions has an intense signal on T2-weighted images that facilitates their characterization and the definition of extent.

Pigmented villonodular synovitis (PVNS) produces soft tissue masses associated with joints, most commonly the large hip and knee joints. The masses are firm and can produce pressure erosions in adjacent bone that can easily be seen and characterized by CT or MRI. PVNS is seen as a heterogeneous, smoothly marginated mass that often fills the synovial space and insinuates itself between the bones of a joint. On CT, it is of muscle density or slightly higher. On MRI, it is low on T1- and irregularly high on T2-weighted images. Often areas of very low signal are distributed throughout the tumor on MRI. These areas are produced by foci of hemosiderin within the lesion (161,176,257,321).

CT also has been used to evaluate a variety of other less common, benign masses, including nodular fasciitis, benign mesenchymoma, intramuscular myxoma, endometriosis, and soft tissue chondroma (388). The CT appearance in these lesions is not specific; however, CT does help identify, localize, and characterize each mass so that the surgical approach can be planned.

Malignant Neoplasms

The value of CT and MRI in the evaluation and staging of soft tissue sarcomas is now widely accepted (275). Current therapy is based on accurate staging of the tumor, which in turn depends on accurate definition of the compartmental and longitudinal extent of the lesion. CT and MRI can provide this information as well as define the relationships of the tumor to adjacent vessels and nerves. Accurate preoperative characterization can facilitate the design and performance of limb surgery that will leave tumor-free surgical margins, preserve function, and lead to few tumor recurrences.

The most common malignant soft tissue neoplasms are relatively indistinguishable by all imaging methods. Malignant fibrous histiocytomas, liposarcomas, and fibrosarcomas all present as heterogeneous masses. They vary from fairly well encapsulated to very invasive. Both CT and MRI can define extent for most lesions on the basis of mass effect and associated distortion or infiltration of the surrounding normal tissues. MRI offers the advantages of increased contrast resolution and additional planes that may make the margins of lesions more conspicuous.

Malignant fibrous histiocytoma, the most common malignant soft tissue neoplasm, generally is a lobulated heterogeneous mass that often is invasive but may be relatively well defined (87) (Fig. 100). Peripheral calcification may be present in some cases. On MRI, the tumor may consist of irregularly shaped regions of both high and low signal intensities, sometimes having areas of hemorrhage. Fibrosarcoma (345), another relatively common soft tissue malignancy, is very difficult to distinguish from infection, hemorrhage, or other invasive neoplasm. It is often infiltrative and may replace muscles and invade bone. Its matrix is irregular and may be quite heterogeneous. Alveolar soft parts sarcoma is a rare sarcoma with an aggressive growth pattern. Its characteristics are indistinguishable from other sarcomas (201).

Liposarcoma (60,61,71,158) usually is a bulky tumor with a pseudocapsule. Margins may be sharp or unsharp, and the matrix mixed or heterogeneous. The amount of fat is variable, with some poorly differentiated tumors containing almost no fat and other tumors contain mostly fat. If any solid or nonfatty component (other than small blood vessels) is present in a predominantly fatty tumor, the possibility of sarcomatous tissue must be considered. Neither CT nor MRI has any advantage in distinguishing benign and malignant fatty tumors (60,71).

Both CT and MRI are effective for identification, characterization, and staging of several less common malignant soft tissue neoplasms, including extraosseous chondrosarcoma, neurofibrosarcoma, leiomyosarcoma, synovial sarcoma, malignant nerve sheath tumors (Fig. 101), and extraskeletal Ewing tumor. Most present as masses similar to the more common malignant lesions and vary in appearance from fairly well defined to infiltrating. Metastases may also be detected.

INFECTION

Computed tomography and magnetic resonance imaging are not generally necessary for initial documentation, localization, or diagnosis of infection because clinical assessment and conventional radiographs are usually adequate (23,314). Radionuclide imaging remains the standard screening method for detection of subradiographic osteomyelitis. CT should be reserved for detailed delineation of bone cavities, sequestra, or cloacae (130,180,329,379) (Fig. 102C, D), for demonstration of inflammatory changes in complex articulations or bones

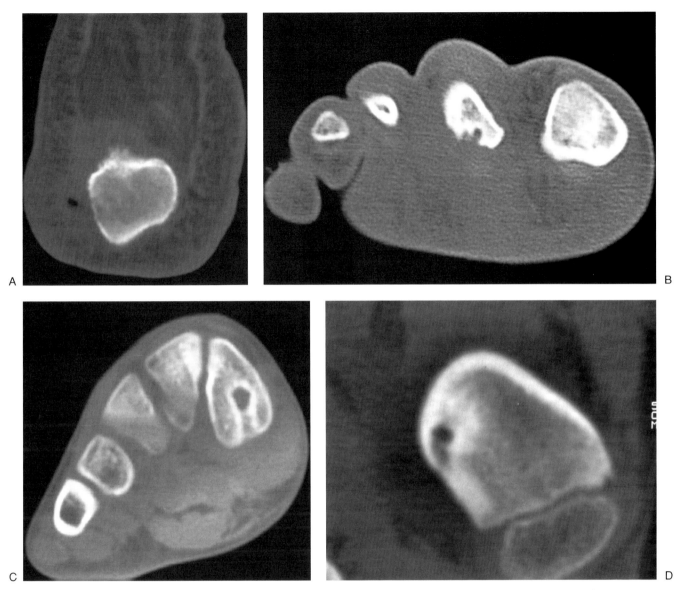

FIG. 102. Osteomyelitis. **A:** Direct coronal CT through posterior calcaneous shows gas in the soft tissue of the medial heel. The adjacent calcaneal cortex in thinned and permeated indicating osteomyelitis. There was a subtle increase in marrow density when compared with the opposite side. **B:** Direct coronal CT through the digits of the foot shows destruction of the undersurface of the second proximal phalanx indicating osteomyelitis. **C:** Direct coronal CT through the midfoot shows a lytic lesion in the first cuniform. The lesion has a sclerotic margin and a tube-like extension ventrally, the cloacae. **D:** CT through the proximal left femur shows a sharply defined lucency with a broad sclerotic rim and no nidus. Biopsy revealed turbid fluid with no microorganisms. These findings are indicative of a chronic infectious process or Brodie abscess.

(1,7,132,135,199,224,228,233,267,291,292,311) (Fig. 102A, B), for demonstration of foreign bodies not visible by conventional radiography (379), and for guiding percutaneous aspiration biopsy or drainage procedures when indicated (135,267,329). These capabilities enable CT to play an important part in the treatment of selected cases of chronic osteomyelitis (135,329,379).

Computed tomography may detect specific signs of osteomyelitis, including cortical destruction (Fig. 102A), intraosseous gas (269,292), intracortical fissuring (290),

and fat–fluid (pus) levels (209). The evaluation of osseous tuberculosis and hydatid disease (echinococcosis) of bone (34,37) has been aided by the use of CT.

Osteomyelitis results in replacement of normal marrow with exudate, fibrosis, and hemorrhage. Fat necrosis and bone proliferation also may be present in varying proportions. CT analysis of the medullary content may detect the alterations in marrow composition that accompany osteomyelitis (180). However, the abnormal marrow of osteomyelitis is better imaged using MRI (23,45,240).

T1-weighted, STIR or fat saturation sequences are used to maximize the contrast between normal and infiltrated bone marrow (93). Normal marrow, with its homogeneous high signal, is replaced by tissues with longer T1 values (and hence decreased signal intensity on T1-weighted sequences). T2-weighted sequences usually will demonstrate increased signal intensity from the areas of marrow abnormality, reflecting prolonged T2 values (probably as a result of increased water and blood in the affected region), but are less sensitive than STIR or fat saturation sequences. By taking advantage of the ability of MRI to image directly in the coronal and parasagittal planes along the long axis of an infected bone, peripheral interfaces of infection with normal marrow and adjacent soft tissues are more clearly demonstrated and the extent of disease more clearly delineated than with alternative methods (93,228,370).

An MRI examination of suspected osteomyelitis should be expected to confirm or exclude marrow abnormality, demonstrate cortical and soft tissue involvement, and characterize the extent of marrow involvement (228,230). An MRI examination showing only normal marrow is a good indication that there is no infection. When conventional radiography and bone scintigraphy are nondiagnostic, MRI may detect or exclude an abnormality.

Both CT and MRI demonstrate soft tissue changes notably better than conventional radiography (23,34,63, 93,180,228,240,267,370,379, 382). They have been useful in evaluating primary soft tissue abscesses, sinus tracts, joint effusions, swelling, edema, necrosis, sterile fluid collections, and infiltrative changes in fat adjacent to soft tissue infections. Also, soft tissue pressure ulcers and their complications have been successfully evaluated (85).

REFERENCES

1. Abbey DM, Hosea SW. Diagnosis of vertebral osteomyelitis in a community hospital by using computed tomography. *Arch Intern Med* 1989;149:2029–2035.
2. Abel MF, Wenger DR, Mubarak SJ, et al. Quantitative analysis of hip dysplasia in cerebral palsy. A study of radiographs and 3-D reformatted images. *J Pediatr Orthop* 1995;14:283–289.
3. Adam P, Labbe JL, Alberge Y, et al. The role of computed tomography in the assessment and treatment of acetabular fractures. *Clin Radiol* 1985;36:13–18.
4. Aisen AM, Glazer GM. Diagnosis of osteoid osteoma using computed tomography. *J Comput Tomogr* 1984;8:175–178.
5. Aisen AM, Martel W, Braunstein EM, McMillin KI, Phillips WA, Kling TF. MRI and CT evaluation of primary bone and soft tissue tumors. *AJR* 1986;146:749–756.
6. Alani WO, Bartal E. Osteoid osteoma of the femoral neck simulating an inflammatory synovitis. *Clin Orthop* 1987;223:308–312.
7. Alexander PW, Shin MS. CT manifestation of sternoclavicular pyarthrosis in patients with intravenous drug abuse. *J Comput Assist Tomogr* 1990;14:104–106.
8. Allon SM, Mears DC. Three dimensional analysis of calcaneal fractures. *Foot Ankle* 1991;11:254–263.
9. Alvarez RE, Macovski A. Energy-selective reconstructions in x-ray computed tomography. *Phys Med Biol* 1976;21:733–744.
10. Amendola MA, Glazer GM, Agha FP, Francis IR, Weatherbee L, Martel W. Myositis ossificans circumscripta: computed tomographic diagnosis. *Radiology* 1983;149:775–779.
11. Anderson IF, Crichton KJ, Grattan ST, et al. Osteochondral fractures of the dome of the talus. *J Bone Joint Surg [Am]* 1989;71A:1143–1152.
12. Atar D, Lehman WB, Grant AD. 2-D and 3-D computed tomography and magnetic resonance imaging in developmental dysplasia of the hip. *Ortho Rev* 1992;21:1189–1197.
13. Bain GI, Bennett JD, Richards RS, et al. Longitudinal computed tomography of the scaphoid: a new technique. *Skeletal Radiol* 1995;24:271–273.
14. Barrow BA, Fajman WA, Parker LM, et al. Tibial plateau fractures: evaluation with MR imaging. *RadioGraphics* 1994;14:553–559.
15. Basett LW, Mirra JM, Cracchiolo AD, et al. Ischemic necrosis of the femoral head. Correlation of magnetic resonance imaging and histologic sections. *Clin Orthop* 1987;223:181–187.
16. Basu P, Beall A, Simmons D. 3-D femoral stress analysis using CT scans and p-version FEM. *Biomed Med Devf Artif Org* 1986;13:163–186.
17. Belsole RJ, Hilbelink D, Llewellyn JA, et al. Scaphoid orientation and location from computed, three-dimensional carpal models. *Orthop Clin North Am* 1986;17:505–510.
18. Beltran J, Gray LA, Bools JC, et al. Rotator cuff lesions of the shoulder: evaluation by direct sagittal CT arthrography. *Radiology* 1986;160:161–165.
19. Beltran J, Noto AM, Chakeres DW, Christoforidis AJ. Tumors of the osseous spine: staging with MR imaging versus CT. *Radiology* 1987;162:565–569.
20. Beltran J, Simon DC, Katz W, Weis LD. Increased MR signal intensity in skeletal muscle adjacent to malignant tumors: pathologic correlation and clinical relevance. *Radiology* 1987;162:251–255.
21. Beltran J, Simon DC, Levy M, Herman L, Weis L, Mueller CF. Aneurysmal bone cysts: MR imaging at 1.5T. *Radiology* 1986;158:689–690.
22. Bernardino ME, Jing BS, Thomas JL, Lindell MM, Zornoza J. The extremity soft tissue lesion: a comparative study of ultrasound, computed tomography, and xeroradiography. *Radiology* 1981;139:53–59.
23. Berquist TH, Brown ML, Fitzgerald RH, May GR. Magnetic resonance imaging: application in musculoskeletal infection. *Magn Reson Imaging* 1985;3:219–230.
24. Bettelli G, Capanna R, van Horn JR, Ruggieri P, Biagini R, Campanacci M. Osteoid osteoma and osteoblastoma of the pelvis. *Clin Orthop* 1989;247:261–271.
25. Billet FP, Schmitt WG, Gay B. Computed tomography in traumatology with special regard to the advances of three-dimensional display. *Arch Orthop Trauma Surg* 1992;111:131–137.
26. Biondetti PR, Vannier MW, Gilula LA, et al. Wrist: coronal and transaxial CT scanning. *Radiology* 1987;163:149–151.
27. Blaquiere RM. Computed tomography in acetabular trauma. *Clin Radiol* 1985;36:5–11.
28. Bloem JL, Bluemm RG, Taminiau AHM, van Oosterom AT, Stolk J, Doornbos J. Magnetic resonance imaging of primary malignant bone tumors. *RadioGraphics* 1987;7:425–445.
29. Bloem JL, Mulder JD. Chondroblastoma: a clinical and radiological study of 104 cases. *Skeletal Radiol* 1985;14:1–9.
30. Blokker CP, Rorabeck CH, Bourne RB. Tibial plateau fractures. An analysis of the results of treatment in 60 patients. *Clin Orthop* 1984;182:193–199.
31. Bogost GA, Lizerbram EK, Crues JR. MR imaging in evaluation of suspected hip fracture: frequency of unsuspected bone and soft tissue injury. *Radiology* 1995;197:263–267.
32. Bohndorf K, Reiser M, Lochner B, Feaux de Lacroix W, Steinbrich W. Magnetic resonance imaging of primary tumours and tumourlike lesions of bone. *Skeletal Radiol* 1986;15:511–517.
33. Bostman OM. Spiral fractures of the shaft of the tibia. Initial displacement and stability of reduction. *J Bone Joint Surgery [Br]* 1986;68B:462–466.
34. Bouras A, Larde D, Mathieu D, Delepine G, Benameur C, Ferrane J. The value of computed tomography in osseous hydatid disease (echinococcosis). *Skeletal Radiol* 1984;12:192–195.

35. Boven F, De Boeck M, Potvliege R. Synovial plicae of the knee on computed tomography. *Radiology* 1983;147:805–809.

36. Boyko OB, Cory DA, Cohen MD, Provisor A, Mirkin D, DeRosa GP. MR imaging of osteogenic and Ewing's sarcoma. *AJR* 1987; 148:317–322.

37. Braithwaite PA, Lees RF. Vertebral hydatid disease: radiological assessment. *Radiology* 1981;140:763–766.

38. Braunstein EM, Silver TM, Martel W, Jaffe M. Ultrasonographic diagnosis of extemity masses. *Skeletal Radiol* 1981;6:157–163.

39. Brown T, Pederson D, Rubin E, Rose E. Global mechanical consequences of bone/cement interface degradation in proximal femoral arthroplasty. *Proc Orthop Res Soc* 1986;11:467.

40. Burk DL Jr, Mears DC, Kennedy WH, et al. Three-dimensional computed tomography of acetabular fractures. *Radiology* 1985; 155:183–186.

41. Bush CH, Gillespy T III, Dell PC. High-resolution CT of the wrist: initial experience with scaphoid disorders and surgical fusions. *AJR* 1987;149:757–760.

42. Campanacci M, Picci P, Gherlinzoni F, Guerra A, Bertoni F, Neff JR. Parosteal osteosarcoma. *J Bone Joint Surg* (Br) 1984;66(B): 313–321.

43. Carrera GF, Foley WD, Kozin F, Ryan L, Lawson TL. CT of sacroiliitis. *AJR* 1981;136:41–46.

44. Castor WR, Miller JDR, Russell AS, Chiu PL, Grace M, Hanson J. Computed tomography of the craniocervical junction in rheumatoid arthritis. *J Comput Assist Tomogr* 1983;7:31–36.

45. Chandnani VP, Beltran J, Morris CS, et al. Acute experimental osteomyelitis and abscesses: detection with MR imaging versus CT. *Radiology* 1990;174:233–236.

46. Chandnani VP, Gagliardi JA, Murnane TG, et al. Glenohumeral ligaments and shoulder capsular mechanism: evaluation with MR arthrography. *Radiology* 1995;196:27–32.

47. Christiansen EL, Thompson JR, Hasso AN, et al. CT number characteristics of malpositioned TMJ menisci. Diagnosis with CT number highlighting (blink-mode). *Invest Radiol* 1987;22:315–321.

48. Coffre C, Vanel D, Contesso G, et al. Problems and pitfalls in the use of computed tomography for the local evaluation of long bone osteosarcoma: a report on 30 cases. *Skeletal Radiol* 1985;13:147–153.

49. Cohen IJ, Hadar H, Schreiber R, et al. Primary bone tumor resectability: the value of serial MRI studies in the determination of the feasibility, timing, and extent of tumor resection. *J Pediatr Orthop* 1997;14:781–787.

50. Cohen JM, Weinreb JC, Redman HC. Arteriovenous malformations of the extremities: MR imaging. *Radiology* 1986;158:475–479.

51. Cohen MD, Weetman RM, Provisor AJ, et al. Efficacy of magnetic resonance imaging in 139 children with tumors. *Arch Surg* 1986; 121:522–529.

52. Coleman BG, Mulhern CB, Arger PH, et al. New observations of soft tissue sarcomas with contrast medium-enhanced computed tomography. *J Comput Tomogr* 1985;9:187–193.

53. Consensus conference. Limb-sparing treatment of adult soft-tissue sarcomas and osteosarcomas. *JAMA* 1985;254:1791–1794.

54. Corbett M, Levy A, Abramowitz AJ, et al. A computer tomographic classification system for the displaced intraarticular fracture of the os calcis. *Orthopedics* 1995;18:705–710.

55. Coumas JM, Waite RJ, Goss TP, et al. CT and MR evaluation of the labral capsular ligamentous complex of the shoulder. *AJR* 1992;158:591–597.

56. Crowninshield RD, Brand R, Johnston R, Milroy J. An analysis of femoral component stem design in total hip arthroplasty. *J Bone Joint Surg (Am)* 1980;62:68–78.

57. Daffner RH, Lupetin AR, Dash N, Deeb ZL, Sefczek RJ, Schapiro RL. MRI in the detection of malignant infiltration of bone marrow. *AJR* 1986;146:353–358.

58. Dawson EG, Clader TJ, Bassett LW. A comparison of different methods used to diagnose pseudarthrosis following posterior spinal fusion for scoliosis. *J Bone Joint Surg (Am)* 1985;67:1153–1159.

59. de Santos LA, Edeiken B. Purely lytic osteosarcoma. *Skeletal Radiol* 1982;9:1–7.

60. de Santos LA, Ginaldi S, Wallace S. Computed tomography in liposarcoma. *Cancer* 1981;47:46–54.

61. de Santos LA, Goldstein HM, Murray JA, Wallace S. Computed tomography in the evaluation of musculoskeletal neoplasms. *Radiology* 1978;128:89–94.

62. de Santos LA, Murray JA. Evaluation of giant cell tumor by computerized tomography. *Skeletal Radiol* 1978;2:205–212.

63. Destouet JM, Gilula LA, Murphy WA, et al. Computed tomography of the sternoclavicular joint and sternum. *Radiology* 1981; 138:123–128.

64. Destouet JM, Gilula LA, Murphy WA. Computed tomography of long-bone osteosarcoma. *Radiology* 1979;131:439–445.

65. Deutsch AL, Resnick D, Berman JL, et al. Computerized and conventional arthrography of the glenohumeral joint: normal anatomy and clinical experience. *Radiology* 1984;153:603–609.

66. Deutsch AL, Resnick D, Campbell G. Computed tomography and bone scintigraphy in the evaluation of tarsal coalition. *Radiology* 1982;144:137–140.

67. Deutsch AL, Resnick D, Mink HH. Computed tomography of the glenohumeral and sternoclavicular joints. *Orthop Clin North Am* 1985;16:497–511.

68. Dias JJ, Stirling AJ, Finlay DB, et al. Computerised axial tomography for tibial plateau fractures. *J Bone Joint Surg (Br)* 1987;69B: 84–88.

69. Dihlmann W. CT analysis of the upper end of the femur: the asterisk sign and ischaemic bone necrosis of the femoral head. *Skeletal Radiol* 1982;8:251–258.

70. Dooms GC, Fisher MR, Hricak H, Higgins CB. MR imaging of intramuscular hemorrhage. *J Comput Assist Tomogr* 1985;9:908–913.

71. Dooms GC, Hricak H, Sollitto RA, Higgins CB. Lipomatous tumors and tumors with fatty component: MR imaging potential and comparison of MR and CT results. *Radiology* 1985;157:479–483.

72. Dorfman HD, Bhagavan BS. Malignant fibrous histiocytoma of soft tissue with metaplastic bone and cartilage formation: a new radiologic sign. *Skeletal Radiol* 1982;8:145–150.

73. Eastwood DM, Gregg PJ, Atkins RM. Intra-articular fractures of the calcaneum. Part I: Pathological anatomy and classification (see comments). *J Bone Joint Surg (Br)* 1993;75B:183–188.

74. Ebraheim NA, Coombs R, Rusin JJ, et al. Reduction of postoperative CT artifacts of pelvic fractures by use of titanium implants. *Orthopedics* 1990;13:1357–1358.

75. Ebraheim NA, Skie MC, Podeszwa DA, et al. Evaluation of process fractures of the talus using computed tomography. *J Orthop Trauma* 1994;8:332–337.

76. Ebraheim NA, Zeiss J, Skie MC, et al. Marginal fractures of the lateral malleolus in association with other fractures in the ankle region. *Foot Ankle* 1992;13:171–175.

77. Ekelund L, Herrlin K, Rydholm A. Comparison of computed tomography and angiography in the evaluation of soft tissue tumors of the extremities. *Acta Radiol* 1982;23:15–28.

78. Engelstad BL, Gilula LA, Kyriakos M. Ossified skeletal muscle hemangioma: radiologic and pathologic features. *Skeletal Radiol* 1980;5:35–40.

79. Enneking WF, Chew FS, Springfield DS, Hudson TM, Spanier SS. The role of radionuclide bone-scanning in determining the resectability of soft-tissue sarcomas. *J Bone Joint Surg (AM)* 1981; 63A:249–257.

80. Enneking WF. Staging of musculoskeletal neoplasms. *Skeletal Radiol* 1985;13:183–194.

81. Epstein RE, Schweitzer ME, Frieman BG, et al. Hooked acromion: prevalence on MR images of painful shoulders. *Radiology* 1993; 187:479–481.

82. Essinger JR, Leyvraz PF, Heegard J, Robertson DD. A mathematical model for the evaluation of the behavior during flexion of condylar-type knee prostheses. *J Biomech* 1989;22:1229–1241.

83. Fairbairn KJ, Mulligan ME, Murphey MD, et al. Gas bubbles in the hip joint on CT: an indication of recent dislocation. *AJR* 1995; 164:931–934.

84. Ferries JS, DeCoster TA, Firoozbakhsh KK, et al. Plain radiographic interpretation in trimalleolar ankle fractures poorly assesses posterior fragment size. *J Orthop Trauma* 1994;8:328–331.

85. Firooznia H, Rafii M, Golimbu C, Lam S, Sokolow J, Kung JS. Computed tomography of pressure sores, pelvic abscess, and osteomyelitis in patients with spinal cord injury. *Arch Phys Med Rehabil* 1982;63:545–548.

86. Firooznia H, Rafii M, Golimbu C. Computed tomography of osteoid osteoma. *J Comput Assist Tomogr* 1985;9:265–268.

87. Fischer HJ, Lois JF, Gomes AS, Mirra JM, Deutsch L-S. Radiology and pathology of malignant fibrous histiocytomas of the soft tissues: a report of ten cases. *Skeletal Radiol* 1985;13:202–206.

88. Fishman EK, Magid D, Mandelbaum BR, et al. Multiplanar (MPR) imaging of the hip. *RadioGraphics* 1986;6:7–54.

89. Fishman EK, Magid D, Ney DR, et al. Three-dimensional imaging and display of musculoskeletal anatomy. *J Comput Assist Tomogr* 1988;12:465–467.

90. Fishman EK, Magid D, Ney DR, et al. Three-dimensional imaging. *Radiology* 1991;181:321–337.

91. Fishman EK, Magid D, Robertson DD, et al. Metallic hip implants: CT with multiplanar reconstruction. *Radiology* 1986;160:675–681.

92. Fishman EK, Wyatt SH, Bluemke DA, et al. Spiral CT of musculoskeletal pathology: preliminary observations. *Skeletal Radiol* 1993;22:253–256.

93. Fletcher BD, Scoles PV, Nelson AD. Osteomyelitis in children: detection by magnetic resonance (work in progress). *Radiology* 1984;150:57–60.

94. Floyd EJ, Ransom RA, Dailey JM. Computed tomography scanning of the subtalar joint. *J Am Podiatr Med Assoc* 1984;74:533–537.

95. Fordyce MJ, Solomon L. Early detection of avascular necrosis of the femoral head by MRI. *J Bone Joint Surg (Br)* 1993;75B:365–367.

96. Frassica FJ, Thompson RC Jr. Evaluation, diagnosis, and classification of benign soft-tissue tumors. *J Bone Joint Surg (Am)* 1996;78A:126–140.

97. Gagliardi JA, Chung EM, Chandnani VP, et al. Detection of chondromalacia patellae: relative efficacies of conventional MR imaging, MR arthrography, and CT arthrography. *AJR* 1994;163:629–636.

98. Garg A, Walker PS, Robertson DD. Theoretical model of knee kinematics using computer simulation. *Proc 11th International Congress Biomech* 1987;151.

99. Garg A. Effect of component design and surgical placement on the mechanics of total knee replacement. Ph.D. Thesis, Massachusetts Institute of Technology, Cambridge, MA 1988.

100. Gebhardt MC, Ready JE, Mankin HJ. Tumors about the knee in children. *Clin Orthop* 1990;255:86–110.

101. Ghelman B. Meniscal tears of the knee: evaluation by high resolution CT combined with arthrography. *Radiology* 1985;157:23–27.

102. Ghelman B. Three methods for determining anteversion and retroversion of a total hip prosthesis. *AJR* 1979;133:1127–1134.

103. Gilula LA, Murphy WA, Tailor CC, Patel RB. Computed tomography of the osseous pelvis. *Radiology* 1979;132:107–114.

104. Ginaldi S, de Santos LA. Computed tomography in the evaluation of small round cell tumors of bone. *Radiology* 1980;134:441–446.

105. Gitelis S, Wilkins R, Conrad EU III. Benign bone tumors. *J Bone Joint Surg (Am)* 1995;77A:1756–1782.

106. Glass RBJ, Poznanski AK, Fisher MR, Shkolnik A, Dias L. Case report. MR imaging of osteoid osteoma. *J Comput Assist Tomogr* 1986;10:1065–1067.

107. Glenn WV, Rhodes ML, Altschuler EM, et al. Multiplanar display computerized body tomography application in the lumbar spine. *Spine* 1979;4:282–352.

108. Glover GH, Pelc NJ. Non-linear partial volume artifacts in x-ray computed tomography. *Med Phys* 1980;7:238.

109. Gould R, Rosenfield AT, Friedlaender GE. Loose body within the glenohumeral joint in recurrent anterior dislocation: CT demonstration. *J Comput Assist Tomogr* 1985;9:404–406.

110. Grasso G, Andreoni A, Romeo N, et al. Recent developments in imaging diagnosis in fractures of the acetabulum: the role of CAT and tridimensional reconstruction. *Ital J Orthop Traumatol* 1990;16:79–91.

111. Greenfield GB, Arrington JA, Kudryk BT. MRI of soft tissue tumors. *Skeletal Radiol* 1993;22:77–84.

112. Gross AE, McKee NH, Farine I, et al. A biological approach to the restoration of skeletal continuity following en bloc excision of bone tumors. *Orthopedics* 1985;8:586–591.

113. Guilford WB, Mintz PD, Blatt PM, Staab EV. CT of hemophilic pseudotumors of the pelvis. *AJR* 1980;135:167–169.

114. Gusmer PB, Potter HG, Schatz JA, et al. Labral injuries: accuracy of detection with unenhanced MR imaging of the shoulder. *Radiology* 1996;200:519–524.

115. Guyer BH, Levinsohn EM, Fredrickson BE, et al. Computed tomography of calcaneal fractures: anatomy, pathology, dosimetry, and clinical relevance. *AJR* 1985;145:911–919.

116. Hall RB, Robinson LH, Malawar MM, Dunham WK. Periosteal osteosarcoma. *Cancer* 1985;55:165–171.

117. Hanna SL, Fletcher BD, Parham DM, Bugg MF. Muscle edema in musculoskeletal tumors: MR imaging characteristics and clinical significance. *J Magn Reson Imaging* 1991;1:441–449.

118. Hansen SJ. CT for pelvic fractures. *AJR* 1982;138:592–593.

119. Harbin WP. Metastatic disease and the nonspecific bone scan: value of spinal computed tomography. *Radiology* 1982;145:105–107.

120. Hatfield MK, Gross BH, Glazer GM, et al. Computed tomography of the sternum and its articulations. *Skeletal Radiol* 1984;11:197–203.

121. Hauman MT, Carlson GH. Three-dimensional computed tomography reconstruction. A presurgical adjunct in the severely traumatized rearfoot. *J Foot Ankle Surg* 1994;33:239–242.

122. Hauzeur JP, Pasteels JL, Schoutens A, et al. The diagnostic value of magnetic resonance imaging in non-traumatic osteonecrosis of the femoral head. *J Bone Joint Surg (Am)* 1989;71A:641–649.

123. Healey JH, Ghelman B. Osteoid osteoma and osteoblastoma. Current concepts and recent advances. *Clin Orthop* 1986;204:76–85.

124. Healey JH, Lane JM. Chondrosarcoma. *Clin Orthop* 1986;204:119–129.

125. Heger L, Wulff K, Seddiqi MS. Computed tomography of calcaneal fractures. *AJR* 1985;145:131–137.

126. Heiken JP, Lee JKT, Smathers RL, Totty WG, Murphy WA. CT of benign soft-tissue masses of the extremities. *AJR* 1984;142:575–580.

127. Heller M, Jend H-H, Bucheler E, Hueck E, Viehweger G. The role of CT in diagnosis and follow-up of osteosarcoma. *J Cancer Res Clin Oncol* 1983;106(suppl):43–48.

128. Helms CA, Cann CE, Brunelle FO, Gilula LA, Chafetz N, Genant HK. Detection of bone-marrow metastases using quantitative computed tomography. *Radiology* 1981;140:745–750.

129. Helms CA, Genant HK. Computed tomography in the early detection of skeletal involvement with multiple myeloma. *JAMA* 1982;248:2886–2887.

130. Helms CA, Jeffrey RB, Wing VW. Computed tomography and plain film appearance of a bony sequestration: significance and differential diagnosis. *Skeletal Radiol* 1987;16:117–120.

131. Helms CA, Kaplan P. Diagnostic imaging of the temporomandibular joint: recommendations for use of the various techniques. *AJR* 1990;154:319–322.

132. Helms CA, Vogler JB III, Morrish RB Jr, et al. Temporomandibular joint internal derangements: CT diagnosis. *Radiology* 1984;152:459–462.

133. Hermann G, Yeh H-C, Gilbert MS. Computed tomography and ultrasonography of the hemophilic pseudotumor and their use in surgical planning. *Skeletal Radiol* 1986;15:123–128.

134. Hermann G, Yeh H-C, Schwartz I. Computed tomography of soft-tissue lesions of the extremities, pelvic and shoulder girdles: sonographic and pathological correlations. *Clin Radiol* 1984;35:193–202.

135. Hernandez RJ, Conway JJ, Poznanski AK, Tachdjian MO, Dias LS, Kelikian AS. The role of computed tomography and radionuclide scintigraphy in the localization of osteomyelitis in flat bones. *J Pediatr Orthop* 1985;5:151–154.

136. Hernandez RJ, Poznanski AK. CT evaluation of pediatric hip disorders. *Orthop Clin North Am* 1985;16:513–541.

137. Hernandez RJ. Evaluation of congenital hip dysplasia and tibial torsion by computed tomography. *J Comput Assist Tomogr* 1983;7:101–108.

138. Hertzanu Y, Glass RBJ, Mendelsohn DB. Sacrococcygeal chordoma in young adults. *Clin Radiol* 1983;34:327–329.

139. Heuchemer T, Bargon G, Bauer G, et al. Advantages in the diagnosis and classification of intra-articular fractures of the calcaneus

using computed tomography (German). *Rofo Fortschr Geb Rontgenstr Neuen Bildgeb Verfahr* 1988;149:8–14.

140. Hinderling R, Rüegsegger P, Anliker M, Dietschi C. Computed tomography reconstruction from hollow projections: an application to in vivo evaluation of artificial hip joints. *J Comput Assist Tomogr* 1979;3:52–57.

141. Hindman BW, Ross SD, Sowerby MR. Fractures of the talus and calcaneus: evaluation by computed tomography. *J Computed Assist Tomogr* 1986;10:191–196.

142. Hodge JC, Ghelman B, O'Brien SJ, et al. Synovial plicae and chondromalacia patellae: correlation of results of CT arthrography with results of arthroscopy. *Radiology* 1993;186:827–831.

143. Holt MD, Williams LA, Dent CM. MRI in the management of tibial plateau fractures. *Injury* 1995;26:595–599.

144. Hudson TM, Galceran M. Radiology of sacrococcygeal chordoma—difficulties in detecting soft tissue extension. *Clin Orthop* 1983;175:237–242.

145. Hudson TM, Hamlin DJ, Fitzsimmons JR. Magnetic resonance imaging of fluid levels in an aneurysmal bone cyst and in anticoagulated human blood. *Skeletal Radiol* 1985;13:267–270.

146. Hudson TM, Hawkins IF. Radiological evaluation of chondroblastoma. *Radiology* 1981;139:1–10.

147. Hudson TM, Manaster BJ, Springfield DS, Spanier SS, Enneking WF, Hawkins IF Jr. Radiology of medullary chondrosarcoma: preoperative treatment planning. *Skeletal Radiol* 1983;10:69–78.

148. Hudson TM, Schakel M II, Springfield DS, Spanier SS, Enneking WF. The comparative value of bone scintigraphy and computed tomography in determining bone involvement by soft-tissue sarcomas. *J Bone Joint Surg (Am)* 1984;66A:1400–1407.

149. Hudson TM, Schakel M II, Springfield DS. Limitations of computed tomography following excisional biopsy of soft tissue sarcomas. *Skeletal Radiol* 1985;13:49–54.

150. Hudson TM, Schiebler M, Springfield DS, Enneking WF, Hawkins IF Jr, Spanier SS. Radiology of giant cell tumors of bone: computed tomography, arthro-tomography, and scintigraphy. *Skeletal Radiol* 1984;11:85–95.

151. Hudson TM, Schiebler M, Springfield DS, Hawkins IF Jr, Enneking WF, Spanier SS. Radiologic imaging of osteosarcoma: role in planning surgical treatment. *Skeletal Radiol* 1983;10:137–146.

152. Hudson TM, Springfield DS, Benjamin M, Bertoni F, Present DA. Computed tomography of parosteal osteosarcoma. *AJR* 1985;144:961–965.

153. Hudson TM, Springfield DS, Spanier SS, Enneking WF, Hamlin DJ. Benign exostoses and exostotic chondrosarcomas: evaluation of cartilage thickness by CT. *Radiology* 1984;152:595–599.

154. Hudson TM, Vandergriend RA, Springfield DS, et al. Aggressive fibromatosis: evaluation by computed tomography and angiography. *Radiology* 1984;150:495–501.

155. Hudson TM. Fluid levels in aneurysmal bone cysts: a CT feature. *AJR* 1984;141:1001–1004.

156. Huiskes R, Chao E. A survey of finite element analysis in orthopedic biomechanics. *J Biomech* 1983;16:385–409.

157. Huiskes R, Vroeman W. A standardized finite element model for routine comparative evaluations of femoral hip prostheses. *Acta Orthop Belg* 1986;52:258–261.

158. Hunter JC, Johnston WH, Genant HK. Computed tomography evaluation of fatty tumors of the somatic soft tissues: clinical utility and radiologic-pathologic correlation. *Skeletal Radiol* 1979;4:79–91.

159. James SE, Richards R, McGrouther DA. Three-dimensional CT imaging of the wrist. A practical system. *J Hand Surg (Br)* 1992;17B:504–506.

160. Janzen DL, Connell DG, Munk PL, et al. Intraarticular fractures of the calcaneus: value of CT findings in determining prognosis. *AJR* 1992;158:1271–1274.

161. Jelinek JS, Kransdorf MJ, Utz JA, et al. Imaging of pigmented villonodular synovitis with emphasis on MR imaging. *AJR* 1989;152:337–342.

162. Joseph PM, Spital RD. A method for correcting bone induced artifacts in computed tomography scanners. *J Comput Assist Tomogr* 1978;2:100–108.

163. Joseph PM, Spital RD. The effects of scatter in x-ray computed tomography. *Med Phys* 1982;9:464.

164. Joseph PM, Spital RD. The exponential edge-gradient effect in x-ray computed tomography. *Phys Med Biol* 1981;26:473.

165. Jurik AG, Albrechtsen J. The use of computed tomography with two- and three-dimensional reconstructions in the diagnosis of three- and four-part fractures of the proximal humerus. *Clin Radiol* 1994;49:800–804.

166. Kälebo P, Swärd L, Karlsson J, et al. Ultrasonography in the detection of partial patellar ligament ruptures (jumper's knee). *Skeletal Radiol* 1991;20:285–289.

167. Kalender WA, Hebel R, Ebersberger J. Reduction of CT artifacts caused by metallic implants. *Radiology* 1987;164:576–577.

168. Kalender WA, Perman W, Vetter J, Klotz E. Evaluation of a prototype-dual-energy computed tomographic apparatus. I. Phantom studies. *Med Phys* 1986;13:334–339.

169. Kaplan PA, Williams SM. Mucocutaneous and peripheral soft-tissue hemangiomas: MR imaging. *Radiology* 1987;163:163–166.

170. Kavanagh BF, Bradway JK, Cofield RH. Open reduction and internal fixation of displaced intra-articular fractures of the glenoid fossa. *J Bone Joint Surg (Am)* 1993;75A:479–484.

171. Kellam JF, Messer A. Evaluation of the role of coronal and sagittal axial CT scan reconstructions for the imaging of acetabular fractures. *Clin Orthop* 1994;305:152–159.

172. Kenney PJ, Gilula LA, Murphy WA. The use of computed tomography to distinguish osteochondroma and chondrosarcoma. *Radiology* 1981;139:129–137.

173. Khouri N, Ducloyer P, Carlioz H. Triplane fractures of the tibia. Apropos of 25 cases and general review. (Review) (French). *Rev Chir Orthop* 1989;75:394–404.

174. Klotz E, Kalender WA, Sokiranski R, Felsenberg D. Algorithms for the reduction of CT artifacts by metallic implants. In: Dwyer SJ, Jost RG, eds. *Medical imaging IV: PACS systems design and evaluation.* SPIE 1234, Bellingham, 1990;624–650.

175. Kode L, Lieberman JM, Motta AO, et al. Evaluation of tibial plateau fractures: efficacy of MR imaging compared with CT. *AJR* 1994;163:141–147.

176. Kottal RA, Vogler JB III, Matamoros A, Alexander AH, Cookson JL. Pigmented villonodular synovitis: a report of MR imaging in two cases. *Radiology* 1987;163:551–553.

177. Koval KJ, Sanders R. The radiologic evaluation of calcaneal fractures. *Clin Orthop* 1993;290:41–46.

178. Kozin F, Carrera GF, Ryan LM, et al. Computed tomography in the diagnosis of sacroiliitis. *Arthritis Rheum* 1981;24:1479–1485.

179. Kuhlman JE, Fishman EK, Ney DR, et al. Two-and three-dimensional imaging of the painful shoulder. *Orthop Rev* 1989;18:1201–1208.

180. Kuhn JP, Berger PE. Computed tomographic diagnosis of osteomyelitis. *Radiology* 1979;130:503–506.

181. Kurosawa H, Walker P, Abe S, Gara A, Hunter T. Geometry and motion of the knee for implant and orthotic design. *J Biomech* 1985;18:487–499.

182. Kuszyk BS, Fishman EK. Direct coronal CT of the wrist: helical acquisition with simplified patient positioning. *AJR* 1996;166:419–420.

183. Laasonen EM, Jokie P, Lindholm TS. Tibial torsion measured by computed tomography. *Acta Radiol Diagn* 1984;25:325–329.

184. Lange TA, Alter AJ. Evaluation of complex acetabular fractures by computed tomography. *J Comput Assist Tomogr* 1980;4:849–852.

185. Lange TA, Austin CW, Seibert JJ, Angtuaco TL, Yandow DR. Ultrasound imaging as a screening study for malignant soft-tissue tumors. *J Bone Joint Surg (Am)* 1987;69A:100–115.

186. Lee KR, Cox GG, Neff JR, Arnett GR, Murphey MD. Cystic masses of the knee: arthrographic and CT evaluation. *AJR* 1987;148:329–334.

187. Lee KR, Tines SC, Yoon JW. CT findings of suprapatellar synovial cysts. *J Comput Assist Tomogr* 1984;8:296–299.

188. Leeson MC, Kay D, Smith BS. Intraosseous lipoma. *Clin Orthop* 1983;181:186–190.

189. Leitch JM, Cundy PJ, Paterson DC. Three-dimensional imaging of a juvenile Tillaux fracture. *J Pediatr Orthop* 1989;9:602–603.

190. Lemerle R, Zucman J, Montagliari C, et al. X-ray computed tomography in the study of fractures of the calcaneus. (Review) *Rev Chir Orthop* 1988;74:378–390.

191. Letournel E. Fractures of the acetabulum. A study of a series of 75 cases. *Clin Orthop* 1994;305:5–9.

192. Levin DN, Herrmann A, Spraggins T, et al. Musculoskeletal tumors: improved depiction with linear combinations of MR images. *Radiology* 1987;163:545–549.

193. Levine E, De Smet AA, Neff JR. Role of radiologic imaging in management planning of giant cell tumor of bone. *Skeletal Radiol* 1984;12:79–89.

194. Levine E, Lee KR, Neff JR, Maklad NF, Robinson RG, Preston DF. Comparison of computed tomography and other imaging modalities in the evaluation of musculoskeletal tumors. *Radiology* 1979;131:431–437.

195. Levine E, Neff JR. Dynamic computed tomography scanning of benign bone lesions: preliminary results. *Skeletal Radiol* 1983;9:238–245.

196. Levine E, Wetzel LH, Neff JR. MR imaging and CT of extrahepatic cavernous hemangiomas. *AJR* 1986;147:1299–1304.

197. Levy RA, Rosenbaum AE, Kellman RM, et al. Assessing whether the plane of section on CT affects accuracy in demonstrating facial fractures in 3-D reconstruction when using a dried skull. *Am J Neuroradiol* 1991;12:861–866.

198. Lindell MM Jr, Shirkhoda A, Raymond AK, Murray JA, Harle TS. Parosteal osteosarcoma: radiologic-pathologic correlation with emphasis on CT. *AJR* 1987;148:323–328.

199. Lopez M, Sauerbrei E. Septic arthritis of the hip joint: sonographic and CT findings. *Can Assoc Radiol J* 1985;36:322–324.

200. Lorigan JG, Libshitz HI, Peuchot M. Radiation-induced sarcoma of bone: CT findings in 19 cases. *AJR* 1989;153:791–794.

201. Lorigan JG, O'Keeffe FN, Evans HL, Wallace S. The radiologic manifestations of alveolar soft-part sarcoma. *AJR* 1989;153:335–339.

202. Lowrie IG, Finlay DB, Brenkel IJ, et al. Computerised tomographic assessment of the subtalar joint in calcaneal fractures. *J Bone Joint Sur (Br)* 1988;70B:247–250.

203. Magid D, Fishman EK, Brooker AJ, et al. Multiplanar computed tomography of acetabular fractures. *J Comput Assist Tomogr* 1986;10:778–783.

204. Magid D, Fishman EK, Ney DR, et al. Acetabular and pelvic fractures in the pediatric patient: value of two- and three-dimensional imaging. *J Pediatr Orthop* 1992;12:621–625.

205. Magid D, Fishman EK, Scott WW Jr, et al. Femoral head avascular necrosis: CT assessment with multiplanar reconstruction. *Radiology* 1985;157:751–756.

206. Magid D, Fishman EK. Imaging of musculoskeletal trauma in three dimensions. An integrated two-dimensional/three-dimensional approach with computed tomography. *Radiol Clin North Am* 1989;27:945–956.

207. Magid D, Michelson JD, Ney DR, et al. Adult ankle fractures: comparison of plain films and interactive two- and three-dimensional CT scans. *AJR* 1990;154:1017–1023.

208. Magid D. Computed tomographic imaging of the musculoskeletal system. Current status. (Review). *Radiol Clin North Am* 1994;32:255–274.

209. Mahboubi S, Horstmann H. Femoral torsion: CT measurement. *Radiology* 1986;160:843–844.

210. Mainwaring BL, Daffner RH, Riemer BL. Pylon fractures of the ankle: a distinct clinical and radiologic entity. *Radiology* 1988;168:215–218.

211. Manaster BJ. Musculoskeletal oncologic imaging. *Int J Radiat Oncol Biol Phys* 1991;21:1643–1651.

212. Mandelbaum BR, Magid D, Fishman EK, et al. Multiplanar computed tomography: a multidimensional tool for evaluation and treatment of acetabular fractures. *J Comput Assist Tomogr* 1987;11:167–173.

213. Mankin HJ, Gebhardt MC. Advances in the management of bone tumors. *Clin Orthop* 1985;200:73–84.

214. Mann FA, Murphy WA, Totty WG. MRI of peripheral nerve sheath tumors: assessment by numerical fuzzy cluster analysis. *Invest Radiol* 1990;25:1238–1245.

215. Mantravadi RVP, Trippon MJ, Patel MK, Walker MJ, Das Gupta TK. Limb salvage in extremity soft-tissue sarcoma: combined modality therapy. *Radiology* 1984;152:523–526.

216. Manzione JV, Katzberg RW, Brodsky GL, et al. Internal derangements of the temporomandibular joint: diagnosis by direct sagittal computed tomography. *Radiology* 1984;150:111–115.

217. Martinez CR, Di PT, Helfet DL, et al. Evaluation of acetabular fractures with two- and three-dimensional CT. (Review). *RadioGraphics* 1992;12:227–242.

218. Martinez S, Herzenberg JE, Apple JS. Computed tomography of the hindfoot. *Orthop Clin North Am* 1985;16:481–496.

219. Martinez S, Korobkin M, Fondren FB, et al. Computed tomography of the normal patellofemoral joint. *Invest Radiol* 1983;18:249–253.

220. Massengill AD, Seeger LL, Eckardt JJ. The role of plain radiography, computed tomography, and magnetic resonance imaging in sarcoma evaluation. *Hematol Oncol Clin North Am* 1995;9:571–604.

221. Mazanet R, Antman KH. Sarcomas of soft tissue and bone. *Cancer* 1991;68:463–473.

222. McEnery KW, Wilson AJ, Murphy WJ. Comparison of spiral computed tomography versus conventional computed tomography multiplanar reconstructions of a fracture displacement phantom. *Invest Radiol* 1994;29:665–670.

223. McEnery KW, Wilson AJ, Pilgram TK, et al. Fractures of the tibial plateau: value of spiral CT coronal plane reconstructions for detecting displacement in vitro. *AJR* 1994;163:1177–1181.

224. Merine D, Fishman EK, Magid D. CT detection of sacral osteomyelitis associated with pelvic abscesses. *J Comput Assist Tomogr* 1988;12:118–121.

225. Michelson JD, Magid D, Ney DR, et al. Examination of the pathologic anatomy of ankle fractures. *J Trauma* 1992;32:65–70.

226. Miller MD, Ragsdale BD, Sweet DE. Posteal lipomas: a new perspective. *Pathology* 1992;24:132–139.

227. Mittlmeier T, Morlock MM, Hertlein H, et al. Analysis of morphology and gait function after intraarticular calcaneal fracture. *J Orthop Trauma* 1993;7:303–310.

228. Modic MT, Feiglin DH, Piraino DW, et al. Vertebral osteomyelitis: assessment using MR. *Radiology* 1985;157:157–166.

229. Modic MT, Pavlicek W, Weinstein MA, et al. Magnetic resonance imaging of intervertebral disk disease: clinical and pulse sequence considerations. *Radiology* 1984;152:103–111.

230. Modic MT, Pflanze W, Feiglin DHI, Behlobek G. Magnetic resonance imaging of musculoskeletal infections. *Radiol Clin North Am* 1986;24:247–258.

231. Monu JUV, Pope TL, Chabon SJ, et al. MR diagnosis of superior labral anterior posterior (SLAP) injuries of the glenoid labrum: value of routine imaging without intraarticular injection of contrast material. *AJR* 1994;163:1425–1429.

232. Moore TM, Patzakis MJ, Harvey JP. Tibial plateau fractures: definition, demographics, treatment rationale, and long-term results of closed traction management or operative reduction. *J Orthop Trauma* 1987;1:97–119.

233. Morgan GJ, Schlegelmilch JG, Spiegel PK. Early diagnosis of septic arthritis of the sacroiliac joint by use of computed tomography. *J Rheumatol* 1981;8:979–982.

234. Moser RP Jr, Kransdorf MJ, Gilkey FW, Manaster BJ. Giant cell tumor of the upper extremity. *RadioGraphics* 1990;10:83–102.

235. Moser RP, Madewell JE. An approach to primary bone tumors. *Radiol Clin North Am* 1987;25:1049–1093.

236. Muller A, Ruegsegger P. Optimal settings for the evaluation of perimenopausal bone loss. *J Comput Assist Tomogr* 1985;9:607–608.

237. Murphey MD, Fairbairn KJ, Parman LM, Baxter KG, Parsa MB, Smith WS. Musculoskeletal angiomatous lesions: radiologic-pathologic correlation. *RadioGraphics* 1995;15:893–917.

238. Murphy S, Kijewski P, Millis M, et al. The planning of orthopedic reconstructive surgery using computer-aided simulation and design. *Comput Med Imaging Graph* 1988;12:33–45.

239. Murphy WA Jr. Imaging bone tumors in the 1990s. *Cancer* 1991;67:1169–1176.

240. Murphy WA, Totty WG. Musculoskeletal magnetic resonance imaging. In: Kressel HY, ed. *Magnetic resonance annual 1986.* New York: Raven Press, 1986:1–35.

241. Nerubay J, Rubinstein Z, Katznelsons A. Technique of building a hemipelvic prothesis using computer tomography. *Prog Clin Biol Res* 1981;99:147–152.

242. Neuhold A, Stiskal M, Kainberger F, et al. Degenerative Achilles

tendon disease: assessment by magnetic resonance and ultrasonography. *Eur J Radiol* 1992;14:213–220.

243. Newberg AH. Computed tomography of joint injuries. (Review). *Radiol Clin North Am* 1990;28:445–460.

244. Ney DR, Fishman EK, Kawashima A, et al. Comparison of helical and serial CT with regard to three-dimensional imaging of musculoskeletal anatomy. *Radiology* 1992;185:865–869.

245. Ney DR, Fishman EK, Magid D, et al. Interactive real-time multiplanar CT imaging. *Radiology* 1989;170:275–276.

246. Ney DR, Fishman EK, Magid D, et al. Three-dimensional volumetric display of CT data: effect of scan parameters upon image quality. *J Comput Assist Tomogr* 1991;15:875–885.

247. Niggebrugge AH, van Heusden HH, Bode PJ, van Vugt AB. Dislocated intra-articular fracture of anterior rim of glenoid treated by open reduction and internal fixation. *Injury* 1993;24:130–131.

248. Nimityongskul P, Hudgens RA, Anderson LD, et al. Ultrasonography in the management of developmental dysplasia of the hip (DDH). *J Pediatr Orthop* 1995;15:741–746.

249. Okada K, Frassica FJ, Sim FH, Beabout JW, Bond JR, Unni KK. Parosteal osteosarcoma. A clinicopathological study. *J Bone Joint Surg (Am)* 1994;76A:366–378.

250. Panicek DM, Gatsonis C, Rosenthal DI, et al. CT and MR imaging in the local staging of primary malignant musculoskeletal neoplasms: report of the radiology diagnostic oncology group. *Radiology* 1997;202:237–246.

251. Passariello R, Trecco F, de Paulis F, et al. Meniscal lesions of the knee joint: CT diagnosis. *Radiology* 1985;157:29–34.

252. Patel RB, Barton P, Green L. CT of isolated elbow in evaluation of trauma: a modified technique. *Comput Radiol* 1984;8:1–4.

253. Peh WCG, Farmer THR, Totty WG. Acromial arch shape: assessment with MR imaging. *Radiology* 1995;195:501–505.

254. Penkava RR. Iliopsoas bursitis demonstrated by computed tomography. *AJR* 1980;135:175–176.

255. Petasnick JP, Turner DA, Charters JR, Gitelis S, Zacharias CE. Soft-tissue masses of the locomotor system: comparison of MR imaging with CT. *Radiology* 1986;160:125–133.

256. Pettersson H, Eliasson J, Egund N, et al. Gadolinium-DTPA enhancement of soft tissue tumors in magnetic resonance imaging-preliminary clinical experience in five patients. *Skeletal Radiol* 1988;17:319–323.

257. Poletti SC, Gates HS III, Martinez SM, Richardson WJ. The use of magnetic resonance imaging in the diagnosis of pigmented villonodular synovitis. *Orthopedics* 1990;13:185–190.

258. Poss R, Robertson DD, Walker PS, et al. Anatomic stem design for press-fit and cemented application. In: Fitzgerald RH, ed. *Noncemented total hip arthroplasty.* New York: Raven Press, 1988; 343–363.

259. Potter HG, Montgomery KD, Heise CW, et al. MR imaging of acetabular fractures: value in detecting femoral head injury, intraarticular fragments, and sciatic nerve injury. *AJR* 1994;163:881–886.

260. Pretorius ES, Fishman EK. Helical (spiral) CT of the musculoskeletal system (review). *Radiol Clin North Am* 1995;33:949–979.

261. Pritchard RS, Shah HR, Nelson CL, FitzRandolph RL. MR and CT appearance of iliopsoas bursal distention secondary to diseased hips. *J Comput Assist Tomogr* 1990;14:797–800.

262. Quinn SF, Sheley RC, Demlow TA, et al. Rotator cuff tendon tears: evaluation with fat-suppressed MR imaging with arthroscopic correlation in 100 patients. *Radiology* 1995;195:497–501.

263. Quint LE, Gross BH, Glazer GM, Braunstein EM, White SJ. CT evaluation of chondroblastoma. *J Comput Assist Tomogr* 1984;8:907–910.

264. Rafii M, Firooznia H, Golimbu C, et al. Computed tomography of tibial plateau fractures. *AJR* 1984;142:1181–1184.

265. Rafii M, Firooznia H, Golimbu C, et al. CT arthrography of capsular structures of the shoulder. *AJR* 1986;146:361–367.

266. Rafii M, Firooznia H, Golimbu C, et al. The impact of CT in clinical management of pelvic and acetabular fractures. *Clin Orthop* 1983;178:228–235.

267. Rafii M, Firooznia H, Golimbu C. Computed tomography of septic joints. *J Comput Assist Tomogr* 1985;9:51–60.

268. Rafii M, Firooznia H, Sherman O, et al. Rotator cuff lesions: signal patterns at MR imaging. *Radiology* 1990;177:817–823.

269. Ram PC, Martinez S, Korobkin M, Breiman RS, Gallis HR, Harrel-

son JM. CT detection of intraosseous gas: a new sign of osteomyelitis. *AJR* 1981;137:721–723.

270. Ramos A, Castello J, Sartoris DJ, Greenway GD, Resnick D, Haghighi P. Osseous lipoma: CT appearance. *Radiology* 1985;157:615–619.

271. Rapperport D, Carter D, Shurman D. Contact finite element analysis of porous ingrowth acetabular cup implantation, ingrowth, and loosening. *J Orthop Res* 1987;5:548–561.

272. Raskin RJ, Schnapf DJ, Wolf CR, et al. Computerized tomography in evaluation of atlantoaxial subluxation in rheumatoid arthritis. *J Rheumatol* 1983;10:33–41.

273. Raymond AK, Surface osteosarcoma. *Clin Orthop* 1991;270:140–148.

274. Reiser M, Rupp N, Biehl TH, et al. MR in diagnosis of bone tumours. *Eur J Radiol* 1985;5:1–7.

275. Reiser M, Rupp N, Heller HJ, et al. MR-tomography in the diagnosis of malignant soft-tissue tumours. *Eur J Radiol* 1984;4:288–293.

276. Reuben J, Rovick J, Walker P, Schrager R. Three-dimensional kinematics of normal and cruciate deficient knees—a dynamic invitro experiment. *Trans Orthop Res Soc* 1986 II:385.

277. Rhodes ML, Azzawi Y, Chu E, Glenn W, Rothman S. Anatomic model and prostheses manufacturing using CT data. *Proc Conf Expo NCGA,* 1985; pp. 110–124.

278. Rhodes ML, Glenn WV, Azzawi YM. Extracting oblique planes from serial CT sections. *J Comput Assist Tomgr* 1980;4:649–657.

279. Rizzo PF, Gould ES, Lyden JP, et al. Diagnosis of occult fractures about the hip. Magnetic resonance imaging compared with bonescanning (see comments). *J Bone Joint Surgery (Am)* 1993;75A:395–401.

280. Roberts D, Schenck J, Joseph P, et al. Temporomandibular joint: magnetic resonance imaging. *Radiology* 1985;155:829–830.

281. Robertson DD, Essinger J, Imura S. Femoral deformity in adults with developmental hip dysplasia. *Clin Orthop* 1996;327:196–206.

282. Robertson DD, Huang HK. Quantitative bone measurements using x-ray computed tomography with second-order correction. *Med Phys* 1986;13:474–479.

283. Robertson DD, Magid D, Poss R, Fishman EK, Brooker AF, Sledge CB. Enhanced computed tomographic techniques for the evaluation of total hip arthroplasty. *J Arthroplasty* 1989;4:271–276.

284. Robertson DD, Seeger L, Mankovich N. The use of CAD/CAM in hip arthroplasty. In: *Hip Arthroplasty,* Amstutz H. ed., New York: Churchill-Livinstone, Inc., (in press).

285. Robertson DD, Walker PS, Fishman E, et al. The application of advanced CT imaging and computer graphics to reconstruction surgery of the hip. *Orthopedics* 1989;12:661–667.

286. Robertson DD, Walker PS, Granholm JW, et al. Design of custom hip stem prostheses using three-dimensional CT modeling. *J Comput Assist Tomogr* 1987;11:804–809.

287. Robertson DD, Walker PS, Hirano SK, Zhou XM, Granholm JW, Poss R. Improving the fit of press-fit hip stems. *Clin Orthop* 1988;228:134–140.

288. Robertson DD, Weiss PJ, Fishman EK, Magid D, Walker PS. Evaluation of CT techniques for reducing artifacts in the presence of metallic orthopedic implants. *J Comput Assist Tomogr* 1988;12:236–241.

289. Robertson DD, Yuan J, Wang G, Vannier MW. Total hip prosthesis metal-artifact suppression using iterative deblurring reconstruction. *J Comput Assist Tomogr* 1997;21:293–298.

290. Rosen RA, Morehouse HT, Karp HJ, Yu GSM. Intracortical fissuring in osteomyelitis. *Radiology* 1981;141:17–20.

291. Rosen RC, Anania WC, Chinkes SL, Gerland JS. Utilization of computerized tomography in osteomyelitis of the foot. A case report. *J Am Podiatr Med Assoc* 1987;77:85–88.

292. Rosenberg D, Baskies AM, Deckers PJ, Leiter BE, Ordia JI, Jablon IG. Pyogenic sacroiliitis: an absolute indication for computerized tomographic scanning. *Clin Orthop* 1984;184:128–132.

293. Rosenberg ZS, Feldman F, Singson RD. Intra-articular calcaneal fractures: computed tomographic analysis. *Skeletal Radiol* 1987;16:105–113.

294. Rosenthal DI, Aronow S, Murray WT. Iron content of pigmented

villonodular synovitis detected by computed tomography. *Radiology* 1979;133:409–411.

295. Rosenthal DI, Schiller AL, Mankin HJ. Chondrosarcoma: correlation of radiological and histological grade. *Radiology* 1984;150:21–26.

296. Rosenthal DI, Scott JA, Mankin HJ, Wismer GL, Brady TJ. Sacrococcygeal chordoma: magnetic resonance imaging and computed tomography. *AJR* 1985;145:143–147.

297. Rosenthal DI, Stauffer AE, Davis KR, et al. Evaluation of multiplanar reconstruction in CT recognition of lumbar disk disease. *AJR* 1984;143:169–176.

298. Rosenthal DI. Computed tomography in bone and soft tissue neoplasm: application and pathologic correlation. *Crit Rev Diagn Imaging* 1982;18:243–278.

299. Rothman SL, Glenn W, Rhodes M, Bruce R, Pratt C. Individualized prosthesis production from routine CT data. *Radiology* 1985;157(P):177.

300. Rougraff BT, Simon MA, Kneisl JS, Greenberg DB, Mankin HJ. Limb salvage compared with amputation for osteosarcoma of the distal end of the femur. *J Bone Joint Surg (Am)* 1994;76A:649–656.

301. Rowell D, Mann R, Hodge A. A computer-aided surgical simulation of femoral and tibial osteotomy. *J Rehabil Res Dev* 1989;26:261–262.

302. Rubenstein J, Kellam J, McGonigal D. Acetabular fracture assessment with computerized tomography. *Can Assoc Radiol J* 1982;33:139–141.

303. Rubin JI, Gomori JM, Grossman RI, Gefter WB, Kressel HY. High-field MR imaging of extracranial hematomas. *AJR* 1987;148:813–817.

304. Saks BJ. Normal acetabular anatomy for acetabular fracture assessment: CT and plain film correlation. *Radiology* 1986;159:139–145.

305. Sanchez RB, Quinn SF, Walling A, Estrada J, Greenberg H. Musculoskeletal neoplasms after intraarterial chemotherapy: correlation of MR images with pathologic specimens. *Radiology* 1990;174:237–240.

306. Sanders R, Gregory P. Operative treatment of intra-articular fractures of the calcaneus. *Orthop Clin North Am* 1995;26:203–214.

307. Sanders R. Intra-articular fractures of the calcaneus: present state of the art. (Review). *J Orthop Trauma* 1992;6:252–265.

308. Sanders WE. Evaluation of the humpback scaphoid by computed tomography in the longitudinal axial plane of the scaphoid. *J Hand Surg (Am)* 1988;13:182–187.

309. Sarno RC, Carter BL, Bankhoff MS, et al. Computed tomography in tarsal coalition. *J Comput Assist Tomogr* 1984;8:1155–1160.

310. Sartoris DJ, Danzig L, Gilula L, et al. Synovial cysts of the hip joint and iliopsoas bursitis: a spectrum of imaging abnormalities. *Skeletal Radiol* 1985;14:85–94.

311. Sartoris DJ, Devine S, Resnick D, et al. Plantar compartmental infection in the diabetic foot. The role of computed tomography. *Invest Radiol* 1985;20:772–784.

312. Sartoris DJ, Kursunoglu S, Pineda C, et al. Detection of intra-articular osteochondral bodies in the knee using computed arthrotomography. *Radiology* 1985;155:447–450.

313. Sartoris DJ, Neumann CH, Riley RW. The temporomandibular joint: true sagittal computed tomography with meniscus visualization. *Radiology* 1984;150:250–254.

314. Sartoris DJ. The role of radiology in orthopaedic sepsis. *Orthop Rev* 1987;16:109–124.

315. Sauser DD, Billimoria PE, Rouse GA, et al. CT evaluation of hip trauma. *AJR* 1980;135:269–274.

316. Schnarkowski P, Redei J, Peterfy CG, et al. Tibial shaft fractures: assessment of fracture healing with computed tomography. *J Comput Assist Tomogr* 1995;19:777–781.

317. Scholten ET, van derLande BA, Willemse AP, et al. Computed tomography with multiplanar reconstruction of acetabular fractures. *Diagn Imaging Clin Med* 1986;55:203–209.

318. Schreiman JS, Crass JR, Wick MR, Maile CW, Thompson RC. Osteosarcoma: role of CT in limb-sparing treatment. *Radiology* 1986;161:485–488.

319. Schreiman JS, McLeod RA, Kyle RA, Beabout JW. Multiple myeloma: evaluation by CT. *Radiology* 1985;154:483–486.

320. Schubiner JM, Simon MA. Primary bone tumors in children. *Orthop Clin North Am* 1987;18:577–595.

321. Schwartz HS, Unni KK, Pritchard DJ. Pigmented villonodular synovitis. A retrospective review of affected large joints. *Clin Orthop* 1989;247:243–255.

322. Schwartz ML, Al-Zahrani S, Morwessel RM, et al. Ulnar collateral ligament injury in the throwing athlete: evaluation with saline-enhanced MR arthrography. *Radiology* 1995;197:297–299.

323. Schwimmer M, Edelstein G, Heiken JP, Gilula LA. Synovial cysts of the knee: CT evaluation. *Radiology* 1985;154:175–177.

324. Seeger LL, Gold RH, Chandnani VP. Diagnostic imaging of osteosarcoma. *Clin Orthop* 1991;270:254–263.

325. Segal D, Marsh JL, Leiter B. Clinical application of computerized axial tomography (CAT) scanning of calcaneus fractures. *Clin Orthop* 1985;199:114–123.

326. Seitz P, Rüegsegger P. Anchorage of femoral implants visualized by modified computed tomography. *Arch Orthop Trauma Surg* 1982;100:261–266.

327. Seitz P, Rüegsegger P. CT bone densitometry of the anchor-age of artificial knee joints. *J Comput Assist Tomogr* 1985;9:621–622.

328. Seitz WJ, LaPorte J. Medial triplane fracture delineated by computerized axial tomography. *J Pediatr Orthop* 1988;8:65–66.

329. Seltzer SE. Value of computed tomography in planning medical and surgical treatment of chronic osteomyelitis. *J Comput Assist Tomogr* 1984;8:482–487.

330. Shapeero LG, Dye SF, Lipton MJ, et al. Functional dynamics of the knee joint by ultrafast, cine-CT. *Invest Radiol* 1988;23:118–123.

331. Shih LY, Chen TS, Lo WH. Limb salvage surgery for locally aggressive and malignant bone tumors. *J Surg Oncol* 1993;53:154–160.

332. Shirkhoda A, Brashear HR, Staab EV. Computed tomography of acetabular fractures. *Radiology* 1980;134:683–688.

333. Simon MA, Finn HA. Diagnostic strategy for bone and soft-tissue tumors. *J Bone Joint Surg (Am)* 1993;75A:622–631.

334. Singson RD, Feldman F, Rosenberg ZS. Elbow joint: assessment with double-contrast CT arthrography. *Radiology* 1986;160:167–173.

335. Solomon MA, Gilula LA, Oloff LM, et al. CT scanning of the foot and ankle. 1. Normal anatomy. *AJR* 1986;146:1192–1203.

336. Solomon MA, Gilula LA, Oloff LM, et al. CT scanning of the foot and ankle. 2. Clinical applications and review of the literature. *AJR* 1986;146:1204–1214.

337. Spanier SS, Shuster JJ, Vander Griend RA. The effect of local extent of the tumor on prognosis in osteosarcoma. *J Bone Joint Surg (Am)* 1990;72A:643–653.

338. Stewart NR, Gilula LA. CT of the wrist: a tailored approach. *Radiology* 1992;183:13–20.

339. Stiles RG, Otte MT. Imaging of the shoulder. *Radiology* 1993;188:603–613.

340. Sundaram M, McGuire MH, Fletcher J, Wolverson MK, Heiberg E, Shields JB. Magnetic resonance imaging of lesions of synovial origin. *Skeletal Radiol* 1986;15:110–116.

341. Sundaram M, McGuire MH, Herbold DR, Wolverson MK, Heiberg E. Magnetic resonance imaging in planning limb-salvage surgery for primary malignant tumors of bone. *J Bone Joint Surg (Am)* 1986;68A:809–819.

342. Sundaram M, McGuire MH, Herbold DR. Magnetic resonance imaging of osteosarcoma. *Skeletal Radiol* 1987;16:23–29.

343. Sundaram M, McGuire MH, Herbold DR. Magnetic resonance imaging of soft tissue masses: an evaluation of fifty-three histologically proven tumors. *Magn Reson Imaging* 1988;6:237–248.

344. Swensen SJ, Keller PL, Berquist TH, McLeod RA, Stephens DH. Magnetic resonance imaging of hemorrhage. *AJR* 1985;145:921–927.

345. Taconis WK, Mulder JD. Fibrosarcoma and malignant fibrous histiocytoma of long bones: radiographic features and grading. *Skeletal Radiol* 1984;11:237–245.

346. Taconis WK, Schutte HE, van der Heul RO. Desmoplastic fibroma of bone: a report of 18 cases. *Skeletal Radiol* 1994;23:283–288.

347. Tanyu MO, Vinee P, Wimmer B. Value of 3D CT imaging in fractured os calcis. *Comput Med Imaging Graph* 1994;18:137–143.

348. Tello R, Suojanen J, Costello P, et al. Comparison of spiral CT

and conventional CT in 3D visualization of facial trauma: work in progress. *Comput Med Imaging Graph* 1994;18:423–427.

349. Thompson JR, Christiansen E, Hasso AN et al. Temporomandibular joints: high-resolution computed tomographic evaluation. *Radiology* 1984;150:105–110.

350. Thompson JR, Christiansen E, Sauser D, et al. Dislocation of the temporomandibular joint meniscus: contrast arthrography vs. computed tomography. *AJR* 1985;144:171–174.

351. Tillie B, Fontaine C, Stahl P, et al. Contribution of x-ray computed tomography to the diagnosis and treatment of fractures of the acetabulum. Apropos of 88 cases. *Rev Chir Orthop* 1987;73:15–24.

352. Totterman SMS, Miller RJ, McCance SE, et al. Lesions of the triangular fibrocartilage complex: MR findings with a three-dimensional gradient-recalled-echo sequence. *Radiology* 1996;199:227–232.

353. Totty WG, Murphy WA, Lee JKT. Soft-tissue tumors: MR imaging. *Radiology* 1986;160:135–141.

354. Totty WG, Vannier MW. Complex musculoskeletal anatomy: analysis using three dimensional surface reconstruction. *Radiology* 1984;150:173–177.

355. Tscherne H, Lobenhoffer P. Tibial plateau fractures. Management and expected results. (Review). *Clin Orthop* 1993;292:87–100.

356. Turcotte RE, Sim FH, Unni KK. Giant cell tumor of the sacrum. *Clin Orthop* 1993;291:215–221.

357. Udupa J, Hung H, Chang K. Surface and volume rendering in three-dimensional imaging: a comparison. *J Digit Imaging* 1994;4:159–168.

358. Unger EC, Glazer HS, Lee JKT, Ling D. MRI of extracranial hematomas: preliminary observations. *AJR* 1986;146:403–407.

359. Unni KK, Dahlin DC, Beabout JW, Ivins JC. Parosteal osteogenic sarcoma. *Cancer* 1976;37:2466–2475.

360. Unni KK, Dahlin DC, Beabout JW. Periosteal osteogenic sarcoma. *Cancer* 1976;37:2476–2485.

361. Van der Werken C, Oostvogel HJ, Appelman PT. The role of computed tomography in fractures of the acetabulum. *Neth J Surg* 1986;38:180–182.

362. Vanel D, Contesso G, Couanet D, Piekarski JD, Sarrazin D, Masselot J. Computed tomography in the evaluation of 41 cases of Ewing's sarcoma. *Skeletal Radiol* 1982;9:8–13.

363. Vanel D, Lacombe MJ, Couanet D, Kalifa C, Spielmann M, Genin J. Musculoskeletal tumors: follow-up with MR imaging after treatment with surgery and radiation therapy. *Radiology* 1987;164:243–245.

364. Vannier MW, Hildebolt CF, Gilula LA, et al. Calcaneal and pelvic fractures: diagnostic evaluation by three-dimensional computed tomography scans. *J Digit Imaging* 1991;4:143–152.

365. Vannier MW, Totty WG, Stevens WG, et al. Musculoskeletal applications of three-dimensional surface reconstructions. *Orthop Clin North Am* 1985;16:543–555.

366. Vogler JB III, Brown WH, Helms CA, et al. The normal sacroiliac joint: a CT study of asymptomatic patients. *Radiology* 1984;151:433–437.

367. Walker PS, Rovick J, Robertson D. The effect of knee brace hinge design and placement on joint mechanics. *J Biomech* 1988;21:965–974.

368. Walker PS, Zhou X-M. The dilemma of surface design in total knee replacement. *Proc Orthop Res Soc* 1987;12:291.

369. Walker PS. Requirements for successful total knee replacements. *Clin Orthop* 1989;20:15–29.

370. Wall SD, Fisher MR, Amparo EG, Hricak H, Higgins CB. Magnetic resonance imaging in the evaluation of abscesses. *AJR* 1985;144:1217–1221.

371. Wang G, Snyder D, O'Sullivan J, Vannier MW. Iterative deblurring for CT metal artifact reduction. *IEE Trans Med Imaging* 1996;16:657–664.

372. Ward WG, Eckardt JJ, Shayestehfar S, Mirra J, Grogan T, Oppenheim W. Osteoid osteoma diagnosis and management with low morbidity. *Clin Orthop* 1993;291:229–235.

373. Wechsler RJ, Wehbe MA, Rifkin MD, et al. Computed tomography diagnosis of distal radioulnar subluxation. *Skeletal Radiol* 1987;16:1–5.

374. Weekes RG, Berquist TH, McLeod Rak, Zimmer WD. Magnetic resonance imaging of soft-tissue tumors: comparison with computed tomography. *Magn Reson Imaging* 1985;3:345–352.

375. Weiner DS, Cook AJ, Hoyt WA Jr, et al. Computed tomography in the measurement of femoral anteversion. *Orthopedics* 1978;1:299–306.

376. Wespe R, Wallin A, Klaue K, Ganz R, Schneider E. Three-dimensional quantitation of established femoral head necrosis. In: Lemke HU, et al, eds. *Computer assisted radiology.* Berlin: Springer-Verlag, 1989;362–368.

377. Westrich GH, Borrelli JJ, Ghelman B, et al. Computerized tomography for the evaluation of posttraumatic multiplane deformities of the tibia. *Am J Orthop* 1995 May Suppl:7–10.

378. White MS. Three-dimensional computed tomography in the assessment of fractures of the acetabulum. *Injury* 1991;22:13–19.

379. Wing VW, Jeffrey RB Jr, Federle MP, Helms CA, Trafton P. Chronic osteomyelitis examined by CT. *Radiology* 1985;154:171–174.

380. Woolson ST, Dev P, Fellingham L, Vassiliadis A. Three-dimensional imaging of bone from computerized tomography. *Clin Orthop* 1986;202:239–248.

381. Woolson ST, Fellingham LL, Dev P, et al. Three dimensional imaging of bone from analysis of computed tomography data. *Orthopedics* 1985;8:1269–1273.

382. Wyatt SH, Fishman EK. CT/MRI of musculoskeletal complications of AIDS. *Skeletal Radiol* 1995;24:481–488.

383. Yiu-Chiu VS, Chiu LC. Complementary values of ultrasound and computed tomography in the evaluation of musculoskeletal masses. *RadioGraphics* 1983;3:46–82.

384. Zatz L, Alvarez R. An inaccuracy in computed tomography: the energy dependence of CT values. *Radiology* 1977;124:91–97.

385. Zimmer WD, Berquist TH, McLeod RA, et al. Bone tumors: magnetic resonance imaging versus computed tomography. *Radiology* 1985;155:709–718.

386. Zimmer WD, Berquist TH, McLeod RA, et al. Magnetic resonance imaging of osteosarcomas. Comparison with computed tomography. *Clin Orthop* 1986;208:289–299.

387. Zinman C, Reis ND. Osteochondritis dissecans of the talus: use of the high resolution computed tomography scanner. *Acta Orthop Scand* 1982;53:697–700.

388. Zlatkin MB, Lander PH, Begin LR, Hadjipavlou A. Soft-tissue chondromas. *AJR* 1985;144:1263–1267.

CHAPTER 23

The Spine

Mauricio Castillo, J. Keith Smith, and Suresh K. Mukherji

Computed tomography (CT) and magnetic resonance (MR) imaging provide complementary information for evaluation of the spine. Computed tomography provides better detailed evaluation of cortical bone, whereas MR is superior for assessment of the soft tissues. This chapter presents an overview of spinal anatomy and common pathologic entities. Congenital abnormalities and disorders that occur primarily in the meninges, subarachnoid spaces, and spinal cord will not be discussed.

NORMAL ANATOMY

Cervical Spine

The cervical spine is composed of seven vertebrae. The first two vertebrae differ in embryologic origin from the rest of the cervical spine and are best considered as part of the craniocervical junction.

The anterior arch of C1 (the atlas) contains a small anterior tubercle to which the anterior longitudinal ligament attaches. The anterior arch continues laterally and joins the superior facets and lateral masses. The bulky lateral masses form the articular surfaces, contain the transverse foramina, and give origin to the transverse processes. The vertebra is completed by a posterior arch.

The second cervical vertebra (the axis) is unique in that it is formed from several different embryologic origins. The tip of the dens is the ossiculum terminale and arises from the proatlantal sclerotome. The midportion of the dens originates from the centrum of C1. The dens is held in apposition to the posterior surface of the anterior arch of C1 by the transverse ligament. The atlantodental space should not exceed 4 to 5 mm in children and 2 mm in adults (55). The body of C2 is derived from the 5th and

6th somites. Laterally, the vertebral body joins the transverse processes, which form the anterior margin of the transverse foramina. The medial and posterior margins of the transverse foramina are formed by the pedicles and the laminae. The laminae join posteriorly at the base of the spinous process (Fig. 1).

Cervical vertebrae C3 through C7 are derived from

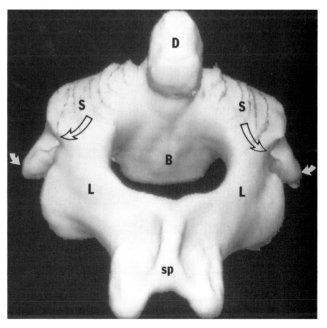

FIG. 1. Normal axis (C2). Three-dimensional reconstruction of C2 vertebra. *Open curved arrows,* foramina transversarium; *small solid curved arrows,* posterior tubercles of transverse processes; D, dens; S, superior articular facets; B, body; L, laminae; SP, spinal processes. (Irregularities in articular surfaces and base of dens represent reconstruction artifacts.)

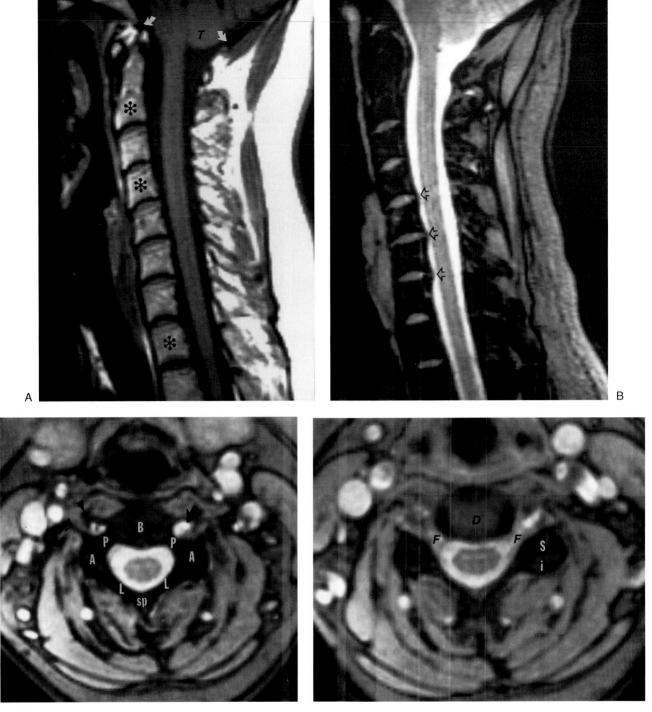

FIG. 2. Normal cervical spine. **A:** Midsagittal T1-weighted image shows normal high signal intensity *(asterisks)* from vertebral bodies due to normal fat contained in marrow. The diameter of spinal cord decreases slightly and progressively from C3 to C7. Cerebellar tonsils are above foramen magnum *(arrows)*. Signal intensity from discs is always less than that of vertebral bodies. T, cerebellar tonsils. **B:** Midsagittal spin echo T2-weighted image shows normal marrow to have decreased markedly in signal intensity. The discs are relatively bright. Spinal cord is normal in diameter and signal intensity. Minimal degenerative changes at C5-C7 *(arrows)* are seen with this sequence. **C:** Transaxial gradient echo T2-weighted image of normal C5 vertebra. *Arrow,* flow-related enhancement in vertebral artery coursing in foramen transversarium; *arrowhead,* anterior tubercle of transverse process; *open arrow,* posterior tubercle of transverse process; B, body; P, pedicles; A, articular pillars; L, laminae; sp, spinous process. Lack of fat in the epidural space of the cervical spine dictates need for utilizing sequences that produce bright CSF and create a myelographic effect. **D:** Transaxial gradient echo T2-weighted image at normal C4-C5 disc space. Neural foramina are oriented in a 45° angle with respect to the vertebral body and therefore not clearly seen in sagittal sequences. The superior facet of C5 is located anteriorly, and the inferior facet of C4 is seen posteriorly. D, disc; F, neural foramina; S, superior articular facet; i, inferior articular facet.

somites 7 to 12, and all have similar anatomic features. The vertebral bodies contain the uncinate processes (which form the uncovertebral joints) in their posterolateral margin. The uncovertebral joints contain loose areolar tissue or a synovial lining. They form the ventromedial margins of the neural foramina. The size of the vertebral bodies increases progressively from C3 to C7 (Fig. 2A,B). In their mid and dorsal portions, the vertebral bodies contain the basivertebral vein canal. All pedicles are short structures formed from cortical bone, which connects the vertebral bodies to the articular pillars (Fig. 2C). The articular pillars are composed of the inferior articular facet of one vertebra and the superior facet of the underlying vertebra. On transaxial images, the anteriorly located facet is the superior facet of the lower vertebra, whereas the posterior one is the inferior facet of the upper vertebra (Fig. 2D). The inferior articular facets join the laminae, which in turn, join the spinous process. The spinous process of C7 is the largest in the cervical spine. All cervical neural foramina are oriented in a 45° plane with respect to the vertebral bodies (20) (Fig. 2D). Although the anteroposterior diameter of the cervical spinal canal decreases from C3 through C7, 12 mm is considered the lower limit of normal throughout the cervical region. It is important to remember that there are eight pairs of cervical nerve roots. Each pair exits cephalad to its respective vertebral body. The C8 nerve roots exit at the C7-T1 neural foramina.

Thoracic Spine

The thoracic spine is composed of 12 vertebrae (Fig. 3A,B). The posterior ribs articulate with the vertebral bodies posterolaterally. The pedicles arise from the superoposterior aspect of the vertebral bodies and form the superior and inferior margins of the neural foramina. The neural foramina are oriented laterally (Fig. 3C). The pedicles continue laterally with the transverse processes, which are located immediately posterior to the corresponding rib. The laminae originate from the dorsal aspect of the transverse processes and join posteriorly to form the spinous process. The superior articular facet is located at the junction between pedicle and lamina. The inferior facet arises from the lateral end of the lamina. The articular surfaces of both facets are flat. On transaxial images, the superior facet of the underlying vertebra is located anteriorly and the inferior facet of the corresponding vertebra is located posteriorly. The spinal canal narrows slightly in the midthoracic region. The anteroposterior diameter of the thoracic spine is abnormal if less than 10 mm (29).

Lumbar Spine

The lumbar spine generally has five vertebrae; however, transitional vertebrae are not uncommon. Therefore the total number of vertebrae may vary between four and six. The vertebral bodies are massive and are larger in the transverse than the anteroposterior dimension. The lumbar vertebral bodies are traversed by one or two venous channels. Thick pedicles are formed from dense cortical bone (Fig. 4A,B). As in the thoracic spine, the pedicles arise from the superodorsal vertebral body and form the superior and inferior margins of the neural foramina. The laminae are flat and join to form the spinous process. The laminae do not overlap each other (as in the thoracic spine) and in flexion they open sufficiently to allow insertion of a needle for lumbar puncture. The transverse processes of L1 and L5 tend to be somewhat larger than those of other lumbar vertebrae. Again, on transaxial images, the superior articular facet of the vertebra below is seen anteriorly, whereas the inferior facet is located posteriorly. The neural foramina are oriented laterally (Fig. 4C,D). The anteroposterior diameter of the spinal canal increases caudally and should be considered abnormal if less than 12 mm.

In the lumbar spine (as in the thoracic region), the nerve roots exit at their corresponding vertebrae. That is, the L3 nerve roots exit at the L3-L4 neural foramina.

Sacrum and Coccyx

The sacrum is formed by five fused vertebrae that contain residual disc spaces between them. The L5 vertebra may be fused to S1. The single median crest is flanked by the smaller intermediate crests. Located lateral to the intermediate crests are four paired neural foramina, which point anteriorly. The coccyx is generally formed by 3 to 5 articulating segments.

Special Imaging Features

By CT, all vertebral bodies are surrounded by well-demarcated cortical bone. The vertebral bodies contain fine bone trabeculae traversing the marrow space. These trabeculae are more prominent in the lumbar region. The pedicles and transverse processes are well corticated and contain little cancellous bone. The laminae and spinous processes in the cervical and thoracic spine contain cancellous bone; however, in the lumbar region, they generally appear as single bony plates. The articular surfaces of the facets, which are dense and smooth (Fig. 4C), generally are biconvex in the cervical spine but flat in the thoracic and lumbar regions. The intervertebral discs are of homogeneous soft-tissue density (50 to 100 HU). On CT scans, the annulus fibrosus cannot be separated from the nucleus pulposus. The ligamentum flavum, also of soft-tissue density, joins the interlaminar spaces (Fig. 4C,D). In the lumbar spine, the ligamentum flavum normally measures 3 to 5 mm and is considered thickened or buckled if larger than 5 mm. The posterior longitudinal

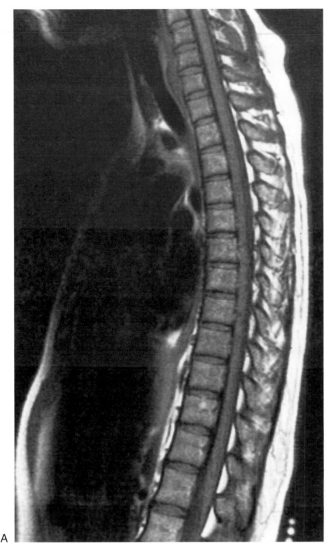

A

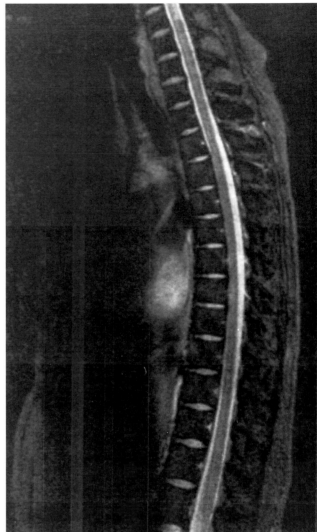

B

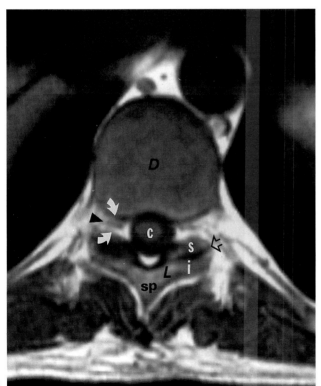

C

FIG. 3. Normal thoracic spine. **A:** Midsagittal T1-weighted image obtained in body coil with high-resolution rectangular matrix (256 × 512) and a 50-cm field-of-view. This sequence allows for adequate visualization of the majority of the spinal cord. In cases of suspected cord compression, the cervical spine is imaged in a different setting with a dedicated surface coil. **B:** Midsagittal T2-weighted image shows normal bright discs, low signal intensity from bone marrow, and normal spinal cord. **C:** Axial T1-weighted image obtained through midthoracic vertebra. C, spinal cord; S, superior articular facet; i, inferior articular facet; L, lamina; sp, spinous process. The neural foramina *(curved arrows)* are oriented laterally. Spinal nerve root *(arrowhead)* is well seen. *Open arrow,* joint space.

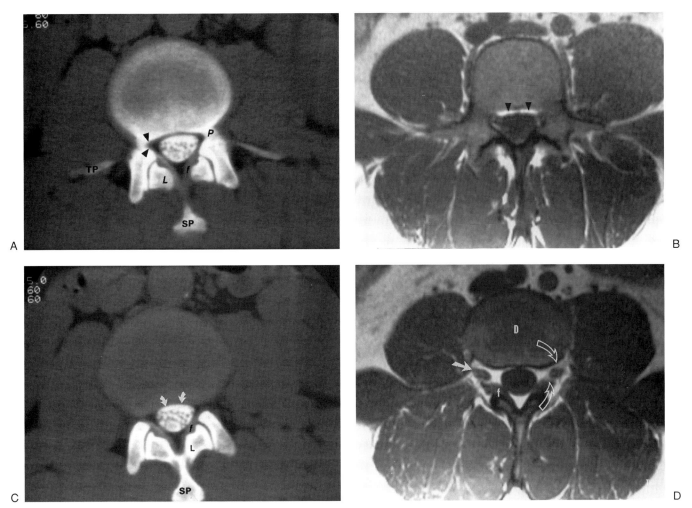

FIG. 4. Normal lumbar spine. **A:** Postmyelogram transaxial CT section (bone windows) at normal L3. Nerve roots are seen as discreet round filling defects floating in opacified CSF. *Arrowheads,* lateral recess; T, pedicle; T, transverse process; L, lamina; SP, spinous process. **B:** Transaxial T1-weighted image at normal L4 shows bright ventral epidural fat *(arrowheads)* creating a contrast between bone and CSF. **C:** Transaxial postmyelogram CT shows normal concavity of L3-L4 disc *(arrows)* in its central portion. SP, spinous process; L, lamina; f, ligamentum flavum. **D:** Transaxial T1-weighted image at normal L3-L4 disc space. The neural foramina *(curved open arrows)* are oriented laterally and, therefore, well imaged in sagittal sequences. The dorsal root ganglia *(solid arrow)* are well seen and will normally enhance after contrast administration. D, disc; f, ligamentum flavum.

ligament is contained in the ventral epidural space together with fat and blood vessels. The fat in the ventral epidural space extends into the lateral recesses, which carry the nerves into the neural foramina. In the lumbar region, the lateral recesses are bordered anteriorly by the vertebral bodies, laterally by the pedicles, and posteriorly by the superior articular facets (Fig. 4A). The lateral recesses normally measure 3 to 5 mm and are considered narrowed if less than 3 mm.

On MR, the vertebral cortex appears as an area of low signal intensity due to lack of mobile protons. On T1-weighted images, cortical bone is inseparable from cerebrospinal fluid (CSF) and ligaments (27). Fatty marrow produces high signal intensity on T1-weighted spin echo and T2-weighted fast spin echo images (63). However,

patchy bone marrow may be seen at any age and by itself should not be considered pathologic (63). On T2-weighted spin echo or gradient echo images, the vertebral bodies are of low signal intensity (Figs. 2B,3B). Normal marrow enhances homogeneously after intravenous administration of gadolinium contrast media. Normal intervertebral discs are of similar or slightly lower signal intensity than marrow on T1-weighted images (17) (Figs. 2A,3A) and of higher signal intensity on T2-weighted images (Fig. 3B). In the normal disc, the annulus fibrosus may be seen as a subtle and peripheral region of lower signal intensity on all T2-weighted sequences (57). The nucleus pulposus is of higher signal intensity and is traversed horizontally by a dark line that represents the normal internuclear cleft (2,57). The internuclear cleft is seen in over 94% of patients 30 years of age or older (2). The ligaments are dark on T2-weighted images (27). The purpose of all T2-weighted sequences (spin echo, gradient echo, and fast-spin echo) is to provide a myelographic effect by making the CSF appear bright (Fig. 2C,D). If fast spin echo sequences are used, the bright CSF may be inseparable from adjacent fat-containing structures, and fat suppression may be needed to distinguish them.

IMAGING PROTOCOLS

Cervical Spine

Computed tomography. For examination of degenerative disorders, 3-mm-thick contiguous sections are obtained from C3 through T1. If thinner sections are needed, 2- or 1.5-mm collimation may be used. Sagittal reformations are performed only in selected instances. All images are filmed using soft tissue and bone window settings.

Magnetic resonance. Sagittal T1-weighted images [500/15/2 (TR/TE/number of excitations)] are obtained initially with a field of view (FOV) of 280 mm, and 4 mm sections with a 10% intersection gap. This is followed by sagittal T2-weighted fast spin echo images (3500/19,93/1) with an echo train of 4 to 8 using the same FOV and section thickness. Transaxial low-flip angle (25°) images (650/20/4/25°) using FOV of 200 mm, and a 4-mm section thickness with a 0.4-mm intersection gap, are also obtained from C3 to T1. In patients with infection, tumor, or prior surgery in this region, sagittal and transaxial T1-weighted images are obtained immediately after intravenous administration of gadolinium.

Thoracic Spine

Computed tomography. Contiguous sections of 3 mm are obtained from one vertebra above to one below the region of interest. Sagittal reformations are optimal. All images are filmed with soft tissue and bone window settings.

Magnetic resonance. Sagittal T1-weighted images (600/16/2) are obtained first with an FOV of 250 to 280 mm, and 4-mm section thickness with 0.4-mm intersection gap. This is followed by sagittal T2-weighted fast spin echo images (3500/19,93/1) with an echo train of 4 to 8, using the same FOV and section thickness. Transaxial low flip angle (20°) images (650/20/4) are obtained with an FOV of 200 mm and 4-mm section thickness with 0.4-mm intersection gap. After intravenous administration of gadolinium, sagittal and transaxial T1-weighted images are obtained.

Lumbar Spine

Computed tomography. Stacked (i.e., no angle) 3-mm contiguous sections are obtained from top of L3 through S1. Sagittal reformations are optional. All images are filmed at both soft tissue and bone window settings.

Magnetic resonance. Sagittal T1-weighted images (600/15/2) are obtained first with an FOV of 250 mm and 4-mm section thickness with 0.4-mm intersection gap. These images are followed by sagittal T2-weighted fast-spin echo images (3500/19,93/1) with an echo train of four, using the identical FOV and section thickness as before. Stacked transaxial T1-weighted images (650/15/2) also are obtained with an FOV of 200 mm and 4-mm section thickness with 0.4-mm intersection gap from L3 through S1. After intravenous administration of gadolinium, transaxial and sagittal T1-weighted images are obtained within 5 to 15 minutes of the injection. If the sacrum is to be studied, transaxial and coronal T1-weighted and T2-weighted sequences are most useful.

If spinal cord compression is a consideration, the entire spine may be screened using a body coil (Fig. 3A,B). Sagittal T1-weighted images (560/18/4) are obtained with an FOV of 500 mm, 4-mm section thickness with 0.4-mm intersection gap and a rectangular matrix of 256 × 512. These images can be obtained in approximately 9.5 minutes and generally include the base of skull through L2. Low flip angle T2-weighted gradient echo images (560/18/4/15°), using the same FOV and section thickness as before, may be obtained in a similar amount of time. If tumor involving bone marrow is suspected, fat suppression is desirable, especially after intravenous gadolinium administration.

For evaluation of extramedullary disease, intravenous gadolinium administration is recommended in patients with suspected infection, tumor, vascular malformations, and failed back surgery syndrome (epidural fibrosis versus recurrent herniated disc) (10,35,48,66,77). Gadolinium-enhanced MR also may be useful for highlighting nerve root abnormalities in unoperated lumbar spines (36). In general, all gadolinium compounds are administered at a standard dose of 0.1 mmol/kg. Increasing the dose of gadolinium to 0.3 mmol/kg may accentuate contrast enhancement of diseased areas (52).

ADVANTAGES AND DISADVANTAGES OF CT AND MRI

All patients with frank and uncomplicated radiculopathy, whose symptoms are not relieved after 6 weeks of conservative treatment, should undergo either CT or MR examination if surgery is being considered. However, if signs of intrinsic spinal cord symptoms are present, MR is the preferred imaging method. In evaluating the postoperative spine, MR imaging (85% accuracy) is superior to CT (43% to 60% accuracy) for separating scar from disc (15). Magnetic resonance is also the method of choice for evaluating infections and congenital anomalies, especially when a tethered cord is suspected. If a soft-tissue tumor is suspected, MR is the preferred imaging technique; if a bone tumor is suspected, CT is usually also obtained.

Overall, CT and MR are comparable in their ability to detect disc herniation. Computed tomography has a greater than 90% accuracy (50). In one series, MR detected 93% of all herniated discs (79).

Minor disadvantages of CT compared with MR include the use of ionizing radiation, the inability to scan in more than one plane, and occasionally, the need for iodinated contrast media. On the other hand, MR may not be readily available, and the examination is generally more expensive and more time consuming. Furthermore, patients with ferromagnetic intracranial aneurysm clips, cardiac pacemakers, cochlear implants, and nerve stimulators cannot undergo MR imaging. In addition, approximately 5% to 10% of the patients complain of claustrophobia and are unable to tolerate MR imaging without medication.

DEGENERATIVE SPINE DISEASE

Pain secondary to degenerative changes of the spine is one of the leading causes of disability among adults. Sixty percent to 80% of working-age adults, at some point in their lives suffer from back pain (39). Most disorders of the spine result from degenerative changes that may arise in the bone, ligaments, or soft-tissue components of the spine.

The intervertebral articulation consists of the intervertebral disc and two posterior facet joints. The major components of the intervertebral disc space consist of the hyaline cartilaginous endplates of the adjacent vertebral bodies, the gelatinous core of the intervertebral disc (nucleus pulposus), and its circumferential thick fibrous ring (annulus fibrosus). Degenerative alterations at any of these sites may alter the normal biomechanical forces and predispose the adjacent articulations to similar changes. Therefore, patients often present with manifestations of degenerative changes in multiple joints.

The degenerative process involving the disc begins as early as the late teens or early twenties. Initially, an increase in the water content of the nucleus pulposus predisposes it to generalized bulges or focal herniations through the cartilaginous endplates of the adjacent vertebra (Schmorl's node) (42) (Fig. 5). With time, the nucleus pulposus undergoes progressive dehydration with resulting loss of height of the disc space. With further loss of water and proteoglycans, the disc becomes brittle and fibrotic and is unable to provide the necessary elasticity for proper support of the vertebral column, a process known as disc desiccation (82). The triad that characterizes disc degeneration includes bulging, loss of height, and loss of water, seen as decreased signal intensity on MR imaging. Almost all of the population over 60 years of age show degenerative disc changes by MR imaging. As the disc degenerates, it becomes hypointense on T2-

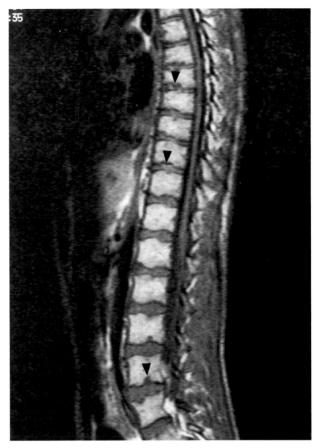

FIG. 5. Schmorl's nodes. Midsagittal T1-weighted image obtained in the body coil with a rectangular matrix in a patient with Scheuermann's disease shows multiple Schmorl's nodes *(arrowheads)*.

weighted sequences. Occasionally, a diseased disc may be bright on precontrast T1-weighted images (Fig. 6). This probably implies the presence of intradiscal calcification (hydrated calcium) and/or hemorrhage. The mechanism by which a degenerated disc produces pain is unclear, but it is probably related to compression and repetitive firing of sensory nerve endings.

The imaging features of progressive degenerative disc disease vary depending on the extent of the abnormality. Computed tomography is unable to detect early disc desiccation; however, it is useful for detecting late changes, such as disc space narrowing and sclerosis of the adjacent cartilaginous endplates. A reliable indicator of disc degeneration is the presence of intradiscal gas, which is referred to as vacuum phenomenon (50) and may be visualized by plain radiographs or CT (62). The gas is predominantly nitrogen and is highly unusual in an infected disc space (50).

Magnetic resonance imaging may show signs of early degenerative changes that are not detected by CT. Early disc desiccation presents as loss of signal intensity on T2-weighted images (Fig. 7). Sagittal images are helpful in determining the degree of disc space narrowing. Magnetic

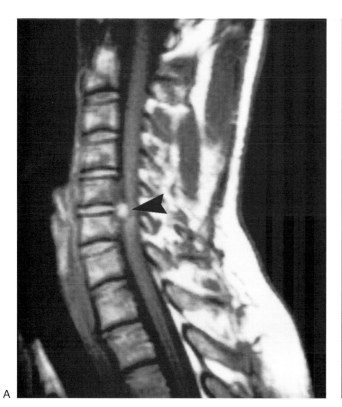 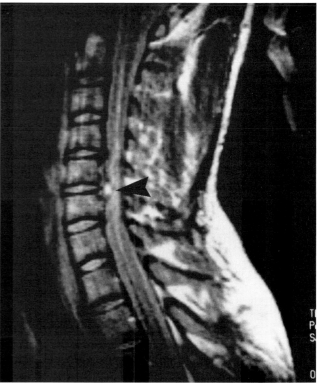

A   B

FIG. 6. Bright disc herniation. **A:** Midsagittal T1-weighted image shows a bright disc herniation at C5-C6 level *(arrowhead)*. **B:** Midsagittal proton-density-weighted fast spin echo image shows that the herniated disc fragment *(arrowhead)* remains hyperintense. Edema, hemorrhage, or hydrated calcium may account for the findings.

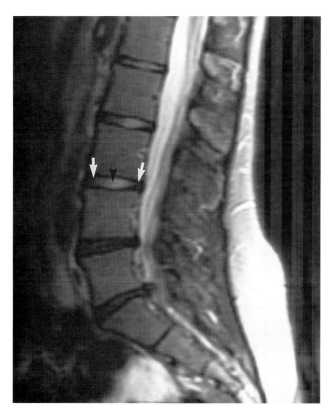

FIG. 7. Degenerated lumbar disc. Midsagittal T2-weighted image shows low signal intensity and decreased height of the L4-L5 and L5-S1 discs. These findings are commonly referred to as degeneration and are probably related to loss of proteoglycans in the disc. The L4-L5 disc bulges posteriorly and there is a probable herniation at the L5-S1 level. Note normal brightness of the L3-L4, L2-L3, and L1-L2 discs. In these normal discs the internuclear cleft (thin central linear hypointensity, *arrowhead*) and the annulus (peripheral zones of hypointensity, *white arrows*) are clearly identifiable.

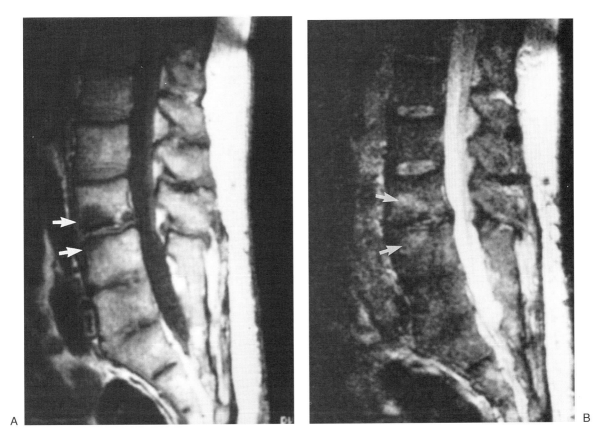

FIG. 8. Type I, Modic changes. **A:** Midsagittal T1-weighted image shows low signal intensity from inferior endplate of L3 and superior endplate of L4 *(arrows)*. The corresponding disc space is narrow. Findings are related to the presence of vascularized fibrous tissue and edema. **B:** Matching conventional spin echo T2-weighted image shows the abnormalities *(arrows)* to be hyperintense.

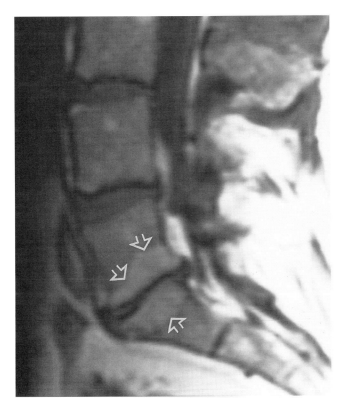

FIG. 9. Type II, Modic changes. Midline sagittal T1-weighted image shows decreased intensity from the L5-S1 disc, which is narrowed. The adjacent vertebral body endplates show hemispherical areas of hyperintensity *(open arrows)*. These areas represent fatty infiltration.

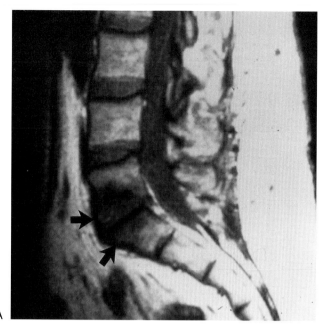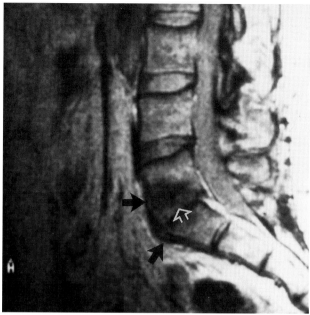

A   B

FIG. 10. Type III, Modic changes. **A:** Midsagittal T1-weighted image shows low signal intensity from the inferior endplate of L5 and superior endplate of S1 *(arrows)*. Corresponding disc space is narrow. **B:** Midsagittal conventional proton-density-weighted image shows that the endplate abnormalities *(solid arrows)* remain hypointense (sclerosis was present on plain radiographs). The L5-S1 disc *(open arrow)* is also of low signal intensity.

resonance imaging also detects marrow changes within endplates adjacent to degenerative discs. These changes are classified into three categories (50). Type I changes show decreased signal on T1-weighted images and increased signal on T2-weighted sequences (Fig. 8). Histologically, these changes correlate with vascularized fibrous tissue, with disruption, fissuring, and edema of the endplate. Type II changes, resulting from yellow (fatty) marrow replacement within the adjacent endplates, are characterized by increased signal on T1-weighted images, with decreased signal intensity on conventional spin echo T2-weighted images, but hyperintensity on fast T2-weighted spin echo images (Fig. 9). Type III changes are advanced changes, characterized by decreased signal on both T1-weighted and T2-weighted images, correlating with extensive bone sclerosis of the involved endplates on plain radiographs and CT (Fig. 10). These changes are best seen on conventional T2-weighted spin-echo images. It is important to recognize the above-described signal intensity changes as resulting from disc degeneration, so as not to confuse them with infection (discitis). There is, however, no correlation between these signal intensity changes and specific symptoms.

Disc Herniation

As the degenerative process progresses, small circumferential fissures develop in the annulus fibrosus, which may later coalesce to form a radial tear. Distinction be-

tween focal extrusion of disc material and a circumferential enlargement is important, as the former is usually treated surgically, whereas the latter may be treated conservatively.

Disc *bulge* refers to a smooth circumferential (global) extension of the disc margin beyond the boundary of the adjacent vertebral end plates (Fig. 11). The annulus fibrosis is intact although weakened. There is usually loss of height of the involved disc space and desiccation of the

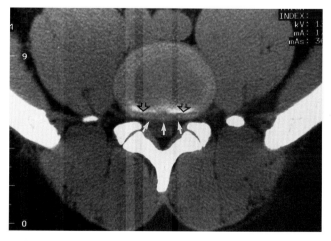

FIG. 11. Disc bulge. Transaxial CT at L4-L5 level shows that the posterior margin of the disc *(solid arrows)* protrudes smoothly and in a generalized fashion posteriorly from the edge of the vertebral body *(open arrows)*. The disc has lost its normal posterior central concavity.

contrast enhancement in the cervical spine has not been determined. In addition, contrast-enhanced imaging may help in excluding other entities in the differential diagnosis of an epidural mass such as neurofibroma, abscess, synovial cyst, and metastatic tumor.

Spondylosis

A common degenerative change of the spine is spondylosis deformans (also called spondylitic ridging or bridging osteophytes), which occurs in 60% to 80% of adults over the age of 50. Spondylosis results from disruption of the peripheral fibers of the annulus fibrosus with minor degrees of displacement of the disc. This change predisposes to the formation of osteophytes at the sites of bony attachments of the ligamentous components of the annulus fibrosus. Spondylosis is usually seen in association with facet joint degeneration, and multilevel disease is the rule. Degenerative spondylosis is the most common cause of spinal canal stenosis in adults (51).

Large bony overgrowths can cause spinal stenosis with resultant compressive myelopathy, especially in the cervical region (Fig. 19). Patients with diffuse spondylitic ridging who are symptomatic may require vertebral corpectomy with anterior cervical fusion for relief of their symptoms. Chronic spinal cord compression is sometimes associated with regions of increased T2 signal in the spinal cord, a finding suggestive of myelomalacia (Fig. 19). A zone of myelomalacia in the presence of multilevel osteophytosis may indicate the need for decompression at that level. However, patients with myelomalacia generally respond less favorably to surgical decompression than those without spinal cord changes.

Spondylolisthesis and Spondylolysis

Spondylolisthesis refers to displacement of a vertebra in relation to an adjacent vertebra, resulting in a malalignment of the spinal column. The displacement can be either anterior (anterolisthesis) or posterior (retrolisthesis). The term *degenerative spondylolisthesis* is used to denote a malalignment that arose as a result of spinal instability due to degenerative changes involving the disc and facet joints. Spondylolisthesis may result from acute trauma, or from congenital or acquired fibrous defects in the pars interarticularis (spondylolysis). The latter are referred to as lytic spondylolistheses.

Spondylolysis occurs in approximately 5% of the population (50). It tends to be bilateral and most commonly involves the lower lumbar spine, but it may also be found in the cervical region. The most widely accepted explanation for spondylolysis is that repeated minor trauma leads to a stress fracture of the pars interarticularis (50). Although both CT and MR imaging readily show the abnormality, CT is preferred when spondylolysis is suspected.

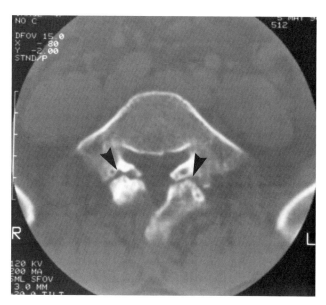

FIG. 20. Spondylolysis. Transaxial CT section at L5, bone window settings, shows bilateral lucent defects *(arrowheads)* involving the pars interarticularis.

Spondylolysis usually affects L5 (90% of cases), with involvement of L4 (10%) and L3 (<1%) much less frequent (50). Computed tomography shows a lucent defect with irregular margins in one or both partes interarticulares (Fig. 20). The presence of "too many facets" in a CT examination should prompt the consideration of pars defects. In cases of unilateral spondylolysis, the contralateral normal articular pillar supports all biomechanical stress at that level and may become sclerotic. If significant slippage of one vertebra over another has occurred, the "double canal" sign may be seen. Spondylolisthesis occurs in over 60% of patients with spondylolysis. Sagittal MR images show pars defects to be oriented perpendicular to the long axis of the adjacent facet joint. At times, the anterior portion of the defective pars interarticularis may show high signal intensity on T1-weighted images. The spondylolisthesis may impinge upon and stretch the nerve roots, producing a radiculopathy that tends to be bilateral.

Facet Joint Disease

Degenerative changes of the facet joints may result from primary osteoarthritis or may be secondary to degenerative changes within the intervertebral disc. When facet joint and intervertebral changes are both present, it is impossible to ascertain which is the primary cause.

The changes that occur with facet joint degeneration are similar to those seen in other osteoarthritides. Although the changes can be seen on MR, they are better demonstrated on CT. The imaging findings consist of joint space narrowing with associated subchondral sclerosis of the articular surfaces, subchondral cyst formation, and hypertrophic new bone formation. In the cervical region, both the uncovertebral and facet joints may degenerate. The former tend to produce stenosis of the neural foramina, whereas the latter result in narrowing of the spinal canal diameter. In the lumbar region, facet degeneration is usually accompanied by buckling ("hypertrophy") of the ligamentum flavum and degenerative disc disease, which in combination, result in spinal canal stenosis.

An additional consequence of facet joint degeneration is the development of synovial cysts, which usually occur in the lower lumbar spine, most commonly at L4-L5. These juxta-articular cysts are lined by synovium and communicate with the joint. They measure 5 to 10 mm in diameter, are more common at the L4-L5 level, are posterolateral in location, may have a completely or partially calcified shell, and contain clear fluid, mucinous fluid, or hemorrhage. Their margins may show enhance-

ment, which is probably related to the presence of granulation tissue (Fig. 21). Ganglion cysts occur in similar location, but they are not lined by synovium, do not communicate with the joint, and are filled with myxoid material. On MR imaging, synovial cysts have a high signal intensity on T2-weighted images. They are always adjacent to a facet joint, which also shows abnormal high signal intensity because of fluid in the intra-articular space.

Spinal Stenosis

Spinal stenosis refers to a reduction in the caliber of the spinal canal. Resultant symptoms depend on the level of involvement. If the cervical portion of the cord is involved, the patient may present with a radiculopathy, myelopathy, or neck or shoulder pain. Stenosis of the lumbar

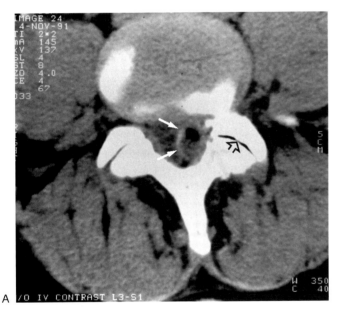

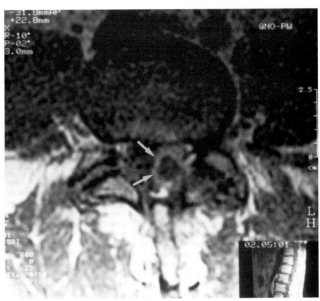

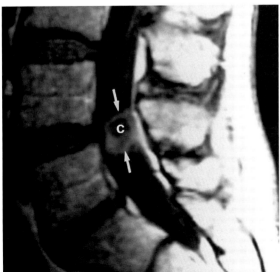

FIG. 21. Synovial cyst. **A:** Transaxial plane CT shows mass *(arrows)* compressing the thecal sac and adjacent to degenerated left facet joint at the L4-L5 level. Note gas *(open arrow)* in facet joint, which extends into the synovial cyst. **B:** Postcontrast transaxial T1-weighted image shows the cyst *(arrows)* to have peripheral enhancement, presumably secondary to granulation tissue formation. **C:** Midsagittal T1-weighted image after contrast in the same patient shows the medial aspect of the cyst (c) to be surrounded by enhancing granulation tissues *(arrows)*.

region may cause neurogenic claudication, back pain, or paresthesia. In cases of superimposed acute lumbar disc herniation, patients may present with an acute cauda equina syndrome.

Spinal stenosis may be either primary or acquired. The most common cause of acquired stenosis is degenerative change. Degenerative spinal stenosis arises from changes occurring in three major locations: the disc space, the facet joints, and the ligamentum flavum. Narrowing of the disc space results in alterations in the mechanical forces on the facet joints and associated ligaments. As a result, the facet joints and ligamentum flavum often hypertrophy. The canal may be narrowed anteriorly by a degenerative disc (bulging or herniated) and posteriorly by hypertrophy of the ligamentum flavum and facet joints. Hypertrophic bone formation of the facet joints also con-

tributes to lateral encroachment on the spinal canal with effacement of the lateral recess. Other rare causes of acquired spinal canal stenosis include epidural lipomatosis and ossification of the posterior longitudinal ligament and/or the ligamentum flavum. Epidural lipomatosis may be seen in cases of endogenous or, more commonly, exogenous hypercortisolism. Epidural lipomatosis may also occur in the setting of morbid obesity. Most cases (70%) involve the thoracic spine and in some instances can produce a myelopathy and polyneuropathy (50). The lumbar region also may be involved.

Ossification of the posterior longitudinal ligament (OPLL) is endemic in Japan, where it is found in 3% of the population with neurologic findings referable to the cervical region (56). It is seen more often in the cervical region (88%), but it also may involve the thoracic region

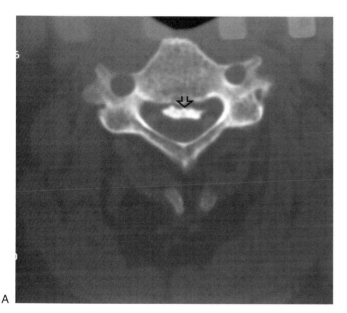

A

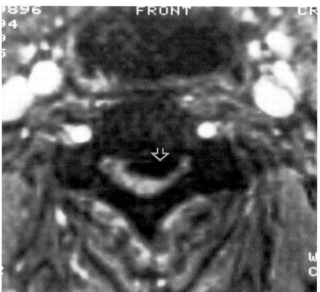

B

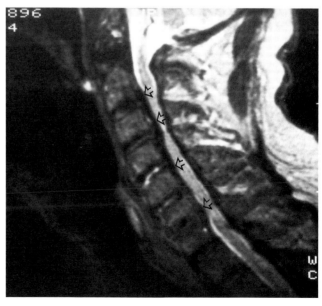

C

FIG. 22. Ossified posterior longitudinal ligament. **A:** Postmyelogram transaxial CT section showing ossified posterior longitudinal ligament *(arrow)* causing spinal cord compression. **B:** Transaxial gradient echo image at the same level shows the ligament *(arrow)* to be hypointense. Note that due to magnetic susceptibility artifact the abnormality appears larger on this sequence. **C:** Midsagittal T2-weighted image shows ossified ligament *(arrows)* extending from C2 to C7. There is spinal canal stenosis at the C3-C4 and C6-C7 levels.

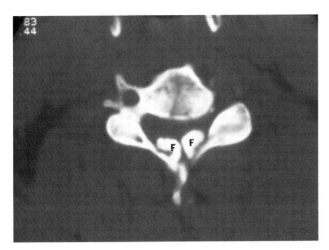

FIG. 23. Ossified ligamentum flavum. Transaxial CT, bone window settings, shows heavily calcified ligamentum flavum (F) bilaterally producing significant narrowing of the spinal canal.

(56). Its incidence is higher in patients with diffuse idiopathic skeletal hyperostosis (DISH). This type of ossification may be continuous or segmental. The ossified ligament is better seen with CT, but MR imaging may show a band of hypointensity posterior to the vertebral bodies (Fig. 22). The ossified ligament is not reliably detected by MR unless it measures more than 3 mm in width. Patchy areas of increased signal intensity, which occasionally are present in the hypertrophied ligament, probably represent areas of bone marrow. Myelopathy is generally manifested when the spinal canal diameter is diminished by 30% (56).

Ossification of the ligamentum flavum is generally seen in the setting of OPLL, but occasionally it occurs in an isolated form (Fig. 23). It is found most commonly in the cervical and thoracic regions (76). An uncommon cause of acquired spinal stenosis is Paget disease (76). Congenital spinal stenosis is usually related to "short" pedicles, but it is seen also in children with achondroplasia and deposition disorders such as Morquio syndrome.

Although absolute measurements are not valuable in all cases, spinal canal stenosis should be considered if the anteroposterior diameter of the cervical and lumbar canals is less than 12 mm. In the thoracic region, an anteroposterior diameter of less than 10 mm is abnormal.

POSTOPERATIVE SPINE

After lumbar spine surgery for disc disease, 10% to 40% of patients report recurrent pain, a condition referred to as failed back surgery syndrome (66). Causes for this pain include recurrent or residual disc herniation (or unrecognized far lateral disc herniation), epidural scar formation, arachnoiditis, postoperative infection, radiculitis, stenoses of the lateral recesses or neural foramina, and

failure of bone fusion. Contrast-enhanced MR is the imaging method of choice for differentiating an epidural scar from a herniated disc.

Herniated disc material is of intermediate signal intensity and blends with the intervertebral disc on T1-weighted images (Fig. 24). Mass effect is seen in up to 69% of cases and may mimic the preoperative findings (66). The substance of the herniated disc should not enhance. Peridiscal scar causes peripheral enhancement in the majority of recurrent/residual disc herniations (10,35) (Fig. 24). Postcontrast MR images should be obtained within 5 to 10 minutes after gadolinium administration, because homogeneous disc enhancement may be seen on images obtained more than 15 minutes after contrast medium administration. This delayed enhancement phenomenon is generally seen at least 3 to 6 weeks after surgery and reflects ingrowth of fibrosis into the disc with proliferation of capillaries which have "leaky" tight junctions (15).

Epidural scar is of intermediate signal intensity on T1-weighted images and of variable signal intensity on T2-weighted images. Although it is generally accepted that scar does not exert mass effect, occasionally it may produce significant compression of the thecal sac or neural structures (13). Scar, which normally contains abundant capillaries with "loose" tight junctions and wide extracellular spaces, enhances markedly, homogeneously, and immediately after MR contrast medium administration. At times, epidural scar may be separated from underlying disc fragments by a thin zone of low signal intensity on the postcontrast T1-weighted images. Scar located in the ventral epidural space may enhance for many years after the surgery, whereas enhancement of scar in the dorsal epidural space is temporary.

Contrast enhancement of the disc space and adjacent bone marrow after discectomy is an abnormal postoperative finding (11). Infection should be strongly considered if the following MR signs are present: complete enhancement of the residual intervertebral disc, enhancement of the vertebral endplates adjacent to the operated disc, and enhancing epidural and/or paravertebral fluid collections.

Arachnoiditis, an inflammatory process involving all three meningeal layers, is an important cause of the failed back surgery syndrome. Causes of arachnoiditis include surgery, infection, intrathecal administration of medications, trauma, subarachnoid hemorrhage, and prior myelography (8). Postmyelogram CT shows lack of nerve root sleeve filling, adhesion of nerve roots to the walls of the thecal sac (the "empty sac" sign), nerve root clumping, and soft-tissue masses that may obliterate the canal (8) (Fig. 25). MR imaging is less sensitive than postmyelogram CT in the detection of arachnoiditis. Magnetic resonance reveals enhancement of thickened meninges in 50% of patients with arachnoiditis shown on myelography (37). Nerve root clumping and enhancement are the most common signs of arachnoiditis by MR imaging.

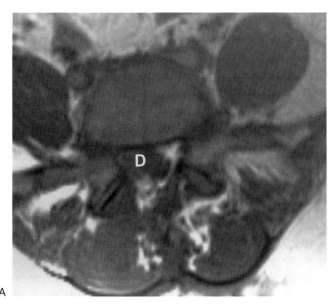 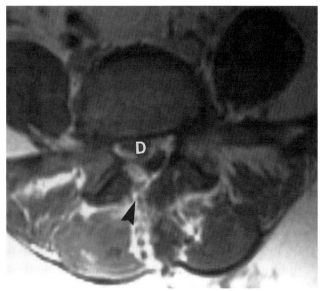

A   B

FIG. 24. Recurrent disc herniation. **A:** T1-weighted image shows ventral and rightward epidural soft tissue (D) at the L5-S1 level in this patient with recurrent symptoms 2 months after surgery. **B:** Image at comparable level immediately after contrast administration shows marginal enhancement of the epidural soft tissue compatible with disc fragment surrounded by granulation tissue. Scar enhances homogeneously. Laminectomy site *(arrowhead)* is clearly seen.

Rare complications of arachnoiditis include intrathecal calcifications and the formation of syringomyelia (8).

Epidural anesthesia rarely induces a severe arachnoiditis that may lead to the formation of arachnoid cysts (72). These cysts can potentially compress the spinal cord. Such anesthesia-related arachnoiditis may result from inadvertent introduction of medication into the subarachnoid space or may be related to the preservatives contained in anesthetic solutions.

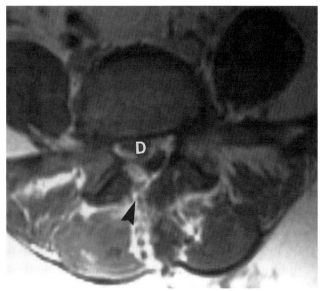

FIG. 25. Arachnoiditis. Transaxial postmyelogram CT shows significant clumping of nerve roots (r) compatible with arachnoidal adhesions.

Intrathecal droplets from prior myelography with Pantopaque (oil-based contrast medium) have a characteristic MR appearance (14). These droplets, primarily localized in the dependent portions of the subarachnoid space, are very bright on T1-weighted images and of very low signal intensity on T2-weighted images (Fig. 26). On proton-density-weighted images, Pantopaque may be isointense to CSF.

INFECTIONS

Infections that begin primarily in the intervertebral disc space are generally caused by staphylococci, enterobacteria, and, less commonly, *Pseudomonas.* Tuberculosis usually involves the vertebral body first. Involvement of the epidural space is usually secondary to discitis or osteomyelitis. Predisposing risk factors include diabetes, intravenous drug use, renal failure, alcoholism, surgery, trauma, and immunosuppression (80). Routes of spread are hematogenous, ascending (via Batson's venous plexus from pelvic infections), and direct implantation. In order of decreasing frequency, the most common sites of infection are the lumbar and thoracic regions, and less commonly the cervical spine (67). Usually, a period of 2 to 8 weeks elapses between the onset of clinical symptoms and the appearance of detectable morphologic changes on imaging studies. Magnetic resonance is the imaging method of choice for evaluation of suspected localized spinal infection. If symptoms are nonlocalizing, a radionuclide bone scan may be used as a screening test. Computed

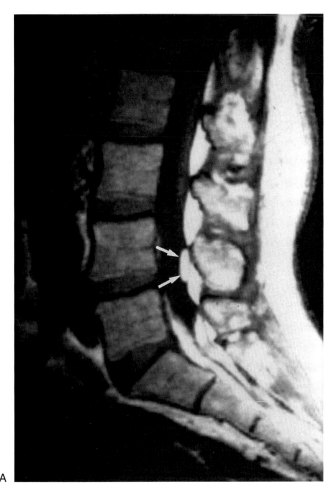 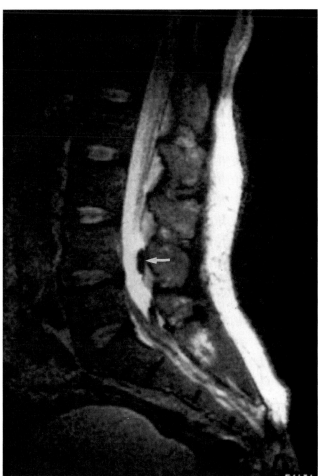

A
B

FIG. 26. Intrathecal Pantopaque. **A:** Midsagittal T1-weighted image shows pill-shaped droplet of Pantopaque *(arrows)* resting in dependent aspect of the subarachnoid space at the L4-L5 level. **B:** Corresponding midsagittal T2-weighted image shows marked hypointensity from the Pantopaque *(arrow)*. Note that on this conventional spin echo image, Pantopaque is less intense than fat.

tomography is less sensitive than radionuclide bone scintigraphy and should be used as a confirmatory test rather than as the initial imaging method.

The earliest CT findings include narrowing of the disc space, erosion of the vertebral body endplates, and vertebral body osteopenia (18). Sagittal reformations are valuable when these findings are present. Later in the process, new bone formation giving rise to osteosclerosis may be seen (18). Extension to the paravertebral soft tissues occurs in approximately 20% of cases and is clearly demonstrated by CT (80). Extension into the epidural or subdural compartments is poorly shown by plain CT. However, lumbar puncture for the introduction of contrast medium is contraindicated in this clinical setting, as it may facilitate spread of infection into the subarachnoid space, thereby resulting in meningitis.

MR imaging is 96% sensitive and 94% accurate in the detection of spinal infection (49). It is more sensitive than myelography and CT in the diagnosis of discitis, osteomyelitis, and epidural abscesses (58). T1-weighted MR images show low signal intensity of the involved

intervertebral disc and the adjacent vertebral bodies (Fig. 27). The cortical bone of the vertebral endplates may be indistinct. On T2-weighted sequences, the disc space and adjacent vertebrae are of increased signal intensity. Occasionally, the intervertebral disc may appear less intense owing to the high signal intensity of the adjacent endplates (59). On T2-weighted images, the normal internuclear cleft is effaced. Extension into the paraspinal soft tissues is seen as focal or confluent areas of low signal intensity on T1-weighted and high signal intensity on T2-weighted images. Epidural infection, which is bright on T2-weighted images and dark on T1-weighted images, may be isointense with CSF and blend with it imperceptibly. Therefore, intravenous gadolinium administration is imperative. The major advantage of a postcontrast study is to separate an epidural abscess from the thecal sac (54,81) (Fig. 27B–E). Separating the enhancing epidural abscess from surrounding fat may necessitate the use of fat suppression techniques. Contrast enhancement of the disc and the adjacent vertebrae are also commonly seen after intravenous administration of gadolinium com-

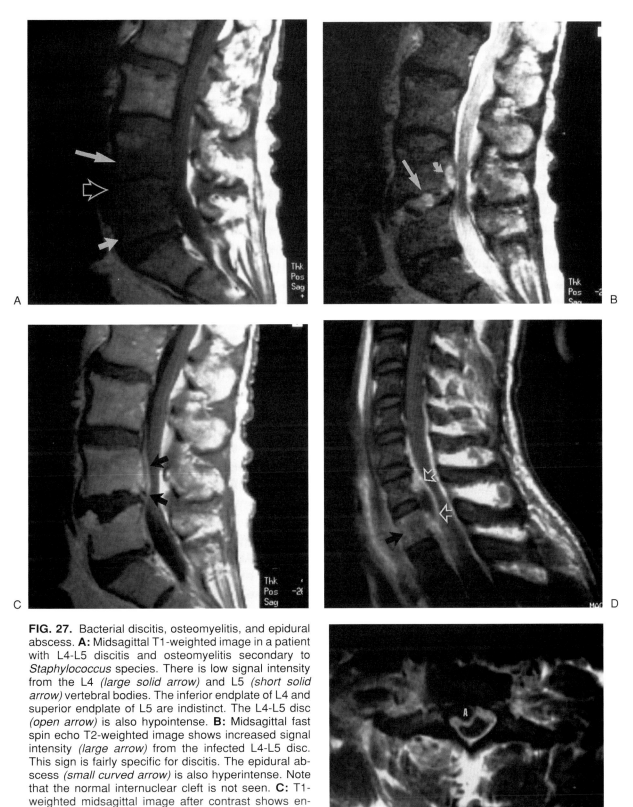

FIG. 27. Bacterial discitis, osteomyelitis, and epidural abscess. **A:** Midsagittal T1-weighted image in a patient with L4-L5 discitis and osteomyelitis secondary to *Staphylococcus* species. There is low signal intensity from the L4 *(large solid arrow)* and L5 *(short solid arrow)* vertebral bodies. The inferior endplate of L4 and superior endplate of L5 are indistinct. The L4-L5 disc *(open arrow)* is also hypointense. **B:** Midsagittal fast spin echo T2-weighted image shows increased signal intensity *(large arrow)* from the infected L4-L5 disc. This sign is fairly specific for discitis. The epidural abscess *(small curved arrow)* is also hyperintense. Note that the normal internuclear cleft is not seen. **C:** T1-weighted midsagittal image after contrast shows enhancement of L4 and L5 vertebral bodies. Small epidural abscess *(arrows)* occurring as consequence of spread of infection from L4 is present and narrows the thecal sac diameter. **D:** In a different patient, midsagittal T1-weighted image after contrast administration shows epidural abscess *(open arrows)* at C7-T1. Note enhancement of T1 vertebral body *(solid arrow)* but intact disc space. The dorsal epidural space from C5 to T2 also enhances and is thickened. Precervical inflammatory changes extending from base of skull to T3 are also present. **E:** Transaxial postcontrast T1-weighted image shows eccentric and rightward location of abscess (A) compressing the spinal cord.

pound (69). After successful treatment, contrast enhancement tends to become less pronounced.

In contradistinction to pyogenic discitis, tuberculosis is said to classically affect the vertebral bodies and the posterior elements (Fig. 28). However, in a large series, tuberculosis was found to cause a variety of lesions, most of them indistinguishable from pyogenic infection (69). Tuberculosis most commonly occurs in the thoracic region in adults. In developing countries, children are primarily affected. The primary source of infection is identified in less than 10% of cases (18). Clinically, spinal tuberculosis is a more insidious process than its pyogenic counterpart. Multilevel disease (generally more than two vertebrae per case) results from a propensity to involve the anteroinferior aspect of the endplates, causing spread beneath the anterior longitudinal ligament (69,80). Destruction of a vertebral body on a chronic basis may lead to a sharply angulated kyphosis, known as a gibbus deformity. Although CT and MR findings are usually nonspecific, the presence of calcifications (on CT) in the paraspinal muscles is characteristic of tuberculosis. Other findings suggestive of tuberculosis include rim enhancement of lesions and of paraspinal abscesses, multilevel involvement, and relative sparing of the intervertebral disc on MR (49). Brucellosis leads to identical findings (80).

Almost all epidural abscesses are the sequelae of adjacent discitis/osteomyelitis. Isolated epidural abscesses are usually from hematogenous spread and seen in diabetics, intravenous drug users, and patients with a chronic illness or an underlying immunodeficiency (69). Dental abscesses and pneumonia also have been implicated. The most common causative microorganism is *Staphylococcus aureus* (60%) (80). If treatment is delayed, paraplegia,

quadriplegia, or death may ensue. Imaging is critical in these patients, as the correct diagnosis is made clinically in only 20% to 25% of patients. Contrast-enhanced MR is the imaging method of choice when an epidural abscess is suspected. If a distinct sensory level is not present, the entire spine should be evaluated. The two most common MR appearances include homogeneous or heterogeneous enhancement of the portion of the abscess and lack of enhancement of the liquefied portions of the abscess (81) (Fig. 27D,E). Follow-up contrast-enhanced MR imaging is extremely helpful if the patient is to be treated primarily with antibiotics, as it can document a decrease in the size of the abscess with successful treatment.

TUMORS AND TUMORLIKE CONDITIONS

Primary Tumors

Hemangioma

Vertebral body hemangiomas are found in more than 10% of all autopsies (46). They are almost always asymptomatic. They occur predominantly in women and are most often located in the thoracic or lumbar region. Hemangiomas are composed of low-pressure, thin-walled vessels with slow flow that are interspersed among thick secondary bone trabeculae and fat. The CT and MR imaging appearance reflects this histology.

On CT, hemangiomas are low in attenuation value and contain thick bone striations, the so-called polka dot pattern. Cortical bone destruction is almost never present. Calcifications within soft tissue extension are detected occasionally. On MR imaging, the lesions are characteristically of high signal intensity on both T1-weighted and T2-weighted sequences (Fig. 29). The main differential diagnosis is that of focal fatty replacement of the vertebral bone marrow. After contrast medium administration, hemangiomas enhance moderately to intensely, whereas fatty replacement does not. In the asymptomatic patient, distinction between these two entities is mostly academic. Occasionally, vertebral body hemangiomas may behave aggressively and lead to compression fractures or soft-tissue masses that may cause spinal cord compression. Such aggressive hemangiomas have been reported to have low signal intensity on T1-weighted images, high intensity on T2-weighted images, and slow enhancement after gadolinium administration (44). On MR imaging, these aggressive hemangiomas are thus indistinguishable from other malignancies.

Aneurysmal Bone Cyst

Aneurysmal bone cysts (ABC) account for only 1% to 2% of all primary bone tumors, and fewer than 25% of all ABCs are found in the spine. Those located in the

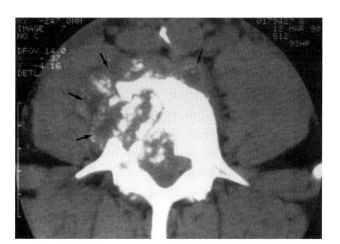

FIG. 28. Tuberculosis. Transaxial CT section in a patient with tuberculosis affecting L4. There is destruction of the right side of the vertebral body with extension of abscesses into right psoas muscle and prevertebral space *(arrows)*. The posterior aspect of the vertebral body is eroded and infection extends into the epidural space (e), producing significant compression of thecal sac.

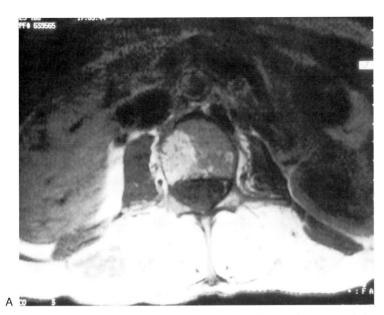
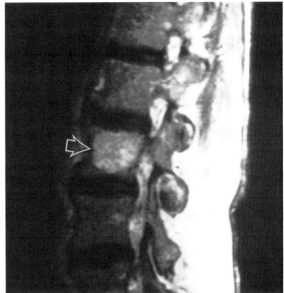

FIG. 29. Vertebral body hemangioma. **A:** Transaxial noncontrast T1-weighted image shows focal area of hyperintensity in right side of the vertebral body. The lesion contains multiple small areas of lower signal intensity which could represent hypertrophic secondary trabeculae or vascular channels. **B:** Right parasagittal T1-weighted image again shows the lesion *(arrow)*.

spine most often involve the neural arch (9). The cervical and thoracic regions are most commonly involved, but the sacrum also may be affected. Most ABCs are found in patients under 20 years of age. Histologically they are benign hamartomas, but biologically they show aggressive behavior. They occur secondary to trauma or at sites of previous lesions such as fibrous dysplasia, chondroblastoma, and osteoblastoma.

On CT, these lesions are typically lytic, expansile, and surrounded by a thin shell of bone. Within the cyst, fluid and blood levels are present (84) (Fig. 30). MR imaging shows similar features. The presence of paramagnetic blood-breakdown products gives rise to fluid levels of varying signal intensities ranging from very bright signal on T2-weighted images (representing extracellular methemoglobin) to very low signal (indicating the presence of intracellular deoxyhemoglobin, cellular debris, or hemosiderin).

Osteoblastoma

Osteoblastoma (giant osteoid osteoma) is another tumor that preferentially involves the neural arch. Approximately 45% of all osteoblastomas occur in the spine. Males in the second to fourth decades of life are primarily affected (43). This lesion may represent reactive changes rather than a true neoplasm. Osteoblastomas generally are larger than 2 cm in diameter when discovered.

Computed tomography shows a well-defined expansile and lytic lesion generally surrounded by a thin rim of calcium. Ossified matrix can be identified in up to 50%

of cases, and extension into neighboring soft-tissue structures also may be seen (43). The MR imaging features are nonspecific. The lesion enhances after intravenous administration of gadolinium (43).

Osteoid Osteoma

Osteoid osteomas are histologically similar to osteoblastomas but smaller, generally measuring less than 2

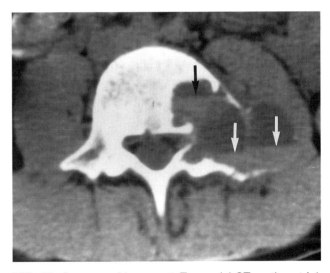

FIG. 30. Aneurysmal bone cyst. Transaxial CT section at L4 shows large aneurysmal bone cyst eroding the vertebral body, pedicle, transverse process, and lamina. The margins of the lesion are well defined and it contains multiple blood/fluid levels *(arrows)*. There is extension into the left psoas muscle.

cm in diameter. They represent approximately 6% of all benign bone tumors. Approximately 10% of osteoid osteomas are found in the spine, most often the lumbar region where they produce scoliosis (7). Within the vertebrae, they most commonly arise in the neural arch (75%), followed by the laminae (33%), articular facets (19%), and the pedicles (15%) (7). The classic symptoms include night pain that is relieved by aspirin, scoliosis, adjacent muscle spasm (particularly torticollis when the cervical spine is affected), and occasionally myelopathy or radiculopathy. Osteoid osteomas are most common in males during the first two decades of life.

The initial localization of the lesion may be accomplished with radionuclide bone scintigraphy. Computed tomography shows a lucent central area (nidus) surrounded by sclerotic reaction. If the osteoid osteoma arises in cancellous bone, the surrounding sclerosis may not be present. Computed tomography is used primarily for precise localization of the lesion before excision. The MR imaging appearance of osteoid osteoma is not characteristic (25).

Giant Cell Tumor

Giant cell tumors comprise fewer than 4% of all bone neoplasms. In the spine, they most often involve the sacrum. Women in their third decade of life are predominantly affected (21). Most giant cell tumors are histologically benign, but up to 25% may show some degree of malignancy. Computed tomography and/or MR imaging studies are often needed for surgical planning. Total resection is the recommended treatment, as treatment with curettage alone results in a 50% recurrence rate (33).

On CT, giant cell tumor is a well-demarcated, expansile and lytic lesion. When it involves the sacrum, it generally is located adjacent to the sacroiliac joint. Cortical disruption may be present. Occasionally, the tumor contains tiny calcifications. In most patients, MR imaging shows the lesion to be of low-to-intermediate signal intensity on T1-weighted images and of heterogeneous intermediate signal intensity on T2-weighted images (33). Focal areas of hemorrhage within the lesions may be seen. Giant cell tumor enhances brilliantly after gadolinium is administered intravenously.

Chordoma

Chordoma accounts for fewer than 4% of bone lesions (78,83). It arises from a notochordal remnant in the vertebral body or within the disc space. Histologically, chordomas are classified as either conventional (having a gelatinous matrix) or chondroid. Half of all chordomas occur in the sacrum (mainly S4 and S5) followed in incidence by the clivus (35%) and one or more vertebrae (15%) (particularly C2) (78). Men between the ages of 40 and 70 years are most commonly affected. Chordomas are slowly growing, locally aggressive tumors. They occasionally produce distant metastases, especially to lungs, lymph nodes, subarachnoid space, and spinal cord (78).

On CT, chordomas are mainly lytic, but sclerotic chordomas are occasionally encountered (Fig. 31). The low-density mass is surrounded by calcium and contains flecks of calcium within it. Low density areas, representing necrosis or gelatinous myxoid material, also may be seen in the tumor. Paravertebral extension is not uncommon. On T1-weighted MR images, chordomas are of intermediate (75%) or low signal (25%) intensity (78). On T2-weighted images, the tumors are of higher signal intensity than CSF. The majority are heterogeneous in signal intensity. After intravenous gadolinium administration, chordomas show marked enhancement (Fig. 31). Although CT better demonstrates the characteristics of the tumor proper, MR imaging is superior in outlining extension into prevertebral and epidural/intradural spaces.

Langerhans Cell Histiocytosis

This group of disorders traditionally has been divided into the eosinophilic granuloma, Hand-Schüller-Christian, and Letterer-Siwe diseases. The solitary form of the disease is the eosinophilic granuloma, which mostly occurs in children. The vertebrae are the primary location (20%) of the lesions (30). Eosinophilic granuloma is a rapidly growing lytic lesion of bone that often leads to a flattened and sclerotic vertebral body (so-called vertebra plana). The diagnosis is easily made from the plain radiograph. Computed tomography and MR imaging are useful in outlining the extension of the lesion if surgery is considered. Lesions are usually lytic (Fig. 32A). The MR imaging appearance of these lesions is nonspecific (Figs. 32B,C). The presence of extension into the adjacent soft tissues by CT or MR imaging is atypical and should prompt histologic confirmation of the lesion. Treatment of eosinophilic granuloma is controversial and ranges from immobilization, curettage, and intratumor injection of steroids, to radiation therapy and surgical excision. Hand-Schüller-Christian is the disseminated form of this disease, involving multiple bones. The spine is affected in 14% to 30% of patients (30). The radiographic features are those of multiple nonspecific lytic lesions. Letterer-Siwe is the fulminant form of the disease. It is seen mainly in the very young and involves multiple organs.

Multiple Myeloma

Multiple myeloma is a disseminated disorder of bone marrow plasma cells (9), occurring mainly in middle- or advanced-age men. Although it may be localized primarily to the spine, it is more often disseminated. The vertebrae are affected in 66% of patients (9). The thoracic and

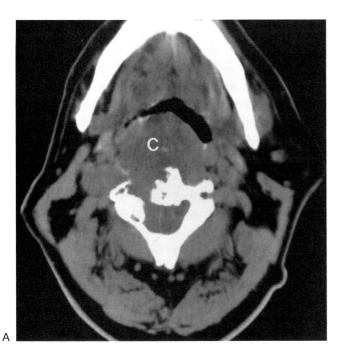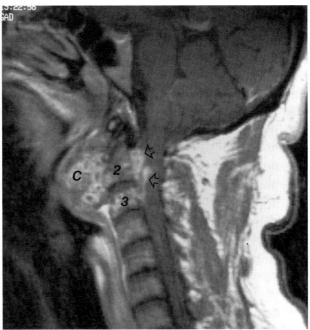

A

B

FIG. 31. Chordoma. **A:** Transaxial CT section at C2 shows chordoma (C) arising in the vertebral body and extending into the precervical region. The vertebral body is partially destroyed. **B:** Postcontrast midsagittal T1-weighted image shows chordoma (C) arising from the axis (2) and also involving C3 vertebral body (3). There is extension into the epidural space *(arrows)* with compression of the upper cervical spinal cord.

lumbar regions are most commonly involved. During the course of the disease, nearly 50% of patients develop neurologic symptoms, most often secondary to compression of the spinal cord due to vertebral body compression fractures and/or epidural spread of the disease. Plasmacytoma refers to the solitary form of the disease and is found in younger patients. Nearly all patients with a plasmacytoma eventually develop multiple myeloma.

CT is very sensitive for detecting and confirming myeloma lesions. The typical CT appearance is that of "punched-out" lytic abnormalities which are devoid of surrounding sclerosis. However, the most common CT manifestation of myeloma is diffuse osteopenia. Magnetic resonance is the most sensitive imaging technique for detecting myeloma lesions (61,71). On MR, the lesions are hypointense on T1-weighted images and hyperintense on T2-weighted images with respect to normal bone marrow (Fig. 33). Therefore, they cannot be distinguished from metastases. After radiation therapy, some lesions become hypointense on both T1-weighted and T2-weighted images, presumably due to fibrosis, but some lesions remain unchanged.

Secondary Tumors

Metastases to the spine are most commonly the result of hematogenous spread. Approximately 20% to 35% of cancer patients develop symptomatic spine metastases (9).

However, at autopsy, 70% of all cancer patients have spinal metastases. The thoracic and lumbar regions are most commonly involved (9). Approximately 5% of affected patients develop symptoms of spinal cord compression due to collapse of one or more vertebrae, or epidural tumor spread. The most common primary tumors to produce spinal metastases are carcinomas of the breast, lung, prostate, kidney, lymphomas, and sarcomas.

CT is used mainly to confirm the presence of lesions suspected from a radionuclide bone scintigram. Depending on their origin, metastases may be lytic (breast), sclerotic (prostate), or, more commonly, mixed (Fig. 34). MR imaging is more sensitive than CT and radionuclide bone scintigraphy for the detection of spinal metastases (24). On T1-weighted images, metastatic foci are usually of low signal intensity (Fig. 35), whereas on T2-weighted images, the lesions are bright. After intravenous contrast medium administration, metastases enhance and their signal intensity may be such that they become isointense with surrounding bone marrow. Therefore, the precontrast sagittal T1-weighted image is most sensitive in the detection of metastases to the vertebrae (including those producing spinal cord compression) (Fig. 36). Intravenous contrast enhancement aids in the evaluation of tumor extension into adjacent paraspinal and epidural compartments. Fat-suppressed T1-weighted images after intravenous contrast medium administration also are useful in demonstrating the lesions. Lymphoma and leukemia in-

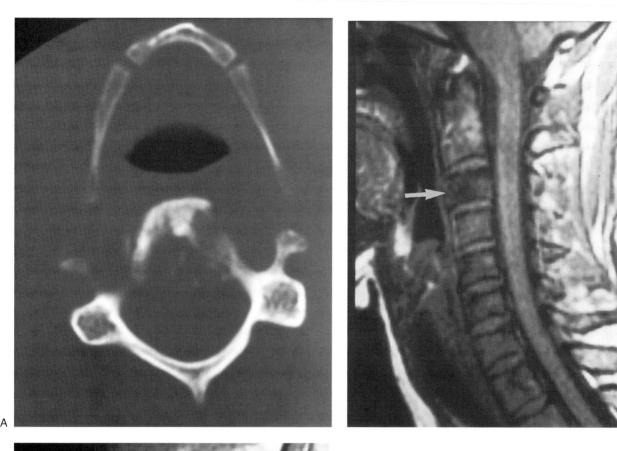

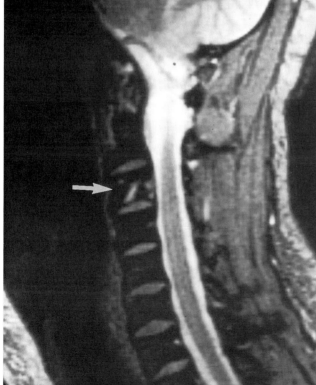

FIG. 32. Eosinophilic granuloma. **A:** Transaxial CT, bone window setting, shows destructive lesion involving the body of C3. **B:** Midsagittal noncontrast T1-weighted image shows low signal intensity from the involved C3 vertebral body *(arrow)*. **C:** Midsagittal T2-weighted image shows inhomogeneous signal intensities from the C3 vertebral body *(arrow)*.

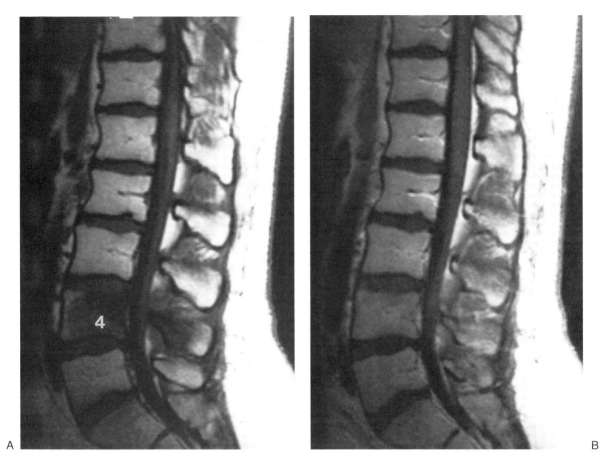

FIG. 33. Plasmacytoma. **A:** T1-weighted image shows low signal intensity from plasmacytoma involving L4 vertebral body (4). The vertebra is of normal height and indistinguishable from a solitary metastasis. **B:** After contrast administration, the lesion enhances and becomes isointense and inseparable from the normal adjacent vertebrae. Precontrast T1-weighted images are the most sensitive sequence for detection of processes that replace the normal bone marrow.

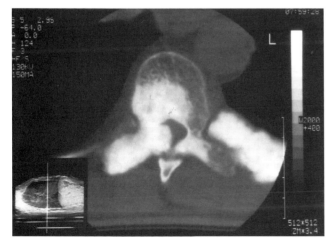

FIG. 34. Sclerotic metastases. Transaxial CT, bone window setting, shows expansile, sclerotic metastases from bronchogenic carcinoid tumor. Note significant narrowing of the spinal canal by involved bone.

volving the spine generally show MR imaging findings identical to metastatic disease. However, lymphoma occasionally dissects the dura from the underlying bone, resulting in a soft-tissue mass that circumferentially compresses the spinal cord (24).

SELECTED VASCULAR DISORDERS

Vascular Malformations

Only radiculomeningeal vascular malformations will be addressed. These malformations consist of a fistula between the radicular arteries and vein. The shunt is located in the surface of the dura mater and drains via one or more dilated radicular veins, which in turn drain to a large venous plexus located on the surface (most commonly dorsal) of the spinal cord. The majority of these malformation are found in men between 30 and 70 years of age (64). The patients may present with the Foix-Alajouanine syndrome (necrotic myelopathy), which is characterized clinically by progressive sensory and motor

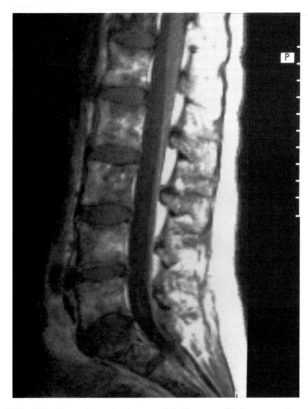

FIG. 35. Breast metastases. Midline sagittal noncontrast T1-weighted image shows multiple areas of low signal intensity in the bone marrow of the vertebral bodies in this patient with diffuse breast cancer. There is no fracture, epidural tumor, or compromise of the spinal canal.

deficits. The etiology of this syndrome is believed to be venous congestion, which leads to compression and ischemia of the spinal cord.

Plain CT is not indicated in these patients. However, postmyelogram CT may show rounded or serpentine filling defects, representing dilated veins, on the surface of the spinal cord. The spinal cord may be atrophic. Spin echo MR imaging demonstrates areas of flow void, mostly on the dorsal surface of the spinal cord. Although this sign is relatively specific, it is not commonly encountered. T2-weighted images in both transaxial and sagittal planes may serve to highlight the areas of signal void against the bright CSF (Fig. 37). The most common MR finding, seen in nearly all patients, is increased signal intensity in the spinal cord. This finding is nonspecific and likely is related to edema and/or gliosis (45). Contrast MR images may show enhancement of some vessels, particularly the veins with slow flow. Enhancement of the spinal cord is not uncommon. Magnetic resonance angiography, preferably using phase contrast techniques, may help document the lesion. Regardless of the CT or MR imaging findings, all patients suspected of harboring a spinal arteriovenous malformation should undergo catheter angiography for pre-embolization or presurgical mapping of feeding vessels.

Epidural Hematoma

The most common cause of an epidural hematoma is trauma. However, spontaneous nontraumatic epidural hematomas also may occur as a result of anticoagulation, vigorous exercise, hypertension, underlying vascular malformations, postintervertebral disc surgery, or collagen vascular disorders (51). Clinically, epidural hematoma is characterized by acute onset of pain and motor and sensory deficits. Epidural hematomas are generally located in the dorsolateral aspect of the spinal canal and most often involve the upper thoracic region. Although the size of hematomas decreases progressively with time, the treatment of choice is surgical decompression. In a series of 18 patients with ventrally located epidural hematomas, two thirds were associated with herniated lumbar spine discs (28). It is therefore conceivable that lumbar epidural hematomas are more common than previously believed and that their progressive resolution accounts for the improvement of symptoms in many patients with lumbar disc herniations.

Unenhanced CT shows a lentiform, high-density collection located adjacent to the neural arch. Magnetic resonance is the imaging method of choice, as CT does not demonstrate the epidural hematoma in all cases. The he-

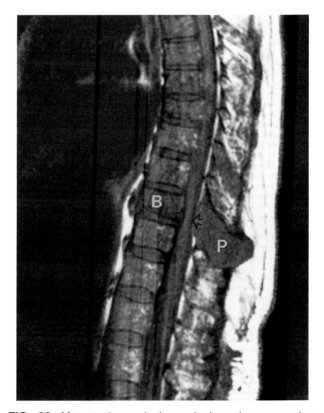

FIG. 36. Metastasis producing spinal cord compression. Midline sagittal T1-weighted image shows breast cancer metastasis involving a midthoracic vertebral body (B) and its posterior elements (P). There is compression of the spinal cord (arrows) by the tumor.

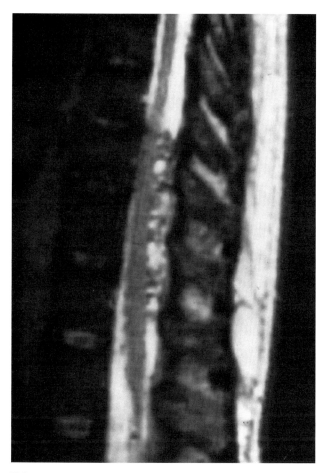

FIG. 37. Vascular malformation. Midline sagittal T2-weighted image shows multiple draining veins in the dorsal subarachnoid space at the level of lower thoracic spinal cord and conus medullaris. These represent venous drainage from a radicular fistula. Signal intensity of cord is normal.

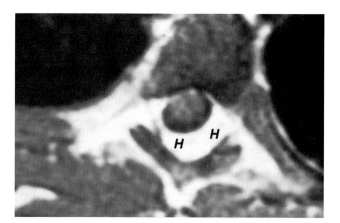

FIG. 38. Epidural hematoma. Transaxial T1-weighted image 3 days after trauma in young patient shows a crescentic region of hyperintensity (H) in the dorsal and lateral epidural compartments. At surgery, an epidural hematoma was evacuated.

elopathy, progressive disability, and death. Atlantoaxial subluxation of more than 8 mm carries an unfavorable prognosis, especially in men. Softening of the base of the skull with upward vertical displacement of the upper cervical segments (basilar invagination) leads to brainstem compression, which occasionally causes death. Basilar invagination is seen in 5% to 8% of patients with rheumatoid arthritis. Erosion of the dens by inflammatory pannus (synovial hypertrophy) is common. If large, the pannus itself may compress the neural elements. Other, less common, types of cervical spine subluxations seen in patients with rheumatoid arthritis include posterior atlantoaxial, lateral, and subaxial. The subaxial type is seen in 40% of patients with rheumatoid arthritis and leads to

matoma is demonstrated best on sagittal and transaxial sections (Fig. 38). The appearance of the blood varies with time. Within the initial 24 to 48 hours, a gradient echo sequence should be used to accentuate the T2 shortening effect of intracellular deoxyhemoglobin. After 48 hours, methemoglobin is well demonstrated and appears as areas of high signal, similar to fat, on T1-weighted images (Fig. 38). Fat-suppression imaging is helpful to distinguish normal epidural fat from methemoglobin. Contrast-enhanced imaging is not routinely indicated.

RHEUMATOID ARTHRITIS

More than 80% of patients with rheumatoid arthritis develop involvement of the cervical spine. In 25% of them, significant subluxations occur. Of the patients with subluxations, compression of the spinal cord or the medulla occurs in 20%. Subluxations are secondary to ligamentous laxity, ligamentous disruption, or local synovitis (38). Atlantoaxial subluxation may lead to chronic my-

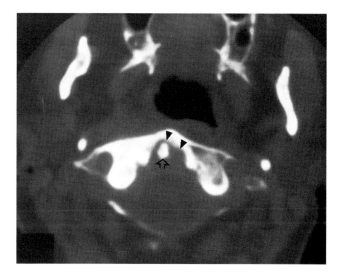

FIG. 39. Rheumatoid arthritis. Transaxial CT section, bone window setting, shows marked thinning of the dens *(open arrow)* secondary to surrounding pannus. The posterior margin of the anterior arch *(arrowheads)* of C1 is also eroded.

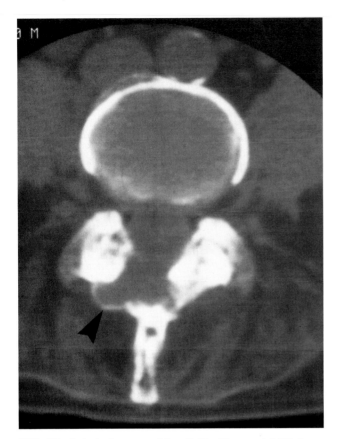

FIG. 40. Ankylosing spondyloarthritis. Transaxial CT, bone window setting, shows marked dural ectasia which has eroded the right lamina (arrow). Also seen are multiple foci of hypodensity in the neural arch, particularly in the vicinity of the facet joints. The joint space is partially obliterated. Bridging syndesmophyte extends along the anterior and lateral borders of the vertebral body.

a "stepladder" appearance of the cervical spine. Occasionally, the subluxations are severe enough to produce compression of the vertebral arteries, which may lead to vascular insufficiency (38).

Atlantoaxial subluxations are best demonstrated by plain radiographs obtained in flexion and extension positions. In adults, a distance greater than 2 mm between the posterior arch of C1 and the anterior surface of the dens is diagnostic of subluxation. Computed tomography may be used to show bone erosions involving the dens, lateral C1-C2 articulations, facet and uncovertebral joints (Fig. 39). CT is also useful in assessing displacements and narrowing of the spinal canal. Pannus occasionally may be identified by CT, but it is better evaluated with MR imaging. Pannus usually is of intermediate signal intensity on T1-weighted images, and it has been reported to be hyperintense on T2-weighted images, probably due to edema (16). Occasionally, it may show low signal intensity on T2-weighted images, probably reflecting its fibrous content. Pannus enhances after intravenous administration of gadolinium. Magnetic resonance imaging readily shows compression of the spinal cord and brain-

stem by pannus. Dynamic, low flip angle imaging with the patient in varying degrees of neck flexion and extension may be helpful in demonstrating atlantoaxial subluxations and compression of the brainstem by pannus.

ANKYLOSING SPONDYLOARTHRITIS

Ankylosing spondylitis (Marie-Strümpell disease) is one of the most common rheumatic diseases of the spine. It most commonly affects young men and is specifically associated with the histocompatibility antigen B27. It affects the sacroiliac joints, spine, and the bone insertions of ligaments. In the spine, it may give rise to ankylosis, subluxations, and fractures (which may produce epidural hematomas). Cauda equina syndrome is an unusual complication seen late in the course of the disease. The etiology of involvement of the cauda equina is uncertain, but it may be secondary to inflammation of the neighboring ligaments, which in turn leads to radiculitis. Dural ectasia, which may be erosive, also may occur (Fig. 40). Destruction of the disc and adjacent vertebrae, without underlying infection, is also a rare complication. Fractures and dislocations secondary to minor trauma are not uncommon. These fractures commonly lead to paralysis.

Plain radiographs are an efficient method to screen the sacroiliac joints for early involvement. Plain radiographs also show the so-called bamboo spine seen in advanced cases. The presence of symmetric sacroiliitis, thin syndesmophytes, squaring of the vertebral bodies ("dog spine"), and fusion of spinal joints establishes the diagnosis. Less common plain radiographic findings are atlantoaxial subluxation, calcification of discs and spinal ligaments, and erosion of posterior elements. Pathologic fractures are identifiable with plain radiographs, but their detailed evaluation requires CT. Computed tomography also is capable of showing obliteration of the sacroiliac joints, erosion

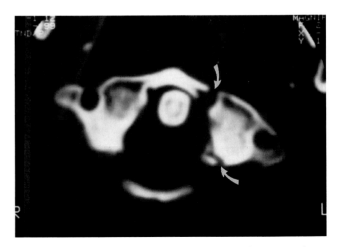

FIG. 41. Jefferson-type fracture. Transaxial CT shows fractures of the anterior and posterior arches of C2 in this unilateral variation of a Jefferson fracture.

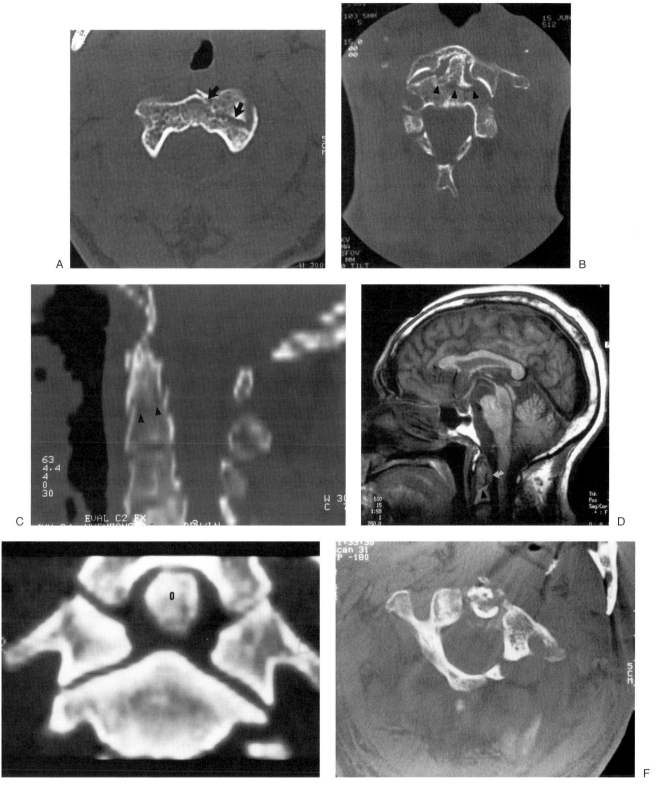

FIG. 42. Dens fractures and os odontoideum. **A:** Transaxial CT section shows fracture *(arrows)* involving the midportion and left lateral mass of C2. **B:** Oblique coronal CT section in the same patient showing the low dens fracture *(arrowheads)*. Hyperextension of the neck should not be done in these patients. Close to coronal images may occasionally be obtained (as in this case) solely by gantry angulation. **C:** Sagittal CT reformation clearly depicts the fracture *(arrowheads)*. **D:** Midline sagittal T1-weighted image of the brain in same patient shows the dens fracture *(arrowhead)* and a small epidural hematoma *(white curved arrow)*. **E:** In a different and asymptomatic patient, coronal CT reformation shows a well-corticated rounded os odontoideum (O). **F:** In a different patient, transaxial CT image shows a rare vertically oriented fracture of the dens with extension into the body of C2. The left lamina is also fractured.

of facet joints, and erosive dural ectasia (1) (Fig. 40). Sterile discitis is better evaluated with MR imaging, which shows destruction of the disc and loss of the vertebral endplate cartilage. The cartilage is replaced by zones of heterogeneous signal intensity. T2-weighted images show decreased signal intensity from the disc and absence of a paraspinal soft-tissue mass (40). These findings are presumed to be related to fibrous tissue replacement, and they serve to distinguish ankylosing spondyloarthritis from infection. Increased signal intensity from the joint space of the facets also may be present. Sterile discitis may lead to kyphosis.

SPINE FRACTURES

Upper Cervical Spine Fractures

The craniovertebral junction is well adapted to provide a remarkable range of motion, with approximately half of the neck rotation occurring at the C1-C2 articulation. This specialized structure also results in patterns of injury after trauma that are specific to the vertebrae in this region. Because of the relatively large spinal canal diameter at this level (approximately twice the spinal cord diameter), neurologic deficits may be mild or absent.

C1 (The Atlas)

A burst fracture of C1 (Jefferson fracture) is the result of transaxial loading, with bilateral outward displacement of the lateral masses of C1 (23). This injury can be diagnosed by recognizing the resultant fractures in both the anterior and posterior arches of C1 (Fig. 41).

An isolated fracture of the posterior arch of C1 may result from hyperextension, with impaction of the poste-rior arch of C1 between the occiput and C2. This injury is distinguished from the C1 burst fracture by involvement of only the posterior arch.

Isolated fracture of the anterior arch of C1 occurs less commonly. It also results from hyperextension, with avulsion of the attachment of the anterior spinal ligament. The small avulsed bone fragment is visible ventral to the anterior arch of C1. The posterior arch of C1 remains intact.

C2 (The Axis)

According to a scheme proposed by Anderson and D'Alonzo (4), fractures of the dens are commonly classified into types I, II, and III. Type II fractures are the most common, consisting of a fracture through the base of the dens at its junction with the body of C2 (Fig. 42). Such fractures have a very high incidence of nonunion if not surgically fused (3). A fracture that extends through the upper body of C2 is classified as type III (31). Type III fractures usually heal completely with external immobilization. A type I fracture is an avulsion of the tip of the dens. This extremely rare injury should be differentiated from an os odontoideum (Fig. 42E). Although most fractures of the dens have a horizontal orientation, vertical fractures of this structure may occur (Fig. 42F).

Traumatic spondylolysis of C2, the so-called hangman's fracture, is the most common fracture of the C2 vertebra. This injury is thought to be caused by hyperextension with resultant bilateral fractures of the pars interarticularis (Fig. 43). (It should be noted that the C2 vertebra is the only cervical vertebra with a true pars interarticularis.) With more severe injuries, the body of the C2 vertebra is displaced anteriorly with respect to the body of C3, and spinal cord injury is more common.

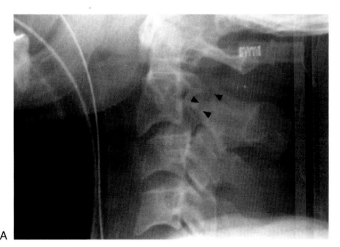
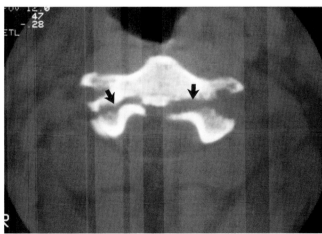

A

B

FIG. 43. Hangman's fracture. **A:** Lateral radiograph shows fractures *(arrowheads)* through the pars interarticularis of C2. The vertebral body of C2 is slightly displaced anteriorly on C3. **B:** CT section in the same patient confirms the presence of bilateral pars interarticularis fractures *(arrows).*

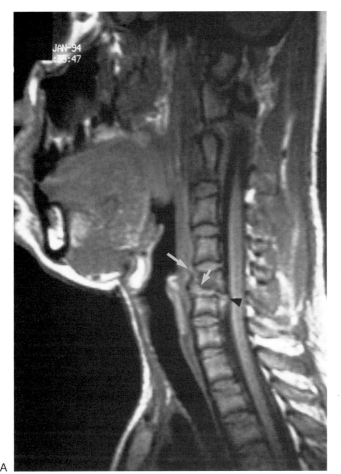

A

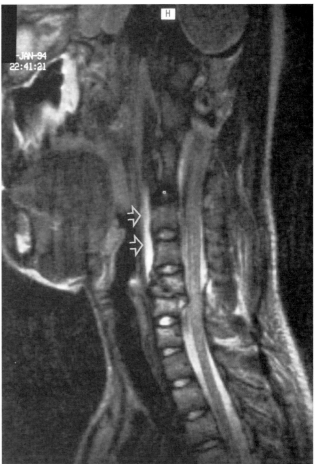

B

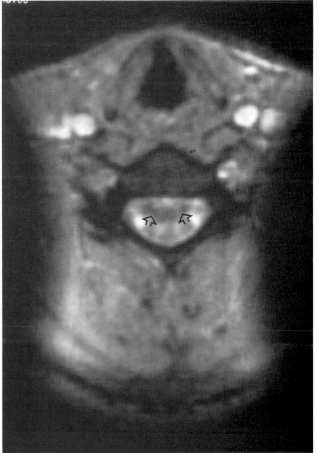

C

FIG. 44. Hyperextension injury. **A:** Midline sagittal T1-weighted image shows a slight posterior displacement of C5 on C6. There is disruption of the anterior longitudinal ligament *(longer white arrow)*, avulsion of the anteroinferior margin of C5 *(short white arrow)*, and a disc herniation *(arrowhead)*. **B:** Corresponding sagittal T2-weighted image shows prevertebral swelling *(arrows)*. **C:** Axial gradient echo image through the superior aspect of C6 shows the disc herniation *(arrows)*.

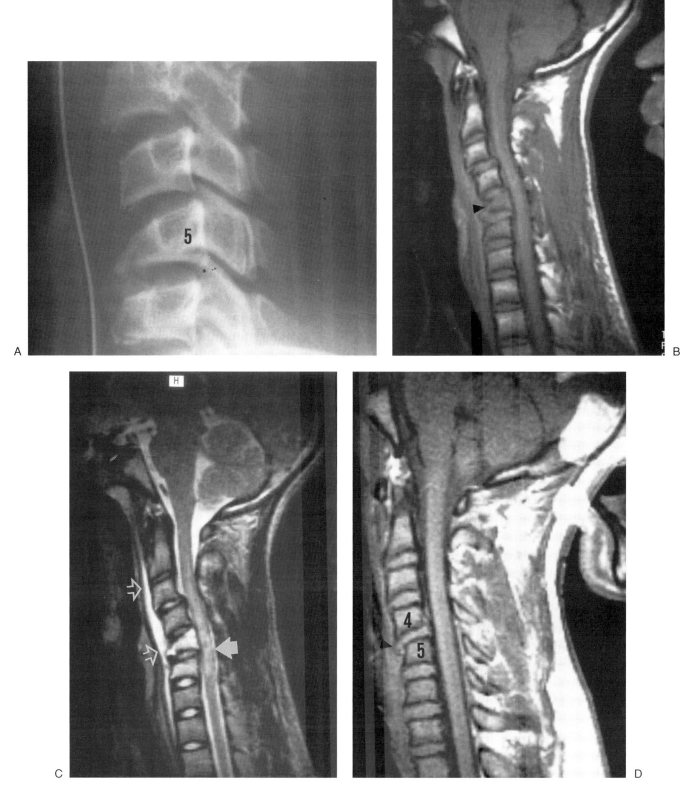

FIG. 45. Hyperflexion injuries. **A:** Lateral radiograph shows wedge fracture of C5 (5) following diving accident. **B:** Sagittal T1-weighted image shows compression fracture of C5 *(arrowhead)*. C5 is displaced posteriorly. C6 is also slightly wedged and its superior endplate is disrupted. Both C5 and C6 vertebral bodies have low signal intensity, suggesting bone marrow edema. **C:** Corresponding T2-weighted image shows prevertebral swelling *(open arrows)* and spinal cord edema *(solid arrow)*. Hyperintensity from C5 and C6 vertebral bodies compatible with bone marrow edema is present. **D:** Midline sagittal T1-weighted image in a different patient with a milder hyperflexion injury. There is slight anterior displacement of C4 (4) on C5 (5). Anterior disc herniation with disruption of the anterior longitudinal ligament *(arrowhead)* is present.

Lower Cervical Spine Fractures

The majority of fractures in adults occur in the lower cervical spine, predominantly at the C6 and C7 levels. The classification of these fractures is conventionally based on the presumed mechanism of injury.

Hyperextension Injuries

Hyperextension injuries, caused by impact to the face or forehead, may result in either dislocation or hyperextension teardrop fracture (34). Hyperextension dislocation is a disruption of the ligaments between adjacent vertebrae, including the anterior longitudinal ligament, annulus fibrosus, and facet capsular ligaments. As there may be no fracture, the plain radiograph or CT may appear nearly normal, except for diffuse thickening of the prevertebral soft tissues (32). Magnetic resonance is the imaging method of choice, because it identifies the prevertebral hematoma and discontinuity of ligaments (Fig. 44). This injury is frequently associated with severe spinal cord contusion, especially in patients with preexisting spondylitic changes. In approximately two thirds of patients with hyperextension dislocation injury, the intact anterior annulus causes an avulsion fracture of the anteroinferior margin of the affected vertebral body (32). This fragment is larger in the transverse dimension than in height, with an almost horizontally oriented fracture line.

Hyperextension teardrop fracture is an avulsion fracture of the anteroinferior margin of the vertebral body caused by excessive stress on the anterior longitudinal ligament (34). This injury occurs most commonly at the C2 level, usually in older, osteoporotic individuals, although it may occur at lower levels in non-osteoporotic patients. The fracture fragment can be distinguished from the avulsion fracture of hyperextension dislocation by the obliquity of the fracture line (approximately 45° from vertical) and the relatively greater height of the fragment.

All hyperextension injuries may be associated with herniated fragments of intervertebral disc, which may cause or worsen the associated spinal cord injury (Fig.

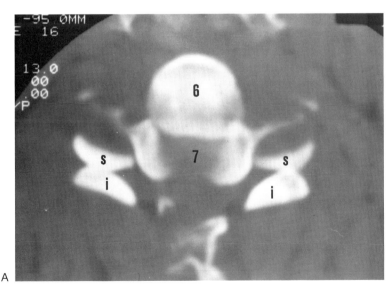

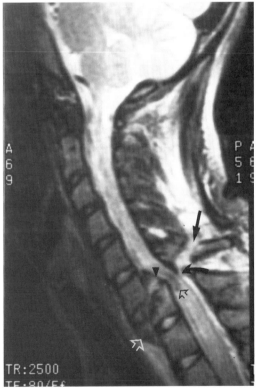

FIG. 46. Bilateral facet dislocation. **A:** Axial CT section shows that the superior facets (s) of C7 lie anterior to the inferior facets (i) of C6 (which is the reverse of normal). The body of C6 (6) is severely anteriorly displaced on the body of C7 (7). The spinal canal is narrow. **B:** Midsagittal T2-weighted image in same patient shows the severe anterior dislocation of C6 on C7. The anterosuperior aspect of C7 is fractured and the fragment *(white open arrow)* displaced anteriorly. Disc herniation *(arrowhead)* is present. The low signal intensity *(black open arrow)* within the spinal cord represents intracellular deoxyhemoglobin in an acute hematoma. The ligamentum flavum *(curved arrow)* is disrupted. The spinous process *(long black arrow)* of C6 is avulsed.

44B) (60). Magnetic resonance imaging provides excellent depiction of these herniated discs.

Hyperflexion Injuries

Hyperflexion injuries result from impact to the top or back of the head, with the neck in flexion (12,41). These injuries, which are especially common in divers, include hyperflexion sprain, wedge fracture, bilateral interfacet joint dislocation, and teardrop fracture.

Hyperflexion sprain refers to disruption of the posterior ligamentous attachments between adjacent vertebrae (the nuchal ligament, interspinous ligaments, facet capsular ligaments, and posterior longitudinal ligament). On plain radiographs, this injury may be recognized by abnormal widening between adjacent posterior elements, and by subtle, acute kyphotic angulation at the level of injury. On T2-weighted MR images, high signal intensity edema and blood products within the posterior ligamentous structures is confirmatory. Diagnosis of this injury is important because it may be associated with chronic neck pain and a high incidence of failed ligamentous healing in patients managed nonsurgically.

Wedge fractures consist of an impaction fracture of the superior endplate of the affected vertebral body in addition to posterior ligament disruption. The inferior endplate remains intact. There is greater loss of vertebral body height anteriorly, resulting in the typical wedge-shaped vertebral body seen on the lateral plain radiograph or sagittal CT reformation (Fig. 45).

Bilateral interfacet joint dislocation requires greater forces than that associated with the hyperflexion injuries described above. In addition to disruption of the posterior ligamentous structures, this injury involves disruption of the anterior longitudinal ligament, the annular fibers of the intervertebral disc, and complete bilateral dislocation of the facet joints (74) (Fig. 46). The inferior articular processes of the upper vertebra become lodged in the neural foramina anterior to the superior articular processes of the lower vertebra, preventing reduction. This injury is thus sometimes referred to as bilaterally locked facets, erroneously implying mechanical stability. On plain radiographs, this injury is diagnosed by anterior displacement of the upper vertebra by one half or more of the width of the lower vertebral. The "naked" articular surfaces of the dislocated facets are usually also visible. Magnetic resonance imaging not only reveals the above features, but it is also useful for detecting the presence of the commonly associated herniated disc or epidural hematoma. Computed tomography may be helpful for detecting fractures of the articular masses, which can interfere with attempts at reduction.

Hyperflexion teardrop fracture occurs with even greater magnitude forces. This injury shares the poste-

rior ligamentous disruption of the other hyperflexion injuries, but it consists additionally of a large triangular fracture fragment of the anterior–inferior margin of the upper vertebral body (41,68) (Fig. 47). Associated severe narrowing of the spinal canal caused by retropulsed bone fragments almost universally produces severe spinal cord injury. This fracture can be distinguished from the similarly named hyperextension teardrop fracture by the larger size of the triangular fragment and distraction of the posterior elements, indicating the flexion mechanism.

Vertical Compression Injuries

Vertical compression injuries result from impact to the top of the head with the spine straight (34). These injuries include the Jefferson fracture of C1, discussed above, and burst fractures of the lower cervical spine.

Vertebral body burst fractures are thought to occur when vertical compressive forces are transmitted through the intervertebral disc, with radial outward forces generated in the vertebral body (75). This type of injury causes a vertical fracture with lateral dispersion of the vertebral body fragments. On plain radiographs, the diagnosis is made by recognizing the widened uncovertebral joints or visualizing the vertical fracture line. Computed tomography may aid in identifying the vertical fracture line and the frequently associated fractures of the pedicles or lami-

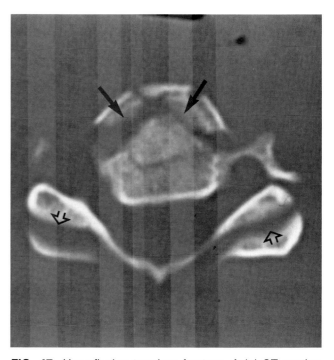

FIG. 47. Hyperflexion teardrop fracture. Axial CT section shows fracture *(arrows)* of anteroinferior margin of C5. The facet joints are splayed *(open arrows)*, indicating rupture of the capsular ligaments.

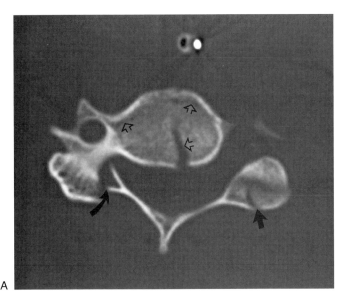 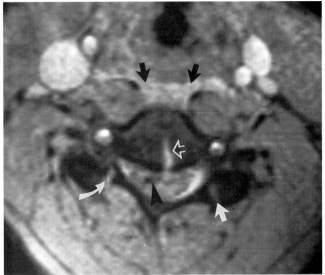

A   B

FIG. 48. Vertical compression fracture. **A:** Axial CT section shows multiple fractures *(open arrows)* in the body of C5. Also seen are fractures of the right lamina *(curved arrow)* and left articular pillar *(arrow)*. **B:** Axial gradient echo image at the same level also shows fractures of vertebral body *(white open arrow)*, right lamina *(white curved arrow)*, and left articular pillar *(white solid arrow)*. Dark signal intensity *(black arrowhead)* in the spinal cord is a result of deoxyhemoglobin in an acute hematoma. Prevertebral edema *(black solid arrows)* is also present.

nae (Fig. 48). MR imaging is helpful in detecting herniated disc fragments, which also commonly accompany this injury.

Other Mechanisms

Less common mechanisms of injury also may lead to recognized fracture patterns. A combination of flexion and rotational forces can result in unilateral facet dislocation (Fig. 49). This injury is distinguished from bilateral facet dislocation by the limited amount of anterolisthesis (approximately 25%, versus 50% for bilateral). Lateral force vectors may lead to isolated fractures of the uncinate processes. Combined extension and rotation forces may result in pillar or pedicolaminar fractures.

Thoracic Spine

The normal thoracic spine is well stabilized by the rib cage, thoracic musculature, and steeply oriented facet joints. Consequently, thoracic spine fractures are uncommon, except with severe trauma. Because of the normal fixed thoracic kyphosis, transaxial forces are transformed into flexion equivalents, with most injuries being related to hyperflexion. The most common of these injuries are wedge-type fractures and flexion fracture dislocations (5). Plain radiographic evaluation of the thoracic spine may be difficult because of superimposition of the shoulder girdle and ribs. Computed tomography is valuable in all cases of suspected thoracic spine fracture (47).

Wedge fractures are considered simple if only the anterior vertebral body is involved. Severe wedge fractures involve the posterior vertebral body as well, with the potential for posterior displacement of bony fragments into the spinal canal (Fig. 50). CT or MR imaging can be used to assess spinal canal narrowing that results from hyperkyphotic angulation or retropulsed fragments.

Fracture dislocations occur with larger magnitude forces, frequently resulting in severe spinal cord injury. Magnetic resonance imaging provides valuable information regarding spinal canal narrowing, cord injury, and the presence of associated epidural hematoma.

Thoracolumbar and Lumbar Spine

The thoracolumbar junction (T12 to L2) is the next most common site of spine fracture after the cervical spine (53). Most of the injuries to the lumbar spine and thoracolumbar junction are related to abnormal flexion or vertical compression forces. Common types of injuries include wedge, burst, and Chance fractures.

Wedge fractures result when flexion forces lead to a fracture of the vertebral body only, without involvement of the posterior elements. Characteristically, the loss of vertebral body height is greater anteriorly than posteriorly. Plain radiographs are diagnostic in most cases. Classification into simple and severe wedge fractures is similar to that of the thoracic spine. If there is a question of posterior element fractures or posterior displacement of fragments, CT provides clarification and assessment of the residual spinal canal diameter (Fig. 51).

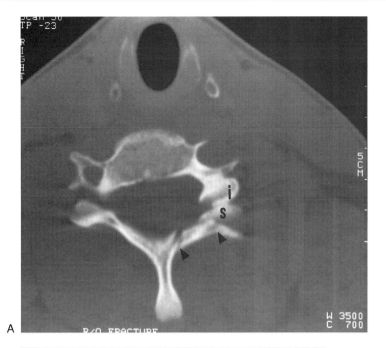

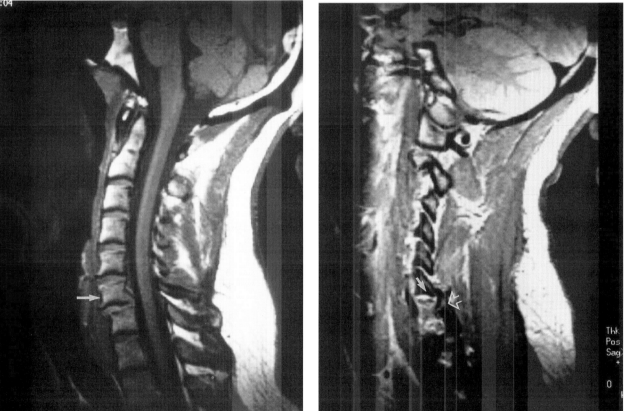

FIG. 49. Unilateral facet dislocation. **A:** Axial CT section shows left-sided facet dislocation. The inferior facet (i) of C6 lies anterior to the superior facet (s) of C7, which is the reverse of normal. The C6 vertebral body is slightly rotated to the right. The left lamina is fractured *(arrowheads).* **B:** Midline sagittal T1-weighted image in the same case shows mild anterior displacement of C6 *(arrow)* on C7. **C:** Parasagittal proton density image through left facet joints shows that the inferior facet of C6 *(solid arrow)* is displaced anteriorly to the superior facet *(open arrow)* of C7. Note the normal arrangement of facet joints in superior levels.

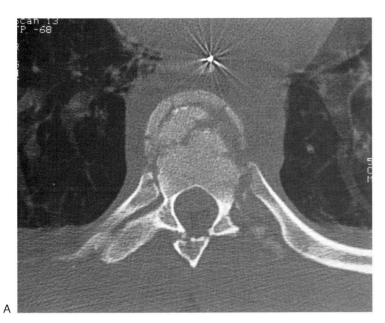

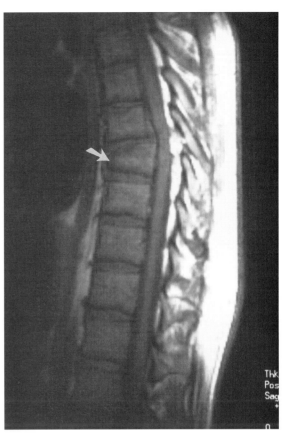

FIG. 50. Thoracic spine compression fracture. **A:** Axial CT section shows compression fracture involving mainly the anterior aspect of the T7 vertebral body. The posterior margin of the body appears intact. **B:** Midsagittal T1-weighted image in same patient showing the wedged T7 vertebral body *(arrow)*. The posterior margin is displaced into the spinal canal producing spinal cord compression.

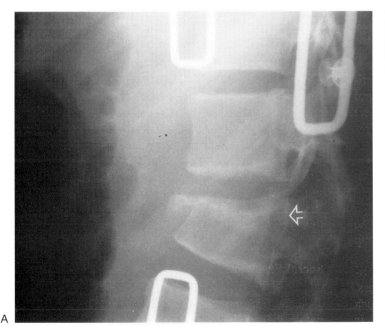

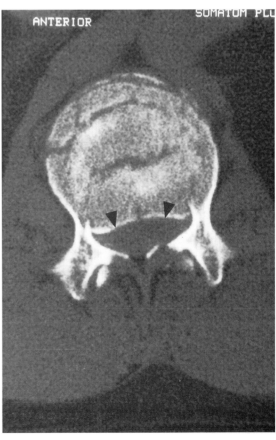

FIG. 51. Lumbar vertebral body wedge fracture. **A:** Lateral radiograph shows typical wedge fracture of L1. Height loss in the anterior aspect of the vertebral body is greater than posteriorly. There is a questionable bone density *(arrow)* in the canal. Patient is in a brace. **B:** Axial CT section shows fractures involving the vertebral body and confirms posterior displacement of dorsal margin *(arrowheads)*, which narrows the canal.

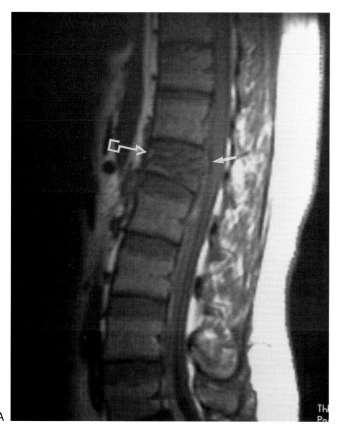

A

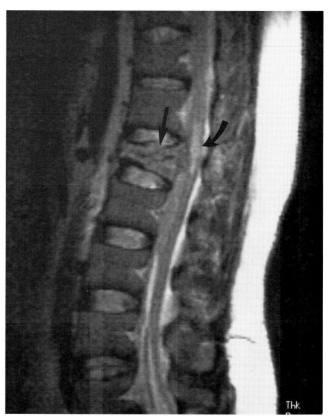

B

FIG. 52. Lumbar burst fracture with edema of conus medullaris. **A:** Midsagittal T1-weighted image shows fracture of L1 *(key arrow)* with posteriorly displaced bone fragment *(straight arrow)*. The vertebral body is of low signal intensity suggesting bone marrow edema. **B:** Corresponding T2-weighted image shows fracture of L1, posteriorly displaced bone fragment, and bone marrow edema (high signal intensity). This sequence shows to better advantage the disruption of the superior endplate *(straight arrow)* of L1 and high signal intensity in the conus medullaris *(curved arrow)* compatible with edema.

Burst fractures in the lumbar spine consist of a vertically oriented fracture of the vertebral body with lateral dispersion of the fracture fragments (6). Usually, there are associated fractures in the posterior elements. This injury can be recognized on plain radiographs by identifying the vertical fracture line or by detecting a widened interpediculate distance. Computed tomography is useful for characterizing the associated posterior element fractures and for assessing spinal canal impingement (70). Magnetic resonance imaging provides assessment of the conus medullaris or spinal nerve roots in patients with neurological deficits (Fig. 52).

The Chance fracture is defined as a horizontally oriented fracture that passes through the spinous process, laminae, and vertebral body (65). This fracture, which occurs exclusively at the thoracolumbar junction, is thought to be the result of distractive forces generated when the spine is flexed about a fulcrum point, such as a car lap seat belt (73). This mechanism has prompted the term *seat belt injury* to describe this and associated injuries. A fracture in which the horizontal plane of disruption passes through the intervertebral disc or posterior ligaments, rather than the vertebral body or posterior bony

elements, is considered a variation of the Chance fracture (Fig. 53). Usually, the fracture lines of the Chance fracture are visible on the plain radiographs. Magnetic resonance imaging may demonstrate the ligamentous components of the various forms of injury, along with any conus medullaris or nerve root injuries. The association of Chance fractures with significant intraperitoneal injuries in up to 50% of patients has prompted some authors to suggest routine CT of the abdomen in all patients with this type of injury (26).

Sacral Fracture

Acute fractures of the sacrum are best considered within the category of pelvic fractures and will not be discussed here.

Insufficiency fractures of the sacrum occur when the elastic strength of the bone is not adequate to withstand the stresses of normal activity (22). Such fractures occur in patients with metabolic bone disease or prior radiation therapy. Although insufficiency fractures of the sacrum are not uncommon, their radiographic diagnosis is fre-

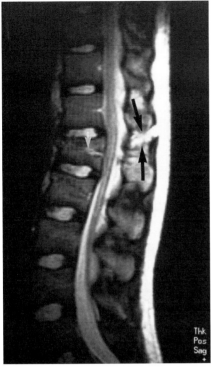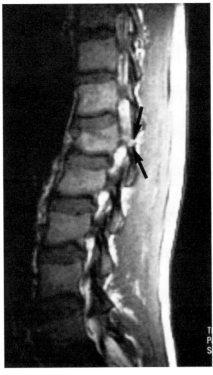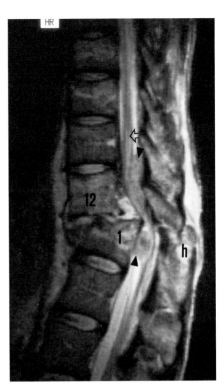

A,B   C

FIG. 53. Chance fracture. **A:** Midline sagittal T2-weighted image in this patient who was involved in a motor vehicle collision while wearing only lap seat belt. There is disruption of the posterior ligament complex with widening of the interspinous space *(long arrows)*. The L1 vertebral body is slightly wedged and there is accentuation of the basivertebral vein canal, suggesting that the fracture line extends through this region *(arrowhead)*. The posterior margins of L1 are minimally displaced dorsally. **B:** Left parasagittal T1-weighted image showing that the facet joints *(arrows)* are separated, implying disruption of the capsular ligaments. The bone marrow within the L1 vertebral body is inhomogeneous. **C:** Different patient after horseback riding accident. Midsagittal T2-weighted image showing severe fracture–dislocation with posterior displacement of L1 (1) on T12 (12). Presence of interspinous hematoma (h) is indicative of disruption in the posterior ligamentous complex. There is total disruption of the disc, with significant posterior displacement of L1 and compression of the cauda equina. Intraspinal epidural hematomas *(arrowheads)* and edema of the conus medullaris *(open arrow)* are present. This constellation of findings may be considered a variant of the Chance type fracture.

quently challenging. The typical plain radiographic finding is linear sclerosis running vertically within the sacral ala, parallel and adjacent to the sacroiliac joint (19). On plain radiographs and radionuclide bone scintigraphy, the fracture may be mistaken for a metastatic lesion. The cross-sectional capability of CT, along with improved contrast resolution of the poorly mineralized bones, aids greatly in the diagnosis. The fracture line usually traverses the sacrum parallel to, and near, the sacroiliac joint. If the diagnosis is equivocal on plain radiographs and CT, a radionuclide bone scan may be used to confirm the presence of the fracture.

REFERENCES

1. Abello R, Rovira M, Sanz MP, et al. MRI and CT of ankylosing spondylitis with vertebral scalloping. *Neuroradiology* 1988;30: 272–275.
2. Aguila LA, Piraino DW, Modic MT, et al. The internuclear cleft of the intervertebral disc: magnetic resonance imaging. *Radiology* 1985;155:155–158.
3. Amyes EW, Anderson FM. Fracture of the odontoid process: report of sixty-three cases. *Arch Surg* 1956;72:377–393.
4. Anderson LD, D'Alonzo RT. Fractures of the odontoid process of the axis. *J Bone Joint Surg Am* 1974;56:1663–1674.
5. Antuaco EJ, Binet EF. Radiology of thoracic and lumbar fractures. *Clin Orthop* 1984;189:43–57.
6. Atlas SW, Regenbogen V, Rogers LF, et al. The radiographic characterization of burst fractures of the spine. *AJR Am J Roentgenol* 1986;147:575–582.
7. Azouz EM, Kozlowski K, Marton D, et al. Osteoid osteoma and osteoblastoma of spine in children. Report of 22 cases with brief literature review. *Pediatr Radiol* 1986;16:25–31.
8. Bangert BA, Ross JS. Arachnoiditis affecting the lumbar spine. *Neuroimaging Clin North Am* 1993;3:517–524.
9. Bazan C. Imaging of lumbosacral spine neoplasms. *Neuroimaging Clin North Am* 1993;3:591–608.
10. Boden SD, Davis DO, Dina TS, et al. Contrast-enhanced MR imaging performed after successful lumbar disc surgery: prospective study. *Radiology* 1992;182:59–64.
11. Boden SD, Davis DO, Dina TS, Sunner JL, Wiesel SW. Postoperative discitis: distinguishing early MR imaging findings from normal postoperative disc space changes. *Radiology* 1992;184:765–771.
12. Braakman R, Penning L. The hyperflexion sprain of the cervical spine. *Radiol Clin Biol* 1968;37:309.
13. Braun IF, Hoffman JC, Davis PC, Landman JA, Tindall GT. Contrast enhancement in CT differentiation between recurrent disc her-

niation and postoperative scar: prospective study. *AJNR Am J Neuroradiol* 1985;6:607–612.

14. Braun IF, Malko JA, Davis PC, Hoffman JC, Jacobs LH. The behavior of Pantopaque on MR: in vivo and in vitro analyses. *AJNR Am J Neuroradiol* 1986;7:997–1001.

15. Bundschuh CV. Imaging of the postoperative lumbosacral spine. *Neuroimaging Clin North Am* 1993;3:499–516.

16. Bunschuh CV, Modic MT, Kearny F, et al. Rheumatoid arthritis of the cervical spine: surface-coil MR imaging. *AJNR Am J Neuroradiol* 1988;9:565–571.

17. Castillo M, Malko JA, Hoffman JC. The bright intervertebral disc: an indirect sign of abnormal spinal bone marrow on T1-weighted MR images. *AJNR Am J Neuroradiol* 1990;11:23–26.

18. Colombo N, Berry I, Norman D. Infections of the spine. In: Manelfe C, ed. *Imaging of the spine and spinal cord.* New York: Raven Press, 1992;489–512.

19. Cooper KL, Beabout JW, Swee RG. Insufficiency fractures of the sacrum. *Radiology* 1985;156:15–20.

20. Czervionke LF, Daniels DL, Ho PSP, et al. Cervical neural foramina: correlative anatomic and MR imaging study. *Radiology* 1988;169:753–759.

21. Dahlin DC, Cupps RE, Johnson EW. Giant-cell tumor: a study of 195 cases. *Cancer* 1970;25:1061–1068.

22. Denis F, Denis S, Comfort T. Sacral fractures: an important problem. Retrospective analysis of 236 cases. *Clin Orthop* 1988;277:67–81.

23. Effendi B, Roy D, Cornish B, et al. Fractures of the ring of the axis: a classification based on the analysis of 131 cases. *J Bone Joint Surg Br* 1981;63:319–327.

24. Enzmann DR, DeLaPaz RL. Tumor. In: Enzman DR, DeLaPaz RL, Rubin JB, eds. *Magnetic resonance imaging of the spine.* St. Louis, MO: CV Mosby, 1990;365–372.

25. Glass RBJ, Poznanski AK, Fisher MR, Shkolnik A, Dias L. MR imaging of osteoid osteoma. *J Comput Assist Tomogr* 1986;10:1065–1067.

26. Green DA, Green NE, Spengler DM, et al. Flexion-distraction injuries to the lumbar spine associated with abdominal injuries. *J Spinal Disord* 1991;4:312–318.

27. Grenier N, Greselle JF, Vital JM, et al. Normal and disrupted lumbar longitudinal ligaments: correlative MR and anatomic study. *Radiology* 1989;171:197–205.

28. Gundry CR, Heithoff KB. Epidural hematoma of the lumbar spine: 18 surgically confirmed cases. *Radiology* 1993;187:427–431.

29. Hackney DB. Magnetic resonance imaging of the spine. Normal anatomy. *Top Magn Reson Imaging* 1992;4:1–6.

30. Haggstrom JA, Brown JC, Marsh PW. Eosinophilic granuloma of the spine: MR demonstration. *J Comput Assist Tomogr* 1988;12:344–345.

31. Harris JH, Burke KT, Ray RD, et al. Low type (III) odontoid fracture: a new radiographic sign. *Radiology* 1984;153:353–356.

32. Harris JH, Yeakley JS. Radiographically subtle soft tissue injuries of the cervical spine. *Curr Probl Diagn Radiol* 1989;25:167–190.

33. Herman SD, Mesgarzadeh M, Bonakdarpour A. The role of magnetic resonance imaging in giant cell tumor of bone. *Skeletal Radiol* 1987;16:635–643.

34. Holdsworth F. Review article: dislocations and fracture–dislocations of the spine. *J Bone Joint Surg Am* 1970;52:1534–1551.

35. Hueftle MG, Modic MT, Ross JS, et al. Lumbar spine: postoperative MR imaging with Gd-DTPA. *Radiology* 1988;167:817–824.

36. Jinkins JR. MR of enhancing nerve roots in the unoperated lumbosacral spine. *AJNR Am J Neuroradiol* 1993;14:193–202.

37. Johnson CE, Sze G. Benign lumbar arachnoiditis: MR imaging with gadopentetate dimeglumine. *AJNR Am J Neuroradiol* 1990;11:763–770.

38. Kawaida H, Sakou T, Morizono Y, Yoshikuni N. Magnetic resonance imaging of upper cervical disorders in rheumatoid arthritis. *Spine* 1989;17:1144–1148.

39. Kelsey JL, White AA, Pastides H, et al. The impact of musculoskeletal disorders in the population of the United States. *J Bone Joint Surg Am* 1979;61:959–964.

40. Kenny JB, Hughes PL, Whitehouse GH. Discovertebral destruction in ankylosing spondylitis: the role of computed tomography and magnetic resonance imaging. *Br J Radiol* 1990;63:448–455.

41. Kim KS, Chen HH, Russell EJ, Roger LF. Flexion tear-drop fractures of the cervical spine: radiographic characteristics. *AJR Am J Roentgenol* 1989;152:319–326.

42. Kirkwood JR. Spine. In: *Essentials of neuroimaging.* New York: Churchill Livingstone, 1990;365–452.

43. Kroon HM, Schurman J. Osteoblastoma: clinical and radiographic findings in 98 new cases. *Radiology* 1990;175:783–790.

44. Laredo JD, Assouline E, Gelbert F, et al. Vertebral hemangiomas: fat content as signal of aggressiveness. *Radiology* 1990;177:467–472.

45. Masaryk TJ, Ross JS, Modic MT, et al. Radiculomeningeal vascular malformations of the spine: MR imaging. *Radiology* 1987;164:845–849.

46. Masaryk TJ. Neoplastic disease of the spine. *Radiol Clin North Am* 1991;4:829–845.

47. McAfee PC, Yuan HA, Fredickson BE, et al. The value of computed tomography in thoracolumbar fractures. *J Bone Joint Surg Am* 1983;65:461–472.

48. Minami S, Sagoh T, Nishimura K, et al. Spinal arteriovenous malformation: MR imaging. *Radiology* 1988;169:109–115.

49. Modic MT, Feiglin DH, Piraino DW, et al. Vertebral osteomyelitis: assessment using MR. *Radiology* 1985;157:157–166.

50. Modic MT, Masaryk TJ, Ross JS, Carter JR. Imaging of degenerative disc disease. *Radiology* 1988;168:177–186.

51. Mohazab HR, Langer B, Spigos D. Spinal epidural hematoma in a patient with lupus coagulopathy: MR findings. *AJR Am J Roentgenol* 1993;160:853–854.

52. Nguyen CM, Haughton VM, Ho KC, An HS. MR contrast enhancement: an experimental study in postlaminectomy epidural fibrosis. *AJNR Am J Neuroradiol* 1993;14:997–1002.

53. Nicoll EA. Fractures of the dorso-lumbar spine. *J Bone Joint Surg Br* 1949;31:376–394.

54. Numaguchi Y, Rigamonti D, Rothman MI, et al. Spinal epidural abscess: evaluation with Gadolinium-enhanced MR imaging. *Radiographics* 1993;13:545–559.

55. Olsen WL, Chakeres DW, Berry I, Richaud R. Spine and spinal cord trauma. In: Manelfe C, ed. *Imaging of the spine and spinal cord.* New York: Raven Press 1992;413–416.

56. Otake S, Marcuo N, Nishizawa S, et al. Ossification of the posterior longitudinal ligament in MR evaluation. *AJNR Am J Neuroradiol* 1992;13:1059–1067.

57. Pech P, Haughton VM. Lumbar intervertebral disc: correlative MR and anatomic study. *Radiology* 1985;156:699–701.

58. Post MJD, Quencer RM, Montalvo BM, et al. Spinal infection: evaluation with MR imaging and intraoperative ultrasound. *Radiology* 1988;169:765–771.

59. Post MJD, Sze G, Quencer RM, et al. Gadolinium-enhanced MR in spinal infection. *J Comput Assist Tomogr* 1990;14:721–729.

60. Pratt ES, Green DA, Sengler DM. Herniated intervertebral discs associated with unstable spine injuries. *Spine* 1990;15:662–666.

61. Rahmouni A, Divine K, Mathieu D, et al. Detection of multiple myeloma involving the spine: efficacy of fat-suppression and contrast-enhanced MR imaging. *AJR Am J Roentgenol* 1993;160:1049–1052.

62. Resnick D, Niwayama G, Guerra J, et al. Spinal vacuum phenomena: anatomical study and review. *Radiology* 1981;139:341–348.

63. Ricci C, Cova M, Kang YS, et al. Normal age-related patterns of cellular and fatty bone marrow distribution in the axial skeleton: MR imaging study. *Radiology* 1990;177:83–88.

64. Rodesch G, Berenstein A, Lasjaunias P. Vasculature and vascular lesions of the spine and spinal cord. In: Manelfe C, ed. *Imaging of the spine and spinal cord.* New York: Raven Press, 1992;565–598.

65. Rogers LF. The roentgenographic appearance of transverse or Chance fracture of the spine: the seat belt fracture. *AJR Am J Roentgenol* 1971;111:844–849.

66. Ross JS, Masaryk TJ, Modic MT, et al. Lumbar spine: postoperative assessment with surface-coil MR imaging. *Radiology* 1987;164:851–860.

67. Sapico FL, Montgomerie JZ. Vertebral osteomyelitis. *Infect Dis Clin North Am* 1990;4:539–551.

68. Schneider RC, Kahn EA. Chronic neurologic sequelae of acute trauma to the spine and spinal cord. Part I: the significance of the acute flexion or ''tear-drop'' fracture–dislocation of the cervical spine. *J Bone Joint Surg Am* 1956;38(A):985.

69. Sharif HS. Role of MR imaging in the management of spinal infections. *AJR Am J Roentgenol* 1992;158:1333–1345.
70. Shuman WP, Rogers JB, Sickler ME, et al. Thoracolumbar burst fractures: CT dimensions of the spinal canal relative to post surgical improvement. *AJR Am J Roentgenol* 1985;145:337–341.
71. Sigimura K, Yamasaki K, Kitagaki H, Tanaka Y, Kono M. Bone marrow diseases of the spine: differentiation with T1- and T2-relaxation time in MR imaging. *Radiology* 1987;165:541–544.
72. Sklar EML, Quencer RM, Green BA, Montalvo BM, Post MJD. Complications of epidural anesthesia: MR appearance of abnormalities. *Radiology* 1991;549–554.
73. Smith WS, Kaufer H. Patterns and mechanisms of lumbar injuries associated with lap seat belts. *J Bone Joint Surg Am* 1969;51:239–254.
74. Sonntag VKH. Management of bilateral locked facets of the cervical spine. *Neurosurgery* 1981;8:150–152.
75. Starr KH, Hanely EN. Junctional burst fractures. *Spine* 1992;17:551–558.
76. Sugimura H, Kakitsubata Y, Suzuki Y, et al. MR of ossification of ligamentum flavum. *J Comput Assist Tomogr* 1992;16:73–76.
77. Sze G, Bravo S, Krol G. Spinal lesions: quantitative and qualitative temporal evolution of gadopentetate dimeglumine enhancement in MR imaging. *Radiology* 1989;170:849–856.
78. Sze G, Uichanco LS, Brant-Zawadzki M, Davis R, et al. Chordomas: MR imaging. *Radiology* 1988;166:187–191.
79. Takahashi M, Shimomura O, Sakae T. Comparison of magnetic resonance imaging with computed tomography—myelography in the diagnosis of lumbar disc herniation. *Neuroimaging Clin North Am* 1993;3:487–498.
80. Van Tassel P. MR imaging of spinal infections. *Top Magn Reson Imaging* 1994;6:69–81.
81. Weaver P, Lifeso RM. The radiological diagnosis of tuberculosis of the adult spine. *Skeletal Radiol* 1984;12:178–186.
82. Yu S, Haughton VM, Sether LA, Wagner M. Annulus fibrosus in bulging intervertebral discs. *Radiology* 1988;169:761–763.
83. Yuh WTC, Flickinger FW, Barloon TJ, Montgomery WJ. MR imaging of unusual chordomas. *J Comput Assist Tomogr* 1988;12:30–35.
84. Zimmer WD, Berquist TH, McLeod RA, et al. Bone tumors, magnetic resonance imaging versus computed tomography. *Radiology* 1985;155:709–718.

CHAPTER 24

Pediatric Applications

Marilyn J. Siegel

Imaging of pediatric diseases has undergone a remarkable evolution with the development of computed tomography (CT) and magnetic resonance imaging (MRI). Both studies have become important imaging techniques in nearly every part of the pediatric body. In fact, CT and MRI have redirected the imaging approach to some pediatric problems. CT is accepted as the primary imaging test to evaluate blunt abdominal trauma. It is commonly used as a secondary test to further evaluate abnormalities of the chest, abdomen, and pelvis detected on conventional radiographic studies or ultrasonography (US). MRI is increasingly utilized as the primary study to evaluate soft tissue and paraspinal masses as well as joint abnormalities, and it is employed as a secondary test to assess abnormalities observed on plain radiographs or CT scans. This chapter will highlight the diagnostic applications of CT and MRI in a wide variety of disease processes of the chest, abdomen, pelvis, and musculoskeletal system in children. General guidelines to assist in appropriately selecting imaging examinations will also be provided.

TECHNIQUE

Sedation

Sedation is required for CT and MRI evaluation of infants and children 5 years of age and younger to prevent motion artifacts during scanning (142,195). Children older than 5 years of age generally will cooperate after verbal reassurance and explanation of the procedure and will not need immobilization or sedation. The drugs most frequently used for sedation are oral chloral hydrate and intravenous pentobarbital sodium (17,103,253). Oral chloral hydrate, 50 to 100 mg/kg, with a maximum dosage of 2000 mg, is the drug of choice for children younger than 18 months. Intravenous pentobarbital sodium, 6 mg/kg with a maximum dose of 200 mg, is advocated in children older than 18 months. It is injected slowly in fractions of one fourth the total dose and is titrated against the patient's response. This is an effective form of sedation with a failure rate of <5%.

Other methods of sedation include intramuscular or rectal barbiturate and a combination of meperidine, chlorpromazine, and promethazine, commonly referred to as a "cardiac cocktail." The failure rate from intramuscular or rectal administration of barbiturates is more than that from the intravenous route of administration. The risks of apnea and respiratory and cardiac depression from narcotic analgesics (e.g., meperidine) are significantly greater than the risks from barbiturate sedation. Because intravenous barbiturate sedation results in fewer failures and has a shorter mean time of duration in young children, it is preferred by most examiners. Regardless of the choice of drug, the use of parenteral sedation requires the facility and ability to resuscitate and maintain adequate cardiorespiratory support during and after the examination. Monitoring sedated or critically ill children in the MR scanner requires magnet-compatible equipment including pulse oximeters, electrocardiographic equipment, and blood pressure monitoring devices.

After being sedated, the infant or child is placed on a blanket on the CT or MRI table. The arms routinely are extended above the head to avoid streak artifacts and to provide an easily accessible route for intravenous injection. The upper arms can be restrained with sandbags, adhesive tape, or velcro straps.

Patients who are to receive parenteral sedation should have no liquids by mouth for 3 hr and no solid foods for 6 hr prior to their examination. Patients who are not sedated but are to receive intravenous contrast medium should be NPO (nothing per mouth) for 3 hr to minimize the likelihood of nausea or vomiting with possible aspiration during a bolus injection of intravenous contrast medium.

After completion of the examination and recovery from sedation, the patient is discharged to either home or the hospital ward. Criteria for discharge include alertness, stable vital signs for 1 hr after the administration of sedation, and the ability to tolerate oral fluids. Children are discharged with an adult who is given verbal and written instructions regarding home care procedures and normal and abnormal behavior after sedation as well as contact telephone numbers for questions that arise later.

CT: SPECIAL TECHNICAL CONSIDERATIONS

Intravenous Contrast Material

Scanning after intravenous administration of iodinated contrast material is helpful to confirm a lesion thought to be of vascular origin, or to establish its relationship to vascular structures, in addition to improving differentiation between normal and pathologic parenchyma, especially in the liver and kidneys. If intravenous contrast material is to be administered, it is helpful to have an intravenous line in place when the child arrives in the radiology department. This reduces patient agitation that otherwise would be associated with a venipuncture performed just prior to administration of contrast material. The largest gauge butterfly needle or plastic cannula that can be placed is recommended. Either low-osmolar or high- osmolar contrast media may be used, usually at a dose of 2 ml/kg (not to exceed 4 ml/kg or 100 ml).

Contrast may be administered by hand injection or via a mechanical injector (140). The latter type of administration should be performed if a 22-gauge or larger plastic cannula can be placed into an antecubital vein. The contrast injection rate is determined by the caliber of the intravenous catheter. Contrast material is infused at 1.2 ml/sec for a 22-gauge catheter, at 1.5 ml/sec for a 20-gauge catheter, and at 2 ml/sec for an 18-gauge needle. The contrast medium should be administered by a hand injection using a bolus technique if intravenous access is through a peripheral access line, a smaller caliber antecubital catheter or butterfly needle, or a central venous catheter.

The scan delay time with spiral scanning is based on the type of examination and the method of contrast administration (e.g., hand versus mechanical injection) (159). For examinations of the chest, spiral scanning should be initiated after 80% of the total volume of contrast has been administered. In the abdomen, scanning should begin after 100% of the contrast dose has been given. There are two exceptions to the above approach for contrast

administration. First, in neonates and very small children in whom small volumes of contrast medium are administered, CT scanning of the chest and abdomen should be delayed at least 30 sec to ensure that there is enhancement of vascular structures. Second, in larger children in whom contrast is given through small-gauge catheters (22- to 24-gauge) with lower flow rates, CT scanning of the abdomen should begin no later than 60 sec after the start of the contrast injection. Adult protocols can be applied to the evaluation of children who weigh more than 45 kg. A uniphasic technique suffices for nearly all spiral CT examinations in children.

Alternatively, an automated bolus tracking technique can be used to monitor contrast enhancement and initiate scanning. This technique allows on-line monitoring of contrast enhancement by acquiring very low milliamperage scans and region of interest measurements at a predetermined level (103). Once an arbitrary threshold level of contrast enhancement has been reached, diagnostic scanning is initiated.

Bowel Opacification

Opacification of the small and large bowel is necessary for most examinations of the abdomen, as unopacified bowel loops can simulate a mass or abnormal fluid collection (142). The exceptions are patients with depressed mental status who are at risk of aspiration and those with acute blunt abdominal trauma where there may be insufficient time for contrast administration. A dilute (1% to 2%) solution of barium or water-soluble, iodine-based oral contrast agent is given by mouth or through a nasogastric tube if necessary. The oral contrast agent can be mixed with Kool-Aid or fruit juice if needed to mask the unpleasant taste.

The gastrointestinal tract from the stomach to the terminal ileum usually can be well opacified if the contrast agent is given in two volumes, one 45 to 60 min before the examination and the other 15 min prior to scanning. The first volume should approximate that of an average feeding. The second volume should be approximately one half that of the first. Appropriate volumes of contrast medium versus patient age are shown in Table 1. Adult protocols can be used in patients older than 15 years of age.

Imaging Techniques

Although either incremental CT or spiral CT scanning may be used in the evaluation of pediatric diseases, spiral CT is recommended (103,233,263). Spiral CT has a number of advantages over conventional CT, including (a) a shortened examination time, (b) elimination of respiratory misregistration, particularly in breath-holding patients, (c) capability of narrow reconstruction intervals, which improves lesion detection, and (d) the ability to optimize vascular

TABLE 1. *Oral contrast vs. patient age*

Age	Amount given 45 min prior to scanning	Amount given 15 min prior to scanning
<1 month	2–3 oz (60–90 ml)	1–1.5 oz (30–45 ml)
1 month–1 year	4–8 oz (120–240 ml)	2–4 oz (60–120 ml)
1–5 years	8–12 oz (240–360 ml)	4–6 oz (120–180 ml)
6–12 years	12–16 oz (360–480 ml)	6–8 oz (180–240 ml)
13–15 years	16–20 oz (480–600 ml)	8–10 oz (240–300 ml)

enhancement as a result of the rapid scan technique. Reformatted multiplanar images also are useful in the preoperative assessment of the extent of thoracic and abdominal tumors. With the spiral technique, an excellent quality study can be obtained even if the patient is breathing quietly.

For optimal examination of children, CT examinations should be performed with scan times of 1 sec or less. Slice thickness and table speed will vary with the area of interest, the age of the patient, and the clinical indication for the examination. Chest examinations are obtained from the thoracic inlet to the subdiaphragmatic region and abdominal examinations from the xiphoid to the symphysis pubis. In general, CT studies in children over 5 years of age are performed with 8-mm collimated sections at 8 mm/sec table speed. Decreased collimation (2 to 4 mm) and reduced table speed (2 to 4 mm/sec) are reserved for areas of maximum interest; for detailed examination such as evaluation of pulmonary nodules, lymphadenopathy, small parts (the thyroid, parathyroid, and adrenal glands), or complex musculoskeletal fractures; and for infants and children under 5 years of age. If the patient is cooperative, sections are obtained with breath holding at suspended inspiration. CT sections are obtained at resting lung volume if the patient is sedated.

MRI: TECHNICAL CONSIDERATIONS

Imaging Parameters

Lesion detectability is dependent on the signal to noise (S/N) ratio, spatial resolution, and contrast resolution. These parameters vary with the size of the receiver coil, slice thickness, field of view (FOV), matrix size, and number of acquisitions. For optimal signal-to-noise ratio and spatial resolution, MRI examinations should be performed with the smallest coil that fits tightly around the body part being studied (41). A head coil usually is adequate in infants and small children, whereas a whole-body coil is needed for larger children and adolescents. Surface coils can be useful in the evaluation of superficial structures, such as the spine, but the drop-off in signal strength with increasing distance from the center of the coil limits the value of these coils in the evaluation of deeper abdominal structures.

Slice thickness varies with patient size and the area of interest. Thinner slices (3 to 4 mm) are used in the evaluation of small lesions and through areas of maximum interest, whereas thicker slices (6 to 8 mm) suffice for a general survey of the chest and abdomen and larger lesions. The FOV can have a square or rectangular shape. A square shape is used when the body part being examined fills the FOV. An asymmetric FOV is ideal for body parts that are narrow in one direction, such as the abdomen in a thin patient. A 128 × 192 matrix and one or two signal acquisitions generally are used in pediatric MRI examinations to shorten imaging time, although 286 × 286 matrix may be needed in areas where more anatomic detail is desired.

Pulse Sequences

Selection of pulse sequences for MRI examinations of the chest, abdomen, and pelvis need to be tailored to the area of interest and the clinical problem (195). As technology advances, the choice of imaging strategies is increasing. The various imaging sequences that have proven useful in children are reviewed below. For a more detailed description of MRI principles and techniques, the reader is referred to Chapter 2.

T1-weighted sequences (short TR, short TE) are obtained in virtually all patients because they increase observer confidence in lesion detection and are useful for minimizing artifacts, especially in the abdomen. Generally, they are acquired with a spin echo technique, which requires a relatively short scanning time and provides excellent anatomic detail, excellent contrast between soft tissue structures and fat, and thinner slices. Fat-suppressed T1-weighted images, such as short tau inversion recovery (STIR) and fat saturation, result in increased signal intensity in water-containing tissues and are useful to improve conspicuity of diseased tissues. Gadolinium administration, especially in combination with fat suppression, is appropriate in the evaluation of tumors to improve contrast between tumor and normal, less vascular tissues. Non-enhanced, out-of-phase gradient echo images are best used to detect fat in the liver and adrenal adenomas.

T2-weighted sequences (long TR, long TE) are used in most examinations of the chest (excluding heart and great vessels), abdomen, and musculoskeletal system. They provide excellent contrast between tumor and adjacent soft tissues and are useful for tissue characterization. The T2-weighted sequences can be acquired with conventional or turbo (fast) spin-echo techniques. Turbo spin echo is useful when decreased imaging time is desired, although these images may lead to a loss of contrast between fat and other similarly intense fluid and tissues. To increase lesion conspicuity, fat suppression techniques should be used in conjunction with T2-weighted fast spin-echo sequences.

Fat-suppressed sequences are useful to increase contrast between normal and pathologic tissue on T2-weighted images. Two basic methods of fat suppression are widely available: STIR and radiofrequency presaturation of the lipid peak (fat saturation). Signal from fat is nulled on STIR and fat-saturated images, whereas most pathologic lesions, with increased free water and prolonged T1 and T2 values, are bright on the fat-suppressed sequences.

The gradient echo (GRE) technique results in high signal in flowing blood and is useful for MR angiography and evaluation of cardiac and vascular abnormalities (215). This technique is most effective in cooperative children who can suspend respiration, but it can be used in children of any age. The evaluation of blood flow with the GRE sequence requires the use of technical parameters that are tailored for vascular imaging (TR/TE of 25–40/8–10, flip angle of 30° to 40°) (215). A two-dimensional (2-D) sequential mode is used for routine MR angiography, whereas a 3-D mode is useful for multiplanar reconstructions.

Chemical shift imaging is a method that is helpful to detect and characterize lesions suspected of containing fat. This technique utilizes GRE images obtained in-phase (TE 4.2 msec, flip angle 70°) and out-of-phase (TE 2.1 or 6.3 msec, flip angle 70°) to exploit differences in relaxation times of fat and water. The presence of fat results in increased signal intensity on in-phase images and decreased signal intensity on out-of-phase images.

Optimizing Image Quality

As a result of the relatively long time required to perform abdominal MRI in children, gross voluntary motion or physiologic motion, such as respiration and blood flow, may produce artifacts that degrade the MR image. Voluntary motion can be minimized or eliminated by the use of sedation, whereas physiologic motion, and its resultant artifacts—ghosting and blurring—can be suppressed by adjusting technical parameters. Gradient echo imaging, described previously, and signal averaging, or increasing the number of excitations in the MRI examination, are two simple methods to reduce respiratory motion artifacts. Spatial presaturation, an additional technique for motion suppression, uses selective radiofrequency pulses to saturate spins that are outside of the area of interest being

imaged. Thus, blood flowing into the imaged section has little signal and consequently produces little or no artifact (28). Presaturation also can eliminate abdominal wall motion artifact even it if is in the same cross-sectional image.

CHEST

CT and MRI have emerged as important imaging techniques in the chest because of their great contrast sensitivity and their ability to provide images unobscured by overlying structures. The cross-sectional CT and MR images are particularly helpful in detecting or clarifying abnormalities in the mediastinum, chest wall, and peridiaphragmatic and subpleural regions of the lung (71,233,235). The information provided by these techniques can directly affect the treatment or aid in determining the prognosis of a patient.

Indications for CT and MRI of the mediastinum include (a) characterization of mediastinal widening or evaluation of a mass suspected or detected on chest radiography; (b) determination of the extent of a proven mediastinal tumor; (c) detection of disease in children who have an underlying disease that may be associated with a mediastinal mass but a normal chest radiograph; and (d) assessment of the response of a mediastinal mass to therapy (220).

Mediastinum

Normal Anatomy

Thymus

In the pediatric population, the normal thymus is seen in virtually every patient. In individuals under age 20,

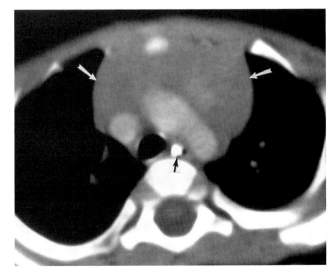

FIG 1. Normal CT appearance of thymus, 9-month-old boy. The thymus (*white arrows*) is quadrilateral in shape with slightly convex lateral borders and a wide retrosternal component. The density of the thymus is equal to that of chest wall musculature. Black arrow, nasogastric tube in esophagus.

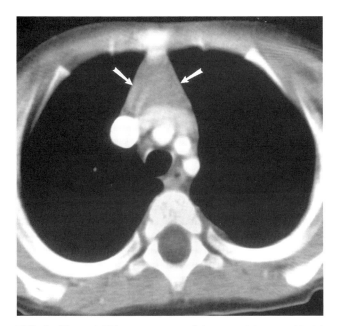

FIG. 2. Normal CT appearance of thymus, 14-year-old girl. The thymus (*arrows*) has assumed a triangular shape, but it still abuts the sternum and has a density equal to that of chest wall musculature.

there are wide variations in size and shape of the normal thymus. Recognition of the various appearances of the normal thymus is important if errors in diagnosis are to be avoided (94,223). In patients under the age of 5 years, the thymus usually has a quadrilateral shape with convex or straight lateral margins (Fig. 1). Later in the first decade the thymus is triangular or arrowhead-shaped with straight

or concave margins, and by 15 years of age, it is triangular in nearly all individuals (209,230) (Fig. 2). In general, in the first two decades of life, the thymus abuts the sternum, separating the two lungs. A distinct anterior junction line between the lungs is usually not seen until the third decade of life.

The thymus in prepubertal children and most adolescents is homogeneous with an attenuation value equal to that of chest wall musculature. In approximately 30% of adolescents, the thymus is heterogeneous, containing low-density areas of fat deposition (94,209). Thymic lobar width (largest dimension parallel to the long axis of the lobe) shows little change with age (94,209). Thymic lobar thickness (the largest dimension perpendicular to the long axis of the lobe) correlates inversely with advancing age, decreasing from 1.50 ± 0.46 (SD) cm for the 0 to 10 year age group to 1.05 ± 0.36 cm for patients between 10 and 20 years of age (209). For infiltrative diseases of the thymus, increased thickness is a fairly sensitive indicator of an abnormality (94,209).

Signal intensity on MR images also varies with patient age. The signal intensity of the normal prepubertal thymus is slightly greater than that of muscle on T1-weighted images and slightly less than or equal to that of fat on T2-weighted images (Fig. 3). After puberty, the signal intensity on T1-weighted images increases, reflecting fatty replacement (Fig. 4). Measurements of thymic thickness are slightly greater on MRI than on CT, probably reflecting the lower lung volumes on MR images (62). MR images are obtained during quiet respiration, whereas CT images generally are obtained in suspended or full

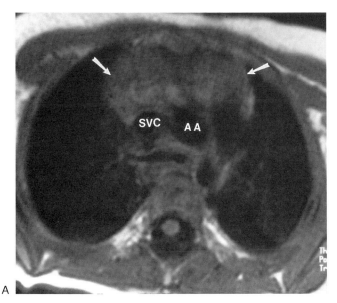

A

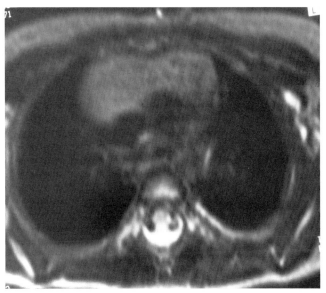

B

FIG. 3. Normal MRI appearance of the thymus, 9-month-old boy. **A:** T1-weighted transaxial MR image (600/15) shows a quadrilateral thymus (*arrows*) anterior to the superior vena cava (SVC) and ascending aorta (AA). The signal intensity is equal to or slightly greater than that of chest wall musculature but less than that of subcutaneous fat. **B:** T2-weighted transaxial MR image (2500/90). The signal intensity of the thymus is equal to that of subcutaneous fat.

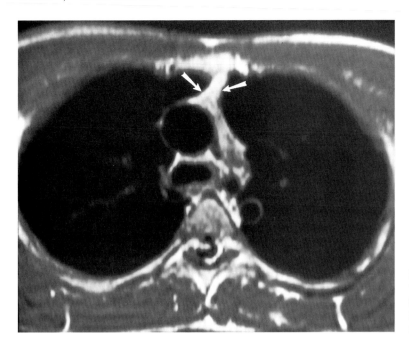

FIG. 4. Normal MRI appearance of the thymus, 17-year-old boy. T1 weighted axial MR image (500/30) shows a high-signal-intensity thymus (*arrows*), indicating the presence of fatty replacement.

inspiration. This difference produces some flattening of the thymus in a craniocaudal dimension on MRI, which increases thickness.

Occasionally, the thymus extends either cranially above the brachiocephalic vessels or into the posterior thorax. The CT or MRI findings of the abnormally positioned thymus are its direct continuity with the thymic tissue in the anterior mediastinum, an attenuation value or signal intensity similar to that of normal thymic tissue, and the lack of compression of adjacent mediastinal vessels or the tracheobronchial tree (50,175,200) (Fig. 5).

Lymph Nodes

Mediastinal lymph nodes generally are not seen on CT scans or MRI in children prior to puberty, and their presence should be considered abnormal. In adolescents, small normal nodes (not exceeding 1 cm in widest diameter) occasionally can be identified. Nodes are of soft tissue attenuation on CT and have a signal intensity between muscle and fat on both T1- and T2-weighted images.

Azygoesophageal Recess

The configuration of the azygoesophageal recess varies with the patient's age. The contour of the recess is convex laterally in children under 6 years, straight in children between 5 and 12 years, and concave in adolescents or young adults (86,171) (Fig. 6). Recognition of the normal dextroconvex appearance in young children is important so that it is not mistaken for lymphadenopathy.

Mediastinal Pathology

A widened mediastinum in infants and children often is due to a mass lesion, usually a lymphoma, neurogenic tumor, teratoma, or cyst of foregut origin. Abundant me-

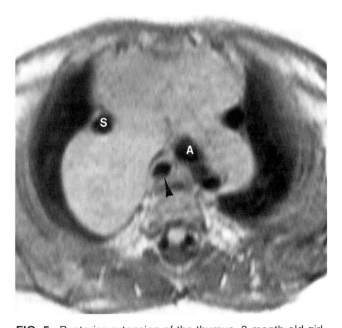

FIG. 5. Posterior extension of the thymus, 3-month-old girl. Proton-density-weighted transaxial MR image (1600/20) shows a normal thymus in the anterior mediastinum. The thymus courses between the superior vena cava (S) and aortic arch (A) as it extends posteriorly. The signal intensity of the posterior thymic extension and the thymus anteriorly are similar. Note the absence of compressive effect on the trachea (*arrowhead*) and the vasculature.

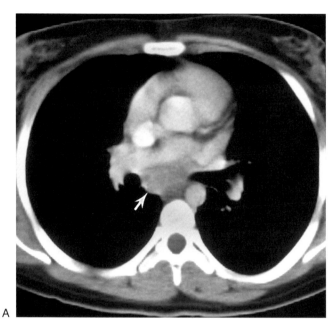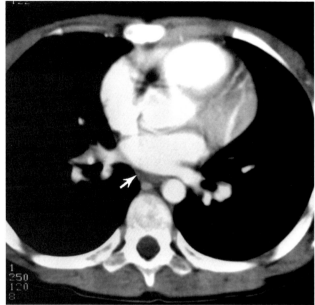

A   B

FIG. 6. Azygoesophageal recess. **A:** In this 4-year-old boy, the recess (*arrow*) has a convex lateral shape, resulting from intrusion of the esophagus into the recess. **B:** A 15-year-old girl has a concave azygoesophageal recess (*arrow*).

diastinal fat, aneurysms, or tortuosity of the mediastinal vessels are rare in children. Approximately 30% of mediastinal masses in children arise in the anterior mediastinum, 30% in the middle mediastinum, and 40% in the posterior mediastinum. CT and MRI have the capability of differentiating among lesions composed predominantly of fat, water, or soft tissues and therefore can provide a more definitive diagnosis than can conventional radiographic techniques.

Fat-containing masses in children usually are teratomas. Rarely, they represent thymolipomas or herniation of omental fat through the foramen of Morgagni. Lesions that can present with attenuation values near that of water include pericardial cysts, thymic cysts, lymphangiomas, and duplication cysts of foregut origin. Rarely, bronchogenic cysts or duplication cysts have a density equal to that of soft tissue because they contain thick viscid contents, rather than simple serous fluid. Vascular causes of mediastinal widening, such as aortic aneurysm or a congenital anomaly of the thoracic vascular system, also can be identified with confidence on MRI or on CT scans.

When a mass has an attenuation value equal to that of soft tissue, CT can be valuable in determining its extent or origin, but a specific pathologic diagnosis generally is not possible. The differential diagnosis, however, can be narrowed by determining the location of the mass in the mediastinum.

The technical parameters for screening the mediastinum with spiral CT are 4- to 8-mm slice thickness, 4- to 8-mm/sec table speed, 1:1 pitch, standard algorithm, and 4- to 8-mm reconstructions. Decreased collimation and table speed should be used in very small children.

Anterior Mediastinal Masses: Soft Tissue Attenuation

Lymphoma

Lymphoma is the most common cause of an anterior mediastinal mass of soft tissue attenuation in children, with Hodgkin disease occurring 3 to 4 times more frequently than non-Hodgkin lymphoma (42). Approximately 65% of pediatric patients with Hodgkin disease have intrathoracic involvement at clinical presentation, and 90% of the chest involvement is mediastinal. In contrast, about 40% of pediatric patients with non-Hodgkin lymphoma have chest disease at diagnosis, and only 50% of this disease involves the mediastinum. CT plays an important role in the identification and staging of disease, the planning of treatment, and the follow-up evaluation of patients with lymphoma (43,158).

Lymphomatous masses in Hodgkin disease are most common in the anterior mediastinum and reflect either infiltration and enlargement of the thymus or lymphadenopathy. The enlarged thymus has a quadrilateral shape with convex, lobular lateral borders (Fig. 7). On CT, the density of the lymphomatous organ is equal to that of soft tissue (122,209). The MR signal intensity is slightly greater than that of muscle on T1-weighted pulse sequences and similar to or slightly greater than that of fat on T2-weighted pulse sequences (175) (Fig. 8). Calcifications or cystic areas, due to ischemic necrosis consequent to rapid tumor growth, can be seen within the tumor (155,184) (Fig. 9). Additional findings include mediastinal or hilar lymph node enlargement, airway narrowing, and compression of vascular structures.

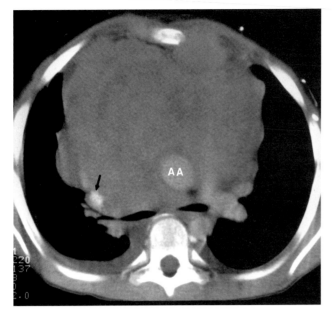

FIG. 7. Thymic Hodgkin disease, nodular sclerosing type, 12-year-old boy. Contrast-enhanced CT scan shows a markedly enlarged thymus with a lobulated contour. The infiltrated thymus displaces the ascending aorta (AA) and superior vena cava (*arrow*) posteriorly. Note the compressive effects on the cava and main stem bronchi and the bilateral pleural effusions.

Lymphadenopathy is the other common intrathoracic manifestation of lymphoma. The appearance varies from mildly enlarged nodes in a single area to large conglomerate soft tissue masses in multiple regions. Typically, the enlarged nodes have well-defined margins and show little enhancement after intravenous administration of contrast medium (Fig. 10). Hodgkin disease usually causes enlargement of the thymus or anterior mediastinal nodes, whereas non-Hodgkin lymphoma predominantly affects middle mediastinal lymph nodes.

Successfully treated lymphomas usually decrease in size, but the mediastinum may not return to normal on serial CT examinations (158). Differential diagnostic considerations in these cases include fibrosis versus persistent or recurrent lymphoma. Serial CT examinations, supplemented by radionuclide studies using gallium, can nearly always distinguish between these two conditions (73). In general, masses due to fibrosis remain stable or decrease in size, whereas tumor is likely to increase in size. MRI may be valuable in assessing treatment response in the instances in which CT and scintigraphy are not diagnostic (76,106,182). Fibrosis displays a low signal intensity on both T1- and T2-weighted images, whereas active neoplasms exhibit a high signal intensity on T2-weighted images. However, relatively high signal intensity on T2-weighted images is not specific for active tumor and also can be seen with infection, hemorrhage, acute radiation pneumonitis, and radiation fibrosis (106,194). In a problematic case, biopsy may be needed.

Thymic Hyperplasia

Thymic hyperplasia is another cause of diffuse thymic enlargement. In childhood, thymic hyperplasia has been associated with myasthenia gravis, red cell aplasia, hyperthyroidism, HIV infection (169), and chemotherapy, with the last being the most common cause. Rebound hyperpla-

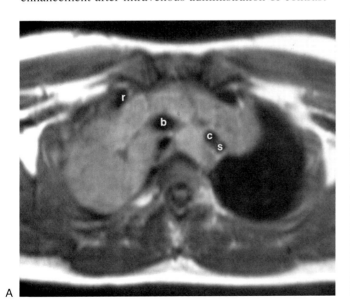

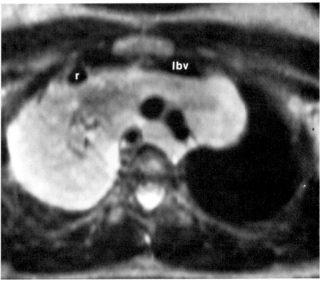

A   B

FIG. 8. Thymic Hodgkin disease, nodular sclerosing type, 12-year-old girl. **A:** T1-weighted transaxial MR image (810/30) shows thymic infiltration with the right lobe affected more than the left lobe. The signal intensity of the infiltrated thymus is slightly greater than that of chest wall musculature and less than that of fat. **B:** On a T2-weighted image (3100/90) the thymus is heterogeneous and has a signal intensity slightly greater than that of subcutaneous fat. r, right brachiocephalic vein; lbv, left brachiocephalic vein; b, brachiocephalic artery; c, left carotid artery; s, left subclavian artery.

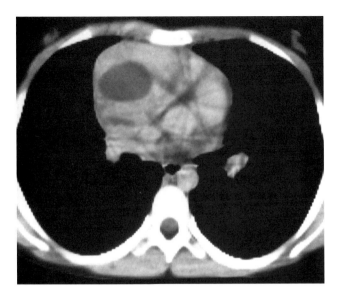

FIG. 9. Thymic Hodgkin disease, nodular sclerosing type with cystic changes, 13-year-old girl. Contrast-enhanced CT scan shows an enlarged right lobe of the thymus with a central cystic component, resulting from necrosis.

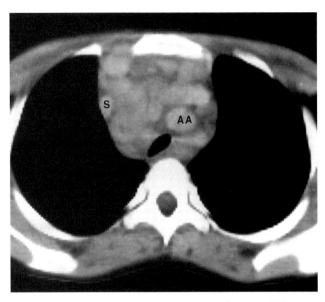

FIG. 10. Lymphadenopathy, Hodgkin disease. CT scan shows multiple enlarged nodes in the superior mediastinum. S, superior vena cava; AA, ascending aorta.

sia may be observed during the course of chemotherapy or after the completion of therapy (45). The mechanism of hyperplasia in these cases is believed to be initial depletion of lymphocytes from the cortical portion of the gland due to high serum levels of glucocorticoids. Thymic hyperplasia results when the cortisone levels return to normal and the cortex is repopulated with lymphocytes.

On CT and MRI, hyperplasia appears as diffuse enlargement of the thymus with preservation of the normal triangular shape (45) (Fig. 11). The attenuation value and the signal intensity of the hyperplastic thymus are similar to those of the normal organ and hence are not helpful in differentiating tumor and hyperplasia (175). It is the absence of other active disease and a gradual decrease in

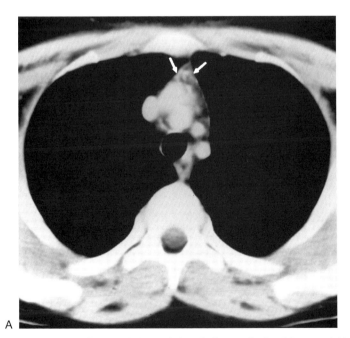

A

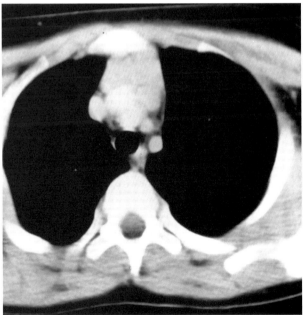

B

FIG. 11. Rebound thymic hyperplasia, 14-year-old boy receiving chemotherapy for Hodgkin disease limited to the cervical lymph nodes. **A:** CT scan of the chest at the time of diagnosis shows a normal thymus (*arrows*) which is partially replaced by fat. **B:** CT scan 6 months later shows symmetric enlargement of both lobes of the thymus. The patient was doing well clinically. A follow-up CT study 4 months later showed spontaneous reduction in the size of the thymus.

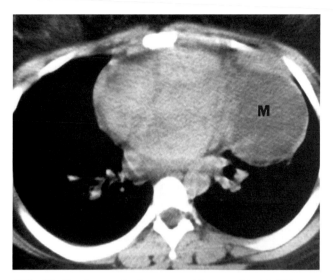

FIG. 12. Benign cystic thymoma, 15-year-old girl. CT scan at the level of the cardiac apex shows a necrotic soft tissue mass (M) in the left hemithorax. At surgery, the mass arose in the left lobe of the thymus.

the size of the thymus on serial CT scans or MRI that supports the diagnosis of rebound hyperplasia as the cause of thymic enlargement.

Thymoma

Thymomas account for less than 5% of all mediastinal tumors in children. The majority of thymomas are benign and occur sporadically, but they can be found in association with myasthenia gravis, red cell aplasia, or hypogammaglobulinemia. Benign thymomas appear as well-defined, round or oval masses in the area of the thymus. On CT, they are of soft tissue density, but sometimes they contain calcifications or lower density areas of necrosis (Fig. 12). On T1-weighted MR images, thymomas have a signal intensity similar to that of muscle; the signal intensity increases on T2-weighted images, approaching that of fat (175). Approximately 10% to 15% of thymomas are invasive, (i.e., malignant). The CT and MRI appearance of invasive thymoma is that of an anterior mediastinal mass associated with metastatic implants along mediastinal, pleural, or pericardial surfaces.

Miscellaneous Lesions

Other differential diagnostic considerations for diffuse thymic enlargement include leukemia, Langerhans cell histiocytosis, and histoplasmosis. Diagnosis requires tissue sampling.

Anterior Mediastinal Masses: Fat Attenuation

Germ Cell Tumors

Germ cell tumors are the second most common cause of an anterior mediastinal mass in children and the most common cause of a fat-containing lesion. They are derived from one or more of the three embryonic germ cell layers and usually arise in the thymus. Approximately 90% are benign and histologically are either dermoid cysts (containing only ectodermal elements) or teratomas (containing tissue from all three germinal layers). On CT, both lesions are well-defined, thick-walled cystic masses containing a variable admixture of tissues: water, calcium, fat, and soft tissue (36,68,205) (Fig. 13). A fat–fluid level and amorphous bone or teeth occasionally can be seen in these tumors (193). On MRI, germ cell tumors are

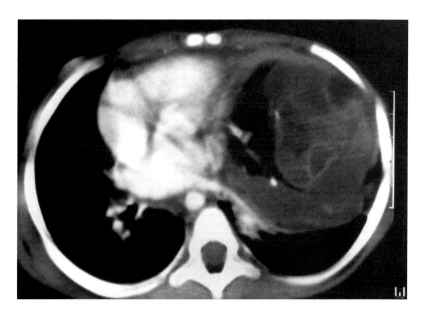

FIG. 13. Benign teratoma. A large, well-circumscribed, heterogeneous mass, containing low-density fluid, calcifications, and fat occupies most of the left hemithorax. The mass displaces but does not invade vascular structures. Pathologic examination showed a benign cystic teratoma that contained sebaceous fluid, a small amount of fat, and embryonic teeth. (Reproduced from Quillin SP, Siegel MJ. CT features of benign and malignant teratomas in children. *J Comput Assist Tomogr* 1992; 16:722–726.)

heterogeneous masses with variable signal intensities depending on the relative amounts of fluid and fat (175). Fluid components usually have a signal intensity less than or equal to that of muscle on T1-weighted images. The signal intensity can be greater than that of muscle if the contents contain blood or proteinaceous material. The signal intensity of fluid usually is hyperintense to fat on T2-weighted images. Fat components have a high signal intensity on both T1- and T2-weighted images. Calcification and bone have low signal intensity on all imaging sequences.

A malignant teratoma generally appears on CT and MRI as a poorly defined, soft tissue mass, sometimes containing calcification and fat. Local infiltration into the adjacent mediastinum with encasement or invasion of mediastinal vessels or airways also is common. Other malignant germ cell tumors arising in the anterior mediastinum are seminoma, embryonal cell carcinoma, choriocarcinoma, and endodermal sinus tumor. These tumors typically are heterogeneous, soft tissue density masses containing some low-density areas of necrosis (Fig. 14). Rarely, they contain calcifications (153,219).

Thymolipoma

Thymolipoma is an uncommon cause of an intrathymic tumor. Most cases in the pediatric population occur in the second decade and are discovered incidentally on plain radiographs. The tumor often is large, extending caudally to the diaphragm. On CT and MRI, it appears as a heterogeneous mass containing fat and some soft tissue elements.

Anterior Mediastinal Masses: Fluid Attenuation

Thymic Cysts

Thymic cysts usually are congenital lesions resulting from persistence of the thymopharyngeal duct, but they can occur after thoracotomy (136). Typically, they are thin-walled, homogeneous masses of near-water density on CT, low signal intensity on T1-weighted MR images, and high signal intensity on T2-weighted sequences. The attenuation value or the signal intensity on T1-weighted images may be higher than that of simple cysts when the cyst's contents are proteinaceous or hemorrhagic rather than serous (175). Multiple thymic cysts have also been described in children with HIV infection and Langerhans cell histiocytosis (75).

Cystic Hygroma

Cystic hygromas are lymphogenous cysts that occur in the antero-superior mediastinum and are almost always inferior extensions of cervical hygromas. On CT, they appear as nonenhancing, thin-walled, multiloculated masses with a near-water attenuation value. The presence of contrast enhancement of the wall or internal septations suggests superimposed infection or a hemangiomatous component. Occasionally, marked dilatation of adjacent veins is noted (139). On MRI, cystic hygroma has a signal intensity equal to or slightly less than that of muscle on T1-weighted images and greater than that of fat on T2-weighted images (Fig. 15). The surrounding fascial planes are obliterated if the tumor infiltrates the adjacent soft

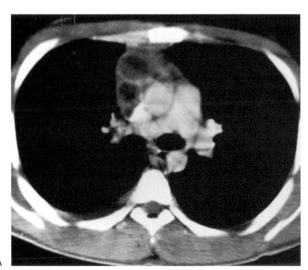
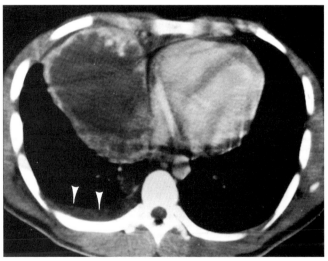

A   B

FIG. 14. Primary thymic choriocarcinoma, 15-year-old boy. **A:** A large, heterogeneous low density mass is seen anterior to the ascending aorta and main pulmonary artery. **B:** On a scan several centimeters caudal, the mass shows an enhancing rim and displaces the heart to the left. Also noted is a right pleural effusion (*arrowheads*). At surgery, the tumor arose from the right lobe of the thymus. (Reproduced from Siegel MJ. Diseases of the thymus in children and adolescents. *Postgrad Radiol* 1993;13:106–132.)

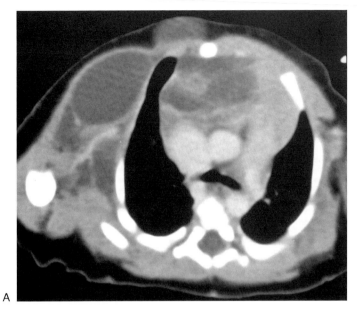

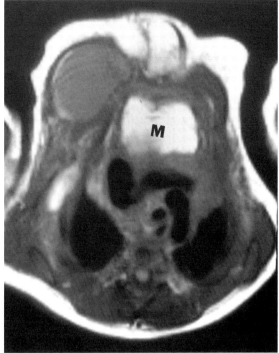

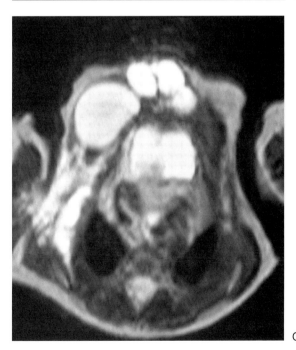

FIG. 15. Cystic hygroma, newborn girl. **A:** CT scan through the superior mediastinum shows a heterogeneous, low density mass infiltrating the superior mediastinum and right axilla. **B:** On a T1-weighted transaxial MR image, the superior mediastinal mass (M) has a homogeneous appearance and a signal intensity higher than that of muscle. The signal intensity of the chest wall components is heterogeneous, with some areas having a signal intensity less than that of muscle and some greater than that of muscle. **C:** On a T2-weighted MR image, the signal intensity of the mediastinal and chest wall masses is greater than that of subcutaneous fat. The high signal intensity on both T1- and T2-weighted images was caused by the presence of acute blood. The planes around the mass are better defined on MRI than on CT.

tissues. Hemorrhage can cause a sudden increase in tumor size and can increase the CT attenuation value or the signal intensity on T1-weighted MR images (229).

Middle Mediastinal Masses

The most common causes of middle mediastinal masses are lymph node enlargement and congenital foregut cysts.

Lymphadenopathy

Lymph node enlargement, as a cause of a middle mediastinal mass, is usually secondary to lymphoma or granulomatous disease. On CT, adenopathy can appear as discrete, round soft tissue masses, or as a single soft tissue mass with poorly defined margins. Calcification within lymph nodes suggests old granulomatous disease, such as histoplasmosis or tuberculosis. On T1-weighted MR

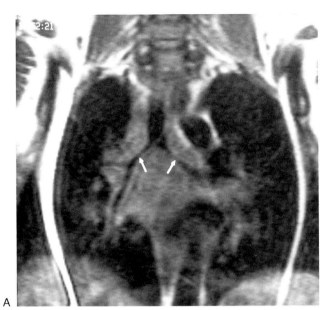 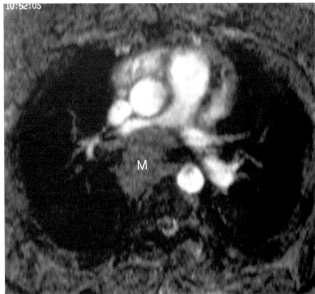

FIG. 16. Fibrosing mediastinitis, 18-year-old boy. **A:** Coronal T1-weighted MR image (630/30) shows paratracheal, hilar, and subcarinal lymph nodes, with secondary narrowing of the mainstem bronchi (*arrows*). **B:** Compression of the right main pulmonary artery by the subcarinal nodal mass (M) is best seen on transaxial gradient-echo image (40/10/40°).

images, lymph nodes involved by infection or tumor have a signal intensity similar to or slightly greater than that of muscle. On T2-weighted MR images, the signal intensity is high, similar to that of fat. Most lymph nodes are homogeneous on MRI, but they can appear heterogeneous, if they contain calcification or necrosis. Neither CT or MRI is able to provide a specific histologic diagnosis, but either can be useful for determining whether mediastinoscopy or thoracotomy would be better to yield a diagnosis.

Mediastinal nodes involved by granulomatous disease usually undergo spontaneous regression, frequently with resultant calcification. In some cases, healing occurs with extensive fibrosis, resulting in airway or vascular (e.g., superior vena caval) obstruction (Fig. 16). CT is superior to MRI for showing calcifications, which are important for establishing the diagnosis of inflammation. MRI, however, can provide complementary information about vascular patency, especially if there is a contraindication to the administration of iodinated contrast media. On MRI, calcifications and fibrotic tissue are of low intensity on both T1- and T2-weighted sequences (197).

Foregut Cysts

Foregut cysts in the middle mediastinum are classified as either bronchogenic or enteric, depending on their histology. Bronchogenic cysts are lined by respiratory epithelium, and most are located in the subcarinal or right paratracheal area. Enteric cysts are lined by gastrointestinal mucosa and are located in a paraspinal position in the

middle to posterior mediastinum. In children, most foregut cysts are discovered because they produce symptoms of airway or esophageal compression; occasionally they are detected incidentally on a chest radiograph.

The CT appearance of a foregut cyst is usually that of

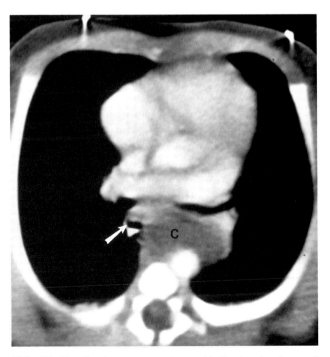

FIG. 17. Duplication cyst, newborn girl. Contrast-enhanced CT shows a homogeneous, near-water-density cyst (C) in the middle mediastinum, adjacent to the esophagus (*arrow*).

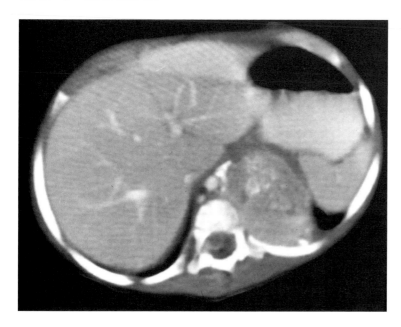

FIG. 18. Neuroblastoma, 2-year-old girl. Contrast-enhanced CT scans show a large left paraspinal soft tissue mass containing scattered calcifications.

a well-defined, round, nonenhancing mass of near-water density, reflecting serous contents (Fig. 17). Air or an air–fluid level can be present when a communication between the cyst and the bronchial tree or gastrointestinal tract develops. On MRI, foregut cysts typically have a low signal intensity on T1-weighted images and a very high signal intensity on T2-weighted images (161). Some cysts have a soft tissue density on CT or a high intensity on T1-weighted images because the fluid is proteinaceous or contains calcium carbonate or oxalate (150).

Posterior Mediastinal Masses

Posterior mediastinal masses are of neural origin in approximately 95% of cases and may arise from sympathetic ganglion cells (neuroblastoma, ganglioneuroblastoma, or ganglioneuroma) or from nerve sheaths (neurofibroma or schwannoma). Rarer causes of posterior mediastinal masses in children include paraspinal abscess, lymphoma, neurenteric cyst, lateral meningocele, and extramedullary hematopoiesis.

On CT, ganglion cell tumors appear as paraspinal masses, extending over the length of several vertebral bodies. They are fusiform in shape, of soft tissue density, and contain calcifications in up to 50% of cases (Fig. 18). Nerve root tumors tend to be smaller, spherical, and occur near the junction of a vertebral body with an adjacent rib (Fig. 19). Both types of tumors may cause pressure erosion of a rib. On MRI, most neurogenic tumors have low signal intensity on T1-weighted images and relatively high signal intensity on T2-weighted images. Some tumors have low attenuation on CT and intermediate to high signal intensity on T1-weighted images because of their myelin content. Because of their origin from neural tissue, neurogenic tumors have a tendency to invade the spinal canal. Intraspinal extension is extradural in location, displacing and occasionally compressing the cord (Fig. 20). Recognition of intraspinal invasion is critical because such involvement usually requires radiation therapy or a laminectomy prior to tumor debulking. MRI is particularly useful in depicting intraspinal tumor extension. It has obviated more invasive techniques, such as CT with myelography, and should be the cross-sectional imaging technique of choice when a neurogenic tumor is suspected to be the cause of a posterior mediastinal mass identified on chest radiography (232).

Vascular Masses

Abnormalities of the aorta and its branches and of the superior or inferior vena cava can cause a mass or medias-

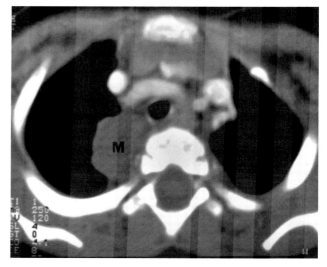

FIG. 19. Neurofibroma. A round, paraspinal mass (M) with an attenuation value slightly lower than that of muscle is identified at the junction of a rib and vertebral body.

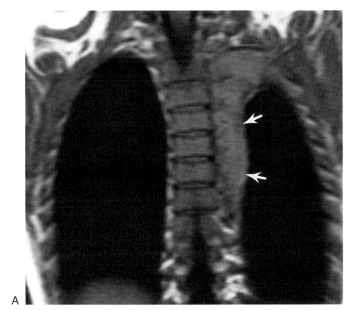

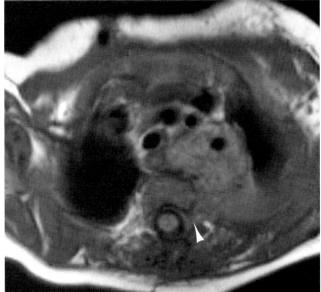

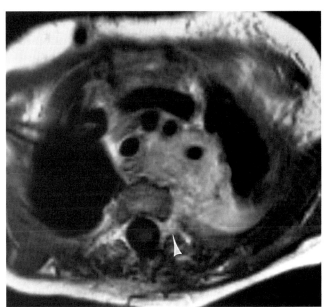

FIG. 20. Neuroblastoma, 10-month-old girl. **A:** Coronal T1-weighted MR image (570/15) shows a large, relatively low signal intensity, paraspinal mass (arrows) extending from the apex of the left hemithorax to the level of midthoracic spine. **B, C:** Transaxial T1-weighted (600/30) and T2-weighted (3000/120) images demonstrate extension of the mass across the midline and invasion of the spinal canal (*arrowhead*), displacing the cord slightly to the right.

tinal widening on plain chest radiography. Either CT, especially with spiral capability, or MRI can be used to detect and characterize vascular anomalies (235). For practical purposes, both provide equivalent anatomic data. Rarely, the multiplanar images provided by MRI yield more relevant information than that provided by CT (14,19,89,92,109,238).

Aortic Arch

The right arch with aberrant left subclavian artery and the double arch are common congenital anomalies of the aorta that produce an abnormal mediastinum on plain chest radiography (14,19) (Fig. 21). The double arch is characterized by two arches that surround the trachea and esophagus. The arches arise from a single ascending aorta and reunite to form a single descending aorta after giving rise to the subclavian and carotid arteries. The right arch component of a double arch anomaly usually is more cephalad and larger than the left arch component. In the right arch with aberrant subclavian artery, the subclavian artery arises as the last branch from the aortic arch and traverses the mediastinum behind the esophagus to reach the left arm.

Aneurysm of the thoracic aorta is another cause of a vascular mediastinal mass. The most common cause of aneurysms in children is Marfan syndrome. Less commonly, bacterial infections or Ehler-Danlos syndrome are the cause.

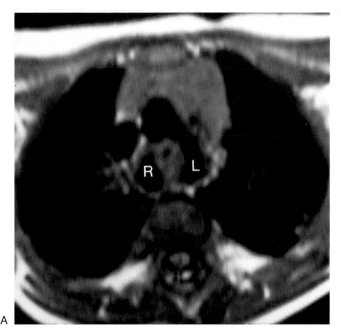

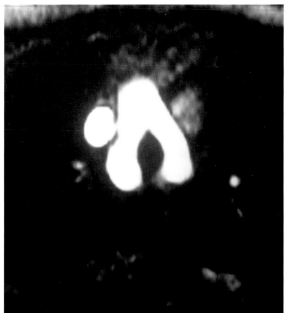

A

B

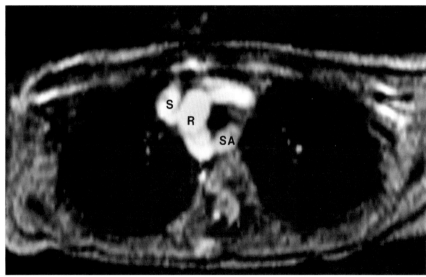

C

FIG. 21. Aortic arch anomalies. **A:** Double arch in an 11-month-old girl. Transaxial T1-weighted MR image (600/25) shows the two limbs of the double arch encircling the trachea and esophagus. R, right arch; L, left arch. **B:** Flow is noted within the two limbs of the double arch on a gradient echo image (30/6/20°). **C:** Right arch with an aberrant left subclavian artery. Transaxial gradient echo image demonstrates a right aortic arch (R) giving rise to the left subclavian artery (SA), which passes behind the trachea and esophagus to reach the left arm. S, superior vena cava.

Most aneurysms are fusiform in configuration. They may be focal or extend the entire length of the vessel.

Superior Vena Cava

Venous anomalies producing mediastinal widening include persistent left superior vena cava and interruption of the inferior vena cava. Persistent left superior vena cava, resulting from failure of regression of the left common and anterior cardinal veins, drains the left jugular and subclavian veins, and, in some cases, the left superior intercostal vein. The persistent vena cava lies lateral to the left common carotid artery and anterior to the left subclavian artery, descends lateral to the main pulmonary artery, and drains into the coronary sinus posterior to the left ventricle.

Dilatation of the azygos or hemiazygos vein is a cause of a posterior mediastinal or right paratracheal mass. When the infrahepatic segment of the inferior vena cava above the renal veins fails to develop, blood from below the renal veins returns to the heart via the azygos or hemiazygos veins, with resultant dilatation of these structures. Typically, the hemiazygos vein crosses behind the aorta to join the dilated azygos vein, which in turn drains into the azygos arch (Fig. 22). The suprarenal portion of the inferior vena cava also is absent, and the hepatic veins drain directly into the right atrium.

Comparative Imaging and Clinical Applications

CT and MRI are both sensitive for detection of mediastinal masses and provide comparable information on the

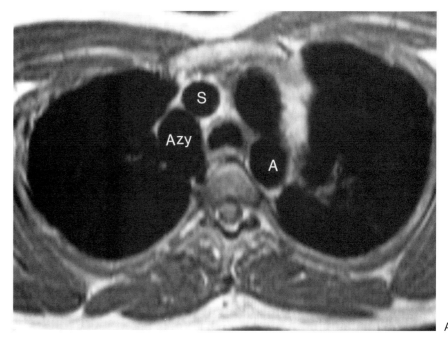

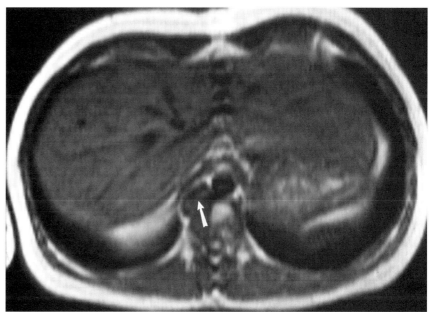

FIG. 22. Azygos continuation of inferior vena cava. **A:** T1-weighted MR image (840/30) at the level of the aortic arch (A) shows a markedly dilated azygos (Azy) vein draining toward the superior vena cava (S). **B:** A dilated azygos vein (*arrow*) is noted at the level of the liver.

presence and size of a lesion. CT is better for demonstrating calcification, whereas MRI is more sensitive than CT in detecting intraspinal extension. Detection of calcification is not clinically relevant, but demonstration of direct intraspinal extension generally is of therapeutic significance because it often necessitates radiation therapy or decompressive laminectomy prior to tumor debulking. We believe that CT is the examination of choice for assessing anterior and middle mediastinal masses with the exception of cystic hygroma. In patients with cystic hygroma, MRI is superior to CT in defining the extent of the tumor, particularly soft tissue infiltration. MRI is the method of choice for evaluating patients with posterior mediastinal masses suspected of being of neurogenic

origin because of the high likelihood of intraspinal extension.

Lungs

Congenital Anomalies

Congenital lung anomalies include a variety of conditions involving the pulmonary parenchyma, the pulmonary vasculature, or a combination of both (70,111,185). Because many of these conditions are associated with either a parenchymal lesion or anomalous vessels, they are well suited for analysis by CT scanning (216,266). In selected

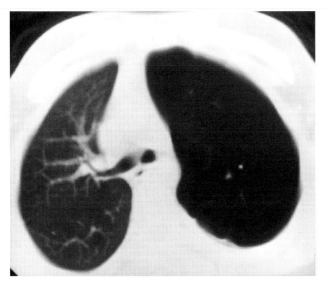

FIG. 23. Congenital lobar emphysema, 13-year-old boy. CT scan through the upper thorax shows a hyperinflated left upper lobe with attenuated vascularity.

cases, MRI can provide complementary information about the presence or absence of an anomalous vessel.

Anomalies with Normal Vasculature

Congenital lobar emphysema, cystic adenomatoid malformation, and bronchial atresia are anomalies resulting from abnormal bronchial development. Chest radiography usually suffices for diagnosis. CT is performed to determine the extent of abnormality in patients in whom surgery is contemplated or to exclude other anomalies, such as bronchogenic cyst or pulmonary sling, which also can cause aeration abnormalities (216). The CT technique for evaluating suspected congenital anomalies should include a general survey scan of the chest using 4- to 8-mm slice thickness and 4- to 8-mm/sec table speed with thinner sections and smaller table incrementation through areas of maximum interest.

Congenital lobar emphysema is characterized by hyperinflation of a lobe. The exact etiology is unknown, but many cases are believed to be due to bronchial obstruction. The affected patient usually presents in the first 6 months of life with respiratory distress. CT shows a hyperinflated lobe with attenuated vascularity, compression of ipsilateral adjacent lobes, and mediastinal shift to the opposite side (Fig. 23). The left upper lobe is involved in about 45% of cases, the right middle lobe in 30%, the right upper lobe in 20%, and two lobes in 5% of cases.

Cystic adenomatoid malformation is characterized by an overgrowth of distal bronchial tissue with formation of a cystic mass. Symptoms of respiratory distress usually occur soon after birth. Histologically, there are three types of cystic adenomatoid malformation: type I (50% of cases) contains a single or multiple large cysts (>10 mm in diameter); type II (41%) contains multiple small cysts (1 to 10 mm in diameter); type III (9%) is a solid lesion to visual inspection but contains microscopic cysts (162,252). The anomaly occurs with equal frequency in both lungs, although there is a slight upper lobe predominance. On CT, cystic adenomatoid malformation appears as a parenchymal mass that may be predominantly cystic or solid or contain an admixture of cystic and solid components (126,204,214). Air–fluid levels occasionally can be seen within the cysts (Fig. 24).

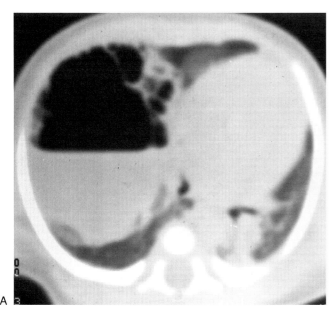
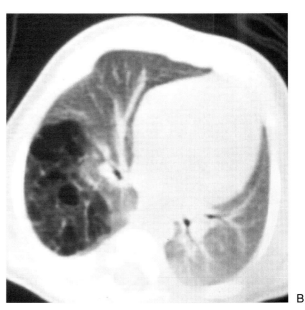

FIG. 24. Cystic adenomatoid malformation. **A:** Type I lesion, a multilocular mass in the right upper lobe containing numerous large cysts, some with air–fluid levels. **B:** Type II malformation, a complex mass in the right lower lobe containing multiple small cysts.

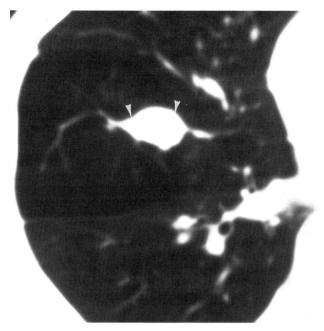

FIG. 25. Bronchial atresia, 13-year-old boy. CT scan shows an ovoid soft tissue nodule (*arrowheads*) in the middle lobe near the right hilum. Note the oligemia distal to the nodule, due to collateral air drift. Mucus-filled bronchocele confirmed at surgery.

Bronchial atresia results from abnormal development of a segmental or subsegmental bronchus. It rarely causes symptoms and is usually discovered on chest radiographs performed for other indications. The CT features of bronchial atresia include overaerated lung distal to the atresia and a round, ovoid, or branching density near the hilum, representing mucoid impaction just beyond the atretic bronchus (47,191) (Fig. 25).

Anomalies with Abnormal Vasculature

Sequestration, hypogenetic lung syndrome, and arteriovenous malformation (AVM) are congenital anomalies with abnormal vasculature. Chronic or recurrent segmental or subsegmental pneumonitis in children, especially at a lung base, is a finding suggestive of sequestration. Pathologically, a sequestered portion of lung has no normal connection with the tracheobronchial tree and is supplied by an anomalous artery, usually arising from the aorta. When the sequestered lung is confined within the normal visceral pleura and has venous drainage to the pulmonary veins, it is termed "intralobar." The sequestered lung is termed "extralobar" when it has its own pleura and venous drainage to systemic veins.

Although plain chest radiography or conventional tomography occasionally may demonstrate an anomalous vessel, CT and MRI are more sensitive for identifying such a vessel (95,127,203). CT scanning after an injection of contrast material demonstrates opacification of the anomalous vessel immediately following enhancement of the descending thoracic aorta (81). The anomalous vessel often can be traced to the sequestered lung. The CT appearance of the pulmonary parenchyma depends on whether or not the sequestered lung is aerated. When the sequestration communicates with the remainder of the lung, usually after being infected, it appears cystic; a sequestration that does not communicate appears as a homogeneous density, usually in the posterior portion of the lower lobe (Fig. 26). On MRI, the feeding vessel appears as an area of signal void on T1-weighted spin-echo images and as a hyperintense area on gradient echo sequences. The parenchymal portion of the sequestration appears as an area of intermediate or high signal intensity (81).

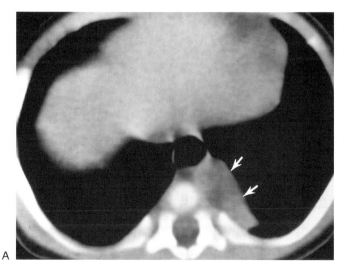
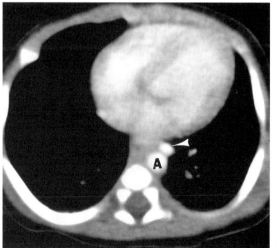

FIG. 26. Extralobar pulmonary sequestration, 2-month-old boy with a left paraspinal mass on chest radiographs. **A:** Unenhanced CT scan demonstrates a soft tissue density (*arrows*) in the lung base. **B:** CT image after bolus injection of intravenous contrast medium demonstrates an anomalous vessel (*arrowhead*) adjacent to the aorta (A).

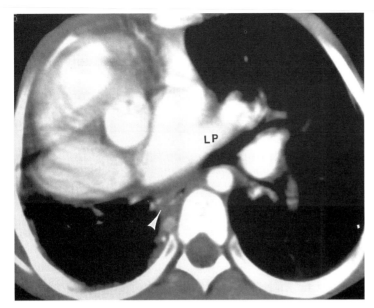

FIG. 27. Pulmonary hypoplasia with congenital absence of the right pulmonary artery, 10-year-old boy. Contrast-enhanced CT scan shows the normal left pulmonary artery (LP) coursing anterior to the left main stem bronchus but no right pulmonary artery. Fibrofatty tissue (*arrowhead*) occupies the space normally filled by the main right pulmonary artery. Also note the small right lung volume and shift of the mediastinal contents to the right.

An additional congenital lung abnormality with vascular anomalies that can be diagnosed by CT or MRI is the hypogenetic lung or scimitar syndrome. CT and MRI findings include a small right lung, ipsilateral mediastinal displacement, a corresponding small pulmonary artery (Fig. 27) and, occasionally, partial anomalous pulmonary venous return from the right lung to the inferior vena cava (Fig. 28). Other associated anomalies include systemic arterial supply to the hypogenetic lung (107), accessory diaphragm, and horseshoe lung. Horseshoe lung is a rare anomaly in which the posterobasal segments of both lungs are fused behind the pericardial sac.

Pulmonary AVM is characterized by a direct communication between a pulmonary artery and vein without an intervening capillary bed. When the diagnosis is suspected on chest radiographs, CT and MRI are useful to establish the definitive diagnosis. However, if surgery or embolization is planned, arteriography may be needed

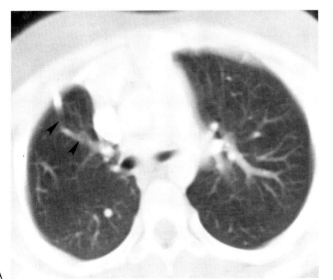

A

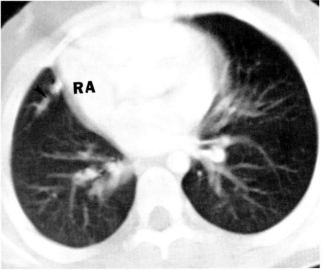

B

FIG. 28. Hypogenetic lung syndrome with partial anomalous venous drainage, 2-month-old girl. **A:** CT scan with lung windows at the level of the arch vessels shows an anomalous pulmonary vein (*arrowheads*). **B:** Several centimeters lower, the anomalous vessel (*arrowhead*) enters the right atrium (RA). Note that the right hemithorax is smaller than the left and that there is mediastinal shift to the right.

to demonstrate the precise vascular anatomy of complex fistulae or the presence of multiple tiny AVMs that may not be visible on CT or MRI. On CT and MRI, AVMs appear as rounded or lobular masses with rapid enhancement and washout after intravenous contrast medium administration. Enhancement typically occurs after enhancement of the right ventricle and before enhancement of the left atrium and left ventricle.

Pulmonary Metastases

Computed tomography is a valuable technique for detection of pulmonary metastases in patients with known malignancies with a high propensity for lung dissemination, such as Wilms tumor, osteogenic sarcoma, and rhabdomyosarcoma (49). Demonstration of one or more pulmonary nodules in such patients, or documentation of additional nodules in a patient with an apparent solitary metastasis for whom surgery is planned, may be critical to treatment planning. In the first instance, such detection may lead to additional treatment (surgery, chemotherapy, or radiation), whereas in the latter setting, demonstration of several metastatic nodules may negate surgical plans. Confusion with benign granulomas does not appear to be as significant a clinical problem in children as it is in adults; in children, almost all noncalcified nodules depicted by CT are due to metastases (Fig. 29) rather than granulomatous disease or a primary neoplasm.

Conventional CT is sensitive for identifying pulmonary nodules, but false negative studies can result from variations in the depth of patient respiration or volume averaging. Spiral CT, which enables contiguous volumetric data acquisition and small overlapping reconstructions (2 to 3 mm), can eliminate or minimize these problems (103,233).

MRI can detect large parenchymal nodules, but it is not as sensitive as CT in detecting nodules that are <1 cm in diameter because of its poorer spatial resolution. Hence, CT remains the imaging method of choice for detecting and characterizing pulmonary nodules.

Diffuse Parenchymal Disease

Chest radiography remains the imaging study of choice for evaluating diffuse parenchymal lung disease. CT, however, can be useful to better define and characterize an abnormality suspected on conventional chest radiography, especially when the CT examination is performed with high-resolution technique using narrow (1 to 2 mm) collimation and a high-spatial-frequency reconstruction algorithm. Indications for high-resolution CT of the lung parenchyma in children include (a) detection of disease in children who are at increased risk for lung disease (e.g., immunocompromised patients) and who have respiratory symptoms but a normal chest radiograph; (b) determination of the extent, distribution, and character of lung diseases; (c) localization of abnormal lung for biopsy; and (d) assessment of the response to treatment (160,167).

Although many lung diseases in children have nonspecific findings, some have characteristic appearances. Cystic fibrosis is characterized by diffuse hyperinflation, bronchiectasis and peribronchial soft tissue thickening (Fig. 30), whereas bronchopulmonary dysplasia is characterized by hyperinflation, cystic airspaces, and septal lines, without bronchiectasis (183) (Fig. 31). Bronchiolitis obliterans is manifested as patchy areas of overinflation with resultant attenuation of pulmonary vessels, sometimes in conjunction with bronchiectasis. In older children who are able to suspend respiration, dynamic CT with

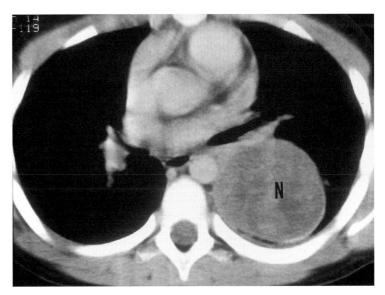

FIG. 29. Metastatic Wilms tumor. A large, soft tissue nodule (N) is seen in the left lower lobe just below the hilar area.

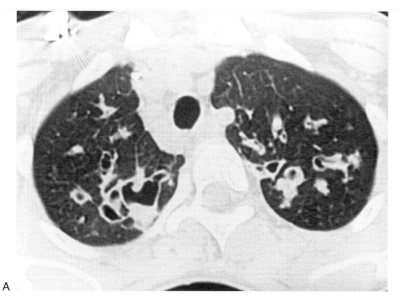

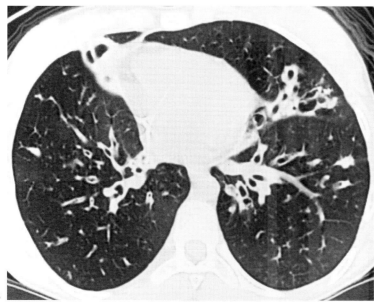

FIG. 30. Cystic fibrosis. **A, B:** High resolution CT sections at two levels demonstrate diffuse cystic bronchiectasis and peribronchial thickening.

inspiratory and expiratory imaging may aid in confirming the diagnosis of focal air trapping (198,210).

Parenchymal or Pleural Disease

In some patients, CT can be helpful in distinguishing between a parenchymal process and a pleural or extra-pleural process. The features of parenchymal lesions are a rounded or oval shape, acute or abrupt angles at the interface with the chest wall, and poorly defined margins with the adjacent lung. The CT features of pleural disease are a lenticular or crescentic shape, obtuse or tapering angles at the interface with the chest wall, and well-defined margins with adjacent lung, bone, and soft tissues.

Extrapleural lesions are lenticular in shape with poorly defined margins and obtuse or tapering angles at the interface with the pleura. Two- and three-dimensional reconstructions in coronal and sagittal planes may be helpful in characterizing a lesion as intraparenchymal or pleural-based.

MRI currently has a limited role in evaluating pulmonary disease, including pleural processes. Although it is sensitive for detection of a variety of pleural and parenchymal disorders, it adds little clinically important information over that gained with CT.

Airway Disease

The tracheobronchial tree, including the trachea, carina, and main and lobar bronchi, are well-depicted by

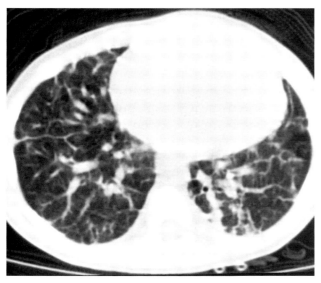

FIG. 31. Bronchopulmonary dysplasia. High-resolution CT shows diffuse septal lines without bronchiectasis.

CT with narrow collimation, especially when performed with spiral technique. The more frequent indications prompting CT of the airway are (a) evaluation of congenital anomalies, (b) detection of posttransplantation complications (Fig. 32), and (c) identification of bronchiectasis (35,100,168,233). By comparison with adults, tracheobronchial neoplasia is a rare indication for CT in children. Typical scan parameters for spiral CT of the airway are slice thickness of 2 to 4 mm, table incrementation of 2 to 4 mm/sec, 1:1 pitch, and 1- to 2-mm reconstructions.

Detection of postoperative complications is im-

proved by the use of multiplanar and three-dimensional reconstructions. Small dehiscences and stenoses can be shown by spiral CT that are not identifiable on conventional CT (233). The length and width of bronchial stenosis and the size and extent of extraluminal gas are shown best by projections rotated to parallel the long axis of the trachea and bronchi (Fig. 32). Three-dimensional images have the advantage of being viewed as a cine loop, allowing depiction of the entire tracheobronchial tree.

A less common indication for airway CT is foreign body aspiration. The foreign body can be precisely localized by spiral CT prior to bronchoscopic retrieval. Dynamic CT with inspiratory and expiratory imaging can show the air trapping distal to the bronchial obstruction.

Cardiac Disease

Most congenital and acquired cardiac lesions are evaluable by echocardiography in combination with Doppler sonography, but MRI can be of use when echocardiography provides inadequate information (14, 15,92,119,124). The major indications for MRI in congenital cardiac anomalies include (a) evaluation of the size and patency of the pulmonary arteries in patients with cyanotic heart disease, such as pulmonary atresia and tetralogy of Fallot, (b) assessment of the extent and severity of aortic coarctation (Fig. 33) and the degree of supravalvar aortic stenosis, (c) determination of the extracardiac anatomy in patients with complex congenital heart disease (e.g., great vessel relationships, bronchial collateral vessels, abdominal situs), and (d) evaluation of surgically created systemic-to-pulmonary

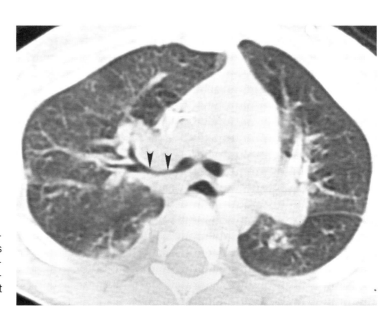

FIG. 32. Bronchial stenosis post lung transplantation. High resolution CT in a 2-year-old boy shows narrowing of the right main bronchus at the anastomotic site (*arrowheads*). The ground glass appearance represents nonspecific inflammation, proven at biopsy.

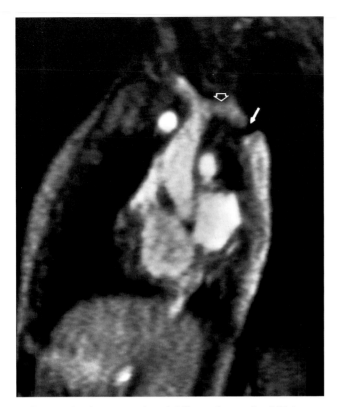

FIG. 33. Aortic coarctation. LAO gradient-echo MR image (40/10/40°) shows mild hypoplasia of the aortic arch (*open arrow*) and flow void in an area of high-grade coarctation (*closed arrow*) just distal to the origin of the left subclavian artery.

artery shunts. MRI also can provide information about acquired lesions, including intra- or pericardial masses (237) (Fig. 34).

ABDOMEN

The appearance of the abdomen on CT and MRI examinations is similar in adults and children, except for the limitations imposed by the small size of the structures being examined and the relative paucity of perivisceral fat. Four major clinical questions usually prompt CT examination of the abdomen: (a) determination of the site of origin, extent and character of an abdominal mass; (b) determination of the extent of a proven lymphoma; (c) evaluation of the extent of injury from blunt abdominal trauma; and (d) determination of the presence or absence of a suspected abscess. Less often, CT is used to evaluate nonneoplastic, parenchymal disease of the kidney, liver, pancreas, and gastrointestinal tract or to assess abnormalities of the major abdominal vessels. Typical scan parameters for screening the pediatric abdomen with spiral CT include 8- to 10-mm slice thickness and table speed with matching reconstruction intervals. MRI is not used as a screening examination. It is most often used to clarify abnormalities seen on ultrasonography or CT (170).

Abdominal masses in the pediatric population are predominantly retroperitoneal in location, with the kidney being the source in more than half of cases. In neonates, most abdominal masses are benign; beyond the neonatal period the percentage of malignant neoplasms increases. CT and MRI have an important role in older infants and children in determining the site of origin, characteristics, and extent of a mass, as well as the presence or absence of metastatic disease (48,49,64,72,225).

Renal Masses

Solid Renal Tumors

Wilms Tumor

Wilms tumor is the most common primary malignant renal tumor of childhood, accounting for approximately 20% of all abdominal masses in children (147). Affected patients generally are under 4 years of age. They present most frequently with a palpable abdominal mass, and less often with abdominal pain, fever, and microscopic or gross hematuria. Approximately, 10% of children have metastatic disease at presentation (83). Metastases are characteristically to the lungs and less frequently to the liver. Bilateral synchronous tumors occur in 5% to 10% of patients.

Wilms tumor appears as a large, spherical, at least partially intrarenal mass with a soft tissue density on CT and an MR signal intensity equal to or lower than normal renal cortex on T1-weighted images and equal to or higher than normal parenchyma on T2-weighted images (11,

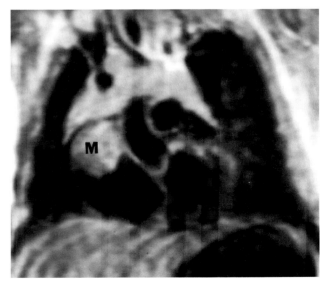

FIG. 34. Rhabdomyoma in a newborn boy with tuberous sclerosis and cardiomegaly. T1-weighted transaxial image shows a large soft tissue mass (M) arising in the lateral wall of the right atrium and encroaching on the right atrial cavity.

26,48,85,110,156,179,225) (Figs. 35 and 36). The tumor enhances after intravenous administration of contrast medium, but usually to a lesser extent than the adjacent parenchyma. Approximately 80% of tumors are heterogeneous because they contain areas of necrosis or hemorrhage (196). Fewer than 15% of Wilms tumors contain calcifications or fat as a minor component. Poor or absent function of the involved kidney occurs in about 10% of patients, resulting from invasion or compression of hilar vessels or the renal pelvis, or from extensive infiltration of tumor throughout the kidney (85,137).

Local spread of tumor may take the form of extension through the capsule into the perinephric space (20% of cases), retroperitoneal lymphadenopathy (20%), or renal vein or inferior vena caval thrombosis (5% to 10%) (83). Perinephric extension may be seen as a thickened renal

capsule or as nodular or streaky densities in the perinephric fat. The diagnosis of lymph node involvement is based on demonstration of perirenal, periaortic, paracaval, or retroperitoneal lymph nodes. Any identified retroperitoneal lymph node, regardless of size, should be regarded with suspicion. Although normal size nodes are commonly demonstrated on abdominal CT and MRI in adults, such nodes are rarely, if ever, seen in infants and young children.

Neither CT nor MRI can detect tumor thrombus in the intrarenal veins, but both imaging techniques are capable of identifying tumor in the main renal vein or inferior vena cava (IVC). The presence or absence of IVC invasion is an important determinant of the surgical approach. A thoracoabdominal approach is required for removal of tumor thrombus extending to or above

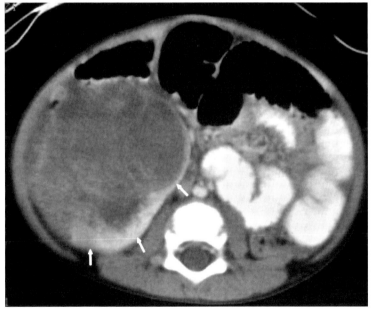

A

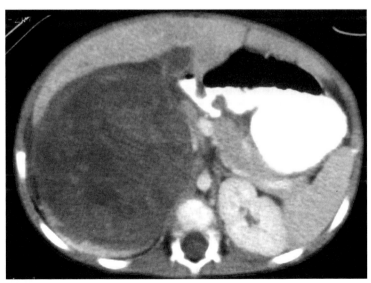

FIG. 35. Wilms tumor in a 2-year-old boy. **A, B:** Two contrast-enhanced CT images demonstrate a large, round, low-density mass that distorts and displaces the enhancing parenchyma (*arrows*) in the lower pole of the right kidney.

B

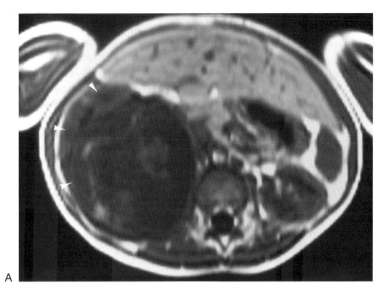

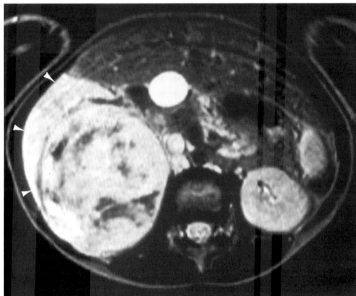

FIG. 36. Wilms tumor in a 2-year-old girl. **A:** T1-weighted transaxial MR image (300/10) shows a large mass replacing most of the right kidney. The predominant signal intensity is similar to that of normal parenchyma (*arrowheads*). Several areas of high signal intensity, representing hemorrhage, are noted in the tumor. **B:** On a T2-weighted (2500/90) transaxial image the signal intensity of the tumor is still equal to that of surrounding renal cortex (*arrowheads*). Also noted are several low intensity areas, corresponding to the high signal intensity areas on the T1-weighted images. (Reproduced from Shady KL, Siegel MJ, Brown JJ. Preoperative evaluation of intraabdominal tumors in children: gradient-recalled echo vs spin-echo MR imaging. *AJR* 1993;161:843–847.)

the confluence of the hepatic veins, whereas an abdominal approach alone is satisfactory for intravascular thrombus below the hepatic veins. On CT, the thrombus may be seen as a low-density intraluminal mass or suggested by renal vein or inferior vena caval enlargement (Fig. 37A). On MRI, tumor thrombus is hyperintense to flowing blood on spin-echo sequences and is hypointense to flowing blood on gradient echo images (Fig. 37B).

After therapy, CT or MRI can be used to detect local recurrence and hepatic metastases. Patients with incomplete resection of tumor, lymph node involvement, and vascular invasion have the highest risk for postoperative recurrence. Features that suggest localized recurrence are a soft tissue mass in the empty renal fossa and ipsilateral psoas muscle enlargement.

Mesoblastic Nephroma

Mesoblastic nephroma, also termed fetal renal hamartoma, is a benign neoplasm usually presenting in the first year of life as an abdominal mass. The CT and MRI findings are those of a fairly uniform intrarenal mass that enhances after intravenous contrast medium injection, although not to the extent of normal renal parenchyma (20). Occasionally areas of cystic degeneration and necrosis are seen as low-density foci within the tumor. Invasion of the vascular pedicle or extension into the renal pelvis is rare, although the tumor can penetrate the renal capsule and invade the perinephric space. Differentiation between Wilms tumor and mesoblastic nephroma usually is not possible without a biopsy.

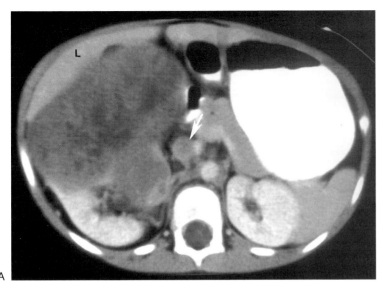
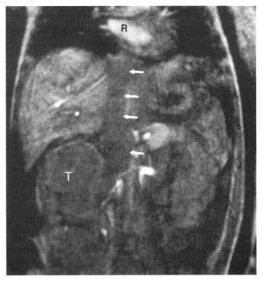

A

B

FIG. 37. Wilms tumor, with extension into the IVC. **A:** CT scan after intravenous contrast medium administration shows a large, heterogeneous, low-density mass in the right kidney posterior to the liver (L). The mass is surrounded by a small amount of normal renal parenchyma posteriorly. Also noted is a dilated inferior vena cava containing tumor thrombus (*arrow*). **B:** Gradient refocused echo image in another patient with a right Wilms tumor (T) shows tumor thrombus filling the inferior vena cava (*arrows*) and extending cranially to the right atrium (R).

Renal Cell Carcinoma

Renal cell carcinoma accounts for <1% of pediatric renal neoplasms. Mean age of presentation of children with renal cell carcinoma is approximately 9 years, in contrast to Wilms tumor with a mean patient age at presentation of 3 years. Presenting signs and symptoms are nonspecific and include mass (60%), pain (50%), and hematuria (30%). On CT and MRI, renal cell carcinoma is indistinguishable from Wilms tumor and appears as a solid intrarenal mass with ill-defined margins (Fig. 38).

After the intravenous administration of contrast medium, the mass enhances, but less than that of the surrounding normal renal parenchyma. Calcification occurs in approximately 25% of tumors. Like Wilms tumor, renal cell carcinoma may spread to retroperitoneal lymph nodes or may invade the renal vein and metastasize to lung and liver (44).

Nephroblastomatosis

Nephroblastomatosis is an abnormality of nephrogenesis characterized by persistence of fetal renal blastema

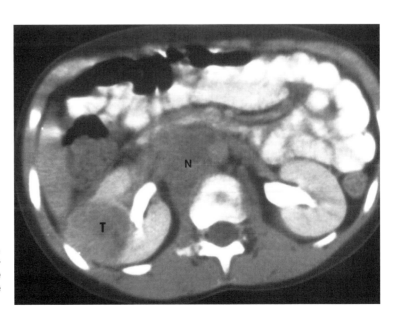

FIG. 38. Renal cell carcinoma, 11-year-old boy. Contrast-enhanced CT scan demonstrates a soft tissue tumor (T) in the right kidney and a conglomerate mass of enlarged lymph nodes (N) adjacent to the renal hilum.

beyond 36 weeks of intrauterine gestation. Nephroblastomatosis itself is not a malignant condition, but it is a precursor to Wilms tumor (9,30). Renal involvement by nephroblastomatosis is usually bilateral. The CT findings of nephroblastomatosis include (a) nephromegaly, (b) low attenuation subcapsular masses or nodules, and (c) poor corticomedullary differentiation (84,179,264) (Fig. 39). On gadolinium-enhanced T1-weighted MR images, nephroblastomatosis is hypointense relative to normal renal tissue (110). On T2-weighted images, nephrogenic rests usually are iso- or slightly hyperintense to renal cortex, but occasionally they can be hypointense. The sensitivity of MRI for detection of nephrogenic rests is 43% on unenhanced images and 58% on gadolinium-enhanced images (110).

Lymphoma

Renal involvement by lymphoma occurs infrequently during the course of disease, but it is not uncommon at autopsy. This complication is more often associated with the non-Hodgkin than with the Hodgkin form of disease and it is often bilateral. In our experience, the most common CT appearance of renal lymphoma in childhood is that of multiple bilateral nodules, occurring in approximately 70% of cases (Fig. 40A and 40B), followed in frequency by direct invasion from contiguous lymph node masses (20% of cases) (Fig. 40C) and solitary nodules (10% of cases). Typically, the intrarenal tumors are hypodense relative to normal renal parenchyma and show minimal enhancement. The CT appearance of solitary renal lymphoma is indistinguishable from that of other solid intrarenal masses, but the diagnosis is possible when there is coexisting splenomegaly or widespread lymph node enlargement. On T1-weighted MR images, lymphomatous nodes have a signal intensity that is slightly higher than that of muscle and lower than that of fat. On T2-weighted images, the signal intensity of lymphomatous nodes is equal to or higher than that of retroperitoneal fat.

Rare Renal Tumors

Clear cell sarcoma and malignant rhabdoid tumor are rare pediatric renal masses. The former tends to affect children between 3 and 5 years of age, whereas the latter is more common in infants with a median age of 13 months (83,239). Presenting signs are similar to those of Wilms tumor. On CT and MRI, these tumors appear as solid intrarenal masses, replacing or compressing the remaining normal kidney. The tumors may involve one or both kidneys. Additional findings include renal capsular thickening and subcapsular or perinephric fluid collection with tumor implants (6,46,239) (Fig. 41). Concomitant primary tumors of the posterior cranial fossa, soft tissues, and thymus occur in association with malignant rhabdoid tumor. Clear cell sarcoma commonly metastasizes to bone.

Renal medullary carcinoma is an unusual tumor associated with sickle cell trait (56). Most patients are diagnosed in the second or third decades of life. The tumor is extremely aggressive, arises centrally within the kidney, grows in an infiltrative pattern, and invades the renal sinus. Contrast enhancement is heterogeneous, reflecting tumor necrosis (56).

Cystic Renal Masses

Multilocular Cystic Nephroma

Multilocular cystic nephroma (also termed benign cystic nephroma, cystic hamartoma, cystic lymphangioma

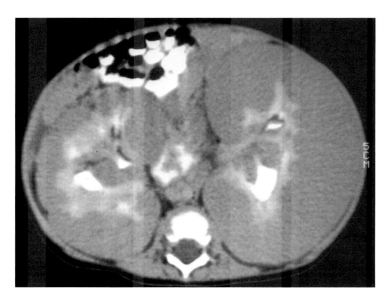

FIG. 39. Nephroblastomatosis, 12-month-old girl. CT scan demonstrates bilateral nephromegaly with a rind of soft tissue in the subcapsular space compressing the enhancing renal cortex.

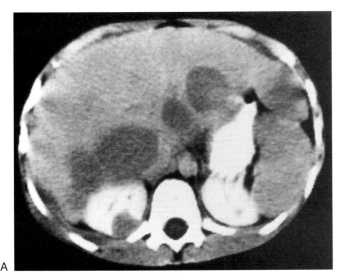

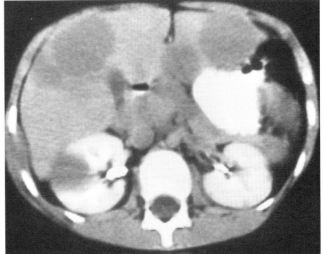

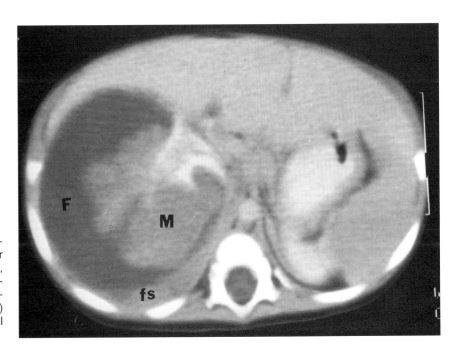

FIG. 40. Renal lymphoma. **A, B:** Contrast-enhanced CT scans in a 11-year-old boy show two nodules in the right kidney as well as multiple hepatic metastases. **C:** CT scan in a 10-year-old boy shows enlarged paraaortic nodes (*arrowheads*) with extension into the left perinephric space (PS). Another nodal mass is seen in the transverse mesocolon (TC).

FIG. 41. Rhabdoid tumor in a 5-month-old boy. CT scan through the upper abdomen demonstrates an irregular, poorly-defined soft tissue mass (M) replacing the parenchyma of the right kidney. Also noted is perirenal fluid (F) and thickening of the posterior renal fascia (fs).

and partial polycystic kidney) is a unilateral, nonhereditary cystic mass. The lesion has a biphasic age and sex distribution, affecting boys under 4 years of age and women over 40 years of age. Presenting signs are a nonpainful abdominal mass or hematuria. On CT and MRI, the lesion appears as a well-defined intrarenal mass with multiple, water density cysts separated by soft tissue septa (7,163) (Fig. 42). The cystic spaces do not communicate with each other and do not enhance, but the septa are vascular and do enhance after intravenous administration of contrast medium. Curvilinear calcifications may be seen in the wall or the septa.

Cystic Disease

Renal cysts in children usually are bilateral and found in association with hereditary polycystic disease. Nonhereditary simple cortical cysts are distinctly uncommon in children. The clinical features of autosomal recessive polycystic disease are dependent on the age of presentation. Infants present with large kidneys, poor renal function, and minimal hepatic disease. In older children, portal hypertension and esophageal varices secondary to hepatic fibrosis predominate. CT or MRI is done to search for collateral vessels, abscess, or hemorrhage. The kidneys are enlarged with smooth margins. The cysts, which represent dilated tubules, usually are centrally located and exhibit near-water attenuation on CT (Fig. 43), low signal intensity on T1-weighted, and high signal intensity on T2-weighted MR images (41,225). Some cysts are hyperdense on CT and hyperintense on T1-weighted MR im-

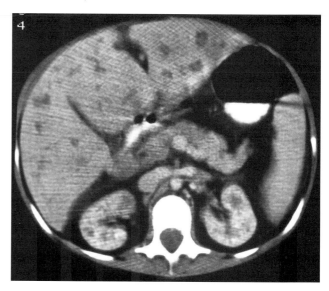

FIG. 43. Autosomal recessive polycystic disease and hepatic fibrosis in a 13-year-old boy. Contrast-enhanced CT scan shows dilated intrahepatic bile ducts and multiple, small renal cysts, representing ectatic tubules.

ages because the contents are mucoid or hemorrhagic. Dilated bile ducts due to hepatic fibrosis also can be seen on CT or MRI.

Autosomal dominant polycystic disease also has age-dependent clinical features. Affected neonates have palpable abdominal masses, whereas children and adolescents present with hypertension or hematuria. The kidneys may be of normal size or enlarged and have lobulated or smooth borders. The cysts are multiple, unequal in size, cortical or medullary in location, and have an attenuation value and signal intensity similar to cysts elsewhere in the body (Fig. 44). Associated hepatic, splenic, and pancreatic cysts also can be identified by CT or MRI.

Fatty Renal Masses

Angiomyolipoma

Angiomyolipoma is a benign renal tumor composed of angiomatous, myomatous, and lipomatous tissue. It is rare as an isolated lesion in the general pediatric population but is present in as many as 80% of children with tuberous sclerosis. The lesions usually are detected as an incidental finding, but some patients present with abdominal pain or anemia secondary to intratumoral or retroperitoneal hemorrhage, or with renal failure because of extensive parenchymal replacement by tumor. On CT, these tumors are small, multiple, bilateral, and of low attenuation, usually containing at least some areas of identifiable fat (Fig. 45). Occasionally, they coexist with cystic renal disease (174). Differentiation with CT usually is possible based

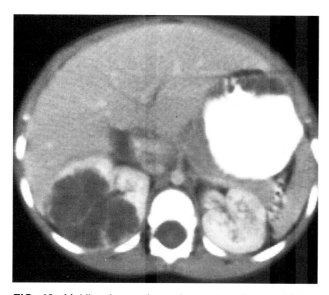

FIG. 42. Multilocular cystic nephroma in a 3-year-old boy. Contrast-enhanced CT scan shows a low-attenuation mass containing several enhancing septations in the upper pole of the right kidney.

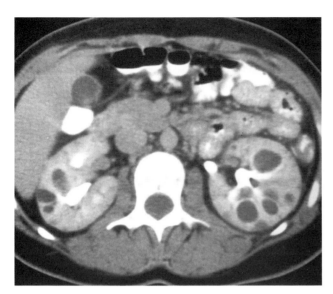

FIG. 44. Autosomal dominant polycystic disease in a 15-year-old boy. CT scan performed for posttraumatic hematuria shows low-attenuation masses in the renal parenchyma.

on differences in the attenuation values of cystic and lipomatous tissue. On MRI, angiomyolipomas demonstrate high signal intensity on T1- and T2-weighted sequences and low signal intensity on fat-suppressed images.

Adrenal Masses

Hemorrhage

Hemorrhage is the most common cause of an adrenal mass in the neonate, occurring as a result of birth trauma, septicemia, or hypoxia. Adrenal hemorrhage is less common in infants and children and usually is the result of trauma (181). The CT attenuation varies with the age of the hematoma. Acute hematoma has a high attenuation, whereas subacute and chronic hematomas are of low attenuation. On MRI, adrenal hemorrhage usually demonstrates a high signal intensity on both T1- and T2-weighted images, reflecting the presence of methemoglobin (34,41,148).

Neuroblastoma

Neuroblastoma is the most common malignant abdominal tumor in children, usually affecting children under the age of 4 years. More than half of all neuroblastomas originate in the abdomen, and two thirds of these arise in the adrenal gland (114). The extraadrenal tumors originate in the sympathetic ganglion cells or paraaortic bodies and may be found anywhere from the cervical region to the pelvis. Neuroblastoma tends to metastasize early and more than half of all patients have bone marrow, skeletal, liver, or skin metastases when initially diagnosed. Lung metastases are rare.

On CT, neuroblastoma appears as a homogeneous or heterogeneous, pararenal or paraspinal, soft tissue mass with lobulated margins (23,27,29,78,156,251). The tumor enhances less than that of surrounding tissues after intravenous administration of contrast material (Fig. 46). Calcifications within the tumor, which may be coarse, mottled, solid or ring-shaped, are observed in approximately 85% of neuroblastomas on CT.

On T1-weighted MR images, neuroblastoma appears either hypointense or isointense relative to the liver. On T2-weighted and gadolinium-enhanced sequences, it ap-

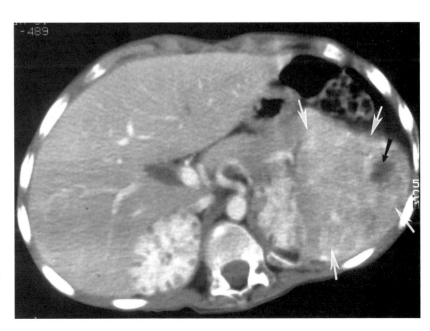

FIG. 45. Angiomyolipomas in a 16-year-old boy with tuberous sclerosis. Contrast-enhanced CT demonstrates multiple, small, bilateral renal masses of low-attenuation, as well as a larger soft tissue mass (*white arrows*) in the left kidney. A focal area of fat (*black arrow*) is noted within the large left angiomyolipoma.

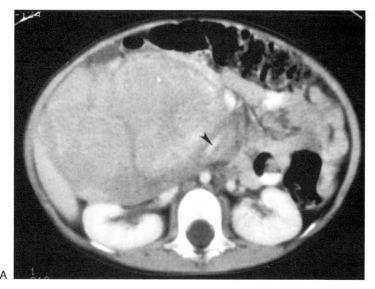

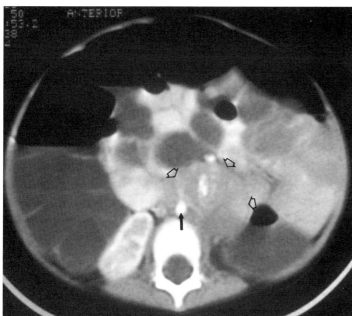

FIG. 46. Neuroblastoma. **A:** Contrast-enhanced CT scan in a 2-year-old girl shows a suprarenal low-density mass extending across the midline in the retroperitoneum and displacing the right kidney posteriorly. The tissue planes around the superior mesenteric artery (*arrowhead*) are obscured due to encasement by tumor. **B:** CT scan in a 2-year-old girl shows a paraspinal soft tissue mass (*open arrows*), with calcifications, surrounding the aorta (*arrow*). The tumor produced vasointestinal peptides which explains the presence of the dilated, fluid-filled bowel loops.

pears slightly to markedly hyperintense relative to liver (Fig. 47). The center of the tumor is often heterogeneous, reflecting the presence of hemorrhage, necrosis, or calcification. Hemorrhage may appear as a low- or high-signal-intensity focus on T1-weighted pulse sequences, depending on the age of the blood; it usually has high signal intensity on T2-weighted images. Focal necrosis produces signal hypointensity on T1-weighted images and hyperintensity on T2-weighted sequences. Calcifications are hypointense on all sequences (26,28,41,67,93). Findings of local spread, such as prevertebral extension across the midline (Fig. 46), vascular encasement (Fig. 46), hepatic metastases, intraspinal extension (Fig. 48), and renal invasion or infarction, can be seen on both MRI and CT (27,59,206). Knowledge of tumor extent is important for

understanding the many appearances of neuroblastoma, for treatment planning, and for prognosis.

Following surgery or chemotherapy, CT or MRI may be used to monitor treatment response and detect recurrent disease. Serial CT examinations after therapy often suffice to determine the adequacy of treatment. In patients with residual masses, MRI may be able to separate fibrosis and tumor involvement. Demonstration of a residual mass with low signal intensity on both T1- and T2-weighted images favors the diagnosis of fibrosis, whereas high signal on the T2-weighted sequence suggests residual tumor.

Adrenocortical Neoplasms

Adrenal lesions, other than neuroblastomas, are rare in childhood, accounting for 5% or less of all adrenal tumors

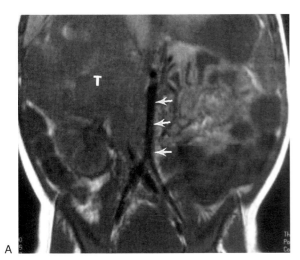

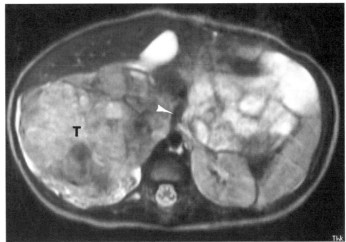

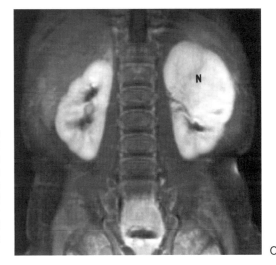

FIG. 47. Neuroblastoma. **A:** T1-weighted (235/10) coronal MR image in a 5-year-old boy shows a large tumor (T) with relatively low signal intensity arising in the right side of the abdomen. The tumor extends to the midline and abuts but does not displace the aorta (*arrows*). **B:** On the axial T2-weighted (2000/80) image, the signal intensity of the tumor (T) is higher than that of the liver. Again noted is extension of tumor to the midline. The tumor abuts but does not encase the superior mesenteric artery (*arrowhead*). **C:** Fat-suppressed T1-weighted MR image after gadolinium administration in a 2-month-old boy shows an enhancing left suprarenal neuroblastoma (N).

(23,53,54). Of these, carcinoma is the most common, followed in frequency by adenoma. The mean ages at presentation of patients with carcinoma and adenoma are approximately 6 years and 3 years, respectively. Adrenal carcinomas are usually hormonally active, producing virilization, feminization or Cushing syndrome. Adenomas can cause Cushing syndrome or primary aldosteronism, but they also may be detected incidentally.

Adrenal carcinomas are typically large masses at the time of presentation, often greater than 4 cm in diameter, with an attenuation value equal to that of soft tissue. Many contain low-density areas from prior hemorrhage and necrosis; some contain calcifications (Fig. 49). Cortisol-producing adenomas range from 2 to 5 cm in diameter, whereas aldosterone-secreting tumors are usually <2 cm in diameter. Both types of adenomas tend to be homogeneous and of low attenuation because of their high lipid content. Carcinomas exhibit a low signal intensity on T1-weighted and high signal intensity on T2-weighted MR images. Adenomas may have a high signal intensity on both pulse sequences.

Pheochromocytoma

Pheochromocytomas are catecholamine-producing tumors that cause paroxysmal hypertension in children (23,53). Approximately 70% to 75% of childhood pheochromocytomas arise in the adrenal medulla; the remainder are extraadrenal, occurring in the sympathetic ganglia adjacent to the vena cava or aorta, near the organ of Zuckerkandl, or in the wall of the urinary bladder. Up to 70% of tumors are bilateral and about 5% are malignant. Most are at least 3 cm in diameter at the time of diagnosis. On CT, pheochromocytomas are of soft tissue density and frequently enhance after intravenous administration of contrast medium. On T1-weighted MR images, they have a signal intensity similar to that of muscle; on T2-weighted images, the signal intensity is equal to or greater than that of fat (Fig. 50). Small pheochromocytomas often are homogeneous, whereas larger tumors appear heterogeneous with both cystic and solid components. Calcifications within the tumor are rare (79).

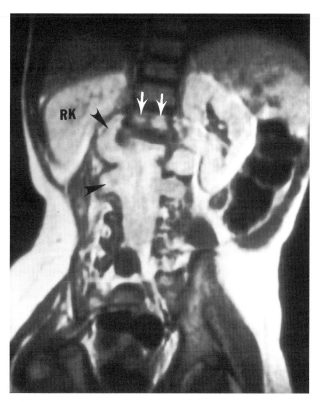

FIG. 48. Neuroblastoma with intraspinal invasion. Coronal T1-weighted MR image shows a small, dumbbell-shaped tumor (*arrowheads*) invading the spinal canal at two levels. The right kidney (RK) is displaced laterally by the tumor. Areas of high signal intensity in the lumbar vertebral body represent metastases (*arrows*).

Retroperitoneal Soft Tissue Masses

Although rare, both benign and malignant primary tumors occur in the retroperitoneal soft tissues. Benign tumors include teratoma, lymphangioma, neurofibroma, and lipomatosis. Teratomas usually arise in the sacrococcygeal region and appear as well-defined, fluid-filled masses with a variable amount of fat or calcium (1,57). Lymphangiomas are well-circumscribed, multiloculated, fluid-filled masses. Neurofibromas are usually well-defined, cylindrical, soft tissue lesions with a characteristic location in the neurovascular bundle. Lipomatosis appears as a diffuse, infiltrative mass with an attenuation value or signal intensity equal to that of fat; it grows along fascial planes and may invade muscle.

Rhabdomyosarcoma is the most common malignant tumor of the retroperitoneum, followed by neurofibrosarcoma, fibrosarcoma, and extragonadal germ cell tumors. These tumors appear as bulky, soft tissue masses with attenuation values slightly less than or equal to that of muscle. On T1-weighted MR images, they appear either hypo- or isointense to liver, kidney, and muscle. On T2-weighted images, rhabdomyosarcoma has a signal intensity equal to or greater than that of fat (88) (Fig. 51). Vessel displacement or encasement sometimes occurs and can be easily seen with gradient echo imaging (215).

Hepatic Masses

Primary Malignant Neoplasms

Primary hepatic tumor is the third most common solid abdominal mass in children, following Wilms tumor and

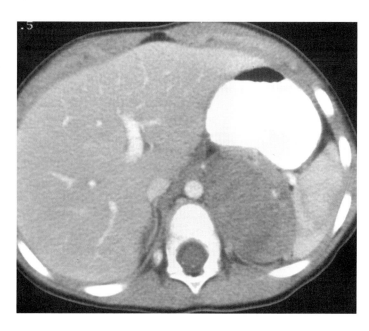

FIG. 49. Adrenal carcinoma in a 10-year-old girl with virilization. A large mass with faint calcifications is present in the left adrenal.

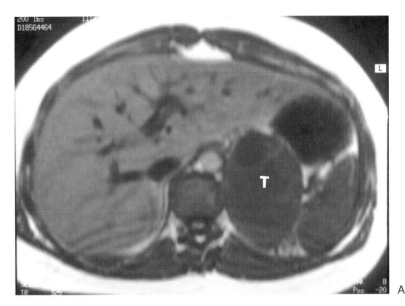

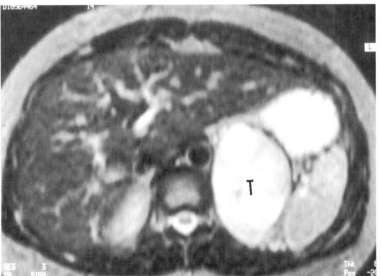

FIG. 50. Adrenal pheochromocytoma in 16-year-old girl with hypertension. **A:** T1-weighted MR image (525/10) shows a low-signal-intensity tumor (T) in the left adrenal gland. **B:** On a T2-weighted image (2000/80) the tumor (T) is markedly hyperintense.

neuroblastoma. Two thirds of hepatic tumors are malignant, with hepatoblastoma and hepatocellular carcinoma accounting for the majority (246,260). The former occurs in children under the age of 3 years, whereas the latter is more common in older children. The tumors are discovered as asymptomatic upper abdominal masses, occasionally associated with anorexia and weight loss.

The CT appearances of hepatoblastoma and hepatocellular carcinoma are similar. Both tumors usually are confined to a single lobe, with the right lobe affected twice as often as the left, but they may involve both lobes or they may be multicentric. They generally have a density lower than that of normal hepatic parenchyma on unenhanced and contrast-enhanced scans (4) (Fig. 52). Less frequently, hepatoblastoma and hepatocellular carcinoma are isodense or hyperdense relative to the adjacent hepatic tissue (51,130,222). Both tumors often are heterogeneous

because they contain hemorrhage, necrosis or focal steatosis. Calcifications occur in approximately 50% of hepatoblastomas and in 25% of hepatocellular carcinomas. Portal vein invasion also is common.

Malignant hepatic lesions are hypointense with respect to liver on T1-weighted MR images and hyperintense on T2-weighted sequences (234) (Fig. 53). Tumor thrombus is seen as a hyperintense focus within a normally signal-free vessel on spin-echo images or as a hypointense area on gradient echo imaging (190) (Fig. 54). Hemorrhage can appear hypo- or hyperintense on T1-weighted pulse sequences, depending on the age of the blood; it usually is hyperintense on T2-weighted images. Focal steatosis produces signal hyperintensity on both T1- and T2-weighted pulse sequences and low signal intensity on fat-suppressed images. Calcifications are hypointense on all sequences. On postcontrast images, both hepatoblastoma

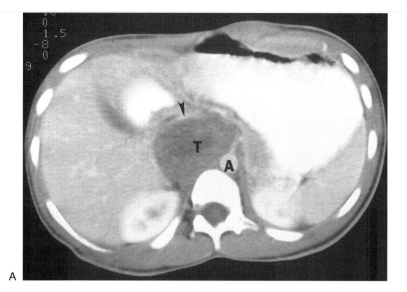

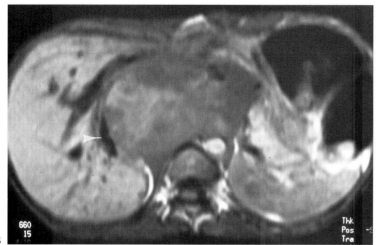

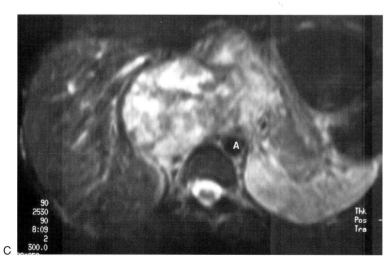

FIG. 51. Retroperitoneal sarcoma. **A:** Contrast enhanced CT scan demonstrates a soft tissue tumor (T) anterior to the vertebral body. The mass displaces the inferior vena cava (*arrowhead*) anteriorly and the aorta (A) to the left. **B:** T1-weighted image (SE, 600 msec, 15) performed 12 months later demonstrates a larger retroperitoneal mass with a predominantly intermediate signal displacing the inferior vena cava (*arrowhead*) to the right. Areas of high signal intensity represent blood. **C:** On a T2-weighted image (SE 2500 msec, 90), the mass is high in signal intensity and appears more heterogeneous. A, aorta.

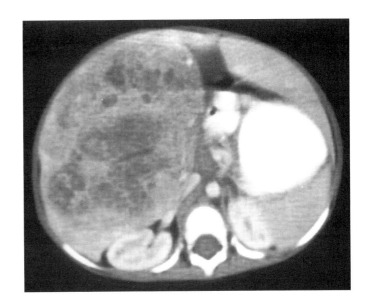

FIG. 52. Hepatoblastoma in a 2-year-old girl with a right upper quadrant mass. Contrast enhanced CT scan shows a large, heterogeneous soft tissue mass occupying the right lobe of the liver. Mild compressive effects are noted on the right kidney.

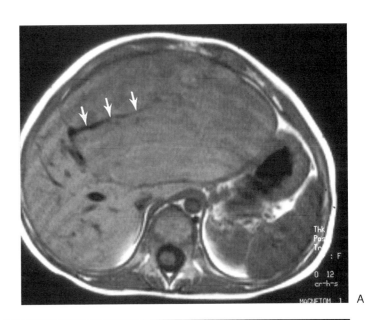

A

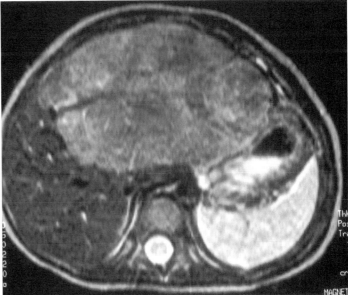

B

FIG. 53. Hepatoblastoma in a 3-year-old boy. **A:** T1-weighted transaxial MR image (525/10) shows a low-signal-intensity mass in the left lobe of the liver. The tumor encases the left portal vein (*arrows*). **B:** On a T2-weighted image (2490/90), the tumor has increased signal intensity relative to normal parenchyma.

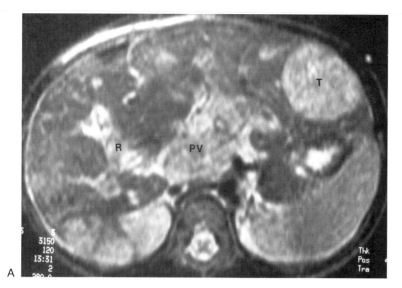

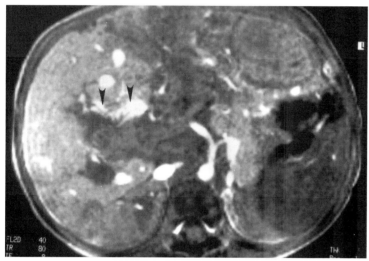

FIG. 54. Hepatoblastoma in a 3-year-old boy. **A:** T2-weighted image (3150/12) shows a high-signal-intensity tumor (T) in the lateral segment of the left lobe of the liver and in the right (R) and main portal vein (PV) due to tumor thrombus. **B:** Gradient echo image (80/8/40°) confirms absence of portal venous blood flow. Flow is noted within a periportal collateral vessel (*arrowheads*).

and hepatocellular carcinoma demonstrate diffuse, heterogeneous enhancement.

MRI and CT are equally sensitive in detecting tumor and in most cases are comparable in demonstrating margins of the tumor. MRI is superior to CT in demonstrating invasion and displacement of portal and hepatic veins.

Fibrolamellar hepatocellular carcinoma, which is a subtype of hepatocellular carcinoma, is a rare malignant tumor in children and adolescents. The prognosis for patients with unresectable tumor is better than that for patients with the usual variety of hepatocellular carcinoma (average survival 32 and 6 months, respectively). On CT and MRI, fibrolamellar hepatocellular carcinoma is usually solitary and well delineated with variable contrast enhancement. Small central calcifications are seen in about 40% of tumors, and a central scar in 30% (99,247). The imaging features of fibrolamellar carcinoma are similar to those of the other malignant hepatic tumors, and so biopsy is needed for definitive diagnosis.

Undifferentiated embryonal sarcoma, also known as

mesenchymal sarcoma, embryonal sarcoma, and malignant mesenchymoma, is the third most common primary malignant tumor in children after hepatoblastoma and hepatocellular carcinoma. It primarily affects older children and adolescents. The usual presenting features are abdominal mass and pain. On CT, the tumor is a multilocular mass with multiple septations and a thick peripheral rim which enhances after injection of contrast medium (201). The MRI appearance is that of a heterogeneous, septated mass with predominantly hypointense contents on T1-weighted images and hyperintense contents on T2-weighted images. The fibrous rim has a low signal intensity on both imaging sequences (190).

Hepatic Metastases

The malignant tumors of childhood that most frequently metastasize to the liver are Wilms tumor, neuroblastoma, and lymphoma. Clinically, patients with hepatic

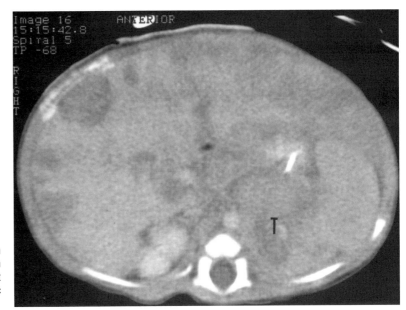

FIG. 55. Hepatic metastases in a neonate with neuroblastoma. Contrast-enhanced CT scan shows a soft tissue tumor (T) arising in the left adrenal gland and multiple low density hepatic metastases.

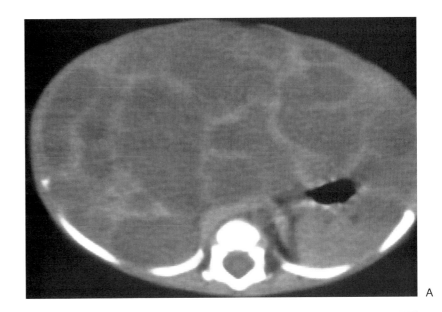

A

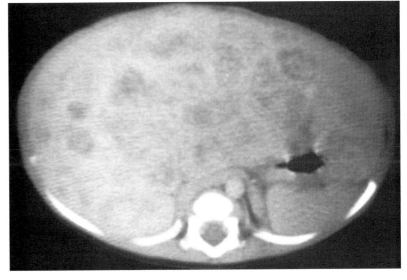

B

FIG. 56. Diffuse hemangioendotheliomatosis in a neonate. **A:** Precontrast CT scan demonstrates multiple hypodense areas in the liver. **B:** CT scan obtained 3 min after a bolus injection of contrast medium demonstrates nearly total opacification of the lesions.

metastases present with hepatomegaly, jaundice, abdominal pain or mass, or abnormal hepatic function tests.

Hepatic metastases are typically multiple, hypodense relative to normal liver on contrast-enhanced CT (Fig. 55), hypointense on T1-weighted images, and hyperintense on T2-weighted images. Although the signal intensity is high on T2-weighted images, it is not as high as that seen with hemangiomas or cysts. Other findings include either a low- or high-signal-intensity capsule and mass effect with displacement of vessels. Hepatic metastases in children may exhibit some degree of heterogeneous central enhancement on postcontrast images.

Benign Neoplasms

Benign tumors account for about one third of all hepatic tumors in children. The majority are of vascular origin and usually hemangioendotheliomas (63,234,246,260). Most patients with hemangioendotheliomas are under 6 months of age and present with hepatomegaly or congestive heart failure due to high-output overcirculation. Occasionally, affected patients present with bleeding diathesis secondary to platelet sequestration (Kasabach-Merritt syndrome) or massive hemoperitoneum due to spontaneous tumor rupture. By comparison with adults, cavernous hemangioma is infrequently found in children, although it is sometimes encountered as an incidental finding.

At gross examination, hemangioendothelioma is a relatively bloodless tumor composed of multiple nodules ranging from 2 to 15 cm in diameter. Histologically, it is composed of vascular channels lined by plump endothe-

lial cells that are supported by reticular fibers. The tumor is usually solitary and has a slight predilection for the posterior segment of the right lobe, but it may be multicentric and involve both lobes. Areas of fibrosis, calcification, hemorrhage, and cystic degeneration are common (52,190).

Hemangioendothelioma and cavernous hemangioma have similar appearances on CT and MRI. On noncontrast-enhanced CT scans, both lesions demonstrate low density relative to the liver (Fig. 56), and on T1-weighted MR images both are hypointense. On T2-weighted images, the lesions are hyperintense (Fig. 57). A heterogeneous appearance may be noted due to areas of fibrosis, necrosis, or hemorrhage. Images after administration of iodinated contrast medium or gadolinium-DTPA demonstrate centripetal enhancement with variable degrees of delayed central enhancement (Fig. 56) (52,82,130,143,157,190,222,249). Small tumors may rapidly become hyperdense without showing peripheral enhancement. Larger lesions, particularly solitary lesions, may not completely enhance on delayed scans (143), reflecting areas of fibrosis or thrombosis. Foci of globular enhancement may be noted in cavernous hemangiomas during dynamic bolus imaging, believed to represent puddling of contrast in vascular lakes.

After the vascular lesions, mesenchymal hamartoma is the next most common benign hepatic tumor of childhood. It is the benign counterpart to the undifferentiated embryonal sarcoma. This tumor usually is found as an asymptomatic mass in boys under 2 years of age. Rarely, the hamartoma has a large vascular component and pro-

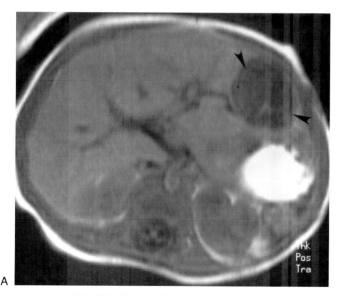
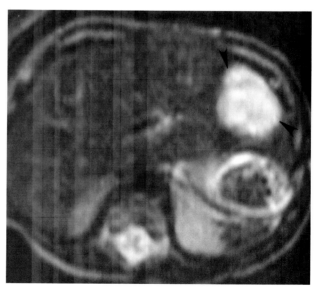

FIG. 57. Hemangioendothelioma in a neonate with cutaneous hemangiomas. **A:** T1-weighted image (325/10) shows a well-defined, hypointense mass (*arrowheads*) in the left lobe of the liver. **B:** On a T2-weighted image (2500/120) the signal intensity of the mass (*arrowheads*) increases and is similar to that of cerebrospinal fluid. (Fig. 57B reproduced from reference Siegel MJ, Luker GD. MR imaging of the liver in children. *MRI Clin North Am* 1996;4:637–656.)

duces arteriovenous shunting, leading to congestive heart failure. On CT, the lesion appears as a well-circumscribed multilocular mass containing multiple low-density areas separated by solid tissue (105,190,250). After intravenous administration of contrast medium, the central contents do not enhance, but the thicker septa may appear more dense. T1-weighted MR images show a low-intensity mass; T2-weighted images demonstrate a hyperintense mass containing septations of low signal intensity (190). Differentiation between mesenchymal hamartoma and undifferentiated embryonal sarcoma by imaging findings is difficult (201). A younger age and absence of symptoms favors a benign hamartoma, but definitive diagnosis requires tissue sampling.

Biliary Masses

Choledochal cyst is the most common mass arising in the biliary ductal tree. Classically, patients present with jaundice, pain, and a palpable abdominal mass, although the complete triad is present in only about one third of patients. CT can enable detection and diagnosis of a choledochal cyst, but it is unnecessary if the diagnosis can be made by sonography supplemented by radionuclide studies using hepatobiliary agents (145,222). If these studies are equivocal, CT can suggest the diagnosis by demonstrating cystic dilatation of both intrahepatic and extrahepatic biliary ducts (Fig. 58). The intrahepatic dilatation is limited to the central portions of the left and right

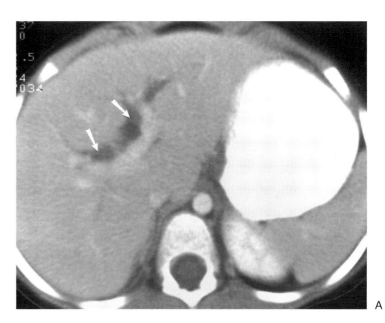

A

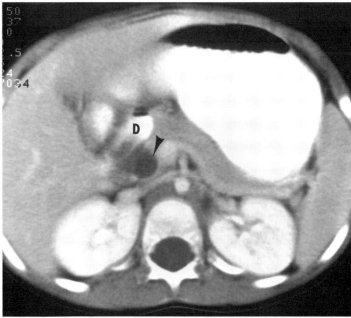

FIG. 58. Choledochal cyst, 5-year-old girl with abdominal pain. **A:** Postcontrast CT scan demonstrates mildly dilated right and left hepatic ducts (*arrows*). The peripheral branches are not dilated. **B:** CT scan 4 cm caudal shows a dilated common bile duct (*arrowhead*), representing the choledochal cyst, medial to the duodenum (D).

B

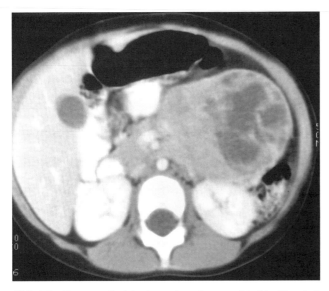

FIG. 59. Pancreaticoblastoma in a 3-year-old girl with a left upper quadrant mass. A 7-cm, heterogeneous mass is present in the tail of the pancreas. Low density areas represent necrosis.

hepatic ducts. Generalized ductal dilatation, with gradual tapering to the periphery, characteristic of acquired obstruction, is absent.

Pancreatic Masses

Pancreaticoblastoma is the most common pancreatic neoplasm in young children (117). It is an encapsulated, epithelial tumor composed of tissue resembling fetal pancreas, has a favorable prognosis, and usually arises in the pancreatic head. On contrast-enhanced CT, the tumor appears as a focal mass of homogeneous or heterogeneous soft tissue density (115,117) (Fig. 59). Secondary signs include hepatic and lymph node metastases and vascular encasement.

Solid and papillary epithelial neoplasm of the pancreas is the most common tumor in adolescent girls (98). The tumor has a low potential for malignancy, is well encapsulated, and usually occurs in the tail. On CT, this neoplasm appears as a large (mean, 11.5 cm), well-defined, thick-walled cystic mass containing papillary projections and occasionally septa.

Splenic Masses

Focal splenic lesions in children include abscess, neoplasms (most commonly lymphoma and rarely hamartoma), vascular malformations (lymphangioma, hemangioma), and cysts. Abscesses, vascular malformations, and cysts have a low attenuation value on CT (Fig. 60), a low signal intensity on T1-weighted MR images, and a signal intensity greater than that of fat on T2-weighted images. Solid tumors are of soft tissue density. On MRI, they show a signal intensity greater than that of muscle and less than that of fat on T1-weighted images, and a signal intensity nearly equal to that of fat on T2-weighted sequences (112). Vascular malformations enhance after intravenous contrast medium administration.

In some children, the spleen is highly mobile, due to failure of fusion of the gastric mesentery with the dorsal peritoneum, and presents as a mass in the anterior abdomen. CT or MRI demonstrates absence of the spleen in the left upper quadrant and a lower abdominal or pelvic soft tissue mass. The mobile spleen enhances after administration of intravenous contrast medium unless it has undergone torsion with resultant vascular compromise (116).

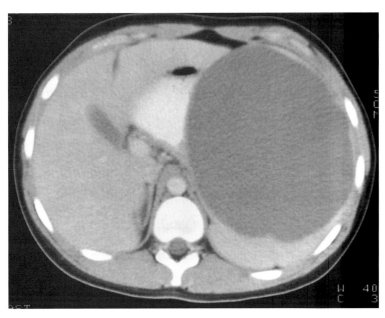

FIG. 60. Epidermoid cyst in a 14-year-old boy with left upper quadrant pain. A large, ovoid, low-density cyst is seen in the spleen on a contrast-enhanced CT scan.

Gastrointestinal and Mesenteric Masses

Lymphangiomatous malformations, also termed mesenteric cysts, and enteric duplications account for most benign gastrointestinal/mesenteric masses, whereas lymphoma is the most common malignant mass (207). On CT, a mesenteric cyst is a near-water-density mass with a barely discernible wall (Fig. 61), whereas an enteric duplication appears as a cystic mass with a thick wall (77,202). Both lesions have a signal intensity equal to or slightly less than that of muscle on T1-weighted MR images, although the signal intensity may be higher if the lesions contain blood or proteinaceous material. On T2-weighted images, the signal intensity is greater than that of fat (229).

The CT features of bowel lymphoma include wall thickening greater than 1 cm in diameter, extraluminal soft tissue mass, and mesenteric invasion (228). On MRI, lymphomatous masses have a signal intensity similar to that of muscle on T1-weighted images and similar to that of fat on T2-weighted sequences.

Comparative Imaging and Clinical Applications

In the evaluation of neuroblastoma, CT has a sensitivity of 100% and can correctly stage the extent of disease in 82%. In comparison, ultrasonography can correctly detect the tumor in 91% and define the stage of disease in 55% (251). In Wilms tumor, CT is as sensitive (100%) as US for detecting the tumor, but it is superior to US for staging (196). The sensitivity and accuracy of MRI in evaluating retroperitoneal tumors has not been evaluated in large series of children, but our experience suggests that MRI is at least as sensitive and accurate as CT.

The choice of examination for evaluation of a patient suspected of having an abdominal mass varies with the age of the patient, the available equipment and expertise at a given institution, and the relative advantages and disadvantages of each imaging method. Plain film radiography often is performed initially in the evaluation of an abdominal mass as it is simple, readily available, inexpensive, and can serve to confirm the presence and position of a mass. Although such information may be helpful in planning other investigative procedures, the plain radiograph usually is not diagnostic. Scintigraphy also has a limited role in diagnosing most abdominal masses, with the exception of hepatobiliary scintigraphy to confirm the diagnosis of a choledochal cyst and ^{131}I-MIBG (metaiodobenzylguanidine) imaging or ^{111}In-pentetreotide, a somatostatin receptor, to diagnose or localize pheochromocytoma and neuroblastoma.

Ultrasonography (US), CT, and MRI provide more detailed information than plain radiography or scintigraphy. Ultrasonography can clearly reveal the location, extent, and solid or cystic nature of a mass. It is especially important in evaluating neonatal abdominal masses because the majority of these are benign. However, it provides no information concerning function, and gas-filled viscera, normally found in young children, can impair sound transmission. CT and MRI are superior to US for assessing tumor extent in the retroperitoneum because they can provide images unobscured by overlying structures, such as gas-filled bowel or bone. However, CT and MRI are not without certain drawbacks. Both require sedation in children under 5 years of age. Other risks related to CT include exposure to ionizing radiation and the need to use oral and intravenous contrast agents because infants and children have little perivisceral fat, making anatomic delineation difficult in many cases.

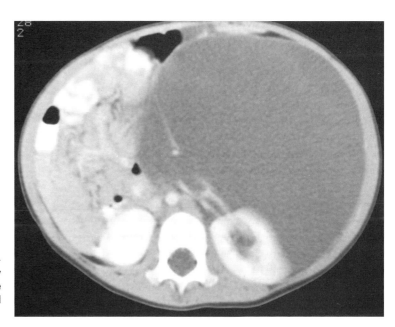

FIG. 61. Mesenteric cyst, 3-year-old girl with abdominal distention. A well-defined, low density mass, containing several septations, is noted in the left abdomen. The lesion involved the small bowel mesentery.

Because of these limitations, US usually is considered the screening technique of choice for evaluation of a pediatric abdominal mass. If the US study is normal, further radiographic evaluation generally is not required. If US cannot yield adequate information or if it suggests a malignant renal or suprarenal mass, CT generally should be considered, particularly to delineate the tumor extent. MRI is the preferred imaging technique in patients with a paraspinal neoplasm, since these tumors have a likelihood of intraspinal extension (66,67,215,232). MRI also can play an important role in determining the extent of hepatic neoplasms, particularly the relationship of a lesion to adjacent vascular structures (25,125,261).

Lymphoma

Intraabdominal lymphoma most often affects the retroperitoneal and mesenteric lymph nodes, bowel, and mesentery. Although CT and MRI occasionally demonstrate normal-size lymph nodes in the retroperitoneum and pelvis in the adult, these are rarely recognized in children. However, lymphoma and metastatic disease of any cause may produce sufficient lymph node enlargement to be demonstrable on CT and MRI (207). The CT appearance of such adenopathy varies from individually enlarged lymph nodes of soft tissue density to a large homogeneous mass obscuring normal structures (Fig. 62). On MRI, lymph nodes involved by lymphoma have a signal intensity greater than or equal to that of muscle on T1-weighted images and close to that of fat on T2-weighted sequences. As in the adult, these imaging studies cannot differentiate normal lymph nodes from those of normal size but replaced with tumor. In addition, it is impossible to distinguish between mild enlargement of lymph nodes due to

inflammatory conditions, such as Crohn disease, giardiasis, tuberculosis, sarcoidosis, and acquired immune deficiency syndrome, and enlargement due to neoplastic involvement.

CT is the initial radiologic procedure of choice for evaluating the abdomen in children with lymphoma, as it is more reliable than ultrasonography for detecting small mesenteric masses. The sonogram is often limited because sound transmission is impaired by gas-filled bowel loops. Differentiation between mesenteric masses and normal bowel is difficult with MRI unless an oral contrast agent is available for bowel opacification.

Abdominal Abscess

Most abdominal abscesses in children are caused by appendicitis, Crohn disease, and/or postoperative complications (69,221). The typical CT appearance of an abscess is that of a mass of relatively low density, with or without a rim that often is enhanced after intravenous administration of contrast material (Fig. 63). Gas is present in slightly more than one third of abscesses and may appear as multiple small bubbles or as a large collection with an air–fluid level. The size and shape are affected by location because abscesses usually are confined to fascial or intraperitoneal compartments, expanding the spaces and displacing contiguous structures. Abscesses commonly produce obliteration of adjacent fat planes and thickening of surrounding muscles, mesentery, or bowel wall.

Ultrasonography and CT are both accurate methods for confirming the presence of intraabdominal abscesses. The choice of examination between CT and US depends on the individual clinical situation. Ultrasonography often is hampered by a large amount of bowel gas; it can also be

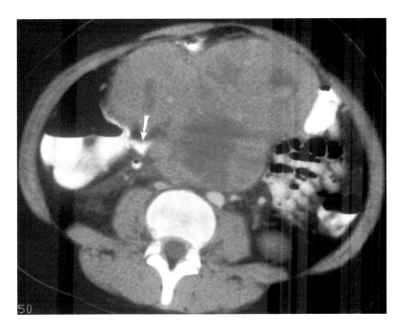

FIG. 62. Lymphoma, 12-year-old boy. A large conglomerate mass of lymphomatous nodes, some with necrosis, extends from the anterior abdominal wall to the retroperitoneum. The mass encases part of the terminal ileum (*arrow*).

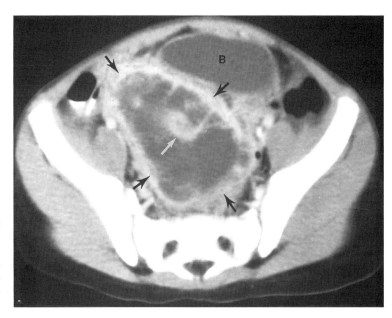

FIG. 63. Appendiceal abscess. Contrast-enhanced CT scan demonstrates a low attenuation mass in the cul-de-sac. The mass is surrounded by an enhancing rim (*black arrows*) and streaky soft tissue densities extending into the adjacent pelvic fat. The soft tissue density (*white arrow*) within the abscess represents the appendiceal stump. B, bladder.

suboptimal in the immediate postoperative period because of the difficulty in imaging the area directly beneath the surgical wound, drainage tubes, and ostomy appliances. Moreover, the left subphrenic area and the lesser sac may be difficult to evaluate by US because of a gas-filled stomach. This is especially true in patients who have had prior splenectomy. Because these areas are readily studied by CT examination, CT is our preferred approach. The right subphrenic and subhepatic areas are at least as well studied by US as by CT; thus, for suspected abnormalities in these locations, US is the initial procedure of choice. CT is considered the method of choice when a retroperitoneal abscess is suspected. If an abscess is detected, CT permits planning of the most appropriate approach for percutaneous or surgical drainage. MRI has no practical role in the evaluation of an intraabdominal abscess.

Blunt Abdominal Trauma

Abdominal injuries in children are most often the result of blunt trauma caused by motor vehicle accidents and are less frequently caused by bicycle, skateboard, and all-terrain vehicle accidents, falls, gunshot injuries, and child abuse (141). The liver is the most commonly injured abdominal organ, followed by the spleen, kidney, adrenal gland, and pancreas (227,242,248,256). CT provides a radiologic display of the entire abdomen following non-penetrating injuries and can document injury to both solid and hollow organs, intraperitoneal or retroperitoneal hemorrhage, sites of active bleeding, and unsuspected thoracic or skeletal injuries (244,248,255,256).

The CT appearance of intraabdominal injuries depends on whether the injury is to a solid or hollow organ. The spectrum of injuries in solid organs, such as the liver, spleen, and kidney, ranges from small intraparenchymal

and subcapsular hematomas to large lacerations or fractures with capsular disruption (141). Typically, hematomas appear on CT as round or oval fluid collections. Fractures and lacerations appear as irregular, linear areas of low density within an organ (Fig. 64). Subcapsular hematomas are lenticular or oval in configuration and flatten or indent the underlying parenchyma. Acute blood generally has a density lower than that of surrounding tissue on contrast-enhanced CT scans. The relatively higher attenuation value of a fresh hematoma will be more apparent on an unenhanced scan. Other CT findings reported with hepatic injuries include subcapsular or intraparenchymal gas due to acute tissue necrosis, and periportal areas of low attenuation (2,186). Periportal low-attenuation zones, presumably representing edema, have been noted in 65% of children with blunt abdominal trauma, and in 30% of patients they are the only CT abnormality (231).

Intra- or extraperitoneal fluid may be seen with fractures or lacerations extending to the surface of an organ. In fact, a localized fluid collection may be more readily appreciated than the underlying parenchymal injury and thus may be a radiologic clue to the diagnosis (241). A large intraperitoneal fluid collection suggests a more severe injury (Fig. 64). Fluid collections in the perirenal and pararenal spaces, interfascial spaces, and psoas space are indicative of injury to retroperitoneal organs (227).

In hollow organ injuries, such as those of the intestine, CT findings include bowel wall or mucosal fold thickening, free intra- or retroperitoneal air, peritoneal fluid, and small bowel obstruction due to an acute hematoma or a subsequent stricture (38,217). Lap-belt ecchymosis occurs in approximately 70% of children with bowel injuries and is a clinical clue to the diagnosis (245). Findings associated with rupture of the urinary bladder include

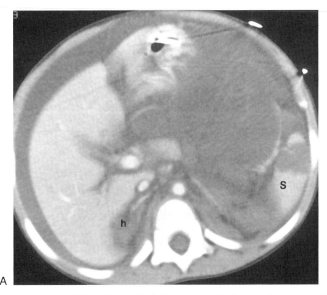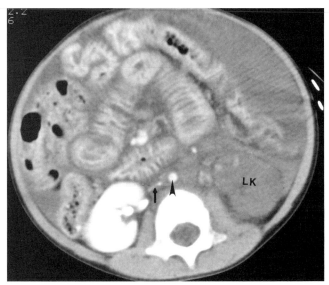

A B

FIG. 64. Splenic fracture with hypovolemic shock. **A:** CT scan through the upper abdomen shows a fragmented spleen (S), hematoma (h) in the posterior segment of the right lobe of the liver, and blood in the subphrenic and perihepatic spaces and gastrosplenic ligament. **B:** A more caudal CT scan reveals blood in the right and left paracolic gutters, dilated small bowel loops with intensely enhancing walls, a small aorta (*arrowhead*) and inferior vena cava (*arrow*), and a dense right nephrogram. Note also absent perfusion of the left kidney (LK) secondary to avulsion of the renal pedicle.

thickening of the bladder wall and leakage of contrast-enhanced urine into the peritoneal or extraperitoneal spaces (240).

Hypoperfusion associated with hypovolemic shock has a characteristic CT appearance, evidenced by diffusely dilated, fluid-filled small bowel loops; intense contrast enhancement of the kidneys, bowel wall, and mesentery; a flattened or collapsed inferior vena cava and a small aorta; and intraperitoneal fluid (243,254) (Fig. 64). It is critical that the radiologist recognize the CT appearance of hypoperfusion, as this is indicative of a severe injury and a poorer prognosis.

Comparative Imaging

In studies comparing CT, US, and scintigraphy for abdominal trauma in children, CT is the most sensitive examination, detecting >95% of traumatic lesions (141,255,256). Additionally, CT has been shown to be superior to the other examinations in defining the extent and severity of injury. An advantage of CT compared with US is that it can be used to assess organ function as well as anatomy. No transducer contact is necessary, and the ileus that is often associated with trauma is not a deterrent to CT. Scintigraphy, unlike CT and US, is organ-specific and therefore limited in the setting of trauma.

CT is employed as the initial imaging procedure for severely traumatized children whose vital signs are stable enough to permit the examination (141,255). Unstable

pediatric patients generally proceed directly to surgery without imaging examinations. Because most trauma patients are treated conservatively, CT also is invaluable for follow-up evaluation (13,37,267).

Diffuse Liver Diseases

Diagnoses of diffuse diseases of the liver can be made with either CT or MRI (222). Cirrhosis is the result of diffuse, irreversible hepatocyte damage and replacement by fibrosis, usually as a consequence of chronic hepatitis, bile stasis, metabolic disorders, congenital hepatic fibrosis, or toxins. Characteristic findings include a small right hepatic lobe and medial segment of the left lobe, enlargement of the caudate lobe and lateral segment of the left lobe, heterogeneous parenchyma, and nodular hepatic margins. Extrahepatic findings, indicative of portal hypertension, include splenomegaly, ascites and dilated collateral vessels in the porta hepatis, umbilical, and splenic regions (Fig. 65).

Attenuation values higher than normal can occur with hepatic iron overload, usually associated with repeated blood transfusions and occasionally with glycogen storage disease. As a result of the increased CT density, the hepatic vessels appear as low-density branching structures against the background of the hyperdense liver on unenhanced scans. Although CT can be used to evaluate iron overload, MRI is more sensitive for the diagnosis. On MRI, the paramagnetic effect of the ferric ions in the

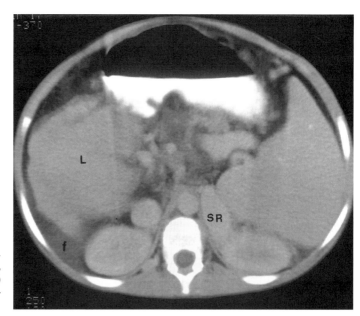

FIG. 65. Cirrhosis in a 10-year-old girl with biliary atresia. CT scan shows a small liver (L) with lobulated borders, ascitic fluid (f), splenomegaly, and a splenorenal (SR) collateral vessel. The density of the mesentery is increased due to edema.

stored iron leads to a low signal intensity on both T1- and T2-weighted images (Fig. 66).

Fatty change, often associated with fulminant liver diseases, severe malnutrition, cystic fibrosis, and chemotherapy, is clearly recognized on CT as diminished hepatic density. The decrease in hepatic attenuation may be focal or diffuse and directly corresponds to the amount of fat deposited in the liver. With diffuse fatty change, the portal veins appear as high-density structures against the background of the lower density hepatic parenchyma. MRI with fat suppression or opposed-phase imaging techniques can be used to corroborate CT findings.

Ultrasonography is the procedure of choice to screen for diffuse infiltrative diseases of the liver. The role of CT and MRI is to clarify equivocal sonographic findings. CT and MRI also are recommended to provide additional information about vascular anatomy in patients who are

scheduled to undergo liver transplantation (18,60). After liver transplantation, US, CT, or MRI can be used to evaluate biliary or vascular complications.

Biliary Tract Obstruction

Biliary tract obstruction in children usually is the result of ductal calculi or acute pancreatitis. A rare cause of ductal obstruction is rhabdomyosarcoma. The CT diagnosis is based on demonstration of dilated intra- or extrahepatic bile ducts of near-water attenuation. Associated findings include ductal calcifications, pancreatic enlargement, or a soft tissue mass in the porta hepatis.

In jaundiced patients, US is the preliminary imaging procedure to detect intrahepatic ductal dilatation associated with obstruction, as well as cystic diseases. This can

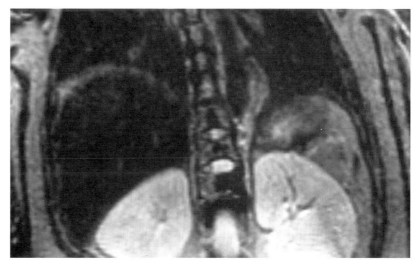

FIG. 66. Hepatic iron overload secondary to multiple transfusions for sickle cell anemia. T2-weighted coronal image (2800/90) demonstrates decreased hepatic signal intensity. The kidneys are enlarged because of sickle cell nephropathy. Also note the biconcave vertebral bodies and the absence of the spleen, which has atrophied following infarction.

be supplemented by radionuclide studies using hepatobiliary imaging agents. Although the ability of CT to document the presence of dilated bile ducts is well known, CT should be reserved for cases in which the level or cause of obstruction cannot be determined by these other radiologic methods (222). MRI can also detect biliary dilatation, but it usually offers no additional information over that provided by US or CT.

Renal Parenchymal Disease

Most renal calcifications in children are associated with obstruction and infection, and less frequently are due to metabolic disorders, cortical necrosis, glomerulonephritis, or adrenocorticotropic hormone (ACTH) therapy. In rare instances, CT may be of value in confirming lithiasis or nephrocalcinosis suspected on sonography.

Acute pyelonephritis can present as uniform enlargement of the kidney. Non-contrast-enhanced scans usually are normal, whereas contrast-enhanced CT scans may show single or multiple low-density areas, presumably related to inflammatory hypovascularity, vasoconstriction, or microabscesses. The term "acute focal bacterial nephritis" has been applied when one or more discrete mass–like areas of poor enhancement, representing inflammatory masses, are present (Fig. 67). More severe renal infection can produce an intrarenal abscess or extend into the perirenal space. A CT diagnosis of chronic pyelonephritis is based on recognition of a small kidney with cortical scars overlying clubbed calyces. Unilateral renal hypoplasia or renal artery stenosis, in contradistinction, is associated with a small, smooth kidney. MRI does not offer additional information over that provided by CT.

A voiding cystourethrogram (VCUG) and US are the initial imaging examinations in a child with an initial urinary tract infection. The VCUG is used to investigate the possibility of reflux. Ultrasonography is preferable to urography to determine if there is coexistent urinary tract dilatation predisposing to infection. CT may be a valuable ancillary examination in patients with acute pyelonephritis suspected of having perinephric extension or a complicating abscess because it provides a better topographic display of the kidney and its adjacent structures than does urography or US.

Pancreatic Disorders

Hereditary Diseases

Hereditary pancreatic diseases include cystic fibrosis (CF) and Shwachman–Diamond syndrome, which are autosomal recessive disorders, and von Hippel–Lindau disease and hereditary pancreatitis, which are autosomal dominant diseases (117). Involvement of the pancreas in cystic fibrosis takes the form of a fatty pancreas, parenchymal calcifications, or single or multiple large cysts, referred to as pancreatic cystosis (117,121) (Fig 68). Shwachman-Diamond syndrome (exocrine pancreatic insufficiency, neutropenia, metaphyseal dysostosis, and dwarfism) also is characterized by fatty replacement of the pancreas, causing a low attenuation value on CT and a high signal intensity on MRI (199). In von Hippel–Lindau disease, the pancreas contains multiple cysts. Findings in patients with hereditary pancreatitis include ductal dilatation, parenchymal and ductal calcifications, and pancreatic atrophy (117).

Pancreatitis

Acute pancreatitis in childhood is most often due to blunt abdominal trauma, but other causes include opera-

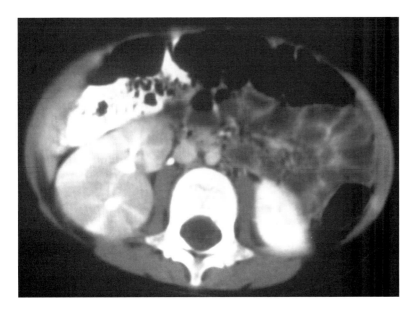

FIG. 67. Acute bacterial pyelonephritis, 3-year-old girl. Contrast-enhanced CT shows an enlarged right kidney with several areas of low density, representing more severe areas of bacterial nephritis. Urine cultures grew *Escherichia coli*.

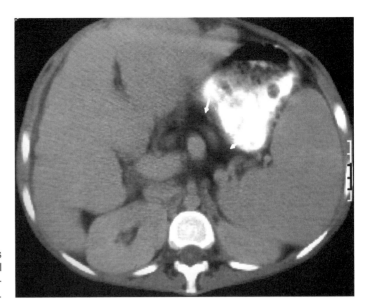

FIG. 68. Cystic fibrosis, 15-year-old boy. The pancreas (arrows) is completely replaced by fatty tissue. A small nodular liver and splenomegaly are complications of cirrhosis, which can be seen with advanced cystic fibrosis.

tive trauma, chemotherapy, cystic fibrosis, mumps, and congenital anomalies, such as pancreas divisum and duplication cyst. CT scans will be normal in approximately 50% of children with acute pancreatitis. The changes of pancreatitis in the remaining patients include diffuse glandular enlargement, contour irregularity, and intrapancreatic or extrapancreatic fluid collections (146). Extrapancreatic fluid in children is seen most often in the anterior pararenal space, followed by the lesser sac, lesser omentum, and transverse mesocolon (146) (Fig. 69). The fluid collections in acute pancreatitis are of water density and variable in size and shape, distending an already existing space in the retroperitoneal or intraperitoneal compartment. They are not considered to be pseudocysts. Pseudocysts have a thick fibrous capsule, are usually found in close proximity to the pancreas, and contain homogeneous fluid of near-water-attenuation value. They are more permanent in nature and unlikely to resolve spontaneously.

Chronic pancreatitis in childhood usually is due to hereditary pancreatitis, and less frequently to malnutrition, hyperparathyroidism, cystic fibrosis, idiopathic fibrosing pancreatitis, or pancreas divisum. CT manifestations of chronic pancreatitis include calcifications, focal or diffuse pancreatic enlargement or atrophy, pancreatic or biliary ductal dilatation, increased density of the peripancreatic fat, and thickening of the peripancreatic fascia.

In patients with good clinical evidence supporting the diagnosis of uncomplicated acute pancreatitis, neither US or CT is necessary. Diagnostic evaluation is reserved for patients suspected of having complications. Ultrasonography is preferred as the screening examination because it does not require ionizing radiation. In cases in which US is suboptimal because of bowel gas, commonly present in patients with acute pancreatitis, CT may be used to provide the needed information. CT is considered the

procedure of choice for displaying calcification in patients suspected of having hereditary pancreatitis. MRI does not contribute useful information in pancreatitis over that provided by CT.

Bowel Diseases

Several congenital and acquired anomalies can affect the bowel in childhood, but only the more common ones evaluated by CT or MRI will be discussed.

Congenital Anomalies

Anorectal malformations are characterized by varying degrees of atresia of the distal hindgut and the levator sling. Preoperative CT and MRI can provide information about the level of atresia and the thickness of the puborectalis muscle and external anal sphincter. Postoperatively, they can show the position of the neorectum in the levator ani sling (149,211,257) (Fig. 70). The neorectum needs to be positioned within both the puborectalis and external sphincter muscles if rectal continence is to be achieved. An additional congenital anomaly that can be diagnosed by CT or MRI is malrotation. CT and MRI findings include inversion of the superior mesenteric vessels, with the artery lying anterior to or to the right of the vein; positioning of the jejunum on the right and the colon on the left; and a whirl-like appearance of the small bowel mesentery.

Inflammation

Crohn disease is the most common inflammatory condition affecting the small bowel in children. CT has been

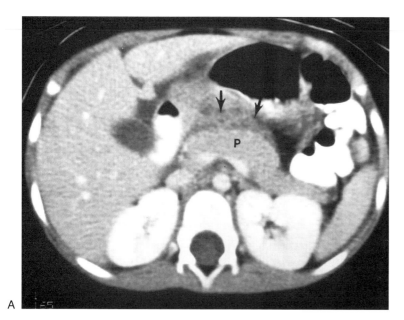

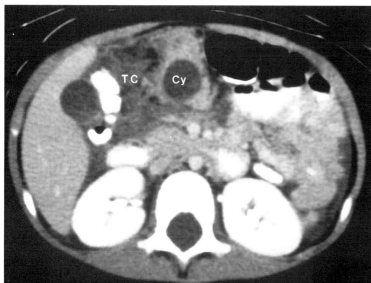

FIG. 69. Acute pancreatitis in a 3-year-old girl with a fistulous communication between the pancreatic duct and a duplication cyst. **A:** CT scan at the level of the pancreatic body and tail shows inflammatory changes in the lesser sac (*arrows*). The pancreas (P) itself appears normal. **B:** CT scan at a more caudal level demonstrates a low density mass, proven to be a duplication cyst (Cy) at surgery. Also noted is inflammation in the transverse mesocolon (TC).

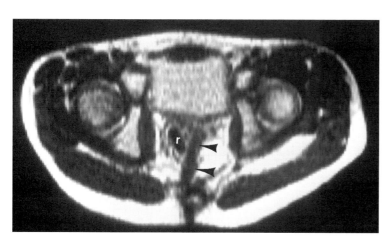

FIG. 70. Congenital anorectal anomaly. A 7-year-old girl with rectal incontinence after a pull-through operation for treatment of an imperforate anus. Transaxial T2-weighted MR image (2100/90) shows the neorectum (r) misplaced outside a hypoplastic puborectalis sling (*arrowheads*) located in the midline.

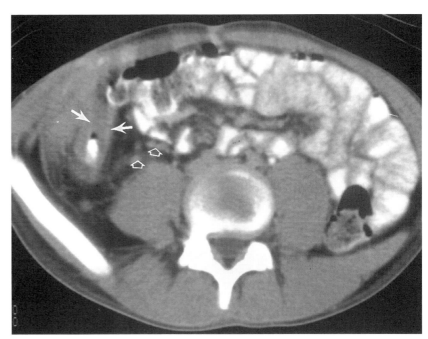

FIG. 71. Crohn disease. A 14-year-old boy with a palpable right lower quadrant mass. CT scan shows circumferential thickening of the wall of the distal ileum (*arrows*), multiple mesenteric nodes (*open arrows*), and an increased amount of mesenteric fat in the right lower quadrant. The inflammatory process extends into the right anterior abdominal wall.

shown to be useful to diagnose extraluminal extension or abscess (128,129). CT findings in the early stage of Crohn disease include circumferential bowel wall thickening, inflammation of the adjacent mesenteric fat, and enlarged regional lymph nodes (128,228) (Fig. 71). Increased amounts of mesenteric fat, segmental narrowed areas of bowel, and fistulas or sinus tracts may be seen in advanced disease. Abscesses appear as well-defined, low-attenuation masses with thick enhancing walls. Other inflammatory small bowel conditions that can be imaged by CT include *Yersinia* ileitis, tuberculosis, and histoplasmosis. The CT appearances of these diseases are similar to those of Crohn disease.

Inflammatory diseases of the colon and appendix also can be easily diagnosed by CT (21). In patients with ulcerative colitis, there is concentric colonic wall thickening, which usually is heterogeneous. The CT findings in granulomatous colitis are similar to those seen in the small bowel, except that the colonic wall tends to be thicker.

Acute appendicitis is manifested by a variety of abnormalities (8,97). In nonperforated appendicitis, the appendix is thickened and dilated, measuring between 8 and 12 mm in diameter. Wall thickness is increased and measures 2 to 4 mm. By comparison, in children without appendicitis, appendiceal diameter ranges between 3 and 8 mm and the appendiceal wall is barely perceptible (97). Other findings of appendicitis include an appendicolith and pericecal inflammation, appearing as streaky opacities in the adjacent fat (Fig. 72). An abscess, as expected, appears as a walled-off fluid collection (see Fig. 63). The sensitivities for diagnosing appendicitis appear to be similar for CT and US, but CT has proven valuable to differentiate between phlegmon and abscess and to aid in planning percutaneous aspiration or drainage.

Obstruction

The most frequent lesions producing obstruction are adhesions, hernias, and intussusception. In obstruction, bowel loops proximal to an obstructing lesion are dilated, and filled with fluid or contrast, compared to loops distal to the site of obstruction. The CT diagnosis of hernia is based on the demonstration of bowel or a combination of

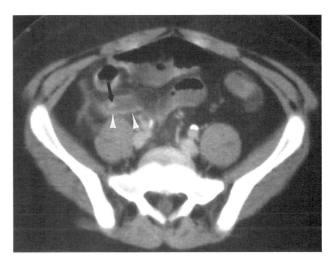

FIG. 72. Acute appendicitis, 7-year-old girl. CT scan demonstrates a dilated, fluid-filled appendix (*arrowheads*) with an enhancing wall and an appendicolith (*arrow*). There are mild inflammatory changes in the periappendiceal area.

bowel, mesenteric fat, and vessels within a hernia sac. The CT appearance of intussusception is that of a doughnut sign, with a collapsed segment of proximal bowel (the intussusceptum) and its surrounding layer of fat-filled mesentery lying within a segment of distal bowel (the intussuscipiens). Regardless of the cause, the bowel loops distal to the site of obstruction are collapsed, whereas those more proximal are dilated and filled with fluid, air, or contrast medium.

Vascular Structures

Aneurysms are rare in children and occur most frequently in association with Marfan syndrome, collagen vascular diseases, sepsis, or trauma. Thrombosis also is uncommon and usually is the result of severe illness associated with intense dehydration, tumor extension, or trauma. In addition, various developmental anomalies of the venous system can occur, and their recognition is important lest they be misinterpreted as pathology. CT or MRI can be used to diagnose congenital anomalies or acquired lesions of the abdominal vascular structures. Congenital vascular anomalies are frequently discovered unexpectedly in patients studied for other clinical concerns.

Ultrasonography is the preferred examination for confirming a suspected aneurysm or venous thrombosis because it can easily demonstrate the dimensions and the effective lumina of the aorta or vena cava and their branches in longitudinal and transverse sections. However, if the abdomen is obscured by bowel gas, CT or MRI can provide the necessary information.

PELVIS

The major indications for CT and MRI examination of the pediatric pelvis are the evaluation of a suspected or known pelvic mass and the determination of the presence or absence of a suspected abscess. In addition to facilitating evaluation of patients suspected of having masses or abscesses, CT and MRI can be useful in characterizing congenital uterine malformations, localizing nonpalpable testes, and evaluating the response of malignant tumors to therapy (24,221,224,226).

Pelvic Masses

Ovarian Masses

Nonneoplastic functional cysts, resulting from exaggerated development of follicular or corpus luteum cysts, are the most common ovarian masses in infant and adolescent girls. An ovarian cyst appears as a large (>3 cm), unilocular, thin-walled mass that has near-water-density contents.

On MRI, the cyst has a very low signal intensity on T1-weighted images and an extremely high signal intensity on T2-weighted images (65,173,224–226). Intracystic bleeding can increase the CT attenuation or the signal intensity on T1-weighted images. In some cases, layering of fluid and high-signal-intensity blood can be observed.

Mature teratomas or dermoid cysts account for two thirds of true pediatric ovarian neoplasms. Patients usually present at between 6 and 11 years with a palpable mass or with pain due to torsion or hemorrhage. The CT diagnosis of teratoma is based on identification of a cystic mass containing fat or a combination of fatty tissue, calcification, ossification, or teeth (39,218) (Fig. 73). Approximately two thirds of teratomas will display characteristic CT features, enabling a specific diagnosis. MRI findings vary depending on the tissue composition. On T1-weighted images, fat appears as an area of high signal intensity, whereas serous fluid and calcifications have low signal intensity. On T2-weighted images, fat and serous fluid show high-signal intensity, whereas calcifications, bone, and hair demonstrate low-signal intensity (224–226).

Malignant ovarian neoplasms are most commonly germ cell tumors (dysgerminoma, immature teratoma, endodermal sinus tumor, embryonal carcinoma, and choriocarcinoma) (60% to 90%) and less commonly stromal tumors

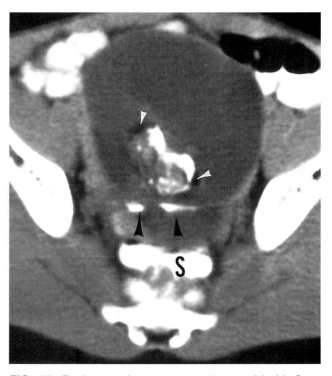

FIG. 73. Benign ovarian teratoma, 10-year-old girl. Contrast-enhanced CT scan shows a low-density teratoma, with an attenuation value close to that of water, lying anterior to the sigmoid (S) colon. The teratoma contains a mural nodule with calcification and fat (*white arrowheads*) and a calcified septum (*black arrowheads*).

(Sertoli-Leydig, granulosa theca) or epithelial carcinomas (33). On CT, malignant tumors are large (average diameter 15 cm), heterogeneous, soft tissue masses, containing low-attenuation areas of necrosis, calcifications, thick septations, or papillary projections (Fig. 74). Cul-de-sac fluid, ascites, peritoneal implants, lymphadenopathy, and hepatic metastases also may be noted. On MRI, malignant ovarian neoplasms appear as heterogeneous masses with intermediate signal intensity on T1-weighted images and intermediate or high signal intensity on T2-weighted images (30,173,224–226).

Other causes of an adnexal mass include ovarian torsion and tubo-ovarian abscess (10). The features of ovarian torsion are an enlarged ovary of soft tissue density on CT. The ovary has a low signal intensity on T1-weighted and very high signal intensity on T2-weighted MR images, reflecting vascular engorgement and edema (224). Abscesses have an appearance similar to abscesses in other parts of the body.

Vaginal/Uterine Masses

Hydrocolpos or hydrometrocolpos is the most common cause of vaginal or uterine enlargement. *Hydrocolpos* refers to dilatation of the vagina, usually by serous fluid or sometimes urine if there is a urogenital sinus; *hydrometrocolpos* refers to dilatation of both the uterus and the vagina. Both conditions are caused by vaginal obstruction, resulting from vaginal atresia or stenosis or an imperforate membrane. The clinical features vary with the patient's age. Affected neonates present with a pelvic or lower abdominal mass or associated anomalies, including imperforate anus, esophageal or duodenal atresia, and congenital heart disease. Adolescent girls present with a pelvic mass or pain. The dilated vagina in this age group often contains blood (e.g., hematocolpos) as a result of physiologic hormonal stimulation.

On CT, the dilated vagina and uterus appear as midline, near- water-density masses. The walls may enhance after administration of intravenous contrast medium. On MRI, they have a low signal intensity on T1-weighted images (Fig. 75) and a high signal intensity on T2-weighted images. The signal intensity is high on T1-weighted images if the contents are hemorrhagic (65,224–226,258). Intraabdominal extension and hydronephrosis due to ureteral compression can be seen in long-standing obstruction.

Rhabdomyosarcoma is the most common malignant uterine and vaginal tumor in childhood. On CT, rhabdomyosarcoma appears as a soft tissue mass with an attenuation value approximating that of muscle. Necrosis or calcification also can be present, along with variable enhancement after intravenous administration of contrast material. Metastases to pelvic lymph nodes can be seen if the involved nodes are enlarged. Rhabdomyosarcoma usually has a low signal intensity on T1-weighted and a high signal intensity on T2-weighted MR images. T1-weighted images are useful for depicting the primary

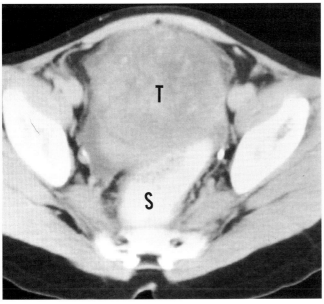
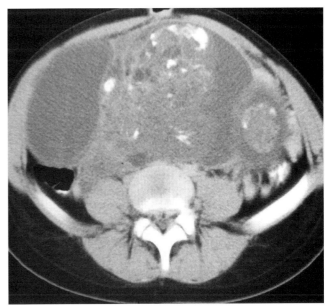

A   B

FIG. 74. Malignant ovarian tumors. **A:** Endodermal sinus tumor, 12-year-old girl. Contrast-enhanced CT shows a solid heterogeneously enhancing tumor (T) anterior to the sigmoid colon (S). The solid nature of this ovarian tumor suggests that it is malignant, but a specific histologic diagnosis cannot be provided based on the CT findings alone. **B:** Malignant teratoma, 13-year-old girl. CT scan shows a complex mass with a large soft tissue nodule containing calcification and fat. The predominance of soft tissue elements should suggest that this lesion is malignant rather than benign.

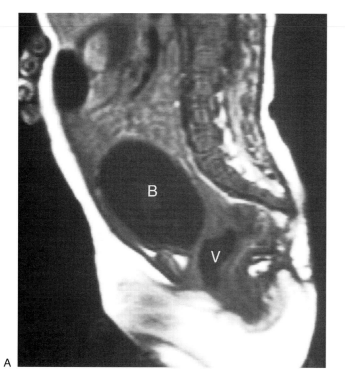

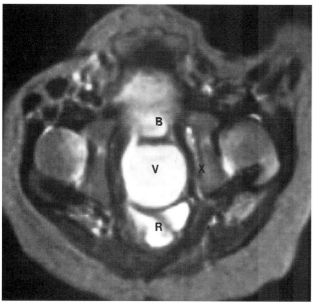

FIG. 75. Neonatal hydrocolpos due to vaginal stenosis. **A:** Sagittal T1-weighted (600/17) MR image shows an enlarged, low-signal-intensity vagina (V). B, bladder. **B:** On an axial T2-weighted (2000/90) the signal intensity of the fluid-filled vagina (V) increases and is equal to that of the urine-filled bladder (B). R, rectum. (Reproduced from Siegel MJ. MRI of the pediatric abdomen. *Magnet Reson Clin North Am* 1995;3:161–182.)

tumor, lymphadenopathy, and invasion of perivesical fat (91).

Bladder and Prostate Masses

Rhabdomyosarcoma accounts for most neoplasms of the bladder and prostate in children. It typically affects children under 10 years of age and usually metastasizes early, either by a lymphatic route to regional lymph nodes or by a hematogenous route to lung, bone, and liver. The CT and MRI features are similar to those of vaginal rhabdomyosarcoma (5,91) (Fig. 76).

Less common bladder neoplasms include hemangioma, neurofibroma, pheochromocytoma, leiomyoma, and transitional cell carcinoma. On CT and MRI, these appear as pedunculated or sessile soft tissue masses, projecting into the bladder lumen (192). Based on CT or MRI findings alone, it is usually impossible to differentiate a benign lesion from a malignant one. However, when there is extension into the perivesical fat or adjacent structures, malignancy should be suspected.

Presacral Masses

Sacrococcygeal teratoma, neuroblastoma, anterior meningocele, and lymphoma are the most frequent presacral masses. Sacrococcygeal teratomas are congenital tumors containing derivatives of all three germinal layers (1). Most teratomas are benign in patients under 2 months of age, but in children beyond the neonatal period they have a higher frequency of malignancy, nearing 90%. Affected children usually present with a large soft tissue mass in the sacrococcygeal or gluteal region and less often with constipation or pelvic pain. On CT, the diagnosis of sacrococcygeal teratoma can be confirmed by identification of a cystic mass containing fat, calcification, bone, or teeth. Usually there are no associated osseous anomalies (262). In general, predominantly fluid-filled teratomas are benign, whereas tumors containing predominantly solid components are more likely to be malignant (144). Fluid-filled, cystic sacrococcygeal teratomas have a low signal intensity on T1-weighted and a high signal intensity on T2-weighted MR images (Fig. 77). Fat appears as high-signal-intensity foci on T1-weighted images, and calcification, bone, or hair as foci of low signal intensity on both T1- and T2-weighted images (262).

Anterior meningoceles are herniations of spinal contents through a congenital defect in the vertebral body (anterior dysraphism) and are most common in the sacral region and at the lumbosacral junction. The mass is termed a myelomeningocele when the contents of the herniated sac contain neural elements in addition to meninges and cerebrospinal fluid, and a lipomeningocele when fat and cerebrospinal fluid are present. Meningoceles or myelomeningoceles are recognized on CT by

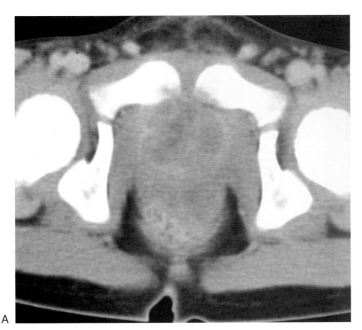

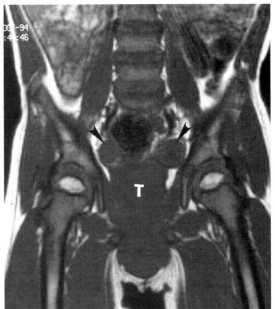

A

B

FIG. 76. Prostatic rhabdomyosarcoma in a 3-year-old boy with urinary retention. **A:** Contrast enhanced CT scan at the level of the pubic symphysis shows a large, heterogeneous soft tissue mass in the expected location of the prostate gland. **B:** Coronal T1-weighted MR image demonstrates extension of the tumor (T) into the lower pelvis as well as enlarged iliac lymph nodes (*arrowheads*). The tumor abuts the pelvic sidewalls.

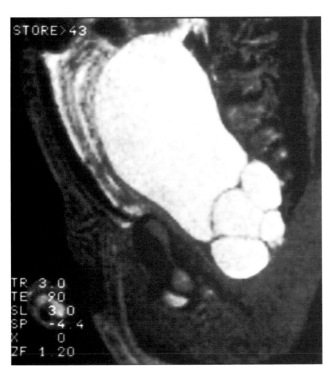

FIG. 77. Benign sacrococcygeal teratoma in a newborn with a palpable pelvic mass. Sagittal T2-weighted (3000/90) MR image shows a presacral mass, with a signal intensity much greater than that of fat. Also noted are internal septations. The sacrum was normal. (Case courtesy of L. Das Narla, M.D., Medical College of Virginia, Richmond, VA.)

their relatively low attenuation values (cerebrospinal fluid or fat), their position anterior to the sacrum, and the associated sacral defects. The soft tissue contents of the herniated sac, especially the presence of a tethered cord, and the communication between the meningocele and the thecal sac can be demonstrated best with MRI (Fig. 78).

Neuroblastoma and lymphoma arise less frequently in the pelvis than in the abdomen or chest. On CT, both appear as presacral soft tissue masses. Neuroblastoma and lymphomas have a signal intensity slightly higher than that of striated muscle on T1-weighted MR images. On T2-weighted images, the signal intensity is close to that of urine or fat (Fig. 79).

Comparative Imaging and Clinical Applications

When a pelvic mass is detected on physical examination or a conventional radiographic study, further characterization of the mass and determination of its etiology and extent are possible with US, CT, and MRI. Ultrasonography is employed initially for the evaluation of most suspected gynecologic masses because it does not use ionizing radiation. However, US is often suboptimal for evaluating the presacral space because of the gas-filled rectum and sigmoid colon. CT and MRI are not degraded by bowel gas and hence are useful for detecting a suspected mass in the presacral area. When a pelvic malignancy has been diagnosed clinically or suggested by US, CT or MRI is warranted to detect the extent of pelvic

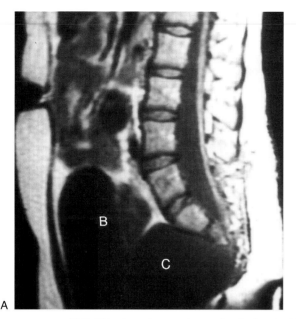

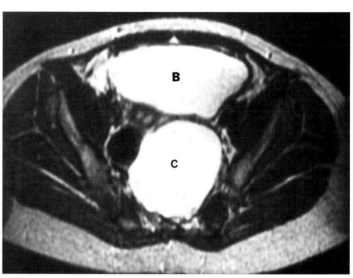

A   B

FIG. 78. Anterior meningocele. **A:** Sagittal T1-weighted MR image shows a low-signal-intensity cyst (C) between the bladder (B) and sacrum. The caudalmost sacral segments are absent. **B:** On an axial T2-weighted image, the signal intensity of the cystic meningocele (C), which is filled with cerebrospinal fluid, increases and is equal to that of the urine-filled bladder (B). (Reprinted from Siegel MJ. Magnetic resonance imaging of the pediatric pelvis. *Semin Ultrasound Comput Magnet Reson Imaging* 1991; 12:475–505).

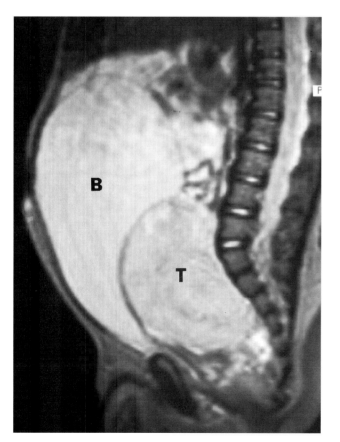

FIG. 79. Presacral neuroblastoma in a 2-year-old boy with constipation. Sagittal T2-weighted MR image (2250/90) shows a presacral soft tissue mass (M) with a signal intensity slightly lower than that of the urine within the bladder (B).

invasion prior to surgery, chemotherapy, or radiation therapy.

Congenital Uterine Malformations

Congenital uterine malformations usually are adequately diagnosed by ultrasonography, but when that study is equivocal, MRI can be more definitive. CT can detect and differentiate congenital anomalies, but it is not performed routinely because it utilizes ionizing radiation and has suboptimal soft tissue contrast compared with MRI.

Uterine Agenesis or Hypoplasia

Uterine malformation occurs in 0.1% to 0.5% of all women. Uterine agenesis or hypoplasia is best displayed on T2-weighted sagittal images. In addition to a small uterus, patients with uterine hypoplasia have poor zonal differentiation and reduced endometrial and myometrial widths.

Uterine Duplication

The spectrum of duplication anomalies includes uterus didelphys (two vaginas, two cervices, and two uterine corpora); uterus bicornuate, either bicollis uterus (single vagina, two cervices, and two uteri) or unicollis uterus (one vagina, one cervix, and two uteri); and uterus septus (single uterus, cervix and vagina with a septum dividing the uterus into two compartments). MRI is particularly

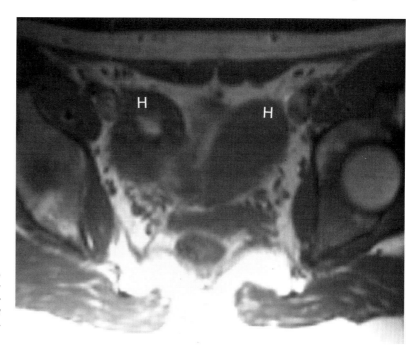

FIG. 80. Uterus didelphys, 18-year old girl. Axial T1-weighted MR image demonstrates duplicated uterine horns (H) with a widened intercornual distance. The high-signal-intensity focus within the right endometrial cavity represents blood.

valuable in differentiating uterus didelphys from a bicornuate or septate uterus. Hydrocolpos or hydrometrocolpos associated with congenital vaginal obstruction also can be evaluated (172,258) (see Fig. 75).

Uterus didelphys and bicornuate uterus have a bilobed shape with a concave fundal contour and myometrium separating the two endometrial cavities (Fig. 80). The appearance of septate uterus is that of a single uterine fundus with a convex fundal contour and a central septum dividing the endometrium into two cavities (Fig. 81).

Impalpable Testes

Identification of an undescended testis or cryptorchidism is important because of the increased risk of infertil-

ity if the testis remains undescended and because of the increased incidence of malignancy, particularly with an intraabdominal testis (96). Early surgery, either orchiopexy in younger patients or orchiectomy in patients past puberty, limits but does not eliminate these risks. Preoperative localization of a nonpalpable testis by CT or MRI is helpful in expediting surgical management and shortening the anesthesia time. The CT and MRI diagnosis of an undescended testis is based on detection of a soft tissue mass, often oval in shape, in the expected course of testicular descent (96) (Fig. 82). The more normal the testis is in size and shape, the lower is its attenuation value or signal intensity on T1-weighted MR images. A very atrophic testis appears as a small focus of soft tissue with a density or signal intensity similar to that of abdominal

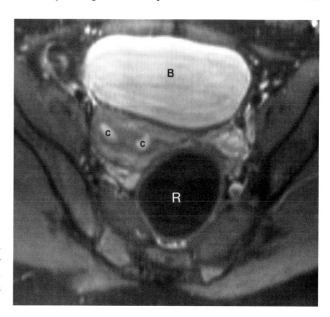

FIG. 81. Septate uterus, 15-year-old girl. T2-weighted MR image shows duplicated uterine cavities (c). The uterine contour is normal, unlike the widened intercornual distance in the bicornuate uterus. The rectum (R) is dilated due to rectal stenosis related to repair of imperforate anus. B, bladder.

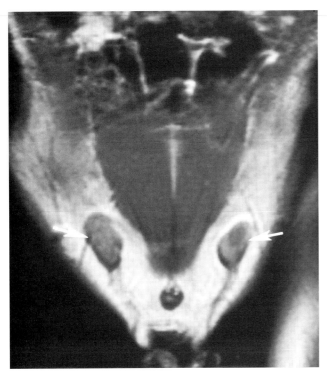

FIG. 82. Undescended testes, 7-year-old boy. Coronal T1-weighted MR image (600/17) demonstrates intermediate signal, ovoid structures (*arrows*) in the inguinal canals bilaterally, representing the undescended testes.

wall musculature. The diagnosis of an undescended testis is easier if the testis is in the inguinal canal or lower pelvis, where structures usually are symmetric. Differentiation of an undescended testis from adjacent structures, such as bowel loops, vessels, and lymph nodes, is more of a problem in the upper pelvis and lower abdomen. In spite of these problems, the accuracy of CT or MRI for localization of nonpalpable testes exceeds 90% (101).

Ultrasonography can detect an impalpable undescended testis when it is in a high scrotal or intracanalicular position, which occurs in about 90% of cases. Because it does not involve ionizing radiation, US is recommended as the initial imaging examination of choice for localizing impalpable testes. However, usually ultrasonography is not reliable for identifying undescended testes located higher in the pelvis or in the abdomen. Therefore, if sonographic findings are equivocal or negative and preoperative localization of the testis is desired, either CT or MRI can be performed, although MRI is preferred because it does not use ionizing radiation.

MUSCULOSKELETAL SYSTEM

Skeletal abnormalities are nearly always first identified by conventional radiography. Scintigraphy is helpful in confirming the presence of a skeletal lesion if the initial radiograph is nonconfirmatory and in determining the

presence of metastatic disease. CT and MRI are used as complementary studies to conventional radiographs and scintigraphy when further definition of an abnormality is needed (212).

Spiral CT is preferred over incremental CT in the evaluation of the skeletal system because of its faster scan times, which help to decrease motion artifact, and its high-quality 2-D and 3-D reconstructions. The frequent indications for spiral CT of the skeleton in children include (a) characterization of congenital abnormalities in areas of complex anatomy, (b) assessment of the extent of complex fractures, and (c) determination of the origin and extent of nidus in osteoid osteoma (233). Depending on the lesion size, spiral CT is performed with 2- to 4-mm collimation and 2- to 4-mm/sec table speed through the area of abnormality. Wider collimation, table speed, and reconstruction intervals are suitable for assessing large joints and lesions, whereas narrower collimation, table speed, and reconstruction intervals are necessary for evaluating small skeletal lesions and regions of the body (e.g., ankle joint, foot, and wrist).

Indications for MRI are more diverse than those for CT and include (a) evaluation of the extent of skeletal and soft tissue neoplasms (3,16,22,31,88,104,134,151, 177,188,189); (b) determination of the extent of infection (12,55,108,166); (c) evaluation of sequela of skeletal trauma (213); (d) assessment of intraarticular derangement (213); (e) definition of anatomy in selected congenital anomalies; (f) assessment of possible bone infarction and osteonecrosis (40,74,133); (g) evaluation of unexplained pain in patients with normal conventional imaging studies (187); and (h) assessment of the response of malignant lesions to treatment (87,90).

Bone Marrow

The appearance of the normal bone marrow varies with the age of the patient (58,176,177,178,236,259,268). At birth, hematopoietic or red marrow predominates. Shortly thereafter, there is conversion of red to yellow marrow. In the shafts of the long bones, this conversion begins in the diaphysis and progresses proximally and distally to the physeal plate. By late adolescence, the appendicular skeleton contains predominantly yellow marrow. Epiphyseal conversion occurs within a few months of the appearance of the ossification center (135). Red marrow has a low signal intensity on T1-weighted MR images and a high signal intensity on T2-weighted images, whereas yellow marrow appears as high signal intensity on both T1- and T2-weighted sequences.

Infiltrative disorders, including tumor, infection and edema alter marrow characteristics on MRI, producing low to intermediate signal intensity on T1-weighted images and high signal intensity on T2-weighted images (177,178,208,236). Abnormalities are easier to identify in bones with predominantly yellow marrow. In bones with a predominance of red marrow, such as those in infants and young children and patients with red cell hyperplasia, differentiation between low signal tumor and red marrow can be difficult. In these individuals, the use of fat suppression techniques can enhance lesion conspicuity. Because the MRI appearance is not specific, a final diagnosis depends on correlation with the patient's history and other clinical information and possibly tissue sampling.

Osseous Neoplasms

Ninety percent of malignant skeletal tumors are osteosarcoma or Ewing sarcoma. Most tumors display a low signal intensity on T1-weighted MR images, high signal intensity greater than that of fat on T2-weighted images (Fig. 83), and variable enhancement on gadolinium-enhanced T1-weighted images depending on the extent of necrosis. Low signal intensity on T2-weighted images suggests sclerosis, partially ossified matrix, tumor hypocellularity or large amounts of collagen, whereas marked hyperintensity suggests highly cellular tumors with a high water content. Fluid–fluid levels due to layering of new and old hemorrhage can be found in telangiectatic osteosarcomas, although they are not specific and also occur in aneurysmal bone cysts, fibrous dysplasia, and giant cell tumors.

Plain skeletal radiography remains the initial technique for the diagnosis of malignant skeletal tumors, but CT and MRI are helpful to further characterize a lesion and to determine its full extent. The soft tissue contrast of MRI makes it superior to CT for detecting bone marrow disease, soft tissue or intraarticular extension and neurovascular encasement, and for monitoring response to treatment (22,87,90). Neurovascular involvement is best

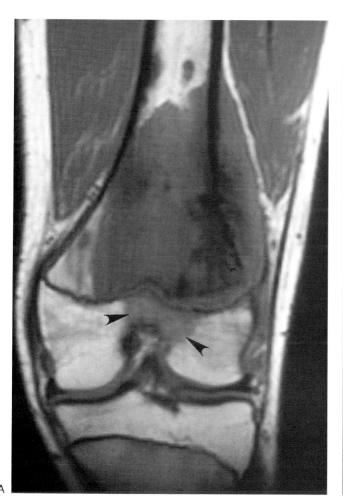
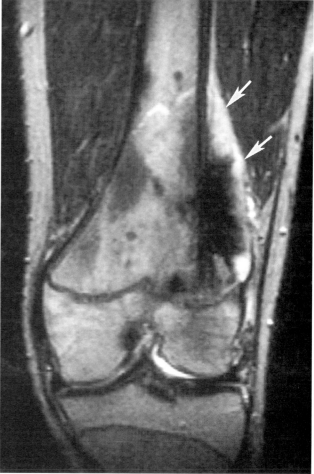

A

B

FIG. 83. Intramedullary osteosarcoma, 13-year-old girl. **A:** Coronal T1-weighted MR image (500/15) shows a low-intensity tumor in the medullary cavity of the distal right femur. The tumor extends into the epiphysis (*arrowheads*) and soft tissues laterally. **B:** Coronal T2-weighted MR image (2300/80) shows increased signal intensity in most of the intramedullary portion of the tumor. Areas of low-signal-intensity corresponded to areas of sclerosis and reactive new bone formation on the plain radiographs. The soft tissue component of the tumor (*arrows*) has a higher signal intensity than the intramedullary component of the tumor.

assessed by sequences that are tailored to blood flow, such as gradient echo images. Slow or absent flow, encasement, and displacement are features suggesting tumor involvement of the neurovascular bundles. MRI and CT are comparable in detecting extensive cortical bone destruction, but CT is more sensitive for diagnosing subtle cortical erosion.

In general, CT and MRI are not needed in the evaluation of most benign osseous neoplasms of the skeleton. However, these examinations can be of value in determining the extent of a lesion or its spatial relationships for preoperative planning (88). Benign osseous lesions usually have well-defined margins on CT and MRI examinations. The attenuation value and signal intensity of the matrix is generally nonspecific, so that correlation with radiographs or tissue sampling is needed for a final diagnosis. Another indication for CT scanning is determination of the precise location of the nidus in osteoid osteomas prior to surgical resection (Fig. 84).

Soft Tissue Neoplasms

The common benign soft tissue masses in childhood are hematoma, abscess, cystic hygroma, hemangioma, and lipoma; the most common malignant mass is rhabdomyosarcoma. Sonography is the initial examination of choice for the study of most soft tissue masses to determine whether they are cystic or solid. MRI, however, has become the examination of choice in large lesions to define

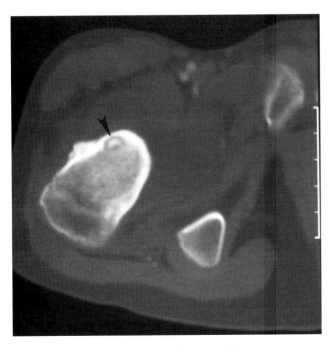

FIG. 84. Osteoid osteoma in a 11-year-old boy. Axial image shows a lytic nidus (*arrowhead*) with faint calcification in the lateral cortex of the proximal right femur. The cortex around the nidus is thickened.

the extent of the mass and its local relationships (3,16,188,189). Small size, well-defined margins with a capsule, homogeneous matrix on T2-weighted MR images, and absence of edema suggest a benign lesion (180). Poorly defined margins and a heterogeneous matrix on T2-weighted images favor an aggressive process. Bone erosion and infiltration of the neurovascular bundles are confirmatory evidence of malignancy. Unfortunately, some acute hematomas, abscesses, and benign neoplasms can have an aggressive appearance, whereas some malignant neoplasms can have a benign appearance (151).

Certain soft tissue lesions have specific MR characteristics (151). Lipomas appear as well-defined masses with a signal intensity equal to that of subcutaneous fat on T1- and T2-weighted images. Intramuscular hemangiomas have an intermediate signal intensity on T1-weighted images and a high intensity on T2-weighted images. The presence of feeding vessels and linear low-signal areas within the mass, reflecting fibrous tissue, support the diagnosis (Fig. 85). Cystic hygromas are complex masses with septations and fluid–fluid levels. Their signal intensity is lower than that of muscle on T1-weighted images and greater than that of fat on T2-weighted and STIR images (see Fig. 15).

Infection

Cross-sectional imaging is useful in children in whom complications of osteomyelitis are suspected or drainage is considered. Both CT and MRI can be used to evaluate osteomyelitis, but MRI is especially well suited for the detection of marrow abnormality and extension into the periosteum and soft tissues (55). Cortical destruction and sequestra are more reliably diagnosed with CT scanning (118).

Bone and Joint Trauma

Traditional radiographs remain the initial examination of choice in the evaluation of acute trauma. When radiographs are not confirmatory, scintigraphy, CT, or MRI can be used to establish the presence and extent of a fracture (Fig. 86), and in particular growth plate injuries, which if unrecognized lead to growth disturbance (80,131,132). CT, with two- or three-dimensional imaging, is especially useful in the evaluation of the axial skeleton and pelvis, which are difficult to evaluate with plain radiographs because of superimposition of osseous parts (164,165).

After the injury has healed, MRI is the preferred study to define the size and location of a posttraumatic bony bridge and the severity of the associated growth deformity (61,113) (Fig. 87). CT is useful in the diagnosis of posttraumatic osteochondral loose bodies.

MRI is the examination of choice for detecting menis-

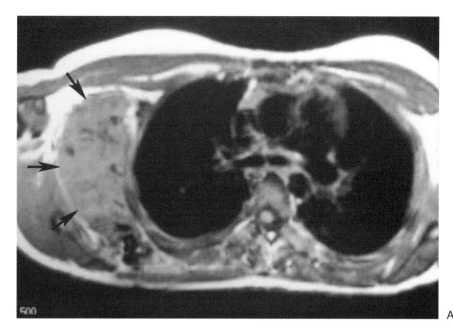

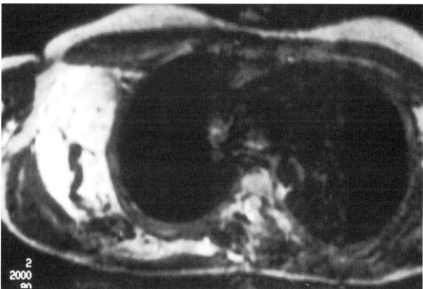

FIG. 85. Chest wall hemangioma, 13-year-old girl. **A:** Transaxial T1-weighted MR image (500/15) shows a soft tissue tumor (*arrows*) with a signal intensity slightly greater than that of muscle in the lateral chest wall. **B:** The tumor is much more intense than muscle on the T2-weighted image (2300/180). Also noted are a large, tortuous vessel and several smaller vascular channels with flow void within the tumor.

A

B

cal and ligamentous tears (269). Tears appear as alterations in morphology and signal intensity within the substance of the meniscus or ligament. MRI has also been shown to be an effective method for evaluating bone marrow edema associated with ligamentous and cartilaginous injuries.

Joint Disorders

The most common arthropathies in childhood are juvenile rheumatoid arthritis (JRA), hemophilia, and pigmented villonodular synovitis (PVNS). MRI is used to demonstrate the extent of cartilaginous and synovial involvement in children in whom surgery is planned. MRI findings of early JRA and hemophilia include thickened synovium which has a low signal on T1-weighted images and mixed intensity on T2-weighted images, reflecting the presence of inflammation and hemosiderin deposition. Late changes include cartilage loss and bony erosions. Gadolinium-enhanced MRI is superior to unenhanced MRI to show cartilage loss, joint effusion, and synovial thickening (123). PVNS appears as an intraarticular mass containing areas of decreased signal intensity on all sequences, corresponding to hemosiderin deposition.

Congenital Anomalies

Developmental hip dysplasia and tarsal coalition are congenital anomalies that are well suited for spiral CT. Plain radiographs can diagnose these conditions, but CT

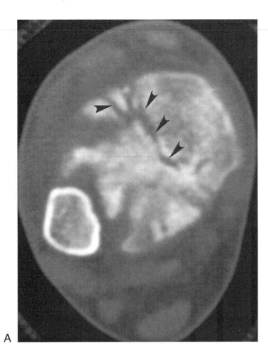

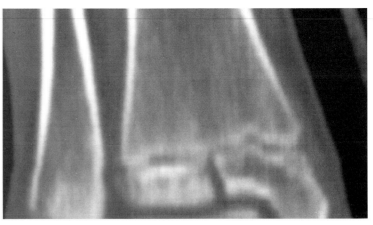

FIG. 86. Epiphyseal fracture in a 11-year-old girl. **A:** Axial CT image of the distal right tibial epiphysis shows a complex linear fracture (*arrowheads*). The relationship of the fracture line to the physis is difficult to appreciate on axial sections. **B:** Coronal multiplanar image (2-mm collimation, 2-mm reconstruction) shows extension of the fracture to the physis and distraction of the fragments, requiring open fixation.

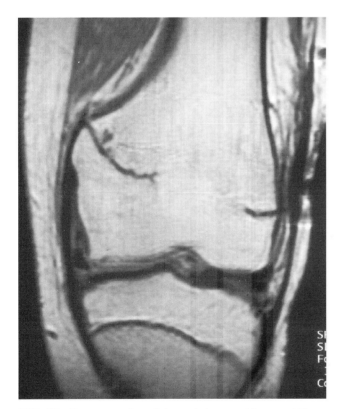

FIG. 87. Posttraumatic epiphyseal closure, 14-year-old boy. Coronal T1-weighted MR image of the left knee obtained 15 months after a condylar fracture shows fusion of the central portion of the physeal plate.

is useful to show the precise relationship between the bony acetabulum and the femoral head or neck (152) (Fig. 88). Three-dimensional reconstructions are particularly useful for assessing acetabular coverage and deformity of the femoral head. In selected cases, MRI can provide information about coverage of the cartilaginous portion of the femoral head (138).

Tarsal coalition is a cause of rigid flatfoot and peroneal spasm in children. Nearly 70% of tarsal coalitions are talocalcaneal and 30% are calcaneonavicular. For talocalcaneal coalitions, scans should be obtained perpendicular to the foot, whereas for calcaneonavicular coalition, scans should parallel the long axis of the foot (154) (Fig. 89). Multiplanar reconstructions can provide an additional display of coalition, but are not essential for diagnosis. Less frequent indications for CT include measurement of the amount of femoral anteversion or tibial torsion (120,265).

Bone Infarction

Bone infarction can involve the subarticular or the metadiaphyseal marrow of long bones. The more common causes in children include sickle cell disease, steroid therapy, and Legg–Calvé–Perthes disease. MRI has become the primary imaging examination for diagnosis of infarction (74,133). Acute avascular necrosis of the femoral head usually exhibits a low signal intensity on T1-weighted images and high signal intensity on T2-weighted images. Varying patterns of devascularization (homogeneous, heterogeneous, and ring) have been described. The

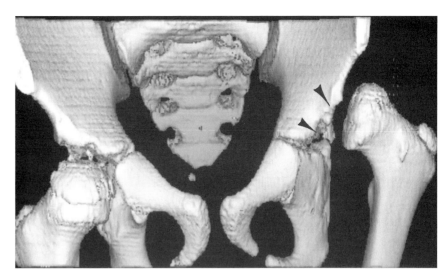

FIG. 88. Developmental dysplasia of the hip, 8-year-old boy. CT scan with three-dimensional reconstruction demonstrates lateral and superior dislocation of the proximal left femur. The femoral head is deformed and the acetabulum (*arrowheads*) is shallow.

sensitivity of MRI for the detection of femoral head ischemic necrosis is approximately 90% (133).

Osteochondritis dissecans is a subarticular osteonecrosis that often involves the femoral condyles, particularly the medial condyle. The necrotic fragment of bone has a heterogeneous low signal intensity on both

T1- and T2-weighted MR sequences and may or may not have intact overlying cartilage. A high-signal-intensity interface on T2-weighted images between the bone fragment and native bone suggests a loose fragment. Knowledge of the stability of the osteochondral fragment is important because a loose fragment may need to be re-

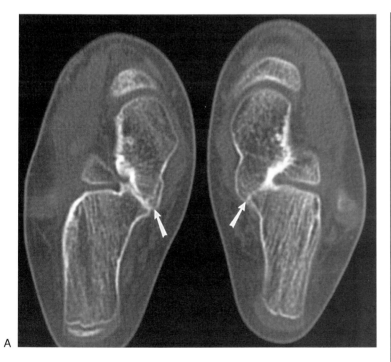

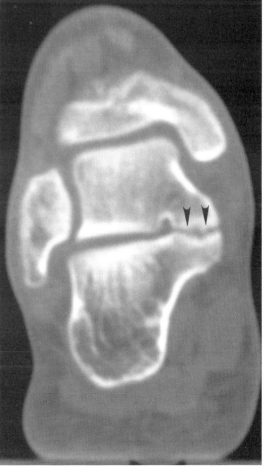

FIG. 89. Tarsal coalition. **A:** CT scan in a 9-year-old boy through the long-axis of the hindfeet shows bilateral calcaneonavicular coalitions (*arrows*). **B:** Short-axis CT scan in a 12-year-old boy shows narrowing and irregularity of the cortical surface of the talocalcaneal joint (*arrowheads*), indicating fibrous coalition.

moved, whereas an attached fragment can be treated conservatively.

Acute medullary bone infarction is seen as a region of low signal intensity on T1-weighted images and high signal intensity on T2-weighted images. A chronic infarct may appear as a central area of high signal intensity, representing fatty marrow, with a surrounding hypointense rim, corresponding to reactive bone.

REFERENCES

1. Ablin A, Issacs H Jr. Germ cell tumors. In: Pizzo PA, Poplack DG, eds. *Principles and Practice of Pediatric Oncology.* Philadelphia: JB Lippincott, 1989;713–731.
2. Abramson SJ, Berdon WE, Kaufman RA, Ruzal-Shapiro C. Hepatic parenchymal and subcapsular gas after hepatic laceration caused by blunt abdominal trauma. *AJR* 1989;153:1031–1032.
3. Aisen AM, Martel W, Braunstein EM, McMillin KI, Phillips WA, Kling TF. MRI and CT evaluation of primary bone and soft-tissue tumors. *AJR* 1986;146:749–756.
4. Amendola MA, Blane CE, Amendola BE, Glazer GM. CT findings in hepatoblastoma. *J Comput Assist Tomogr* 1984;8:1105–1109.
5. Argons GA, Wagner BJ, Lonergan GJ, Dickey GE, Kaufman MS. Genitourinary rhabdomyosarcoma in children: radiologic-pathologic correlation. *RadioGraphics* 1997;17:919–937.
6. Argons GA, Kingsman KD, Wagner BJ, Sotelo-Avila C. Rhabdoid tumor of the kidney in children: a comparison of 21 cases. *AJR* 1997;168:447–451.
7. Argons GA, Wagner BJ, Davidson AJ, Suarez ES. Multilocular cystic renal tumor in children: radiologic-pathologic correlation. *RadioGraphics* 1995;15:654–669.
8. Balthazar EJ, Megibow AJ, Siegel SE, Birnbaum BA. Appendicitis: prospective evaluation with high-resolution CT. *Radiology* 1991;180:21–24.
9. Beckwith JB, Kiviat NB, Bonadio JF. Nephrogenic rests, nephroblastomatosis, and the pathogenesis of Wilms tumor. *Pediatr Pathol* 1990;10:1–36.
10. Bellah RD, Griscom NT. Torsion of normal uterine adnexa before menarche: CT appearance. *AJR* 1989;152:123–124.
11. Belt TG, Cohen MD, Smith JA, et al. MRI of Wilms tumor: Promise as the primary imaging method. *AJR* 1986;146:955–961.
12. Beltran J, Noto AM, McGhee RB, et al. Infections of the musculoskeletal system: high-field strength MR imaging. *Radiology* 988;168:151–156.
13. Benya EC, Bulas DI, Eichelberger MR, Sivit CJ. Splenic injury from blunt abdominal trauma in children: follow-up evaluation with CT. *Radiology* 1995;195:685–688.
14. Bisset GS III. Magnetic resonance imaging of the pediatric thorax. *Semin Ultrasound Comput Tomogr Magnet Reson Imaging* 1991;12:429–447
15. Bisset GS III. Magnetic resonance imaging of congenital heart disease. *Radiol Clin North Am* 1991;29:279–291
16. Bisset GS III. MR imaging of soft tissue masses in children. *Magnet Reson Clin North Am* 1996;4: 697–719.
17. Bisset GS, Ball WS. Preparation, sedation and monitoring of the pediatric patient in the magnetic resonance suite. *Semin Ultrasound Comput Tomogr Magnet Reson Imaging* 1991;12:376–378.
18. Bisset GS III, Strife JL, Balistreri WF. Evaluation of children for liver transplantation: value of MR imaging and sonography. *AJR* 1990;155:351–356
19. Bisset GS III, Strife JL, Kirks DR, Bailey WW. Vascular rings: MR imaging. *AJR* 1987;149:251–256
20. Bitter JJ, Harrison DA, Kaplan J, Irwin GA. Mesoblastic nephroma. *J Comput Assist Tomogr* 1982;6:180–183.
21. Blickman JG, Boland GWL, Cleveland RH, Bramson RT, Lee MJ. Pseudomembranous colitis: CT findings in children. *Pediatr Radiol* 1995;25:S157–159.
22. Bloem JL, Taminiau AH, Eulderink F, Hermans J, Pauwels EK. Radiologic staging of primary bone sarcoma: MR imaging, scintig-

23. raphy, angiography, and CT correlated with pathologic examination. *Radiology* 1988;169:805–810.
23. Boechat MI. Adrenal glands, pancreas and retroperitoneal structures. In: Siegel MJ, ed. *Pediatric body CT.* New York: Churchill Livingstone, 1988;177–217.
24. Boechat MI. MR imaging of the pediatric pelvis. *Magnet Reson Clin North Am* 1996;4:679–696.
25. Boechat MI, Hooshang K, Ortega J, et al. Primary liver tumors in children: Comparison of CT and MR imaging. *Radiology* 1988; 169:727–732.
26. Boechat MI, Kangarloo H. MR imaging of the abdomen in children. *AJR* 1989;152:1245–1250.
27. Boechat MI, Ortega J, Hoffman AD, Cleveland RH, Kangarloo H, Gilsanz V. Computed tomography in stage III neuroblastoma. *AJR* 1985;145:1283–1287.
28. Borrello JA, Mirowitz SA, Siegel MJ. Neuroblastoma. In: Siegel BA, Proto AV, eds. *Pediatric Disease (Fourth Series) Test and Syllabus.* Reston, VA: American College of Radiology, 1993;640–665.
29. Bousvaros A, Kirks DR, Grossman H. Imaging of neuroblastoma: an overview. *Pediatr Radiol* 1986;16:89–106.
30. Bove KE, McAdams AJ. The nephroblastomatosis complex and its relationship to Wilms tumor: a clinicopathologic treatise. *Persp Pediatr Pathol* 1976;3:185–223.
31. Boyko OB, Cory DA, Cohen MD, Provisor A, Mirkin D, DeRosa GP. MR imaging of osteogenic and Ewing's sarcoma. *AJR* 1987; 148: 317–322.
32. Brammer HM, Buck JL, Hayes WS, Sheth S, Tavassoli FA. Malignant germ cell tumors of the ovary: radiologic-pathologic correlation. *RadioGraphics* 1990;10:715–724.
33. Breen JL, Bonamo JF, Maxson WS. Genital tract tumors in children. *Pediatr Clin North Am* 1981;28:355–367
34. Brill PW, Jagannath A, Winchester P, et al. Adrenal hemorrhage and renal vein thrombosis in the newborn: MR imaging. *Radiology* 1989;170:95–98.
35. Brody AS, Kuhn JP, Seidel FG, Brodsky LS. Airway evaluation in children with use of ultrafast CT: pitfalls and recommendations. *Radiology* 1991;178:181–184.
36. Brown LR, Muhm JR, Aughenbaugh GL, Lewis BD, Hurt RD. Computed tomography of benign mature teratomas of the mediastinum. *J Thorac Imaging* 1987;2:66–71.
37. Bulas DI, Eichelberger MR, Sivit CJ, Wright CJ, Gotschall CS. Hepatic injury from blunt trauma in children: follow-up evaluation with CT. *AJR* 1993;160:347–351.
38. Bulas DI, Taylor GA, Eichelberger MR. The value of CT in detecting bowel perforation in children after blunt abdominal trauma. *AJR* 1989;153:561–564.
39. Buy JN, Ghossain MA, Moss AA, et al. Cystic teratoma of the ovary: CT detection. *Radiology* 1989;171:697–701.
40. Caron KH, Bisset GS III. Magnetic resonance imaging of pediatric atraumatic musculoskeletal lesions. *Top Magnet Reson Imaging* 1990;3:43–60.
41. Caron KH. Magnetic resonance imaging of the pediatric abdomen. *Semin Ultrasound Comput Tomogr Magnet Reson Imaging* 1991; 12:448–474.
42. Castellino RA. Hodgkin disease: practical concepts for the diagnostic radiologist. *Radiology* 1986;159:305–310.
43. Castellino RA, Blank N, Hoppe RT, et al. Hodgkin disease: contributions of chest CT in the initial staging evaluation. *Radiology* 1986;160:603–605.
44. Chan HSL, Daneman A, Gribbin M, Martin DJ. Renal cell carcinoma in the first two decades of life. *Pediatr Radiol* 1983;13: 324–328.
45. Choyke PL, Zeman RK, Gootenberg JE, Greenberg JN, Hoffer F, Frank JA. Thymic atrophy and regrowth in response to chemotherapy: CT evaluation. *AJR* 1987;149:269–272.
46. Chung CJ, Lorenzo R, Rayder S, et al. Rhabdoid tumors of the kidney in children: CT findings. *AJR* 1995;164:6976–700.
47. Cohen AM, Solomon EH, Alfidi RJ. Computed tomography in bronchial atresia. *AJR* 1980;135: 1097–1099.
48. Cohen MD. Kidneys. In: Siegel MJ, ed. *Pediatric body CT.* New York: Churchill Livingstone, 1988;135–175.
49. Cohen MD. Commentary: imaging and staging of Wilms' tumors: problems and controversies. *Pediatr Radiol* 1996;26:307–311.

50. Cory DA, Cohen MD, Smith JA. Thymus in the superior mediastinum simulating adenopathy: appearance on CT. *Radiology* 1987; 162:457–459.

51. Dachman AH, Pakter RL, Ros PR, Fishman EK, Goodman ZD, Lichtenstein JE. Hepatoblastoma: radiologic-pathologic correlation in 50 cases. *Radiology* 1987;164:15–19.

52. Dachman AH, Lichtenstein JE, Friedman AC, Hartman DS. Infantile hemangioendothelioma of the liver: a radiologic-pathologic-clinical correlation. *AJR* 1983;140:1091–1096.

53. Daneman A. Adrenal neoplasms in children. *Semin Roentgenol* 1988;23:205–215.

54. Daneman A, Chan HSL, Martin J. Adrenal carcinoma and adenoma in children: a review of 17 patients. *Pediatr Radiol* 1983; 13:11–18.

55. Dangman BC, Hoffer FA, Rand FF, O'Rourke EJ. Osteomyelitis in children: gadolinium-enhanced MR imaging. *Radiology* 1992; 182:743–748.

56. Davidson AJ, Choyke PL, Hartman DS, Davis CJ. Renal medullary carcinoma associated wtih sickle cell trait: radiologic findings. *Radiology* 1995;195:83–85.

57. Davidson AJ, Hartman DS, Goldman SM. Mature teratoma of the retroperitoneum: radiologic, pathologic, and clinical correlation. *Radiology* 1989;172:421–425.

58. Dawson KL, Moore SG, Rowland JM. Age-related marrow changes in the pelvis: MR and anatomic findings. *Radiology* 1992; 183:47–51.

59. Day DL, Johnson RT, Odrezin GT, Woods WG, Alford BA. Renal atrophy or infarction in children with neuroblastoma. *Radiology* 1991;180:493–495.

60. Day DL, Letourneau JG, Allan GT, Ascher NL, Lund G. MR evaluation of the portal vein in pediatric liver transplant candidates. *AJR* 1986;147:1027–1030.

61. DeCampo JF, Boldt DW. Computed tomography of partial growth plate arrest: initial experience. *Skeletal Radiol* 1986;15:526–529.

62. DeGeer G, Webb WR, Gamsu G. Normal thymus. Assessment with MR and CT. Radiology 1986;158:313–317.

63. Dehner LP, Ishak KG. Vascular tumors of the liver in infants and children. A study of 30 cases and review of the literature. *Arch Pathol* 1971;92:101–111.

64. Dietrich RB, Kangarloo H. Kidneys in infants and children: Evaluation with MR. *Radiology* 1986;159:215–221.

65. Dietrich RB, Kangarloo H. Pelvic abnormalities in children: assessment with MR imaging. *Radiology* 1987;163:367–372.

66. Dietrich RB, Kangarloo H. Retroperitoneal mass with intradural extension: Value of magnetic resonance imaging in neuroblastoma. *AJR* 1986;146:251–254.

67. Dietrich RB, Kangarloo H, Lenarsky C, Feig SA. Neuroblastoma: the role of MR imaging. *AJR* 1987;148:937–942.

68. Dobranowski J, Martin LFW, Bennett WF. CT evaluation of posterior mediastinal teratoma. *J Comput Assist Tomogr* 1987;11:156–157.

69. Donaldson JS, Gilsanz V. CT findings in rectal cuff abscess following surgery for Hirschsprung disease. *J Comput Assist Tomogr* 1986;10:151–153.

70. Donaldson JS, Siegel MJ. Lungs, pleura, and chest wall. In: Siegel MJ, ed. *Pediatric body CT*. New York: Churchill Livingstone, 1988;81–102.

71. Donaldson JS. Mediastinum. In: Siegel MJ, ed. *Pediatric body CT*. New York: Churchill Livingstone, 1987;29–79.

72. Donaldson JS, Shkolnik A. Pediatric renal masses. *Semin Roentgenol* 1988;23:194–204.

73. Drossman SR, Schiff RG, Kronfeld GD, et al. Lymphoma of the mediastinum and neck: evaluation with Ga-67 imaging and CT correlation. *Radiology* 1990;174:171–175.

74. Egund N, Wingstrand H. Legg-Calvé-Perthes disease: imaging with MR. *Radiology* 1991;179:89–92.

75. Eftekhari F, Shirkhoda A, Cangir A. Cavitation of a mediastinal mass following chemotherapy for histiocytosis X: CT demonstration. *J Comput Assist Tomogr* 1986;101:130–132.

76. Elkowitz SS, Leonidas JC, Lopez M, et al. Comparison of CT and MRI in the evaluation of therapeutic response in thoracic Hodgkin disease. *Pediatr Radiol* 1993;23:301–304.

77. Faerber EN, Balsara R, Vinocur CD, de Chadarevian JP. Gastric duplication with hemoptysis: CT findings. *AJR* 1993;161:1245–1246.

78. Farrelly C, Daneman A, Chan HSL, Martin DJ. Occult neuroblastoma presenting with opsomyoclonus: utility of computed tomography. *AJR* 1984;142:807–810.

79. Farrelly CA, Daneman A, Martin DJ, Chan HSL. Pheochromocytoma in childhood: the important role of computed tomography in tumor localization. *Pediatr Radiol* 1984;14:210–214.

80. Feldman F, Singson RD, Rosenberg ZS, Berdon WE, Amodio J, Abramson SJ. Distal tibial triplane fractures: diagnosis with CT. *Radiology* 1987;164:429–435.

81. Felker RE, Tonkin ILD. Imaging of pulmonary sequestration. *AJR* 1990;154:241–249.

82. Fellows KE, Hoffer FA, Markowitz RI, O'Neill JA Jr. Multiple collaterals to hepatic infantile hemangioendotheliomas and arteriovenous malformations: effect on embolization. *Radiology* 1991; 181:813–818.

83. Fernbach DJ, Hawkins EP, Pokorny WJ. Nephroblastoma and other renal tumors. In: Fernbach DJ, Vietti TJ, eds. *Clinical pediatric oncology*, 4th ed. St. Louis: Mosby Year Book, 1991:465–489.

84. Fernbach SK, Feinstein KA, Donaldson JS, Baum ES. Nephroblastomatosis: comparison of CT with US and urography. *Radiology* 1988;166:153–156.

85. Fishman EK, Hartman DS, Goldman SM Siegelman SS. The CT appearance of Wilms tumor. *J Comput Assist Tomogr* 1983;7:659–665.

86. Fitzgerald SW, Donaldson JS. Azygoesophageal recess: normal CT appearance in children. *AJR* 1992;158:1101–1104.

87. Fletcher BD. Response of osteosarcoma and Ewing sarcoma to chemotherapy: imaging evaluation. *AJR* 1991;157:825–833.

88. Fletcher BD. Pediatric musculoskeletal lesions simulating neoplasms. *Magnet Reson Clin North Am* 1996;4:721–747.

89. Fletcher BD, Dearborn DG, Mulopulos GP. MR imaging in infants with airway obstruction: preliminary observations. *Radiology* 1986;160:245–249.

90. Fletcher BD, Hanna SL, Fairclough DL, Gronemeyer SA. Pediatric musculoskeletal tumors: use of dynamic contrast-enhanced MR imaging to monitor response to chemotherapy. *Radiology* 1992; 184:243–248.

91. Fletcher BD, Kaste SC. Magnetic resonance imaging for diagnosis and follow-up of genitourinary, pelvic, and perineal rhabdomyosarcoma. *Urol Radiol* 1992;14:262–272.

92. Fletcher BD, Jacobstein MD. MRI of congenital abnormalities of the great arteries. *AJR* 1986;146:941–948.

93. Fletcher BD, Kopiwoda SY, Strandjord SE, Nelson AD, Pickering SP. Abdominal neuroblastoma: magnetic resonance imaging and tissue charaterization. *Radiology* 1985;155:699–703

94. Francis IR, Glazer GM, Bookstein FL, Gross BH. The thymus: re-examination of age-related changes in size and shape. *AJR* 1985; 145:249–254.

95. Frazier AA, Rosado de Christenson ML, Stocker JT, Templeton PA. Intralobar sequestration: radiologic-pathologic correlation. *RadioGraphics* 1997;17:725–745.

96. Friedland GW, Chang P. The role of imaging in the management of the impalpable undescended testis. *AJR* 1988;151:1107–1111.

97. Friedland JA, Siegel MJ. CT appearance of acute appendicitis in childhood. *AJR* 1997;168:439–442.

98. Friedman AC, Lichtenstein JE, Fishman EK, et al. Solid and papillary epithelial neoplasm of the pancreas. *Radiology* 1985;154:333–337.

99. Friedman AC, Lichtenstein JE, Goodman Z, Fishman EK, Siegelman SS, Dachman AH. Fibrolamellar hepatocellular carcinoma. *Radiology* 1985;157:583–587.

100. Frey EE, Smith WL, Grandgeorge S, et al. Chronic airway obstruction in children: evaluation with cine-CT. *AJR* 1987;148:347–352.

101. Fritzche PJ, Hricak H, Kogan BA, Winkler ML, Tanagho EA. Undescended testis: value of MR imaging. *Radiology* 1989;164:169–173.

102. Frush DP, Bisset GS III, Hall SC. Pediatric sedation in radiology: the practice of safe sleep. *AJR* 1996;1667:1381–1387.

103. Frush D, Siegel MJ, Bisset GS III. Challenges of pediatric spiral CT. *RadioGraphics* 1997;17:939–959.

104. Gillespy T III, Manfrini M, Ruggieri P, Spanier SS, Pettersson H,

Springfield DS. Staging of intraosseous extent of osteosarcoma: correlation of preoperative CT and MR imaging with pathologic macroslides. *Radiology* 1988;167:765–767.

105. Giyanani VL, Meyers PC, Wolfson JJ. Mesenchymal hamartoma of the liver: computed tomography and ultrasonography. *J Comput Assist Tomogr* 1986;10:51–54.

106. Glazer HS, Lee JKT, Levitt RG, et al. Radiation fibrosis: differentiation from recurrent tumor by MR imaging. *Radiology* 1985;156:721–726.

107. Godwin JD, Tarver, RD. Scimitar syndrome: Four new cases examined with CT. *Radiology* 1986;159: 15–20.

108. Gold RH, Hawkins RA, Katz RD. Bacterial osteomyelitis: findings on plain radiography, CT, MR, and scintigraphy. *AJR* 1991;157:365–370.

109. Gomes AS, Lois JF, George B, Alpan G, Williams RG. Congenital abnormalities of the aortic arch: MR imaging. *Radiology* 1987;165:691–695.

110. Gylys-Morin V, Hoffer HA, Kozakewich H, Shamberger RC. Wilms tumor and nephroblastomatosis: imaging characteristics at gadolinium–enhanced MR imaging. *Radiology* 1993;188:517–521.

111. Haddon MJ, Bowen A. Bronchopulmonary and neurenteric forms of foregut anomalies. Imaging for diagnosis and management. *Radiol Clin North Am* 1991;29: 241–254.

112. Hahn PF, Weissleder R, Stark DD, et al: MR imaging of focal splenic tumors. *AJR* 1988;150:823–827.

113. Havranek P, Lizler J. Magnetic resonance imaging in the evaluation of partial growth arrest after physeal injuries in children. *J Bone Joint Surg (Am)* 1991;73:1234–1241.

114. Hayes FA, Smith EI. Neuroblastoma. In: Pizzo PA, Poplack DG, eds. *Principles and practice of pediatric oncology.* Philadelphia: JB Lippincott, 1989:607–622.

115. Herman TE, Siegel MJ. CT of pancreaticoblastoma derived from the dorsal pancreatic anlage. *J Comput Assist Tomogr* 1994;18:648–650.

116. Herman TE, Siegel MJ. CT of acute splenic torsion in children with wandering spleen. *AJR* 1991;156:151–153.

117. Herman TE, Siegel MJ. CT of the pancreas in children. *AJR* 1991;157:375–379.

118. Hernandez RJ. Visualization of small sequestra by computerized tomography: report of 6 cases. *Pediatr Radiol* 1985;15:238–241.

119. Hernandez RJ. Cardiovascular MR imaging of children. *Magnet Reson Clin North Am* 1996;4:615–636.

120. Hernandez RJ, Tachdjian MO, Poznanski AK, Dias LS. CT determination of femoral torsion. *AJR* 1981;137:97–101.

121. Hernanz-Schulman M, Teele RL, Perez-Atayde A, et al. Pancreatic cystosis in cystic fibrosis. *Radiology* 1986;158:629–631.

122. Heron CW, Husband JE, Williams MP. Hodgkin disease: CT of the thymus. *Radiology* 1988;167:647–651.

123. Hervé-Somma CMP, Sebag GH, Prieur AM, Bonnerot V, Lallemand DP. Juvenile rheumatoid arthritis of the knee: MR evaluation with Gd-DOTA. *Radiology* 1992;182:93–98.

124. Ho VB, Kinney JB, Sabn DJ. Contributions of newer MR imaging strategies for congenital heart disease. *RadioGraphics* 1996;16:43–60.

125. Hubbard AM, Meyer JS, Mahboubi S. Diagnosis of liver diseases in children: value of MR angiography. *AJR* 1992;159:617–621.

126. Hulnick DH, Naidich DP, McCauley DI. Late presentation of congenital cystic adenomatoid malformation of the lung. *Radiology* 1984;151:569–573.

127. Ikezoe J, Murayama S, Godwin JD, Done SL, Verschakelen JA. Bronchopulmonary sequestration: CT assessment. *Radiology* 1990;176: 375–379.

128. Jabra AA, Fishman EK, Taylor GA. Crohn disease in the pediatric patient: CT evaluation. *Radiology* 1991;179:495–498.

129. Jabra AA, Fishman EK, Taylor GA. CT findings in inflammatory bowel disease in children. *AJR* 1994;162:975–979.

130. Jabra AA, Fishman EK, Taylor GA. Hepatic masses in infants and children: CT evaluation. *AJR* 1992;158:143–149.

131. Jaramillo D. Hoffer FA. Cartilaginous epiphysis and growth plate: normal and abnormal MR imaging findings. *AJR* 1992;158:1105–1110.

132. Jaramillo D, Hoffer FA, Shapiro F, Rand F. MR imaging of fractures of the growth plate. *AJR* 1990;155:1261–1265.

133. Jaramillo D, Kasser JR, Villegas-Medina OL, Gaary E, Zurakowski D. Cartilaginous abnormalities and growth disturbances in Legg-Calvé-Perthes disease: evaluation with MR imaging. *Radiology* 1995;197:767–773.

134. Jaramillo D, Laor T, Gebhardt MC. Pediatric musculoskeletal neoplasms. *Magnet Reson Clin North Am* 1996;4:749–770.

135. Jaramillo D, Laor T, Hoffer FA, et al. Epiphyseal marrow in infancy: MR imaging. *Radiology* 1991;180:809–812.

136. Jaramillo D, Perez-Atayde A, Griscom NT. Apparent association between thymic cysts and prior thoracotomy. *Radiology* 1989;172:207–209.

137. Johnson KM, Horvath LJ, Gaisie G, Mesrobian HG, Koepke JF, Askin FB. Wilms tumor occurring as a botryoid renal pelvicalyceal mass. *Radiology* 1987;163:385–386.

138. Johnson ND, Wood BP, Jackman KV. Complex infantile and congenital hip dislocation: Assessment with MR imaging. *Radiology* 1988;168: 151–156.

139. Joseph AE, Donaldson JS, Reynolds M. Neck and thorax venous aneurysm: association with cystic hygroma. *Radiology* 1989;170:109–112.

140. Kaste SC, Young CW. Safe use of power injectors with central and peripheral venous access devices for pediatric CT. *Pediatr Radiol* 1995;26:499–501.

141. Kaufman RA. CT of blunt abdominal trauma in children: a five-year experience. In: Siegel MJ, ed. *Pediatric body CT.* New York: Churchill Livingstone, 1986;313–347.

142. Kaufman RA. Technical aspects of abdominal CT in infants and children. *AJR* 1989;153:549–554.

143. Keslar PJ, Buck JL, Selby DM. Infantile hemangioendothelioma of the liver revisited. *RadioGraphics* 1993;13:657–670.

144. Keslar PJ, Buck JL, Suarez ES. Germ cell tumors of the sacrococcygeal region: radiologic-pathologic correlation. *RadioGraphics* 1994;14:607–620.

145. Kim OH, Chung HJ, Choi BG. Imaging of the choledochal cyst. *RadioGraphics* 1995;15:69–88.

146. King LR, Siegel MJ, Balfe DM. CT of pancreatitis in childhood: intra-and extrapancreatic fluid collections. *Radiology* 1995;195:196–200.

147. Kirks DR, Merten DF, Grossman H, Bowie JD. Diagnostic imaging of pediatric abdominal masses: an overview. *Radiol Clin North Am* 1981;19:527–545.

148. Koch KJ, Cory DA. Case Report: Simultaneous renal vein thrombosis and bilateral adrenal hemorrhage: MR demonstration. *J Comput Assist Tomogr* 1986;10:681–683.

149. Kohda E, Fujioka M, Ikawa H, Yokoyama J. Congenital anorectal anomaly: CT evaluation. *Radiology* 1985;157:349–352.

150. Kramer SS, Blum EE. CT of bronchogenic cysts. In: Siegelman SS, ed. *Computed tomography of the chest.* Churchill Livingstone: New York, 1984;219–231.

151. Kransdorf MJ, Jelinek JS, Moser RP Jr, et al. Soft tissue masses: Diagnosis using MR imaging. *AJR* 1989;153: 541–547.

152. Lang P, Steiger P, Genant HK, et al. Three-dimensional CT and MR imaging in congenital dislocation of the hip: clinical and technical considerations. *J Comput Assist Tomogr* 1988;12:459–464.

153. Lee KS, Im J-G, Han CH, Han MC, Kim C-W, Kim WS. Malignant primary germ cell tumors of the mediastinum: CT features. *AJR* 1989;153:947–951.

154. Lee MS, Harcke HT, Kumar SJ, Bassett GS. Subtalar joint coalition in children: new observations. *Radiology* 1989;172:635–639.

155. Lindfors KK, Meyer JE, Dedrick CG, Hassell LA, Harris NL. Thymic cysts in mediastinal Hodgkin disease. *Radiology* 1985;156:37–41.

156. Lowe RE, Cohen MD. Computed tomographic evaluation of Wilms tumor and neuroblastoma. *RadioGraphics* 1984;4:915–928.

157. Lucaya J, Enriquez G, Amat L, Gonzalez-Rivero MA. Computed tomography of infantile hepatic hemangioendothelioma. *AJR* 1985;144:821–826.

158. Luker GD, Siegel MJ. Mediastinal Hodgkin Disease in children: response to therapy. *Radiology* 1993;189:737–740.

159. Luker GD, Siegel MJ. Hepatic spiral CT in children: scan delay time-enhancement analysis. *Pediatr Radiol* 1996;26:337–340.

160. Lynch DA, Brasch RC, Hardy KA, Webb WR. Pediatric pulmo-

nary disease: assessment with high-resolution ultrafast CT. *Radiology* 1990;176:243–248.

161. Lyon RD. McAdams HP. Mediastinal bronchogenic cyst: demonstration of a fluid-fluid level at MR imaging. *Radiology* 1993;186: 427–428.

162. Madewell JE, Stocker JT, Korsower JM. Cystic adenomatoid malformation of the lung. Morphologic analysis. *AJR* 1975;124: 436–448.

163. Madewell JE, Goldman SM, Davis CJ, et al. Multilocular cystic nephroma: a radiologic-pathologic correlation of 58 patients. *Radiology* 1983;146:309–321.

164. Magid D, Fishman EK, Dey DR, Kuhlman JE, Frantz KM, Sponseller PD. Acetabular and pelvic fractures in the pediatric patient: value of two- and three-dimensional imaging. *J Pediatr Orthop* 1992;12:621–625.

165. Magid D, Fishman EK, Sponseller PD, Griffin PP. 2D and 3D computed tomography of the pediatric hip. *RadioGraphics* 1988; 8:901–934.

166. Mazur JM, Ross G, Cummings J et al. Usefulness of magnetic resonance imaging for the diagnosis of acute musculoskeletal infections in children. *J Pediatr Orthop* 1995;15:144–147.

167. Medina LS, Siegel MJ, Glazer HS et al. Diagnosis of pulmonary complications associated with lung transplantation in children: value of CT vs histopathologic studies. *AJR* 1994;162:969–974.

168. Medina LS, Siegel MJ. CT of complications in pediatric lung transplantation. *RadioGraphics* 1994;14:1341–1349.

169. Mercado-Deane MG, Sabio H, Burton EM, Hatley R. Cystic thymic hyperplasia in a child with HIV infection: imaging findings. *AJR* 1996;166:171–172.

170. Meyer JS. Retroperitoneal MR imaging in children. *Magnet Reson Clin North Am* 1996:657–678.

171. Miller FH, Fitzgerald SW, Donaldson JS. CT of the azygoesophageal recess in infants and children. *RadioGraphics* 1993;13:623–634.

172. Mintz MC, Grumbach K: Imaging of congenital uterine anomalies. *Semin Ultrasound Comput Tomogr Magnet Reson Imaging* 1988; 9:167–174.

173. Mitchell DG, Mintz MC, Spritzer CE, et al. Adnexal masses: MR imaging observations at 1.5T, with US and CT correlation. *Radiology* 1987;162:319–324.

174. Mitnick JS, Bosniak MA, Hilton S, Raghavendra BN, Subramanyam BR, Genieser NB. Cystic renal disease in tuberous sclerosis. *Radiology* 1983;147:85–87.

175. Molina PL, Siegel MJ, Glazer HS. Thymic masses on MR imaging. *AJR* 1990;155:495–500.

176. Moore SG, Dawson KL. Red and yellow marrow in the femur: age-related changes in appearance at MR imaging. *Radiology* 1990;175:219–223.

177. Moore SG, Bisset GS, Siegel MJ, Donaldson J. Pediatric musculoskeletal MR imaging. *Radiology* 1991;179:345–360.

178. Moore SG, Sebag GH. Primary disorders of bone marrow. In: Cohen MD, Edwards MK, eds. *Magnetic resonance imaging of children.* Philadelphia: BC Decker, 1990;765–824.

179. Morello FP, Donaldson JS. Nephroblastomatosis. In: Siegel BA, Proto AV, eds. *Pediatric disease (Fourth Series) test and syllabus.* Reston, VA: American College of Radiology, 1993;584–615.

180. Moulton JS, Blebea JS, Dunco CM, Braley SE, Bisset GS, Emery KH. MR imaging of soft tissue masses: diagnostic efficacy and value of distinguishing between benign and malignant lesions. *AJR* 1995;164:1191–1199.

181. Nimkin K, Teeger S, Wallach MT, DuVally JC, Spevak MR, Kleinman PK. Adrenal hemorrhage in abused children: imaging and postmortem findings. *AJR* 1994;162:661–663.

182. Nyman RS, Rehn SM, Glimelius BLG, et al. Residual mediastinal masses in Hodgkin disease: prediction of size with MR imaging. *Radiology* 1989;170:435–440.

183. Oppenheim C, Mamou-Mani T, Sayegh N, de Blic J, Scheinmann P, Lallemand D. Bronchopulmonary dysplasia: value of CT in identifying pulmonary sequelae. *AJR* 1994;163:169–172.

184. Panicek DM, Harty MP, Scicutella CJ, Carsky EW. Calcification in untreated mediastinal lymphoma. *Radiology* 1988;166:735–736.

185. Panicek DM, Heitzman ER, Randall PA, et al. The continuum of pulmonary developmental anomalies. *RadioGraphics* 1987;7: 747–772.

186. Patrick LE, Ball TI, Atkinson GO, Winn KJ. Pediatric blunt abdominal trauma: periportal tracking at CT. *Radiology* 1992;183: 689–691.

187. Pay NT, Singer WS, Bartal E. Hip pain in three children accompanied by transient abnormal findings on MR images. *Radiology* 1989;171:147–149.

188. Petasnick JP, Turner DA, Charters JR, Gitelis S, Zacharias CE. Soft tissue masses of the locomotor system: comparison of MR imaging with CT. *Radiology* 1986;160: 125–133.

189. Pettersson H, Gillespy T III, Hamlin DJ, et al. Primary musculoskeletal tumors: examination with MR imaging compared with conventional modalities. *Radiology* 1987;164: 237–241.

190. Powers C, Ros PR, Stoupis C, Johnson WK, Segel KH. Primary liver neoplasms: MR imaging with pathologic correlation. *RadioGraphics* 1994;14:459–482.

191. Pugatch RD, Gale ME. Obscure pulmonary masses: bronchial impaction revealed by CT. *AJR* 1983;141: 909–914.

192. Quillin SP, McAlister WH. Transitional cell carcinoma of the bladder in children: radiologic appearance and differential diagnosis. *Urol Radiol* 1991;13:107–109.

193. Quillin SP, Siegel MJ. CT features of benign and malignant teratomas in children. *J Comput Assist Tomogr* 1992;16:722–726.

194. Rahmouni A, Tempany C, Jones R, Mann R, Yang A, Zerhouni E. Lymphoma: monitoring tumor size and signal intensity with MR imaging. *Radiology* 1993;188:445–451.

195. Rawson J, Siegel MJ. Techniques and strategies in pediatric body MR imaging. *Magnet Reson Clin North Am* 1996;4:589–613.

196. Reiman TAH, Siegel MJ, Shackelford GD. Abdominal CT and sonography in children with Wilms tumor. *Radiology* 1986;160: 501–505.

197. Rholl KS, Levitt RG, Glazer HS. Magnetic resonance imaging of fibrosing mediastinitis. *AJR* 1985;145:255–259.

198. Ringertz HG, Brasch RC, Gooding CA, Wikstrom M, Lipton MJ. Quantitative density-time measurements in the lungs of children with suspected airway obstruction using ultrafast CT. *Pediatr Radiol* 1989;19:366–370.

199. Robberecht E, Nachtegaele P, Van Rattinghe R, et al. Pancreatic lipomatosis in the Shwachman-Diamond syndrome. Identification by sonography and CT-scan. *Pediatr Radiol* 1985;15:348–349.

200. Rollins NK, Currarino G. MR imaging of posterior mediastinal thymus. *J Comput Assist Tomogr* 1988;12:518–520.

201. Ros PR, Olmsted WW, Dachman AH, etal. Undifferentiated (embryonal sarcoma) of the liver: radiologic-pathologic correlation. *Radiology* 1986;160:141–145.

202. Ros PR, Olmsted WW, Moser R Jr, Dachman AH, Hjermstad BH, Sobin LH. Mesenteric and omental cysts: histologic classification with imaging correlation. *Radiology* 1987;164:327–332.

203. Rosado-de-Christenson ML, Frazier AA, Stocker JT, Templeton PA. Extralobar sequestration: radiologic-pathologic correlation. *RadioGraphics* 1993;13:425–441.

204. Rosado-de-Christenson ML, Stocker JT. Congenital cystic adenomatoid malformation. *RadioGraphics* 1991;11: 865–886.

205. Rosado-de-Christenson ML, Templeton PA, Moran CA. Mediastinal germ cell tumors: radiologic and pathologic correlation. *RadioGraphics* 1992;12:1013–1030.

206. Rosenfield NS, Leonidas JC, Barwick KW. Aggressive neuroblastoma simulating Wilms tumor. *Radiology* 1988;166:165–167.

207. Ruess L, Frazier AA, Sivit C. CT of the mesentery, omentum, and peritoneum in children. *RadioGraphics* 1995;15:89–104.

208. Ruzal-Shapiro C, Berdon WE, Cohen MD, Abramson SJ. MR imaging of diffuse bone marrow replacement in pediatric patients with cancer. *Radiology* 1991;181:587–589.

209. St. Amour TE, Siegel MJ, Glazer HS, Nadel SN. CT appearance of the normal and abnormal thymus in childhood. *J Comput Assist Tomogr* 1987;11:645–650.

210. Sargent MA, Cairns RA, Murdoch MJ, Nadel HR, Wensley D, Schultz KR. Obstructive lung disease in children after allogeneic bone marrow transplantation: evaluation with high-resolution CT. *AJR* 1995;164:693–696.

211. Sato Y, Pringle KC, Bergman RA et al. Congenital anorectal anomalies: MR imaging. *Radiology* 1988;168:157–162.

212. Schlesinger AE, Hernandez RJ. Diseases of the musculoskeletal system in children: imaging wth CT, sonography, and MR. *AJR* 1991;158:729–741.

213. Seeger LL, Hall TR. Magnetic resonance imaging of pediatric musculoskeletal trauma. *Top Magnet Reson Imaging* 1990;3: 61–72.

214. Shackelford GD, Siegel MJ. CT appearance of cystic adenomatoid malformation. *J Comput Assist Tomogr* 1989;13:612–616.

215. Shady KL, Siegel MJ, Brown JJ. Preoperative evaluation of intraabdominal tumors in children: gradient-recalled echo vs spin-echo MR imaging. *AJR* 1993;161:843–847.

216. Shady K, Siegel MJ, Glazer HS. CT of focal pulmonary masses in childhood. *RadioGraphics* 1992;12: 505–514.

217. Shalaby-Rana E, Eichelberger MR, Kerzner B, Kapur S. Intestinal stricture due to lap-belt injury. *AJR* 1992;158:63–64.

218. Sheth S, Fishman EK, Buck JL, Hamper UM, Sanders RC. The variable sonographic appearances of ovarian teratomas: correlation with CT. *AJR* 1988;151:331–334.

219. Shin MS, Odrezin GT, Van Dyke JA, Ho KJ. Unusual initial calcification of primary and metastatic seminomas. Detection by computed tomography. *Chest* 1991;99:1543–1545.

220. Siegel MJ. Chest applications of magnetic resonance imaging in children. *Top Magnet Reson Imaging* 1990;3:1–23.

221. Siegel MJ. Pelvic organs and soft tissues. In: Siegel MJ, ed. *Pediatric body CT*. New York: Churchill Livingstone, 1988;219–251.

222. Siegel MJ. Liver and biliary tract. In: Siegel MJ, ed. *Pediatric body CT*. New York: Churchill Livingstone, 1988;103–134.

223. Siegel MJ. Diseases of the thymus in children and adolescents. *Postgrad Radiol* 1993;13:106–132.

224. Siegel MJ. Magnetic resonance imaging of the pediatric pelvis. *Semin Ultrasound Comput Tomogr Magnet Reson Imaging* 1991; 12:475–505.

225. Siegel MJ. MRI of the pediatric abdomen. *Magnet Reson Clin North Am* 1995;3:161–182.

226. Siegel MJ. Pelvic tumors in childhood. *Radiol Clin North Am*. 1997. In press.

227. Siegel MJ, Balfe DM. Blunt renal and ureteral trauma in childhood: CT patterns of fluid collections. *AJR* 1989;152:1043–1047.

228. Siegel MJ, Evans SJ, Balfe DM. Small bowel disease in children: diagnosis with CT. *Radiology* 1988;169:127–130.

229. Siegel MJ, Glazer HS, St. Amour TE, Rosenthal DD. Lymphangiomas in children. MR imaging. *Radiology* 1989;170:467–470.

230. Siegel MJ, Glazer HS, Wiener JI, Molina PL. Normal and abnormal thymus in childhood: MR imaging. *Radiology* 1989;172:367–371.

231. Siegel MJ, Herman TE. Periportal low attenuation at CT in childhood. *Radiology* 1992;183:685–688.

232. Siegel MJ, Jamroz GA, Glazer HS, Abramson CL. MR imaging of intraspinal extension of neuroblastoma. *J Comput Assist Tomogr* 1986;10:593–595.

233. Siegel MJ, Luker GD. Pediatric applications of helical (spiral) CT. *Radiol Clin North Am* 1995;33:997–1022.

234. Siegel MJ, Luker GD. MR imaging of the liver in children. *Magnet Reson Clin North Am* 1996;4:637–656.

235. Siegel MJ, Luker GD. Pediatric chest MR imaging. *Magnet Reson Clin North Am* 1996;4:599–613.

236. Siegel MJ, Luker GD. Bone marrow imaging in children. *Magnet Reson Clin North Am* 1996;4:771–796.

237. Siegel MJ, Weber CK. Cardiac and paracardiac masses. In: Gutierez FR, Brown JJ, Mirowitz SA. *Cardiovascular magnetic resonance Imaging*. St. Louis: Mosby Year Book, 1992;112–123

238. Simoneaux SE, Bank ER, Webber JB, Parks WJ. MR imaging of the pediatric airway. *RadioGraphics* 1995;15:287–298.

239. Sisler CL, Siegel, MJ. Malignant rhabdoid tumor of the kidney: radiologic features. *Radiology* 1989;172:211–212.

240. Sivit CJ, Cutting JP, Eichelberger MR. CT diagnosis and localization of rupture of the bladder in children with blunt abdominal trauma: significance of contrast material extravasation in the pelvis. *AJR* 1995;164:1243–1246.

241. Sivit CJ, Eichelberger MR, Taylor GA, et al. Blunt pancreatic trauma in children: CT diagnosis. *AJR* 1992;158:1097–1100.

242. Sivit CJ, Ingram JD, Taylor GA, et al. Post-traumatic adrenal hemorrhage in children: CT findings in 34 patients. *AJR* 1992; 158:1299–1302.

243. Sivit CJ, Taylor GA, Bulas DI, Kushner DC, Potter BM, Eichel-

berger MR. Posttraumatic shock in children: CT findings associated with hemodynamic instability. *Radiology* 1992;182:723–726.

244. Sivit CJ, Taylor GA, Eichelberger MR. Chest injury in children with blunt abdominal trauma: evaluation with CT. *Radiology* 1989; 171:815–818.

245. Sivit CJ, Taylor GA, Newman KD, et al. Safety belt injuries in children with lap-belt ecchymosis: CT findings in 61 patients. *AJR* 1991;157:111–114.

246. Smith WL, Franken EA, Mitros FA. Liver tumors in children. *Semin Roentgenol* 1983;18:136–148.

247. Soyer P, Roche A, Levesque M, Legmann P. CT of fibrolamellar hepatocellular carcinoma. *J Comput Assist Tomogr* 1991;15:533–538.

248. Stalker HP, Kaufman RA, Towbin RB. Patterns of liver injury in childhood: CT analysis. *AJR* 1986;147:1199–1205.

249. Stanley P, Geer GD, Miller JH, Gilsanz V, Landing BH, Boechat IM. Infantile hepatic hemangiomas. Clinical features, radiologic investigations, and treatment of 20 patients. *Cancer* 1989;64:936–949.

250. Stanley P, Hall TR, Woolley MM, Diament MJ, Gilsanz V, Miller JH. Mesenchymal hamartomas of the liver in childhood: sonographic and CT findings. *AJR* 1986;147:1035–1039.

251. Stark DD, Moss AA, Brasch RD, deLorimier AA, Albin AR, London DA, Gooding CA. Neuroblastoma: diagnostic imaging and staging. *Radiology* 1983;148:101–105.

252. Stocker JT, Madewell JE, Drake RM. Congenital cystic adenomatoid malformation of the lung. Classification and morphologic spectrum. *Hum Pathol* 1977;8:155–171.

253. Strain JD, Harvey LA, Foley LC, et al. Intravenously administered pentobarbital sodium for sedation in pediatric CT. *Radiology* 1986; 161: 105–108.

254. Taylor GA, Fallat ME, Eichelberger MR. Hypovolemic shock in children: abdominal CT manifestations. *Radiology* 1987;164:479–481.

255. Taylor GA, Fallat ME, Potter BM, Eichelberger MR. The role of computed tomography in blunt abdominal trauma in children. *J Trauma* 1988;28:1660–1664.

256. Taylor GA, Guion CJ, Potter BM, Eichelberger MR. CT of blunt abdominal trauma in children. *AJR* 1989;153:555–559.

257. Vade A, Reyes H, Wilbur A, Gyi B, Spigos D. The anorectal sphincter after rectal pull-through surgery for anorectal anomalies: MRI evaluation. *Pediatr Radiol* 1989;19:179–183.

258. Vainright JR, Fulp CJ, Schiebler ML. MR imaging of vaginal atresia with hematocolpos. *J Comput Assist Tomogr* 1988;12:891–893

259. Waitches G, Zawin JK, Poznanski AK. Sequence and rate of bone marrow conversion in the femora of children as seen on MR imaging. Are accepted standards accurate? *AJR* 1994;162:1399–1406.

260. Weinberg AG, Finegold MJ. Primary hepatic tumors of childhood. *Hum Pathol* 1983;14:512–537.

261. Weinreb JC, Cohen JM, Armstrong E, Smith T. Imaging the pediatric liver: MRI and CT. *AJR* 1986;147:785–790.

262. Wells RG, Sty JR. Imaging of sacrococcygeal germ cell tumors. *RadioGraphics* 1990;10:701–713.

263. White KS. Invited article: helical/spiral CT scanning: a pediatric radiology perspective. *Pediatr Radiol* 1996;26:5–14.

264. White KS, Kirks DR, Bove KE. Imaging of nephroblastomatosis: an overview. *Radiology* 1992;182:1–5.

265. Widjaja PM, Ermers JWLM, Sijbrandij S, Damsma H, Klinkhamer AC. Technique of torsion measurement of the lower extremity using computed tomography. *J Comput Assist Tomogr* 1985;9: 466–470.

266. Woodring JH, Howard TA, Kanga JF. Congenital pulmonary venolobar syndrome revisited. *RadioGraphics* 1994;14:349–369.

267. Yale-Loehr AJ, Kramer SS, Quinlan DM, La France ND, Mitchell SE, Gearhart JP. CT of severe renal trauma in children: evaluation and course of healing with conservative therapy. *AJR* 1989;152: 109–113.

268. Zawin J, Jaramillo D. Conversion of marrow in the humerus, sternum and clavicle: changes with age on MR images. *Radiology* 1993;188:159–164.

269. Zobel MS, Borrello J, Siegel MJ, Stewart NR. Pediatric knee MR imaging: pattern of injuries in the immature skeleton. *Radiology* 1994;190:397–401.

Subject Index

Page numbers followed by *f* refer to figures and page numbers followed by *t* refer to tables.

I-1

Cavernous hemangioma, of rectum, 681, 680*f*
Cavernous lymphangiomatoid tumor, hepatic, 727
CBD. *See* Common bile duct
CCK stress technique, 780, 784
CEA (carcinoembryonic antigen), 70, 900
Cecostomy, percutaneous drainage, 95
Cecum, fluid-filled, simulating abscess, 984, 984*f*
Celiac artery, encasement, 903
Celiac ganglion block, CT-guided, 97–98, 97*f,* 98*f*
Cervical carcinoma
  incidence, 1229
  staging, 1229–1230, 1229*t*
    clinical applications of, 1234
    CT imaging for, 1230–1232, 1230*f,* 1231*f*
    MR imaging for, 1232–1234, 1232*f*–1234*f*
Cervical space
  anatomy, 111*f,* 112, 112*f*
    buccal, 112*f,* 114
    parotid, 114–117, 116*f*–118*f*
    sublingual, 111*f,* 112–113, 112*f*–115*f*
    submandibular, 111*f,* 112*f,* 113–114
    masticator, 112*f,* 120–121, 121*f*–123*f*
    parapharyngeal, 112*f,* 118, 118*f*
    pharyngeal mucosal, 112*f,* 121–125, 123*f*–125*f*
    posterior, 152, 152*f,* 153*f*
    prevertebral, 112*f,* 153, 153*f*
    retropharyngeal, 112*f,* 150–152, 151*f,* 152*f*
    visceral, 112*f,* 125 *See also specific visceral space structures*
Cervical spine
  anatomy, normal, 1449, 1451, 1449*f,* 1450*f*
  CT imaging
    advantages/disadvantages of, 1454–1455
    protocols, 1454
    special features, 1451, 1453–1454, 1453*f*
  degenerative disease, 1455, 1456*f*
  disc herniation, 1460, 1460*f*
  fractures
    lower, 1483–1485, 1481*f*–1486*f*
    upper, 1480, 1478*f*–1480*f*
  MR imaging
    advantages/disadvantages of, 1454–1455
    protocols, 1454
    special features, 1451, 1453–1454, 1453*f*
Cervical triangle, 111–112, 111*f*
Cervix
  anatomy, normal, 629, 631, 629*f*–631*f*
  MR imaging, 1216–1217, 1217*f*
Chamberlain procedure, for lymph node sampling, 230, 231*t*
Chance fractures, of lumbar spine, 1488, 1489*f*
Charcot's triad, 822
CHD. *See* Common hepatic duct
Chemical shielding, 26
Chemical shift artifacts
  bladder, 1214, 1214*f*
  causes, 51–52, 51*f,* 52*f*
  chest, 199
  mediastinal, 320
Chemical shift imaging, for pediatric patients, 1496
Chemical shifts, 26
Chest. *See also* Chest wall
  CT imaging
    for cross-sectional view, 181–182

    for differentiation of radiographic abnormality, 181–183, 182*f*
    field of view for, 185
    indications for, 183
    interslice spacing for, 185
    intravenous contrast administration, 187–189, 188*f*–190*f*
    patient positioning for, 184–185
    preliminary digital radiograph for, 185, 185*f,* 186*f*
    preparation for, 183–184
    radiation dose, 185, 187
    scan collimation for, 185, 186*f*
    window settings, 187
  disease
    computed tomography of, 181–182
    magnetic resonance imaging of, 181–182
  MR imaging
    artifacts, 198–199
    indications for, 183
    limitations of, 183
    preexam screening for, 184
    preparation for, 183–184
    protocol for, 184
  trauma, blunt, 1275–1276
Chest radiography
  abnormalities, CT differentiation of, 181–183, 182*f*
  aortic aneurysms, 302
  breast mass, 182*f*
Chest tube
  drainage, for empyema, 466, 466*f*
  malpositioned, 474–475, 475*f,* 476*f*
Chest wall
  anatomy, normal, 211–212, 214, 211*f*–213*f*
  axilla, 502–503, 502*f,* 503*f*
  collateral vessels, 490, 492
  disease
    clavicle involvement, 487–489, 488*f,* 489*f*
    CT imaging, 486–487, 487*f*
    MR imaging, 510–511
    rib involvement, 489–490, 490*f*
    sternal involvement, 487–489, 488*f,* 489*f*
  hemangioma, in pediatric patient, 1552, 1553*f*
  hematoma, 1276, 1277*f*
  infections, 492
  invasion, by breast cancer, 500–502, 501*f,* 502*f*
  MR imaging, 510–511
    brachial plexus, 511–512, 512*f*
    intrathoracic malignancies/neoplasms, 512–513, 513*f*
  postsurgical changes, 498, 500, 500*f*
  primary neoplasms, MRI, 514, 513*f*
  trauma, blunt, 1276–1278, 1277*f,* 1278*f*
  tumors, 492–493
    bone, 493–496, 494*f*–496*f*
    neurogenic, 496–497, 497*f*
    soft-tissue, 497–498, 497*f,* 498*f*
Chiba needle, 71, 72*f*
Children. *See* Pediatric patients
Cholangiocarcinoma
  CT imaging, 830–831, 831*f*–834*f*
  incidence, 829–830
  intrahepatic, 734–735, 735*f,* 736*f*
  morphologic patterns, 830
  MR imaging, 831, 833, 834*f,* 835*f*
  predisposing factors, 829

  survival rate, 830
  unresectability criteria, 831
Cholangiography, direct, 780
Cholangiohepatitis, oriental, 822, 824, 825*f*
Cholangiopathy, AIDS-related, 825–826, 826*f*
Cholangitis
  ascending, 822, 823*f*
  hepatic-artery-infusion-chemotherapy-related, 829, 830*f*
  primary sclerosing, 782–783, 783*f,* 794, 796, 796*f*
Cholecystectomy, complications, 837–838, 837*f,* 838*f*
Cholecystitis
  acalculous, 809
  acute, 803, 806–808, 806*f,* 810*f*
  chronic, 810, 810*f*
  complicated, 808–809, 807*f*
  CT imaging, 803, 806–809, 806*f*–809*f*
  emphysematous, 808, 808*f,* 809*f*
  gangrenous, 808, 807*f,* 808*f*
  MR imaging, 809–810, 810*f*
  xanthogranulomatous, 809
Cholecystokinin stress technique, 780, 784
Choledochal cysts
  classification, 813, 815, 815*f,* 816*f*
  in pediatric patients, 1533–1534, 1533*f*
Choledocholithiasis
  CT imaging, 819–821, 819*f*–821*f*
  incidence, 818
  MR imaging, 821, 822*f*
  signs/symptoms, 818–819
Cholelithiasis, 802–803, 804*f,* 805*f*
Cholesterol stones, 783, 786*f,* 802
Chondroblastomas, 1425
Chondromas, 143, 335
Chondrometaplasia, 143
Chondrosarcomas
  chest wall, 496
  differential diagnosis, 143
  laryngeal, 143, 143*f*
  MR imaging, 514, 513*f*
  musculoskeletal, 1427, 1428*f*
Chordoma, spinal, 1472, 1473*f*
Choriocarcinoma, thymic, 265–266, 267*f,* 1503, 1503*f*
Choristoma, 1138–1139. *See also* Angiomyolipomas, renal
Chronic obstructive pulmonary disease (COPD), neck scanning, 107
Chylothorax, 459
Cicatrization atelectasis, 384
Cine magnetic resonance imaging
  heart valve disease, 552
  velocity-encoded or phase contrast, of heart, 523–524
Cirrhosis
  causes, 750
  CT arterial portography of, 714, 714*f*
  CT imaging, 750–751, 750*f,* 751*f*
  extrahepatic features, 752–753, 755*f*
  hepatic fibrosis and, 751–752, 753*f,* 754*f*
  hepatocellular carcinoma in, 732, 734*f*
  MR imaging, 751, 752*f,* 753*f*
  in pediatric patient, 1538, 1539*f*
Claustrophobia, of MRI patients, 110
Clavicle
  anatomy, normal, 1347–1348, 1347*f*
  benign tumors, 488–489
  dislocation, 1278
Clear cell sarcoma, in pediatric patients, 1520